A PRACTICE OF

ANAESTHESIA

A PRACTICE OF ANAESTHESIA

EDITED BY

W. D. WYLIE

M.A., M.B. (Cantab), F.R.C.P., F.F.A.R.C.S., Hon. F.F.A. R.C.S.I.

Consultant Anaesthetist, St. Thomas's Hospital and The Royal Masonic Hospital, London

and

H. C. CHURCHILL-DAVIDSON

M.A., M.D. (Cantab.), F.F.A.R.C.S.

Consultant Anaesthetist, St. Thomas's Hospital and The Chelsea Hospital for Women

Third Edition

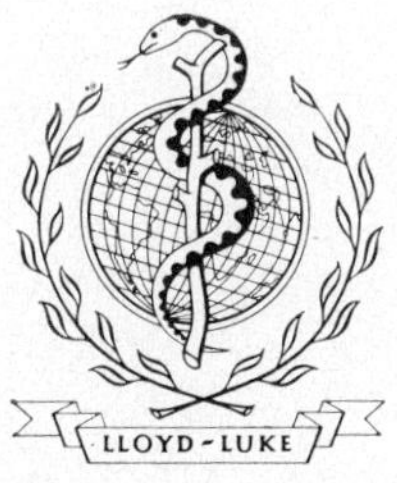

LLOYD-LUKE (MEDICAL BOOKS) LTD

49 NEWMAN STREET

LONDON

1972

FIRST EDITION . . .	1960
Reprinted	1960
Reprinted	1962
Polish translation . . .	1962
SECOND EDITION . . .	1966
Spanish translation . . .	1969
Italian translation . . .	1969
Reprinted	1970
THIRD EDITION . . .	1972

PRINTED AND BOUND IN ENGLAND BY
HAZELL WATSON AND VINEY LTD
AYLESBURY, BUCKS

ISBN 0 85324 094 9

ASSOCIATE EDITORS

M. A. BRANTHWAITE, B.A., M.B., B.Chir. (Cantab.), M.R.C.P., F.F.A.R.C.S.
Consultant Anaesthetist, The Brompton Hospital, London; late Senior Registrar, Department of Clinical Physiology, St. Thomas's Hospital, London.

A. J. CLEMENT, M.B., B.S. (London), F.F.A.R.C.S.
Consultant Anaesthetist to the Cardio-Thoracic Department, St. Thomas's Hospital, London

R. M. M. FORDHAM, B.A., M.B., B.Chir. (Cantab.), F.F.A.R.C.S.
Consultant Anaesthetist, United Oxford Hospitals; late Senior Registrar, Department of Anaesthetics, St. Thomas's Hospital, London

C. A. FOSTER, E.R.D., M.B., B.S. (London), F.F.A.R.C.S.
Consultant Anaesthetist, St. Thomas's Hospital, London

P. J. HORSEY, M.B., B.S. (London), F.F.A.R.C.S.
Consultant Anaesthetist, Southampton Group of Hospitals; late Senior Registrar, Department of Anaesthetics, St. Thomas's Hospital, London

J. R. NICHOLSON, M.B., B.S. (London), F.F.A.R.C.S.
Consultant Anaesthetist, King's College Hospital, London; late Senior Registrar, Department of Anaesthetics, St. Thomas's Hospital, London

S. E. SMITH, M.A. (Oxon.), Ph.D. (London), B.M., B.Ch. (Oxon.), D.A.
Reader in Applied Pharmacology and Therapeutics, St. Thomas's Hospital Medical School, London

R. P. WISE, M.B., B.S. (London), F.F.A.R.C.S.
Consultant Anaesthetist, St. Thomas's Hospital, London

CONTRIBUTORS

Special chapters have been contributed by the following:

T. H. S. BURNS, M.A., B.M., B.Ch. (Oxon.), F.F.A.R.C.S.
Consultant Anaesthetist, St. Thomas's Hospital and the Royal Northern Hospital, London

Andrew DOUGHTY, M.B., B.S. (London), F.F.A.R.C.S.
Consultant Anaesthetist, Kingston Group of Hospitals and St. Teresa's Maternity Hospital, Wimbledon; late Senior Registrar, Department of Anaesthetics, St. Thomas's Hospital, London

W. W. HOLLAND, B.Sc., M.D. (London), M.R.C.P., F.S.S.
Professor of Clinical Epidemiology and Social Medicine, St. Thomas's Hospital Medical School, London

H. S. KASAP, A.I.S., F.S.S.
Lecturer in the Department of Clinical Epidemiology and Social Medicine, St. Thomas's Hospital Medical School, London

D. D. B. MORRIS, M.B., B.S. (London), F.F.A.R.C.S.
Consultant Anaesthetist, the Bournemouth and East Dorset Group of Hospitals; late Senior Registrar, Department of Anaesthetics, St. Thomas's Hospital, London

Felicity REYNOLDS, M.D. (London), F.F.A.R.C.S.
Lecturer in the Department of Pharmacology, St. Thomas's Hospital Medical School; late Registrar, Department of Anaesthetics, St. Thomas's Hospital, London

I. Z. ROTH, C.Sc., Dip.Stat.
Head, Division of Medical Statistics, Medical Research Institute, University of Prague, Czecho-Slovakia; late Lecturer in the Department of Clinical Epidemiology and Social Medicine, St. Thomas's Hospital Medical School, London

G. T. SPENCER, M.B., B.S. (London), F.F.A.R.C.S.
Consultant Anaesthetist, St. Thomas's Hospital, London

FOREWORD

"WHAT shall I read?" is a question posed again and again to every teacher of anaesthetics. The answer will vary of course with the needs of the individual. Several books are available for those requiring either an introduction to the subject or concentrated factual information. When the question is put by a man of some experience, however, who wants a book which will supply in large measure his needs for, say, the F.F.A.R.C.S. diploma, teachers have in the past had to direct his attention to a host of papers and monographs—and even to weighty tomes—dealing with particular aspects of the specialty. There seemed, therefore, to the authors of this book a real need for gathering within the covers of one volume the greater part of that widely scattered knowledge which the anaesthetist of today is expected to possess. To this end, the subjects of physics, anatomy, and pathology—as they bear upon the specialty—have been touched upon; the relevant portions of physiology and pharmacology treated in detail; and the clinical aspect repeatedly emphasised.

The authors are recognised teachers and acknowledged authorities in anaesthesia, and they have called upon other members of the Anaesthetic Department and experts in particular fields at St. Thomas's Hospital to contribute a few special chapters. The composition has been handled in a novel way; contrary to usual anaesthetic custom, the subject has been arranged in sections devoted to the various systems of the body. Frequent repetition—so difficult to avoid in a work of such magnitude—has been obviated by cross-reference, and the comprehensive index is there to be used.

In presenting the practical aspects of anaesthesia some basic experience has been assumed. Special techniques used in those branches of the specialty which the trainee may not have had the good fortune to come across in a general hospital have been described in the fullest detail. There are always more ways than one of tackling every anaesthetic problem; for the sake of clarity, however, attention has largely been confined to those approaches which have proved themselves of greatest value in the hands of the authors and which are in current use at St. Thomas's Hospital, and each chapter ends with a list of references to the relevant literature.

Having watched it grow and having been given the opportunity of reading the greater part of it, I have no doubt that this book will bring to the established anaesthetist a ready source of reference to recent work on this rapidly expanding specialty and that the herculean labours of the authors will materially ease the burden for those still in training.

M. D. NOSWORTHY

PREFACE TO THE THIRD EDITION

THE problems associated with bringing up to date and constantly striving to improve a postgraduate textbook are considerable. Five years have passed since the publication of the second edition and during this period there have been many advances in clinical anaesthesia and in the sciences from which anaesthesia stems. We have become increasingly aware of the need to widen the field of editorship to ensure a thorough and expert revision of the subject matter, but we have been equally anxious to maintain the style of the original editions and the scientific foundations upon which they were built. Throughout we have been particularly careful to make the whole work relevant to clinical practice.

We want to pay tribute to our Associate Editors. They will deserve most of the credit for any success that this edition may achieve, for as well as revising a large part of the text and contributing many new sections, they have been our constant advisers and ever-helpful colleagues. Once again we thank those experts who have contributed special chapters for this edition or who have brought up to date or remodelled their earlier chapters.

We are very grateful to the following anaesthetists who, either currently or during the past three years, have been working as Senior Registrars or Registrars in the Department of Anaesthetics at St. Thomas's Hospital. They have each played a most helpful and active role in the formation of this Third Edition by reading critically parts of the Second Edition in conjunction with the relevant up-to-date literature and by setting down on paper their own ideas for improvement.

J. C. Edwards
C. D. G. Evans-Prosser
G. J. J. Fuzzey
P. Furniss
I. C. Gregory
Jennifer Jones
J. A. Mathias
J. S. Paddle
H. R. Waters

Many other people have made this edition possible and we are most grateful to them. Miss Joan Dewe, Miss Jean Davenport, Mrs. Diana Hayton and Mr. D. P. Hammersley for diagrams and illustrations, Mr. T. W. Brandon for our photographs, and Mr. R. A. Pyne for comments on methods of sterilizing equipment. The burden of secretarial assistance has been borne by Miss Jean Davenport but much help has come from Miss Coral Brandon, Mrs. Mary Blake, Mrs. Helen Ferrelly and Mrs. Norah Wilmot. Finally, it is a pleasure to record once again our indebtedness to Mr. Douglas Luke, our publisher, for his consistent help and advice at all stages of the preparation of this edition.

W. D. WYLIE
H. C. CHURCHILL-DAVIDSON

August, 1971

PREFACE TO THE FIRST EDITION

PHYSIOLOGICAL and pharmacological principles now govern the choice of anaesthetic drugs and techniques; and, although many patients can be safely dealt with by routines born of experience, a sound understanding of the background of a particular patient enables the proper and best choice to be made.

In a sense anaesthesia is simply the application of a knowledge of the pharmacological action of drugs to known physiology and pathology, and for this reason the student of anaesthesia must be well-versed in the basic sciences and their application to anaesthesia. Moreover, he must be aware of the modern trends in the medical and surgical care of patients.

We have deliberately assumed that our readers are familiar with the elementary practice of anaesthesia, and practical methods are not always dealt with in great detail, unless they are either of special value though rarely performed, or likely to be required by only a small proportion of practitioners. By the addition of a little more than the bare requirements for competent anaesthesia in the operating theatre, and in some places by the description of a particular disease, pathological process or therapeutic measure, it is hoped to give the reader a broader view of the subject and a better foundation from which to assess the value of the specialty.

The preparation of a book of this nature has necessitated frequent reference to standard and specialised texts and papers in the world literature. These are acknowledged in the relevant parts of this work, but we wish to express our indebtedness to their authors since they have been the foundations upon which we have built, and to crave indulgence should any acknowledgement—through oversight—have been omitted.

A very special word of thanks must be made to Dr. M. D. Nosworthy, who first interested and instructed us in the art and science of anaesthesia. Not only has he read and corrected the greater part of the manuscript, and contributed a foreword to it, but he has never failed to give us helpful advice. We are very grateful to the contributors of special chapters, and to Dr. C. A. Foster for his continuous industry and unstinted aid during each stage of the preparation of the book. We also wish to thank Dr. K. G. Lupprian for so carefully checking all the formulae and being kind enough to write for us the resumé of work on 5-hydroxytryptamine, and Dr. B. R. Whittard for his helpful proof-reading. We are indebted to the following who have read chapters, drawn illustrations, taken photographs, provided radiographs, sought out references, or generally given advice: Mr. T. W. Brandon and the staff of the Photographic Department at St. Thomas's Hospital, Miss Joan Dewe, Mr. L. G. Donnellon, Dr. W. J. Griffith, Dr. Bjørn Ibsen, Dr. Christine John, Miss A. M. Jones, Mr. A. F. Masson, Mr. I. K. R. McMillan, Dr. A. T. Richardson, Miss Gladys Storey, Mrs. M. F. Toole Stott, Dr. J. Sutcliffe, Dr. R. P. Wise and Miss I. M. Young.

It is a very great pleasure to acknowledge the help of Mr. Douglas Luke, our publisher, who, despite the many years that have passed during the preparation of this work, has never failed to understand the difficulties that beset medical authors.

Finally, without the expert secretarial care and continuous aid of Miss Jean Davenport and her assistants, it is very doubtful whether this book would ever have been completed.

W. D. WYLIE
H. C. CHURCHILL-DAVIDSON

May, 1959

ACKNOWLEDGEMENTS

WE wish to express our thanks to the many individuals, editors, publishers and manufacturers who have so kindly helped us in numerous ways, but principally by allowing reproduction of their own illustrations or material, and by supplying photographs or blocks.

The following grateful acknowledgements are made in detail for each chapter.

Section One

Chapter 1—Figs. 2, 3 and 4, Dr. J. D. K. Burton and the Editor of *The Lancet*; Fig. 5, Dr. N. G. Toremalm and the Editor of *Acta Anaesthesiologica Scandinavica*; Fig. 6, The Bird Corporation; Fig. 7, Dr. P. Herzog, Dr. O. P. Norlander and Dr. C. G. Engstrom and the Editor of *Acta Anaesthesiologica Scandinavica*; Fig. 10, based on two illlustrations in a chapter by W. J. Hampton and R. J. Hamilton in *Disease of the Ear, Nose and Throat*, Vol. 1, by W. B. Scott-Brown, published by Butterworth and Co.; Fig. 16, Dr. G. H. Bush and John Sherratt and Son, publishers of the *British Journal of Anaesthesia*; Fig. 17, photographs of the original drawings belonging to Mr. M. Meredith Brown; Fig. 19, based on two figures in the *Anatomy of the Bronchial Tree* by Lord Brock and published by the Oxford University Press; Fig. 21, reproduced from William Snow Miller's *The Lung*, courtesy of Charles C. Thomas, publisher, Springfield, Illinois, and Fig. 22, based on reconstruction models illustrated in the same book; Fig. 23, Dr. J. A. Clements and *Scientific American*; Fig. 24, Dr. R. E. Brooks; Fig. 25, Dr. G. Corssen and the Editor, *Journal of the American Medical Association*; Fig. 27, redrawn from figures in an article by Drs. M. Ambiavagar, E. Sherwood Jones and D. N. Roberts published in *Anaesthesia*; Table 7 from *Lung Function* by Dr. S. E. Cotes, published by Blackwell Scientific Publications.

Chapter 2—Fig. 1, based on a figure in *Anatomy for the Anaesthetist* by Professor H. Ellis and Miss McLarty and published by Blackwell Scientific Publications; Fig. 2, based on anatomical dissections made available by Professor R. J. Last of the Royal College of Surgeons of England; Fig. 3, Dr. B. R. Fink and John Sherratt and Son, publishers of the *British Journal of Anaesthesia*; Figs. 6, 7, 8 and 9, Dr. H. J. V. Morton and the Editor of *Anaesthesia.*

Chapter 3—Fig. 2, Professor B. Delisle Burns and the Editor of the *British Medical Bulletin*; Figs. 3 and 7, Professor J. W. Severinghaus and The American Physiological Society; Fig. 4 redrawn from a figure in a chapter by C. J. Lambertsen in *Pharmacology in Medicine* edited by V. Drill and used by permission of McGraw-Hill Book Company; Fig. 5, Dr. J. Weldon Bellville and the Editors of *Anesthesiology*; Figs. 6 (*a*) and (*b*), Drs. C. P. Larson, Jr., E. I. Eger II, M. Muallem, D. R. Buechel, E. S. Munson and J. H. Eisele, and the Editors of *Anesthesiology*; Figs. 9 and 11 are adapted from two figures in *The Physiological Basis of Medical Practice* by C. H. Best and N. B. Taylor published by Williams and Wilkins Co.; Fig. 12, Professor H. Prystowsky and the Editor of the *Bulletin of the Johns Hopkins Hospital*; Fig. 13, the C. V. Mosby Co., publishers of the *American Journal of Obstetrics and Gynecology*; Fig. 14 is an adaptation of a figure in *The Physiology of the Newborn Infant* by C. A. Smith, published by Blackwell Scientific Publications; Fig. 15, Dr. C. E. Flowers and the C. V. Mosby Co.; Fig. 16, Professor K. W. Cross and the Editors of the *Journal of Physiology*; Fig. 18, Professor G. V. R. Born, Dr. G. S. Dawes and the Editor of *Cold Spring Harbor Symposia on Quantitative Biology*; Fig. 19, Professor W. W. Holland and the Editor of the *British Medical Journal*; Fig. 20, Dr. H. Barrie and the Editor of *The Lancet.*

Chapter 4—Figs. 1 and 6, from *Respiration in Health and Disease* by R. M. Cherniack and L. Cherniack, published by W. B. Saunders Co.; Fig. 5 (*c*), Dr. H. A. Fleming and the Editors of *Thorax*; Figs. 7(*a*) and (*b*), Professor J. B. West and the Editor of *The Lancet*; Fig. 7(c), Professor J. B. West, Professor C. T. Dollery and Dr. A. Naimark and the Editor of the *Journal of Applied Physiology*; Fig. 8, Dr. J. Panday and Professor J. F. Nunn and the Editor of *Anaesthesia*; Fig. 10, Dr. B. E. Marshall and the Editor of the *Journal of Applied Physiology*; Fig. 12 from a *Textbook of Medical Physiology* by A. C. Guyton published by W. B. Saunders

Co.; Fig. 13 from *The ABC of Acid-Base Chemistry* by H. W. Davenport published by the University of Chicago Press; Fig. 15, J. & A. Churchill Ltd.; Fig. 17, the Editor of the *Scandinavian Journal of Clinical and Laboratory Investigation*; Fig. 18, Professor T. C. Gray and John Sherratt and Son, publishers of the *British Journal of Anaesthesia*; Figs. 19 and 20 are adapted from illustrations in *Physics for the Anaesthetist* by Sir Robert Macintosh, Professor W. W. Mushin and Dr. H. E. Epstein published by Blackwell Scientific Publications; Fig. 21 is reproduced from the same work; Figs. 22, 23 and 24, Dr. E. S. Munson and the Editors of *Anesthesiology*; Fig. 26, Dr. M. L. Kain and Professor J. F. Nunn and the Honorary Editors of the *Proceedings of the Royal Society of Medicine*; Fig. 27, Dr. S. N. Steen and the Editor of *Current Researches in Anesthesia and Analgesia*; Fig. 28, Dr. H. B. Sandiford; Fig. 30, Dr. G. J. Rees.

Chapter 5—Fig. 1, adapted from a figure in *The Physiological Basis of Medical Practice* by C. H. Best and N. B. Taylor published by Williams and Wilkins Co.; Fig. 2, British Oxygen Co. Ltd.; Figs. 3 and 5, Oxygenaire Ltd.; Fig. 4, Bakelite Xylonite Ltd.

Chapter 6—Fig. 1(*a*) and (*b*), Dr. C. A. Foster; Fig. 1(*c*), (*d*) and (*e*), Dr. K. G. Williams and Vickers Research Ltd.

Chapter 7—Fig. 4 is from a chapter by Professor J. W. Severinghaus and Fig. 8 from one by Dr. E. I. Eger II, both in *Uptake and Distribution of Anesthetic Agents*, edited by E. M. Papper and R. J. Kitz, and both used by permission of McGraw-Hill Book Company; Fig. 5 is based on an original by Dr. S. S. Kety and published in *Anesthesiology*; Fig. 6 is based on a figure by Dr. J. G. Bourne and published in *Anaesthesia*; Fig. 7, Dr. E. I. Eger II and John Sherratt and Son, publishers of the *British Journal of Anaesthesia*; Fig. 11, The American Society of Biological Chemists, Inc.

Chapter 8—Figs. 1 and 2, Dr. L. McArdle, Dr. G. W. Black and John Sherratt and Son, publishers of the *British Journal of Anaesthesia.*

Chapter 9—Figs. 2 and 3 are reproduced from *Physics for the Anaesthetist* by Sir Robert Macintosh, Professor W. W. Mushin and Dr. H. G. Epstein, published by Blackwell Scientific Publications; Fig. 4, Dr. G. W. Black, Dr. L. McArdle, Dr. H. McCullough and Dr. V. K. N. Unni and the Editor of *Anaesthesia*; Fig. 5 is reproduced from *Trichlorethylene Anaesthesia* by Gordon Ostlere, published by E. & S. Livingstone Ltd.; Figs. 6, 7 and 8, Dr. G. W. Black, Dr. L. McArdle and John Sherratt and Son, publishers of the *British Journal of Anaesthesia*; Fig. 9, Cyprane Ltd.; Fig. 10, Dr. G. M. Paterson, Dr. G. H. Hulands and Professor J. W. Nunn and John Sherratt and Son, publishers of the *British Journal of Anaesthesia.*

Chapter 10—Fig. 9, Longworth Scientific Instrument Co. Ltd.

Chapter 12—Figs. 1, 2 and 3, Dr. V. Goldman and Dr. P. W. Thompson and John Sherratt and Son, publishers of the *British Journal of Anaesthesia*; Fig. 4, Medical and Industrial Equipment Ltd.

Chapter 13—Fig. 14(*d*), British Oxygen Company Ltd.; Fig. 16, Professor T. C. Gray and the Editors of *Thorax.*

Chapter 14—Fig. 2 is adapted from a diagram in *Thoracic Surgery for Physiotherapists* by Miss G. M. Storey, published by Faber and Faber Ltd.

Chapter 15—Fig. 1, Dr. M. H. Brook and the Editor of the *British Medical Journal*; Figs. 2 and 5, Medical and Industrial Equipment Ltd.; Fig. 3(*a*) British Oxygen Company Ltd.; Fig. 3(*b*) Ambu International; Fig. 4, The Laerdal Resusci Folding Bag is marketed by Vickers Limited Medical Engineering who kindly supplied the illustration; Figs. 6 and 7, Dr. W. H. Kelleher; Fig. 9, Portex Ltd.; Fig. 14, Mr. G. Kent Harrison; Fig. 15, Oxygenaire Ltd.; Fig. 17, Littlemore Engineering Co., Oxford.

Chapter 16—Figs. 1 and 2, H. G. East & Co. Ltd.; Fig. 3, The Cape Engineering Co. Ltd.; Fig. 4, Mivab, Stockholm; Fig. 5, W. Watson and Sons Ltd.; Fig. 6, Dr. R. A. Beaver; Fig. 7, Blease Anaesthetic Equipment Ltd.; Fig. 8, The Bird Corporation; Fig. 9, Puritan Medical Gases and Equipment.

Chapter 18—Figs. 2 and 3, The United States Bureau of Mines; Fig. 4, Dr. A. Quinton, from a diagram in *Radio-isotope Conference*, 1954, Vol. II, published by Butterworth Scientific Publications.

Section Two

Chapter 19—Figs. 1 and 9 are reproduced from *Principles of Clinical Electrocardiography* by Mervyn J. Goldman, published by Lange Medical Publications; Figs. 2 and 3, Dr. Peter Stock and the Editor of the *British Journal of Hospital Medicine*; Fig. 6 is adapted from an illustration in *The Lung* by J. H. Comroe, Jr., R. E. Forster II, A. B. Dubois, W. A. Briscoe and E. Carlson, published by the Year Book Medical Publishers, Inc.; Fig. 8 is reproduced from *Unipolar Lead Electrocardiography and Vectorcardiography* by E. Goldberger, published by Lea and Febiger; Figs. 18(*a*) and (*b*), 23(*a*) and (*b*), 25, 26 and 28 are reproduced from *A Primer of Electrocardiography* by G. E. Burch and T. Winsor, published by Lea and Febiger; Fig. 24, Dr. J. J. Osborn and the Editor of the *American Journal of Physiology*; Fig. 27, reproduced from *Electrocardiography* by M. Bernrieter, published by J. B. Lippincott Co.

Chapter 20—Fig. 1, the Editor of the *British Medical Bulletin*; Fig. 4 is reproduced from *Applied Physiology* by Samson Wright, published by Oxford Medical Publications.

Chapter 22—Fig. 3, Professor P. R. Bromage and the Honorary Editors of the *Proceedings of the Royal Society of Medicine.*

Chapter 23—Figs. 1 and 2, Dr. G. E. Hale Enderby and the Editor of *The Lancet.*

Chapter 25—Figs. 1, 2, 3, 5, 6, 8, 9, 10, 11 and 12, Dr. J. S. Fleming, Mr. M. V. Braimbridge and Blackwell Scientific Publications; Fig. 4, Dr. A. Devloo and the Mayo Clinic; Fig. 7, Dr. G. Melrose and Honeywell Controls Ltd.

Chapter 26—Fig. 1 is adapted from a figure in a paper by Dr. M. A. Hayes published in the *New England Journal of Medicine.*

Chapter 27—Fig. 1, Ethicon Ltd.

Section Three

Chapter 29—Figs. 3 and 5(*a*) and (*b*), Professor Sir Bernard Katz and the Editors of the *Journal of Physiology*; Fig. 4, the Editors of the *Journal of Biophysical and Biochemical Cytology* and the Pergamon Press Ltd.; Fig. 6, Professor Sir Bernard Katz and the Royal Society; Figs. 7 and 8, Professor Peter G. Waser and the Editor of the *Journal of Pharmacy and Pharmacology*; Fig. 10, the Honorary Editors of the *Proceedings of the Royal Society of Medicine*; Figs. 12 (*a*) and (*b*), Dr. S. Page and the Editor of the *British Medical Bulletin*; Fig. 13, Dr. P. Furniss and the Honorary Editors of the *Proceedings of the Royal Society of Medicine*; Fig. 14, Dr. P. Furniss.

Chapter 30—Fig. 2, Dr. Raymond Greene and the Editor of *The Lancet*; Figs. 3 and 15, Professor Eleanor Zaimis and the Editors of the *Journal of Physiology*; Figs. 7, 18, 19 and 20, the Honorary Editors of the *Proceedings of the Royal Society of Medicine*; Figs. 8, 10, 11, 12, 13, 16 and 17, Dr. C. L. Hewer and J. & A. Churchill Ltd.; Figs. 21 (*a*) and (*b*), Drs. P. O. Bridenbaugh and M. D. Churcher, and the Editor of *Anesthesia and Analgesia*; Figs. 24 (*a*) and (*b*), Drs. E. N. Cohen, H. W. Brewer, D Smith, and the Editors of *Anesthesiology*; Fig. 25, the Editors of *Anesthesiology*; Fig. 26, the Editor of the *Canadian Anaesthetists' Society Journal.*

Chapter 31—Figs. 1, 12 and 14, Dr. E. N. Cohen, Dr. N. Hood and Dr. R. Golling and the Editors of *Anesthesiology*; Fig. 4, Dr. H. H. Birch and the Editor of the *Journal of the American Medical Association*; Fig. 5, Professor J. Crul; Fig. 9, the Editors of *Anesthesiology*; Figs. 13 (*a*) and (*b*), Drs. E. N. Cohen, H. W. Brewer, D. Smith and the Editors of *Anesthesiology.*

Chapter 33—Fig. 2, Professor D. Elmquist, Drs. W. W. Hofman, J. Kugelburg and D. M. J. Quastel and the Editors of the *Journal of Physiology*; Fig. 7 is reproduced from a chapter by Dr. E. H. Lambert in *Myasthenia Gravis*, courtesy of Charles C. Thomas, publisher; Fig. 8, Dr. A. Goldberg and the Editors of the *Quarterly Journal of Medicine.*

Chapter 34—Fig. 3, Dr. B. B. Brodie, Dr. T. B. Binns and E. & S. Livingstone; Fig. 6 is adapted from a figure previously printed in the *British Journal of Pharmacology*; Fig. 7, Professor W. D. M. Paton and the Honorary Editors of the *Proceedings of the Royal Society of Medicine*; Fig. 8 is adapted from a table in a paper by N. F. Paxson published in *Current Researches in Anesthesia and Analgesia.*

Chapter 35—Fig. 1, Professor M. Jouvet and the Administrator of the *Archives Italiennes de Biologie*; Fig. 2, Dr. B. B. Brodie and the Editor of *Federation Proceedings*.

Chapter 37—Fig. 1, Charles C. Thomas, publisher; Fig. 3, Dr. J. C. White and the Williams and Wilkins Company; Fig. 4, Professor R. Melzack and Professor P. D. Wall.

Chapter 38—Figs. 1 and 2 are redrawn from originals in *Regional Block* by D. C. Moore, published by Charles C. Thomas; Fig. 4, from *Functional Neuroanatomy*, edited by N. B. Everett and published by Lea and Febiger.

Chapter 39—Figs. 1 and 6, Dr. E. H. Burrows and the Wessex Neurological Centre; Fig. 7, the late Dr. Christine John; Fig. 8, Sir Wylie McKissock and the Editor of the *British Medical Journal*.

Chapter 41—Fig. 2, Dr. L. Ekblom and Dr. B. Widman and the Editors of *Acta Anaesthesiologica Scandinavica*.

Chapter 42—Fig. 4 is adapted from an illustration in *A Method of Anatomy: Descriptive and Deductive*, by J. C. Boileau Grant, published by the Williams and Wilkins Co.; Fig. 9, Professor Sir Robert Macintosh and Dr. R. Bryce Smith and E. & S. Livingstone.

Chapter 43—Fig. 2, C. R. Bard International Ltd.; Fig. 3, Lloyd-Luke (Medical Books) Ltd.

Chapter 44—Figs. 1, 2 and 3 are reproduced from *Anatomy for the Anaesthetist* by Professor H. Ellis and Miss M. McLarty published by Blackwell Scientific Publications.

Chapter 45—Fig. 1, Dr. C. L. Hewer and A. K. Hawkins & Co. Ltd.

Section Four

Chapter 46—Fig. 1 is reproduced from *The Lung* by J. H. Comroe, Jr., R. E. Forster II, A. B. Dubois, W. A. Briscoe and E. Carlson, published by the Year Book Medical Publishers, Inc.; Fig. 4, Dr. David Benazon and the Editor of *Anaesthesia*; Fig. 5, Dr. J. D. Michenfelder and the Editors of *Anesthesiology*.

Chapter 47—Fig. 1 is based on a figure in a paper by Drs. B. Creamer and J. W. Pierce, published in *Thorax*. Parts of the section on regurgitation and vomiting are reprinted from articles by Dr. H. J. V. Morton and one of us, and are published here by kind permission of Dr. Morton and the Editor of *Anaesthesia*. Other parts are based on an article by one of us in the *British Journal of Anaesthesia* and are reproduced by kind permission of John Sherratt and Son, publishers of this journal.

Section Five

Chapter 50—Figs. 1 and 2 adapted from figures in a chapter by Drs. J. J. Brown, A. F. Lever and J. I. S. Robinson published in the 15th edition of *Recent Advances in Medicine*, J. & A. Churchill Ltd.

Section Six

Chapter 51—Figs. 1 and 4, Lloyd-Luke (Medical Books) Ltd.

Chapter 52—Fig. 1, Dr. R. C. Nainby-Luxmoore and the Editor of *Anaesthesia*; Figs. 3, 4 and 5, British Oxygen Company Ltd.; Fig. 6, Medical and Industrial Equipment Ltd.; Figs. 7 and 8, Cyprane Ltd.

Chapter 53—Fig. 1, Lloyd-Luke (Medical Books) Ltd.; Table 1, H.M. Stationery Office; Table 2, Dr. M. J. Rorke, Dr. D. A. Davey and Dr. H. J. Du Toit, and the Editor of *Anaesthesia*.

Appendices

Appendix II—Figs. 2, 5, 6, 7 and 8, I.B.M. United Kingdom Ltd.; Figs. 3 and 4, Mr. R. Corkhill.

CONTENTS

Section Two—THE CARDIOVASCULAR SYSTEM

Section Three—THE NERVOUS SYSTEM

APPENDICES

Section One

THE RESPIRATORY SYSTEM

Chapter 1

ANATOMY OF THE RESPIRATORY TRACT IN RELATION TO ANAESTHESIA

THE NOSE

Functions

The nose has five important functions to perform:—

1. The adult patient breathes through his nose, unless there is some form of obstruction caused, for example, by nasal polypi or a severe catarrhal condition. In normal subjects the resistance created by breathing through the nose is $1\frac{1}{2}$ times greater than mouth breathing. Deflection of the nasal septum may diminish the lumen of the respiratory air-way and in some cases it is sufficiently severe to prevent the passage of all but the smallest of endotracheal tubes. Before attempting nasal intubation it is advisable to test the patency of each nostril in turn by listening for the sound that indicates a free flow of air, and to choose the side where the obstruction is greatest anteriorly. One of the disadvantages of nasal intubation as compared with the oral route is that it usually necessitates using an endotracheal tube of small diameter.

2. The stiff hairs in the anterior part of the nasal fossa together with the spongy mucous membrane and the ciliated epithelium comprise a powerful defence against the invasion of any organism. In reserve lie the flushing action of the watery secretions, the bactericidal properties of these secretions, and the extensive lymph drainage of the whole area.

3. Warming and humidifying the inspired air or gases is probably the most important work the nose performs. The enormity of the task can only be realised if it is recalled that 10,000 litres of air pass through every twenty-four hours. The great vascularity of the mucosa helps to maintain a constant temperature: inspired air at 17° C is heated to approximately 37° C during its passage through the nose and variations in external air temperature ranging from 25–0° C produce less than 1° C change in the temperature of air reaching the laryngeal inlet.

The supply of moisture comes partly from transudations of fluid through the mucosal epithelium and to a less extent from secretions of glands and goblet cells in the nasal mucous membrane. The daily volume of nasal secretions is about 1 litre, of which about three-quarters is utilised in saturating the inspired air. Moisture is also obtained from the air or gases that are inhaled.

The optimum relative humidity of air is 45–55 per cent but the bronchi and alveoli require 95 per cent for adequate function.

As a result of endotracheal intubation, or after tracheostomy, only relatively dry gases or air reach the lower part of the trachea, thus compelling the mucosa in this area to perform the duties of the nasal mucous membrane. Although in time the mucosa can adapt itself to the changed conditions, to begin with it becomes dry, and the absence of moisture, even for a few minutes, leads to a cessation of ciliary activity. When adaptation is slow there may be degeneration of the mucosal cells. Endotracheal anaesthesia is in fact frequently followed by a mild tracheitis; this incidence is accentuated when gases, which have had almost all their moisture removed before storage in cylinders, are used in an anaesthetic system that has a relatively low humidity.

Even the nasal inhalation of dry gas can be dangerous if it is prolonged, and when oxygen therapy is ordered the gas should always be humidified.

4. Vocal resonance is influenced by the patency of the nasal passages.
5. The nose detects smells.

The Nasal Mucous Membrane

Anatomically this covers three areas:

The vestibule, in front, is lined by stratified squamous epithelium. Anteriorly, the epithelium has a superficial horny layer from which many stout hairs (vibrissae) protrude into the lumen of the nares. Posteriorly, these hairs are absent and the stratified epithelium gives way to ciliated columnar cells in the region of the turbinates and the inferior meatus.

The respiratory region covers the major part of the walls of the nasal cavities and accessory nasal sinuses. The mucous membrane is ciliated columnar epithelium with tall cells which extend through the entire depth of the layer.

The olfactory region is where the terminal filaments of the olfactory nerve reach the surface and is lined by stratified squamous epithelium.

The blood supply to the nasal mucosa is controlled by an elaborate autonomic reflex which enables the mucosa to swell or shrink on demand. There is a dual nerve supply to this area. Parasympathetic fibres pass via the facial, greater superficial petrosal and vidian nerves to relay in the spheno-palatine ganglion. Sympathetic fibres reach the ganglion from the plexus surrounding the internal carotid artery, via the vidian nerve, while sensory fibres come from the maxillary nerve. From the ganglion palatine and naso-palatine branches travel in the septum and lateral walls of the nose to the mucosa. A small area of mucosa is supplied by the anterior ethmoidal nerve, a branch of the ophthalmic nerve.

In animals a notable reflex from this area is that known as the "Kratschmer" reflex in which stimulation of the anterior part of the nasal septum leads to constriction of the bronchioles. When a patient's nose is plugged with gauze after an operation in it, intense restlessness often occurs during the recovery period even though the oral airway is adequate and there is no pain. This situation is frequently encountered in adolescents who have had a fractured nasal septum remodelled. It suggests a reflex from the nasal mucous membrane.

Ciliary Activity

Throughout the respiratory tract the continuous activity of the cilia is probably the most important single factor in the prevention of the accumulation of secretions. In the nose the flow of material is swept towards the pharynx, whereas in the bronchial tree the flow is carried towards the entrance to the larynx.

Each cilia consists of a very fine hair-like structure approximately 7μ long and $0{\cdot}3\mu$ thick, in which the tip is always bent towards the direction of the flow of mucus (Fig. 1). The co-ordinated movement of numerous cilia is capable of moving large quantities of material but their activity is greatly assisted by their mucous covering, which consists of two layers: an outer layer of thick viscous mucus which is designed to entrap particulate matter such as dust, soot, or micro-organisms, and an inner layer of thin serous fluid designed to lubricate the action of the ciliary mechanism. The tips of the cilia come just in contact with the outer layer with each beat. Acting in unison, they set the outer mucous

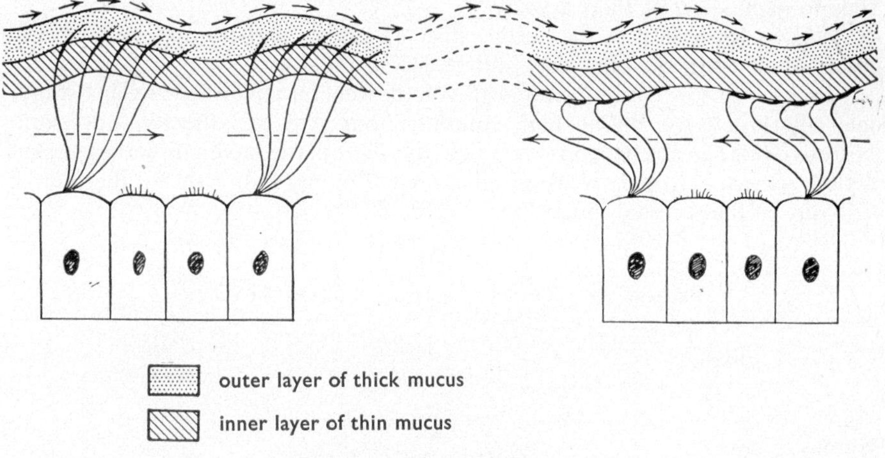

1/Fig. 1.—Ciliary movement.

layer in motion and with gathering momentum this flows towards the pharynx and larynx.

Ciliary movement consists of a rapid forward thrust followed by a slow recoil which occupies about four-fifths of the cycle. At 30° C the cilia of the nasal mucosa beat about 10–15 times per second. The streaming movement of the overlying mucus has been estimated at 0·25–1·0 centimetre per minute, the slowest speeds being in the bronchioles. The entire contents of the nose can thus be emptied into the pharynx every 20–30 minutes.

Factors Influencing Ciliary Activity

Temperature.—The optimum range of temperature for ciliary movement in excised human nasal mucosa is 28°–33° C, while the average nasal temperature is about 32° C. Ciliary activity ceases when the temperature of the mucosa falls to 7°–10° C and is depressed by temperatures rising above 35° C; however, only these extreme variations in temperature have much effect on ciliary action and any changes that do occur are largely caused by alterations in the amount of mucus secreted rather than by any direct influence on the ciliated epithelium.

Mucus.—Cilia cannot work without a blanket of mucus. Negus (1949) has compared their action to that of a conveyor belt system in which the platform on which the packages rest corresponds to the blanket of mucus and the propulsive force underneath is represented by the cilia. In all probability the volatile general anaesthetics not only slow the propelling mechanism but also limit the production of suitable secretions. If a patient has an inadequate secretion of mucus after the use of atropine, or breathes dry gases for a long period, then evaporation will result in drying of the mucosa and ciliary activity will cease.

Changes in pH.—Cilia prefer a dilute alkaline solution and are readily paralysed by acid solutions with a pH of 6·4 or less (Negus, 1934). A rise of pH to 8·0 or more leads to swelling of the columnar cells bearing the cilia and thus to depression of their activity.

Sleep.—Natural sleep has little effect on ciliary activity and even several hours after death the cilia may still be found moving.

Drugs.—In low concentrations all volatile general anaesthetic agents stimulate ciliary activity, but in high concentrations they are directly depressant. Nitrous oxide has no effect on ciliary activity. The opiates have a direct depressant action, whereas atropine weakens ciliary activity only indirectly by altering the viscosity of the secreted mucus.

1/Table 1

Effects of Various Agents on Ciliary Activity

Drugs		*Low concentrations*	*High concentrations*
Nitrous oxide		0	0
Ether		+	− −
Chloroform		+	− −
Cyclopropane		+	− −
Morphia		−	− −
Atropine		−	− −
Cocaine	10 per cent	− − −	
,,	5 per cent	− −	
,,	2½ per cent	+	
Ephedrine	½ per cent	+	
Adrenaline	(1:10,000)	− − −	

− = inhibition of ciliary movement. 0 = no effect on ciliary movement. + = stimulation of ciliary movement.

Posture.—Gravity appears to have no effect on ciliary action and the flow always continues in the same direction whatever the patient's position.

Anaesthesia and Humidity

Importance of humidity.—The importance of humidifying the inspired gases is well-known to all those responsible for the management of patients on intermittent positive-pressure respiration. The anaesthetised patient undergoing a routine operation usually breathes virtually dry gases for long periods of time. With an artificial airway in position the gases tend to flow through the mouth so that the functions of the nose are largely short-circuited, while with an endotracheal tube, the whole role of providing adequate humidification falls on the lower respiratory tract. This situation may influence the incidence of tracheitis, bronchitis and pulmonary collapse in the post-operative period.

Physical principles.—The quantity of water needed to saturate air with water vapour increases with the temperature (Fig. 2).

Thus, the warmer the air becomes the more vapour it can hold. For example, if warm air is breathed out on to the surface of a mirror (at room temperature) then this air is cooled and can no longer hold so much water vapour, consequently the water vapour condenses on the glass. On the other hand, if a mirror is warmed to body temperature or above (as in indirect laryngoscopy) then condensation does not occur.

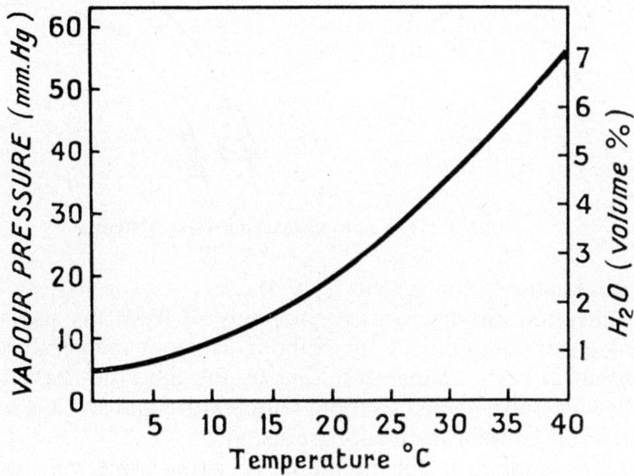

1/Fig. 2.—The relationship of water vapour tension in air to temperature.

At a room temperature of 17° C the air contains 2 volumes per cent of water when fully saturated. At a body temperature of 37° C the air in the trachea contains 6 volumes per cent of water vapour. The nose and respiratory tract, therefore, not only have the task of warming the inspired air but also of adding large quantities of water vapour. The value of this mechanism is appreciated to the full by anyone who runs rapidly on a cold dry morning. The increased inhalation of air through the mouth leads to drying of the tracheal mucous membrane and an uncomfortable "soreness" in the chest.

Anaesthetic Apparatus

In most anaesthetic systems the temperature of the gases reaching the patient is approximately the same as the room temperature. This is because the room air warms the gases during their passage through a long length of flexible rubber breathing tubing. The principal exception to this rule is in the to and fro' system where the temperature of the cannister (near the patient's mouth) may rise to as high as 45° C and in which no time is available for the cooling of gases en route to the patient. This system, therefore, provides very efficient humidification but it has other disadvantages (see p. 204).

Two other principal types of anaesthetic system should be considered:

(*a*) The non-rebreathing valve system (Fig. 3).

The inspired air is always at room temperature (17° C) and therefore even if fully saturated it can only hold about 2 volumes per cent of water. Because there is no rebreathing the expired air (at 37° C and fully saturated) passes out through the valve and is lost to the atmosphere.

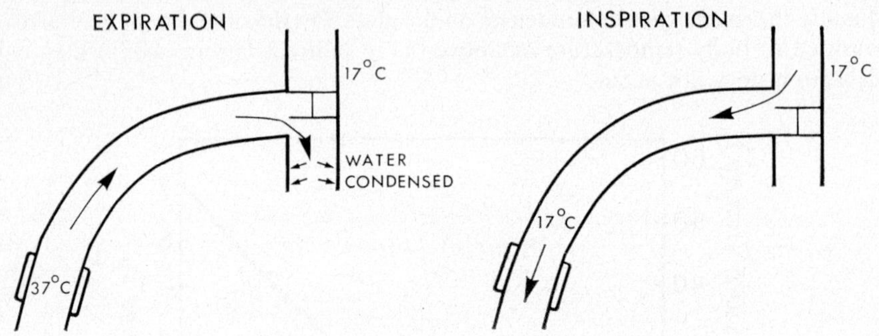

1/Fig. 3.—The non-rebreathing valve system.

(*b*) The circle absorption system (Fig. 4).

Here the inspired mixture consists not only of fresh dry gases but also of some expired gases containing water vapour at room temperature. The latter leave the patient at body temperature, but by the time they have traversed the apparatus they will have cooled to room temperature and so have lost the major part of their water content in the apparatus.

Approximate values for the humidity of gases using various anaesthetic systems are shown in Table 2.

1/Table 2

The Relative Humidity of Gases in the Various Anaesthetic Systems

Anaesthetic system	*Percentage humidity of gases*
Non-rebreathing valve	0
T-piece	0
To and fro'	40–100
Closed circle	40–60
Human nose	100

Effect of Premedication, Intubation and Dry Gases

Burton (1962) studied the effects of premedication, the endotracheal tube, and dry anaesthetic gases on ciliary activity by observing the movement of an ink marker placed at the carina of anaesthetised dogs. Under pentobarbitone anaesthesia alone the ink passed up the trachea and out through the vocal cords within 20–30 minutes.

After atropine premedication, the rate of movement of the ink was slowed to 10 cm. in 30 minutes and normal movement was not resumed for some 4–5 hours. The endotracheal tube by itself had little untoward action if the gases were

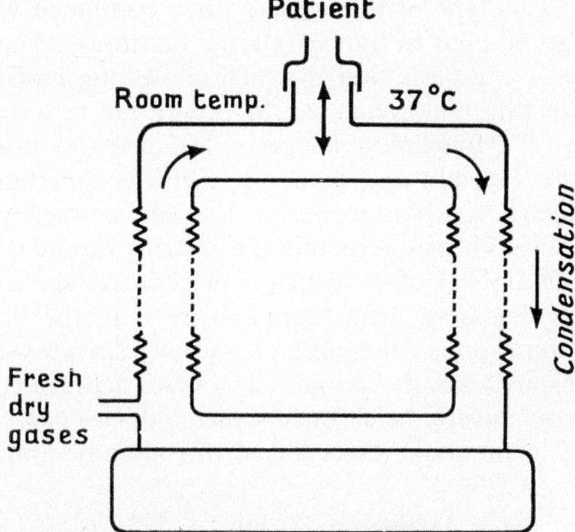

1/FIG. 4.—The loss of water by condensation in a circle absorption system.

humidified, but the inflation of a cuff immediately produced a complete barrier to the passage of the marker ink. Dry anaesthetic gases, as delivered direct from a cylinder, produced gross reduction in ciliary movement. Thus, after 4½ hours anaesthesia using a Rubens non-rebreathing valve the maximal movement of the marker was only 2.5 cm. in 30 minutes.

It is hardly surprising, therefore, that after a prolonged period of anaesthesia the mucosa of the trachea and lower respiratory tract shows evidence of dryness and an inflammatory reaction.

The whole process may be summarised as follows:

Atropine + Dry gas } → Dry mucosa → Inflammatory reaction → Excessive mucus

Inflammatory reaction ↓ Tracheitis & Bronchitis

Excessive mucus ↓ ? Pulmonary collapse

Methods of Humidification

1. **Direct instillation.**—Water or saline may be administered by slow drip directly into a tracheostomy. This technique is not very effective, but it is probably better than nothing at all.

2. **Water-bath.**—The gas mixture is blown across the surface of a heated, thermostatically controlled, water-bath. This may be used in conjunction with an artificial ventilator, when the humidifier must be placed on the inspiratory side of the system, and the gases led to the patient by the shortest possible route.

The tubing should be insulated to prevent heat loss, with consequent condensation. By raising the temperature in the humidifier slightly above body-temperature it is possible to deliver gases to the patient which are at 37°C and completely saturated with water-vapour. The exact temperature setting of the water-bath will depend on the surface area of water exposed to the gases, the flow rate of these gases and the amount of cooling and condensation taking place in the inspiratory tubing.

This type of humidifier, when combined with a fan to blow air through it, can be used to humidify a tracheostomy. The attachment to the tracheostomy. is of a T-piece design which allows the moistened air to flow freely across the opening. The weight of the tubing can be a serious disadvantage to the patient.

3. **Moisture exchanger.**—The heat and moisture exchanger (Toremalm, 1960) offers a light and moderately efficient method of humidification for a patient breathing spontaneously through a tracheostomy or endotracheal tube. It consists of two aluminium foil strips wound together and covered by a plexiglass container (Fig. 5), which is placed over the tracheostomy or endotracheal tube. As it is at a lower temperature than the body, part of the water vapour of expiration is condensed on its inner surface where it is available to humidify the inspired air. It cannot, of course, achieve full saturation owing to the lower temperature. Nevertheless such a device can considerably improve the humidity of inspired air, especially if this already contains a little water vapour.

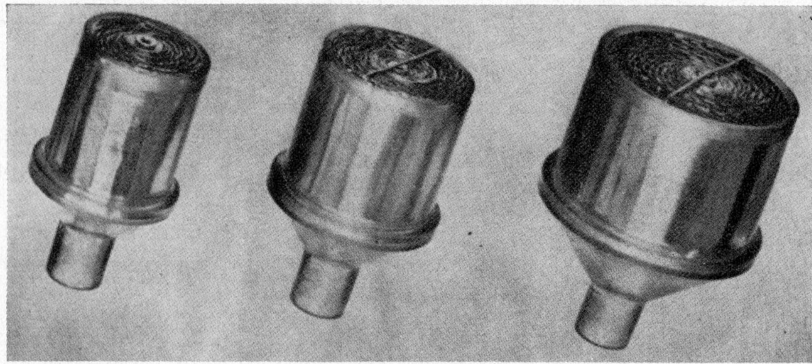

1/Fig. 5.—The heat and moisture exchanger of Toremalm. It comprises two aluminium foil strips (one of which is corrugated) wound together and covered by a plexiglass cylinder.

4. **Mechanical nebuliser.**—This is a pneumatic device which breaks up a liquid into small particles. Water, when placed in the nebuliser passes up a capillary tube at the summit of which it is nebulised by a jet of gas. The droplet leaving the capillary tube then crashes into the side of a ball where it is fractured into numerous small particles. Most particles of 5 microns and above cling to the ball, coalesce, and fall back into the reservoir. Those particles of 4 microns or less tend to float out and join the inspired gases. In this type of nebuliser 80 per cent of the particles are in the range 2–4 microns and the remainder are smaller. Most of these particles are deposited around the pharynx, and only a small percentage reach the bronchial level, but for many patients this is sufficient. Because it is compact this nebuliser can conveniently be placed in

close proximity to the patient's airway (Fig. 6). It can also be used pre- or post-operatively with a face mask for the improvement of lung function, or it can be attached directly to a tracheostomy tube.

5. **Ultrasonic nebuliser.**—All the methods so far described have various disadvantages, and they may interfere with ventilator treatment.

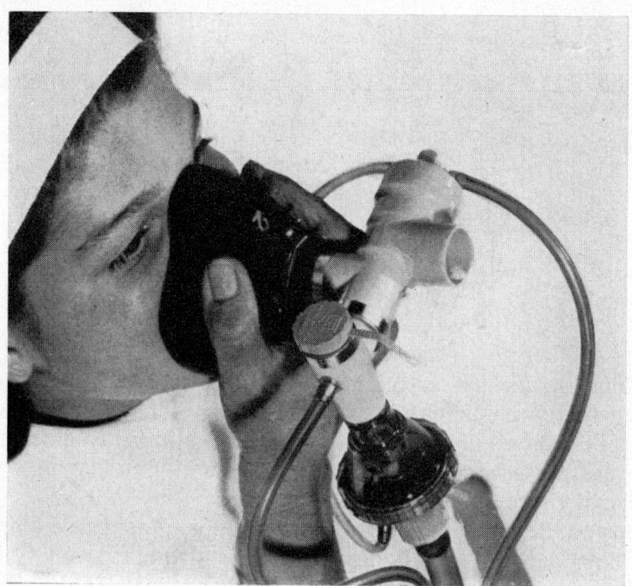

1/FIG. 6.—Mechanical nebuliser (Bird).

In 1964 Herzog and his colleagues introduced to clinical practice an ultrasonic nebuliser consisting of a plexiglass container to hold 150 ml. of fluid and with a vibrating transducer head at its base. The transducer head is activated by a high-frequency (3 megacycle) generator and is fed with drops of fluid by a capillary tube which passes through the top of the container. The nebuliser should be connected to the inspiratory side of a ventilator (Fig. 7).

Each drop of fluid is completely nebulised to an aerosol in which 70 per cent of the particles have a size of 0·8 to 1 micron, the actual size being dependent on the frequency of the transducer head (Matauschek, 1961). Most particles of 1 micron or less are deposited in the lower airways and alveoli of the lungs. At the maximum rate of 12 drops per minute dripping on to the transducer head and with a ventilator delivering 10 litres of gas per minute, 72 mg. water are provided with each litre of gas. This corresponds to a relative humidity of 164 per cent at 37°C. No other method of humidification can achieve more than a fifth of this amount.

Ultrasonic nebulisers produce satisfactory humidification in patients who have very dry airways at the start of treatment (e.g. children with tracheo-bronchitis) and they can be used for the administration of water-soluble aerosol drugs, but they are not without dangers. Their extreme efficiency makes over-hydration possible, especially in children, and they are difficult to sterilise by conventional

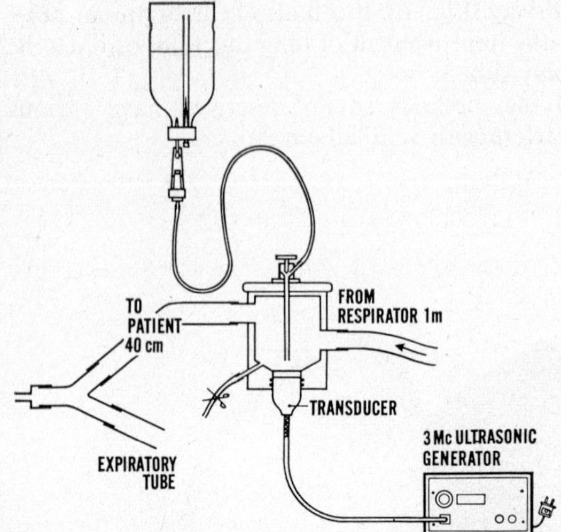

1/FIG. 7.—Diagram of an ultrasonic nebuliser (Herzog *et al.*, 1964).

methods. Ringrose and his colleagues (1968) have described how outbreaks of infection can follow inadequate cleaning of ultrasonic nebulisers. When used for a long time continuously on the same patient an ultrasonic nebuliser will increase the airway resistance (Cheney and Butler, 1968), and may cause pulmonary collapse (Modell, 1968).

Variations on the design of Herzog's nebuliser, such as the de Vilbis and the Elmed, are in production, their main difference being the frequency of the transducer head and hence an alteration in the size of the particles of fluid produced.

An ultrasonic nebuliser can be used to sterilise a ventilator by producing an aerosol of alcohol (Spencer *et al.*, 1968).

PHARYNX

The pharynx extends from the posterior aspect of the nose at the base of the skull down to the level of the lower border of the cricoid cartilage where it becomes continuous with the oesophagus, and the respiratory tract through the larynx. The soft palate partially divides the pharynx into two—an upper nasopharyngeal portion and a lower orolaryngeal portion.

In the nasopharyngeal part a collection of lymphoid tissue—the nasopharyngeal tonsil or "adenoids"—lies embedded in the mucous membrane at the junction of the roof with the upper and posterior part of the pharynx. Lying close to the base of the nasopharyngeal tonsil is a small recess—the pharyngeal bursa. These structures often impede the passage of an endotracheal tube; if force is used the tube may penetrate the mucosa and create a false passage which can lead to trouble from sepsis and collection of secretions during the post-operative period.

The lymph drainage of the pharynx is often of clinical importance because enlargement of the lymphatic glands and swelling of the overlying mucosa may, in some instances, lead to partial obstruction of the airway. These lymph glands are numerous and are arranged in a circular fashion—the ring of Waldeyer (Fig. 8).

In essence the ring consists of the large palatine tonsils (P) lying between the pillars of the fauces; the smaller lingual tonsil (L) at the base of the tongue on each side of the middle line and in front of the vallecula, the Eustachian tonsil (E) which is an accumulation of lymphoid follicles sometimes found on the posterior lip of the orifice of the Eustachian tube, and the nasopharyngeal tonsil (NP) which is a group of follicles united in one mass on the posterior wall of the nasopharynx. On the posterior wall of the pharynx at the level of the large palatine tonsils some small lymph nodes are often found. These are of particular importance when sepsis occurs in this neighbourhood because they swell up to form a retropharyngeal abscess. This may either occur in conjunction with sepsis tracking inwards from the spinal column or with a

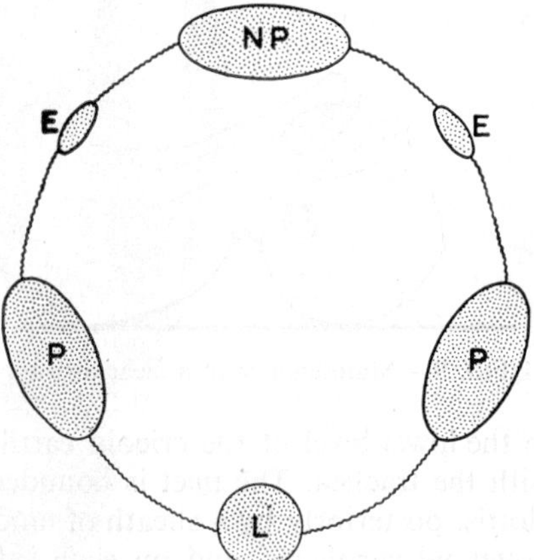

1/FIG. 8.—PHARYNGEAL AND TONSILLAR GLANDS (RING OF WALDEYER)
P = Palatine tonsil.
L = Lingual tonsil.
E = Eustachian tonsil.
NP = Nasopharyngeal tonsil or "adenoids".

peritonsillar abscess ("quinsy"). The presence of a large retropharyngeal abscess makes nasal intubation extremely difficult and dangerous because the endotracheal tube may be deflected sharply forwards or it may impinge on and rupture the abscess.

Pharyngeal obstruction and the airway.—One of the principal duties of an anaesthetist is to learn the art of maintaining a completely unobstructed airway in an unconscious patient. The introduction of endotracheal intubation enables the lazy anaesthetist to circumvent this duty. Nevertheless, the fact that intubation may lead to a sore throat, infection, or—rarely—laryngeal lesions is a reason why it should only be used when indicated.

The principal difficulty in maintaining a perfect airway in an unconscious patient is the tendency of the tongue to fall backwards and obstruct the laryngeal opening. This occurs as soon as consciousness is lost and the muscles supporting the tongue start to relax. If the tongue is brought forward then the laryngeal opening once again is cleared.

The recent interest in teaching lay members of the public the various methods of artificial respiration has highlighted the importance of correct positioning of the head and neck if a clear airway is to be obtained.

Two separate manoeuvres are required to provide the perfect airway in the unconscious patient. First, the lower jaw must be carried forwards and upwards

lengthen the vocal cords and the thyro-arytenoid muscles which shorten them.

The tension of the vocal cords is altered by the vocales, which are a part of the thyro-arytenoid muscles.

Nerve Supply to the Larynx

The mucous membrane receives its nerve supply from both the superior and recurrent laryngeal nerves. The superior laryngeal nerve arises from the inferior ganglion of the vagus but receives a small branch from the superior cervical sympathetic ganglion. This nerve descends in the lateral wall of the pharynx, passing posteriorly to the internal carotid artery, and at the level of the greater horn of the hyoid divides into an internal and an external branch.

The internal laryngeal branch, which is entirely sensory apart from a few motor filaments to the arytenoid muscles, descends to the thyrohyoid membrane, pierces it above the superior laryngeal artery and then divides again into two branches. The upper branch supplies the mucous membrane of the lower part of the pharynx, epiglottis, vallecula and vestibule of the larynx. The lower branch passes medial to the pyriform fossa beneath the mucous membrane and supplies the ary-epiglottic fold and the mucous membrane of the posterior part of the rima glottidis.

The external laryngeal branch carries motor fibres which innervate the cricothyroid muscle.

The recurrent laryngeal nerve accompanies the laryngeal branch of the inferior thyroid artery and travels upwards, deep to the lower border of the inferior constrictor muscle of the pharynx immediately behind the cricothyroid joint. Apart from sensory fibres which supply the mucous membrane of the larynx below the level of the vocal cords, this nerve innervates all the muscles of the larynx except the cricothyroid, and a small part of the arytenoid muscles.

Cord Palsies

The cords can be visualised either indirectly by means of a mirror or—and this is the more familiar method for the anaesthetist—directly with a laryngoscope. This description of normal and abnormal cord movements is, therefore, written and illustrated from the point of view of direct laryngoscopy.

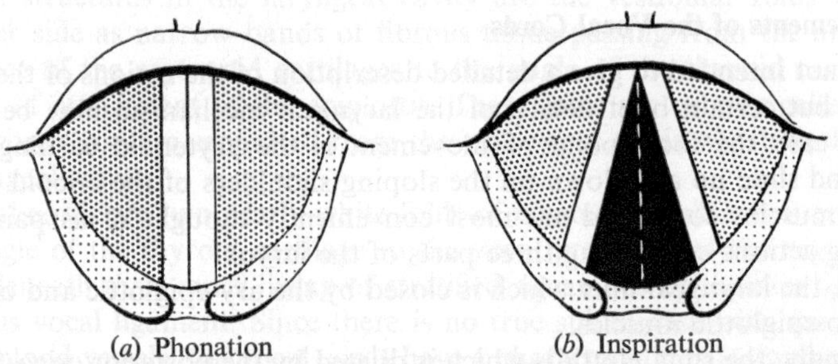

(*a*) Phonation (*b*) Inspiration

1/FIG. 11.—The vocal cords.

During phonation the vocal cords meet in the mid-line (Fig. 11*a*). On inspiration they abduct (Fig. 11*b*), returning to the mid-line on expiration, but leaving a small gap between them. The opening into the trachea between the vocal cords is maximal at the end of a deep inspiration. In order, therefore, to minimise the risk of any possible trauma to the cords, intubation and extubation should be carried out during inspiration. When laryngeal spasm is present, both the false and the true cords are held tightly in apposition.

Topical analgesia of the throat and larynx blocks the sensory nerve endings of the superior and recurrent laryngeal nerves. Following this procedure, an occasional patient is unable to phonate clearly and develops a "gruff" voice—an effect which is probably due to some local analgesic solution reaching and blocking the external branch of the superior laryngeal nerve. This nerve carries motor fibres to the cricothyroid muscle, which is the principal tensor of the cords. Paralysis of the cricothyroid muscle produces visible alterations in the shape of the glottis and vocal cords—effects that must be remembered should they follow topical analgesia for diagnostic laryngoscopy. The superior laryngeal nerve itself may be traumatised during thyroidectomy when the superior thyroid artery is tied. Since the only motor fibres of the nerve are those that run on into its external branch, exactly similar effects to those just described will follow.

Damage to the recurrent laryngeal nerve may take the form of complete section or merely bruising. This nerve carries both the abductor and the adductor motor fibres of the vocal cords. The abductor fibres, however, are more vulnerable so that moderate trauma usually leads to a pure abductor paralysis. Severe trauma or section of the recurrent laryngeal nerve causes both abductor and adductor paralysis. A pure adductor paralysis does not occur as a clinical entity.

It is not always easy to differentiate between the various types of cord palsy but the main points are illustrated diagrammatically below. Unilateral lesions are assumed to exist on a patient's left side. The position of the cords during both phonation and inspiration is diagnostic.

Pure abductor palsy—left.—On phonation both cords meet in the mid-line because the adductor fibres on the left (damaged) side are still active. It will be noticed, however, that the right false cord tends to lie slightly anterior to that

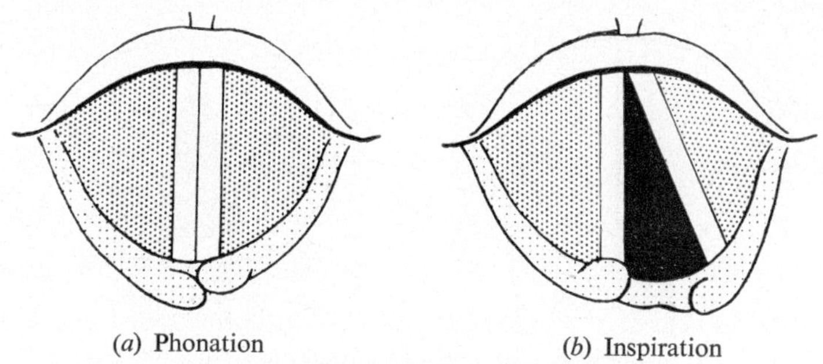

(*a*) Phonation (*b*) Inspiration

1/FIG. 12.—Pure abductor palsy—Left.

on the left (Fig. 12 *a*). On inspiration the cord on the side of the injury remains in approximately the same position, but the cord on the unaffected side moves into full abduction (Fig. 12 *b*).

Abductor and adductor palsy—left.—In this case both types of fibre are no longer functioning on the left, so that the cord tends to rest in a slightly more abducted position. On phonation, the right cord crosses the mid-line in an attempt to meet its opposite number (Fig. 13*a*). As it is forced to move in the arc of a circle, the right false cord appears to lie in front of the left. On inspiration, the unaffected cord moves back again into full abduction (Fig. 13 *b*).

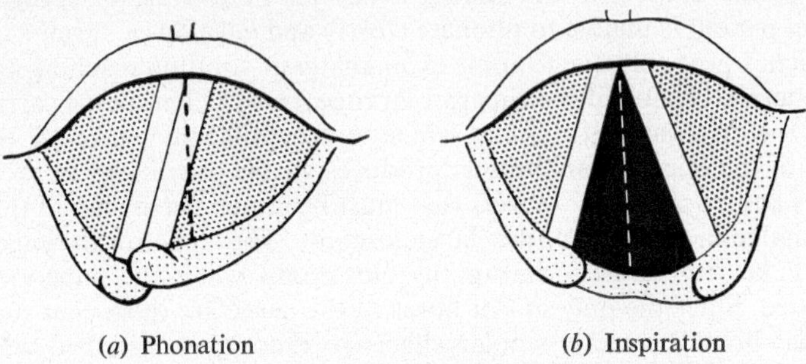

(*a*) Phonation (*b*) Inspiration

1/Fig. 13.—Abductor and adductor palsy—Left.

Bilateral damage to the recurrent laryngeal nerves.—This may occur during removal of the thyroid gland. The position of the vocal cords will depend upon the severity of the damage.

When the trauma is mild on both sides, then a bilateral abductor paralysis may result. Severe trauma, or complete section, on both sides affects both abductor and adductor fibres. It is important to differentiate between these two conditions because they have differing effects on the laryngeal airway. After partial damage the vocal cords lie near the mid-line because the adductor fibres are still functioning, and the airway is reduced to a mere chink (Fig. 14 *a*). A patient in this condition usually rapidly shows signs of severe respiratory obstruction, particularly when respiration is active due to fear or other causes.

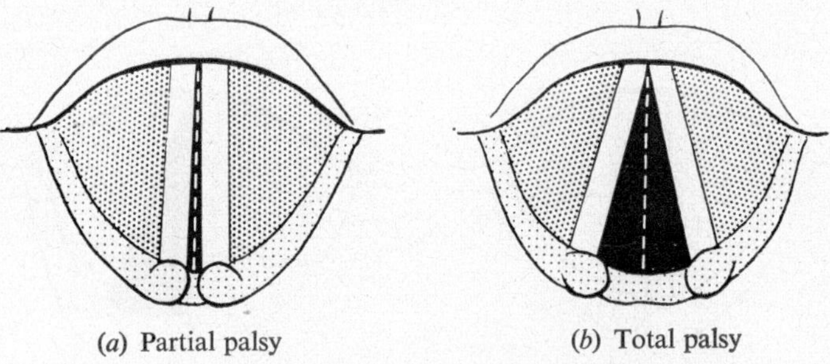

(*a*) Partial palsy (*b*) Total palsy

1/Fig. 14.—Bilateral damage to the recurrent laryngeal nerve.

When both nerves are severely damaged, or cut across, the vocal cords lie stationary in the mid position with a fair-sized lumen between them (Fig. 14 *b*). Now, the airway is fairly adequate unless respiratory effort is very marked, when the cords tend to be sucked in with each inspiration.

Bilateral palsy of the recurrent laryngeal nerves with palsy of the external branch of the superior laryngeal nerve.—Total paralysis of the cords is now associated with paralysis of the cricothyroid muscles. The vocal cords are no longer tensed and the antero-posterior diameter of the glottis is reduced. This is the true cadaveric position. With complete relaxation, such as may be obtained by one of the muscle relaxants, exactly the same position is seen (Fig. 15).

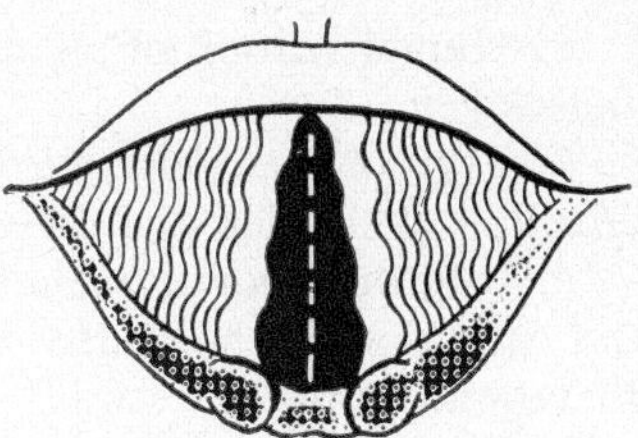

1/FIG. 15.—Bilateral palsy of the recurrent laryngeal nerves with palsy of the external branch of the superior laryngeal nerve.

Laryngeal Trauma and Oedema (see also Chapter 10)

Trauma to the larynx during intubation of the trachea may lead to oedema (particularly in small children) and to a granuloma of the cords at a later date.

TRACHEA AND BRONCHIAL TREE (Figs. 17 and 18)

The trachea is a tube formed of rings of cartilage which are incomplete posteriorly. It is about 10–11 cm. long, extending downwards from the lower part of the larynx opposite the level of the 6th cervical vertebra to the point of its bifurcation into a right and left main bronchus at the carina, about the upper border of the 5th thoracic vertebra. It is lined by ciliated columnar epithelium.

The trachea moves with respiration and with alterations in the position of the head. Thus on deep inspiration the carina can descend as much as 2·5 cm. The significance of this movement is not known but it may facilitate expansion of the apical parts of the lung. Similarly extension of the head and neck—the ideal position in which to maintain an airway in an anaesthetised patient—can increase the length of the trachea by as much as 23 to 30 per cent. Clinically, if a patient is intubated with the head in a flexed position at the atlanto-occipital joint, and the endotracheal tube is so short that it just reaches beyond the vocal cords, the subsequent hyperextension of the head may withdraw the tube into the pharynx.

Tracheostomy is always performed at a level below the first tracheal ring cartilage as section of this structure may lead later to the development of a stricture. One of the principal problems following a tracheostomy is the prevention of drying and encrustation of the mucous membrane in the trachea and main bronchi. This may develop rapidly despite humidification of the air and occasionally it may lead to complete respiratory obstruction and death.

Encrustation of the tracheal mucosa, of the inner tracheostomy tube and of the main bronchi can be prevented in the following ways (see also Chapter 15):

1. The material used in the tracheostomy tube is important because rubber is an irritant to the mucosa whereas silver or plastic tubes are not. Metal tracheostomy tubes have an inner tube which can be removed, inspected, cleaned

and replaced. Rubber and plastic tracheostomy tubes are more comfortable and can be provided with a cuff which may be blown up to provide an airtight fit in the trachea. When these are used a sharp watch must be kept to see that they do not become blocked. Suction alone may not prevent the gradual accumulation of crusts and it is advisable to remove the tube at regular intervals (every other day) at first to be certain that all is well. Later the tube can be left for longer periods.

2. Humidification of all air entering through the tracheostomy tube must be undertaken.

3. Trypsin is an enzyme which hydrolyses proteins and when used as an aerosol it can soften and digest the inspissated secretions.

4. Isopropyl noradrenaline (1:100–1:200 solution) is miscible with trypsin and can therefore be added to the aerosol mixture to produce local broncho-dilatation.

5. Promethazine (25 mg. q.d.s.) can be used as a parenteral broncho-dilator.

A variety of names has been given to the divisions of the bronchial tree and this has for many years past been a constant source of confusion. In 1948 an international committee agreed on a generally acceptable nomenclature which is shown in diagrammatic and schematic form in Fig. 17 and Table 3. In the description that follows the English nomenclature will be used throughout.

Right Bronchial Tree.

The *right main bronchus* is wider and shorter than the left, being only 2·5 cm. long. As it is more nearly vertical than the left main bronchus there is a much greater tendency for either endotracheal tubes or suction catheters to enter this

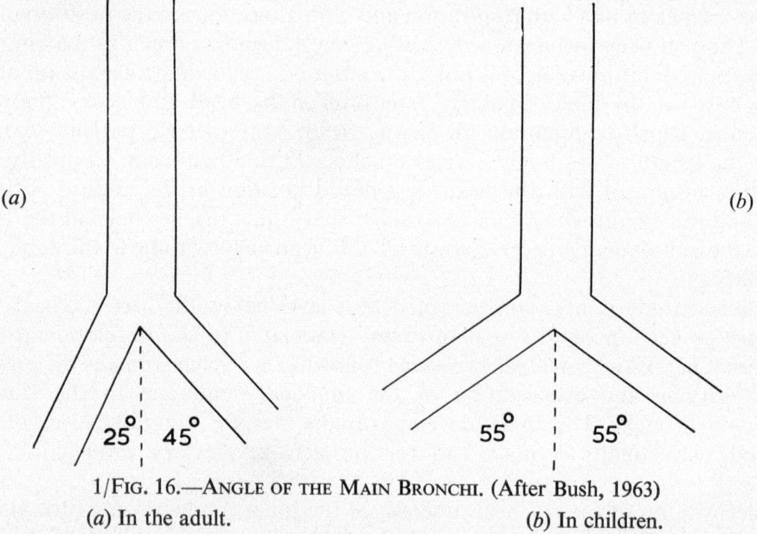

1/Fig. 16.—Angle of the Main Bronchi. (After Bush, 1963)
(*a*) In the adult. (*b*) In children.

lumen. Adriani and Griggs (1954) have pointed out that in small children under the age of three years the angulation of the two main bronchi at the carina is equal on both sides (Fig. 16). In the event of an endotracheal tube being inserted

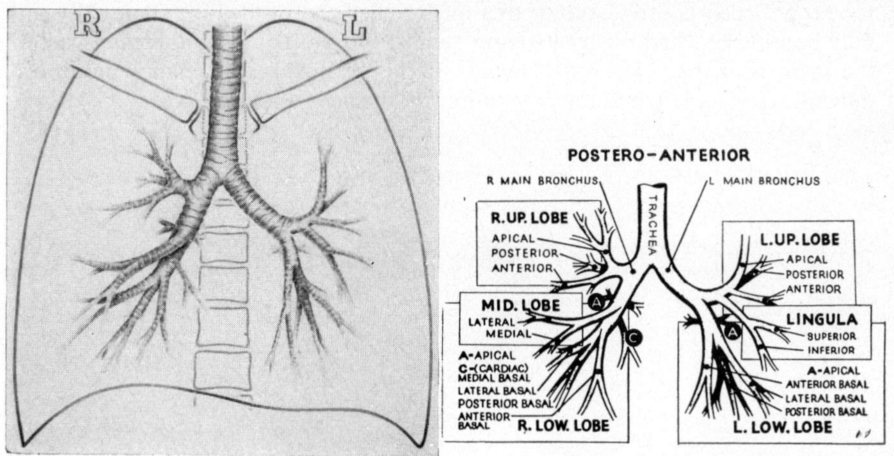
R
L
POSTERO–ANTERIOR
R MAIN BRONCHUS
L MAIN BRONCHUS
TRACHEA
R. UP. LOBE
APICAL
POSTERIOR
ANTERIOR
MID. LOBE
LATERAL
MEDIAL
A-APICAL
C-(CARDIAC) MEDIAL BASAL
LATERAL BASAL
POSTERIOR BASAL
ANTERIOR BASAL
R. LOW. LOBE
L. UP. LOBE
APICAL
POSTERIOR
ANTERIOR
LINGULA
SUPERIOR
INFERIOR
A-APICAL
ANTERIOR BASAL
LATERAL BASAL
POSTERIOR BASAL
L. LOW. LOBE

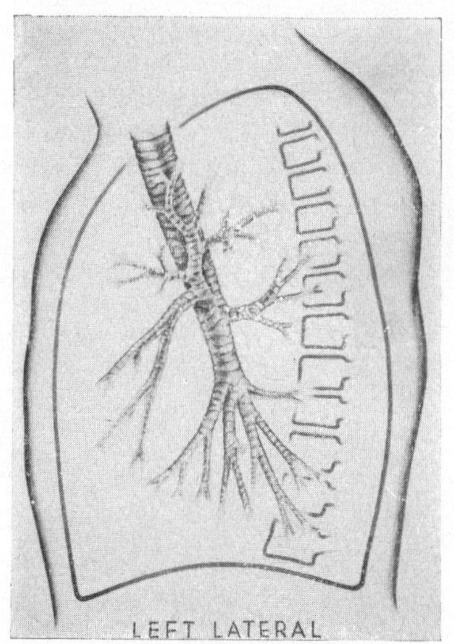
LEFT LATERAL

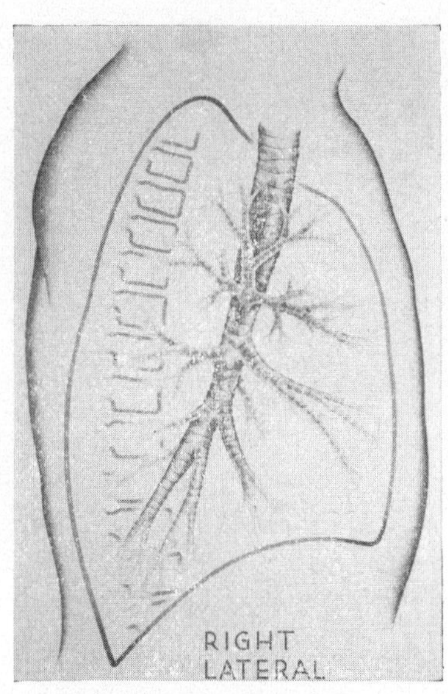
RIGHT LATERAL

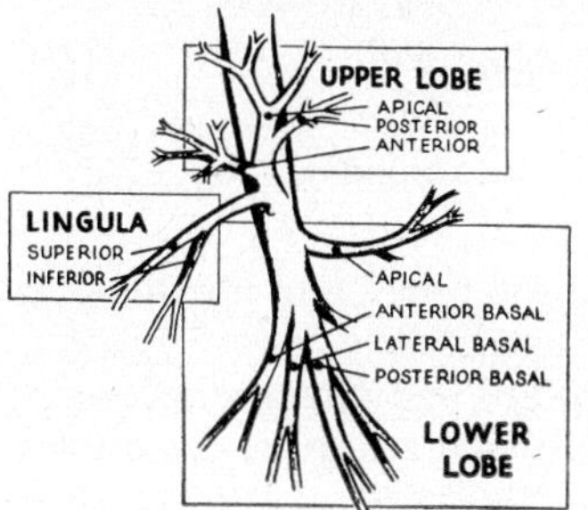
UPPER LOBE
APICAL
POSTERIOR
ANTERIOR
LINGULA
SUPERIOR
INFERIOR
APICAL
ANTERIOR BASAL
LATERAL BASAL
POSTERIOR BASAL
LOWER LOBE

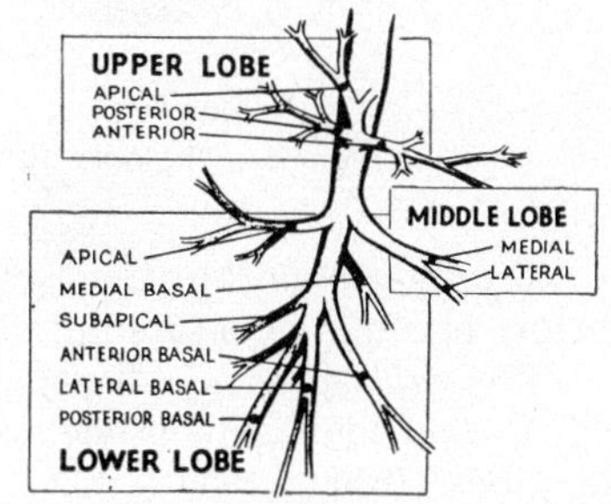
UPPER LOBE
APICAL
POSTERIOR
ANTERIOR
MIDDLE LOBE
MEDIAL
LATERAL
APICAL
MEDIAL BASAL
SUBAPICAL
ANTERIOR BASAL
LATERAL BASAL
POSTERIOR BASAL
LOWER LOBE

1/Fig. 17

too far a further complication is that the bevelled end of the tube (as usually cut) may become blocked off by its lying against the mucosa on the medial wall of the main bronchus. The short length of this bronchus also makes the lumen difficult to occlude when this is required in thoracic anaesthesia.

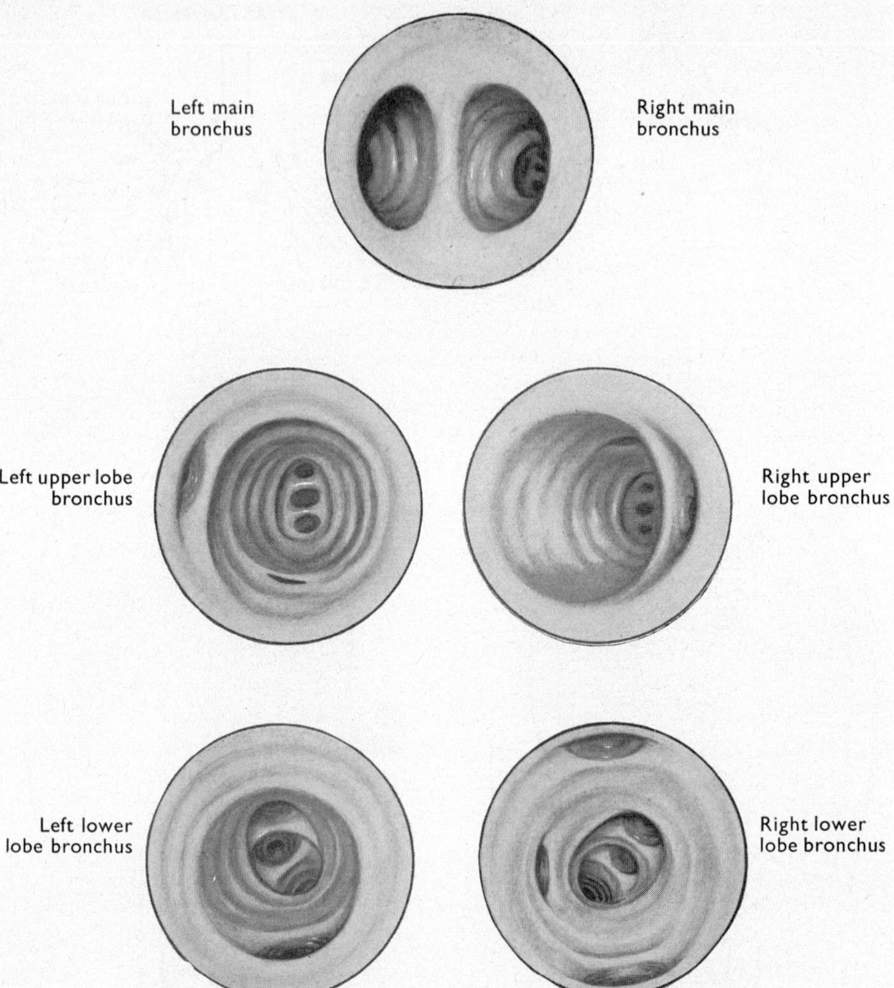

1/FIG. 18.—The normal bronchial tree as seen down a bronchoscope.

The right main bronchus gives off branches to the upper and middle lobes before becoming continuous with the lower lobe bronchus.

The *right upper lobe* bronchus passes in an upward and lateral direction at 90° to the right main bronchus for 1 cm. before dividing into its three main divisions (Brock, 1954).

The apical bronchus runs upwards with a lateral inclination and after about

1 cm. usually gives off a lateral branch and then almost immediately divides into anterior and posterior branches.

The posterior bronchus runs in a backward, lateral, and slightly upward direction. After about 0·5–1·0 cm. it gives off an important lateral branch and then ends by dividing into superior and inferior divisions.

The anterior bronchus runs in a downward, forward and slightly lateral direction. Soon after its origin it also gives off a lateral branch.

Each of these bronchi supplies a segment of the upper lobe. The posterior segment of the upper lobe, together with the apical segment of the lower lobe, is one of the common sites for the development of a lung abscess. When a patient is lying wholly or partly on his side, inhaled material tends to gravitate into the lateral portion of the posterior segment of the upper lobe—particularly on the right side (Fig. 19 *a*). Alternatively, if the patient lies on his back the material accumulates in the apical segment of the lower lobe (Fig. 19 *b*). The incidence of lung abscess is nearly twice as high in the upper lobes as in the lower ones. Surgery offers some of the most favourable conditions for aspiration of infected material, since if the anaesthetised patient is placed on his side either during or after operation then the upper lobe bronchus acts as the most dependent drain. The accumulation of secretions here, together with an inadequate cough reflex,

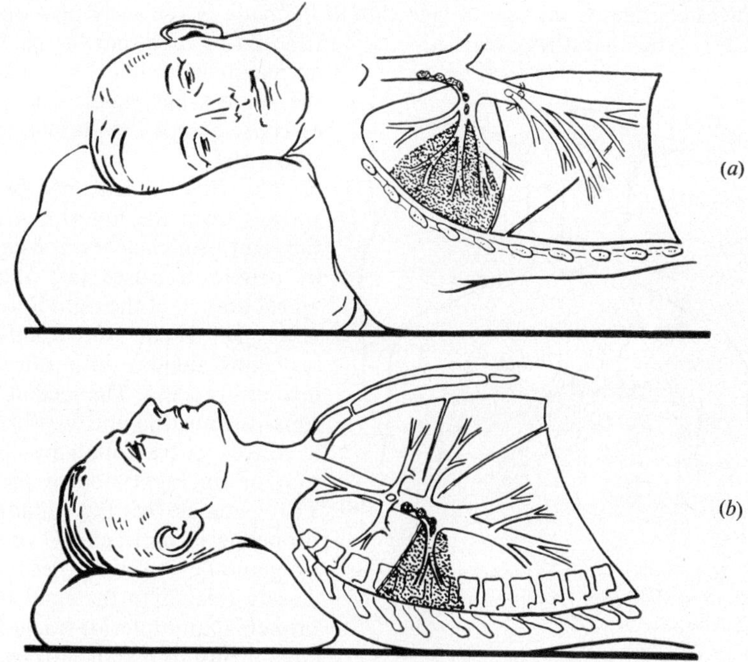

1/Fig. 19.—Diagrams to Illustrate the Relationship between Posture and the Focal Incidence of Lung Abscess

(*a*) Patient lying on side: inhaled material collects in posterior segment of right upper lobe.
(*b*) Patient lying on back: inhaled material collects in apical segment of right lower lobe.

results in an area of pulmonary collapse which may later suppurate to form a lung abscess. Although the posterior segment of the upper lobe is the commonest to be involved, it is the most difficult segment to examine radiographically or clinically, because being situated in the upper part of the axilla, it is almost completely hidden by the scapula.

In an attempt to avoid this complication the following measures may be used. (*a*) The main bronchi, trachea and nasopharynx should be cleared of mucus by suction at the end of a long operation; (*b*) the patient should be placed in the lateral position with a slight head down tilt after operation, thus encouraging mucus to flow into the pharynx rather than accumulate in a lobe of a lung. Frequent changes from side to side should be made in the early post-operative period; (*c*) the anaesthetic technique chosen should be such that the patient has an adequate cough reflex soon after the surgery has ended. On recovery of consciousness he should be urged to cough.

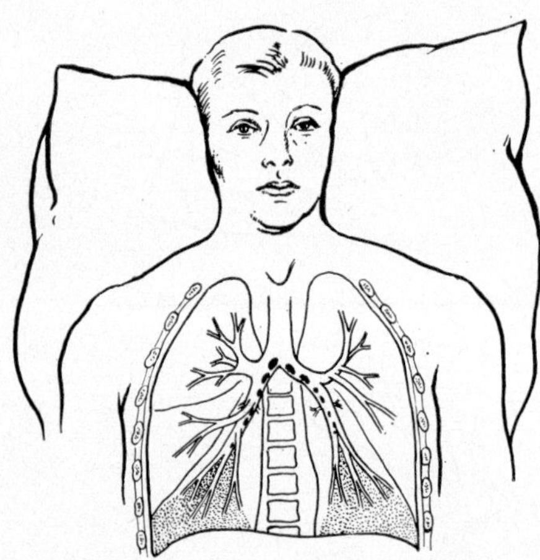

1/FIG. 20.—Figure to show the accumulation of secretions in the lower lobes of a patient in the sitting position.

The *right middle lobe* bronchus springs from the anterior aspect of the right bronchus about 3 cm. from its origin. It arises just above the apical branch of the right lower lobe. After 1–1·5 cm. the middle lobe bronchus divides into lateral and medial branches. The medial branch runs downwards and forwards with a convex curve following the contour of the right side of the heart. The patency of the middle lobe bronchus is particularly vulnerable to glandular swelling because it is closely related to the right tracheobronchial and inferior tracheo-bronchial group of glands (Brock, 1943).

The *right lower lobe* bronchus is the continuation of the right main bronchus and has five, or occasionally six, divisions. The apical branch comes off 0·5–1·0 cm. below the origin of the middle lobe but slightly more laterally (Fig. 17 *c*). About 1·5 cm. below the apical bronchus the cardiac or medial basal branch arises from the medial side of the lower lobe stem and passes downwards for 2·5 cm. before dividing into its two terminal branches—anterior and posterior. Sometimes there is a subapical branch which comes off the posterior wall of the main bronchus just below the cardiac branch. After giving off these branches the main stem divides into the basal bronchi—the anterior, lateral and posterior branches to supply the appropriate segments.

The apical segment of either of the lower lobes is particularly vulnerable to inhaled material when the patient lies supine (Fig. 19 *b*), and the right and left sides provide an approximately similar incidence of lung abscess. When a patient is propped up in bed in the post-operative period, secretions tend to gravitate to the lower lobes (Fig. 20).

Left Bronchial Tree

The *left main bronchus* is narrower than the right and is nearly 5 cm. long. It terminates at the origin of the upper lobe bronchus becoming the main stem to the lower lobe. It should be noted that this is in direct contrast to the right lung, where the branches to the upper lobe and middle lobes are offshoots of the parent main bronchus. The presence of 5 cm. of bronchial lumen uninterrupted by any branching makes the left main bronchus particularly suitable for intubation and "blocking" during thoracic surgery.

The *left upper lobe bronchus* is unlike that of the right upper lobe, for it does not arise as an offshoot of the left main bronchus but as one part of the bifurcation of the main trunk. After its origin it begins to curve rapidly to the lateral side. The angle that it forms when visualised from within the main bronchial lumen often makes it possible to insert in it a very small bronchial blocker. The upper lobe bronchus continues for 1–1·5 cm. before bifurcating into an upper and a lower division. The upper division curves upwards in line with the main stem bronchus before dividing into apical, posterior and anterior branches. The lower division descends as the *lingular bronchus.*

The *left lower lobe* bronchus arises as a continuation of the left main bronchus and runs in a downward, backward and lateral direction. About 1 cm. below its origin it gives off the apical branch from its posterior wall. This branch is important because, when the patient is lying on his back, inhaled material tends to flow through it into the apical segment of the lower lobe. The apical branch runs backwards as a short stem before dividing into three branches.

Sometimes, the left lower lobe bronchus gives off a subapical branch from its posterior wall about 1–1·5 cm. below the origin of the apical branch before finally dividing into its main terminations—the basal bronchi. The anterior basal branch arises from the antero-lateral aspect of the lower lobe stem and runs downwards, forwards and slightly laterally. About 1 cm. below its origin it may give off a small branch from its medial side which corresponds to the cardiac bronchus on the right side. The lateral basal bronchus runs in a downward and lateral direction. The posterior basal bronchus is the largest of three and sometimes appears as a continuation of the main stem running downwards, backwards and slightly laterally.

All three basal bronchi may give off lateral branches soon after their origin. These branches are often found to play an important part in the surgical anatomy of lung abscess.

Bronchioles

Before the introduction of the new nomenclatures shown in Table 3 considerable confusion existed in any description of this area.

1/TABLE 3

B.N.A.	*English*
Bronchioli	Bronchiole (incl. terminal bronchiole)
Bronchioli Respiratorii	Respiratory bronchiole
Ductuli Alveolaris	Alveolar ducts; alveolar passages
Atria	Atria
Sacculi Alveolares	Air sacs
Alveoli Pulmonum	Air cells

As a bronchiole is traced distally the cartilaginous rings gradually recede, forming irregular plates which occur sporadically until the diameter of the bronchiole is approximately 0·6 mm., when they disappear completely. Continuing the progress down the bronchial tree the tubular outline of the bronchiole wall changes and small projections in increasing numbers appear on all sides. This area is now termed a respiratory bronchiole and the small projections are alveolar ducts leading to the air sacs (Fig. 21). The name "terminal bronchiole" has arisen in the English nomenclature and usually denotes that area of the bronchiole not containing cartilage which lies just before the origin of the respiratory bronchiole.

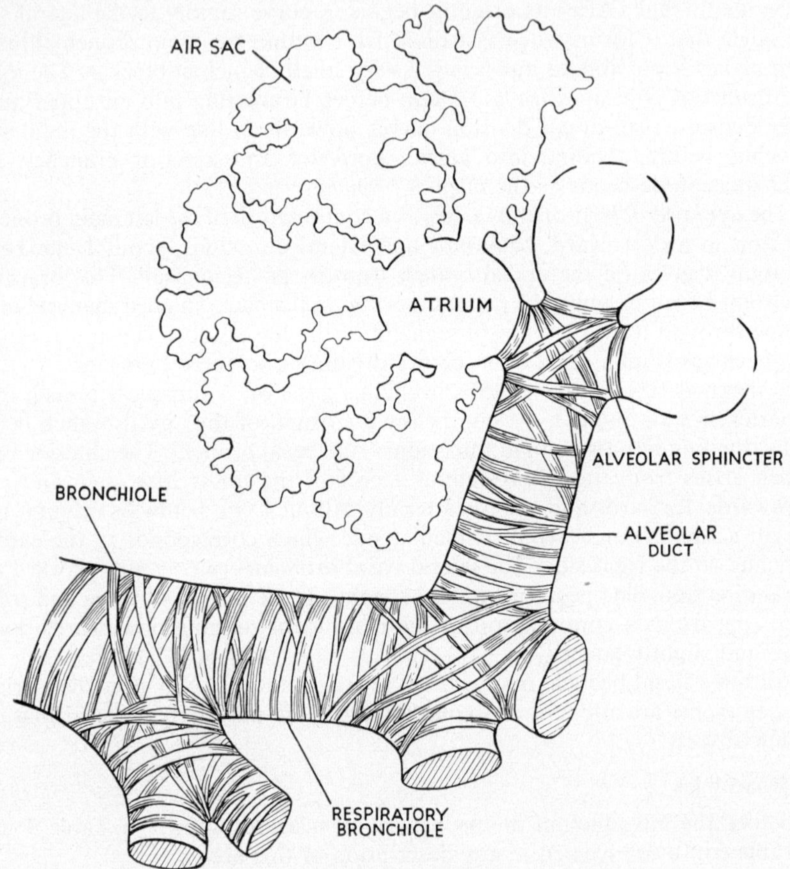

1/FIG. 21.—Diagram of alveoli and bronchiole.

The Bronchial and Bronchiolar Musculature

As long ago as 1822 Reisseissen, using a small hand-lens, dissected fresh material to show that a muscle-layer could be traced down to the finer bronchioles. So great was his contribution to the anatomy of the lung that later investigators often refer to the bronchial musculature as the "muscle of Reisseissen."

The fundamental purpose of this muscle is to permit alterations in the length and width of the bronchial tube with the various phases of respiration. The particular arrangement of the muscle fibres is of great importance, for the muscle-pattern is best described as a "geodesic network" (a geodesic line on any surface is the one of shortest distance, e.g. an arc of a circle on a sphere). A geodesic pattern, therefore, is the ideal method of withstanding or producing pressures in a tubular structure without there being a tendency for the fibres to slip along the surface (Fig. 22).

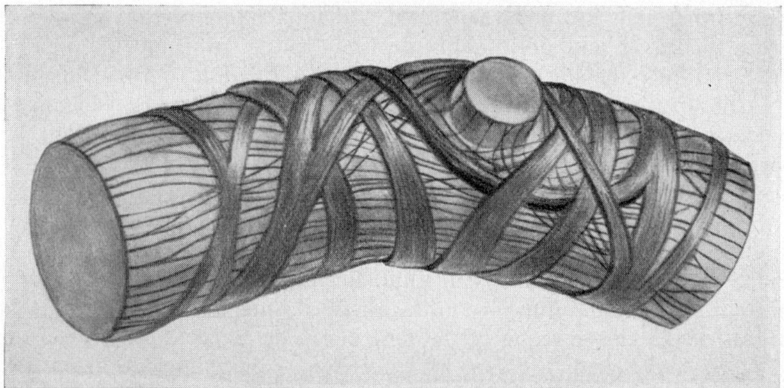

1/FIG. 22.—Diagram to show the geodesic arrangement of the musculature in a bronchiole.

As the muscle layer is followed down the bronchial tree so it becomes thinner, but the relative thickness of this layer in relation to that of the wall as a whole increases. Thus in a bronchiole of 1 mm. diameter the muscle bands are relatively five times as strong as in a bronchus of 10 mm. The terminal bronchiole, which has the narrowest lumen, has therefore relatively the thickest muscle layer.

Elastic fibres run lengthwise between the mucosal and muscle layers. In general their course is longitudinal, but at the points where branching of the bronchioles occur the fibres swing over and encircle each branch as it leaves (Fig. 22). Since the smooth muscle fibres also undergo this arrangement the origin of each branch is reinforced by a series of interlacing fibres. So close is the admixture of elastic and muscle fibres that some authorities refer to this layer as a "myo-elastic layer".

Bronchial and Bronchiolar Epithelium

The trachea down to the beginning of the respiratory bronchiole is lined by ciliated columnar epithelium freely interspersed with goblet cells lying on an intermediate layer of spindle-shaped cells; these are derived from the basal cells with round nuclei found in the deepest layer. In the lower part of the bronchial tree the ciliated cells far outnumber the other forms, but at the beginning of the respiratory bronchiole they give way to a cuboidal cell without any cilia.

Alveolar Epithelium

For many years past the question whether there is an epithelial lining to the alveolar walls has been a matter of controversy. William Snow Miller (1947) was the chief protagonist of the theory that the air sacs were lined by a layer of epithelial cells which were in direct continuity with the epithelial lining of the respiratory bronchiole. His evidence was based on the pathological changes sometimes seen in the alveolar wall in cases of acute lobar pneumonia. The introduction of the electron microscope has gone far to elucidate this problem. Low (1952 and 1953) has shown that the capillaries are not "naked" but are covered by a specialised membranous layer. It closely resembles the endothelium of the underlying alveolar capillaries. Two types of cells are found (Avery, 1968). The first type consists of large vacuolated cells with some lipoidal material, while the other cells are non-vacuolated and look like connective tissue cells. Covering this layer and presumably derived from it, is a mucoid film, with functions that may include the removal of fine living and dead particular matter, the control of alveolar surface tension, the facilitation of gaseous exchange and the protection of the underlying tissue from desiccation (Macklin, 1954).

Surfactant.—It was originally believed that retraction of the lungs during passive expiration was due entirely to their elastic tissue. However, Von Neergaard (1929) noted that when lungs were distended to peak capacity with air, the transpulmonary pressure was two to three times as great as when they were distended to the same volume with fluid. Because the only difference was the presence of an air-liquid interface in the air-filled lung, he concluded that up to two-thirds of the elastic recoil of the lung could be ascribed to surface forces. Mead (1957) confirmed this, and also noted that the contribution of surface forces to the elastic recoil was less at low lung volumes. This was surprising in view of the formula of Laplace (an 18th century mathematician) which states that the pressure across a curved surface is equal to twice the surface tension at the air-liquid interface divided by the radius.

$$\text{Pressure} = \frac{2\ (\text{Surface Tension})}{\text{Radius}}$$

For the average alveolus, with its minute size, a very considerable pressure could thus be exerted by the fluid lining it; in fact, if pure water lined it, this pressure would equal 20,000 dynes per cm., or 20 cm. of water.

Laplace's formula implies that as the alveoli decrease in size during expiration, the pressure tending to collapse them increases and a vicious circle is established. The fact that this does not happen must mean that the surface tension has, in some way, altered during expiration.

Measurement of surface tension.—The simplest method of measuring the surface tension of a liquid is with the aid of a Maxwell frame (Fig. 23). This is a U-shaped wire with the open end of the U closed by a cross-wire that can slide along the edges of the frame. A film of liquid placed in the frame tends to pull the cross-wire downwards so that the force necessary to resist this pull is a measure of surface tension. The surface tension of a liquid varies with temperature, that of pure water at 37°C being about 70 dynes per centimetre.

Clements (1962) used a surface balance that permitted the measurement of surface tension at different surface areas (which is not possible with the Maxwell frame). He studied washings of minced lungs, and found that a reduction of the surface area to 20 per cent was associated with a reduction in surface tension from about 40 dynes per cm. to 30 dynes per cm. Ordinary biological fluids, such as plasma, showed very little change in surface tension with change in area.

He concluded that the change in surface tension, as well as the ability to achieve a very low tension, was essential to the stability of the alveoli; in other

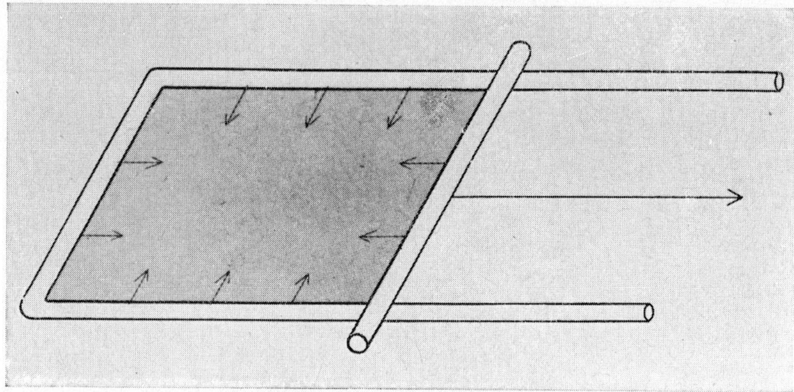

1/FIG. 23.—The Maxwell frame.

words, the substance at the alveolar-air interface (surfactant) is a kind of anti-atelectasis factor.

Nature of surfactant.—Chemical analysis has shown that surfactant is a lipoprotein, which is a compound molecule made up of protein and fatty constitutents. Only the phospho-lipid fraction is strongly active, the other constituents—neutral lipids and protein—playing no part. One particular phospholipid, namely dipalmitoyl lecithin, has been isolated from the lung fluid (Brown, 1962) and made synthetically. This is known to produce high surface activity and is probably the principal surface-acting material in human lung.

Production of surfactant.—Recent studies, particularly with the electron microscope, have demonstrated that the vacuolated alveolar lining cells contain peculiar osmiophilic inclusions, and the evidence suggests that these inclusions are a storage site for surfactant. In addition the use of isotopically tagged glucose has indicated that these large vacuolated cells may also be the site of the synthesis of phospholipids, an important component of surfactant. Macklin (1954) postulated that the large alveolar cells were secretory, and he showed, on electron micrographs, osmiophilic inclusions entering the airspace (Fig. 24). This process is probably the way in which surfactant is secreted into the alveoli.

The time of appearance of surfactant in sufficient quantities to stabilise airspaces has been studied intensively in the lamb, where it appears between the 120th and 130th days of a 147-day gestation (Avery, 1968). It is not known with certainty when it appears in the human.

Clinical significance.—Absence of this material in the infant at birth is believed to be one of the primary causes of the 'respiratory distress syndrome' (see p. 117). Attempts have been made to aerosolise one component of the surfactant (dipalmitoyl lecithin) into the airways of infants with the syndrome but have not proved life-saving (Robillard, 1964; Chu, 1967).

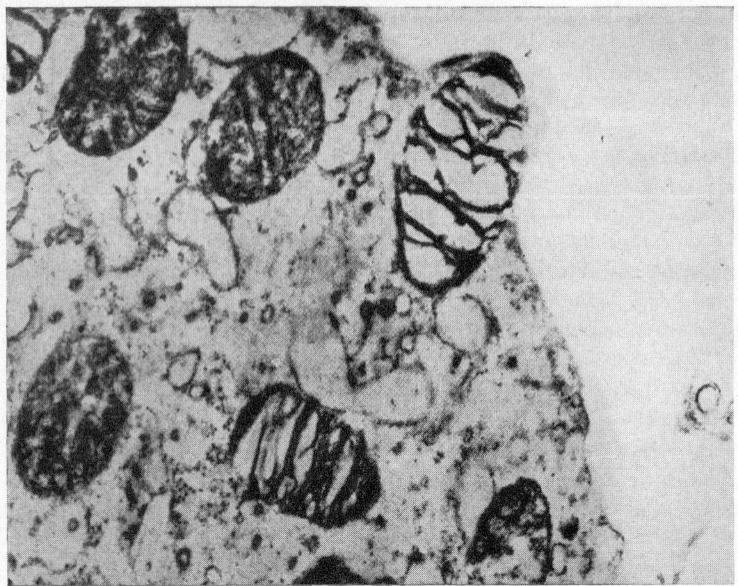

1/FIG. 24.—A transformed mitochondria passing into the alveolar air space.

There seems little doubt that oxygen therapy may lead to a reduction in surfactant (Norlander, 1968), and hence it should be used in the lowest possible concentration, and for the shortest time, necessary to achieve the desired effect. Hill (1967) found that intermittent positive pressure ventilation at normal pressures and volumes did not produce a fall in surfactant, but when abnormally high pressures were used there was a marked reduction, with consequent atelectasis. It is apparent, therefore, that in some situations, for example the respiratory distress syndrome (see above), there is an antagonism between the high inflation pressures and high concentrations of oxygen that are needed, initially at any rate, to expand the lungs and to oxygenate the infant, and which if continued may lead to a reduction of an already low quantity of surfactant.

Pulmonary collapse, whether occurring on its own or in association with a reduction in the pulmonary circulation—as from embolism or ligation (Chernick *et al.*, 1966),—may well be associated with too little surfactant (see p. 45). Deficiency of it may also account for some of the respiratory difficulties that are encountered in patients who have been artificially perfused with a pump oxygenator (Tooley *et al.*, 1961). Guest *et al.* (1966) investigating both humans and dogs following such perfusion found an absent or decreased surfactant level in many cases. In the humans this was always associated with valve replacement procedures. Evidence of the action of anaesthetic drugs on surfactant is scanty. Nishimura and Metori (1967) examined the effects of halothane, methoxyflurane and ether on rabbits and humans. In the former they found there was definite evidence of increased surfactant action, but in the latter the changes were extremely variable. On balance they concluded that such agents will lower surface tension in clinically used concentrations.

Cilia. See page 4 *et seq.*

Alveolar Muscle-fibres

Baltisberger (1921) studied the lungs of recently executed criminals and found numerous smooth muscle fibres coursing throughout the interstitial tissue. These fibres are arranged partly as a fenestrated membrane overlying the interlobular septa and partly as a mantle surrounding and accompanying the lymph vessels of the interstitial tissue. Many bundles also occur in the perivascular tissue, especially around the veins, having no definite structure but occurring simply as interlacing fibres. The exact anatomical significance of these fibres has not yet been decided but Baltisberger suggested that vagal stimulation might produce contraction of the interstitial musculature and so compress the

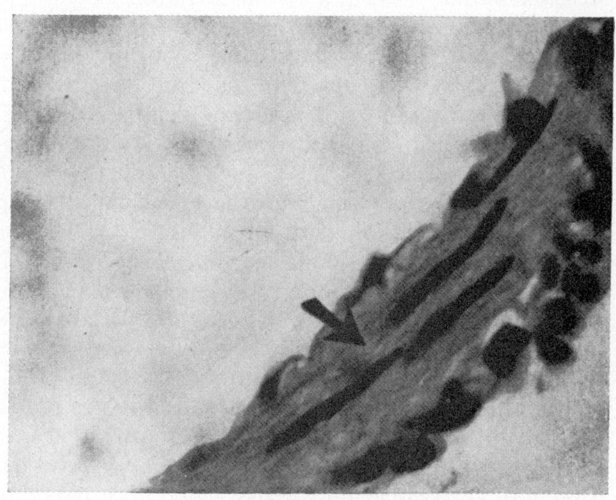

1/FIG. 25.—Smooth muscle cells in alveolar wall.

lung, squeezing it like a sponge. Corssen (1963) (Fig. 25) has confirmed the presence of smooth muscle fibres within the lung structure but points out that they are found predominantly in diseased tissue, e.g. bronchitis, emphysema and, particularly, pulmonary hypertension. He considers that the human lung parenchyma is capable of active contraction, a factor that helps to explain some cases of pulmonary collapse without bronchial obstruction.

Alveolar Pores

Kohn (1893) described the presence of fibrinous threads running through the walls of the alveoli in cases of lobar pneumonia but many investigators considered these pores were only artefacts occurring in a pathological state. More recently, however, the demonstration of collateral respiration has supplied confirmatory evidence of the normal presence of these pores.

Collateral respiration.—Adams in 1930 found that if the bronchus of a dog was permanently obstructed by painting the mucosa with silver nitrate, collapse of the distal pulmonary tissue only occurred when the main bronchus was occluded. Obstruction of a secondary bronchus was not followed by collapse.

He concluded, therefore, that there must be a communication between the alveoli involving adjacent lobules. Since then collateral respiration has been demonstrated in man and the amount of air which can pass via this channel has been measured (Baarsma, *et al.* 1948). During a thoracotomy, particularly if the lingular bronchus (of the left upper lobe) is clamped, it is often possible to see the lingular lobe inflating freely as fresh gases pass into the clamped-off lobe from the surrounding tissues. More often, collateral respiration is clearly seen during a segmental lobectomy.

Bronchial Vessels

There are usually three bronchial arteries, one for the right and two for the left lung, each taking its origin from the ventral side of the aorta, although occasionally they arise as a common trunk.

On entering the lung the bronchial arteries embed themselves in the layer of connective tissue surrounding the bronchus. Usually two or three branches of the bronchial artery run with the larger bronchi and bronchioli until finally each bronchial sub-division is accompanied by a corresponding division of the artery. In this manner the arteries continue until the distal end of the terminal bronchiole is reached.

Anastomotic branches from the bronchial artery pierce the outer fibrous coat of the bronchi and form an arterial plexus in the adventitia around the muscle layer. From this outer arterial plexus, branches pierce the muscle layer to enter the submucosa. The vessels run for a short distance parallel with the muscle fibres before splitting up into a fine capillary plexus which supplies the mucous membrane. From this capillary network venous radicles arise which in their turn pierce the muscle layer to reach a venous plexus in the outer adventitia. From this second plexus veins arise and form one of the sources of the pulmonary vein. It is evident, therefore, that an arterial and venous plexus lies on the outside of the muscle layers, whilst a capillary plexus lies on the inside (Fig. 26). A point of great importance is that blood must pass through the muscle layer in its passage between the various plexuses.

Therefore, when the muscle layer contracts, it is probable that whilst the arterial plexus with its higher pressure can maintain a flow to the capillary plexus, the latter is unable to empty into the outer venous plexus. This must lead to swelling of the mucosa with a further narrowing of the lumen.

When the respiratory bronchiole is reached the bronchial arteries disappear as a distinct set of vessels. The internal capillary plexus, however, fuses with that of the pulmonary artery in the walls of the alveoli. It appears that the pulmonary artery supplies the respiratory bronchiole in a similar manner to the bronchial artery supplying the terminal bronchiole.

This junction of the bronchial and pulmonary circulations has an important clinical significance. For operations within the heart it may be necessary to use an extra-corporeal circulation—the inferior and superior vena cavae are clamped so that the heart and lungs are isolated from the general circulation. Fresh blood is then pumped into the aorta (see Chapter 25). Despite the fact that theoretically no blood is now entering the lungs, when the pulmonary vein is opened blood will still flow from it. The explanation lies in this junction between the bronchial and pulmonary systems. Blood passes from the aorta, down the bronchial arteries and then through this anastomosis of vessels in the region of the respiratory bronchioles to reach the pulmonary vein.

True bronchial veins are only seen at the hilum of the lung and do not play a significant part in the venous drainage of the bronchioles. They arise at the level of the first divisions of the main bronchial tree and usually drain into the azygos, hemi-azygos and intercostal veins. The pulmonary vein arises from the venous plexus in the terminal bronchiole wall, from that in the wall of the respiratory bronchiole down to and including the alveoli, and finally from the plexus underlying the pleura.

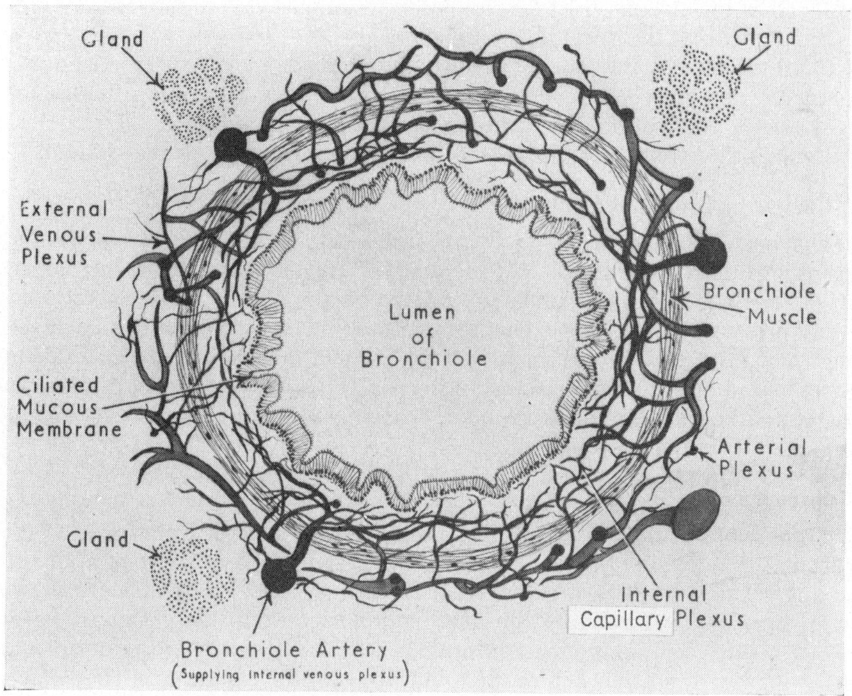

1/Fig. 26.—Diagrammatic Representation of the Blood Supply of a Respiratory Bronchiole.

Below the ciliated mucous membrane lies a capillary plexus. The arterial supply reaches it by piercing the muscle layer. Venous drainage also has to pass back through this muscle layer.

Innervation of the Bronchial Tree

The lung receives innervation from both sympathetic and parasympathetic sources. The sympathetic nerve fibres are derived from the 1st–5th thoracic ganglia along with branches from the inferior cervical ganglion, though some fibres may also be received from the middle cervical ganglion (Fontaine and Herrmann, 1928; Larsell and Dow, 1933). The vagus nerve supplies the parasympathetic fibres, joining with the sympathetic fibres to form the posterior pulmonary plexus at the root of the lung. Fibres from this plexus pass round the root of the lung to form the anterior pulmonary plexus.

The posterior pulmonary plexus divides into a peri-arterial and peri-bronchial plexus. The latter again divides into an extrachondrial and intra-chondrial plexus in relation to cartilaginous plates in the bronchial wall. On reaching the non-cartilaginous parts of the lung the two plexuses again unite and continue distally as one. Ganglia are to be found at all levels of the bronchial tree so that short post-ganglionic fibres reach the bands of smooth muscle in which they break up into individual fibres. These fibres give off twigs to supply the individual smooth muscle fibres of the geodesic network and at the distal end of the alveolar duct delicate motor terminals pass to the muscle fibres of the sphincter at the atrial openings.

In all probability the mucous glands are innervated solely by the vagus. As regards the nervous control of the vessel walls, recent evidence suggests that the vagus carries cholinergic dilator fibres whilst the thoraco-lumbar nerves carry predominantly adrenergic constrictor fibres to the bronchial arterial system.

Control of Bronchial Calibre

The bronchi dilate and retract passively with each phase of respiration. On inspiration the pressure in the air ducts is greater than that in the pleural cavity—consequently the bronchi are dilated by the pull of the negative intra-pleural pressure. As the lung expands, therefore, the bronchial tree is dilated and lengthened, and as it diminishes in size the bronchi shorten and contract due to the retraction of the elastic tissue in their walls (Ellis, 1936). In man, it is known that sympatho-mimetic drugs produce bronchial relaxation whilst cholinergic drugs lead to muscular constriction.

Bronchomotor Tone

Bronchomotor tone is a continuous and variable state of contraction of the bronchial musculature which is present during both phases of respiration. In the dog, section of the sympathetic nerves has no effect on bronchial calibre, while vagal section produces considerable alterations. In fact, bilateral vagal section results in the bronchi opening more widely during inspiration and narrowing to a greater degree than normal during expiration. These facts strongly suggest that it is predominantly the vagi that carry impulses influencing the diameter of the bronchial lumen and that they are responsible for normal bronchial tone.

Apart from the vagi, there is evidence that the baroceptors in the carotid sinus and aortic arch, together with reflexes from other vasosensory areas, play an important role in this matter. Thus—in dogs under chloralose anaesthesia—a severe and rapid haemorrhage leading to a fall in blood pressure to 40 mm. Hg will be accompanied by bronchodilatation. This will change to constriction as the pressure rises again (Daly and Schweitzer, 1952).

On the other hand the chemoreceptors do not appear to play any role in controlling bronchomotor tone and their inactivation leaves the bronchial lumen unaffected in size. Carbon dioxide does, however, play some part in the maintenance of normal tone, but probably through an entirely central effect. Perfusion of a dog's brain with blood containing a high concentration of carbon dioxide causes bronchoconstriction but, when a low concentration is used, bronchodilatation follows (Daly *et al.*, 1953). The role of oxygen is imperfectly understood (Nicholson and Trimby, 1940; Ellis, 1936), but hypoxia leads to bronchial dilatation.

Respiratory Tract Reflexes

Because of the immense difficulties involved, most of the studies of respiratory reflexes have been made in animals rather than in man, yet these reflexes play a significant role in the control of the respiratory and the cardio-vascular systems.

(a) Inflation.—Hering and Breuer in 1868 showed that the inflation of the lungs inhibited the spontaneous contraction of the diaphragm in anaesthetised animals, and Adrian (1933) concluded that the pulmonary stretch receptors were responsible for this inflation reflex. These receptors are unencapsulated and without end-organs. The nerve fibrils splay out in the underlying mucosa, and are found mainly in the walls of the bronchi and bronchioles rather than in the alveoli or pleura. They are generally believed to be responsible for signalling changes in the mechanical state of the lungs to the brain.

Whitteridge and Bulbring (1944) first suggested that while the increased excitability of the pulmonary stretch receptors was largely responsible for the reduction in depth of ventilation during inhalation of volatile anaesthetics, other changes might be contingent upon excitation of a second set of pulmonary stretch receptors. Coleridge *et al.* (1968) found that high concentrations (e.g. 5–20 per cent halothane) produced a marked activity in slowly conducting vagal fibres which were normally only stimulated by hyper-inflation. They suggested that these nerve endings are responsible for the gross bradycardia sometimes seen in the non-atropinised subject when anaesthetised with halothane. This agrees with Johnstone (1961) who found that this only occurred when hyper-inflation of the lungs was associated with a high concentration of halothane (e.g. 10 per cent).

Barbiturate anaesthesia depresses the inflation reflex, but only abolishes it completely with very high doses (May and Widdicombe, 1954).

A weak inflation reflex has been demonstrated in man, but it may be absent in the anaesthetised subject (Widdicombe, 1961). It may be responsible for the apnoea produced in inflation of the newborn baby's lung, though this response only persists for the first few days of life.

(b) Deflation.—During expiration the tonic discharge of the stretch receptors diminishes so that soon inspiration can start again. Nevertheless, there is evidence that a deflation reflex exists in its own right; the receptors are sited differently in that they lie principally in the alveoli and terminal bronchioles. Sensitisation of these receptors leads to an increase in the rate and force of the inspiratory effort and its role may be designed primarily to protect the individual by increasing ventilation in the event of pulmonary collapse. Paintal (1964) has shown that these receptors are stimulated by inhalational anaesthetics.

(c) Paradoxical reflex.—This reflex was described by Head in 1889 and can only be demonstrated when the vagus nerve is *partially* blocked. Inflation of the lungs under this condition leads to a strong diaphragmatic contraction. It does not occur if the vagus nerve is intact or completely blocked, and because it is the opposite response of the normal inflation reflex it has been termed "paradoxical". This reflex may account for the primitive gasp observed in newborn babies when the lungs are first inflated (Cross, 1961).

(d) Irritant reflexes.—Afferent nerve endings responding to both mechanical and chemical irritants have been described lying beneath the epithelium and sending out their terminal branches between the mucosal cells. They are concentrated mainly at the carina and at the points of branching of the bronchial tree. These nerve endings are excited by particulate matter and are paralysed by ether and local analgesic sprays (Widdicombe *et al.*, 1962). (See p. 40.)

Aspiration of fluid, whether it be fresh water, sea water, or vomit with a hydrochloric acid content, always leads to reflex closure of the glottis and bronchoconstriction. Animal experiments have demonstrated that even after both vagi have been sectioned atropine, neostigmine and isopropyl-noradrenaline are all capable of influencing the bronchial response (Colebatch and Halmagyi, 1962). This suggests that aspiration of fluid invokes a reflex response of the parasympathetic nervous system, but there is not only a central component acting via the vagus nerve, but also a peripheral fraction which is intrinsic within the bronchial wall.

(e) Pulmonary vascular reflexes.—In animals, pulmonary congestion sensitises the stretch receptors and leads to rapid, shallow breathing. This reflex is mediated by the vagus nerve and is often associated with reflex hypotension and bradycardia (Widdicombe, 1963).

Jesser and de Takats (1942) demonstrated that an embolism of the pulmonary artery in dogs produced constriction of the whole bronchial tree. If the vagi were previously cut, this did not occur. They concluded, therefore, that the mortality and morbidity of a pulmonary embolus was not solely due to mechani-

1/TABLE 4

Reflex	*Response*			
	Respiratory	*Blood Pressure*	*Heart rate*	*Bronchial Calibre*
Inflation	Inhibition of inspiration	? Hypertension	? Tachycardia	? Dilatation
Deflation	Increase of inspiration	? Hypotension	? Bradycardia	? Constriction
Paradoxical	Increase of inspiration	—	—	—
Irritant	Hyperpnoea	? Hypotension	? Bradycardia	Constriction
Pulmonary embolism	Apnoea and rapid shallow breathing	Hypotension	Bradycardia	Constriction

(After Widdicombe, 1962)

cal plugging of the pulmonary artery, but also partly due to the reflex effects on other thoracic viscera, including generalised bronchoconstriction.

The introduction of small emboli into the pulmonary artery at first causes apnoea, followed by a period of rapid, shallow breathing. The blood pressure and pulse rate fall whilst pulmonary vasoconstriction and oedema can occur throughout the lung. As the injection of 5-hydroxytryptamine produces almost identical changes it has been suggested that the release of this substance from the intravascular thrombus may be partly responsible for the signs observed (Widdicombe, 1963).

A summary of the possible responses (where known) to the principal respiratory reflexes in animals is given in Table 4.

Relation of Respiratory Tract Stimulation to Cardiac Arrhythmias

Intubation of the trachea under light general anaesthesia is consistently accompanied by a pressor response, tachycardia, and occasionally cardiac arrhythmias. Nevertheless, an interesting finding is that though these circulatory changes are not affected by atropine, they can be prevented by the prior administration of phentolamine (Devault *et al.*, 1960). This suggests that the reflex pathway is not entirely through the vagus nerve and that part of it is mediated through the sympathetic-adrenal system, though clearly an alteration in the carbon dioxide level of the blood may sensitise this reflex.

Bronchospasm

This condition is occasionally encountered during anaesthesia. The term denotes spasm of the bronchi, but a better name would be bronchiolar spasm, as this is the area of the respiratory tree which is mainly involved. Stimulation can be initiated by chemical, mechanical or neurogenic methods. It is most commonly encountered in patients who have an "irritable" bronchial tree, i.e. chronic bronchitics. The constriction of the bronchiole is greater during expiration than inspiration. The unfortunate patient rapidly shows signs of respiratory embarrassment with his chest fixed in a postion of inspiration, while an inspiratory and expiratory wheeze can be heard on auscultation. In anaesthetised patients, progressively increasing resistance to positive pressure inspiration occurs, but before a presumptive diagnosis of bronchospasm is made it is essential to eliminate a mechanical obstruction of the airway due to kinking of an endotracheal tube or the presence of secretions. A tension pneumothorax can readily simulate severe bronchospasm, and Galloon and Rosen (1965) have shown how the use of a negative phase during intermittent positive pressure ventilation for patients with normal lungs may lead to bronchiolar narrowing and wheezing. Bronchospasm is a diagnosis that only should be made when all other causes of ventilatory insufficiency have been excluded. The treatment of this condition is broadly the same as the treatment of an attack of asthma in an unanaesthetised patient (see below).

Respiratory pressure changes can be plotted against resulting lung volume changes to produce a pressure-volume "loop" (Ambiavagar *et al.*, 1967). Such "loops" may be of value in illustrating the progress of some acute chest illnesses in which intermittent positive pressure ventilation is required. Figure 27 (A) shows a normal loop, where a volume change of 1150 ml. takes place for a total pressure change of less than 10 mm. Hg. Figure 27 (B) is from a patient in an acute asthmatic attack, where a volume change of only 280 ml. is produced by a pressure change of 45 mm. Hg. Marked variations in the intrathoracic pressure lead to considerable fluctuation in the venous return to the heart, the stroke volume of the heart, and thus in the level of aortic pressure. Changes in these parameters may therefore be useful as an indication of the degree of cardiac embarrassment.

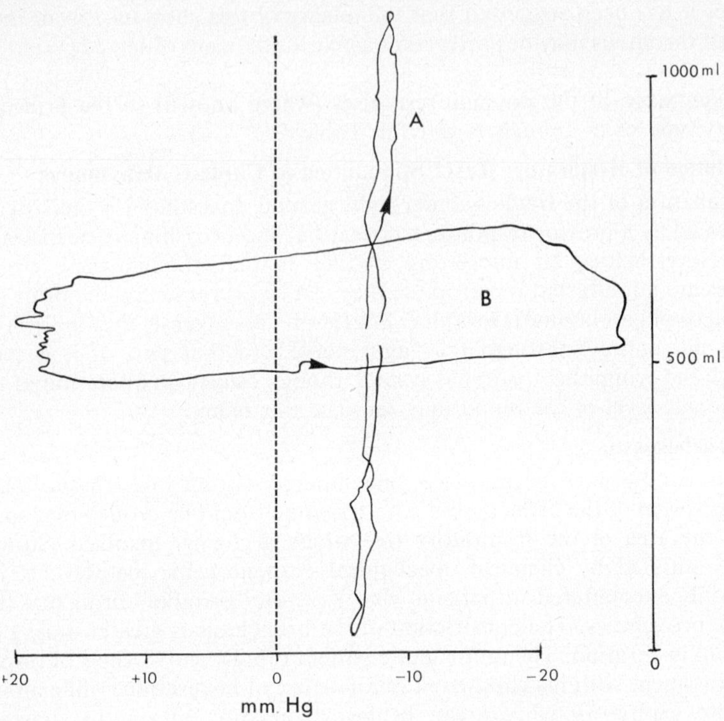

1/FIG. 27.—Pressure volume loops.

Asthma

Until recently, there has been no clear indication of just how commonly bronchospasm or asthma developed during routine anaesthesia. Shnider and Papper (1961), however, report that an incidence of wheezing of 6.5 per cent was found in a group of unselected patients with a clear chest pre-operatively. The only incriminating factor appeared to be endotracheal intubation. Regional analgesia in the conscious subject was associated with the same incidence of wheezing as general anaesthesia without endotracheal intubation. Simonsson *et al.* (1967) have found that the intravenous administration of atropine prior to irritation of the bronchial tree by a catheter or a chemical dust prevents bronchoconstriction in patients with obstructive airway disease. This may not appear in accord with the clinical experience of many anaesthetists, but it is possible that an adequate dose of atropine given in advance of stimulation is more valuable than one given after the bronchial constriction has been produced.

Pre-operative preparation.—The prevention of an attack of asthma, or improvement of ventilation in a patient suffering from asthma, requires careful pre-operative treatment. Whenever possible elective surgery should be performed only under optimum conditions, i.e. in the summer months, or a season when chest infections are rare. Antibiotic therapy is indicated in severe cases and the sputum should be cultured to ascertain the sensitivity of the organism concerned. In an emergency a broad-spectrum antibiotic can be used. Bronchodilator drugs combined with active physiotherapy can considerably improve the patient's ventilation; isopropyl noradrenaline given as an aerosol is particularly useful and the effectiveness of this therapy can be observed by such routine tests as maximal expiratory flow rate or timed vital capacity. Antihistamines, especially promethazine, may be found effective in producing bronchodilatation, drying of secretions, and general sedation. In very severe cases the adrenal cortical steroids may relieve wheezing where other agents fail. Several cases of sudden death have been recorded following the use of aerosols, and they should not be prescribed indiscriminately (Committee on Safety of Drugs, 1967).

Anaesthesia.—Thiopentone (or other intravenous barbiturate anaesthetics), though once incriminated as a cause of bronchospasm, is preferable to induction with an inhalational anaesthetic agent because asthmatic patients are usually extremely nervous and fear alone is capable of inducing an attack. Halothane is probably the agent of choice for maintenance of anaesthesia because it is relatively non-irritating to the respiratory tract and may also produce some bronchodilatation.

In the event of a severe attack of bronchospasm developing during anaesthesia the *slow* intravenous injection of 250 to 500 mg. of aminophylline (i.e. given over five minutes) will often improve ventilation and this should be combined with assisted respiration. It should be remembered, however, that the rapid injection of aminophylline may increase the rate and amplitude of contraction of cardiac muscle in the same manner as an injection of adrenaline; thus, in combination with hypoxia the result might prove fatal. An intravenous injection of hydrocortisone (100 mg.) remains the most effective treatment of a severe and protracted attack of bronchospasm. A new drug, disodium cromoglycate ("Intal") has been introduced for the treatment of allergic asthma, and represents an important advance in the treatment of the disease (Howell and Altounyan, 1967; Smith and Devey, 1968).

Treatment of the moribund asthmatic.—Such patients are invariably resistant to isoprenaline and adrenaline, though they may be temporarily improved by aminophylline. The institution of intermittent positive pressure ventilation at this stage may save a patient's life. If, however, retained bronchial secretions are leading to marked airway plugging with increasing tachycardia and cyanosis, then bronchial lavage must be carried out as well. Intermittent positive pressure ventilation is maintained with nitrous oxide—oxygen—halothane and gallamine triethiodide, and during a short pause, 10 ml. of sterile, isotonic saline warmed to body temperature are poured down the endotracheal tube, following which the trachea and major bronchi are sucked out. This manoeuvre is repeated at five-minute intervals for up to an hour, during which time the arterial oxygen tension may be expected to rise rapidly.

Ambiavagar and Jones (1967) emphasise the importance of applying topical analgesia to the larynx (4 per cent lignocaine) before introduction of an endotracheal tube. They describe a short period of "total bronchospasm" in one patient during which intermittent positive pressure ventilation was impossible and this was thought to be due to the process of endotracheal instrumentation without prior topical analgesia of the respiratory tract. Ambiavagar and Jones also report that bronchial lavage via a bronchoscope is no more effective than through an endotracheal tube, and that they have abandoned bronchoscopy as part of their treatment.

The effect of some commonly known drugs on the bronchial musculature is given below (Table 5).

1/TABLE 5

EFFECT ON THE BRONCHIAL MUSCULATURE OF DRUGS USED IN ANAESTHESIA

Dilatation	*Constriction*
1. Drugs reducing the sensitivity of the bronchial mucosa	1. Drugs stimulating vagal nerve endings
Cocaine	Physostigmine
Lignocaine	Neostigmine
Decicaine	Pilocarpine
	Muscarine
	Acetylcholine
2. Drugs paralysing vagal ganglia	2. Drugs stimulating vagal ganglia
Atropine	Lobeline (small doses)
Hyoscine	Nicotine (small doses)
Pethidine	
Lobeline (large doses)	
Nicotine (large doses)	
3. Drugs directly relaxing bronchial musculature	3. Drugs directly stimulating bronchial musculature
Ether	Histamine (including histamine released by the injection of other drugs, e.g. certain muscle relaxants)
Ethyl chloride	Pituitrin
Divinyl ether	Morphine (large doses)
Halothane	
Amyl nitrite	
4. Drugs stimulating sympathetic nerve endings	4. Drugs paralysing sympathetic ganglia or nerve endings
Ephedrine	Hexamethonium
Adrenaline	Pentamethonium
Isopropyl noradrenaline	Thiophanium derivatives ("Arfonad")
l-noradrenaline	
5. Drugs acting centrally via the respiratory centre	5. Drugs acting centrally via the respiratory centre
Chloroform	Cyclopropane
Morphine (small doses)	Barbiturates
Codeine	Paraldehyde
Tribromethanol	Thiopentone

Nitrous oxide and ethylene are generally believed not to affect the size of the bronchial lumen.

Cold gases produce dilatation and hot gases constriction of the bronchial musculature, whereas oxygen lack and carbon dioxide excess cause bronchial dilatation.

Exchange of Gases in the Lungs

The transfer of a gas from the alveoli to the blood occurs by a process of diffusion when the tension exerted by the gas in the alveoli differs from that in the blood. The total surface area of the alveoli is about 50–100 square meters and that of the pulmonary vascular bed about 40 square meters. Under resting conditions about 500 mls. of blood are present in this vascular bed at any one time. The gases in the alveoli are separated from the blood stream by four extremely thin layers—a layer of surface-active material which is responsible for the low surface tension in this area, an alveolar epithelium consisting of molecules of lipoprotein in the form of a net (probably with water-repelling properties which accounts for the lack of water in the alveoli), an interstitial layer, and the endothelial lining of the capillaries. The thickness of all four layers together—*the alveolar-capillary membrane*—is no more than 1–2 microns.

Composition of the Respiratory Gases

The average percentage compositions of atmospheric air, alveolar air and expired air are as follows:—

Gas	*Inspired air*	*Alveolar air*	*Expired air*
Oxygen	20·94 per cent	14·2 per cent	16·3 per cent
Carbon Dioxide ..	0·04 per cent	5·5 per cent	4·0 per cent
Nitrogen (inc. the rare gases)	79·02 per cent	80·3 per cent	79·7 per cent

Atmospheric air contains less than 1 per cent. water vapour whilst air in the alveoli is fully saturated, containing about 6·2 per cent. The tension exerted by this water vapour is 47 mm. Hg and should always be remembered when calculating the partial pressure of any gas in the alveoli. Thus:

Barometric pressure − Water vapour pressure
760 mm. Hg − 47 mm. Hg = 713 mm. Hg.

Tension of oxygen in alveoli is therefore:

$$713 \times \frac{14{\cdot}2}{100} = 103 \text{ mm. Hg approx.}$$

Tension of carbon dioxide

$$713 \times \frac{5{\cdot}5}{100} = 40 \text{ mm. Hg.}$$

Tension of nitrogen

$$713 \times \frac{80{\cdot}3}{100} = 570 \text{ mm. Hg.}$$

Rate of Exchange

The rate of transfer of a gas is a function of the diffusion characteristics of the alveolar-capillary membrane for the gas in question, but is also, and mainly, proportional to the difference in the tensions of the gas on the two sides of the membrane. Thus, the partial pressure of oxygen in venous blood reaching the pulmonary capillaries is about 40 mm. Hg, whereas in the alveoli it is approximately 100 mm. Hg. Oxygen is then driven across the membrane into the blood in an attempt to equalise the difference in partial pressures (Table 6).

1/TABLE 6

COMPARISON OF GAS TENSIONS IN ATMOSPHERIC AND ALVEOLAR AIR AND IN THE BLOOD

Gas	*Air* *mm. Hg*	*Alveolus* *mm. Hg*	*Arterial blood* *mm. Hg*	*Venous blood* *mm. Hg*
Oxygen	158·2	103	100	40
Nitrogen ..	596·5	570	573	573
Carbon dioxide ..	0·3	40	40	46
Water vapour ..	5·0	47	47	47
Tota	760·0	760·0	760·0	706·0

The diffusion characteristics of the alveolar capillary membrane are determined partly by its physical properties and partly by those of the diffusing gas. Among the former, the total area of the gas-to-blood interface is an important variable in health and disease. Thus in emphysema it may be considerably reduced, while in pneumonia the alveolar walls become thickened. Bronchial secretions, such as may be present in some disease states or as a result of inadequate atropinisation may also impede gaseous exchange.

The aqueous solubility and molecular weight of the individual gas affects its rate of diffusion in the following manner:—

$$\text{Rate of diffusion} \propto \text{solubility} \div \sqrt{\text{molecular weight of gas}}$$

Table 7 lists the rate of diffusion of some gases relative to that of oxygen, and demonstrates that the rate of diffusion of a gas is determined much more by its solubility than by its molecular weight. Carbon dioxide, which is about 25 times more soluble in water than oxygen under the same conditions diffuses 20 times as fast.

The uptake and distribution of inhalational anaesthetics and of other gases is considered in detail in Chapter 7.

1/TABLE 7

DIFFUSION RATES OF GASES RELATIVE TO OXYGEN (COTES, 1968)

Substance	*Molecular weight*	*Solubility at 37°C*	*Partition coefficient*	*Rate of diffusion*
Oxygen	32	0·0239	5·0	1·00
Acetylene	26	0·749	—	34·8
Argon	40	0·0259	5·3	0·97
Carbon dioxide ..	44	0·567	1·6	20·3
Carbon monoxide ..	28	0·0184	—	0·83
Ethylene	28	0·0784	14·4	3·43
Helium	4	0·0085	1·7	1·01
Krypton	85*	0·0449	9·6	1·15
Nitrogen	28	0·0123	5·2	0·55
Nitrous oxide ..	44	0·388	3·2	13·9
Xenon	133*	0·085	20·0†	1·75

* Radioactive isotope
† Fat-to-blood partition coefficient 8·0–9·8:1

Pulmonary Collapse and Gas Absorption

The rate of absorption of gases in pulmonary collapse is affected by many factors. This probably explains the wide variations in the literature describing the time taken for the entrapped gases to become absorbed. Coryllos and Birnbaum (1928), working on dogs, reported that it took six hours for the lung to collapse after obstruction of the main bronchus, but others have reported, also in dogs with an open chest, an almost phenomenally rapid speed of gas absorption (Table 8).

1/TABLE 8

Carbon dioxide ..	1 min. 6 seconds
Oxygen	1 min. 20 seconds
Nitrous oxide ..	1 min. 42 seconds
Air	9 min. 21 seconds
Nitrogen ..	12 min. 6 seconds

(Lemmer and Rovenstine, 1935)

One lung is filled with 600 c.c. of the gas to be tested and the animal is respired on the other lung. The time taken for the lung to collapse to $\frac{7}{8}$ of its original size is recorded.

The rate of gas absorption can be varied more than 60-fold by alteration in the partial pressures of the blood gases as well as by changes in the initial gas composition. If the composition of the gases in the occluded lobe is analysed it will be found that a state of constant composition between the blood and alveolar gases is rapidly attained (Dale and Rahn, 1952).

In man there are no figures available but clinical observation suggests that such rapid rates of absorption are only applicable to the condition of the open chest. In the closed chest the negative intrapleural pressure opposes the elastic recoil of the lung and thus tends to retard the rate of collapse. (See also Chapter 2.) During anaesthesia for thoracic surgery it is often necessary to occlude one of the main bronchi before commencing a thoracotomy. If the affected lung is filled with oxygen by hyperventilation prior to the introduction of the "blocker" it can be assumed that the entrapped gases contain a high percentage of oxygen, which will be rapidly absorbed, but at the moment of opening the chest twenty minutes or so later, no evidence of gross pulmonary collapse will be seen. Two to three minutes later partial collapse becomes evident and very quickly the whole process becomes complete. However, Nilsson *et al.* (1965) have shown that, in spite of an apparently total collapse obtained in such circumstances, the circulation is still partly maintained through the collapsed lung. This is shown by a marked reduction in the patient's systemic arterial oxygen tension which indicates a shunt of from 20 per cent to 40 per cent. When the branch of the pulmonary artery supplying the collapsed lung was clamped, there was an immediate rise in systemic arterial oxygen tension. Thus the occlusion of a main bronchus may impair the oxygenation of vital organs, and there is a case for clamping the supplying artery of the collapsed lung as soon as possible when this is feasible. Otherwise oxygenation should be maintained at as high a level as possible to compensate for the shunt.

The following factors are concerned in the rate of onset of pulmonary collapse:

Intrapleural pressure.—This opposes the elastic recoil of the lung and also any attempt on the part of the pulmonary tissue to reduce its volume. It is to a certain degree offset by movement of the mediastinum and falling-in of the surrounding soft tissues.

Position of the obstruction in the bronchial tree.—"Collateral respiration" makes it necessary for the obstruction to be present in the main bronchus.

Respiratory movements.—The abolition of the cough reflex and impairment of respiratory movements as in profound anaesthesia or in the presence of large abdominal tumours greatly accelerate the speed of pulmonary collapse.

Partial pressure of the entrapped gases.—Assuming that at the moment the block occurs the entrapped gases are in equilibrium with those in the blood stream, then the process begins by oxygen or some other rapidly diffusible gas —such as an anaesthetic agent—being taken up by the circulation. This is because the gas in the alveolus is at a higher partial pressure than that in the mixed venous blood returning to the lung. As the gas enters the circulation so the elastic tissue of the lung retracts to fill this hypothetical space and the total pressure of the retained gases thus remains the same. Each individual gas is, however, now at a slightly higher pressure than that in the circulation, so that the process is repeated again, and indeed repeatedly, until finally the alveolar walls are in opposition and the lung completely collapsed. The rate of collapse will be rapid if the lung is filled with oxygen and very slow if filled with nitrogen.

Several attempts have been made to reduce the incidence of post-operative atelectasis by ventilating the lungs with a gas of low solubility (such as air) at the end of anaesthesia, in order to wash out oxygen which, because of its rapid rate of absorption, has been thought to predispose to this condition. Results are conflicting, and different workers have reached diametrically opposite conclusions (Dery *et al.*, 1965; Stevens *et al.*, 1966; Cotes, 1968).

Ciliary activity.—Little is known of the force that can be exerted by ciliary activity in man, but the isolated trachea and bronchi of the hen are capable of pushing a bolus of mucus towards the larynx with a propulsive force of 30 to 40 mm. of water. Baetjer (1967) has shown that the rate of removal of mucus by cilia ranges from 7–17 mm. per minute, being increased by ventilation with warm moist air (as occurs in a closed or semi-closed system), and decreased with cold dry air (as occurs with a high flow open system). If, therefore, a plug of mucus obstructs the lumen of a bronchiole, the affected area will rapidly become collapsed, but during this time the cilia in the region of the plug will constantly be trying to push the plug towards the larger bronchi, thereby creating a negative pressure in its wake which will increase the rate of the collapse.

Circulation through the collapsed lung.—Under normal conditions about half the output of the right side of the heart passes through each lung, and continues to do so for the first few hours after blockage of the main bronchus, provided the chest wall remains intact and the lung inflated. By twenty-four hours this flow of blood to the blocked lung has begun to diminish, and at the end of the first week it represents only a very small proportion of the output from the right heart. This circulation of blood is important since on it depends the absorption of gases from an affected lung. If the lung contains air, the oxygen is rapidly removed, leaving the nitrogen to be slowly absorbed. In this state the affected lung represents a large venous shunt, as nearly half the output of the right side of the heart is no longer oxygenated. The patient may develop cyanosis. When the pleural cavity is opened the lung collapses, the pulmonary circulation diminishes rapidly and the arterial saturation improves again. It is advisable, therefore, to attempt to wash out the nitrogen and replace it with oxygen before placing a "blocker" in the main bronchus.

Surface tension of the alveolar epithelium.—As explained on p. 28, the presence of surfactant is essential to prevent alveoli progressively collapsing as they periodically decrease in size during ventilation. A reduction in surfactant would, therefore, be a potent predisposing cause of pulmonary collapse. Imrie *et al.* (1966) described a case of acute massive collapse of one lung seen during thoracotomy. The lung was completely airless, like a lobe of the liver, which suggests a primary alveolar collapse rather than one secondary to an obstruction when some air trapping would have taken place. Their patient suffered from a disordered pulmonary capillary circulation (known to affect the production of surfactant) which was probably made worse by surgical manipulation, thus accounting for the sudden massive collapse. Re-expansion of the lung was very slow and required inflation pressures far in excess of normal.

Ball-valve action.—If the obstruction in the bronchus is arranged in such a manner that the entrapped gases can partially escape with each expiration but no fresh gases can enter again on inspiration, the affected part of the lung will collapse rapidly.

REFERENCES

ADAMS, W. E. (1930). Further studies in obstructive pulmonary atelectasis. *Proc. Soc. exp. Biol. (N.Y.)*, **27**, 982.

ADRIAN, E. D. (1933). Afferent impulses in the vagus and their effects on respiration. *J. Physiol. (Lond.)*, **79**, 332.

ADRIANI, J., and GRIGGS, T. S. (1954). An improved endotracheal tube for pediatric use. *Anesthesiology*, **15**, 466.

Ambiavagar, M., and Sherwood Jones, E. (1967). Resuscitation of the moribund asthmatic. *Anaesthesia*, **22,** 375.

Ambiavagar, M., Sherwood Jones, E., and Roberts, D. V. (1967). Intermittent positive pressure ventilation in severe asthma. *Anaesthesia*, **22,** 134.

Avery, M. E. (1968). *The Lung and its Disorders in the Newborn Infant*, 2nd edit., pp. 7, 170. Philadelphia: W. B. Saunders.

Baarsma, P. R., Dirken, M. N. J. and Huizinga, E. (1948). Collateral ventilation in man. *J. thorac. Surg.*, **17,** 252.

Baetjer, A. M. (1967). Effect of ambient temperature and vapor pressure on cilia-mucus clearance rate. *J. appl. Physiol.*, **23,** 498.

Baltisberger, W. (1921). Ueber die glatte Muskulatur der menschlichen Lunge. *Z. Anat. Entwickl. Gesch.*, **61,** 249.

Brock, R. C. (1943). Observations on the anatomy of the bronchial tree, with special reference to the surgery of lung abscess. Part III: The middle lobe. *Guy's Hosp. Rep.*, **92,** 82.

Brock, R. C. (1954). *Anatomy of the Bronchial Tree, with Special Reference to the Surgery of Lung Abscess*, 2nd edit. London: Oxford Univ. Press.

Brown, E. S. (1962). Chemical identification of a surface-active agent. *Fed. Proc.*, **21,** 438.

Burton, J. D. K. (1962). Effects of dry anaesthetic gases on the respiratory mucous membrane. *Lancet*, **1,** 235.

Bush, G. H. (1963). Tracheo-bronchial suction in infants and children. *Brit. J. Anaesth.*, **35,** 322.

Cheney, F. W., and Butler, J. (1968). The effects of ultrasonically-produced aerosols on airway resistance in man. *Anesthesiology*, **29,** 1099.

Chernick, V., Hudson, W. A., and Greenfield, L. J. (1966). Effect of chronic pulmonary artery ligation on pulmonary mechanics and surfactant. *J. appl. Physiol.*, **21,** 1315.

Chu, J., Clements, J. A., Cotton, E. K., Klaus, M. H., Sweet, A. Y., and Tooley, W. H. (1967). Neonatal pulmonary ischaemia. *Pediatrics* (Suppl.), **40,** 709.

Clements, J. A. (1962). Studies of surface phenomena in relation to pulmonary function. *Physiologist*, **5,** 11.

Colebatch, H. J. H., and Halmagyi, D. F. J. (1962). Reflex airway reaction to fluid aspiration. *J. appl. Physiol.*, **17,** 787.

Coleridge, H. M., Coleridge, J. C. G., Luck, J. S., and Norman, J. (1968). The effect of four volatile anaesthetic agents on the impulse activity of two types of pulmonary receptor. *Brit. J. Anaesth.*, **40,** 484.

Committee on Safety of Drugs (1967). Bulletin, June.

Corssen, G. (1963). Pulmonary atelectasis. *J. Amer. med. Ass.*, **183,** 314.

Coryllos, P. N. and Birnbaum, G. L. (1928). Obstructive massive atelectasis of the lung. *Arch. Surg. (Chicago)*, **16,** 501.

Cross, K. W. (1961). Respiration in the new-born baby. *Brit. med. Bull.*, **17,** 163.

Dale, W. A. and Rahn, H. (1952). Rate of gas absorption during atelectasis. *Amer. J. Physiol.*, **170,** 606.

Daly, M. de B., Lambersten, C. J. and Schweitzer, A. (1953). The effects upon the bronchial musculature of altering the oxygen and carbon dioxide tensions of the blood perfusing the brain. *J. Physiol. (Lond.)*, **119,** 292.

Daly, M. de B. and Schweitzer, A. (1952). The contribution of the vasosensory areas to the reflex control of bronchomotor tone. *J. Physiol. (Lond.)*, **116,** 35.

Dery, R., Pelletier, J., Jacques, A., Claret, M., and Houde, J. (1965). Alveolar collapse induced by denitrogenation. *Canad. Anaesth. Soc. J.*, **12,** 531.

Devault, M., Greifenstein, F. E., and Harris, L. C., Jr. (1960). Circulatory responses to endotracheal intubation in light general anesthesia—the effect of atropine and phentolamine. *Anesthesiology*, **21,** 360.

ELLIS, M. (1936). Mechanism of rhythmic changes in calibre of bronchi during respiration. *J. Physiol.* (*Lond.*), **87,** 298.

FONTAINE, R. and HERRMANN, L. G. (1928). Experimental studies on denervated lungs. *Arch. Surg.* (*Chicago*), **16,** 1153.

GALLOON, S., and ROSEN, N. (1965). Changes in airway resistance and alveolar trapping with positive-negative ventilation. *Anaesthesia,* **20,** 429.

GUEST, J. L., SEKULIC, S. M., YEH, T. J., ELLISON, L. T., and ELLISON, R. G. (1966). Role of atelectasis in surfactant abnormalities following extracorporeal circulation. *Circulation* (Suppl. I), **33–34,** 65.

HEAD, H. (1889). On the regulation of respiration. *J. Physiol.* (*Lond.*), **10,** 1.

HERING, E., and BREUER, J. (1868). Die Selbsteuerung der Athmung durch den Nervus Vagus. *S.-B. Akad. Wiss. Wien,* **57,** 672.

HERZOG, P., NORLANDER, O. P., and ENGSTROM, C. G. (1964). Ultrasonic generation of aerosol for the humidification of inspired gas during volume-controlled ventilation. *Acta anaesth. scand.,* **8,** 79.

HILL, D. W. (1967). *Physics Applied to Anaesthesia,* p. 87. London: Butterworth.

HOWELL, J. B. L., and ALTOUNYAN, R. E. C. (1967). A double-blind trial of disodium cromoglycate in the treatment of allergic bronchial asthma. *Lancet,* **2,** 537.

IMRIE, D. D., MCCLELLAND, R. M. A., and SHARDLOW, W. B. (1966). Massive pulmonary collapse during thoracotomy. *Brit. J. Anaesth.,* **38,** 973.

JESSER, J. H. and DE TAKATS, G. (1942). Bronchial factor in pulmonary embolism. *Surgery,* **12,** 541.

JOHNSTONE, M. (1961). Halothane-oxygen: a universal anaesthetic. *Brit. J. Anaesth.,* **33,** 29.

KOHN, H. N. (1893). Zur Histologie der indurirenden fibrinösen Pneumonie. *Münch. med. Wschr.,* **40,** 42.

LARSELL, O., and DOW, R. S. (1933). The innervation of the human lung. *Amer. J. Anat.,* **52,** 125.

LEMMER, K. E. and ROVENSTINE, E. A. (1935). Rate of absorption of alveolar gases in relation to hyperventilation. *Arch. Surg.* (*Chicago*), **30,** 625.

LOW, F. N. (1952). Electron microscopy of the rat lung. *Anat. Rec.,* **113,** 437.

LOW, F. N. (1953). The pulmonary alveolar epithelium of laboratory mammals and man. *Anat. Rec.,* **117,** 241.

MACKLIN, C. C. (1954). The pulmonary alveolar mucoid film and the pneumonocytes. *Lancet,* **1,** 1099.

MATAUSCHEK, J. (1961). *Einführung in die Ultraschalltecknik.* Berlin: Veb. Verlag Techn. Aug.

MAY, A. J., and WIDDICOMBE, J. G. (1954). Depression of the cough reflex by pentobarbitone and some opium derivatives. *Brit. J. Pharmacol.,* **9,** 338.

MEAD, J., WHITTENBERGER, J. L., and RADFORD, E. P. (1957). Surface tension as a factor in pulmonary volume-pressure hysteresis. *J. appl. Physiol.,* **10,** 191.

MILLER, W. S. (1947). *The Lung,* 2nd edit. Springfield, Ill.: Charles C. Thomas.

MODELL, J. H., MOYA, F., RUIZ, B. C., SHOWERS, A. V., and NEWBY, E. J. (1968). Blood, gas and electrolyte determinations during exposure to ultrasonic nebulised aerosols. *Brit. J. Anaesth.,* **40,** 20.

NEGUS, V. E. (1934). The action of cilia and the effect of drugs on their activity. *J. Laryng.,* **49,** 571.

NEGUS, V. E. (1949). Ciliary action. *Thorax,* **4,** 57.

NICHOLSON, H. C. and TRIMBY, R. H. (1940). Attempt to detect reflex changes in bronchial calibre synchronous with respiration. *Amer. J. Physiol.,* **128,** 276.

NILSSON, E., SLATER, E. M., and GREENBARG, J. (1965). Cost of the quiet lung: fluctuations in PaO_2 when Carlens tube is used in pulmonary surgery. *Acta anaesth. scand.,* **9,** 49.

NISHIMURU, N., and METORI, S. (1967). Effect of gaseous anaesthetic agents on pulmonary compliance. *Anaesth. et Analg.*, **46,** 187.

NORLANDER, O. (1968). The use of respirators in anaesthesia and surgery. *Acta anaesth. scand.*, (Suppl. 30), p. 35.

PAINTAL, A. S. (1964). Effects of drugs on vertebrate mechano-receptors. *Pharmacol. Rev.*, **16,** 341.

REISSEISSEN, R. D. (1822). Ueber den Bau der Lungen (Thesis), Berlin. (Quoted by Macklin, C. C. (1929). *Physiol. Rev.*, **9,** 1.)

ROBILLARD, E., ALARIE, Y., DAGENAIS-PERUSSE, P., BARIL, E., and GUILBEAULT, A. (1964). Microaerosol administration of syntheticβ-γ- dipalmitoyl-L-α Lecithin in the respiratory distress syndrome. A preliminary report. *Canad. med. Ass. J.*, **90,** 55.

RINGROSE, R. E., MCKOWN, B., FELTON, F. G., BARCLAY, B. O., MUCHMORE, H. G., and RHOADES, E. R. (1968). A hospital outbreak of serratia marcescens associated with ultrasonic nebulizers. *Ann. intern. Med.*, **69,** 719.

SHNIDER, S. M., and PAPPER, E. M. (1961). Anesthesia for the asthmatic patient. *Anesthesiology*, **22,** 886.

SIMONSSON, B. G., JACOBS, F. M., and NADEL, J. A. (1967). Role of autonomic nervous system and the cough reflex in increased responsiveness of airways in patients with obstructive airways disease. *J. clin. Invest.*, **46,** 1812.

SMITH, J. M., and DEVEY, G. F. (1968). Clinical trial of disodium cromoglycate in treatment of asthma in children. *Brit. med. J.*, **2,** 340.

SPENCER, G. T., RIDLEY, M., EYKYN, S., and ACHONG, J. (1968). Disinfection of lung ventilators by alcohol aerosol. *Lancet*, **2,** 667.

STEVENS, W. C., GOSSETT, J. A., HAMILTON, W. K., and MOORHEAD, R. T. (1966). Relation of postoperative atelectasis to solubility of gases filling lungs at termination of anaesthesia. *Anesthesiology*, **27,** 163.

TOOLEY, W. H., FINLEY, T. N., and GARDNER, R. (1961). Some effects on the lungs of blood from a pump oxygenator. *Physiologist*, **4,** 124.

TOREMALM, N. G. (1960). Heat and moisture exchanger for post-tracheostomy care. *Acta oto-laryng.* (*Stockh.*), **52,** Fasc. 6.

VON NEERGAARD, K. (1929). Neue Auffassungen ueber einen Grundbegriff der Atemmechanik, abhaenzig von der Oberglaichen spannung in der Alveolen. *Z. ges. exp. Med.*, **66,** 373.

WHITTERIDGE, D., and BULBRING, E. (1944). Changes in activity of pulmonary receptors in anaesthesia and their influence on respiratory behaviour. *J. Pharmacol. exp. Ther.*, **81,** 340.

WIDDICOMBE, J. G. (1961). Respiratory reflexes in man and other mammalian species. *Clin. Sci.*, **21,** 163.

WIDDICOMBE, J. G. (1962). Clinical significance of reflexes from the respiratory system. *Anesthesiology*, **23,** 4.

WIDDICOMBE, J. G. (1963). Respiratory reflexes from the lung. *Brit. med. Bull.*, **19,** 19.

WIDDICOMBE, J. G., KENT, D. C., and NADEL, J. A. (1962). Mechanism of bronchoconstriction during inhalation of dust. *J. appl. Physiol.*, **17,** 613.

Chapter 2

THE MECHANICS OF RESPIRATION

THE RESPIRATORY MUSCLES

THE diaphragm is the principal muscle of respiration, but many other muscles, including the intercostals, the abdominals, the scalenes, the sternomastoids and even some of the back muscles, have their part to play. All of these muscles have one thing in common—they are attached to the thoracic cage. Each group will now be considered in turn.

THE DIAPHRAGM

Anatomy

The diaphragm (Fig. 1) consists of a central tendon which is arched on both sides to form a cupola. Muscle fibres radiate from each portion of the tendon and can be traced to their origin in three distinct regions. First, the spinal or crural portion in which the fibres arise from the upper three or four lumbar vertebrae and from the arcuate ligaments. This division is inserted into the posterior margin of the central tendon. Secondly, the costal portion which arises by a series of digitations from the inner surface of the lower six ribs and cartilages. Finally there is a small contribution arising from the back of the ensiform process. The central or tendinous part of the diaphragm is domed upwards into the chest, partly due to the higher intra-abdominal pressure and partly due to the negative pressure pull exerted by the elastic recoil of the lung.

The motor innervation of the diaphragm is largely supplied by the phrenic nerves whose fibres are 90 per cent motor and 10 per cent sensory and autonomic. The two crura receive a motor supply from the 11th and 12th intercostal nerves. Peripheral parts of the diaphragm receive a sensory and autonomic innervation from the lower six intercostal nerves.

Movements

The diaphragm moves in a vertical plane and in quiet respiration it is almost wholly responsible for the tidal exchange, thus fully deserving the title of the principal muscle of respiration. The exact extent to which it moves has been studied radiologically. Wade (1954) gives it a range of about 1·5 cm. upwards or downwards during quiet respiration, but this distance may be extended to 6–10 cm. with deep breathing. Extension of the spine and lifting of the whole thoracic cage are associated with maximal respiratory effort and account for part of this extended movement.

Contrary to popular belief, the range of movement of the diaphragm does not alter with a change of posture from the standing to the supine position. The resting level, however, is higher when the subject is lying down.

It is sometimes claimed that diaphragmatic excursion can be aided by nursing patients in the upright position after an operation, thus avoiding undue

The function of the intercostal muscles is in doubt. Campbell (1958) believes that this action is determined by the incline of the structures to which they are attached. Thus those fibres which are parasternal lie between costal cartilages and slope upwards, paralleling therefore the external intercostal muscles in both direction and action during inspiration, while the fibres that lie between the ribs slope backwards as well as downwards and contract during expiration. These inter-osseous fibres also contract during speech.

Abdominal Muscles

There are four principal groups of abdominal muscles that influence respiration—namely the external and internal obliques, the transversi and the recti muscles (Fig. 2).

Anatomy

The *external oblique* muscle arises from the outer surface of the lower eight ribs and the fibres pass downwards in a fan-shape to be inserted into the iliac

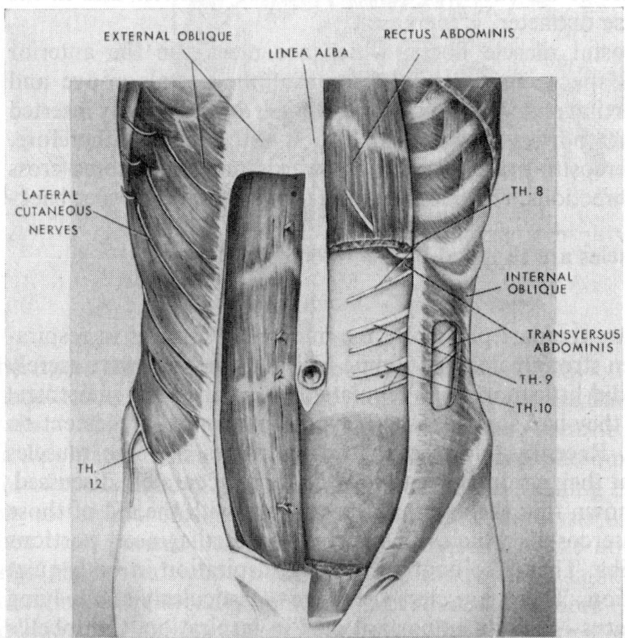

2/Fig. 2.—The muscles of the abdominal wall.

crest posteriorly and into a fibrous aponeurosis blending with the rectus sheath anteriorly. The lower border of this aponeurosis forms the inguinal ligament.

In contrast, the *internal oblique* arises from the iliac crest, lumbar fascia and inguinal ligament, and the fibres pass vertically upwards to be inserted into the lower three ribs posteriorly and into the aponeurosis forming part of the rectus sheath anteriorly. The *transversus abdominis* muscle arises from the costal cartilages of the lower six ribs, the lumbar fascia, the iliac crest and a small portion of the inguinal ligament. The fibres run horizontally and are attached to the aponeurosis forming part of the rectus sheath. Finally, the *rectus abdominis* muscle arises from the pubic symphysis and crest and the fibres pass vertically upwards to become attached to the 5th, 6th and 7th costal cartilages. During their passage these fibres are enclosed in an aponeurosis or sheath which is closely related to the three abdominal muscles already mentioned.

Movements in Conscious People

During quiet respiration, and any increase in ventilation up to 40 litres a minute (i.e. about five times the resting minute volume), the abdominal muscles remain inactive in the conscious subject when supine, and often even when the body is erect (Campbell and Green, 1953). As the volume of respiration increases further so the abdominal muscles gradually start to take an active part. By the time forceful abdominal contractions can be seen, ventilation will have risen to 90 litres per minute—the equivalent of strenuous exercise. These muscles also contract when a forced expiratory effort is made.

The time at which abdominal muscle activity starts in relation to the respiratory cycle is interesting, for the earliest movements are seen at the end of expiration. This finding may be connected with their function, and may perhaps be explained as follows:—The maximum intra-abdominal pressure that can be maintained by a conscious patient for more than a few seconds is 110 mm. Hg, yet Gordh and Silferkiold (1943) found that intra-abdominal pressures of 150–200 mm. Hg were reached during electro-convulsive therapy. Campbell (1958) believes that the function of the abdominal muscles in the conscious subject is to preserve a steady intra-abdominal pressure and that, for this purpose, there are reflex pathways which tend to prevent too rapid or too great a rise. Thus, during inspiration the diaphragm descends and causes an increase in intra-abdominal pressure; then early in expiration it starts to ascend again, due to the elastic recoil of the lungs. This leads to a fall in pressure in the abdomen and the muscles of the abdomen now start to contract in a reflex attempt to keep the intra-abdominal pressure stable. These facts help to explain why the abdominal muscles start to contract at the end of expiration. The abdominal muscles, therefore, play no part in inspiration. In expiration they maintain the stability of the intra-abdominal pressure and thus indirectly assist the ascent of the diaphragm.

In the past various people have argued that the abdominal muscles have an inspiratory function on the basis that they contract during inspiration, so fixing the lower ribs and allowing the diaphragm a greater range of movement. Campbell (1958) made electromyographic studies of the abdominal muscles in over thirty subjects during increased breathing and found an inspiratory contraction in only two patients. He feels that the elastic property of the abdominal wall, rather than muscular contraction, is the more important factor in producing the intra-abdominal tension of inspiration.

To summarise, the abdominal muscles are muscles of expiration. Essentially they have two functions during expiration—one to raise the intra-abdominal pressure, and the other to draw the lower ribs downwards and medially. In normal quiet respiration they play no part at all, but when ventilation becomes more vigorous, they contract during expiration and thus aid the ascent of the diaphragm. They are the major muscles concerned in developing the enormously high expulsive pressures of defaecation and coughing.

Movements in Anaesthetised Patients

Fink (1961), using an electromyographic technique, has studied the movements of both the abdominal muscles and the diaphragm during anaesthesia. Under all types of light anaesthesia some electrical activity can always be detected in the abdominal musculature (oblique-transverse group) during expiration. This can be abolished by the use of a muscle relaxant.

In anaesthetised patients under light anaesthesia the diaphragm contracts with inspiration and the abdominal muscles with expiration (see Fig. 3*a*). On the other hand, if the patient is now ventilated manually until spontaneous respiration is abolished, then activity ceases in the diaphragm during the period of apnoea but persists as continuous activity in the abdominal muscles (Fig. 3*b*).

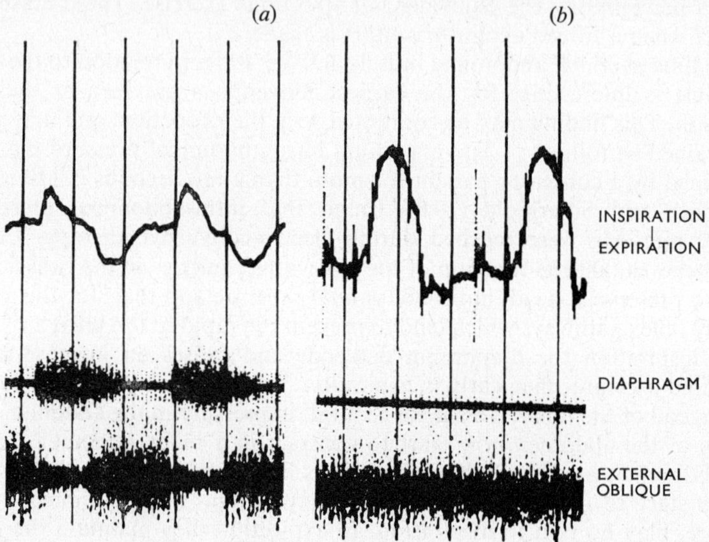

2/Fig. 3.—Electromyogram of diaphragmatic and abdominal muscle activity in an anaesthetised patient.

(*a*) Spontaneous respiration under halothane/nitrous oxide/oxygen anaesthesia.
(*b*) Controlled respiration (i.e. apnoea) under same anaesthesia.

Such an observation does not support Campbell's theory that the role of the abdominal muscles is to preserve an even intra-abdominal tension because there is no obvious reason why such a reflex should be abolished by light anaesthesia. Fink favours the view that the diminished abdominal activity during a spontaneous inspiration is due to a direct inhibition of these muscles brought about by the respiratory centre. During apnoea this inhibition is removed, so that they enter a state of continuous activity.

Other Accessory Muscles of Respiration

The *scalene muscles* contract during quiet inspiration and as such are almost entitled to be considered as a principal muscle of respiration. Their total contribution to the amount inspired, however, is not considered to be great. They also are believed to contract during violent expiratory motions such as coughing, presumably in an attempt to support the apex of the lung (Campbell, 1958).

The *sternomastoid muscles*, on the other hand, are inactive during quiet breathing but become vigorous as ventilation increases. They then contract during inspiration and are regarded as important accessory muscles and their action can be seen well in patients with dyspnoea.

There are many other muscles attached to the thoracic cage which have, at one time or another, been considered as important accessory muscles of respiration. Campbell (1954), using electromyography, has studied many of them, including the trapezius, serratus anterior, latissimus dorsi and pectoralis muscles. He failed to find any evidence that they play a significant part in respiration. Many of them contract during the act of coughing. The latissimus dorsi is important in this respect as it may become paralysed following section of its nerve supply at a radical amputation of the breast or division of the muscle fibres at a thoracotomy incision. As a result there is sometimes a serious limitation of the power to expel sputum. A posterior incision for thoracotomy alone may, by dividing the latissimus dorsi, cause a permanent reduction of lung function.

Normal Lung Movements

Those parts of the lung lying in direct relation to the mobile or expansile parts of the thoracic cage—i.e. the ribs and diaphragm—are expanded in direct contact with their neighbouring wall. The peripheral parts of the lung thus undergo a greater degree of expansion than those nearer the hilum. There are three areas of the lung which are not expanded directly, the mediastinal surface in contact with the pericardium, the dorsal surface in contact with the spinal segments of the ribs, and the posterior apical surface lying close to the deep cervical fascia of Sibson. At each inspiration the capacity of the chest is increased in its transverse, antero-posterior and vertical diameters; the converse applies during expiration. As the chest wall expands, so the glottis opens more widely and air enters the lungs.

The movements of the lungs are best considered in relation to the change in position of the chest wall and diaphragm.

I. *The apex.*—The thoracic inlet, formed by the first two ribs, the vertebral column, and the manubrium sterni, moves upwards and forwards on inspiration to increase the antero-posterior diameter of the chest wall. In this manner the anterior part of the apex of the upper lobe is expanded directly. In later life (60 years and over) the manubrio-sternal junction becomes ankylosed and this part of the lung ceases to expand.

II. *The thoracic cage.*—This is best divided into two parts, the upper stretching from the second to the sixth ribs and the lower from the seventh to the tenth. The ribs move outwards and upwards on inspiration; in the upper portion it is the antero-posterior diameter of the thoracic cage that is chiefly increased, whereas in the lower portion the main enlargement lies in the transverse diameter.

III. *The diaphragm.*—The diaphragm has already been mentioned as the principal muscle of respiration. In quiet breathing it can account for the whole of the inspired air, whilst in a maximal inspiratory effort it can still claim over

60 per cent. It is hardly surprising, therefore, that the bases of the lung are the parts which undergo the greatest movement. Radiographically the position of the diaphragm can be seen to vary markedly with changes in posture. In the supine position the abdominal muscles are relaxed and the intestines push the diaphragm up to its highest level. In this position, therefore, the diaphragm possesses its greatest potential powers of contraction. In the erect posture, on the other hand, the weight of the intestines falls away and the level of the diaphragm descends. Frequently, however, the abdominal muscles are contracted, presumably in an attempt to maintain an even intra-abdominal pressure. A similar set of circumstances prevails in the sitting position because the cupola lies at a low level and the abdominal muscles may be contracting if the ventilation is large.

Patients with severe dyspnoea adopt the sitting posture for comfort. This is not due to any change in position of the diaphragm, which would tend to be detrimental rather than beneficial, but to a reduction in the pulmonary congestion and also an improved action of the accessory muscles of respiration. The most satisfying position is often found to be with the trunk bent forward and the head and arms fixed on a support.

IV. *Other factors.*—Vertical movements of the thoracic cage occur in some subjects, mainly at the end of deep inspiration, and are usually most marked in the standing position. These movements are caused by flexion and extension of the vertebral column, but they do not appear to play an important part in ventilating the lungs. They are especially marked during voluntary hyperventilation and thus may aid the contractions of the diaphragm (Wade, 1954).

To summarise, during normal ventilation those parts of the lung near the diaphragm are better ventilated than their relatively static cousins near the apex.

Abnormal Chest and Lung Movements

When the stability of the thoracic cage is destroyed either by trauma or surgical intervention, then abnormal movements of both chest wall and the underlying lung may occur. There are three principal conditions that must be considered, paradoxical respiration, pendelluft and mediastinal flap.

Paradoxical Respiration

In the presence of a crush injury of the chest wall or the deliberate surgical removal of part of the rib cage (as in a thoracoplasty), the affected part of the chest wall collapses inwards. On inspiration the unaffected side will expand in the normal fashion but the injured side will be sucked in. On expiration, the reverse takes place. This type of respiration—paradoxical respiration—is only seen in patients breathing spontaneously and is abolished by controlled ventilation. The objective of a thoracoplasty operation is to remove part of the chest-wall to allow the underlying lung to collapse; the presence of paradoxical respiration is an indication to apply external pressure (in the form of a pad) over the wound site to prevent this abnormal movement of the chest wall.

Pendelluft

This signifies the pendulum-like movement of air that occurs from one lung to the other in the presence of an open pneumothorax in a patient breathing spontaneously. Thus, when the chest is opened the underlying lung partially deflates as the negative intrapleural pressure is lost. On inspiration, the lung on the normal side fills with air partly from the trachea and partly from the partially deflated lung on the affected side. On expiration, the converse takes place and some expired air from the normal lung passes over into the other side (Fig. 4). The physiological result of this pendulum-like flow of air is that the alveolar carbon dioxide tension rises.

Previously, this condition was always believed to occur in the presence of paradoxical respiration, but Maloney and his associates (1961) have shown that

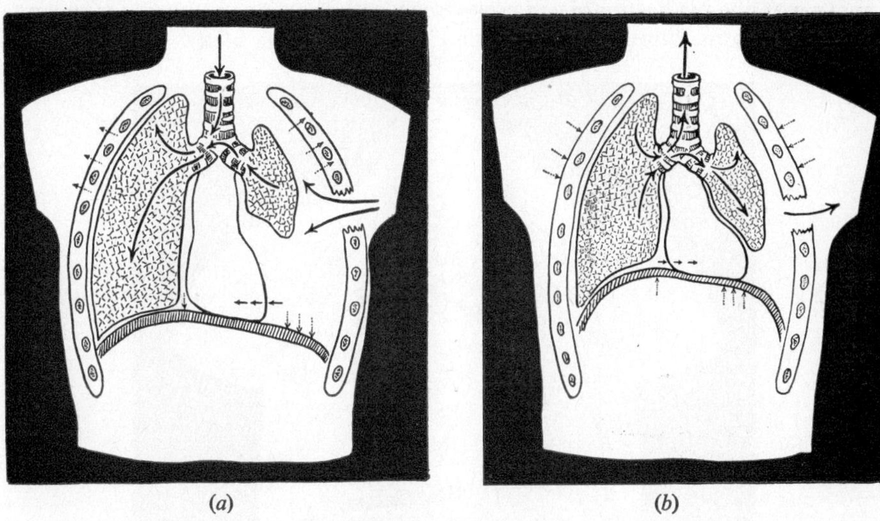

(*a*) (*b*)

2/FIG. 4.—PENDELLUFT
a) Inspiration. (*b*) Expiration.

this conception is untrue. In a study of dogs using a bronchospirometric technique together with gas analysis they were able to prove that pendelluft does not occur in the presence of paradoxical respiration provided the pleural cavity is not open to the atmosphere.

In the presence of an open pneumothorax, pendelluft does not necessarily occur; much will depend on the size of the opening in the chest wall and the volume of the ventilation. If the size of the hole in the chest wall is less than the diameter of the trachea, then it is easier for air to enter via the trachea, so very little air will be sucked into the affected side and both lungs will expand on inspiration. Similarly, a patient breathing spontaneously can often tolerate a large opening in his pleural cavity provided he is breathing quietly. The moment ventilation increases both paradoxical respiration and pendelluft may result.

Pendelluft is most likely to occur during anaesthesia in a patient who breathes spontaneously in the presence of an open pneumothorax. The presence of a distended reservoir bag in a carbon dioxide absorption system will tend to aggravate pendelluft. For example, when the patient makes a spontaneous effort at inspiration some gas will pass into the lung on the unaffected side. This will reduce the tension in the reservoir bag and the alveolar pressure on both sides will fall. The reduction in alveolar pressure on the side with the open pneumothorax will result in the lung getting smaller, so as one lung expands the other shrinks. The reverse takes place on expiration. However, this situation is hardly likely to arise in good clinical practice as the presence of an open pneumothorax under anaesthesia is an indication for intermittent positive-pressure ventilation. Neither paradoxical respiration nor pendelluft can occur in the presence of adequate controlled respiration.

Mediastinal Flap

In man the mediastinum can move freely with the different phases of respiration. It remains, however, approximately in the middle of the thorax because

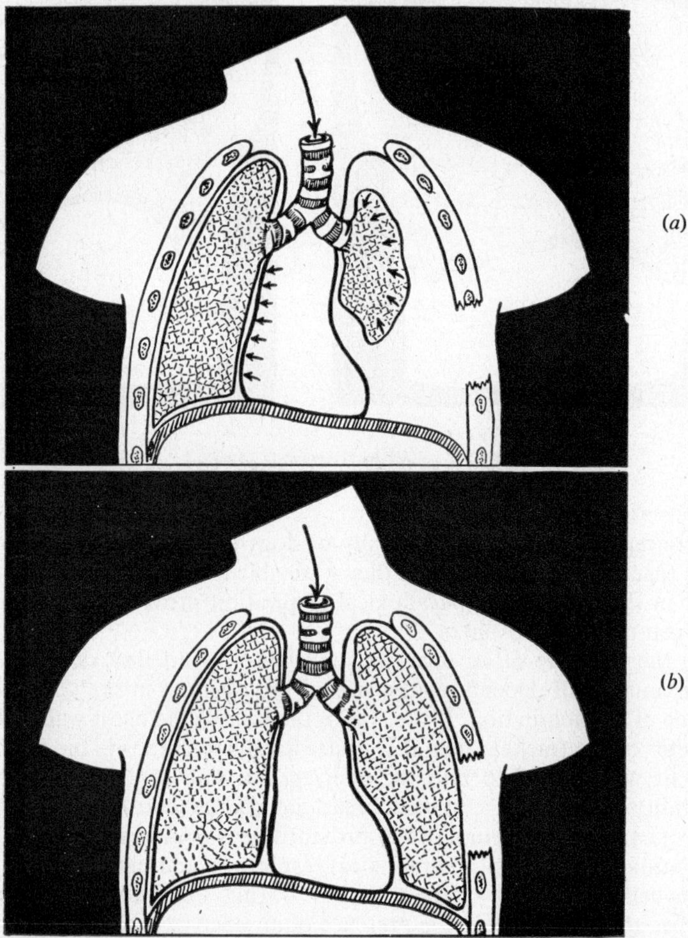

2/Fig. 5.—Effect of Pneumothorax on Mediastinum (Inspiration)

(*a*) Mediastinal flap + weight of heart and great vessels (spontaneous respiration).
(*b*) These factors corrected by positive-pressure ventilation.

the negative pressure in the pleural cavities balance each other. When the pleural cavity is opened, so that the lung collapses and the pressure around it becomes atmospheric, the negative intrapleural pressure on the other side will pull the heart and great vessels in the mediastinum towards the sound lung. This negative pull reaches its maximum during inspiration and, therefore, the mediastinum comes furthest over at this time (Fig. 5*a*). On expiration the intrapleural pressure becomes less negative and the mediastinum passes back to its original position.

During quiet breathing, even in the presence of a large hole in the chest wall, the mediastinum merely moves with a slight to and fro' motion. As the volume of ventilation increases so the flapping movement becomes more obvious. Its presence tends to embarrass respiration because it impairs the filling of the lung on the normal side. The actual range of movement is greatest when the patient is in the supine position but it is more dangerous in the lateral position because, then, the whole weight of the mediastinal contents is compressing the dependent normal lung. In addition, mediastinal flap interferes with the filling of the great veins, leading to a fall in cardiac output.

Paradoxical respiration, pendelluft, mediastinal flap and the disturbances caused by the weight of the mediastinal viscera, can all be prevented during anaesthesia by assisted or controlled respiration (Fig. 5*b*).

Assisted and Controlled Respiration

In a conscious patient breathing spontaneously, the carbon dioxide tension of the blood varies between 36 and 44 mm. Hg, and only rarely can values outside this range be recorded. Under the conditions of anaesthesia, when spontaneous respiration is maintained, the effective tidal exchange can be impaired by anaesthetic, analgesic and relaxant drugs, so that the level of carbon dioxide in the body will consequently rise. Moreover the patient's efforts may be further impeded by the resistance of the anaesthetic system.

Since oxygen is usually added to anaesthetic mixtures the tidal volume may well be sufficient to ensure oxygenation of the patient, yet inadequate to carry away all this carbon dioxide. There is no simple method available for measuring the carbon dioxide tension of blood or alveolar air and, as a result, the anaesthetist must estimate the balance and effectiveness of the tidal exchange on a purely empirical basis. When there is any doubt about this, respiration must be assisted.

Assisted Respiration

With this, the patient spontaneously commences inspiration and the anaesthetist then assists with positive-pressure down the trachea until the lungs are fully expanded. Expiration is then allowed to take place passively. Assisted respiration is useful when respiratory activity is temporarily depressed or hampered by such things as a small dose of central depressant like pethidine or a peripherally acting drug of the muscle relaxant type. It is, however, not easy to match spontaneous activity satisfactorily in this way, especially for long periods, and when it is possible to carry it out efficiently, apnoea tends to result as the carbon dioxide tension in the blood falls. Respiration is now said to be controlled. In other words efficient assisted respiration soon becomes controlled respiration.

Controlled Respiration

Controlled respiration can be initiated in three different ways:

1. Paralysis of the muscles of respiration.
2. Depression of the respiratory centre.
3. Removal of the carbon dioxide stimulus to the respiratory centre.

In practice a combination of all three methods can be used, but nowadays the first—nearly always by muscle relaxants—is normally made to account for the greatest proportion of the apnoea. The effects of a raised threshold to the respiratory centre and a decreased stimulus are valuable adjuncts—which enable the total dose of relaxant to be restricted. Provided the respiratory centre has not been heavily depressed by analgesic drugs then spontaneous respiratory activity can be resumed at will, even though the carbon dioxide tension of the blood has been reduced to a very low level.

The dangers of a high carbon dioxide tension are far greater than those of a low one, and during controlled respiration the anaesthetist should err, if at all, on the side of hyperventilation. This is particularly important during thoracotomy when a partially collapsed lung may cause gross defects of gas distribution and elimination.

Apart from its value to ensure adequate ventilation of the lungs in certain circumstances, controlled respiration can be made to provide ideal conditions for the surgeon working either in the chest or abdominal cavity. The smooth, rhythmical inflation of the lungs and the movement of the diaphragm with controlled respiration is preferable to the jerky, and often gross, movement frequently seen during spontaneous respiration under anaesthesia for abdominal and thoracic operations. The anaesthetist can also help the surgeon by momentarily preventing movement of the lungs and diaphragm during some critical manoeuvre.

The principal disadvantage of controlled respiration is the risk of persistent apnoea, which has become prominent since the introduction of muscle relaxant drugs. The effects of both controlled and assisted respiration on the circulation are discussed in Chapter 15.

Diffusion Respiration

In a normal person the interchange of gases at the alveolar capillary membrane depends upon physical diffusion, while at tidal volumes smaller than 1 litre the movement of gas molecules from the alveolar ducts to the alveoli is almost entirely by diffusion. Some movement is caused by the contraction of the heart and by the ejection of blood from it leading to a pulsatile flow in the pulmonary vessels. If the nitrogen in the lungs is replaced by oxygen then these factors are sufficient to maintain an adequate uptake of oxygen in the blood in the absence of respiratory muscle activity. This process is known as diffusion respiration, but during it carbon dioxide is not removed from the blood. In fact the tension of carbon dioxide in the alveoli rises rapidly to equal that of the mixed venous blood (46 mm. Hg) but thereafter more slowly.

Diffusion respiration can be produced in an anaesthetised patient following the use of a muscle relaxant and the endotracheal administration of oxygen, and is often deliberately practised during bronchoscopy (see Chapter 10).

Respiratory Movements in Anaesthesia

During the induction of anaesthesia the respiratory pattern undergoes a whole series of changes. When ether is used, increasing concentrations of the drug in the body are only gradually achieved, so that the consequent effects on respiration are produced as a relatively slow and orderly process, and are classical of the progressively increasing depth of anaesthesia. These have been well-described by Guedel (1951) and are briefly reviewed here.

The movement of the thoracic cage on inspiration passes steadily from one of expansion during light anaesthesia to one of retraction in the late stages of ether anaesthesia. This transition occurs gradually and must be related to the paralysis of the various muscle groups. Thus, in light anaesthesia the abdominal muscles probably act as synergists and exert a steady isometric pull on the lower costal margin. The chest and abdominal wall rise and fall in unison (Stage III, Planes I and II). As the depth of anaesthesia increases so the synergistic muscles of respiration drop out one by one. In the second plane (Stage III, Plane II) respiratory rate, rhythm, and depth are similar to those found in the first plane, but when the third plane (Stage III, Plane III) is reached a characteristic expiratory pause may occur together with an absence of movement in the upper part of the thoracic cage. At the same time, the abdominal element of respiration becomes more marked and the abdomen begins to protrude just before the lower part of the thoracic cage moves outwards. Chest movements are in fact starting to lag behind those of the abdomen.

When the anaesthesia is deepened to the fourth plane (Stage III, Plane IV) the inspiratory phase is marked by a quick jerky protrusion of the abdominal wall as the diaphragm descends, followed immediately by a similar jerky retraction of the chest wall. This is often called diaphragmatic respiration (p. 65) and is characterised by paradoxical movements of the abdomen and thoracic cage. At this point, almost all the muscles of respiration, except the diaphragm, have ceased to function; thus, as the diaphragm descends, the intra-abdominal pressure is raised, and the abdominal wall is thrust out in a forceful manner. At the same time the descent of the diaphragm creates a relatively negative intrathoracic pressure and the intercostal muscles and ribs are sucked inwards. Expiration, by comparison, is a slow, prolonged movement during which the muscles return to their former positions. It is followed by a slight pause.

In the fourth stage of anaesthesia (Stage IV) this expiratory pause grows longer, inspiration becomes more jerky and irregular, until finally respiratory activity ceases altogether.

Tracheal Tug

In deep anaesthesia (Stage III, Plane III or IV) inspiration is associated with a tracheal tug. This is a sharp downward movement of the trachea on inspiration. The exact mechanism is obscure but there are two theories which deserve serious attention. Harris (1951) believes it is associated with the dual origin of the muscle fibres of the diaphragm. In deep anaesthesia there is a general loss of muscle tone so that the sterno-costal fibres of the diaphragm are no longer supported by a rigid costal margin when they contract on inspiration. In consequence, these costal fibres contract ineffectively leaving the crural fibres alone to appear to be functioning. The result is that a sharp contraction of the central part of the diaphragm on inspiration is transmitted to the whole mediastinum. The root of the lung and trachea is then pulled downwards with each inspiration. This explanation, however, does not account for the occurrence of this condition in dyspnoea.

Another approach has been made on the basis of the part played by the elevating muscles of the larynx. In rats, the sterno-thyroid and sterno-hyoid muscles contract during inspiration and are directly controlled by the respiratory centre. In man, these muscles may help to raise the sternum as accessory muscles of respiration but their size and mobility make it unlikely they play an important role. In normal breathing the larynx remains stationary in both phases of respiration. This is due to the pull of its stabilising muscles (mylohyoid, stylohyoid, styloglossus and the posterior belly of the digastric), all of which are elevators of the larynx. It has been suggested that "tracheal tug" is due to a failure of these stabilising muscles to stand up to the forceful traction of the diaphragm (Campbell, 1958).

Apart from deep anaesthesia, tracheal tug may be noticed in partially curarised patients and in the presence of respiratory obstruction. It also occurs in shock states and, in the past, often signified moribundity. In most cases it can be cured by returning full power to the muscles of respiration or removing the cause of the respiratory obstruction. Tracheal tug at the end of anaesthesia—in the absence of muscular paralysis—may be an indication for endotracheal suction or bronchoscopy, as the cause is not infrequently inadequate ventilation of one lung due to an accumulation of mucus.

Respiratory Patterns

The different wave forms of respiration can be visualised from tracings made either by a spirometer (tidal flow) or by a pneumograph (chest expansion and deflation). These offer a useful method for teaching the various patterns that may occur during anaesthesia.

Expiratory phase.—During quiet breathing in a conscious subject the duration of expiration is usually 1·3–1·4 times longer than that of inspiration. A pause at the end of expiration is present as a constant feature in both conscious and anaesthetised subjects, provided the rate of respiration is slow enough and the tidal volume sufficiently large (Morton, 1950). An increase in the rate and a diminution in the tidal volume lead to an abolition of this pause (Fig. 6). The presence of the pause in the third plane (Stage III, Plane III) of ether anaesthesia is largely related to the use of premedication. It may not occur, even in fourth plane anaesthesia, if no central respiratory depressant has been used, yet is a marked feature in all patients who have previously received morphine. It is interesting to recall that this expiratory pause was not included by Guedel in his original description of respiratory activity under ether anaesthesia.

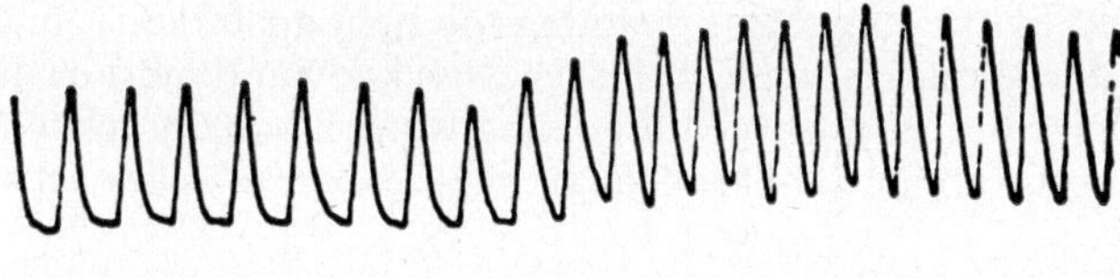

2/FIG. 6.—Respiratory tracing. Expiratory pause. Increasing the rate and volume of respiration abolishes this pause in both conscious and anaesthetised subjects.

Inspiratory pause.—A pause at the end of inspiration is seen during diaphragmatic respiration due to the use of muscle relaxants. This type of respiration has been described as "truncated" (Morton, 1950) because of the turret-shaped manner in which inspiration is suddenly interrupted by the prolonged pause (Fig. 7). Just as with the expiratory pause, an increase in the rate of

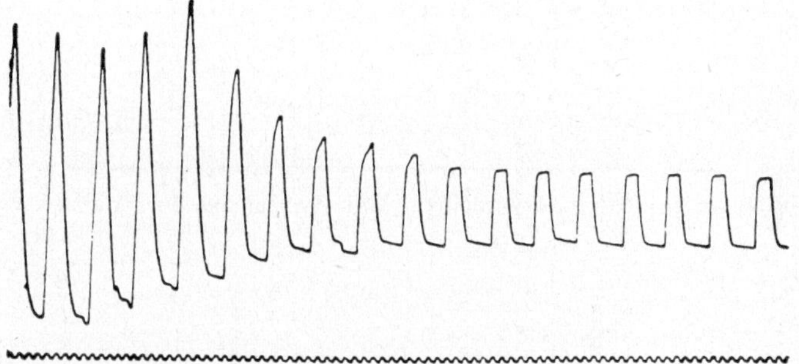

2/FIG. 7.—Respiratory tracing. Spirometer: Time in 1 and 4 seconds. Truncated respiration.

respiration tends to diminish it. In deep anaesthesia or in the presence of good muscle relaxation, a small superadded inspiratory effort may also sometimes be seen, giving a sort of step-ladder effect. The cause of "truncated" respiration still remains unknown. The respiratory pattern is almost identical with normal respiration in which the "peaks" have been neatly sliced off. The reason for this plateau is more difficult to understand. Morton (1950) suggests that it may be due to partial paralysis of the muscles of respiration. There is no reason to believe that impulses do not continue to flow down the phrenic nerves when muscle relaxants are used. If only half of the usual number of muscle fibres in the motor unit responded to this stimulus, then inspiration would commence in the normal manner but might be only half completed. Nevertheless, these fibres would remain in a state of contraction until the impulses from the phrenic nerve ceased. A step-ladder pattern is most commonly observed in the presence of a high carbon dioxide tension and when decamethonium is used as the relaxant. Again, its cause is obscure.

Sigh.—A deep sigh (Fig. 8) is occasionally seen in both conscious and anaesthetised subjects. In the latter it is commonly associated with deep anaesthesia, particularly when open ether is administered. Its occurrence may be misinterpreted by the surgeon as denoting too light anaesthesia, but in practice it is unrelated to surgical stimuli, nor is its cause known. It must be distinguished from the inspiratory gasp or breath-holding which is clearly related to surgical stimulation in the presence of inadequate suppression of reflex activity (Fig. 9).

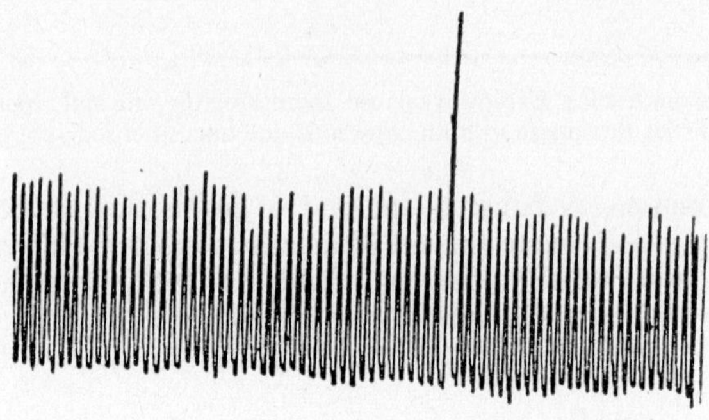

2/FIG. 8.—Sigh. Respiratory tracing to show typical sigh during anaesthesia.

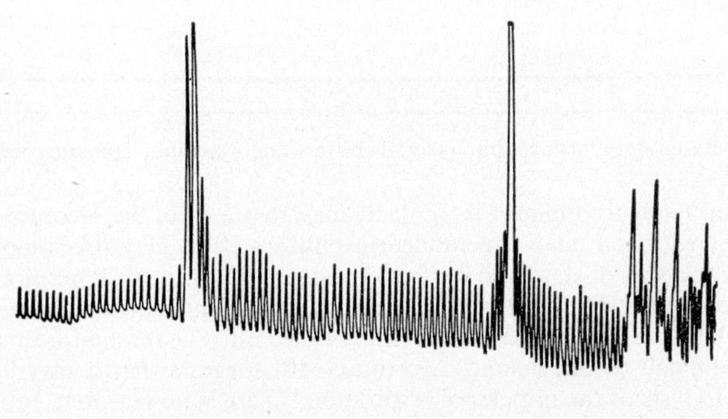

2/FIG. 9.—Inspiratory gasp. Result of surgical stimulation under too light anaesthesia.

Sighing in a conscious person is thought to be a mechanism by which during quiet respiration an occasional deep breath prevents underventilated alveoli from collapsing. However, Fletcher and Barber (1966) investigated conscious subjects breathing spontaneously and found that sighing was not followed by any change in lung mechanisms or in lung compliance. They were also unable to demonstrate any changes when sighing was almost completely abolished by intravenous morphine.

Diaphragmatic Respiration

This type of respiration generally occurs under three conditions, and all should be readily distinguishable:

1. Deep ether anaesthesia (Stage III, Plane IV).
2. Curarisation (used in its widest sense) just short of total paralysis.
3. Respiratory obstruction.

A combination of any of these may occur in the same patient. Nevertheless, squeezing the rebreathing bag will quickly differentiate between the deeply anaesthetised or paralysed and the obstructed patient. In all these conditions respiratory activity may appear to take on an "inverted" pattern in which the abdomen contracts and moves in whilst the chest moves out. Attempts to measure an actual increase in the diameter of the chest reveal no change because a reduction in the antero-posterior measurement is exactly compensated for by an equal increase in the lateral one. Nevertheless this "see-saw" type of respiration is very characteristic. The mechanism in the paralysed patient has already been discussed (see "truncated" respiratory pattern).

The movements of the abdomen and chest wall in respiratory obstruction are more complex and there is little experimental evidence available. For descriptive purposes there would appear to be two distinct types of respiratory obstruction. One is *mechanical*, in which, for example, the tongue falls back and partially obstructs the glottis. The other is *reflex*, occurring in conjunction with laryngeal or bronchial spasm when the level of anaesthesia is insufficient to combat the stimulation of surgery.

In mechanical respiratory obstruction the patient continues to breathe in an entirely normal manner, but the expiratory pause disappears the moment the obstruction starts. In fact this is such a constant finding that it could be used as a method of diagnosing its presence. The explanation may well be that the restriction of the airway causes a prolongation of the duration of both expiration and inspiration, thus abolishing the expiratory pause.

Reflex obstruction is more complicated, since the effects of surgical or anaesthetic stimulation in the presence of inadequate reflex suppression may not only lead to laryngeal spasm (when the trachea is not intubated) but also to breath-holding and contraction of the abdominal muscles. The patient behaves as though impulses fan out from the spinal cord causing numerous muscle groups to contract. The carbon dioxide tension rises until, depending upon the threshold of the respiratory centre, an inspiratory effort occurs as the glottis partially or completely opens. At the same time the abdominal muscles momentarily relax. Thus in cases of partial reflex obstruction, the vocal cords open and the abdominal muscles relax on inspiration, only to contract again in the expiratory phase. The jerky movements of the abdominal musculature in this type of case give the impression of "see-saw" respiration, but in actual practice the movement is almost entirely abdominal and the chest wall remains relatively steady.

Hiccup

Hiccup is an intermittent clonic spasm of the diaphragm, of reflex origin. With each contraction the bronchial lumen is constricted and, in unintubated patients, the glottis closed. Fitzgerald (1967) has questioned the commonly accepted sequence of events. From a consideration of the anatomy of the central nervous system connections that are involved, he argues that the reverse is more likely, glottic closure preceding phrenic nerve stimulation through the respiratory centre. In mild cases, unassociated with anaesthesia, the spasm is usually a unilateral contraction of the diaphragm which, if the condition persists, gradually spreads across the whole muscle (Samuels, 1952). The left side is more often affected than the right.

Afferents can arise from almost any part of the body, including the central nervous system, but during anaesthesia are most frequently associated with visceral stimulation, usually in the upper abdomen, and probably transmitted through the vagus. Hiccup may also be caused by inflation of the stomach with anaesthetic gases, or from irritation below the diaphragm due to extraneous fluids, such as blood, pus or gastric juice.

Hiccup is not a common complication of deep anaesthesia but rather a product of modern methods when relaxation is produced by motor paralysis, and sensory reflex activity is by comparison relatively undepressed. It can be regarded as a reflex response of the partially anaesthetised respiratory centres and incompletely paralysed peripheral musculature to vagal stimulation.

Treatment.—Careful appraisal of the surgeon's technique will usually enable the anaesthetist to suppress reflex activity in advance of stimulation so that hiccup is prevented. A deeper level of anaesthesia than that previously maintained, or the addition of a further dose of relaxant just before a procedure which is known to be particularly stimulating, are often successful. Such preventive measures may be necessary even when the surgical conditions, in terms of relaxation, are satisfactory. Hiccup is often associated with the slow return of diaphragmatic activity as the degree of relaxation wears off, when it is no more than attempted forceful respiratory movement and should be treated as such. It also often occurs "out of the blue" in the presence of very adequate relaxation of the abdominal muscles.

Total paralysis will always prevent or stop hiccup, but the very large dose of muscle relaxant that this may entail in some patients is not always advisable, and may complicate the situation at the end of the operation. Vagal block, either by infiltration in the neck, or beneath the diaphragm by the surgeon after the peritoneum has been opened, has been recommended as a preventive measure, but the results are not impressive.

A large number of individual drugs, ranging from the administration of amyl nitrite to the addition of a sudden blast of ether vapour to the anaesthetic mixture, have been tried at one time or another. Salem *et al.* (1967) found that stimulation of the mid-pharynx behind the uvula, and opposite the second cervical vertebra, by gentle movement with the end of a catheter inserted through the nose stopped hiccups in 84 out of 85 patients. Such methods presumably act by reflex inhibition, and even though many of them stop the disturbance, they are usually only temporarily effective.

The best and most rational treatment for hiccup during anaesthesia is to block the reflex pathways concerned by a deeper level of anaesthesia than can be produced with nitrous oxide alone (supplementation with analgesic, hypnotic or more potent inhalational anaesthetic) or by incremental doses of a muscle relaxant.

In the post-operative period a cause for hiccup must be sought before special treatment is advised. Uraemia, subphrenic abscess and grossly distended bowels are some of the conditions which must be excluded, but in many patients no specific factor can be incriminated. Then, adequate sedation together with large doses of chlorpromazine and similar phenothiazine compounds should be tried. A method of treatment which often proves successful is initiation of the swallowing reflex with both ears blocked. The patient drinks repeatedly from a glass of water while his external auditory meatae are obstructed. The success of this manoeuvre presumably depends on the afferent stimulus in the middle ear from fluctuating pressure waves being stronger than that which initiates the hiccup.

An oesophageal tube and suction are helpful to relieve distension. Carbon dioxide inhalation occasionally inhibits an attack. For prolonged and severe cases, after screening the patient to decide which side is affected, infiltration with local analgesic of a phrenic nerve in the neck should be considered.

The Work of Breathing

As the term suggests, the work of breathing comprises all the energy required to ventilate the lungs. Unfortunately the task of the respiratory muscles is not simply the inflation of a passive balloon (the lungs). Certain forces which tend to prevent the lungs being inflated must be overcome. There are three essential components in this opposition: (*a*) the force needed to overcome the elastic resistance of the lung; (*b*) the force to move non-elastic tissues (structural resistance); and finally (*c*), the force to overcome resistance to the flow of air through the tracheo-bronchial tree.

The **elastic resistance** of the lung is defined as the force tending to return the lung to its original size after stretching. It should not be thought of as the force required to expand the lung, as this is also a measure of the rigidity of the lung which varies with pulmonary congestion. The *compliance of the lung* is a measure of its change in volume per unit of pressure change. In cardiac and pulmonary disease the congestion and fibrosis which are frequently present lead to a fall in the "compliance" of the lung.

The **structural resistance** is composed of the thoracic wall, the diaphragm and the abdominal contents. It is related to the speed of the flow of air so that when this is maximal so is the structural resistance.

The **air resistance** is important because it is dependent on the length and size of the lumen of the bronchial tree. The anaesthetist adds an extra air resistance when he inserts an endotracheal tube. This matter is of particular importance in the intubation of a young child for whom too small an endotracheal tube may increase the air resistance enormously.

The flow of air through the bronchial tree may be laminar (streamlined) or turbulent. In this latter condition the air pursues an erratic course with the creation of many eddy-currents. The air resistance in laminar flow can be lowered by reducing the *viscosity*, whereas in turbulent flow it is the *density* that must be lowered. Anaesthetists sometimes use a mixture of helium and oxygen (79 per cent: 21 per cent) in certain cases of upper respiratory obstruction with the object of improving the patient's oxygenation. As the viscosity of this mixture is slightly *greater* than air, the resistance to laminar flow will be increased. On the other hand, its density is less than that of air, so the resistance to turbulent flow is decreased. As partial upper respiratory obstruction sets up turbulent flows the rationale of this therapy appears to be soundly based.

Compliance

The lungs and thoracic wall function as a single unit. and provided the tidal volume is in the normal range there is a linear relationship between the volume change and the pressure that produces it. If it is measured when the flow of air has ceased, as during breath holding or during apnoea in anaesthesia, it is known as *static compliance.*

$$\text{Static compliance} = \frac{\text{Volume change in litres}}{\text{Pressure change in cm. of } H_2O}$$

The compliance of the lungs and of the thoracic wall in a normal person are approximately the same, namely 0·2 litres/cm. H_2O. Thus a volume change of 0·2 litres in the thorax is obtained by a pressure of 1 cm. of H_2O exerted against the lungs in conjunction with a pressure of 1 cm. of H_2O against the thoracic wall, giving a total thoracic compliance of 0·1 litre/cm. H_2O (Comroe *et al.*, 1962).

When the volume change of the thorax in relation to pressure changes is measured during respiration it is known as *dynamic compliance.*

Measurement of total thoracic compliance.—The pressure gradient to be measured is that between the airway and the atmosphere, but it is difficult to obtain a reliable result unless the patient is able to relax completely. Thus the measurement of total thoracic compliance is best made in a patient who is relaxed and ventilated, either with the aid of a tank ventilator (conscious patient) or an endotracheal tube (unconscious patient).

(a) *Tank ventilator.*—The conscious patient is placed in the ventilator so that the transthoracic pressure can be measured. The volume of air inspired at each level of subatmospheric pressure within the tank reveals the data for a pressure-volume curve.

(b) *Endotracheal method.*—In the anaesthetised patient an endotracheal tube is inserted. This tube is then occluded and the pressure within the system during a period of apnoea is measured. After this the tube is unclamped and the volume of air or gas expired is collected in a spirometer. Again, a pressure-volume curve is plotted.

Measurement of lung compliance.—The pressure gradient to be measured is that between the airway and the pleural space. Direct measurements by placing the tip of a sampling needle (connected to a manometer) within the pleural space are dangerous. This disadvantage has been overcome by the method of Dornhorst and Leathart (1952) who have shown that the intrapleural pressure is transmitted directly through the thin-walled oesophagus to its lumen. Thus changes in oesophageal pressure represent alterations in intrapleural pressure. Since this measurement is a static one, it is made with the patient holding his breath after having inspired a known volume of air from a spirometer. The procedure is then repeated many times with different volumes so that a pressure-volume curve can be constructed. This is usually linear provided large volumes are not used, and will give an average value for lung compliance.

Measurement of thoracic wall compliance.—This is obtained by subtraction of lung compliance from total thoracic compliance.

Measurement of dynamic compliance.—This requires a very sensitive technique for the measurement of the pressure, volume and air flow.

Discussion

Values for compliance should always be related to the predicted normal value for a person of the same sex, age, height, weight and lung volume, and are preferably related to the functional residual capacity (FRC). For example, a simple change in posture can alter the FRC and thus produce a change in compliance.

One of the principal factors causing the elastic recoil of the lungs is the presence of elastic fibres within the pulmonary tissue. The important role of the surface tension of the fluid lining the alveolar walls has also been emphasised (see p. 28). This tends to draw the opposing walls closer together and so collapse the alveoli. If this fluid were pure water it would exert the very considerable pull of about 70 dynes/cm., but fortunately it contains a "detergent-like" agent (surfactant) which reduces the surface tension to as little as 2–8 dynes/cm.

Von Neergaard (1929) was the first to observe this effect. He demonstrated that much less pressure was required to inflate lungs filled with saline than those filled with air, the difference being due to abolition of the elastic pull of the surface tension exerted by the alveolar lining membrane. The detergent-like agent is believed to be absent in hyaline membrane disease of the newborn, and therefore to account for the very high inflationary pressures that are needed to expand the lungs in this condition.

Pulmonary oedema (altered surface tension with fluid in the alveoli), emphysema (destruction of elastic fibres) and mitral stenosis (increased pulmonary vascular congestion) are but some of the conditions that decrease the compliance of the lungs.

Under the conditions of anaesthesia so many factors are operating at the same time, and the situation changes so often, that it is frequently impossible to relate any change in compliance to a single agent or procedure. For example, a drug may affect the muscles of the thorax, the secretions in the respiratory tract, alter the cardiac output, constrict the bronchioles or dilate the pulmonary vessels.

However, very many investigations have been carried out and nearly all agree with Mead and Collier (1959) that there is a progressive fall in compliance during anaesthesia. This is almost entirely accounted for by changes in lung compliance, which decreases with time and with any action which tends to deflate the lungs. This has been accounted for by the absence of the periodic deep sighs that a conscious person takes unknowingly. Thus Gliedman *et al.* (1958) found that lung compliance fell more during ventilation with an automatic ventilator, which provides regular, even tidal volumes, than in those ventilated by hand. Particularly with a pressure preset ventilator, a reduction in compliance will lead to a reduction in tidal volume which will tend to cause a further reduction in compliance.

Egbert and his colleagues (1963) showed that occasional deep breaths during anaesthesia with intermittent positive pressure ventilation will prevent or lessen the occurrence of falls in compliance, and Sykes *et al.* (1965) have produced similar results by the use of large tidal volumes. Norlander *et al.* (1968), however, using the Engstrom ventilator at normal tidal volumes throughout, found no decrease in compliance and they believe this is due to the special flow-pressure pattern of that ventilator which—with an accelerating gas flow and a variable end-inspiratory pressure plateau—offers breath-to-breath mini-sighs.

Breathing and Oxygen-Consumption

In a normal resting subject the work of breathing uses up approximately 0·5 ml. oxygen for every litre of ventilation. Thus at average minute volume of 8 litres about 4 ml. of oxygen are required, or about 1·5 per cent of the total oxygen consumption each minute. Increasing respiratory activity leads to a disproportionately high rate of oxygen consumption.

Respiratory Work and Disease

Just as in health, so it has been found in *heart disease* (e.g. mitral stenosis) that the metabolic needs of the body are met with the minimal amount of respiratory work (Marshall *et al.*, 1954). In patients with mitral stenosis the severity of the dyspnoea is directly proportional to the degree of pulmonary rigidity, which presumably is due to vascular congestion. Thus more work is required to inflate the lungs. It is this increase in respiratory work that makes the patient short of breath. When the respiratory work rises from a normal value of about 0·3 kg.m./minute to as high as 2–3 kg.m./minute, then dyspnoea is usually present. The exact increase necessary to make the patient actually conscious of the respiratory effort varies from individual to individual.

Anaesthetists who commonly come in contact with cases of heart disease have often commented on the general improvement in the circulatory condition that frequently follows the induction of anaesthesia. This is particularly true when assisted or controlled respiration is used. The explanation may lie in the removal of this extra respiratory work by the mode of anaesthesia and the improved ventilation of the lungs.

In chest diseases, especially chronic ones, there is always an upset in respiratory mechanics with an increased work load. In pulmonary fibrosis the lung compliance is decreased, but to a small extent this is offset by a reduction in airway resistance which may occur because the traction exerted by the parenchymal tissue on the lung airways is increased. In diseases affecting the thoracic cage, such as ankylosing spondylitis or kyphoscoliosis, the chest wall compliance may be much reduced.

In obstructive lung conditions, such as severe asthma, chronic bronchitis, and emphysema there is an increased airway resistance and a reduced dynamic compliance. In emphysema marked changes take place in the structure of the lungs, associated with an increase in tissue rigidity leading to a complete loss of elasticity. This lack of elasticity markedly reduces the radial support of the peripheral airways and, combined with a possible intrinsic narrowing as well, means that during expiration the small bronchioles collapse before the alveoli distal to them have emptied completely, and air-trapping ensues. The lung-volume is increased, the intrathoracic pressure becomes less negative, and there is no lung-recoil when a pneumothorax is induced. The chest wall gradually becomes fixed in a position of inspiration.

All these changes make the emphysematous patient work harder to ventilate his lungs, and, owing to the fixed chest wall, put the respiratory muscles at a mechanical disadvantage. This increase in respiratory work leads to the onset of dyspnoea and the limitation of the maximal breathing capacity (McIlroy and Christie, 1954).

In the conscious state, the emphysematous patient can partially compensate for the loss of elastic tissue in the lung by actively contracting the abdominal muscles on expiration. It has already been pointed out that these muscles are the principal muscles of expiration. Anaesthesia, however, is frequently designed to relax them, so that while providing the surgeon with ideal conditions to explore the abdomen it deprives the emphysematous patient of his principal means for emptying the alveoli. In such circumstances, if spontaneous respiration is allowed, the level of carbon dioxide in the blood must necessarily rise. Therefore, on both theoretical and practical grounds, when marked abdominal relaxation is produced during general anaesthesia for an emphysematous patient, respiration should be controlled or assisted. Although intermittent positive-pressure respiration permits the anaesthetist to allow an adequate time for expiration to take place in these patients, it does not otherwise help to empty the alveoli, and, whenever possible, should be combined with a negative pressure suction phase during expiration. (See also Chapter 15, p. 488). A mechanical ventilator is necessary for this purpose. In crush injuries of the chest the use of intermittent positive pressure ventilation ensures that both or all segments of the thoracic cage move uniformly without the varying pull of the external muscles. This eliminates the work of breathing and the possibility of paradoxical respiration, corrects the pathological changes consequent on the abnormal mechanics of breathing, and is the most efficient way of obtaining a normal gas exchange. It also reduces pain, and by splinting the damaged chest wall permits speedier healing of the fractures.

The Pleural Cavity

Each lung is invested with a thin serous covering on its outer surface (visceral pleura) and this is reflected on to the inner aspect of the chest wall and the upper surface of the diaphragm (parietal pleura). The potential space between these two layers is the pleural cavity and under normal conditions the two surfaces are in apposition save for a small quantity of lymph which acts as a lubricant. In disease, adhesions form between the two surfaces, but if the underlying lung is not involved there is no appreciable change in respiratory function.

At the apex of the pleural cavity the outer surface is surrounded by loose areolar tissue (extrapleural or Sibson's fascia) in which small fibrous bands can sometimes be demonstrated coursing over the dome of the lung (bands of Sebalot).

Intrapleural Pressure

Owing to the continual retractive force exerted by the elastic recoil of the lung, the intrapleural pressure under normal conditions is always negative. When the pleural cavity is opened the negative pressure returns to atmospheric, the lung collapses, and the mediastinum moves over towards the unaffected side.

The elastic recoil of the lung is made up of three factors:

1. The elastic tissue in the bronchial wall and also that coursing throughout the interstitial tissue of the lungs.
2. The arrangement of the muscle fibres of the bronchi and bronchioles in a "geodesic" network so that on contraction the bronchial tree not only becomes reduced in diameter but also shortened in length.
3. The surface tension of the fluid lining the alveolar walls (see p. 28).

In man the intrapleural pressure ranges from −5·6 mm. Hg on inspiration to −2·6 mm. Hg on expiration. It is less negative at the bottom than at the top of the lung. In normal circumstances the force required to separate the two pleural surfaces is prodigious unless air or fluid enters the pleural cavity. During a strong inspiratory effort with the glottis closed, pressures of −40 mm. Hg have been recorded, whereas forced expiration under similar conditions may lead to pressures as high as +50 mm. Hg. These variations in pressure have little bearing on the thoracic cage, but are reflected on the thin walled surrounding structures, namely the heart and great vessels. A rise of intrathoracic pressure impedes the venous return and expels blood from the large veins into the neck and abdomen.The intra-abdominal (intragastric) pressure rises and falls with respiration in the conscious subject. The pressure reaches its highest point at the end of inspiration and falls to a minimum at the end of expiration (Mills, 1951).

Intrapleural Pressure-changes in Pulmonary Collapse

With the pleura intact, collapse of lung can take place only if the surrounding soft tissue structures such as those at the apex of the lung, the diaphragm, and the mediastinum move inwards to fill the vacant space. In practice, as the lung collapses, so the negative pressure in the intrapleural space rises. This is then reflected on the entire thoracic cavity but only the soft tissues can yield. When they do so, the intrapleural pressure falls and the lung can then collapse a little further. This cycle is repeated over and over again. The diaphragm is the principal tissue to be affected and, in cases with a large area of pulmonary collapse, it will be found to be raised.

In cases of severe post-operative pulmonary collapse, negative intrapleural pressures four times greater than normal have been recorded (Habliston, 1928).

Pneumothorax

Air can enter the pleural cavity in a number of ways. If there is a free communication with the atmosphere, whether through a broncho-pleural fistula or a wound of the chest wall, the pneumothorax is described as *open*, whereas if there is no communication it is *closed.* A particularly dangerous type of pneumothorax is that in which air can enter but cannot escape (ball-valve), leading to a *tension* pneumothorax. Thus in an anaesthetised patient a pneumothorax may be found to be open, closed, or under tension.

It is important to remember in any discussion of the physiological changes occurring under these conditions that the pleural cavity in the experimental animal often differs profoundly from that in man. For example, the commonest animal to be used for such investigations is probably the dog, and in this animal the parietal and visceral pleura are of almost diaphanous texture, the mediastinum extremely mobile, and the two pleural cavities are often in direct communication. The extremely thin and lax pleural membranes permit pressure changes in one cavity to be rapidly transmitted to the other. In man, however, the pleural membrane is thicker and the mediastinum represents a fairly solid mass separating the two cavities, which have no communication. Thus a change of pressure in one cavity is only partially reflected in the other cavity.

Norris and his colleagues (1968) have shown a correlation between the extent of a pneumothorax as judged from a radiograph and the size of the anatomical shunt producing arterial oxygen desaturation. When the ratio of lung to intrapleural space is greater than 75 per cent the shunt does not exceed the normal value of 2 per cent of the cardiac output. Below 65 per cent the shunt increases as the size of the lung decreases. When the air is removed from the pleural space a delay of several hours occurs before the ventilation-perfusion upset in the lung improves, and this despite an early increase in the size of the lung. This delay is probably due to the relatively greater pressure required to open a ventilatory unit which is completely closed, than that needed for one that has remained at least partially open.

Open pneumothorax.—In the presence of a pneumothorax the size of the opening in relation to the diameter of the trachea will determine how much air enters the lungs. But patients breathing quietly under local analgesia can tolerate large openings in their chest wall although there is no negative intrapleural pressure and the lung is partially collapsed. The reason for this is that in the resting state only a small volume of air—the tidal air—is required, and this is a small fraction of the vital capacity. If, however, the patient becomes alarmed and attempts deep respirations, more air is sucked into the pleural space, the lung collapses further, and dyspnoea and cyanosis result. It must be clear, therefore, that those patients with a reduced vital capacity tolerate a pneumothorax badly. Under anaesthesia the detrimental effects of a pneumothorax are countered by intermittent positive-pressure respiration when the opening is between the pleura and the chest wall. If the opening is via a bronchopleural fistula this treatment may lead to a tension pneumothorax unless special precautions are taken (see Chapter 13, p. 429).

The degree of collapse of lung with the chest open and in the presence of a free airway depends on a number of factors which are altered in both health and disease:

1. Size of opening in the pleura.
2. The elastic recoil of the lung.
3. Bronchial calibre. A continuous bronchomotor tone is maintained in the bronchial tree during both phases of respiration, and bronchial calibre is altered by the action of certain drugs (see Chapter 1, p. 34 *et seq.*).
4. Pulmonary resistance. This is the force that air encounters on its passage through the bronchial tree to the alveoli.

Closed pneumothorax.—This may be accidentally acquired or result during the closure of a thoracotomy wound, or be induced for therapeutic reasons. An accidental pneumothorax may arise when an emphysematous bulla ruptures and partially fills the pleural space with air. As a thoracotomy wound is closed, a certain amount of air will remain entrapped in the pleural cavity. This volume can be considerably reduced if the anaesthetist ensures that the lung is fully distended just prior to complete closure of the wound. After such operations as lobectomy and pneumonectomy, a potential space is created which it is often impossible to fill with the surrounding soft tissues. In order to allow the remaining lung tissue to function adequately a negative intrapleural pressure must be re-established. Gases may be removed from this space in the following ways:

1. *Absorption.*—Any gas—including air—when introduced into the pleural cavity, is absorbed by the blood stream, because the visceral pleura is permeable to these gases. The rate of absorption of the contained gases depends largely on their respective partial pressures. Thus, air will be absorbed slowly, for the partial pressure of nitrogen is high in both the pleural space and the blood stream. Oxygen, however, is rapidly removed, and according to Dalton's Law this then raises the partial pressure of nitrogen so that it is now higher than that in the circulation; thus some nitrogen is absorbed. This process continues until all the air has been removed but, depending on the amount entrapped, may take up to three or four days to be completed.

2. *Aspiration.*—A pneumothorax apparatus may be used to take off small amounts of air in the operating theatre so that the patient returns to the ward with a normal negative intrapleural pressure.

3. *Water seal.*—This has two main functions—one to act as a drainage tube for any blood that may collect in the pleural cavity; the other to allow air to leave the cavity and to prevent its return. It is an efficient and simple type of unidirectional valve. A litre of sterile water is placed in a large glass bottle and the height of the water level is noted. A glass column starting just below the surface of the water is connected by a length of rubber tubing directly with the intrapleural space via a leakproof circuit. On inspiration water is sucked up the glass column and falls again on expiration. If the patient coughs, or the lung is distended on expiration by increasing the respiratory resistance, then air is driven out of the chest and bubbles out into the bottle, which is in direct communication with the atmosphere. Using this method, provided there are no leaks either from the lung surface or bronchus, it is possible to re-establish a negative intrapleural pressure almost immediately after closure of the thoracic wound.

4. *Suction through a water seal.*—In order to be certain that all the air is removed from the pleural space suction may be applied to the air in the glass bottle. This will be transmitted via the drainage tube to the pleural cavity and thus rapidly establish a negative intrapleural pressure. It is an extremely useful method of treatment after segmental resection of lung, particularly where the remaining portion of lung continues to leak air into the pleural space. It must be remembered, however, that the indiscriminate use of suction may continue to keep open channels which might otherwise seal off.

Artificial pneumothorax.—The introduction of air under sterile conditions into the pleural cavity has been widely used in cases of tuberculous lesions of the lung. The collapse may be directed towards resting the whole or only a lobe of the lung (termed selective collapse). This method of resting the lung requires frequent refills, often for a number of years, as the air is rapidly absorbed. Air may also be introduced into the peritoneal cavity to cause a pneumoperitoneum and, by raising the diaphragm, collapse part of the lung. The positive intra-abdominal pressure pushes the diaphragm upwards and reduces pulmonary expansion. This form of therapy is now rarely used.

The presence of large quantities of air in one of the body cavities, i.e. pleura or peritoneum, has a twofold importance in anaesthesia. First, the positive-pressure on the lung reduces the potential respiratory capacity of the patient so that the danger of anoxia is increased, and secondly, when volatile anaesthetic agents are used, equilibrium is gradually established between the concentration in the lungs, the blood stream, and the air in the body cavity. In these circumstances, the total pressure of the gases in the pneumothorax cavity may rise to a level that will compress the normal lung tissue and great veins (Hunter, 1955). Eger and Saidman (1965) have shown that nitrous oxide-oxygen causes a fairly rapid increase in intrapleural pressure, but that halothane-oxygen is relatively safe. Also when the anaesthetic gases are withdrawn at the close of the operation, the concentration of vapour in the enclosed space may be responsible for prolonging the duration of unconsciousness.

When air enters the intrapleural space but cannot leave it, a tension pneumothorax results. It may arise spontaneously or during anaesthesia, especially when intermittent positive pressure ventilation is used. In the earlier instance a bulla may rupture or a broncho-pleural fistula may be present. A quite normal lung may rupture if unduly high inflation pressures are allowed during anaesthesia.

A simple valve-system usually causes the pressure in the enclosed space to rise sometimes as high as +20 mm. Hg—thus displacing the mediastinum and compressing the great veins and auricles.

Tension pneumothorax should be suspected during anaesthesia if inflation becomes increasingly difficult and the patient's condition steadily deteriorates. An unanaesthetised patient presents with cyanosis, hypotension and dyspnoea. Whether anaesthetised or not, tachycardia or bradycardia, depending on how far the condition has progressed, may be present. Pneumomediastinum and subcutaneous emphysema may or may not be present. In two recorded cases (Vance, 1968; Rastogi and Wright, 1969) the onset of marked respiratory wheezing led to the mistaken diagnosis of severe bronchospasm, and consequent ineffective treatment with bronchodilator drugs. Bronchospasm may be reflexly produced through the pulmonary plexuses and initiated by the mediastinal shift produced by the pneumothorax, or it may be directly caused by bronchiolar compression (Martin and Patrick, 1960). Rarely a tension pneumothorax may occur due to the rupture of a bulla during an asthmatic attack when bronchospasm will also be present. Once a tension pneumothorax is suspected percussion of the chest wall will usually reveal the side which is affected. A wide-bore needle should be passed into the pleural space on that side and this should be connected to an underwater seal. A tension pneumothorax may occasionally be bilateral (Golding *et al.*, 1966; Rastogi and Wright, 1969). In case of doubt a chest X-ray should be taken at once, or bilateral pleural drainage instituted.

Pleural Shock

This rare condition has been reported following aspiration of the pleural cavity. On insertion of the needle through the parietal pleura the patient suddenly collapses. The blood pressure falls, the heart rate slows and the skin becomes cold and pale. The whole picture strongly resembles a vasovagal attack. Death may result. There are two principal suggestions as to the cause of this condition. First, that stimulation of the visceral pleura or underlying lung sets up afferent impulses which pass to the brain and then down the vagus to result in inhibition of the heart. A more popular theory is that the injection leads to the introduction of air into a small vein, and this air embolus then tracks along an intercostal vein, up the vertebral vein and so reaches the cerebral circulation. Neither of these two theories takes into account a toxic reaction to any local analgesic solution that may have been used.

REFERENCES

CAMPBELL, E. J. M. (1954). The muscular control of breathing in man. (Ph.D. Thesis), Univ. London.

CAMPBELL, E. J. M. (1955). An electromyographic examination of the role of the intercostal muscles in breathing in man. *J. Physiol.* (*Lond.*), **129,** 12.

CAMPBELL, E. J. M. (1958). *The Respiratory Muscles and the Mechanics of Breathing.* London: Lloyd-Luke (Medical Books).

CAMPBELL, E. J. M., and GREEN, J. H. (1953). The variations in intra-abdominal pressure and the activity of the abdominal muscles during breathing: a study in man. *J. Physiol.* (*Lond.*), **122,** 282.

COMROE, J. H., FORSTER, R. E., DUBOIS, A. B., BRISCOE, W. A., and CARLSEN, E. (1962). *The Lung: Clinical Physiology and Pulmonary Function Tests*, p. 172, 2nd edit. Chicago: Year Book Medical Publishers, Inc.

DORNHORST, A. C., and LEATHART, G. L. (1952). A method of assessing the mechanical properties of lungs and air passages. *Lancet*, **2,** 109.

EGBERT, L. D., LAVER, M. B., and BENDIXEN, H. H. (1963). Intermittant deep breaths and compliance during anaesthesia in man. *Anesthesiology*, **24,** 57.

EGER, E. I., II, and SAIDMAN, L. J. (1965). Hazards of nitrous oxide anaesthesia in bowel obstruction and pneumothorax. *Anesthesiology*, **26,** 61.

FINK, B. R. (1961). Electromyography in general anaesthesia. *Brit. J. Anaesth.*, **33,** 555.

FITZGERALD, P. (1967). The anatomy of hiccough. *Irish J. med. Sci.*, **6,** 529.

FLETCHER, G., and BARBER, J. L. (1966). Lung mechanics and physiologic shunt during spontaneous breathing in normal subjects. *Anesthesiology*, **27,** 638.

GLIEDMAN, M. L., SIEBENS, A. A., VESTAL, B. L., TIMMES, J. J., GRANT, R. N., MURPHY, J. L., and KARLSON, K. E. (1958). Effect of manual versus automatic ventilation on the elastic recoil of the lung. *Ann. Surg.*, **148·,** 899.

GOLDING, M. R., URBAN, B. J., and STEEN, S. N. (1966). Sub-cutaneous emphysema pneumomediastinum and pneumothorax. *Brit. J. Anaesth.*, **38,** 482.

GORDH, T., and SILFERKIOLD, B. P. (1943). Body plethysmograph in infants. *Acta med. scand.*, **113,** 183.

GREEN, J. H., and HOWELL, J. B. C. (1955). Correlation of respiratory airflow with intercostal muscle activity. *J. Physiol.* (*Lond.*), **130,** 33P.

GUEDEL, A. E. (1951). *Inhalation Anesthesia*, 2nd edit. New York: The Macmillan Co.

HABLISTON, C. C. (1928). Intrapleural pressures in massive collapse of the lung, with report of cases. *Amer. J. med. Sci.*, **176,** 830.

HARRIS, T. A. B. (1951). *The Mode of Action of Anaesthetics.* Edinburgh: E. & S. Livingstone.

HUNTER, A. R. (1955). Problems of anaesthesia in artificial pneumothorax. *Proc. roy Soc. Med.*, **48,** 765.

LITTLE, D. M. (1956). *Controlled Hypotension in Anesthesia and Surgery*. Springfield, Ill.: Charles C. Thomas.

MCILROY, M. B., and CHRISTIE, R. V. (1954). The work of breathing in emphysema. *Clin. Sci.*, **13,** 147.

MALONEY, J. V., Jr., SCHMUTZER, K. J., and RASCHKE, E. (1961). Paradoxical respiration and "pendelluft". *J. thorac. cardiovasc. Surg.*, **41,** 291.

MARSHALL, R., MCILROY, M. B., and CHRISTIE, R. V. (1954). The work of breathing in mitral stenosis. *Clin. Sci.*, **13,** 137.

MARTIN, J. R., and PATRICK, R. T. (1960). Pneumothorax, its significance to the anesthesiologist. *Curr. Res. Anesth.*, **39,** 420.

MEAD, J., and COLLIER, C. (1959). Relation of volume history of lungs to respiratory mechanics in anaesthetized dogs. *J. appl. Physiol.*, **14,** 669.

MILLS, J. N. (1951). Intra-abdominal pressures during quiet breathing. *J. Physiol.* (*Lond.*), **112,** 201.

MORTON, H. J. V. (1950). Respiratory patterns during surgical anaesthesia. *Anaesthesia*, **5,** 112.

NORLANDER, O., HERZOG, P., NORDEN, I., HOSSLI, G., SCHAER, H., and GATTIKER, R. (1968). Compliance and airway resistance during anaesthesia with controlled ventilation. *Acta anaesth. scand.*, **12,** 135.

NORRIS, R. M., JONES, J. G., and BISHOP, J. M. (1968). Respiratory gas exchange in patients with spontaneous pneumothorax. *Thorax*, **23,** 427.

PRIMROSE, W. B. (1952). Chest movements and the intercostal muscles. *Brit. J. Anaesth.*, **24,** 3.

RASTOGI, P. N., and WRIGHT, J. E. (1969). Bilateral tension pneumothorax under anaesthesia. *Anaesthesia*, **24,** 249.

SALEM, M. R. (1967). An effective method for the treatment of hiccups during anesthesia. *Anesthesiology*, **28,** 463.

SAMUELS, L. (1952). Hiccup. A ten year review of anatomy, etiology, and treatment. *Canad. med. Ass. J.*, **67,** 315.

SYKES, M. K., YOUNG, W. E., and ROBINSON, B. E. (1965). Oxygenation during anaesthesia with controlled ventilation. *Brit. J. Anaesth.*, **37,** 314.

VANCE, J. P. (1968). Tension pneumothorax in labour. *Anaesthesia*, **23,** 94.

VON NEERGAARD, K. (1929). Neue Auffassungen ueber einen Grundbegriff der Atemmechanik, abhaengig von der Oberglaechen Spannung in der Alveolen. *Z. ges. exp. Med.*, **66,** 373.

WADE, O. L. (1954). Movements of the thoracic cage and diaphragm in respiration. *J. Physiol.* (*Lond.*), **124,** 193.

Chapter 3

THE PHYSIOLOGY OF RESPIRATION

NERVOUS CONTROL OF BREATHING

The Respiratory Centres

Situated in the pons and medulla are nerve cells which are responsible for the automatic rhythm of breathing. These cells are arranged in functional groups called respiratory centres. The concept of a single respiratory centre is untenable because of the multiplicity of factors and parts of the brain which can influence respiratory activity.

The medullary centres. Section of the brain stem at the lower end of the pons (Fig. 1, Section 4) results in the complete cessation of respiration. A section across the junction between the pons and the medulla (Fig. 1, Section 3) does not abolish breathing but instead leads to a gasping type of respiration which is irregular both in depth and rhythm, and which is not influenced by vagal afferent impulses. Therefore, somewhere in the medulla there must be a group of neurones which is capable of maintaining a primitive type of respiratory rhythm. These cells are the medullary centre and have been localised to an area in the reticular formation beneath the caudal end of the floor of the IVth ventricle. The medullary centre has been divided into two different parts, the inspiratory and expiratory centres. The most important evidence for this is as follows:— (1) Records of neuronal activity in various parts of the medulla have

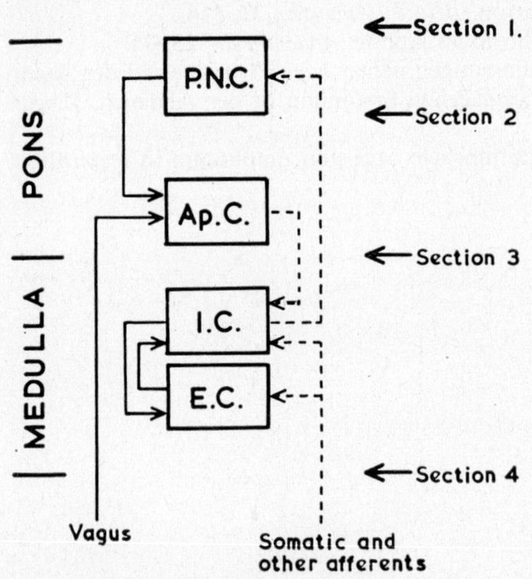

3/Fig. 1.—Schematic diagram of the possible organisation of the respiratory centres.

revealed electrical activity which coincides with either inspiration or with expiration. (2) Electrical stimulation of these two areas causes either inspiration or expiration, and indeed rhythmic respiration can be produced by stimulating them alternately. Anatomically the expiratory centre has been described as being situated in the reticular substance under the floor of the IVth ventricle, the inspiratory centre lying more caudal and deep to the expiratory centre (Fig. 3) (Pitts, 1946), although other workers have not been able to locate anatomically separate centres (Burns and Salmoiraghi, 1960). The medullary centres have connections with the higher respiratory centres, the reticular activating system and the hypothalamus.

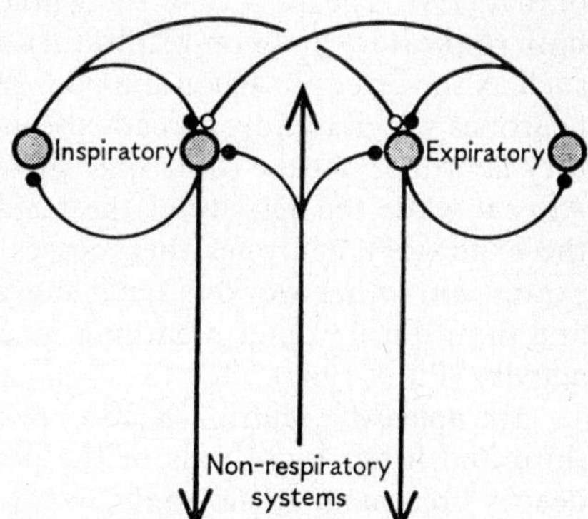

3/FIG. 2.—Brain stem respiratory system (see text).

Records of neuronal activity within the inspiratory or expiratory centres indicate that stimulation of one part of the centre results in a spread of activity throughout the whole group of cells, and that activity in one group causes reciprocal inhibition of the other. Alter-

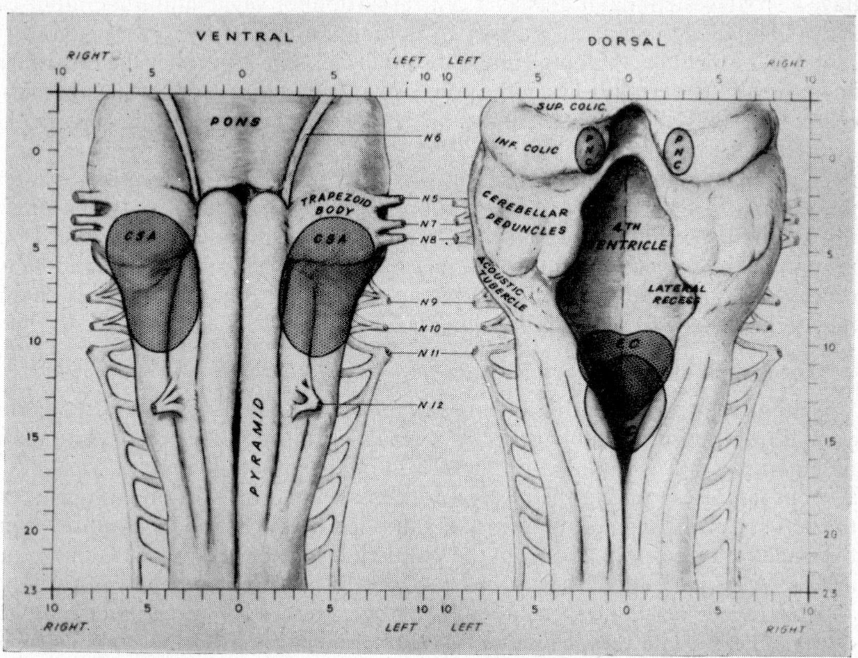

3/FIG. 3.—The ventral and dorsal surfaces of the brain in the region of 6th–12th cranial nerves. The central chemoreceptor (CSA) is seen lying superficially on the ventral surface. The respiratory centre (EC & IC) lies deep in the medulla oblongata in the floor of the 4th ventricle.

nating activity of the two centres can be explained by a system such as that shown in Fig. 2 (Burns, 1963). The respiratory neurones belong to one of two different classes concerned either with the act of inspiration or of expiration. They are so arranged that when excitation starts in one class it spreads to all members of that class. The activity of the whole system depends on initial excitation from both respiratory and non-respiratory sources, and possibly from chemical stimuli such as the arterial carbon dioxide. Inspiration begins with the activity of a few neurones which rapidly spreads through the network of interconnecting inspiratory neurones. At the same time there is inhibition of the expiratory neurones. After a while the activity of the inspiratory neurones wanes and inhibition of the expiratory neurones then ceases. The whole process is then repeated for expiration. Other workers have suggested that expiration is a passive process and that, during quiet breathing, occurs because of the absence of inspiratory activity (Pitts, 1946).

The apneustic centre.—Section of the brain stem at the junction of the upper third and lower two-thirds of the pons (Fig. 1, Section 2) leads to slower and deeper breathing. If the vagus nerves on both sides are also divided a state of inspiratory spasm appears (Apneusis), which is interrupted by expiratory gasps (Apneustic Breathing). The inference is that uninhibited action of the apneustic centre causes prolonged activation of the inspiratory centre in the medulla, but that its action can be interrupted by afferent vagal impulses, and to a lesser extent by the pneumotaxic centre (see below) (Wang *et al.*, 1957). These workers have also suggested that it acts as a central station for vagal inhibitory impulses. Pitts (1946) held that apneusis arises from uninhibited activity of the inspiratory centre in the medulla. Although afferent stimuli can influence apneustic breathing, its origin almost certainly lies in the pons. It has been suggested that the apneustic centre provides the initial stimulus which begins inspiratory activity in the medulla.

The pneumotaxic centre.—Section of the brain stem at the upper limit of the pons (Fig. 1, Section 1) has no effect on respiration, so that in the upper third of the pons must lie a further respiratory centre which is capable of inhibiting the apneustic centre. Stimulation of this centre – the pneumotaxic centre – results in tachypnoea. The pneumotaxic centre has no inherent rhythmicity, but seems to act by controlling the other centres.

The Origin of Respiratory Rhythm

Although a primitive rhythmicity lies in the medullary centres, in the intact animal respiration probably arises as a result of outside influences acting upon them. Inspiration is initiated by the action of the apneustic centre and somatic afferent impulses exciting the inspiratory centre. Once inspiration is in progress the activity of the inspiratory centre is inhibited by the action of impulses from the pneumotaxic centre and from the pulmonary stretch receptors via the vagus nerves. A series of feedback loops probably exist. For example, inspiratory activity causes nerve impulses to pass up the brain stem to the pneumotaxic centre. These excite the pneumotaxic centre which in turn causes inhibition of inspiration and allows expiration to take place. A similar negative feedback loop involving the vagus nerve also tends to terminate inspiration. The relative importance of the pneumotaxic centre and the vagus varies from species to species, and indirect evidence suggests that vagal inhibitory reflexes are of little importance in man.

The Stimulant Effect of Wakefulness on Respiration

Hyperventilation in the anaesthetised patient will lead to apnoea. This occurs at various levels of carbon dioxide tension in the blood and is partly dependent on the anaesthetic technique used. Thus with thiopentone and nitrous oxide a Pa_{CO_2} of approximately 38·5 mm. Hg may be obtained before apnoea occurs in contrast to33·0 to 37·0 mm. Hg with halothane (Fink *et al.*, 1960; Hanks *et al.*, 1961). Fink (1961), however, found that in *conscious* healthy volunteers the Pa_{CO_2} could be reduced to a mean of 22 mm. Hg $\pm$ 4 without apnoea developing at the end of the period of hyperventilation. On the contrary in the first minute of recovery, ventilation was usually greater than before the test. Subsequently the minute volume fell to about two-thirds of the control value. Thus wakeful subjects do not develop apnoea but continue to breathe rhythmically. It would appear from these observations that rhythmic respiration can be maintained by wakefulness in the presence of a reduced blood carbon dioxide, or by an increased carbon dioxide level in the blood in an anaesthetised patient, but not when both wakefulness and the carbon dioxide level of blood are abnormal.

The stimulant effect of wakefulness on respiration can be ascribed tentatively to the brain stem reticular system. The depression of respiration at the onset of natural sleep may be due to lack of wakefulness.

Other Centres Affecting the Respiratory Centre

Many of the higher centres exert some influence on respiration—for example, the acts of swallowing, speaking and coughing require a careful integration of the mechanical systems. These changes are due to impulses arising in the cerebral cortex. Similarly, impulses from the cortical and thalamic areas influence the respiratory pattern during crying and laughing. The temperature-regulating centre in the region of the hypothalamus can influence respiration, as is shown by the increased pulmonary ventilation during a pyrexia.

Effect of Anaesthetic Agents on the Respiratory Centres

Little is known of the effects which anaesthetic agents have on the respiratory centres, although it seems likely that their activity is depressed in common with other parts of the brain. Katz and Ngai (1962) observed in decerebrate cats that the inhalation of ether raised the electrical intensity required to produce inspiration on stimulation of the inspiratory centre, and that deepening the level of anaesthesia raised the threshold. This finding suggests that the medullary centres are depressed by ether. The possibility that trichloroethylene stimulates the pneumotaxic centre, thus producing tachypnoea, has also been suggested (Ngai *et al.*, 1963). Reports that other areas of the brain associated with respiration in animals are depressed during anaesthesia have also been published.

THE CHEMICAL CONTROL OF BREATHING

The Response to Carbon Dioxide

Since the primary function of the respiratory system is to maintain satisfactory partial pressures of O_2 and CO_2 in the arterial blood, it is not surprising to find that these pressures exert an influence on ventilation. The volume of ventilation is affected by both the arterial P_{O_2} and P_{CO_2}, and is especially responsive to changes in carbon dioxide. When a subject is presented with a step increase in inhaled CO_2 concentration, the arterial P_{CO_2} rises, but takes some minutes to reach a steady value. This is because the body can absorb large volumes of CO_2 and it therefore takes a little time for a new equilibrium to be reached. Both the rate and depth of ventilation increase steadily, and after about 10 to 20 minutes reach constant values. Similarly, after the withdrawal of inhaled CO_2 ventilation takes some minutes to return to control values. The test is performed by stressing the patient either with step increases in CO_2 in inhaled gas mixtures, and then measuring ventilation and arterial or alveolar P_{CO_2} at each step when a steady ventilatory state has been reached, or by allowing CO_2 to accumulate during rebreathing. The advantages of rebreathing are that it is rapid, less distressing to the subject, is easy to perform and can readily be repeated. Higher P_{CO_2} values can be obtained than with the steady state method, since patients will tolerate a very high P_{CO_2} for a short time. Disadvantages are that equilibrium is not attained, and there is no time for any appreciable change of C.S.F. P_{CO_2} to occur, so that the full ventilatory response at any given P_{CO_2} is not obtained. The main disadvantages of the steady state method are that it is more uncomfortable for the patient, especially at high P_{CO_2} values, and not so many points on the curve can be obtained. Even with this method the full ventilatory response is not always reached. Once the test is complete the minute or alveolar ventilation can be plotted against the corresponding arterial or alveolar (end-tidal) P_{CO_2}, and the *Carbon Dioxide Response Curve* obtained. The most accurate plot is that of alveolar ventilation against arterial P_{CO_2}. However, plots of total ventilation, which is simpler to measure than alveolar ventilation because dead-space changes need not be taken into account, against end-tidal CO_2 are often used, and give essentially the same results. Reduced accuracy of end-tidal CO_2 measurements at low tidal volumes is a possible source of error, and may in part account for alinearity of the plotted curve at its lower end. The results of such a test show that ventilation is exquisitely responsive to rises in P_{CO_2}. A rise in ventilation can be detected for an increase in arterial P_{CO_2} of as little as 1 to 2 mm. Hg, and it is approximately doubled for a rise of 5 mm. Hg. For moderate rises in P_{CO_2} the

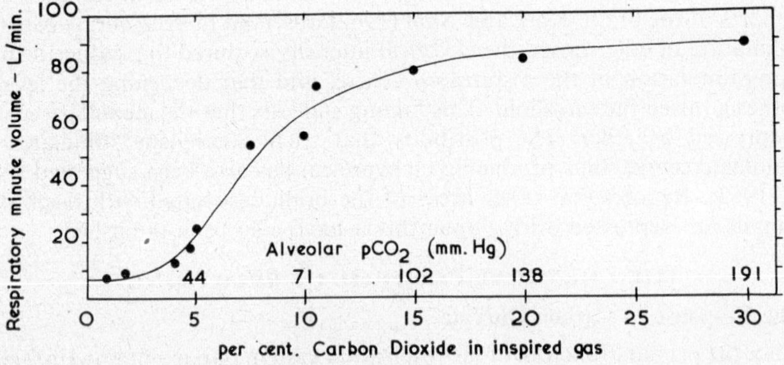

3/FIG. 4.—The carbon dioxide response curve.

ventilation increases in nearly a linear fashion, although the curve may be a little flatter at its lower end. Also, at very high P_{CO_2} values ventilation reaches a maximum, although the P_{CO_2} may continue to rise. There is, however, a very large variation in the response of different individuals to inhaled CO_2, and even in the same individual from time to time. The test must therefore be performed under carefully controlled conditions, as changes in the environment can alter the response to CO_2. Furthermore, it takes some 10 to 20 minutes for ventilation to reach a steady state after the introduction of a new inhaled CO_2 concentration, and errors can arise if enough time is not given for equilibration to be attained.

Since the CO_2 response curve is initially almost linear, it is possible to express the sensitivity of any individual to CO_2 in terms of the change in ventilation for each mm. Hg rise in P_{CO_2}. Bearing in mind that the individual variation is large, an average normal value of 2·5 l/min./mm. Hg rise in P_{CO_2} can be quoted using the steady state method.

The carbon dioxide response curve, properly performed, is a sensitive index of respiratory depression, and is regarded as more valuable than isolated measurements of arterial P_{CO_2}. It has been extensively used in the study of the respiratory effects of narcotic drugs (Bellville and Seed, 1960).

Factors Influencing the Carbon Dioxide Response Curve

Alterations in the CO_2 response curve may be of two types. (a) The *slope* may be increased or decreased, sometimes termed as an alteration in CO_2 sensitivity, or (b) the curves may be displaced either to the left or to the right. Both types may of course be seen together. Some of the factors which influence the CO_2 response are as follows:

(1) *Individual responses* vary widely from person to person, and in the same individual from time to time (*Environmental Factors*), as mentioned previously.

(2) *Hypoxia.* In the presence of hypoxia the CO_2 response curve becomes steeper. Hypoxia therefore reinforces the ventilatory response to CO_2 (Lloyd *et al.*, 1958).

(3) *Metabolic acidosis and alkalosis.* Metabolic acidosis shifts the curve to the left and alkalosis shifts it to the right, although the slopes remain unchanged. When the ventilation is plotted as a function of C.S.F. pH, however, no displacement occurs (Fencl *et al.*, 1969).

(4) *Chronic bronchitis.* In chronic bronchitis or other lung diseases causing chronic diffuse airway obstruction the slope of the curve is flattened, and is displaced to the right in the presence of CO_2 retention. If the increase in respiratory *work*, rather than the ventilation, is plotted against the P_{CO_2}, in some patients the increase in work when breathing CO_2 is close to normal, and in others it is reduced. It has been suggested that these different responses may characterise "blue bloaters" (reduced work response) and "pink puffers" (normal work response) (Lane, 1970).

(5) *Drugs.* Two methods have been used to assess the effect of drugs on respiration. One is to measure the arterial P_{CO_2} and/or the ventilation before and after the administration of the drug under study. A rise in P_{CO_2} or a fall in ventilation indicates that respiration has been depressed. Alternatively, a full CO_2 response curve can be performed. The latter is more sensitive than the former, and may show a depressed response to CO_2 inhalation in spite of there having

been no change in the resting arterial P_{CO_2}. Analgesic drugs depress the ventilatory response to CO_2. For example, morphine shifts the response curve to the right, but its slope is not usually affected (Fig. 5). Pethidine depresses the slope as well as moving it to the right, although the dose of the drug which has been

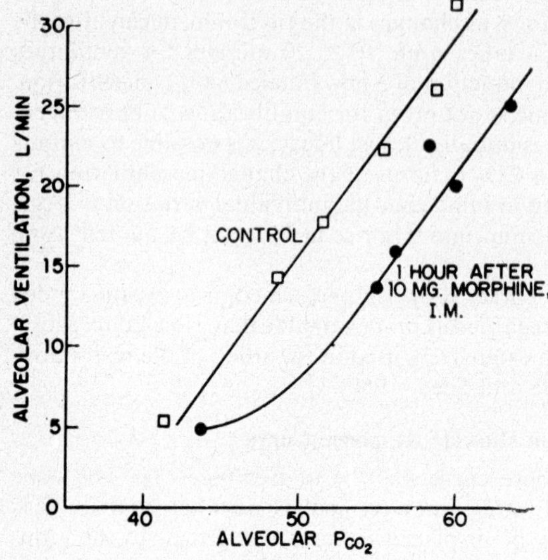

3/Fig. 5.—Carbon dioxide response curve after 10 mg. of morphine sulphate.

administered is probably important as regards its precise effect. In Table 1 are listed the doses of a number of analgesic drugs which depress the CO_2 response curve an equivalent amount to 10 mg. of morphine.

It is interesting to note that the administration of an analgesic + antagonist mixture causes the same amount of respiratory depression as does the analgesic when given alone, although the depressant effect, once developed, can readily be reversed by the subsequent administration of an antagonist.

3/Table 1

Doses of some Analgesic Drugs which have the same Respiratory Depressant Effect as Morphine 10 mg. (Compiled from Various Sources)

Pethidine	— 75 mg.
Dihydrocodeine	— 60 mg.
Codeine	— 100 to 120 mg.
Methadone	— 10 mg.
Oxymorphone	— 0·68 mg.
Phenazocine	— 1·5 mg.
Pentazocine	— 20 mg.
Phenoperidine	— 2 mg.

(6) *Inhalation Anaesthetics.* Recently a number of studies into the effects of anaesthetic agents on the ventilatory response to inhaled CO_2 have appeared in the literature (Munson *et al.*, 1966; Dunbar *et al.*, 1967; Larson *et al.*, 1969). The use of the Minimum Alveolar Anaesthetic Concentration (MAC) to describe the depth of anaesthesia has enabled several different agents to be compared. Cyclopropane, halothane, fluroxene and methoxyflurane all cause a fall in

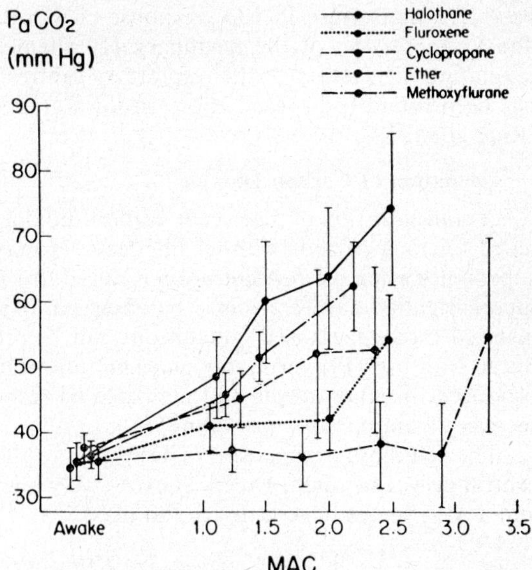

3/Fig. 6(*a*).—Alterations in P_{CO_2} with increasing depth of anaesthesia, the latter expressed as multiples of the Minimum Alveolar Anaesthetic Concentration (MAC). Note that with diethyl ether the P_{CO_2} remains around normal until deep levels of anaesthesia, and the wide variations in P_{CO_2} about the mean values. P_{CO_2} plotted as means $\pm$ one Standard Deviation. (Larson *et al.*, 1969).

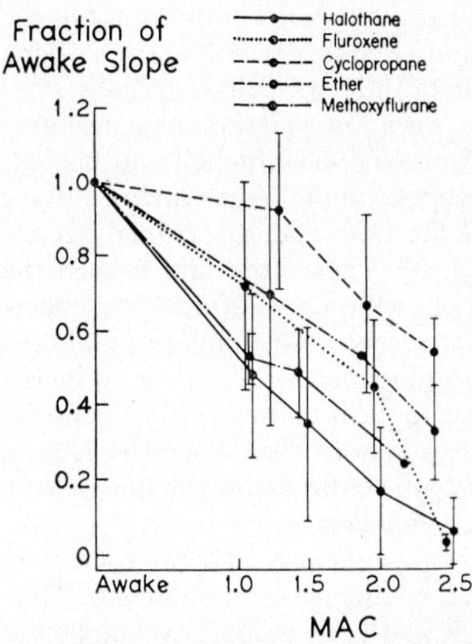

3/Fig. 6(*b*).—Alterations in the response to CO_2 inhalation with deepening anaesthesia. The slope of the ventilatory response to administering CO_2 in the inspired gases is plotted as a fraction of the slope obtained before the induction of anaesthesia. Note that as anaesthesia is deepened the response to CO_2 progressively falls and that, as in the conscious subject, there is a wide variation in the individual response. CO_2 response plotted as mean values $\pm$ one Standard Deviation. (Source: as for Fig. 6*a*)

ventilation and a rise in arterial P_{CO_2}, these changes increasing with the depth of anaesthesia (Fig. 6). The ventilatory response to inhaled CO_2 is also progressively reduced as anaesthesia becomes deeper with these agents, and eventually becomes almost flat. The effects of diethyl ether are slightly different to those described above. With this agent ventilation and arterial P_{CO_2} are maintained at or near normal levels until deeper levels of anaesthesia are obtained, although the response to inhaled CO_2 progressively diminishes as with the other anaesthetic agents, even at light levels of anaesthesia. In a study on dogs Muallem *et al.* (1969) concluded that this effect was due to a central effect of the drug rather than to its irritant effect on the lining of the respiratory tract, as has been suggested in the past. The alterations in CO_2 response curves during anaesthesia are probably due to depression of the medullary H^+ chemoreceptor, or of its influence in regulating the activity of the respiratory centres. *d*-Tubocurarine in small doses has been found to have no effect on the CO_2 response curve in conscious man (Rigg *et al.*, 1970).

Inhalation of Carbon Dioxide

A concentration of 5 per cent carbon dioxide, though unpleasant, can be inhaled for long periods without ill-effects. However, unconsciousness inevitably supervenes when the concentration is raised to 15 per cent or above. At this level, muscle rigidity and tremor may be observed. If 20–30 per cent carbon dioxide is inspired then generalised convulsions can be produced. Thus, the acidosis produced by a high P_{CO_2} probably plays an important part in deepening anaesthesia produced by other agents and may also be responsible for part of the delay in recovery from narcotic poisoning.

The ventilatory response to CO_2 is due to the stimulation of cells within the central nervous system. Except at excessively high arterial P_{CO_2} values the carotid and aortic bodies have little part to play.

The Central H^+ Chemoreceptor

The pioneer studies by Leusen first suggested the possible importance of the cerebrospinal fluid in the control of ventilation (Leusen, 1954 *a* and *b*). Using anaesthetised animals he showed that perfusion of the ventriculo-cisternal system with mock C.S.F. containing either a high P_{CO_2} or a low bicarbonate concentration (low pH) caused an increase in ventilation. In 1963 Mitchell and his colleagues located a bilateral superficial chemoreceptor on the ventro-lateral surface of the medulla in the region of the origins of the IXth and Xth cranial nerves, extending partially towards the mid-line (Fig. 3). These areas are termed the *Medullary H^+ Chemoreceptor*. The topical application to these sites of pledgets soaked in cerebrospinal fluid with a raised H^+ concentration leads to an almost immediate increase in ventilation which is proportional to the increase in H^+ concentration above normal. Furthermore, the application of a pledget containing a very low concentration of procaine causes apnoea even when the arterial P_{CO_2} is high. The area of the medullary respiratory centre below the floor of the IVth ventricle does not react to any of these manoevres.

In a series of most elegant experiments Pappenheimer and his colleagues (1965) examined the responses mediated by the medullary chemoreceptor. They used normal unanaesthetised goats into which had been chronically implanted nylon catheters leading to the lateral ventricles and the cisterna magna. The ventriculo-cisternal system could then be perfused with artificial C.S.F. of any desired composition. The goats were trained to tolerate masks for long periods, and samples of arterial blood could be withdrawn at will from carotid artery loops. The respiratory responses of the animals to various alterations in the H^+ concentration of both blood and C.S.F. could then be studied. The main conclusions they reported were: (1) The sensitivity of the chemoreceptor in normal animals to changes in C.S.F. pH was two to seven times that found when the animals were anaesthetised. (2) The P_{CO_2} in the outflow of C.S.F. was constantly about 10mm. Hg higher than that in the arterial blood, irrespective of the P_{CO_2}

in the infused artificial C.S.F. The P_{CO_2} of the C.S.F. is therefore controlled by the P_{CO_2} in the brain tissue adjacent to the walls of the ventricular cavities. (3) During the inhalation of CO_2 the difference between the P_{CO_2} in C.S.F. and arterial blood decreased, and this effect was thought to be secondary to an increase in cerebral blood flow at this time. (4) CO_2 response curves were slightly more linear when referred to C.S.F. P_{CO_2} than when referred to arterial blood P_{CO_2}. (5) Ventilation was increased when the C.S.F. H^+ concentration was raised by perfusing the cerebral ventricles with mock C.S.F. containing a low bicarbonate concentration. This response to a "metabolic acidosis" within the C.S.F. was much reduced if the increase in ventilation was allowed to cause a reduction in the P_{CO_2} of the C.S.F. outflow. (6) During CO_2 inhalation it was estimated that about 40 per cent of the ventilatory response was due to the alteration of the C.S.F. H^+ concentration, the remaining 60 per cent being the result of changes in P_{CO_2} or H^+ concentration elsewhere. Other estimates of the contribution of the medullary H^+ chemoreceptors to the response to the inhaled CO_2 vary from 30 per cent to over 80 per cent.

From these and other experiments there has emerged the concept of the medullary H^+ chemoreceptor and the factors which affect it. It is situated superficially near the surface of the medulla, and is sensitive to the H^+ concentration of the interstitial fluid bathing it. Because CO_2 combines with water to form H^+, it also reacts to changes in P_{CO_2} via this reaction. There is no convincing evidence that it is sensitive to changes in P_{CO_2} *per se*. The H^+ concentration of the all-important interstitial fluid is determined by its P_{CO_2} and bicarbonate concentration. These in turn are influenced by the P_{CO_2} of the C.S.F. and the cerebral capillary blood and by the bicarbonate concentration of the C.S.F. The bicarbonate concentration in the blood has no immediate effect on the medullary H^+ chemoreceptor due to the diffusion barrier for bicarbonate ions which exists between blood and C.S.F. and between blood and brain, although there appears to be free diffusion of bicarbonate between the C.S.F. and the interstitial fluid bathing the receptor. Carbon dioxide, being rapidly diffusible throughout blood, tissues and C.S.F., provides the means whereby rapid changes in the H^+ concentration of the C.S.F. and the fluid surrounding the receptor can be produced. Slower adjustments are mediated through alterations in the C.S.F. bicarbonate concentration and the processes involved are probably more than diffusion alone. The evidence suggests that there is an active transport mechanism between blood and C.S.F. which is capable of adjusting the C.S.F. pH, although whether this involves the transport of bicarbonate or hydrogen ions is not clear (Severinghaus *et al.*, 1963; Mitchell, 1968).

The normal values for the pH, P_{CO_2} and bicarbonate concentration in arterial plasma and cerebrospinal fluid in man are shown in Table 2 (Bradley and Semple, 1962). Because the bicarbonate system is the only buffer in the cerebrospinal fluid, its chemical buffering power is small, and for a given rise in P_{CO_2} the C.S.F. pH will, therefore, fall more than that of blood. Because of this the influence of the C.S.F. on the activity of the medullary H^+ chemoreceptors is increased in response to changes in CO_2 in the body. In spite of this poor buffering capacity the C.S.F. pH is kept remarkably constant in a wide variety of acid-base disturbances. Thus, it is normal or near normal in patients with chronic metabolic acidosis and alkalosis, moderate long-standing respiratory acidosis, and

3/TABLE 2
NORMAL VALUES FOR pH, P_{CO_2} AND $[HCO_3^-]$ IN ARTERIAL PLASMA AND C.S.F. IN MAN. MEANS AND STANDARD DEVIATIONS (IN BRACKETS).

	pH	P_{CO_2}	$[HCO_3^-]$
Arterial Plasma	7·397 (0·022)	41·1 (3·6)	25·3 (1·8)
C.S.F.	7·307 (0·027)	50·5 (4·9)	23·3 (1·4)

(Modified from Bradley and Semple, 1962)

following acclimatisation to high altitude (respiratory alkalosis). Only in severe chronic respiratory acidosis is the C.S.F. pH below normal, and also in acute respiratory changes before compensation has had time to occur.

FACTORS REGULATING C.S.F. pH

C.S.F. pH
- P_{CO_2}
  - Arterial P_{CO_2}
  - Cerebral blood flow
  - Tissue metabolism
- HCO_3
  - Bulk secretion of C.S.F.
  - Active transport mechanisms
  - Slow passive diffusion

As CO_2 is rapidly diffusible throughout the brain and C.S.F., and because the C.S.F. P_{CO_2} is controlled by the P_{CO_2} of adjacent brain tissue, changes in arterial P_{CO_2} are followed by only slightly less rapid changes in C.S.F. P_{CO_2}, and therefore in its pH. Bradley *et al.* (1965) have studied the changes in P_{CO_2} in blood and C.S.F. following the sudden administration of 5 per cent CO_2 to anaesthetised patients for a period of 20 minutes. The arterial P_{CO_2} rose rapidly over 4–6 minutes and then became stable. There was a delay of 2–3 minutes before the C.S.F. P_{CO_2} began to increase, and thereafter the rise was rather slower than that which occurred in the arterial blood so that after 20 minutes the C.S.F. P_{CO_2} and pH lagged behind those in arterial and jugular venous blood, the time difference being measured in minutes. During the time of these experiments the plasma and C.S.F. bicarbonate rose by the amount expected from the rise in P_{CO_2}. In conscious man Bradley *et al.* (1965) found that ventilatory changes lagged behind the rising P_{CO_2} in arterial and jugular venous blood, so that after 15 minutes ventilation was still increasing slowly, although both blood P_{CO_2} values were now constant. Opposite, but equally rapid changes in P_{CO_2} and pH occur in both blood and C.S.F. following the institution of hyperventilation. However, if alterations in P_{CO_2} in either direction are maintained beyond the acute stage, the C.S.F. bicarbonate slowly alters so that the changes in C.S.F. pH are minimised.

even though there is no further change in the blood bicarbonate. In contrast to the changes in P_{CO_2} this change in bicarbonate is slow, and its time course can be measured in hours. McDowall and Harper (1970) have reported on the changes occurring in the C.S.F. during hyperventilation to an arterial P_{CO_2} of 19–20 mm. Hg in baboons. They found that the C.S.F. pH rose rapidly from an average value of 7·32 to 7·49 following the institution of hypocapnia. Over the next 3 hours the C.S.F. pH fell slowly to an average value of 7·41, and during this time the C.S.F. bicarbonate concentration fell from 21·4 mEq./litre to 17·5 mEq./litre. The C.S.F. P_{CO_2} remained stable at 29 $\pm$ 2 mm. Hg during the whole period.

Practical Implications

When a patient inspires a high concentration of carbon dioxide, the raised P_{CO_2} of the blood reaching the brain causes an increased number of CO_2 molecules to diffuse into the extracellular fluid and stimulate respiration. If this inhalation continues for a time, the H^+ ion concentration of the cerebrospinal fluid is decreased by a compensatory rise of HCO_3^-. A sudden withdrawal of the inhaled CO_2 will be accompanied by a diminution of ventilation below normal because the stimulus of a high H^+ ion content is no longer present in the cerebrospinal fluid.

The practical significance of this mechanism can best be illustrated by taking a few hypothetical examples:

Normal patient breathing air:

BLOOD			C.S.F.		
P_{CO_2} (mm. Hg)	pH	Bicarb. mEq/l.	Bicarb. mEq/l.	pH	P_{CO_2}
40	7·4	25	23	7·32	48

N.B. Under resting conditions the P_{CO_2} of C.S.F. is about 8 mm. Hg higher than that found in blood.

Patient hyperventilated for 30 *minutes under anaesthesia:*

20	7·60	19·5	22	7·55	28

N.B. The time interval is too short for any significant change to have occurred in the bicarbonate level of the C.S.F.

After 6 *hours of hyperventilation:*

20	7·55	17·0	14	7·32	28

N.B. The pump mechanism is now in full force in an attempt to return the C.S.F. pH to normal.

Return to spontaneous respiration

23	7·51	18·0	14	7·28	31

N.B. At first the large amount of H^+ ions together with the low level of bicarbonate in the C.S.F. stimulates ventilation, but soon the bicarbonate level starts to creep up as the pump mechanism reduces the amount of H^+ ions in the C.S.F. There is less stimulus to breathe so the P_{CO_2} of the blood rises. This cycle of events repeats itself over and over again until normal values for both blood and C.S.F. have been reached. However, in the anaesthetised patient who has been on positive-pressure ventilation for, say, six hours, it may take at least that period of time again before the blood level of arterial P_{CO_2} has returned to the normal level of 40 mm. Hg.

The effect of this central chemoreceptor reflex is probably of even greater significance in the patient who is underventilating during anaesthesia for a long time. For example:

At start of anaesthesia:

BLOOD			C.S.F.		
P_{CO_2}	pH	Bicarb. mEq/l.	Bicarb. mEq/l.	pH	P_{CO_2}
40	7·4	25	23	7·32	48

After 30 *minutes of hypoventilation*

80	7·20	30	26	7·07	88

After 6 *hours of hypoventilation*

80	7·20	30	32	7·19	88

N.B. The pump mechanism now attempts to raise the bicarbonate level of the C.S.F. so that the pH may return to its normal level.

At the end of anaesthesia (patient breathing normally on room air)

BLOOD			C.S.F.		
P_{CO_2}	pH	Bicarb. mEq/l.	Bicarb. mEq/l.	pH	P_{CO_2}
52	7·33	26	32	7·35	60

N.B. At this time, although the P_{CO_2} of the blood is falling, the patient's central chemoreceptor mechanism has ceased to act due to the low level of H^+ or the high level of HCO_3^- ions in the C.S.F. In these circumstances, the patient will continue to underventilate despite the fact that the level of blood P_{CO_2} appears to be improving towards normal. The activity of the respiratory centre is influenced purely by hypoxic drive acting through the peripheral chemoreceptors. The sudden administration of oxygen may abolish this drive and lead to apnoea.

Such an example helps to emphasise the dangers of hypoventilation under anaesthesia, because the hypoxia may be avoided during the administration by increasing the inspired oxygen concentration, but when the reduced ventilation persists in the post-operative period with the patient breathing room air, then chronic hypoxia may supervene. In the presence of a surgical metabolic acidosis the patient may have a normal blood level of P_{CO_2} yet be underventilating. Though such a state of affairs must be highly unusual, it can only arise if the hypoventilation during anaesthesia has been very prolonged. The only satisfactory treatment is a period of normal ventilation on a mechanical ventilator to allow the homeostatic mechanisms to regain control.

The theory of the chemical control of respiration is shown diagrammatically in Fig. 7.

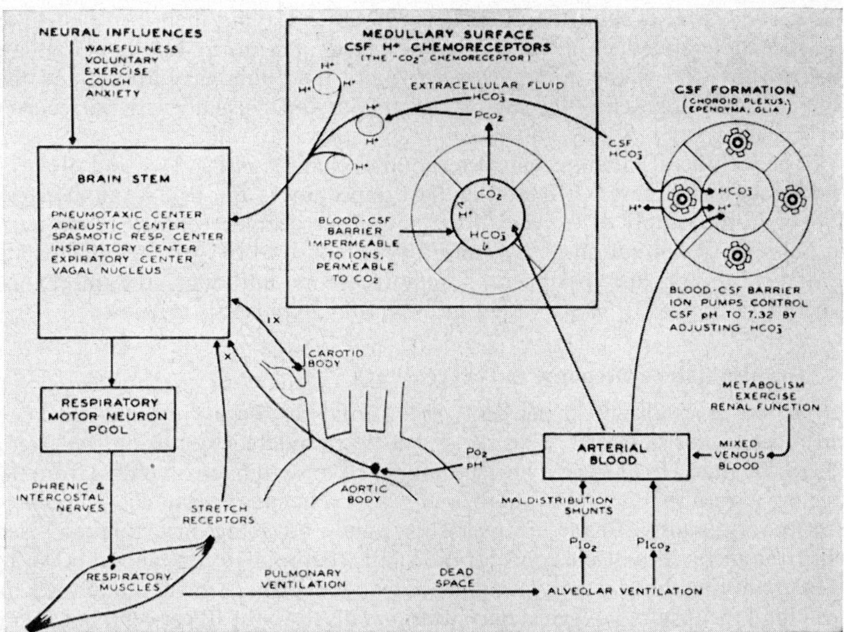

3/FIG. 7.—DIAGRAM OF THE THEORY OF THE CHEMICAL CONTROL OF RESPIRATION.

The medullary surface CO_2 chemoreceptor responds to the extracellular hydrogen ion concentration. The latter is controlled by (*a*) the local P_{CO_2}, which in turn, is determined by arterial P_{CO_2}, local blood flow and metabolism; and (*b*) by the bicarbonate ion concentration in the C.S.F. which is unaffected by sudden changes in the P_{CO_2} of arterial blood, but is determined by active transport in the formation of C.S.F. and is adjusted in an attempt to keep the pH of the C.S.F. constant (Severinghaus and Larson, 1965).

Effects of Anaesthetic Agents on the Medullary H^+ Chemoreceptor

Although the ventilatory response to inhaled CO_2 is depressed during general anaesthesia, the mechanism of this phenomenon is unknown. Experiments in which the central chemoreceptor have been stimulated by the application of pledgets to the medulla have shown that the ventilatory response to a given pH change is much less in anaesthetised animals than has been found in other experiments in conscious animals and man. This suggests that the chemoreceptor itself may be depressed by anaesthesia. The response of the central respiratory mechanisms to chemoreceptor activity may also be depressed. In total spinal analgesia the action of the local analgesic at this site may well explain the cessation of respiration which occurs. It has also been observed that the direct application of *d*-tubocurarine to this site stimulates respiration.

THE PERIPHERAL CHEMORECEPTORS

The peripheral chemoreceptors, the carotid and aortic bodies, consist of small masses of glandular-looking cells, richly supplied with blood vessels and nerves. The carotid bodies are located between the origins of the external and internal carotid arteries. They lie adjacent to the carotid sinus, but are completely different both in structure and function. They receive a lavish blood supply from the carotid arteries, and the afferent nerve fibres leaving them run first in the carotid nerve and then in the glossopharyngeal. The aortic bodies are situated next to the arch of the aorta, between it and the pulmonary artery, and their afferent nerve fibres enter the vago-sympathetic trunks, usually with the recurrent laryngeal nerves.

The peripheral chemoreceptors respond to changes in P_{O_2}, P_{CO_2} and pH of the blood supplying them. Of these the most important is the P_{O_2}. A fall in arterial P_{O_2}, or in the supply of oxygen to the peripheral chemoreceptors, causes a rise in pulmonary ventilation. The respiratory response to oxygen lack is mediated entirely through the peripheral chemoreceptors, although the mechanism whereby a fall in P_{O_2} is converted into nervous impulses is unknown.

The Ventilatory Response to Oxygen Lack

At sea level about 20 per cent of the total respiratory drive arises in the carotid and aortic bodies. This drive can be eliminated by raising the arterial P_{O_2} to 200 mm. Hg or over. The ventilatory response to hypoxia differs from that due to a rise in P_{CO_2} in a number of ways. The peripheral chemoreceptors are not very sensitive to a fall in arterial P_{O_2}. Thus, no change in ventilation is seen until the inspired oxygen concentration falls to about 16 per cent and then the increase in breathing is only marginal. Obvious increases in ventilation are not seen until the inspired oxygen concentration falls to about 10 per cent, but at concentrations below this, ventilation increases steeply as the oxygen concentration falls. At these low inspired oxygen percentages there is a marked individual variation in the response to hypoxia. If the arterial P_{CO_2} is kept constant while breathing low oxygen mixtures, ventilation is approximately doubled at an arterial P_{O_2} of 45 mm. Hg. However, if the arterial P_{CO_2} is allowed to fall naturally as a result of increasing ventilation, the full hypoxic response is masked by the change in P_{CO_2}, and at a P_{CO_2} of 45 mm. Hg only a 10 per cent increase in ventilation is seen. The response to hypoxia is more sensitive in the presence of acidaemia, hypotension or sympathetic activity. Ventilatory responses which arise in the peripheral chemoreceptors are rapid, the full response being seen almost from breath to breath. Also, unlike the respiratory response to a high P_{CO_2}, the response to hypoxia is relatively unaffected by narcotic drugs, barbiturates or by anaesthetic agents.

The Response of the Peripheral Chemoreceptors to Changes in Arterial P_{CO_2} and pH

The carotid and aortic bodies are not of great importance in the normal regulation of ventilation in response to changes in P_{CO_2}. No part of this response is mediated through them unless the arterial P_{CO_2} rises more than 10 mm. Hg, and even then the response is considerably less than in the whole animal.

The addition of acid to the blood causes an increase in pulmonary ventilation. So does the perfusion of the carotid bodies with blood containing a high hydrogen ion concentration, although hyperventilation still occurs in the whole animal following the addition of acid to the blood even after the carotid and aortic bodies have been completely denervated. It therefore appears that the peripheral chemoreceptors are responsible for some part of the ventilatory response to a metabolic acidosis, although this has been denied (Fencl *et al.*, 1969). However, in metabolic acidosis down to a pH of about 7·3 the hyperventilation is probably mediated through the peripheral chemoreceptors alone. At pH values below 7·3, hydrogen ions may leak into the C.S.F., thus stimulating the medullary H^+ chemoreceptor as well (Mitchell, 1965).

Reflex Control of Respiration

Pulmonary Reflexes

Although physiology has made great strides in the past few years, many of the present-day views on the nervous control of respiration are based on observations made many years ago in animals. Classical amongst these is the concept of the automatic control of the rhythm of respiration postulated by Hering and Breuer in 1868, who showed in cats that a sudden inflation immediately made the lungs come to rest in the position of expiration, while a sudden deflation led to a sharp inspiratory effort. From this they concluded that there are stretch receptors in the lung which signal the volume changes in the alveoli to the respiratory centre. Later in 1933, Adrian, also working with cats, demonstrated a stream of nerve impulses passing up the vagus nerve as the lungs increased in size. The number of these impulses passing at any one moment bore a direct relationship to the degree of distension of the lung. This evidence, while emphasising the importance of the inflation receptors, left deflation as a purely passive movement. Later writers drew attention to the role of deflation receptors. It was generally agreed that the vagus nerve played a vital part in the control of respiration, since section of it resulted in slow deep respiratory activity, whilst stimulation of the central end led to apnoea.

In man, despite the fact that numerous nerve filaments are known to exist in the lungs and can be traced right down to the bronchial tree to their final terminations, nerve fibres have never been successfully demonstrated in the alveolar walls. Widdicombe (1961) studied the inflation and deflation reflexes in a number of mammalian species, including conscious and anaesthetised man, and concluded that in man the reflexes were relatively weak when compared to the other species which he studied. In conscious man bilateral vagal blockade causes no change in the pattern of respiration, making man unique in this respect, but has been found to effect the sensation of breathlessness. In patients anaesthetised with nitrous oxide and halothane Guz *et al.* (1964) found that (i) Bilateral vagal blockade caused no alteration in the respiratory pattern, arterial P_{CO_2} heart rate or blood pressure. (ii) Sudden lung inflation only caused a period of apnoea when large volumes, 1 litre or more, were used. This effect was abolished by vagal block. (iii) Vagal stimulation, when intense, was capable of causing apnoea. They concluded that, although vagal afferent impulses were able to affect respiration in anaesthetised man, their influence was weak and probably of little physiological importance. In 1968 Paskin *et al.* attempted to excite the inflation reflex in humans during the administration of various anaesthetic agents—halothane, methoxyflurane, fluroxene and cyclopropane—but were unable to find any evidence that the reflex was active under these conditions. The action of diethyl ether on the respiration is also unaffected by vagal blockade in dogs, and Ngai *et al.* (1961) showed that the tachypnoea caused by trichloroethylene in decerebrate cats continued even after division of the vagi. It appears, therefore, that the suggestion made by Whitteridge and Bülbring (1944 and 1946) that anaesthetic agents lead to sensitisation of the inflation reflex cannot be applied to man.

The cause of the tachypnoea which is so often seen under anaesthesia remains undecided, although many suggestions have been put forward. These include sensitisation of the pulmonary stretch receptors, irritation of the respiratory tract, stimulation of extrapulmonary receptors, mobilisation of catecholamines and the development of acidosis in either blood or C.S.F. Studying the effects of diethyl ether on respiration in the dog Muallem *et al.* (1969) found no change in the pattern of breathing following vagal blockade, high spinal analgesia (up to cervical level), carotid body denervation or a combination of all three, and neither could they detect any difference in the acid base status of the C.S.F. between halothane and ether anaesthesia, although the respiratory effects of the two drugs were quite different. They concluded that ether asserts its characteristic action on breathing through a central action on respiratory control.

There are, however, instances during anaesthesia when the lung receptors may influence the character of the respiratory pattern: for example, if a patient's breathing is depressed by too much cyclopropane or pethidine, apnoea will follow. On manual compression of the breathing bag, as the lung starts to become inflated the patient may suddenly check the inspiration and then go on to make a full deep inspiratory movement of his own accord. The slightest increase in intratracheal pressure appears to trigger-off a complete inspiration, yet, without some manual assistance, the patient remains in apnoea for long periods. This type of respiration is often believed to be due to stimulation of the stretch receptors, but this seems an inadequate explanation. Stimulation would be expected to arrest rather than to complete respiration.

Another interesting inspiratory pattern is sometimes seen when controlled respiration has been used for a considerable time, and the carbon dioxide tension kept within normal limits. Although nearly awake and perhaps moving his arms and legs, the patient still does not breathe. He will, however, take a long deep inspiration when told to breathe—but only when asked. Such a patient has usually received relatively large doses of a general analgesic during the course of the anaesthetic. It is possible that in such a case the stretch receptors have been over-stimulated and are exhausted, but both these types of respiratory pattern are difficult to explain on the basis of the present conception of the lung receptors. It is also interesting to note that an increase in the carbon dioxide tension plays an important part in returning both these respiratory patterns to normal.

Another variation, which may well be concerned with the lung receptors, is sometimes seen in conscious patients placed in a tank ventilator. Despite a normal arterial oxygen saturation, a low carbon dioxide tension, and a raised pH, the patient may feel inadequately ventilated, frequently requesting greater ventilation—which only results in a further rise in the pH. Also, if respiration becomes severely depressed in the cat or dog under nembutal or chloroform anaesthesia, it is often possible to initiate a full deep inspiration by squeezing the

3/TABLE 4

GAS TENSIONS IN ALVEOLAR AIR AND BLOOD IN MM. HG

	Alveolar air	*Arterial blood*	*Venous blood*
Oxygen	103	100	40
Carbon dioxide ..	40	40	46
Water vapour ..	47	47	47
Nitrogen	570	573	573

Oxygen consumption.—In a conscious but premedicated adult a total of 200–225 ml. of oxygen are utilised per minute. During anaesthesia the oxygen consumption is about 85 per cent of that found in the awake "basal" subject.

Transport of carbon dioxide in the blood.—The tissues produce carbon dioxide and this is then given up to the blood circulating through the capillaries. It rapidly enters the plasma and then passes into the red cells. On reaching the pulmonary capillaries the tension of carbon dioxide (P_{CO_2}) in the venous blood is 46 mm. Hg; in the alveoli the tension is 40 mm. Hg. There is, therefore, a pressure gradient of 6 mm. Hg driving carbon dioxide across the alveolar membrane. In normal circumstances each 100 ml. of blood carries 3 ml. of carbon dioxide.

Carbon dioxide is distributed in the blood in the following manner:

(*a*) *In solution in the plasma.*—Only a small yet very important proportion of the total carbon dioxide (i.e. 6 per cent) is carried in this manner. As with oxygen, this quantity is responsible for determining the tension of the gas in blood and also acts as the intermediary between the air in the alveoli and the inside of the red cell. The majority of the carbon dioxide is present in physical solution in the plasma, but a small proportion is combined with water to form carbonic acid—H_2CO_3.

(*b*) *As bicarbonate* (70 per cent).—Except for the small proportion that is physically dissolved in the plasma, most of the carbon dioxide passes to the red cells where the enzyme *carbonic anhydrase* aids its rapid union with water to form carbonic acid (H_2CO_3) (Fig. 10). This enzyme is not found outside the red cell, and is destroyed both by heat and cyanide. Normally carbon dioxide combines with water very slowly, but in the presence of carbonic anhydrase the whole process is greatly speeded up. Similarly, this enzyme has the remarkable property of accelerating the same process in the reverse direction when the pulmonary capillaries are reached. Recent studies have revealed that premature babies, neonates and young infants have a very low level of carbonic anhydrase enzyme activity. They, therefore, are particularly dependent on adequate ventilation for the elimination of carbon dioxide (Boutros and Woodford, 1963).

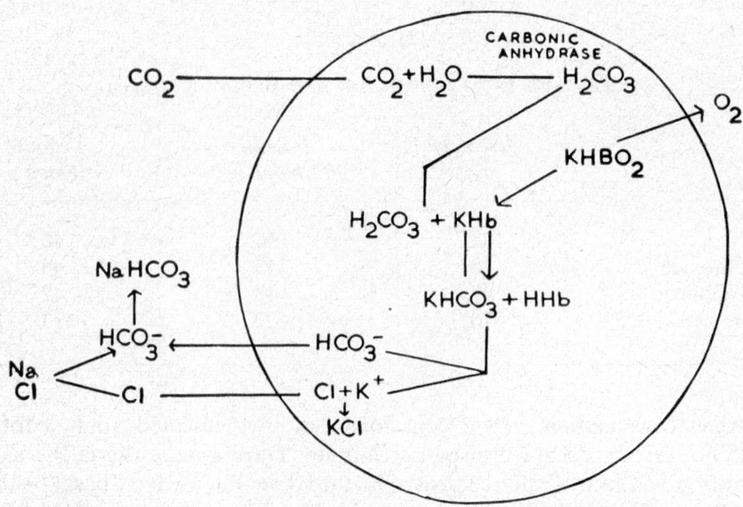

3/Fig. 10.—Chloride shift.

The role of carbonic anhydrase and haemoglobin is depicted in Fig. 10. The key to the whole process is the liberation of oxygen, thus:

$$K\,Hb\,O_2 \longrightarrow K\,Hb + O_2$$

As the carbon dioxide enters the red cell it is rapidly converted to H_2CO_3. The presence of KHb provides a ready source of base to combine with the carbonic acid. Thus the liberation of oxygen actually aids the take-up of carbon dioxide. The K^+ ions now combine with the HCO_3^- ions to form potassium bicarbonate. This ability to form bicarbonate is largely limited to the red cells. The red cell membrane, however, is only permeable to anions, e.g. Cl^- and HCO_3^- and to positively charged H^+ ions. In this manner K^+ ions are entrapped within the cell, whereas Na^+ ions abound in the plasma. When the concentration of $KHCO_3$ starts to build up within the cell ionic equilibrium is disturbed, so HCO_3^- ions pass out into the plasma and Cl^- ions pass in to take their place. The HCO_3^- ions rapidly combine with the Na^+ ions in the plasma to form sodium bicarbonate; in fact this combination is only a loose one as both ions remain almost completely ionised. Nevertheless a large proportion of the carbon dioxide is carried in this manner.

The whole process involving the transport of both oxygen and carbon dioxide together with the formation of bicarbonate ions is sometimes colloquially referred to as the *Hamburger phenomenon* or *chloride shift* (Fig. 10).

When the blood reaches the capillaries of the lung there is a pressure difference of 6 mm. Hg (46—40 mm.) of carbon dioxide on either side of the alveolar membrane, and as it diffuses across this barrier very rapidly this is quite sufficient to ensure an adequate interchange of gases. The process is the reverse of that already described for the uptake of carbon dioxide. First the small percentage physically dissolved in the plasma falls, then as the pressure gradient of dissolved carbon dioxide between the red cell and the plasma widens, so the carbon dioxide leaves the red cell and allows bicarbonate ions to enter. Thus the sodium bicarbonate in the plasma splits again so that the bicarbonate can pass back into the red cell and chloride ions move out into the plasma again. Following the formation of carbonic acid the enzyme carbonic anhydrase aids the breakdown to carbon dioxide and water so that finally carbon dioxide passes out into the plasma and from thence across the alveolar membrane.

Plasma bicarbonate, therefore, plays a very important role as the principal storehouse and carrier of carbon dioxide in the blood.

(*c*) *As a carbamino compound* (24 per cent).—Carbon dioxide can combine with the amino groupings of the haemoglobin to form carbamino-haemoglobin:

$$Hb.NH_2 + CO_2 \rightleftarrows Hb.NH.COOH$$

A smaller amount combines in a similar manner with the plasma proteins. The combination takes place directly between the carbon dioxide and the haemoglobin or plasma protein, as no enzyme—such as carbonic anhydrase—is required. The amount formed is influenced mainly by the degree of oxygen saturation of the blood and not by the carbon dioxide tension.

Christian and Greene (1962) have demonstrated that both ether and thiopentone-nitrous oxide-oxygen anaesthesia decrease the activity of carbonic anhydrase in blood, whereas cyclopropane is without effect.

Carbon Dioxide Dissociation Curve

The total amount of carbon dioxide dissolved in the blood varies in direct proportion to the tension to which it is exposed. It is possible, therefore, to express this relationship graphically as a dissociation curve (Fig. 11). However, there is a third factor concerned, namely the degree of oxygenation of the blood, so that there is a slightly different curve for each change in percentage oxygenation. As the oxygen content of the blood falls so the curve moves over to the left. The result is that the more reduced the haemoglobin becomes, the greater the quantity of carbon dioxide it can carry. Conversely, the higher the oxygenation of haemoglobin, the less carbon dioxide it can transport. Thus, taking as an example the arterial tension of carbon dioxide at 40 mm. Hg, the blood contains approximately 52 volumes per cent of this gas, but if it is fully reduced, then at the same tension it contains as much as 57 volumes per cent. This peculiar property of blood, or more strictly of haemoglobin, is partly due to the greater acidity of oxyhaemoglobin and partly to its great power of combining directly with the carbon dioxide.

The clinical significance of this curve is that more carbon dioxide can be taken up from the tissues where the oxygenation of the blood is low, but when the blood reaches the lung capillaries the reverse takes place and the tendency is for the amount of carbon dioxide held in the blood to fall.

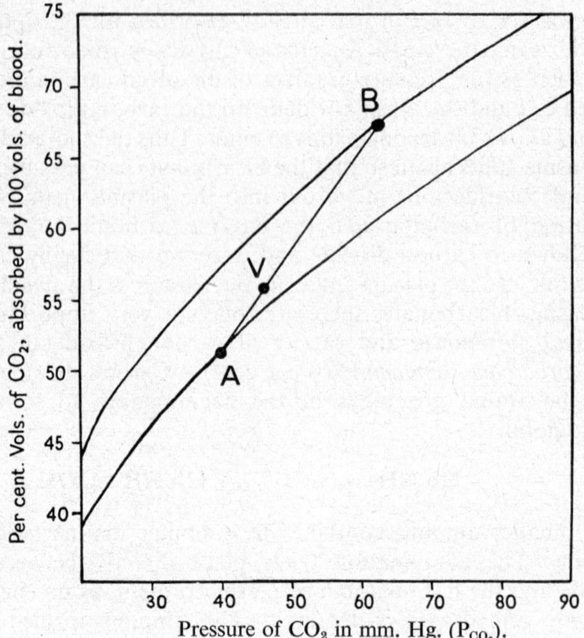

Pressure of CO_2 in mm. Hg. (P_{CO_2}).

3/FIG. 11.—CARBON DIOXIDE DISSOCIATION CURVE.

Upper line = Fully reduced human blood.
Lower line = Fully oxygenated human blood.
A = volume and tension of CO_2 in arterial blood.
V = volume and tension of CO_2 in venous blood.
B = Conditions in fully reduced blood.

Line AV is the dissociation of CO_2 in human blood. A rise in the respiratory quotient moves it to the right. A fall in the respiratory quotient moves it to the left.

PLACENTAL FUNCTION AND CARRIAGE OF OXYGEN AND CARBON DIOXIDE IN THE FOETUS

The human placenta consists of numerous maternal sinuses into which project the thin villi carrying the capillaries of the foetal circulation. Maternal blood in the intervillous spaces bathes the outside of these villi, so that there are only three layers of tissue separating the two circulations and these are all on the foetal side. They consist of the endothelial lining of the capillaries, the surrounding connective tissue and the epithelium lining the villi.

Most of the data available on the transfer of oxygen across the placental barrier is derived from a study of sheep with a five-layered placenta. Prystowsky (1957), however, devised a method for studying the pressure gradients in a human subject. Samples were obtained simultaneously from the maternal intervillous space and also from the umbilical artery and vein of the foetus. In a series of normal pregnancies the oxygen tension in the intervillous space averaged 40 mm. Hg (saturation of 75 per cent). The P_{O_2} in the umbilical vein of the infant immediately after delivery was 20 mm. Hg (saturation of 40 per cent).

This signifies an effective pressure gradient for oxygen of 20 mm. Hg between the maternal and foetal circulations (Fig. 12).

Bartels and his colleagues (1962) have summarised the data available for blood-gas levels in the human infant at birth. These figures are slightly different from those reported by Prystowsky (1957). The oxygen tension in the arterial

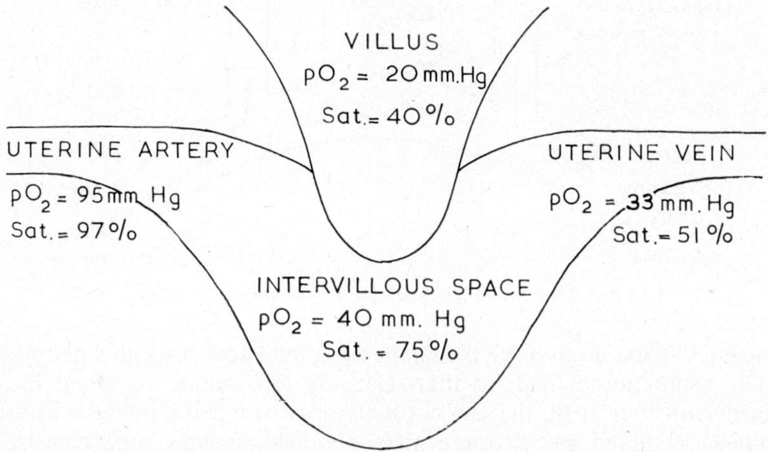

3/FIG. 12.—The placental circulation.

blood of the mother has been variously reported as 91 mm. Hg and 96 mm. Hg (Wulf, 1958; Vasicka *et al.*, 1960). In the uterine veins this tension has dropped to an average of 33 mm. Hg. However, it is important to emphasise that blood from the maternal uterine vein is not representative of the pressures in the foetal villae because maternal shunts exist resulting in the admixture of venous blood from uterine musculature. This will tend to give a falsely low value for foetal villus oxygenation. In fact, measurement of gas content of blood taken from the intervillous space showed an average tension for oxygen of 38–40 mm. Hg (range 28–54 mm. Hg) and a carbon dioxide tension of 38 mm. Hg.

The approximate values of the blood-gas tensions in the human foetus are summarised in Fig. 13. However, the actual values of the P_{O_2} in umbilical vein blood depend to some extent on the P_{O_2} and P_{CO_2} of maternal arterial blood. Rorke (1970) has reported that as maternal arterial P_{O_2} rises so does the P_{O_2} in the umbilical vein of the foetus, but only up to a point. Once the maternal P_{O_2} rises above about 300 mm. Hg, when the umbilical vein P_{O_2} is approximately 50 mm. Hg, although with a wide scatter around this value, the latter begins to fall even though the maternal P_{O_2} is increased further. At very high maternal P_{O_2} values the umbilical vein P_{O_2} approached those figures found when the mother was breathing 21 per cent oxygen.

It will be observed that there appears to be a foetal shunt in the placenta and this has been confirmed by injection studies of the human placenta (Bøe, 1954). The influx of this shunted blood would tend to lower the concentration of oxygen and raise that of carbon dioxide in the foetal umbilical vein.

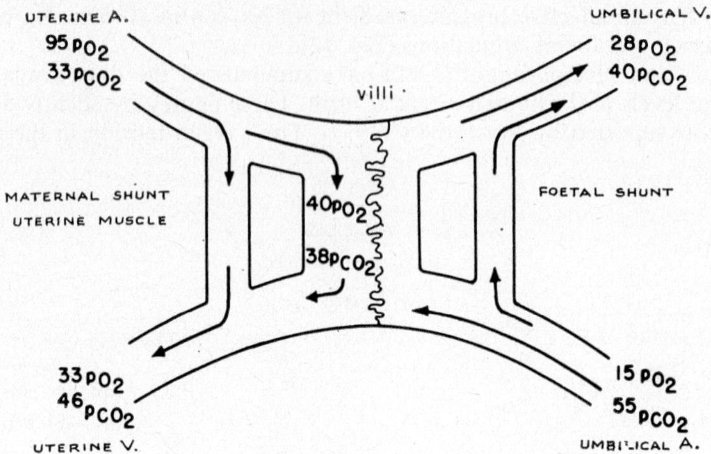

3/FIG. 13.—Blood gas tensions in the human placenta.

During the first hour of life the infant has a mild acidosis with a pH of about 7·3. The ventilation is high so that relatively low values for blood P_{CO_2} are obtained soon after birth. In cases of prematurity or foetal asphyxia a metabolic component is added and a severe metabolic acidosis may supervene in such cases.

There is little doubt that the transfer of gases across the placental barrier is nothing like so efficient as that found in the lungs. Clearly, the thickness of the chorionic tissue is sufficient to explain this discrepancy. The foetus, however, offsets this disadvantage in two principal ways:

1. *Foetal haemoglobin.*—Foetal haemoglobin has a different type of dissociation curve from that observed in the adult (Fig. 14). This differentiation can be made by means of a spectroscope. The most striking characteristic is the greater affinity of the foetal red cell for oxygen at the same partial pressure levels. For example, at a tension of 22 mm. Hg maternal haemoglobin is only 33 per cent saturated, whereas foetal haemoglobin reaches a value of 50 per cent saturation.

An interesting finding is that in solutions of foetal and adult haemoglobin (i.e. in the absence of red cells) the oxygen dissociation curves are the same. The difference in these curves, therefore, is probably related to some factor like the thickness of the red-cell wall rather than to any specific change in the haemoglobin molecule itself (Allen *et al.*, 1953).

With the progress of pregnancy, adult haemoglobin begins to appear, so that the concentration of this type rises from 6 per cent at the twentieth week to just over 20 per cent at birth. After birth, foetal red cells, and with them foetal haemoglobin, rapidly disappear, so that by the fourth month they can no longer be detected in the blood. Abramson (1960) considers that foetal haemoglobin is present as part of the process of development and, in his opinion, it performs no special role relative to the state of oxygenation of the foetus.

2. *Increased haemoglobin concentration.*—As pregnancy nears its termination so the concentration of haemoglobin rises, increasing the total amount

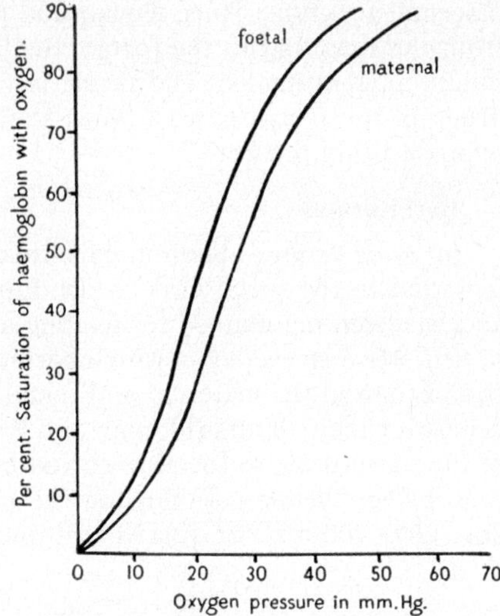

3/FIG. 14.—OXYGEN DISSOCIATION CURVES OF HUMAN INFANT AT BIRTH (UPPER LINE) AND PREGNANT WOMAN (LOWER LINE).

Note the large difference in oxygen saturation of foetal and maternal blood at an oxygen pressure of 22 mm. Hg.

of oxygen that can be carried. At birth 100 ml. of blood contains 23 g. of haemoglobin (adult 13·4 g.); in other words approximately 180 per cent of the maternal haemoglobin concentration, but by the end of the third month of life the figure has fallen to 10·5 g. (approximately 80 per cent). From then on it gradually recovers to reach 12·5 g. (approximately 90 per cent) by the end of the first six months.

The clinical significance of these various findings lies in the low oxygen tension with which the foetus carries on life. These are counteracted by the factors discussed above, and by an apparent ability on the part of the foetus to withstand hypoxia better than the adult. A small amount of oxygen is absorbed through the skin. Thus if an average-sized newborn infant is placed in an atmosphere of 100 per cent oxygen it will absorb about 1 ml. of oxygen per minute through its skin surface. As its total requirements are somewhere in the region of 25 ml. per minute this route obviously plays an insignificant part in the normal oxygenation process. Anaerobic metabolism may also take place in certain circumstances. Nevertheless, a drop in maternal oxygen tension produces a marked degree of hypoxia in the foetus.

PLACENTAL TRANSMISSION OF DRUGS

Striking developments in the field of placental perfusion have enabled studies to be made on the transmission of various drugs. It now seems likely that any substance found in maternal blood will ultimately penetrate the placental barrier unless it is altered or destroyed during its passage; the question remains only to gauge the rate and mechanism of the transfer (Page, 1957). The various factors and theories involved in this mechanism, together with evidence for specific drug transmission, have been reviewed by Moya and Thorndike (1962). The efficiency of drug transfer across the placental barrier must depend to a large extent on placental function. Thus, if placental function is impaired the transfer of drugs from the maternal to the foetal circulation is less rapid than if the placenta is functioning normally. The result is fortuitous as the build-up of anaesthetic drugs in the foetus is least when there is the greatest chance of severe foetal hypoxia being present.

Barbiturates

(*a*) *Long acting.*—Sodium barbitone has been found to pass rapidly from the maternal to the foetal circulation. Equilibrium is reached within four minutes and has been maintained for as long as fifteen hours (Flowers, 1957).

(*b*) *Medium acting.*—Amylobarbitone sodium has been found to reach equilibrium in the maternal and foetal circulations within thirty minutes and to persist for many hours (Ploman and Persson, 1957). There was an accumulation of the barbiturate in foetal liver and brain tissue.

(*c*) *Short acting.*—Following the maternal intravenous injection of a large dose (200–300 mg.) of quinalbarbitone sodium this barbiturate was detected in

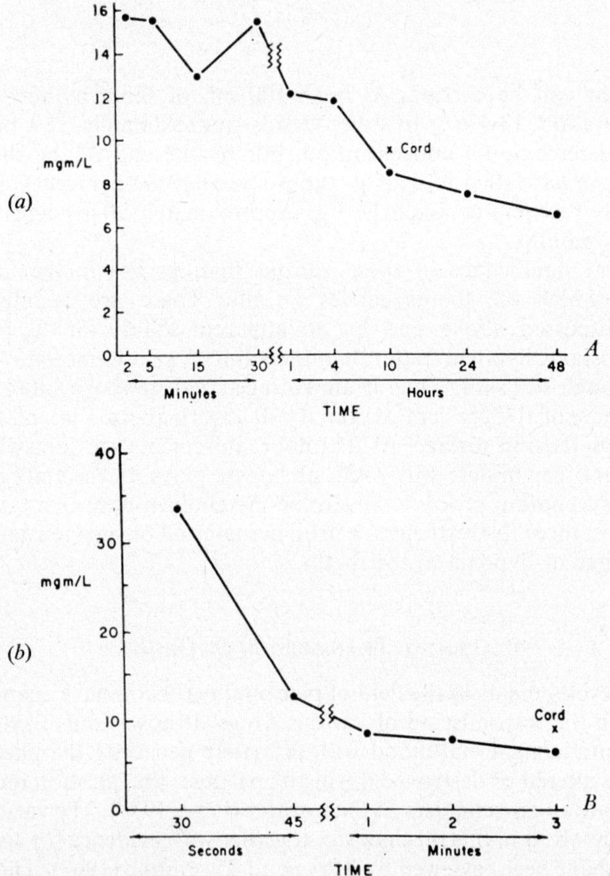

3/Fig. 15.—Decay curves of long (*a*) and short-acting (*b*) barbiturates.

the cord of the newborn after one minute, and equilibrium was established within three to five minutes (Root *et al.*, 1961).

(*d*) *Ultra short acting*.—It is now firmly established that thiopentone sodium crosses the placental barrier within seconds of its injection into the maternal circulation. Furthermore, though the concentration in the foetal circulation soon after injection equals that in the mother, it wanes rapidly in the next few minutes as the maternal concentration falls, and within five minutes has fallen to a small fraction of that observed thirty seconds after injection (Fig. 15) (Flowers, 1959; McKechnie and Converse, 1955). Some authors have suggested a preferential absorption of this drug by the foetal liver but work in animals suggests that the newborn is not capable of metabolising it (Ploman and Persson, 1957; Fouts and Adamson, 1959).

Methohexitone crosses the placental barrier with ease.

Tranquillisers

Chlorpromazine has been shown to cross the placental barrier, and its presence in foetal urine and tissues has been demonstrated, but to date all attempts at assaying the concentration in the foetal circulation have been unsuccessful. Promethazine rapidly crosses the placental barrier and can be found in the foetal circulation within two minutes of injection. Similarly, promazine can be detected in the foetal circulation within two minutes of its intravenous injection into the mother, with a maximum foetal level at about five minutes. Foetal blood concentrations are always lower than maternal, and only about 0·5 per cent of the total dose passes into the baby (Crawford and Rudofsky, 1965).

Paraldehyde

This drug has been used widely in obstetrics and particularly in the treatment of toxaemia in pregnancy. The concentrations in the maternal and foetal circulation remain parallel for many hours after an oral or rectal dose to the mother (Gardner *et al.*, 1940). A dose sufficient to produce amnesia in the mother is believed to produce neonatal depression in a large percentage of infants.

Atropine and Hyoscine

Both drugs are believed to cross the placental barrier but no quantitive studies are available. Atropine has been shown to increase the foetal pulse rate six minutes after its injection into the mother (Hon *et al.*, 1961). Complete vagal blockade in the foetus is reported fifteen minutes after the intravenous injection of 1 mg. of atropine into the mother (Hellman *et al.*, 1962). John (1965) suggested that the response of the foetal heart rate to a maternal intravenous injection of atropine might be used as a test of placental function.

Morphine and Pethidine

Despite the almost universal use of these drugs in the control of labour pains there is very little evidence to prove one drug is better than the other. However, there is general agreement that both drugs cause depression of foetal respiration (Taylor *et al.*, 1955; Roberts *et al.*, 1957). Apgar and Papper (1952) studied blood levels of pethidine in the umbilical cord and maternal circulation and found foetal plasma levels up to 70 per cent of the maternal level. Nevertheless, there is general agreement that if the infant is born within one hour or more than six hours after administration there will be a minimal depression of respiration. Furthermore, nalorphine and levallorphan, which are weak narcotics in themselves, have been found readily to cross the placental barrier and stimulate respiration of the newborn. They can either be given intravenously to the mother just prior to delivery or injected into the neonate immediately after birth.

Ethyl Alcohol

Following slow maternal intravenous injection, the level of alcohol detected in the foetal circulation is about 20 per cent less than that found in the mother (Belinkoff and Hall, 1950).

Anaesthetic Agents

Diethyl ether readily crosses the placenta and equilibrium between the maternal and foetal circulations is soon established. The degree of depression of the infant is believed to be directly related to the depth and duration of the maternal anaesthesia (Smith and Barker, 1942).

Studies have revealed that cyclopropane appears in the foetal circulation within 1½ minutes after administration to the mother, and the concentration is about 60 per cent of the maternal circulation (Apgar *et al.*, 1957). There would appear to be a direct relationship between the duration of cyclopropane anaesthesia prior to birth and the incidence of depression of the newborn.

No foetal depression has been demonstrated following the use of nitrous oxide and oxygen mixtures. However, there appears to be some impediment to the passage of nitrous oxide across the placenta, because the concentration in the foetal circulation rarely rises above 50 per cent of that found in the maternal circulation (Cohen *et al.*, 1953).

Trichloroethylene passes readily across the placenta within a few minutes and rapidly reaches equilibrium with the maternal concentration. It is believed that foetal blood has a greater capacity than maternal blood for trichloroethylene.

Halothane readily passes across the placenta but the time taken to reach equilibrium between maternal and foetal circulations is not as yet known (Sheridan and Robson, 1959).

Muscle Relaxants

There is now abundant evidence that *d*-tubocurarine chloride does not cross the placental barrier in significant amounts in man following the intravenous injection of a clinically paralysing dose to the mother, i.e. 15–25 mg. (Buller and Young, 1949; Crawford and Gardiner, 1956). Animal experiments suggest that very high concentrations of *d*-tubocurarine allow sufficient quantities to cross and cause neuromuscular block.

Crawford and Gardiner (1956) found significant levels of gallamine triethiodide in the foetal circulation three minutes after the injection of 80 mg. to the mother. The concentration in some cases even equalled that found in the mother. More recently, Schwarz (1958) has measured iodine levels of cord blood samples and noted significant levels soon after the injection of 80 mg. gallamine.

Moya and Kvisselgaard (1961) have shown with the aid of a frog rectus bioassay method that no suxamethonium could be found in the infant when clinical doses (up to 100 mg.) of the relaxant were given to the mother. These results have been confirmed by Schmermund *et al.* (1961). After a single dose of 300 mg. suxamethonium, small but detectable levels of the drug could be found in the infants, though none of them appeared to be affected by the relaxant.

The placenta appears to form a relative, rather than an absolute, barrier to the passage of muscle relaxants, so that in clinical dosage these drugs do not pass across in sufficient quantity to affect the foetus. The only exception seems to be gallamine, following which clinically detectable amounts are found in the foetal circulation.

Local Analgesic Drugs

It is generally believed that provided there is no systemic disturbance in the maternal circulation (Marx, 1961), these drugs have no direct effect on the foetus, even when they are given intravenously to the mother (Allen, 1945). Maternal hypotension of 80 mm. Hg or less almost always results in foetal bradycardia due to hypoxia, and this is commonly experienced with spinal analgesia if a vasopressor is not used (Downs and Morrison, 1963). Nyirjesy and his colleagues (1963), in a review of the hazards of paracervical block analgesia in obstetrics, could only explain their complications on the basis that large amounts of lignocaine were absorbed into the maternal and foetal circulation. Thomas and his colleagues (1968) studying the placental transfer of lignocaine following lumbar epidural administration, observed that within 15 minutes the drug was present in the foetal circulation in quite high concentrations. They found that the foetal blood concentration varied between 25 per cent and 100 per cent of the maternal concentration. Reynolds and Taylor (1970) observed an average foetal blood concentration of lignocaine of 57 per cent of the maternal concentration. They compared the placental transfer of bupivacaine with that of lignocaine after extradural injection and found that the average foetal concentration of bupivacaine was 30 per cent of the maternal blood concentration, or about half that of lignocaine.

Respiration in the Newborn

Intra-Uterine Respiration

In 1946 Barcroft showed that small and feeble foetal respiratory movements can be detected in animals during pregnancy. Working on sheep, he was able to produce movement of the foetal head by tactile stimulation of it as early as the thirty-fourth day—a stage when the organism is only a little larger than a human thumb-nail. Gradually over the next few days this response to stimulation spread to involve other muscle groups, including those of respiration.

The movements are slow and prolonged, while at about the fiftieth day respiratory activity becomes distinct from that of other muscle groups. Up to this stage, however, the foetus responds only to tactile stimulation, and not until the fifty-fifth day does it enter a "quiescent" phase in which steadily decreasing sensitivity to this type of stimulation is coupled with increasing responsiveness to chemical factors. Asphyxia, for instance, produced by clamping the cord rapidly evokes respiratory activity.

Deep general anaesthesia of the mother inhibits the response of the foetus to tactile stimulation. At birth following such anaesthesia, instead of smooth, rhythmical respirations developing at once there is a delay during which asphyxia progresses until finally a gasping type of respiration commences. On the other hand, after light general anaesthesia or spinal analgesia regular and rhythmical breathing rapidly ensues.

It seems, therefore, that there are two main factors which may prevent rhythmic respiration at birth—anaesthesia and asphyxia. Smith (1951) suggests that there are two possible keys which will release respiratory activity in the newborn infant. One is sensory, the other is chemical. Sensory stimuli may produce regular rhythmic respiration, whereas chemical stimuli (provided by asphyxia) act as an emergency mechanism leading to a gasping type of respiration.

There is considerable difference of opinion as to whether rhythmical respiration is present or not in the human foetus just prior to birth, and as yet there is insufficient data available to allow any definite statement to be made. Movements of the trunk, arms and legs have been observed at the 55th day, and respiratory movements following temporary asphyxia have been reported at the 84th day (Windle *et al.*, 1938). The injection of a radio-opaque medium into the amniotic cavity between the 15th and 20th weeks has revealed that enough respiratory activity takes place to draw the contrast medium deeply into the lungs (Davis and Potter, 1946). The evidence for similar activity just prior to birth is less convincing.

In summarising our knowledge of human foetal activity, both from available data and in the light of animal experiments, it seems probable that muscular movements develop at an early stage. A rhythmical type of respiration soon becomes segregated from these generalised movements (phase of segregation) but is later inhibited as the central nervous system develops. This is the stage of quiescence, and in it the foetus becomes less sensitive to tactile stimulation but increasingly responsive to the effects of oxygen lack.

Onset of Breathing

The precise mechanism by which the newly-born child takes its first breath is still debated. Barcroft (1946) considered asphyxia was the most potent stimulus to respiratory movement at birth in lambs. Dawes (1961) believes the fall in oxygen saturation due to the delivery, coupled with the chemoreceptor reflexes and sensory stimuli from the skin, reinforce the effects of pre-existing hypoxia and are sufficient to initiate respiration.

The average oxygen saturation in the umbilical vein at birth is between 50 and 60 per cent, whereas it falls to between 15 and 30 per cent in the umbilical artery. Soon after birth the saturation starts to rise so that it reaches about 70 per cent after 15 minutes, 80 per cent at one hour, and 90 per cent three hours after delivery (Brandfass, 1959).

Oxygen Lack and Carbon Dioxide Excess

Oxygen lack depresses the respiratory centre by direct action, but it also stimulates the chemoreceptors in the carotid and aortic bodies. These organs are believed to be the dominant factors in the start of respiration because they are known to function even after the oxygen tension has fallen to zero (Schmidt, 1956). In the severely hypoxic infant, respiration starts in the form of gasps with the accessory muscles of respiration playing a major role. In most instances, the first few breaths of the newborn are of this type and then rhythmical respiration with both intercostal and diaphragmatic movement soon develops.

The neonate is usually regarded as being relatively unresponsive to carbon dioxide. This is probably true only when a very low oxygen saturation is present, because hypoxia depresses the activity of the respiratory centre. Cross and his co-workers (1953) have shown that the well-oxygenated newborn infant is extremely sensitive to changes in inspired carbon dioxide, a rising concentration resulting in an increase in both rate and depth of respiration.

Chemoreceptor Reflexes

The general picture of the regulation of respiration in the newborn through control by pH and P_{CO_2} is similar to that in the adult. The oxygen tension is believed to be regulated largely through chemoreceptor activity in the carotid and aortic bodies. Evidence for this activity is provided by the response of the neonate to hypoxia (Fig. 16).

When an infant breathing air is suddenly exposed to an atmosphere with a low oxygen concentration (i.e. 15 per cent) the immediate response is hyperventilation, resulting in an increased minute volume. After a minute this response starts to fall and returns to its previous values after about three or four minutes. This increase in ventilation is believed to be due to chemoreceptor activity, because when pure oxygen is administered (see Fig. 16) there is a sharp reduction in ventilation. This is explained on the basis that hypoxia now no longer evokes chemoreceptor activity.

There is very suggestive evidence, therefore, that chemoreceptor activity is present in the newborn infant and that the control of respiration is similar to the adult pattern, with the possible exception that the neonatal respiratory centre may more easily be depressed by hypoxia. Lobeline (3·0 mg.) is believed to stimulate respiration by acting on the chemoreceptors in the aortic and carotid bodies.

Expansion of the Lungs at Birth

Considerable pressures are required to expand the lungs at birth. Karlberg and his colleagues (1957) placed a catheter in the oesophagus of newborn infants before the first breath and found that the intra-oesophageal pressure (reflecting intrapleural pressure) was as high as 60 to 80 cm. H_2O. Furthermore, the first breath often had a volume as high as 80 ml. It is also known that pressures as high as 35 cm. H_2O must be applied to the trachea in order to expand the lungs at birth (Smith and Chisholm, 1942; Donald and Lord, 1953). Nevertheless, the finding that a high intratracheal pressure, when maintained for an indefinite period of time, invariably led to rupture of the lungs, has led to extreme caution in the use of intermittent positive-pressure ventilation in infants. In clinical practice pressures as high as 30–35 cm. H_2O can be used with safety provided they are only applied for a brief period of time (Day *et al.*, 1952).

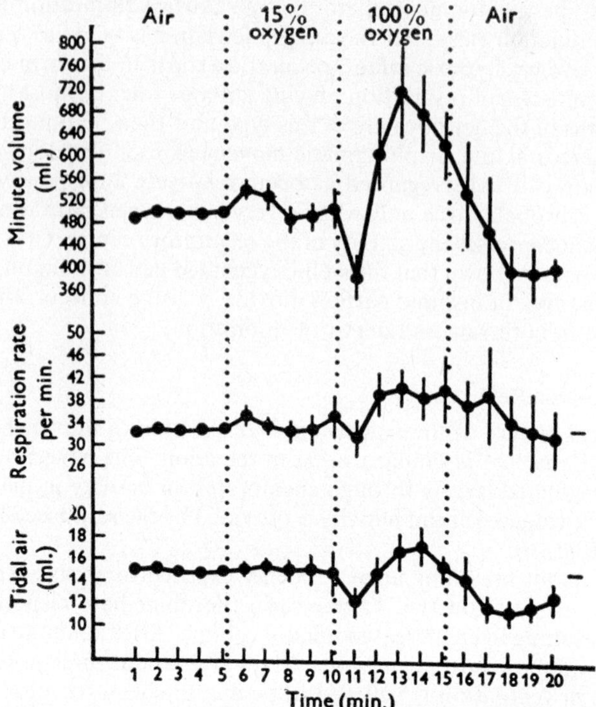

3/FIG. 16.—Effect of low (hypoxia) and high (hyperoxia) oxygen tension on the minute volume, respiration rate and tidal air of normal full-term infants. Note the temporary rise in minute volume caused by hypoxia; also the fall followed by the rise in minute volume caused by hyperoxia.

Another reason for the reluctance to use positive pressure to expand the neonatal lung has been based on a false concept derived from observations of rubber balloons (Abramson, 1960). It is well-known that if a person blows down the end of a Y-piece connection to which are attached two balloons, then one balloon inflates preferentially (Fig.17*a*). If now further air is blown down the connection, one might reasonably expect that the deflated balloon would expand. This is not the case. The already expanded balloon expands even further (Fig. 17*b*).

This phenomenon is due to the law of Laplace*. If this law applied strictly in the case of the lung, then theoretically a small segment of collapsed tissue could never be re-expanded as any further pressure would only continue to expand the already distended alveoli.

Experience with thoracic anaesthesia has shown that this law cannot be applied rigidly. There is no doubt that alveoli which already contain air are easier to expand than those that are completely collapsed. However, prolonged positive pressure will reinflate all portions of the lung. The reasons why the lungs are not

* The tangential tension in the wall of a hollow structure is proportional to the internal pressure and to the radius.

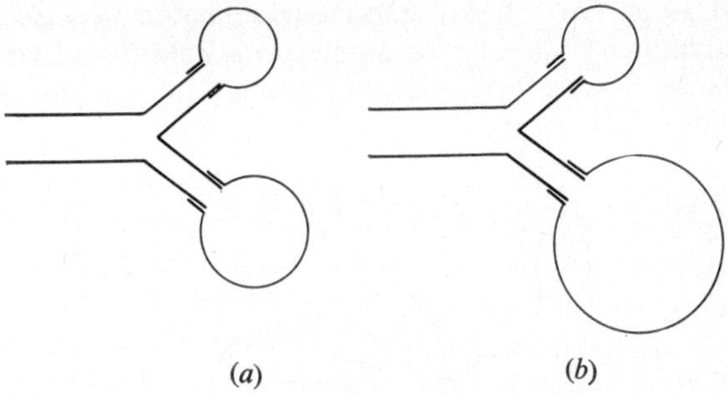

3/FIG. 17.—Diagram to illustrate the law of Laplace.

(*a*) (*b*)

strictly comparable with a rubber balloon are threefold. First, the presence of elastic fibres in the interstitial tissue, second, the effect of the surface tension of the fluid lining the alveolar wall (see Chapter I). The remarkable quality of this fluid is that its surface tension varies directly with the amount of surface area exposed. Thus, as an alveolus contracts, the tension of the lining secretion automatically decreases. If it were not for this unusual property an alveolus, once collapsed, would require greater force to re-expand it and persistant collapse would result. Finally the lack of elasticity in the visceral pleura.

Lung inflation reflex.—In the sleeping baby, sudden inflation of the lungs leads to an obvious period of apnoea (Cross *et al.*, 1960). During the first 24 hours of life there is an initial "inspiratory gasp" before the onset of the apnoea. The exact significance of this reflex is unkown, but it may be related to the expansion of the lungs at birth.

Circulatory Changes at Birth

The foetal circulation is a complex one. However, with the aid of cine-radiography and blood-gas analysis it has been possible to obtain much valuable information about it in animals (Dawes, 1961). One of the principal findings is that the flow of blood in the inferior vena cava appears to move in two almost distinct streams. Oxygenated blood coming from the placenta via the umbilical vein and the ductus venosus passes along the inside track of the inferior vena cava and through the foramen ovale into the left atrium (Fig. 18).

The other stream, consisting of blood coming from the lower limbs and viscera, passes along the outside track of the inferior vena cava to join blood from the superior vena cava and pass to the right atrium. This division of the vena cava into two streams is achieved by a ridge termed the crista dividens.

The ductus venosus.—Apart from acting as a by-pass channel, the role of this structure is uncertain. It has smooth muscle in its wall and is innervated by the vagus. Dawes (1961), working with foetal lambs, has shown that tying the ductus venosus does not change the pressure either in the umbilical vein or in the inferior vena cava. Barcroft (1946) believed that it was less important for the ductus venosus to remain patent during foetal life than that it should close during life.

The ductus arteriosus.—This is a by-pass channel allowing blood from the right side of the heart to pass from the pulmonary artery into the aorta. At birth, it does not close at once. It constricts rapidly at first, so that in lambs its lumen is considerably narrowed within 10–30 minutes of adequate ventilation

(Dawes, 1961). Because of the rise in systemic vascular resistance and the fall of pulmonary vascular resistance with inflation of the lungs, the direction of the blood flow normally reverses and a loud murmur may be detected over the left side of the heart.

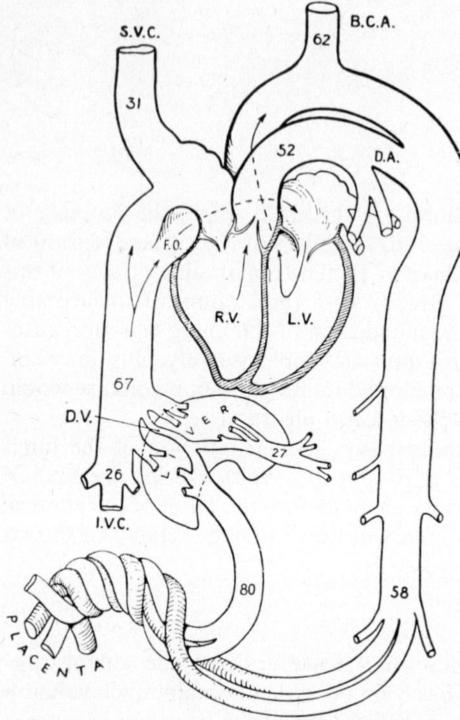

3/FIG. 18.—THE FOETAL CIRCULATION IN THE LAMB.

I.V.C.: Inferior vena cava.
R.V.: Right ventricle.
D.V.: Ductus venosus.
D.A.: Ductus arteriosus.
S.V.C.: Superior vena cava.
L.V.: Left ventricle.
F.O.: Foramen ovale.
B.C.A.: Brachiocephalic artery.

The figures indicate the mean O_2 percentage saturation in samples of blood withdrawn simultaneously and averaged from estimations on six lambs.

The closure of the ductus arteriosus is believed to be directly related to the high oxygen saturation of the blood. The effect of an increased P_{CO_2} is the same and is probably due to a direct action on the muscle wall of the vessel. Adrenaline and noradrenaline have a similar effect.

The foramen ovale.—This is the principal by-pass channel allowing blood to pass almost directly from the inferior vena cava, through the right atrium into the left atrium.

Before birth the pressure in the right atrium is higher than in the left atrium, but as soon as the lungs are expanded the quantity of blood entering the left atrium is increased, so that the higher pressure in this chamber now tends to keep the foramen ovale closed. However, this closure does not become permanent for several weeks, so that in the event of a rise in right atrial pressure for some reason or other, the foramen ovale may re-open.

Cardiac Output and the Pulmonary Circulation

The moment the lung expands there is a tremendous increase in the size of the pulmonary vascular bed, so that the lungs can now accept the whole output of the right heart. The act of expansion of the lungs uncoils the capillaries so that the vascular resistance falls, with the result that the right atrial pressure now falls below the left and the foramen ovale tends to close.

Vasomotor Tone

During the first three days of life there is little evidence of vasomotor control in the skin vessels, but after this time there is increasing evidence of both constrictor tone and sympathetic vasodilator activity. The time-delay in the onset of this activity may be due to the lower than normal body temperature during this period (Young, 1962).

The blood pressure of the neonate is difficult to measure. In the past, large inflatable cuffs on the arm have tended to give falsely low readings. A 2·5 cm. wide cuff of 8 to 10 cm. length is the most suitable. At birth the mean systemic pressure is around 60–70 mm. Hg and this gradually rises over the next few days and weeks (Young, 1961. See Fig. 19). The fact that the cardiac output (on a

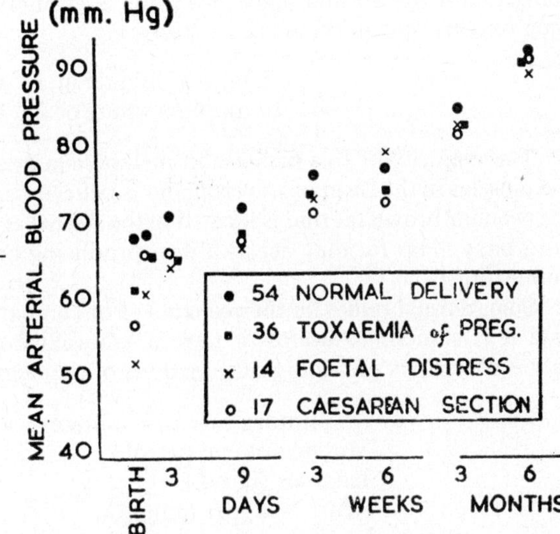

3/FIG. 19.—Arterial blood pressure at birth and soon after.

body-weight basis) is about double that of the adult and the peripheral blood flow to the extremities is also high, suggests that the lower mean systemic pressure of the newborn is due to a lower peripheral resistance. This may be due to the infant's poorly developed vasomotor tone.

Temperature Control

The newborn infant has a lower body temperature than its mother, but the reason for this is uncertain. It may be due to a generally lower metabolism or it may be due to hypoxia. Cross and his associates (1958) have suggested that an infant responds to a lowered intake of oxygen by deliberately reducing its oxygen consumption, resulting in a fall in body temperature. This emphasises that raising oxygen intake is equally important to raising environmental temperature.

The optimum temperature for the newborn infant, and particularly the premature baby, is still debated. Wagner (1958) found that many premature infants can survive—and indeed thrive—when kept at low body temperatures for long periods. Other workers, however, using a controlled study, found that babies maintained at a temperature of 28·9° C did not do as well as those at 31·7° C (Silverman *et al.*, 1958).

The danger of heat loss during anaesthesia and surgery in this class of patient is now fully realised. Previously unsuspected hypothermia was believed to be one of the principal causes of post-operative morbidity and death (Farman, 1962). It has been found very much easier to prevent the fall in body temperature in the anaesthetised infant than it has been to treat the hypothermia once it has occurred.

Metabolism

The average newborn child has an oxygen consumption of 5 ml./kg./minute for the first twelve hours of life, and this rises to 6 ml./kg./minute during the first two days of life. Raising the environmental oxygen has no effect on oxygen consumption of the normal baby, but if the environmental temperature is lowered then oxygen consumption rises rapidly, e.g.:

6 ml./kg./minute at 34° C.
10 ml./kg./minute at 28° C.

The majority of this increase in metabolism does not come from activity in the muscles in the form of shivering but is believed to be related to metabolism of the peculiar brown fat that is located in the sternal and cervical region of the newborn baby. This fat may act as a heat-producing organ (Cross—personal communication).

Some normal values for the neonate.—For comparison with other pathological data it is sometimes useful to have a knowledge of the approximate normal values of various physiological functions of the neonate. Thus:

Respiratory rate (per minute)	33
Minute volume (in ml.)	500
Tidal air (in ml.)	15
Heart rate (per minute)	140
Body temperature (° C)	34
Oxygen consumption (ml./kg.)	6
Blood pressure (mean—mm. Hg)	65

NEONATAL ASPHYXIA

Neonatal asphyxia is said to be present when efficient pulmonary ventilation does not start in the first few minutes after birth. Even if the lungs of a mature and normal infant become fully aerated within a few seconds of the onset of breathing, ventilation may still be inadequate owing to both central and peripheral factors (Table 6). Moreover, these factors may prevent or limit expansion of the lungs or lead to collapse some time after aeration has taken place. Failure of the lung to expand at birth is known as neonatal atelectasis, but cases of partial or complete expansion followed by collapse in a matter of minutes or hours are usually included under the same heading. The more premature the infant, the less likely is respiration to be efficient at birth and the more vulnerable will it be to these abnormal factors. Atelectasis is, in fact, a most important cause of death in premature infants.

Causes of Neonatal Asphyxia

Central causes.—Intra-uterine anoxia, the effects of analgesic and anaesthetic drugs, and trauma, either directly or indirectly affecting the respiratory centre, are the commonest conditions. There is little evidence that prematurity alone, and a consequently immature respiratory centre, is likely to be a factor of great importance, although without doubt the premature infant is very susceptible to anoxia and narcotic drugs (Potter, 1954).

Intra-uterine anoxia—persisting after birth—may follow obstetrical complications such as separation or infarction of the placenta, cord prolapse and prolonged labour, or the effects of analgesia and anaesthesia. Foetal asphyxia leads to premature attempts at respiration *in utero*, and amniotic fluid or meconium may then be aspirated into the respiratory tract.

Donald (1954*a*) has described how asphyxia may cause intraventricular haemorrhage in the brain of a premature infant from the rupture of a small ependymal vessel on the surface of the thalamus. This must be differentiated from the effects of trauma which produce a subdural haematoma, classically from a tear of the tentorium.

Peripheral causes.—Mucus or aspirated material such as meconium or amniotic fluid may obstruct the airway at all levels of the respiratory tract. In very premature infants the peripheral mechanisms may be too weak to produce adequate pulmonary ventilation.

Neonatal asphyxia is most often a combination of factors, and in all cases the possible presence of congenital abnormalities must not be overlooked.

Respiratory Distress Syndrome (Hyaline Membrane Disease) (Scopes, 1970)

Incidence.—About five in every thousand live infants die with respiratory failure in the first few days of life. The majority of these deaths are due to the respiratory distress syndrome, or hyaline membrane disease. This condition accounts for 50 per cent of the mortality in premature infants and in those weighing from 1000 to 1500 g. (2¼ lb. to 3¼ lb.) whereas it is only found in 5 per cent of those weighing 2000 to 2500 g. (4¾ lb. to 5½ lb.). As the syndrome is usually evident within a few hours of birth, it is believed to develop *in utero*.

Aetiology.—This is unknown, but it is now believed to be intimately associated with a failure of production of the surface-acting material normally lining the alveolar walls (see p. 28). The condition is associated with prematurity, maternal diabetes mellitus, delivery by caesarean section, or following an episode of intra-uterine asphyxia, such as occurs after an antepartum haemorrhage or in toxaemia of pregnancy. Avery and Mead (1959) studied the lung washings from a series of premature infants who died of hyaline membrane disease and found that the lungs from these infants lacked the normal surface properties. They suggested that the association of changes in surface tension observed in cases of congenital atelectasis and hyaline membrane disease could be the primary cause of the pulmonary collapse. Clements (1962) described the detergent-like property of the fluid which lines the alveolar wall. Subsequently,

Pattle (1963) studied the time of appearance of lung surface-acting material in foetal rats, mice and guinea-pigs and found that it only appeared when the larger alveoli ceased to be lined by cuboidal epithelium. Present day opinion as to the aetiology of the condition has been summarised by Reynolds *et al.* (1968), who state that "the crucial factors in determining whether an infant will develop hyaline membrane disease is the state at birth of the mechanism responsible for the synthesis of surfactant and that the illness will arise either because this mechanism is too immature to supply the demand for surfactant, or because it has been damaged by asphyxia before, during or immediately after birth, or because of the interaction of these two influences".

An interesting observation related to the absence of this pulmonary detergent or surface-acting material is that whereas pulmonary oedema fluid in normal children and adults forms a remarkable foam in the respiratory passages, this does not occur with the secretions of infants with hyaline membrane disease.

Absence of this surface-acting material is believed to increase the surface tension in the lungs. This means that very high pressures—pressures which may adversely affect the circulation—will be required to expand the lungs of these infants. The normal balance of osmotic pressure within the pulmonary bed is destroyed and fluid passes into the alveoli. Although lacking in foam-producing properties, this fluid is rich in eosinophilic material and fibrin, and it lines the alveoli, alveolar ducts and terminal bronchioles.

The principal cause of this condition is prematurity, but it is also commonly associated with maternal diabetes and toxaemia of pregnancy, both of which are prominent causes of an early delivery.

Lung changes.—There is a marked fall in compliance so that the baby has to work very hard to breathe. The tidal volume falls and the dead-space increases, and an attempt is made to maintain alveolar ventilation by increasing the respiratory rate. In moderate and severe cases the baby is unable to maintain sufficient ventilation and the arterial P_{CO_2} rises. As alveoli close off venous admixture increases, resulting in arterial hypoxia. The ductus ateriosus commonly remains patent. At autopsy the characteristic findings are widespread atelectasis, hyaline membranes with oedema and haemorrhage within the lung substance. A well-formed hyaline membrane is unusual in babies dying within a few hours of birth.

Clinical course.—The diagnostic signs of the respiratory distress syndrome are chest retraction, expiratory grunting and diminished air entry on auscultation, all of which are usually present soon after birth. With each inspiration the rib cage is sucked in and during each expiration there is a characteristic grunting sound arising in the larynx. Radiological examination shows fine "ground glass" mottling throughout the lung fields. The respiratory rate gradually increases to about 75 per minute at 24 hours of age and the pulse rate rises to between 130 and 170 per minute. Pitting oedema of the hands and feet may develop and sometimes this is the precursor of sclerema in the tissues. Apnoeic spells lasting only a few seconds or as long as a minute frequently occur.

Biochemical changes.—An infant with the respiratory distress syndrome is usually born with an uncomplicated respiratory acidosis (i.e. P_{CO_2} 50–80 mm. Hg: pH 7·00–7·25—Normal values: P_{CO_2} 45 mm. Hg: pH 7·30). As time progresses, a metabolic acidosis develops and gradually the signs of a rise in plasma potassium and non-protein nitrogen appear. These signs are probably due to a progressively diminishing oxygen supply to the tissues with an accumulation of lactic acid. Hypoglycaemia may occur.

Treatment.—Unfortunately there is no really effective therapy for this condition, but two main measures should be considered. First, the oxygenation of the infant must be improved. The use of an incubator with humidity, temperature and oxygen control is essential. Second, the metabolic disturbances may be ameliorated with intravenous glucose and sodium bicarbonate solutions administered soon after birth (Usher, 1961). Good nursing and general care is of vital importance. There is great divergence of opinion as to the exact indications for controlled respiration, especially because of the practical difficulties associated with this form of treatment. As a general rule artificial ventilation should be commenced for the following reasons: (i) apnoea (ii) progressive deterioration in the face of conservative treatment.

Clinical Diagnosis of Neonatal Asphyxia

Classically, cases have been divided into the two extremes of blue and white asphyxia, but it is rare to get a clear-cut picture and in any event the condition is a progressive one, usually commencing *in utero* or during the act of birth. For this reason it may often be expected from a history of the pregnancy and labour, the type and dosage of narcotics, and the maturity of the child. The importance of the background to the case cannot be overstressed when considering treatment.

Blue asphyxia is typified by an infant with good muscle tone: indeed this may be more than normal, and convulsions occasionally occur. The heart beat is slow but of good power. The normal heart rate varies from 130 to 160 a minute, and bradycardia is the invariable response to oxygen lack. The effect is precipitated by anoxia of the medulla. When anoxia is progressive or very severe, irregularity of the heart beat supervenes on bradycardia. There is little, if any, respiratory effort and even when respiration starts each breath must be carefully observed until regular and rhythmical activity is established. Until the respiratory centre is fully oxygenated the respirations are usually gasping in character, and irregular and infrequent in occurrence. There are often obvious signs of mucus in the respiratory tract, or even of atelectasis. A narcotised child may breathe more actively with the stimulus of birth, but gradually lapse into shallow respiration with relaxed muscles soon after; while a child with intracranial damage may respond to resuscitative measures but fail later as the central disease progresses. If the condition progresses, white asphyxia supervenes and the infant begins to suffer from the extreme results of oxygen lack and carbon dioxide retention. It becomes shocked, cold and clammy. There is no muscle tone and no response to external stimuli. The heart beat is weak and the rate rapid and irregular in the final stage.

In the first group treatment will probably lead to adequate respiration, and if it does not the need for further measures can be assessed over a minute or two; while in the second, even though some respiratory activity is present, active resuscitation is necessary at once. As would be expected, it is with premature infants that difficulty may be experienced in deciding whether special treatment should be undertaken or not, since respiration may appear adequate at birth but gradually fail later.

The Apgar Score

A more objective method of evaluating the state of a newborn infant is by means of scoring, using five signs noted sixty seconds after birth, but disregarding the cord and placenta (Apgar, 1953; Apgar *et al.*, 1958). The signs are heart rate, respiratory effort, muscle tone, reflex irritability, and colour. Each sign is given a score of 0, 1 or 2. A total score of 10 shows that the infant is in the best possible condition. Active resuscitation is necessary below 5. Details of this Apgar score are given in Table 5.

Treatment of Neonatal Asphyxia

Before dealing with more specialised methods, the routine treatment of a newborn child must be described, for the first four minutes are of great importance. Furthermore, particular attention is drawn to the value of preventive therapy during labour and birth. In this sense careful selection and estimation of dosage of drugs—particularly in the presence of obstetric abnormalities—must be made, and anoxia of mother or child avoided at all costs. When necessary the mother should be given oxygen during labour.

Routine Care after Birth

As soon as the child is delivered it should be held by the obstetrician with its head hanging down. The mouth must be cleared of all mucus before the cord is clamped, and there is much to be said for keeping the child hanging upside down for a minute or two at this stage to ensure that as much amniotic fluid as possible

3/Table 5

The Apgar Score

Sign	*Score*		
	0	1	2
Heart rate	absent	slow (below 100)	over 100
Respiratory effort	absent	weak cry hypoventilation	good strong cry
Muscle tone	limp	some flexion of extremities	well flexed
Reflex irritability (response of skin stimulation to feet)	no response	some motion	cry
Colour	blue pale	body pink extremities blue	completely pink

3/TABLE 6
THE CAUSES OF NEONATAL ASPHYXIA

	Central	*Peripheral*
During pregnancy and labour	Anoxia from: Placental infarction or separation Toxaemia Prolapse and knots of the cord Maternal hypotension caused by: Drugs Haemorrhage Maternal anoxia	
During labour	Anoxia from: Uterine dysfunction Prolonged labour Trauma from: Instrumental delivery Depression from: Effects of drugs i.e. Morphine Pethidine Certain anaesthetics	Premature respiration and aspiration Trauma to thoracic cage
After labour	Residual effects of factors occurring during labour, such as drugs	Failure to relieve the airway Immaturity

drains out of the respiratory tract, while the delay in clamping the cord allows the child to receive all the blood from the placenta. This is particularly essential when the infant is premature. The child should then be placed on its side, in the head-down position, in a cot. Excessive warmth is detrimental as it increases metabolism and oxygen consumption, and a cot-temperature of 36–37°C is probably optimal.

At this stage it may be necessary to clear the airway again by suction through the nares and over the back of the tongue with a special catheter or a rubber air bulb, but unnecessary and misapplied suction by irritating the glottis only inhibits respiration and must be avoided. The primary object is to allow air, and therefore oxygen, to enter the infant so that rhythmic respiration can start as soon as possible. Finally, and very important, the child should not be disturbed unnecessarily once breathing has started.

Resuscitation

When considering active methods for treating asphyxia, personal experience and knowledge of the background of a particular case condition the choice of method. It is impossible to be dogmatic about what must be done, or indeed when anything should be done, although in practice the decision is seldom difficult since the majority of mature infants respond to the simple routine already outlined, aided perhaps by the administration of oxygen. In extreme cases of asphyxia active measures must be instituted at once, but in those cases of doubtful origin, or in those which progressively deteriorate, a decision may be difficult. In such a situation the Apgar score is most helpful. The primary object is to prevent the vicious circle of hypoxia. Whatever the cause of the failure to breathe, the respiratory centres are depressed and the hypoxia which follows depresses them further.

It is always assumed that the newborn infant has a far greater tolerance to oxygen-lack than the adult, but unfortunately there is no data available on this point. Throughout uterine life foetal blood is relatively unsaturated with oxygen when compared with the adult, and the foetus is adapted to contend with the poor rate of diffusion of oxygen between the maternal placental circulation and its own. Moreover, during pregnancy there is a continuous reduction in this oxygen saturation, and finally in labour periods of acute hypoxia occur each time the uterus contracts. Several factors counteract these natural handicaps, but most important is the oxygen capacity of foetal blood which is greater than that of maternal blood. This is acquired by the increased affinity of foetal haemoglobin for oxygen (see carriage of oxygen in foetus, p. 104). After birth a high percentage of this haemoglobin remains for a week or more. There is also evidence that anaerobic metabolism can take place in foetal life and that this may persist for some time after birth. Clinically it has been shown that the heart will continue to beat for as long as 50 minutes after birth in the absence of breathing.

Many practitioners argue that little is to be lost by active treatment at an early stage in all doubtful cases, and indeed since our knowledge of the ultimate morbidity that may accrue from neonatal hypoxia is slight, much might be gained. The late effects of asphyxia are difficult to assess but include an increase in the immediate postnatal complications and the production of neurological damage. Despite the capacity of foetal and neonatal tissues to tolerate oxygen lack, this is no excuse for allowing hypoxia to persist and to risk the brain suffering damage. Hibbard (1955) has described the effective resuscitation by endotracheal aspiration and insufflation of oxygen, commencing 15 minutes after delivery, of a mature infant in white asphyxia but with a fair heart beat. When followed up one year later the infant was blind, spastic, and suffering from convulsions. If cerebral damage may be the result, as well as the cause, of asphyxia, it can only be prevented by efficient and *immediate* resuscitation—no one can estimate how much hypoxia a particular infant can tolerate. Moreover, such a case underlines the necessity for a simple means of oxygenating the baby which can be utilised by the midwife when the more skilled help needed for tracheal intubation is not at once available. Intubation of the trachea, the administration of oxygen by this and other routes, and assisted respiration, are not necessarily dangerous or traumatic procedures when carried out carefully, although no one would wish to recommend their routine use. The neonatal mortality rate has fallen in the past few years, but the fall hardly compares with that for maternal mortality, and the number of deaths from asphyxia is still large enough to suggest that ample room exists for improvement in our treatment of this condition of the newborn. The greatest field undoubtedly lies in the care of the premature infant.

The various methods of resuscitation are described individually.

Intubation

The indication for intubation in neonatal asphyxia can be broadly summarised in four groups. First, when there is suspected inhalation of amniotic or other material: this is particularly likely after Caesarean section. Secondly, when a full-term infant is born severely asphyxiated and in a state of shock. Thirdly, when a premature infant is born in poor condition, after foetal distress. Fourthly, when a full-term infant at one minute has not established regular respirations.

The principal object of intubation is to clear the respiratory passage of foreign material which may impede the normal passage of air. Oxygen can be administered directly once this has been done, and neither spontaneous nor artificial respiration is necessary to make the method effective. But, as will be described, there are other simple methods of getting oxygen into the blood stream, so that unless there is a strong reason—such as respiratory obstruction—or an indication for attempted artificial respiration through an endotracheal tube, intubation solely for this purpose is rarely justified. In mature infants the lungs can be easily expanded and rhythmically ventilated by intermittent positive pressure when spontaneous respiration has not started. A pressure of between 15 and 30 cm. of water is required. In fact a mature newborn infant is capable of developing by its own muscular power much greater negative pressures than these. In practice the act of intubation often provides a stimulus which starts respiration if it has not already commenced, so that it is difficult to be dogmatic about the overall value of artificial respiration in starting respiration, though it may aid complete and rapid pulmonary expansion. On the other hand, the dangers of intubation and intermittent positive-pressure respiration in the mature newborn infant have been exaggerated. With normal skill and care glottic trauma and rupture of lung tissue should not occur.

If spontaneous respiration does not start within a minute or two after intubation, clearing of the airway, and the use of oxygen in mature infants, then it is unlikely to do so, whether intermittent positive-pressure is used or not. The presumption must be made that extensive damage to the central or peripheral mechanism has occurred sometime before or during the actual birth.

Delayed intubation, some hours or so after birth, to relieve obstruction which is preventing complete expansion, is rarely justified, because the offending material will almost certainly have already been sucked into the peripheral bronchial tree where it is inaccessible. Furthermore, at this stage the infant will have full muscle tone and the act of laryngoscopy will be more traumatic.

Technique of intubation and artificial respiration.—The infant should be placed on its back on a flat padded board. Intubation is most easily performed with a small straight-bladed laryngoscope so that the curled epiglottis can be lifted, and the tube passed through the glottis. The choice of tube is largely a matter of personal preference, but the Portsmouth neonatal resuscitation tube (Tunstall and Hodges, 1961) and the St. Thomas's Hospital tube designed and described by Barrie (1963) have much to recommend them. They are made of vinyl and can, if necessary, be left in the trachea for long periods without the risk of causing oedema or ulceration. Both are available in sterile disposable packs and the latter is small enough to accommodate a very premature baby, and has a right-sided bevel which lessens the risk of total respiratory obstruction should it enter the right main bronchus. Immediately after intubation suction should be applied to the tube. This is efficient and safe, provided the suction pressure is gentle and that spontaneous respiration has not commenced. When there is a considerable amount of mucus present, it may be necessary to remove the endotracheal tube and after clearing it, reinsert it in the trachea. This process may be repeated several times to produce a clear airway.

As an alternative, a small sterile vinyl catheter of 1 mm. diameter can be passed down the tube, but this is of little value if the secretions are viscid. Oxygen should be given at a flow of 2 litres per minute by means of the simple device described by Barrie (1963) and illustrated in Fig. 20. Intermittent positive pres-

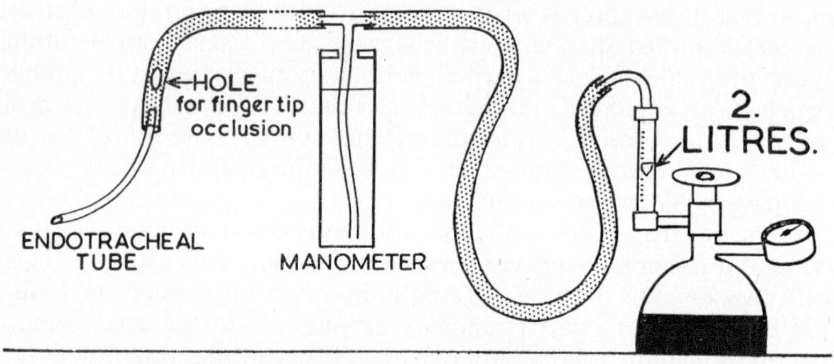

3/FIG. 20.—Neonatal resuscitation equipment.

sure can be built up in the infant's lungs by alternately opening and closing the outlet hole in the system. Essentially, the apparatus consists of a source of oxygen (with reducing valve), an endotracheal tube or face-mask, and a water-bubble safety-valve in the circuit. The latter is merely a wide-bore hollow tube the end of which is inserted to a prescribed depth in a jar of water. If it is placed 30 cm. below the surface then the infant's lungs can be inflated to a maximum pressure of 30 cm. of water. As soon as this figure is reached the excess oxygen escapes harmlessly to the atmosphere. This simple and inexpensive device will avoid over-inflation of the child's lungs. A pressure of 40 cm. of water should never be exceeded because of the risk of causing pulmonary damage. Normally a flow rate of 2 litres/minute of oxygen should be delivered into the apparatus. However, if large flows are inadvertently used, pressures of as high as 90 cm. H_2O can be produced. This circumstance can be avoided by using an under-water tube of at least 8 mm. internal diameter, and ensuring that the outlet vent from the bottle is adequately large (Mathias, 1966). If these simple precautions are observed the pressure delivered to the child with the tube set 40 cm. below the surface of the liquid will not rise above 45 cm. H_2O even with an oxygen flow-rate as high as 25 litres/minute. It is generally believed that a sharp rise in pressure is less likely to cause injury to the lung than a sustained one.

The lungs can also be inflated by manual squeezing of a breathing bag filled with oxygen and connected to a small mask which accurately fits the infant's face. Distension of the stomach must be avoided by gentle pressure beneath the costal margin. Mouth to mouth respiration and compression of the thoracic cage are inadequate and time-wasting practices which should be avoided if resuscitation is really essential, unless they are the only methods available.

Oxygen Therapy

Oxygen is the first need in asphyxia. But the giving of oxygen or oxygen-rich mixtures is of little value if they do not reach the vital centres. The child must have a clear airway,* adequate respiratory movement, and an effective circulation if simple methods of administration are to succeed. If these conditions are fulfilled then oxygen can best be given through a small catheter, the tip of which should lie just behind the tongue. The catheter can be passed through the mouth or through the nose and a flow of 2 litres per minute of the gas should be supplied. In the absence of respiratory activity oxygen must be administered either via a mask and intermittent positive pressure as described above, or intratracheally to ensure that some is absorbed into the blood stream and reaches the vital centres. Intragastric oxygen is of no value at all.

Endotracheal oxygen.—When oxygen is administered intratracheally absorption occurs, irrespective of spontaneous respiration, from the bronchial mucosa. If respiration has commenced or commences soon after intubation, an oxygen-rich mixture may then be given by the intratracheal route. Nevertheless great care should be taken in the selection of apparatus to ensure that the infant's lungs are not subjected to a high pressure of oxygen.

Hyperbaric oxygen.—A detailed discussion of this form of oxygen therapy is contained in Chapter 6. Hutchison and his colleagues (1963) describe the use of hyperbaric oxygen for the treatment of asphyxia neonatorum and consider that it is an effective method of making oxygen quickly available to anoxic tissues. Whether it is overall a better method than those previously described remains to be proven, but at the time of writing it cannot be considered a substitute for intubation and inflation of the infant's lungs. Hyperbaric oxygenation can also relieve the hypoxia associated with the respiratory distress syndrome, but it is ineffective in the treatment of the associated respiratory acidosis (Hutchison *et al.*, 1962).

Danger of oxygen therapy in newborn infants.—The principal danger of oxygen therapy is the uncontrolled use of oxygen flows at high pressure. Oxygen should never be administered without some device to avoid the possible build-up of

* "A clear airway" in this context implies freedom from the presence of foreign material rather than simple obstruction from the tongue. The latter can, however, occur and may be an indication for the use of tongue forceps so that the tongue can be held well forward. The occasions on which such a form of treatment is necessary are very rare indeed, and the routine use of tongue forceps is to be deprecated.

pressure within the respiratory tract. A special reducing valve designed to limit the pressure and flow of gas obtainable from the cylinder is of great value. Safety can be further assured when the trachea is intubated, by the use of an outlet hole to release the excess gas should an unduly high pressure start to build up.

Retrolental fibroplasia.—The administration of oxygen to premature babies may lead to the production of retrolental fibroplasia unless the special precautions outlined later are observed.

This disease is characterised by the formation of a fibrovascular membrane behind the lens. It is incurable and almost exclusively confined to premature babies.

Ashton *et al.* (1953), from experimental work on kittens, have shown how exposure to oxygen may produce the disease. They used kittens for their work because the degree and type of vascularisation of the retina of these animals at birth, and for some weeks afterwards, is comparable to that of a premature baby. If kittens are kept in a high concentration of oxygen at atmospheric pressure for a day or two after birth, the ingrowing retinal vessels become vasoconstricted and eventually obliterated. This vascular closure is permanent and when the animals are returned to air only a few vessels are likely to be open, and these only partly so. Severe anoxia develops and leads to an extensive and abnormal proliferation of vessels, producing a picture like that of retrolental fibroplasia. Oxygen concentrations below 35 per cent do not have any deleterious effect.

The connection between retrolental fibroplasia and oxygen has been noted clinically by several observers (Campbell, 1951; Ryan, 1952; Crosse and Evans, 1952; Patz *et al.*, 1952), but cases have been reported in infants who have had no oxygen therapy at all. It is not infrequently associated with other cerebral defects and is often part of a general cerebral disorder resulting from anoxaemia (Scott, 1954). Moreover, vaso-proliferation might well be initiated by other factors. Prolonged oxygen administration will certainly aggravate the situation by producing vasoconstriction, and the more frequent use of this form of therapy in recent years perhaps accounts for the higher incidence of the disease.

Oxygen should only be administered to premature babies when it is essential, and then for the shortest time possible. It must be emphasised that oxygen is only dangerous if it raises the saturation of arterial blood above the normal level (i.e. 95 per cent). There is no risk, therefore, in using oxygen in premature babies when cyanosis is present. Nevertheless, once equilibrium has been restored the excessively high concentration of oxygen should be withdrawn in order to prevent the occurrence of retrolental fibroplasia. Concentrations above 35 per cent should be avoided unless for very brief periods. Forrester *et al.* (1954) and Gordon *et al.* (1954) have reported that the use of measured concentrations of oxygen of 40 per cent or less for the shortest possible time eliminate the occurrence of retrolental fibroplasia, and do so without affecting the survival rate of the infants.

Measurement of oxygen concentration in incubators.—When oxygen is administered for anything but the briefest period of time the actual flow used should be recorded by the use of a rotameter and the concentration received by the infant measured at regular intervals. Oxygen concentration in the air of an incubator can be measured by a simple analyser, and Banister *et al.* (1954) have described an instrument for obtaining continuous records.

Stimulants and Antidotes

Carbon dioxide should not be given to a newborn baby. In the presence of neonatal asphyxia the concentration in the infant will already be higher than normal, and any addition to it is more likely to depress rather than stimulate respiration. Excess of carbon dioxide accounts for much of the circulatory collapse in white asphyxia.

Respiratory stimulants such as lobeline and camphor are generally to be avoided. Work by Barrie *et al.* (1962) has shown that nikethamide and vanillic acid diethylamide ("Vandid") produce a consistent stimulant action on respiration and that they are equally effective administered lingually as when they are injected intravenously. Barrie and his co-workers consider that these drugs are useful in less severe degrees of asphyxia neonatorum, when their prior use may avoid the need for intubation. The recommended doses are either nikethamide 125 mg. (0·5 ml. of a 25 per cent solution) or "Vandid" 25 mg. (0·5 ml. of a 5 per cent solution) dropped on to the tongue. Half these doses should be used for premature infants. Failure of the infant to respond within one minute to either of these drugs suggests severe respiratory depression.

Specific antidotes are often very useful. The respiratory depressant effects of morphine and its related analogues such as pethidine can be offset by N-allylnormorphine. If the mother has had a large dose of a depressant analgesic within an hour or two of delivery, the antidote may be given to her either intravenously or intramuscularly about ten to fifteen minutes before the expected delivery to allow time for it to reach the foetus. The dose varies from 1–10 mg. but 5 mg. is generally sufficient. Large doses may produce undesirable reactions such as nausea, sickness and mental confusion in the mother. Alternatively, N-allylnormorphine may be given to the child by injection into the umbilical cord immediately after birth. In this case the solution must be diluted so that 1 mg. can be given slowly. It should be injected three to four inches away from the umbilicus and massaged towards the infant. N-allylnormorphine and similar compounds only offset the respiratory depression due to morphine and like drugs. If the concentration of morphine in the baby is too low to affect respiration there is a danger that the antidotes themselves may cause depression, and in these circumstances they must never be used. It also seems probable that effective antagonism of the respiratory depression will lead to removal of some analgesia, so that if they are given to the mother, the last few minutes of labour may require inhalational analgesia or anaesthesia to compensate.

The synthetic antagonist amiphenazole may also be used. It is claimed that this will relieve the severe respiratory depression of morphine and its analogues without impairing the analgesia. The adult dose is 20–40 mg. and for neonates is 3 mg.

Treatment of Metabolic Abnormalities

Severely asphyxiated infants may suffer from a metabolic acidosis and hypoglycaemia. Therefore once respiration is established consideration should be given to correcting these metabolic abnormalities. As soon as is practical after initial resuscitation blood should be taken for assessment of acid-base status and blood sugar (the latter can be rapidly and conveniently estimated using Dextrostix). Suitable intravenous correction can then be undertaken. When deciding whether this is necessary it must be borne in mind that the administration of hypertonic solutions can rapidly expand the intravascular volume, and that their use in the asphyxiated infant, especially the premature, could lead to or aggravate intraventricular haemorrhage.

Early Postnatal Care of Premature Babies

By definition any child weighing less than 5½ pounds (2·5 kg.) at birth is considered to be premature. Prematurity does not cause harmful effects on the future growth of the child and there is no evidence to suggest that either physical or mental development differs from those who were mature at birth.

Premature infants not only have the disadvantage of a low arterial oxygen saturation at birth, but also difficulty in oxygenating blood after birth. The reason is twofold. First, the alveolar membrane in the lungs of the premature infant is thicker and therefore the transfer of gases is slower; secondly, the number of pulmonary capillaries per unit area is fewer so that the total vascular bed is smaller.

Mortality and morbidity are high in premature infants, and since most deaths occur during the first 24 hours after birth, the immediate and correct care of the child is most important. Everything must be prepared in advance. Particular care must be taken to limit the use of depressant drugs given to the mother during labour, while anoxia must be scrupulously avoided (see Chapter 52). Generally, because of the size of the foetus, labour is relatively easy and pain-free, so that neither analgesic nor anaesthetic agents are needed in more than minimal dosage, while in exceptional cases it may be possible and preferable to dispense with them altogether.

After birth the child should be nursed in a warm and humid atmosphere. A special incubator will supply the optimum conditions which are needed according to the body size and the condition of the child. The temperature of the premature infant is very unstable, since the regulating mechanisms are undeveloped; it is usually subnormal and must be adjusted by varying the temperature of the external environment. Room temperatures of 18–24° C and an incubator temperature of 31–34° C are desirable, while the humidity of the incubator should be between 55 and 65 per cent. The abdominal skin temperature of the child should be 36–36·5° C.

The addition of oxygen to the air breathed in the incubator may be essential to maintain life, but the potential dangers of this therapy to premature infants must be remembered and avoided by never allowing concentrations above 40 per cent to reach the infant, and then only for the shortest time necessary (see p. 126). The immature peripheral respiratory mechanism may also need help, and although premature babies usually breathe spontaneously, the ventilation they produce is often insufficient to prevent the onset of asphyxia. The effect of drugs and aspiration of amniotic fluid accentuate this inadequacy.

To some extent poor ventilation can be offset by the more active use of oxygen therapy, giving it by the intratracheal route. Although good oxygenation may lead to regular respiration, atelectasis often persists and hyaline membrane is very likely present. On the other hand, if adequate and vigorous respiratory activity occurs soon after birth the risk of a fatality from hyaline membrane is greatly diminished (Donald, 1954). For all these reasons assisted or augmented respiration may be of great value in the period soon after birth and for some time afterwards.

REFERENCES

ABRAMSON, H. (1960). *Resuscitation of the Newborn Infant*, pp. 41 and 51. St. Louis: C. V. Mosby Co.

ADRIAN, E. D. (1933). Afferent impulses in the vagus and their effect on respiration. *J. Physiol.* (*Lond.*), **79,** 332.

ALLEN, D. W., WYMAN, J., Jr., and SMITH, C. A. (1953). The oxygen equilibrium of foetal and adult haemoglobin. *J. biol. Chem.*, **203,** 81.

ALLEN, F. M. (1945). Intravenous obstetrical anesthesia. *Amer. J. Surg.*, **70,** 283.

APGAR, V. (1953). A proposal for a new method of evaluation of the newborn infant. *Curr. Res. Anesth.*, **32,** 260.

APGAR, V., HOLADAY, D. A., JAMES, L. S., PRINCE, C. E., and WEISBROT, I. M. (1957). Comparison of regional and general anesthesia in obstetrics with special reference to transmission of cyclopropane across the placenta. *J. Amer. med. Ass.*, **165,** 2155.

APGAR, V., HOLADAY, D. A., JAMES, L. S., WEISBROT, I. M., and BERNERS, C. (1958). Evaluation of the newborn infant. *J. Amer. med. Ass.*, **168,** 1985.

APGAR, V., and PAPPER, E. M. (1952). Transmission of drugs across the placenta. *Curr. Res. Anesth.*, **31,** 309.

ASHTON, N., WARD, B. and SERPELL, G. (1953). Role of oxygen in the genesis of retrolental fibroplasia. A preliminary report. *Brit. J. Ophthal.*, **37,** 513.

AVERY, M. E., and MEAD, J. (1959). Surface properties in relation to atelectasis and hyaline membrane disease. *Amer. J. Dis. Child.*, **97,** 517.

BANISTER, P., KAY, R. H., and COXON, R. V. (1954). Continuous gas analysis in the control of oxygen therapy for infants. *Lancet*, **2,** 777.

BARCROFT, J. (1946). *Researches in Prenatal Life*. Springfield, Ill.: Charles C. Thomas.

BARRIE, H. (1963). Resuscitation of the newborn. *Lancet*, **1,** 650.

BARRIE, H., COTTOM, D., and WILSON, B. D. R. (1962). Respiratory stimulants in the newborn. *Lancet*, **2,** 742.

BARTELS, H., MOLL, W., and METCALFE, J. (1962). Physiology of gas exchange in the human placenta. *Amer. J. Obstet. Gynec.*, **84,** 1714.

BELINKOFF, S., and HALL, O. W. (1950). Intravenous alcohol during labour. *Amer. J. Obstet. Gynec.*, **59,** 429.

BELLVILLE, J. W., and SEED, J. C. (1960). The effect of drugs on the respiratory response to carbon dioxide. *Anesthesiology*, **21,** 727.

BØE, F. (1954). Vascular morphology of the human placenta. The mammalian fetus. Physiological aspects of development. *Cold Spr. Harb. Symp. quant. Biol.*, **19,** 29.

BOUTROS, A. R., and WOODFORD, V. R. (1963). Blood carbonic anhydrase activity. A possible role in the production of acid-base imbalance in children and infants. *Canad. Anaesth. Soc. J.*, **10,** 428.

BRADLEY, R. D., and SEMPLE, S. J. G. (1962). A comparison of certain acid-base characteristics of arterial blood, jugular venous blood and cerebrospinal fluid in man, and the effect on them of some acute and chronic acid-base disturbances. *J. Physiol.* (*Lond.*), **160,** 381.

Bradley, R. D., Spencer, G. T., and Semple, S. J. G. (1965). In *Cerebrospinal Fluid and the Regulation of Ventilation.* Eds. Brooks, C. McC., Kao, F. F. and Lloyd, B. B. Oxford: Blackwell.

Brandfass, R. T. (1959). Oxygen-saturation determination of the newborn in vaginal and caesarean delivery using various anesthetics. *W. Va. med. J.*, **55,** 161.

Buller, A. J., and Young, I. M. (1949). The action of *d*-tubocurarine chloride on foetal neuromuscular transmission and the placental transfer of this drug in the rabbit. *J. Physiol.* (*Lond.*), **109,** 412.

Burns, B. D. (1963). The central control of respiratory movements. *Brit. med. Bull.*, **19,** 7.

Burns, B. D., and Salmoiraghi, G. C. (1960). Repetitive firing of respiratory neurones during their burst activity. *J. Neurophysiol.*, **23,** 27.

Campbell, K. (1951). Intensive oxygen therapy as a possible cause of retrolental fibroplasia: a clinical approach. *Med. J. Aust.*, **2,** 48.

Christian, G., and Greene, N. M. (1962). Blood carbonic anhydrase activity in anesthetized man. *Anesthesiology*, **23,** 179.

Clements, J. A. (1962). Studies of surface phenomena in relation to pulmonary function. *Physiologist*, **5,** 11.

Cohen, E. N., Paulson, W. J., Wall, J., and Elert, B. (1953). Thiopental, curare and nitrous oxide anesthesia for cesarian section with studies on placental transmission. *Surg. Gynec. Obstet.*, **97,** 456.

Crawford, J. S., and Gardiner, J. E. (1956). Some aspects of obstetric anaesthesia. Part II. The use of relaxant drugs. *Brit. J. Anaesth.*, **28,** 154.

Crawford, J. S., and Rudofsky, S. (1965). Placental transmission and neonatal metabolism of promazine. *Brit. J. Anaesth.*, **37,** 303.

Cross, K. W., Hooper, J. M. D., and Oppé, T. E. (1953). The effect of inhalation of carbon dioxide in air on the respiration of the full-term and premature infant. *J. Physiol.* (*Lond.*), **122,** 264.

Cross, K. W., Klaus, M., Tooley, W. H., and Weisser, K. (1960). The response of the new-born baby to inflation of the lungs. *J. Physiol.* (*Lond.*), **151,** 551.

Cross, K. W., Tizard, J. P. M., and Trythall, D. A. H. (1958). The gaseous metabolism of the new-born infant breathing 15 per cent oxygen. *Acta paediat.* (*Uppsala*), **47,** 217.

Crosse, V. M., and Evans, P. J. (1952). Prevention of retrolental fibroplasia. *Arch. Ophthal.* (*N.Y.*), **48,** 83.

Davie, I., Scott, D. B., and Stephen, G. W. (1970). Respiratory effects of pentazocine and pethidine in patients anaesthetised with halothane and oxygen. *Brit. J. Anaesth.*, **42,** 113.

Davis, M. E., and Potter, E. (1946). Intra-uterine respiration of the human fetus. *J. Amer. med. Ass.*, **131,** 1194.

Dawes, G. S. (1961). Changes in the circulation at birth. *Brit. med. Bull.*, **17,** 150.

Day, R., Goodfellow, A. M., Apgar, V., and Beck, G. I. (1952). Pressure-time relationships in safe correction of atelectasis in animal lungs. *Pediatrics,* **10,** 593.

Donald, I. (1954). Atelectasis neonatorum. *J. Obstet. Gynaec. Brit. Emp.*, **61,** 725.

Donald, I., and Lord, J. (1953). Augmented respiration: studies in atelectasis neonatorum. *Lancet*, **1,** 9.

Donald, I., and Steiner, R. E. (1953). Radiography in the diagnosis of hyaline membrane. *Lancet*, **2,** 846.

Downs, H. S., and Morrison, P. H. (1963). Effect of spinal anesthesia on foetal heart rate. *Calif. Med.*, **99,** 374.

Dunbar, B. S., Ovassapian, A., and Smith, T. C. (1967). The effects of methoxyflurane on ventilation in man. *Anesthesiology*, **28,** 1020.

FARMAN, J. V. (1962). Heat losses in infants undergoing surgery in air-conditioned theatres. *Brit. J. Anaesth.*, **34,** 543.

FENCL, V., VALE, J. R., and BROCH, J. A. (1969). Respiration and cerebral blood flow in metabolic acidosis and alkalosis in humans. *J. appl. Physiol.*, **27,** 67.

FINK, B. R. (1961). Influence of cerebral activity in wakefulness on regulation of breathing. *J. appl. Physiol.*, **16,** 15.

FINK, B. R., HANKS, E. C., HOLADAY, D. A., and NGAI, S. H. (1960). Monitoring of ventilation by integrated diaphragmatic electromyogram: determination of carbon dioxide (CO_2) threshold in anesthetized man. *J. Amer. med. Ass.*, **172,** 1367.

FLOWERS, C. E. (1957). Transfer of materials across the human placenta. *Amer. J. Obstet. Gynec.*, **74,** 705.

FLOWERS, C. E. (1959). The placental transmission of barbiturates and thiobarbiturates and their pharmacological action on mother and infant. *Amer. J. Obstet. Gynec.*, **78,** 730.

FORRESTER, R. M., JEFFERSON, E., and NAUNTON, W. J. (1954). Oxygen and retrolental fibroplasia. A seven-year study. *Lancet*, **2,** 258.

FOUTS, J. R., and ADAMSON, R. H. (1959). Drug metabolism in the newborn rabbit. *Science*, **129,** 897.

GARDNER, H. L., LEVINE, H., and BODANSKY, M. (1940). Concentration of paraldehyde in the blood following its administration during labor. *Amer. J. Obstet. Gynec.*, **40,** 435.

GORDON, H. H., LUBCHENCO, L., and HIX, I. (1954). Observations on the etiology of retrolental fibroplasia. *Bull. Johns. Hopk. Hosp.*, **94,** 34.

GUZ, A., NOBLE, M. I. M., TRENCHARD, D., COCHRANE, H. L., and MAKEY, A. R. (1964). Studies on the vagus nerves in man: their role in respiratory and circulatory control. *Clin. Sci.*, **27,** 293.

HANKS, E. C., NGAI, S. H., and FINK, B. R. (1961). The respiratory threshold for carbon dioxide in anesthetized man. Determination of carbon dioxide threshold during halothane anesthesia. *Anesthesiology*, **22,** 393.

HELLMAN, L. M., JOHNSON, H. L., TOLLES, W. E., and JONES, E. H. (1962). Some factors affecting the fetal heart rate. *Amer. J. Obstet. Gynec.*, **82,** 1055.

HERING, E. (1868). Die Selbststeuerung der Athmung den Nervus vagus. *S.B. Akad. Wiss. Wien., II. Abth.*, **57,** 672.

HERING, E., and BREUER, J. (1868). Die Selbststeuerung der Athmung durch den Nervus vagus. *S.B. Akad. Wiss. Wien., II. Abth*, **58,** 909.

HIBBARD, B. M. (1955). Late result of prolonged endotracheal insufflation in asphyxia neonatorum. *Brit. med. J.*, **2,** 183.

HOFF, H. E., and BRECKENRIDGE, C. G. (1955). Regulation of respiration. *In* Fulton, J. F. *A Textbook of Physiology*, pp. 867–886. Philadelphia: W. B. Saunders.

HON, E. H., BRADFIELD, A. H., and HESS, O. W. (1961). The electronic evaluation of the fetal heart rate. V: The vagal factor in fetal bradycardia. *Amer. J. Obstet. Gynec.*, **82,** 291.

HUTCHISON, J. H., KERR, M. M., MCPHAIL, M. F. M., DOUGLAS, T. A., SMITH, G., NORMAN, J. N., and BATES, E. H. (1962). Studies in the treatment of the pulmonary syndrome of the newborn. *Lancet*, **2,** 465.

HUTCHISON, J. H., KERR, M. M., WILLIAMS, K. G., and HOPKINSON, W. I. (1963). Hyperbaric oxygen in the resuscitation of the newborn. *Lancet*, **2,** 1019.

JOHN, A. H. (1965). Placental transfer of atropine and the effect on foetal heart rate. *Brit. J. Anaesth.*, **37,** 57.

KARLBERG, P., ESCARDO, F., CHERRY, R. B., LIND, J., and WEGELIUS, C. (1957). Studies of the respiration of the newborn in the first minutes of life. *Acta paediat. (Uppsala)*, **46,** 396.

KATZ, R. L., and NGAI, S. H. (1962). Respiratory effects of diethyl ether in the cat. *J. Pharmacol. exp. Ther.*, **138,** 329.

LANE, D. J. (1970). D. M. Thesis, University of Oxford.

LARSON, C. P., JR., EGER, E. I., II, MAULLEM, M., BUECHEL, D. R., MUNSON, E. S., and EISELE, J. H. (1969). Effects of diethylether and methoxyflurane on ventilation. II. A comparative study in man. *Anesthesiology*, **30,** 174.

LEUSEN, I. R. (1954*a*). Chemosensitivity of the respiratory centre. Influence of CO_2 in the cerebral ventricles on respiration. *Amer. J. Physiol.*, **176,** 39.

LEUSEN, I. R. (1954*b*). Chemosensitivity of the respiratory centre. Influence of changes on the H^+ and total buffer concentrations in the cerebral ventricles on respiration. *Amer. J. Physiol.*, **176,** 45.

LLOYD, B. B., JUKES, M. G. M., and CUNNINGHAM, D. J. C. (1958). The relation between alveolar oxygen pressure and the respiratory response to carbon dioxide in man. *Quart. J. exp. Physiol.*, **43,** 214.

MCDOWALL, D. G., and HARPER, A. M. (1970). Cerebral blood flow and CSF pH during hyperventilation. In *Progress in Anaesthesiology. Proceedings of the Fourth World Congress of Anaesthesiologists*, p. 542. Amsterdam: Excerpta Medica Foundation.

MCKECHNIE, F. B., and CONVERSE, J. G. (1955). Placental transmission of thiopental. *Amer. J. Obstet. Gynec.*, **70,** 639.

MARX, G. (1961). Placental transfer and drugs used in anesthesia. *Anesthesiology*, **22,** 294.

MATHIAS, J. (1966). Resuscitation of the newborn. *Lancet*, **1,** 262.

MITCHELL, R. A. (1965). In *Cerebrospinal Fluid and the Regulation of Ventilation*, p. 109. Eds. Brooks, C. McC., Kao, F. F. and Lloyd, B. B. Oxford: Blackwell.

MITCHELL, R. A. (1966). In *Advances in Respiratory Physiology*. p. 1. Ed. Caro, C. G. London: Edward Arnold.

MITCHELL, R. A., LOESCHCKE, H. H., MASSION, W. H., and SEVERINGHAUS, J. W. (1963). Respiratory responses mediated through superficial chemosensitive areas on the medulla. *J. appl. Physiol.*, **18,** 523.

MOYA, F., and KVISSELGAARD, N. (1961). The placental transmission of succinylcholine. *Anesthesiology*, **22,** 1.

MOYA, F., and THORNDIKE, V. (1962). Passage of drugs across the placenta. *Amer. J. Obstet. Gynec.*, **84,** 1778.

MUALLEM, M., LARSON, C. P., JR. and EGER, E. I., II (1969). The effects of diethyl ether on Pa_{CO_2} in dogs with and without vagal, somatic and sympathetic block. *Anesthesiology*, **30,** 185.

MUNSON, E. S., LARSON, C. P., JR., BABAD, A. A., REGAN, M. J., BUECHEL, D. R. and EGER, E. I., II (1966). The effects of halothane, fluroxene and cyclopropane on ventilation: a comparative study in man. *Anesthesiology*, **27,** 716.

NGAI, S. H., FARHIE, S. E., and BRODY, D. C. (1961). Effects of trichloroethylene, halopropane and methoxyflurane on respiratory regulatory mechanisms. *J. Pharmacol. exp. Ther.*, **131,** 91.

NYIRJESY, I., HAEKS, B. L., HEBERT, J. E., HOPWOOD, H. G., and FALLS, H. C. (1963). Hazards of the use of paracervical block anesthesia in obstetrics. *Amer. J. Obstet. Gynec.*, **87,** 231.

PAGE, E. W. (1957). Transfer of materials across the human placenta. *Amer. J. Obstet. Gynec.*, **74,** 705.

PAPPENHEIMER, J. R., FENCL, V., HEISEY, S. R., and HELD, D. (1965). Role of cerebral fluids in control of respiration as studied in unanesthetized goats. *Amer. J. Physiol.*, **208,** 436.

PASKIN, S., SKOVSTED, P., and SMITH, T. C. (1968). Failure of the Hering-Breuer reflex to account for tachypnoea in anesthetized man. *Anesthesiology*, **29,** 550.

PATTLE, R. E. (1963). The lining layer of the lung alveoli. *Brit. med. Bull.*, **19,** 41.

PATZ, A., HOECK, L. E., and DE LA CRUZ, E. (1952). Studies on the effect of high oxygen administration in retrolental fibroplasia. I. Nursery observations. *Amer. J. Ophthal.*, **35,** 1248.

PITTS, R. F. (1946). Organisation of the respiratory center. *Physiol. Rev.*, **26,** 609.

PLOMAN, L., and PERSSON, B. H. (1957). On the transfer of barbiturates to the human foetus and their accumulation in some of its vital organs. *J. Obstet. Gynaec. Brit. Emp.*, **64,** 706.

POTTER, E. L. (1954). The trend of changes in causes of perinatal mortality. *J. Amer. med. Ass.*, **156,** 1471.

PRYSTOWSKY, H. (1957). Fetal Blood Studies. VII. The oxygen pressure gradient between the maternal and fetal bloods of the human in normal and abnormal pregnancy. *Bull. Johns Hopk. Hosp.*, **101,** 48.

REYNOLDS, E. O. R., ROBERTSON, N. R. C., and WIGGLESWORTH, J. S. (1968). Hyaline membrane disease, respiratory distress, and surfactant deficiency. *Pediatrics*, **42,** 758.

REYNOLDS, F., and TAYLOR, G. (1970). Maternal and neonatal blood concentrations of bupivacaine (A comparison with lignocaine during continuous extradural analgesia). *Anaesthesia*, **25,** 14.

RIGG, J. R. A., ENGEL, L. A., and RITCHIE, B. C. (1970). The ventilatory response to carbon dioxide during partial paralysis with tubocurarine. *Brit. J. Anaesth*, **42,** 105.

ROBERTS, H., KANE, K. M., PERCIVAL, N., SNOW, P., and PLEASE, N. W. (1957). Effects of some analgesic drugs used in childbirth, with special reference to variation in respiratory minute volume of the newborn. *Lancet*, **1,** 282.

ROOT, B., EICHNER, E., and SUNSHINE, I. (1961). Blood secobarbital levels and their clinical correlation in mothers and newborn infants. *Amer. J. Obstet. Gynec.*, **81,** 948.

RORKE, M. J. (1970). Maternal oxygenation and the unborn foetus. In *Progress in Anaesthesiology. Proceedings of the Fourth World Congress of Anaesthesiologists*, p. 654. Amsterdam: Excerpta Medica Foundation.

RYAN, H. (1952). Retrolental fibroplasia: a clinicopathologic study. *Amer. J. Ophthal.*, **35,** 329.

SCHMERMUND, H. J., KITTEL, E., and SCHMOLLING, E. (1961). Placental penetration of short-acting relaxants. *Arch. Gynäk.*, **195,** 288.

SCHMIDT, C. F. (1956). in *Medical Physiology*. Ed. P. Bard. St. Louis: C. V. Mosby Co.

SCHWARZ, R. (1958). Untersuchungen zur diaplacentaren Passage von Gallamin. *Anaesthesist*, **7,** 299.

SCOPES, J. W. (1970). Idiopathic respiratory distress syndrome. *Brit. J. Hosp. Med.*, **3,** 579.

SCOTT, G. I. (1954). Discussion on the neuro-ophthalmological aspects of failure of vision in children. *Proc. roy. Soc. Med.*, **47,** 491.

SEVERINGHAUS, J. W., and LARSON, C. P. (1965). "Respiration in Anesthesia." In *Handbook of Physiology—Respiration II*, Chap. 49, p. 1223. Washington, D.C.: American Physiological Society.

SEVERINGHAUS, J. W., MITCHELL, R. A., RICHARDSON, B. W., and SINGER, M. M. (1963). Respiratory control at high altitude suggesting active transport regulation of CSF pH. *J. appl. Physiol.*, **18,** 1155.

SHERIDAN, C. A., and ROBSON, J. G. (1959). Fluothane in obstetrical anaesthesia. *Canad. Anaesth. Soc. J.*, **6,** 365.

SILVERMAN, W. A., FERTIG, J. W., and BERGER, A. P. (1958). Effect of environmental temperature on premature infants. *Pediatrics*, **22,** 876.

SMITH, C. A. (1951). *Physiology of the Newborn Infant*, 2nd edit. Springfield, Ill.: Charles C. Thomas.

SMITH, C. A., and BARKER, R. H. (1942). Ether in the blood of the newborn infant. *Amer. J. Obstet. Gynec.*, **43,** 763.

SMITH, C. A., and CHISHOLM, T. C. (1942). Intrapulmonary pressures in new born infants. *J. Pediat.*, **20,** 338.

TAYLOR, E. S., VON FUMETTI, H. H., ESSIG, L. L., GOODMAN, S. N., and WALKER, L. C. (1955). Effects of demerol and trichlorethylene on arterial oxygen saturation in newborn. *Amer. J. Obstet. Gynec.*, **69,** 348.

THOMAS, J., CLIMIE, C. R., and MATHER, L. E. (1968). Placental transfer of lignocaine following lumbar epidural administration. *Brit. J. Anaesth.*, **40,** 965.

TUNSTALL, M. E., and HODGES, R. J. H. (1961). A sterile disposable neonatal tracheal tube. *Lancet*, **1,** 146.

USHER, R. (1961). "Respiratory distress syndrome of prematurity". In *Pediatric Clinics of North America*, p. 525. Ed. R. James Mackay. Philadelphia: W. B. Saunders Co.

VASICKA, A., QUILLIGAN, E. J., AZNAR, R., LIPSITZ, P. J., and BLOOR, B. M. (1960). Oxygen tension in maternal and fetal blood, amniotic fluid and cerebrospinal fluid of mother and baby. *Amer. J. Obstet. Gynec.*, **79,** 1041.

WAGNER, H. (1958). Zum warm-oder Kaltbehandlung von frühgeborenen: Vergleiche zweier verschieden gepflegter Kollektive. *Z. Kinderheilk.*, **81,** 261.

WANG, S. C., NGAI, S. H., and FRUMIN, M. J. (1957). Organization of central respiratory mechanisms in the brain stem of the cat: genesis of normal respiratory rythmicity. *Amer. J. Physiol.*, **190,** 333.

WHITTERIDGE, D., and BÜLBRING, E. (1944). Changes in activity of pulmonary receptors in anaesthesia and their influence on respiratory behaviour. *J. Pharmacol.*, **81,** 340.

WHITTERIDGE, D., and BÜLBRING, E. (1946). Changes in activity of pulmonary receptors in anaesthesia and their influence on respiratory behaviour. *Brit. med. Bull.*, **4,** 85.

WIDDICOMBE, J. G. (1961). Respiratory reflexes in man and other mammalian species. *Clin. Sci.*, **21,** 163.

WIDDICOMBE, J. G. (1963). Respiratory reflexes from the lungs. *Brit. med. Bull.*, **19,** 15.

WINDLE, W. F., DROGSTADT, C. A., MURRAY, D. E., and GREENE, R. R. (1938). Note on respiration-like movements of the human fetus. *Surg. Gynec. Obstet.*, **66,** 987.

WULF, H. (1958). Blutgaswerte und Neugeborenenatmung (Blood gas values and respiration of newborn). *Klin. Wschr.*, **36,** 234.

YOUNG, I. M. (1957). Adrenaline Hyperpnoea. (Ph.D. Thesis), Univ. London.

YOUNG, I. M. (1961). Blood pressure in the new-born baby. *Brit. med. Bull.*, **17,** 154.

YOUNG, I. M. (1962). Vasomotor tone in the skin blood vessels of the newborn infant. *Clin. Sci.*, **22,** 325.

FURTHER READING

BROOKS, C. MCC., KAO, F. F., and LLOYD, B. B. (Eds.) (1965). *Cerebrospinal Fluid and the Regulation of Ventilation.* Oxford: Blackwell.

COMROE, J. H. (1965). *Physiology of Respiration. An Introductory Text.* Chicago: Year Book Medical Publishers.

CRAWFORD, J. S. (1965). *Principles and Practice of Obstetric Anaesthesia*, 2nd. edit. Oxford: Blackwell.

Chapter 4

PULMONARY GAS EXCHANGE AND ACID-BASE BALANCE

THE function of the respiratory system is to maintain the partial pressures of oxygen (P_{O_2}) and carbon dioxide (P_{CO_2}) in the arterial blood as near to normal as possible under widely varying circumstances. The lungs are one link in a complex chain of systems, and provide the mechanisms which allow the transfer of oxygen and carbon dioxide between blood and air. Three principal factors are concerned in their function, namely: ventilation, diffusion, and pulmonary blood flow. Ventilation must not only be sufficient to move an adequate volume of air, but its distribution throughout the lungs must be related to the distribution and quantity of pulmonary blood flow. Finally, each gas must be able to diffuse across the alveolar membrane with ease.

VENTILATION

The terminology used in this chapter to describe the lung volumes and capacities was introduced by a group of American physiologists in an attempt to simplify the subject, and has now gained general acceptance (Table 1 and Fig 1). (Pappenheimer, 1950).

Tidal Volume and Minute Volume

The tidal volume is the amount of air passing in and out of the lungs and respiratory passages during each respiratory cycle. The quantity, therefore, varies with the size and age of the individual and the depth of respiration. It ranges from 19 ml. in the average newborn infant (less in premature infants) to

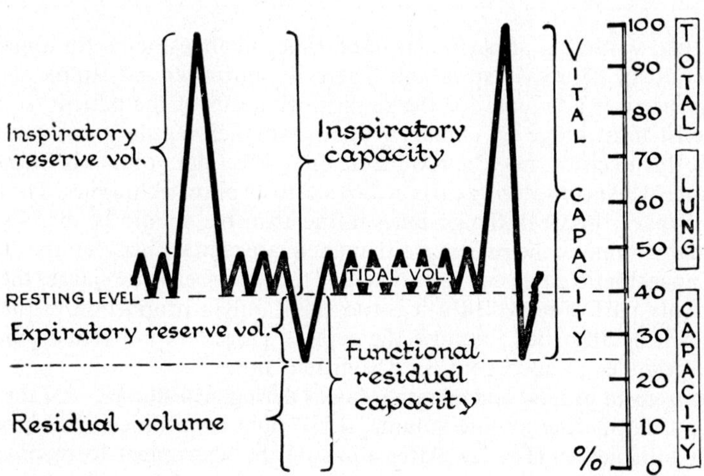

4/FIG. 1.—Spirometer record showing lung volumes and capacities.

between 450 and 750 ml. in resting adults. The tidal volume multiplied by the respiratory rate (breaths per minute) gives the minute volume.

4/TABLE 1

NOMENCLATURE FOR LUNG VOLUMES AND CAPACITIES, with normal values in adults. Normal values have been taken from Needham *et al.* (1954). The figures are mean values, with the standard deviation in brackets. 98 per cent of the population will lie within ± two standard deviations of the mean.

Terminology	*Explanation*	*Normal Values* M.	F.
Tidal volume	Volume of air inspired or expired at each breath.	660 (230)	550 (160)
Inspiratory reserve volume	Maximum volume of air that can be inspired after a normal inspiration	2240	1480
Expiratory reserve volume	Maximum volume of air that can be expired after a normal expiration.	1240 (410)	730 (300)
Residual volume	Volume of air remaining in the lungs after a maximum expiration.	2100 (520)	1570 (380)
Vital capacity	Maximum volume of air that can be expired after a maximum inspiration	4130 (750)	2760 (540)
Total lung capacity	The total volume of air contained in the lungs at maximum inspiration	6230 (830)	4330 (620)
Inspiratory capacity	The maximum volume of air that can be inspired after a normal expiration	2900	2030
Functional residual capacity	The volume of gas remaining in the lungs after a normal expiration	3330 (680)	2300 (490)

The tidal volume is of particular importance in anaesthesia, for almost every anaesthetic can depress respiration. There is, moreover, no simple device for ensuring that it is adequate for the respiratory needs of the patient, so that the anaesthetist must judge on clinical grounds whether ventilation is satisfactory. At times this decision may be a difficult one. The tidal volume is of particular importance when considering carbon dioxide absorption techniques. The capacity of the air spaces between the granules in the absorber should be directly related to the tidal volume of the patient, so that adequate contact between the absorbent and the anaesthetic gases can take place. If the absorber is too large, the patient will use only part of it, whilst if it is too small only a proportion of the carbon dioxide will be absorbed, because the expired gases will not remain in contact with the granules of absorbent for a sufficient time.

Measurement of tidal and minute volumes during anaesthesia.—Of the various methods of measuring minute volume, the Wright respirometer has been found the most satisfactory (Fig. 2). After allowing the instrument to record for one minute, the minute volume can be read directly, and the tidal volume then calculated from this reading and the respiratory rate. A rough estimate of the tidal volume can also be made for each breath. The instrument is compact and light; it under-reads at low flow rates and over-reads at high flow rates, but in practice the respiratory waveform and the nature of the anaesthetic gases tend to minimise these errors. For clinical purposes the instrument offers an accurate assessment of the patient's minute volume ($\pm$ 10 per cent) within the range of 3·7 to about 20 l./minute (Nunn and Ezi-Ashi, 1962). A falsely high reading (+ 10 to 20 per cent) will be obtained if the instrument is connected directly to

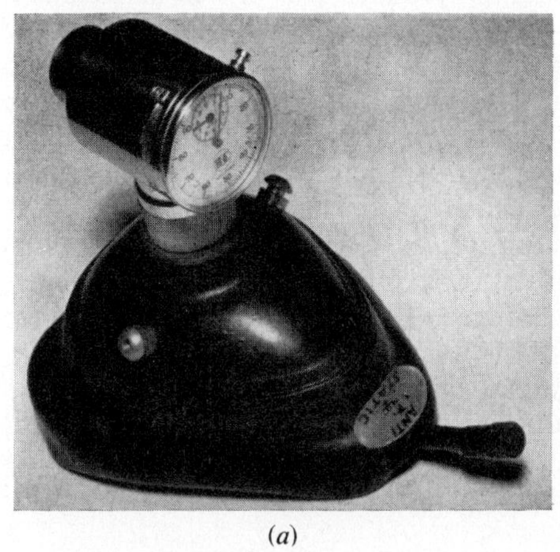

(*a*)

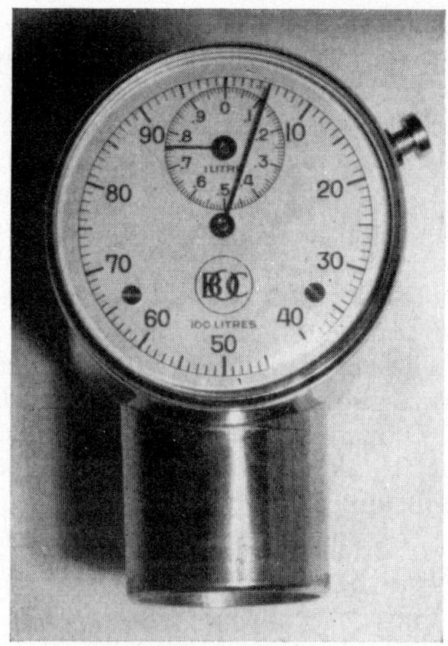

(*b*)

4/Fig. 2.—The Wright respirometer.

the catheter mount unless the baffled connecting piece provided by the manufacturers is also inserted into the circuit. This is done to avoid channelling of gases.

Some Abnormalities of Ventilation

Tachypnoea.—Tachypnoea means an increase in the rate of respiration. The rate of respiration in any given situation is such that the work of breathing is at a minimum.

Hyperpnoea.—Hyperpnoea means an increase in ventilation which is in proportion to an increase in carbon dioxide production. The arterial P_{CO_2} therefore remains near normal. The commonest example of this situation is the hyperpnoea which occurs on exercise. In hyperthyroid states the general body metabolism is raised, and the pulmonary ventilation may be increased by as much as 50–100 per cent.

Hyperventilation.—Hyperventilation is an increase in ventilation out of proportion to carbon dioxide production. It is a common occurrence during controlled ventilation. Another example is the hyperventilation which accompanies a metabolic acidosis, such as occurs in renal failure and especially in diabetic coma. It can also be due to psychological factors or it may follow brain damage.

Hypoventilation.—This means a decrease in ventilation so that the arterial

P_{CO_2} rises. Some degree of hypoventilation is the rule rather than the exception during anaesthesia with spontaneous respiration.

Dyspnoea.—Dyspnoea is a subjective sensation which is difficult to define. It is best described as an awareness of respiration which is unpleasant or distressing. This description does not include "breathlessness", which is not distressing, and may indeed be mildly pleasureable, such as is experienced after mild or moderate exercise.

The physiological mechanisms leading to dyspnoea are not well defined, and the most satisfying theory is that of Campbell and Howell (1963), who have suggested that the sensation arises when there is an inappropriate result (i.e. volume of inspiration) for a given muscular effort, or that a greater effort than expected is required to produce a given ventilation. They describe this as "length-tension inappropriateness", the normal situation being "learnt" by experience. The abnormal sensation of dyspnoea can then be recognised.

Dyspnoea is a common symptom of disease, and is the presenting symptom in many pulmonary and cardiac abnormalities. Its severity is very variable from person to person, so that in two patients with disease of apparently similar severity one may complain of crippling dyspnoea while it is of much less importance to the other.

Increased ventilation during anaesthesia.—During anaesthesia with spontaneous respiration, an increase in ventilation is usually due to one of four causes; (1) Oxygen lack; (2) Carbon dioxide excess; (3) Irritation of the respiratory tract by an anaesthetic vapour or other stimulating procedure; (4) Reflex surgical stimulation.

The stimulant effect of *oxygen lack* (acting via the chemoreceptors) on the respiratory centre has already been discussed (Chapter 3).

Carbon dioxide, acting through the medium of a change in the acid-base balance of the blood bathing the respiratory centre, brings about an increase mainly in the depth of respiration. In the past some anaesthetists deliberately added 5 per cent of carbon dioxide to produce a hyperpnoea when inducing with an agent such as ether. Provided this practice is only continued for a short time, and that once a physiological response has been obtained the concentration is gradually diminished, then little harm can follow in normal subjects. The danger, however, of the ill-advised use of carbon dioxide has led some people to dispense with it entirely, except through the medium of rebreathing. The continued increase in concentration that follows its prolonged use leads to an alteration in the response of the respiratory centre so that a sudden withdrawal of the stimulus causes a depression of the centre, possibly resulting in Cheyne-Stokes respiration or apnoea.

Ether, being a *respiratory irritant*, stimulates the bronchial mucosa, bringing about an increase in respiratory rate and depth together with the production of copious secretions. Premedication and induction with such respiratory depressants as the short-acting barbiturates tend to diminish all these effects.

Hyperventilation as a result of *reflex stimulation* from the operation site or stimulation of bronchial mucosa has already been discussed. Pulling on the mesentery, or dilating the anal sphincter under too light anaesthesia—in other words, inadequate reflex suppression—results in an increase in the depth of respiration. If the stimulus is even more severe or the depth of anaesthesia totally inadequate, then laryngeal spasm may result.

The tidal volume and minute volume are made up from two components, the dead space and the alveolar ventilation.

Dead Space

1. **Anatomical dead space** (V_D anat) comprises the volume of the respiratory passages, extending from the nostrils and mouth down to (but not including) the alveoli. The term "dead space" is used since in it there is no exchange of gases between blood and air. Its capacity varies with age and sex, the figure normally quoted being 150 ml., but in young women it may be as low as 100 ml., whereas in old men it can rise to as much as 200 ml. The position of the lower jaw can influence dead space. Depression of the jaw with flexion of the head (a common cause of respiratory obstruction in the anaesthetised patient) reduces dead space by 30 ml. On the other hand, protrusion of the jaw with extension of the head increases dead space by 40 ml. (Nunn *et al.*, 1959). Pneumonectomy or tracheostomy clearly reduces the volume of dead space.

2. **Physiological dead space** (V_D phys) is defined as that fraction of the tidal volume which is not available for gaseous exchange. It includes therefore not only the anatomical dead space, but also the volume of gas which ventilates alveoli that are not being perfused, as in these alveoli gaseous exchange does not occur. This ventilation is therefore wasted, appearing as an increase in physiological dead space. This second component is called "alveolar dead space". The actual situation is not so clear cut as has been outlined above, because if areas of lung are overventilated, although normally perfused, they also contribute to an increase in dead space. The relationships between ventilation and perfusion of alveoli are further discussed on page 158. In normal man, anatomical and physiological dead space are numerically almost equal, and amount to about one-third of the tidal volume. Because the relationship between physiological dead space (V_D phys) and tidal volume (V_T) remains fairly constant when tidal volume is altered, the physiological dead space is often expressed as a fraction of the tidal volume (V_D/V_T ratio; normal 0·25 to 0·4).

Physiological dead space is increased in old age, in the upright position when compared with supine subjects, with large tidal volumes or high respiratory rates, after the administration of atropine, if inspiratory time is reduced to 0·5 seconds or less during controlled ventilation, and in the presence of lung disease whenever ventilation-perfusion relationships are altered. For instance, in chronic bronchitis or asthma the physiological dead space may rise to 50–80 per cent of the tidal volume; it is also found to be high following pulmonary embolism. It is increased following haemorrhage (Freeman and Nunn, 1963) and during controlled hypotension, especially if the patient is tilted head up (Askrog *et al.*, 1964).

The effect of anaesthesia on the physiological dead space appears to be very variable, but as a general rule it can be taken that both V_D phys and V_D/V_T are increased during anaesthesia, after taking into account any changes due to apparatus dead space. During intermittent positive pressure respiration, this increase in V_D phys is approximately compensated for by intubation (which reduces dead space by about 70 ml.); thus for ventilated, intubated and anaesthetised patients V_D/V_T is found to be 0·3–0·45, but if the effect of intubation is corrected for, then V_D/V_T appears to be in the 0·4–0·6 range. In one recent study the effects of intubation on total functional dead space during halothane anaesthesia during spontaneous ventilation has been studied (Kain *et al.*, 1969). These workers found that, using a mask and Frumin valve, the total dead space was increased considerably (mean $V_D/V_T = 0{\cdot}68$; SD $= 0{\cdot}062$), being reduced by intubation (mean $V_D/V_T = 0{\cdot}51$; SD $= 0{\cdot}073$), representing in absolute terms an average difference in total functional dead space of 82 ml. between intubated patients and those anaesthetised with a mask. These subjects were able to compensate for changes in dead space by altering their tidal volumes.

As a general rule it may be said that the dead space is increased during anaesthesia, although the changes are very variable. Cooper (1967) has suggested that the physiological dead space during anaesthesia with passive ventilation can be roughly estimated from the formula:

$$V_D/V_T = 33 + \frac{\text{Age}}{3} \text{ per cent}$$

Measurement of physiological dead space.—This is usually done by utilising Enghoff's modification of Bohr's equation;

$$V_D \text{ phys} = \frac{(Pa_{CO_2} - P\bar{E}_{CO_2})\, V_T}{Pa_{CO_2}} - V_D \text{ apparatus}$$

where Pa_{CO_2} = tension of carbon dioxide in arterial blood (assumed to be equal to alveolar carbon dioxide tension); $P\bar{E}_{CO_2}$ = tension of carbon dioxide in mixed air; and V_T = Tidal volume. The method requires the collection of a sample of mixed expired air into a Douglas bag over a known number of breaths, and measurement of its carbon dioxide content and total volume. The arterial P_{CO_2} must also be measured in a blood sample taken during the period of gas collection. The values obtained for Pa_{CO_2}, $P\bar{E}_{CO_2}$ and V_T are then substituted in the equation, and V_D phys calculated as a fraction of the tidal volume. Since the latter is known, the absolute value for V_D phys can also be calculated, and also the ratio $\frac{V_D \text{ phys}}{V_T}$

3. **Apparatus dead space** consists of the volume of gas contained in any anaesthetic apparatus between the patient and that point in the system where rebreathing of exhaled carbon dioxide ceases to occur (e.g. the expiratory valve in a Magill system, or the side-arm in an Ayre's T-piece). The importance of apparatus dead space is so well known as hardly to need further emphasis, especially when anaesthetising small children. The interior volume of an adult face-piece and the connections up to the point of the expiratory valve in a Magill system may be as much as 125 ml. of dead space to the patient. This problem is further discussed below and on page 205 (section on paediatric anaesthetic apparatus).

Alveolar Ventilation

Alveolar ventilation is defined as that proportion of the tidal or minute volume which takes part in gas exchange. The normal value for alveolar ventilation is 2·0 to 2·4 l./minute/square metre B.S.A.*, or about 3·5 to 4·5 l./minute in adults. Its importance lies in the fact that it is the pulmonary factor controlling

*Body surface area.

the excretion of carbon dioxide by the lungs (see 3/Fig. 5), and it is directly related to the tidal volume, physiological dead space and respiratory rate.

Alveolar Ventilation/Min. = (Tidal Volume − Physiological Dead Space) × Respiratory Rate.

$$\text{or } \dot{V}_A = (V_T - V_D \text{ phys}) \times f$$

From this relationship it can be seen that a rise in physiological dead space or a fall in the respiratory rate will lead to a reduction in the alveolar ventilation provided the other factors remain fairly constant. So too will a fall in the tidal volume, although in normal man the physiological dead space also decreases, so that the effect on the alveolar ventilation is lessened.

For example, if we calculate the alveolar ventilation under various circumstances we find the following figures are obtained:

1) *Normal*

$(450 - 150) \times 13 = 3{\cdot}9$ l./min. (P_{CO_2} normal)

2) *Tidal Volume Reduced*

$(300 - 100) \times 13 = 2{\cdot}6$ l./min. (P_{CO_2} raised)

3) *Physiological Dead Space Increased by Anaesthetic Apparatus*

$(450 - 225) \times 13 = 2{\cdot}7$ l./min. (P_{CO_2} raised)

4) *Respiratory Rate Decreased*

$(450 - 150) \times 8 = 2{\cdot}4$ l./min. (P_{CO_2} raised)

These simple calculations, although useful as a guide, do not always represent the true state of affairs. For instance, the addition of apparatus dead space of 100 ml. (measured by filling the relevant volume with water) may represent a rather smaller addition when in clinical use. This is due to patterns of gas flow and channelling of gases within the apparatus. For example, the central core of the gas stream may move rapidly whilst gas in the periphery moves relatively slowly. Thus the central element represents the major portion of the ventilation, so reducing the role of the dead space. It should also be noted that in practice physiological mechanisms react to any of these changes and tend to return the P_{CO_2} towards normal values, so that the alterations in alveolar ventilation are not as great as those indicated above. However, under the influence of sedative or anaesthetic drugs these physiological responses may be depressed, so that any alteration in alveolar ventilation due to the addition of apparatus dead space may not be compensated fully. Deep anaesthesia, respiratory depressant drugs and the muscle relaxants all tend to depress alveolar ventilation. The resulting rise in alveolar carbon dioxide tension will produce a fall in alveolar oxygen tension unless extra oxygen is added to the inspired air. The explanation of this phenomenon is as follows: in very general terms, and provided that no great exchange of inert gases is occurring in the lungs, the alveolar oxygen tension can be calculated from the following equation, which is a simplification of the Alveolar Air Equation (Comroe *et al.*, 1962):

$$\text{Alveolar oxygen tension} = \text{Inspired oxygen tension} - \frac{\text{Alveolar carbon dioxide tension}}{\text{Respiratory quotient}}$$

$$\text{or } P_{A_{O_2}} = P_{I_{O_2}} - Pa_{CO_2}/R$$

3. **Space-occupying lesions in the chest.**—Neurofibromata and other extra-pleural tumours, kypho-scoliosis, pericardial and pleural effusions, pneumothorax, and some diseases—such as carcinoma of the lung with infiltration or consolidation—will reduce the vital capacity.

4. **Abdominal tumours which impede the descent of the diaphragm.**—The addition of 1 litre of water to the stomach brings about no significant change in the vital capacity, but if another litre is added a slight fall occurs, which returns to normal again on emptying the stomach (Mills, 1949). Although the gravid uterus displaces the diaphragm upwards, the vital capacity of a pregnant woman is not decreased. On the contrary, it is increased on average 10 per cent over the normal, since the thoracic cage is enlarged transversely and antero-posteriorly and there is marked splaying of the subcostal angle.

5. **Abdominal pain.**—The pain experienced after an operation involving the abdominal musculature leads to a reduction in vital capacity of 70–75 per cent in upper abdominal and 50 per cent in lower abdominal operations (Churchill, 1925).

These figures have been confirmed more recently by Simpson and his associates (1961), who advocated the use of a continuous thoracic epidural technique for the relief of post-operative pain. Using this method, they were able to produce not only complete freedom from pain, but also a very substantial improvement in the vital capacity (see Table 3). It is interesting to note, however, that in very few patients in their series was the vital capacity restored to the pre-operative level. It might be argued, therefore, that the epidural itself was responsible for limiting some respiratory activity, but Moir (1963) in a similar study, concluded that no important degree of respiratory paresis was produced by epidural blockade.

4/TABLE 3

VITAL CAPACITY READINGS EXPRESSED AS A % OF THE PRE-OPERATIVE VALUE

	Before epidural (In pain)			*1 hour after epidural (Pain-free)*			*24 hours after epidural (Pain-free)*		
	Range %	*Mean %*	*No. of Cases*	*Range %*	*Mean %*	*No. of Cases*	*Range %*	*Mean %*	*No. of Cases*
Upper Abdominal	20–56	35·2	54	44–139	69·0	54	61–139	83·2	50
Lower Abdominal	37–69	55·5	6	80–91	84·8	6	92–96	94·7	3

Vital capacity readings in 60 patients undergoing abdominal surgery (Simpson *et al.*, 1961).

There seems to be little doubt that a continuous epidural technique provides the most effective form of pain relief in combination with the maximum ventilatory function. Nevertheless, such techniques are time-consuming and require a high degree of technical skill if the thoracic level is used (in order to reduce the incidence of hypotensive complications). For these reasons this technique is best reserved for the special case.

Morphine and allied substances, although they relieve pain, act as respiratory depressants and therefore themselves tend to reduce the vital capacity. Intravenous procaine, however, reduces the pain sensation without depressing respiration, yet the results show that under the influence of procaine there is only about a 10–12 per cent improvement in the post-operative vital capacity overestimated values (Pooler, 1949). Specific nerve block is likely to be more effective.

6. **Abdominal splinting.**—Tight abdominal binders, strapping, or bandaging limit the range of respiratory movement. Elastic strapping applied in the vertical plane allows the greatest freedom of respiration in the post-operative period.

7. **Alterations in posture.**—Changes in posture in the conscious subject lead to considerable alterations in the vital capacity, and these are mainly related to positions which are calculated to alter the volume of blood in the lungs. Thus the capacity is greater when standing than when sitting or lying. It increases by as much as $\frac{1}{4}$–$\frac{1}{2}$ litre if there is an accumulation of blood in the legs. The inhalation of amyl nitrite causes an increase of about $\frac{1}{4}$ litre. The latter is probably mainly due to increased depth of inspiration.

The various positions in which an anaesthetised patient may be placed on the operating table have been shown to have a considerable effect on the vital capacity of the unanaesthetised subject. For example:

	Loss of Vital Capacity
Trendelenburg position (20°)	14·5 per cent
Lithotomy	18·0 per cent
Left lateral	10·0 per cent
Right lateral	12·0 per cent
Bridge in dorsal position	12·5 per cent
Prone position, unsupported	10·0 per cent

(Case and Stiles, 1946)

Residual Volume and Functional Residual Capacity

Residual volume is the amount of air that still remains in the lungs after the patient has made a maximal expiration. Normal average values range from 2,100 ml. for males to 1,570 for females. Functional residual capacity is the amount of air remaining in the lungs after a normal expiration. Normal average values range from 3,300 ml. for males to 2,300 ml. for females.

Unfortunately neither of these two measurements can be made directly. There are, however, two indirect methods which use a known concentration of a relatively insoluble gas, i.e. one that does not readily traverse the alveolar membrane and become dissolved in the plasma.

Nitrogen technique.—The principle is to collect all the nitrogen that can be washed out of the patient's lungs. Following a maximal expiration (if residual volume is required) or a normal expiration (if functional residual capacity is required) the patient inspires oxygen from a special source and then expires into a spirometer which is known to be free of nitrogen. Over some minutes almost all the alveolar nitrogen is washed out of the lungs. In healthy adults this may be achieved after only two minutes, but in patients with severe emphysema at least 7–20 minutes may be needed. At the beginning of the test all the nitrogen is in the lungs and at the end it has all passed to the spirometer. The concentration of nitrogen in the spirometer can now be measured. The total volume of gases in the spirometer is known so that the total volume of nitrogen in the mixture can be calculated. As air contains 80 per cent nitrogen a suitable correction will reveal the total alveolar gas volume at the moment the test began.

Helium technique.—In this case a spirometer with carbon dioxide absorption is used. This is filled with a mixture of 10 per cent helium and 90 per cent oxygen and the patient then breathes in and out of it. At first, there is no helium in the patient's lungs, but gradually mixing takes place until after a few minutes the concentration of helium in the patient's lungs and in the spirometer is the same. Again, the volume of gas in the alveoli can then be calculated.

Significance.—As the residual volume represents the amount of air remaining in the lungs at the end of a maximal expiration, any increase in it signifies that the lung is larger than usual and cannot empty adequately. Increases in residual volume are usually associated with emphysematous changes in the lungs, but may occur temporarily without any actual structural change. For example, obstruction to the airway, as in asthma or over-inflation of the lungs after a thoracic operation, may cause an increase. If there is a marked increase in residual air the act of respiration may be difficult, since by implication the patient is unable to reduce the volume even by forced expiration, and it is likely that respiration is carried out with the mechanical disadvantage of a thorax already larger than normal.

In severe emphysema some air is 'trapped' completely in the alveoli and never comes in contact with the respired gases. In emphysematous patients it is impossible to obtain a true reading of the residual volume by either of the methods mentioned above. This can only be obtained in a highly specialised respiratory unit where a body plethysmograph is available. Such an instrument measures the thoracic gas volume whether it is in free communication with the airway or not.

Thoracic Gas Volume

The principle of measuring the total volume of air contained in the thorax is based on a change of the air pressures inside and outside the thorax when the patient's airway is suddenly obstructed. First, the patient is enclosed in a body plethysmograph in a special chamber, and permitted to breathe the air within the chamber. The airway pressure and the plethysmograph pressure are noted. At the desired moment (usually at the end of a normal expiration) the airway is suddenly occluded by an electrical shutter. The patient will then attempt to inspire against a total obstruction. The chest expands, the intrathoracic pressure falls whilst the pressure in the plethysmograph rises. Alveolar pressure is assumed to equal mouth pressure under these circumstances, so that the pressure differences now enable the original thoracic gas volume to be calculated.

This method is rapid and relatively simple. It is often used in combination with the dilution methods of nitrogen and helium for in this manner it is easy to determine the amount of 'non-ventilated' areas of lung in a particular patient.

In a patient with severe emphysema these tests may reveal that as much as 1–3 litres of air are trapped within the alveoli.

Discussion.—All these tests must be interpreted with caution because there is a wide margin for normal values even in the healthy adult. Nevertheless, an increase in functional residual capacity is usually assumed to denote structural emphysematous changes in the lung. In reality it represents hyperinflation of the lung during quiet breathing and though this is commonly caused by emphysema and partial obstruction of the airway, it could in rare cases be due to a deformity of the thorax.

Minimal Air

Even after the pleural cavities have been opened and the lungs have collapsed, there still remains a very small, but nevertheless important, quantity of air entrapped in the lungs—the minimal air. In medico-legal circles the presence of air in the lungs of a newborn child suggests that it has breathed after birth, but this deduction does not hold if the lungs have been positively inflated during resuscitation. A piece of aerated lung when placed in water will float, whereas a piece of atelectatic lung (i.e. one which has not been aerated) will sink to the bottom.

Dynamic Tests of Ventilation

The tests of ventilatory function so far discussed are more or less static in nature. However, ventilation is essentially a dynamic process, and other function tests have been devised which attempt to quantitate ventilatory function in terms of the *rate* at which ventilation can take place, rather than in terms of volumes.

1. **Maximum breathing capacity** (MBC).—This test, introduced by Hermannsen in 1933, is designed to measure the speed and efficiency of filling and emptying the lungs during increased respiratory effort, and is defined as the maximum volume of air that can be breathed per minute. It is usually measured for 15 seconds and the result expressed in flow per minute. It is therefore a dynamic test, as opposed to the static measurement of vital capacity. As age increases there is a large reduction in the maximum breathing capacity, but it is in patients with pulmonary emphysema that it shows the most impairment. It also falls in the presence of bronchospasm and bronchiolar obstruction and the test has been used, therefore, to judge the effectiveness of broncho-dilators in the treatment of bronchoconstriction. Cournand and Richards (1941) reported that the maximum breathing capacity is reduced by 15 per cent after a five-rib thoracoplasty but that this functional loss is considerably greater if a pronounced scoliosis develops.

A disadvantage of the maximum breathing capacity test is that results are apt to differ in the hands of separate workers; this is largely due to variations in technique, and to the different types of apparatus used for measurement. The instrument may introduce errors in certain circumstances, such as by adding resistance to respiration or influencing the rate of breathing. Furthermore the test is a tiring procedure and not without risk in severely disabled subjects, and the results can be fairly accurately predicted from the timed vital capacity (forced expiratory volume) (Needham *et al.*, 1954). For these reasons it has fallen into disrepute at the present time. Average values for normal subjects range from 100–200 litres per minute depending upon the mode of measurement, but there is a big difference between these figures and those for abnormal subjects.

2. **Forced expiratory volume (FEV).**—The patient makes a maximal inspiration, expires as forcefully and rapidly as he can into a spirometer, and the total amount of air expelled over a given time is measured. The time intervals at which the total amount of air expelled is measured are 0·5, 1, 2 and 3 seconds. However, as there seems to be little advantage between the results taken at each of these intervals, it is customary to take only the volume expired at 1 second, called the $FEV_{1\cdot0}$. This volume is expressed as a percentage of the forced vital capacity. In normal young subjects 83 per cent of the vital capacity should be expired during the first second. The lower limit of normal is normally taken as 70 per cent. In a patient with chronic bronchitis the $FEV_{1\cdot0}$ may be only 50 per cent or less.

Recently the dry spirometer has come into common use to measure the vital capacity and $FEV_{1\cdot0}$. One such instrument is the Vitalograph (Fig. 3). Expiring

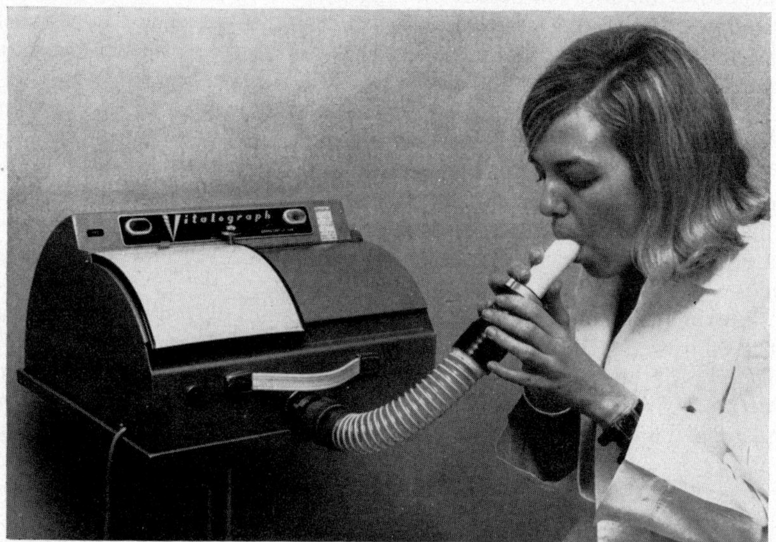

4/FIG. 3.—The "Vitalograph".

into it causes a bellows to expand and results in the vertical deflection of a pen writing on a calibrated chart. The initial act of expiration activates a pressure switch, and the whole chart is then moved sideways at a constant speed by an electric motor. A graph is drawn out on the chart, in which the vertical axis is expressed in litres, and the horizontal axis as time in seconds (see Fig. 4). The result is a graphical analysis of the rate and volume of the patient's forced vital capacity, from which the $FEV_{1\cdot0}$ can be calculated. One of the main advantages of this type of instrument is that the records are produced on a small flat sheet of paper which can be filed away for reference, and subsequent tests can then be compared with previous records. A rough estimate of the peak expiratory flow rate can be obtained by measuring the slope of the steepest part of the curve.

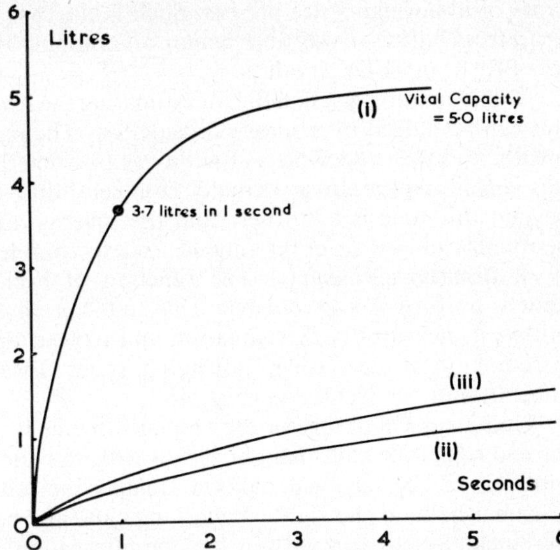

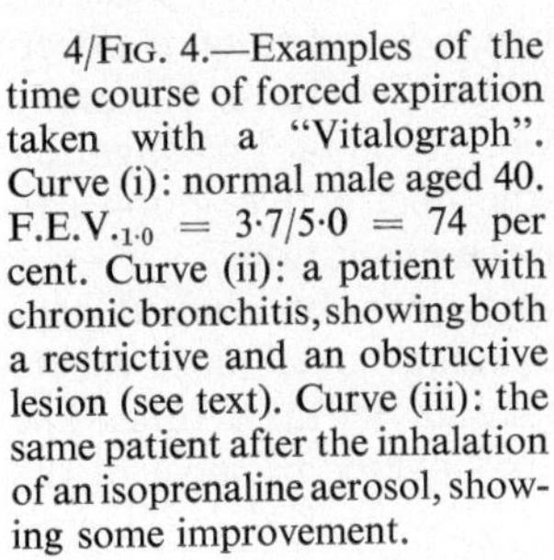
4/Fig. 4.—Examples of the time course of forced expiration taken with a "Vitalograph". Curve (i): normal male aged 40. F.E.V.$_{1\cdot0}$ = 3·7/5·0 = 74 per cent. Curve (ii): a patient with chronic bronchitis, showing both a restrictive and an obstructive lesion (see text). Curve (iii): the same patient after the inhalation of an isoprenaline aerosol, showing some improvement.

3. **Peak expiratory flow rate (PEFR).**—After a maximal inspiration, the patient expires as forcefully as he can, and the maximum flow rate of air is measured. The measurement can be made either into a pneumotachograph, or by a specially designed instrument, such as the Wright Peak Flow Meter. The normal limits for the PEFR are taken as 450–700 l./minute in men, and 300–500 l./minute in women, although like all tests of ventilatory function the normal value varies with the age and build of the subject.

Discussion.—The results from measurement of both the $FEV_{1\cdot0}$ and the PEFR can be improved with a little practice on the patient's part. For this reason it is customary to perform the test five times, and then to take the average of the last three readings as the final result. Alternatively, the best of the five readings can be taken. It is of great importance to use apparatus with a low resistance to high gas flow rates.

Low values for the $FEV_{1\cdot0}$ and PEFR usually indicate a higher than normal resistance to gas flow within the conducting airways (i.e. a diffuse airways obstruction). This type of abnormality is termed "obstructive" and is found in such conditions as asthma, chronic bronchitis, and bronchitis with bronchospasm. The response to the inhalation of a bronchodilator aerosol can readily be tested. If reversible bronchoconstriction is present, then both the PEFR and $FEV_{1\cdot0}$ improve after aerosol inhalation (see Fig. 4). This gives a guide as to whether bronchodilator drugs will or will not be an effective form of treatment, for example in combination with physiotherapy during the preoperative preparation of such a patient. Some patients are found to have a reduced vital capacity, although their PEFR and $FEV_{1\cdot0}$ values are within normal limits. This type of ventilatory defect is described as "restrictive" and is found in some of the conditions which are listed on p. 143. Although this distinction between obstructive and restrictive abnormalities of ventilation has been made, it is usual to find that both the vital capacity and the tests of flow rate are reduced so that both types of abnormality are present. Such is the case in chronic bronchitis where, apart from diffuse airway obstruction, air-trapping also contributes to abnormally low PEFR and $FEV_{1 \cdot 0}$ values.

If no apparatus is available for estimating the severity of an obstructive lesion, this can be judged by a simple bedside test. The patient is asked to take a deep breath, and then to exhale as forcibly as possible through his mouth. Normally this forced expiration is virtually complete after three seconds. Prolongation beyond this time is abnormal, and the severity of the obstructive lesion can be roughly judged from the time it takes to complete the expiration.

4. **Broncho-spirometry.**—The function of each lung can be studied separately by broncho-spirometry. This test has an advantage over most others in that it measures both ventilation and oxygen uptake at the same time. The introduction of the Carlens catheter (Carlens, 1949) has overcome most of the difficulties of the technique (Fig. 5*a*).

Under topical analgesia the special catheter is placed in the trachea so that the end rests in the left main bronchus with the hook over the carina (Fig. 5*b*). Inflation of the terminal balloon isolates the left lung and inflation of the proximal balloon the right. Each lung can then be connected separately to a spirometer fitted with carbon dioxide absorption, and a simultaneous record obtained from both lungs. In a normal subject one would expect 55 per cent of both the ventilation and the oxygen consumption to be carried out by the right lung and 45 per cent by the left. Figure 5*c* illustrates how disease in one lung may be suggested by a considerable alteration in this ratio.

This test is most useful when used to estimate the function of one or other lung when pneumonectomy or lobectomy on the opposite side is being considered.

5. **Uneven ventilation.**—The way in which inspired air is distributed to the alveoli may be influenced by local changes in airways resistance or pulmonary elasticity. The simplest method for detecting abnormal distribution of pulmonary ventilation involves studying the elimination of nitrogen from the alveoli when breathing 100 per cent oxygen. The subject inhales pure oxygen for a period of seven minutes, and at the end of this time the nitrogen concentration in a sample of alveolar air is measured using a nitrogen meter. If the concentration is above 2 per cent, it is considered to be an indication of abnormal distribution of ventilation, as washout of nitrogen has not been achieved in those alveoli which are being poorly ventilated. It should be remembered that the rate of nitrogen washout can also be affected by (1) the tidal and minute volumes and (2) the functional residual capacity.

DIFFUSION

The exchange of gases within the lung occurs through a process of passive diffusion across the alveolar-capillary membrane. This membrane consists of the alveolar membrane, interstitial fluid, and the capillary endothelium. In the case of oxygen, the plasma, red cell membrane and intracellular fluid must also be considered, as the rate of reaction of oxygen with haemoglobin plays an important part in determining the rate of diffusion. The rate of transfer of a gas is directly proportional to the area of the membrane, the solubility of the gas in liquid, and the partial pressure gradient across the membrane; and is inversely

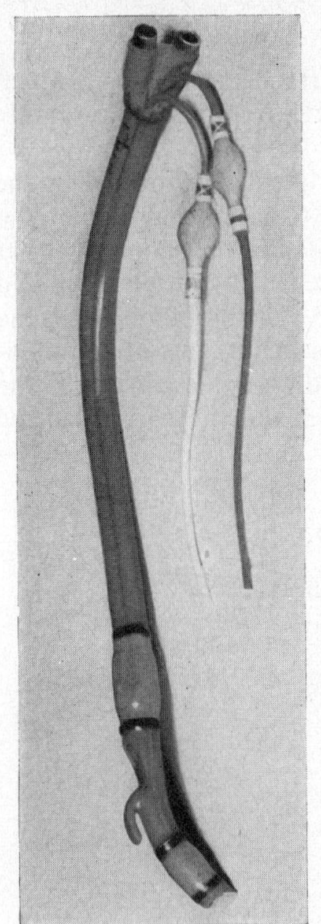

(*a*)

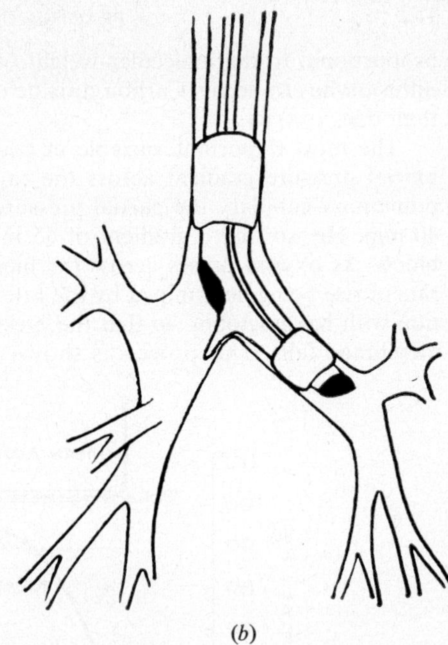

(*b*)

4/Fig. 5.—(*a*) Carlens catheter. (*b*) Carlens catheter *in situ* (diagrammatic).

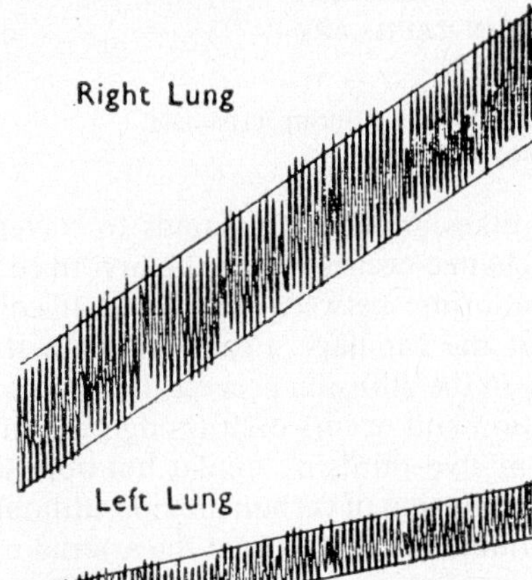

4/Fig. 5(*c*).—Broncho-Spirometry

Spirometer tracings of individual lungs during broncho-spirometry (31-year old woman with diseased left lung).

Right lung

O_2 uptake . .	210 ml./min. (77 per cent)
Ventilation . .	6·0 l./min. (73 per cent)

Left lung

O_2 uptake . .	63 ml./min. (23 per cent)
Ventilation . .	2·16 l./min. (27 per cent)

proportional to the molecular weight of the gas and the distance across which diffusion has to occur. Carbon dioxide diffuses some twenty times more rapidly than does oxygen.

The most important variable in considering the diffusion of oxygen is the partial pressure gradient across the capillary wall. At the arterial end of the pulmonary capillary the partial pressure of oxygen (P_{O_2}) in the blood is about 40 mm. Hg, so that a gradient of 65 mm. Hg is present between alveolus and blood. As oxygen passes across the membrane, the P_{O_2} of the blood rises, the rate of rise being determined by the rate of gas transfer and its rate of combination with haemoglobin, so that the pressure gradient driving the gas across the membrane falls. This process is shown in Fig. 6. From this diagram it can be

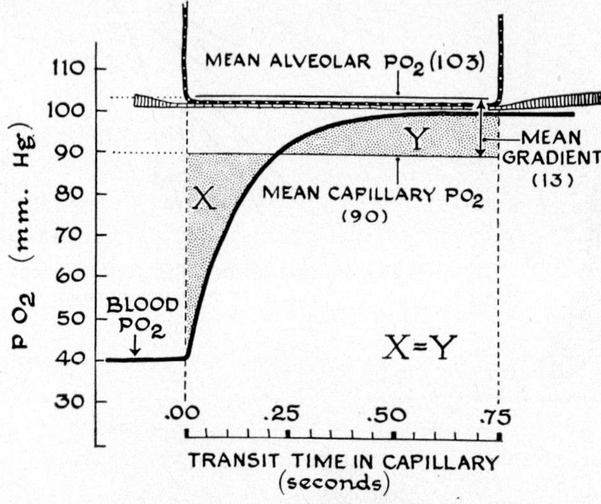

4/FIG. 6.—The change in oxygen tension of blood during its passage through a pulmonary capillary.

seen that an average red blood corpuscle takes about 0·75 seconds to traverse a capillary, that the majority of the gas exchange occurs within the first third of this time, and that virtually complete equilibrium between blood and alveolus has been established at the venous end of the capillary. From this data it is evident that there is a great reserve capacity in the diffusion process. For example during exercise almost complete equilibration still occurs even though the time available for gas transfer may be reduced by two-thirds. A similar but opposite and much more rapid process occurs during diffusion of carbon dioxide, although the driving pressures are much lower (maximum of 6 mm. Hg at the arterial end of the capillary).

The alveolar-capillary membrane can be seen to be thickened in certain diseases, such as sarcoidosis, asbestosis, pulmonary fibrosis, and infiltrating carcinoma, and this thickening can produce defects in the diffusion process. This state of affairs has been given the name "alveolar-capillary block", and is characterised clinically by dyspnoea and profound cyanosis, especially on exercise, associated with a low arterial P_{CO_2}. However, it has been shown that the supposed diffusion defect in these conditions is not nearly so severe as was once supposed, and that most of the hypoxia is due to ventilation/perfusion abnormalities (see below). At present it is considered that impairment of diffusion does not play nearly such an important role in clinical practice as was at one time suspected.

Measurement

The diffusing capacity of the lungs is assessed by measuring the rate of uptake of carbon monoxide while breathing a low concentration of the gas (0·2 per cent) (Comroe *et al.*, 1962). The normal rate of uptake is 15–30 ml./min./mm. Hg of CO. Because of the difference in the diffusing characteristics of carbon monoxide and oxygen, the diffusing capacity of oxygen is approximately 1·23 times that of carbon monoxide.

The interpretation of diffusing capacities is difficult, because the values obtained may be affected by other factors, such as abnormal distribution of ventilation, and inequalities of ventilation and perfusion. Hence a low figure for carbon monoxide uptake might be interpreted as being due to a diffusion defect, when it is actually due to some other cause.

THE PULMONARY CIRCULATION

The pulmonary circulation consists of the pulmonary artery and its branches, the precapillary vessels (which unlike those in the systemic circulation are thin-walled and easily distended), the pulmonary capillaries, the pulmonary venous system and the left atrium. It is a low pressure system, easily distensible, with a low resistance to blood flow, and accepts all the blood that leaves the right side of the heart. The normal pulmonary artery pressure curve is similar in shape to the aortic pressure curve, but with a systolic pressure of 20–30 mm. Hg, a diastolic pressure of 8–12 mm. Hg, and a mean pressure of 12–15 mm. Hg at rest. The normal mean left atrial pressure is about 8 mm. Hg, with an upper limit of 15 mm. Hg. The system is very flexible in adapting itself to changes in blood flow and blood volume, its adaptability being almost entirely passive in nature. Thus, immediately after blocking the pulmonary artery to one lung, the pressure in the other only rises by about 5 mm. Hg. Also, the low pulse pressure in the pulmonary artery, when compared to that in the aorta, is due to the high distensibility and low resistance of the system. The compliance of the entire pulmonary vascular tree resembles that of a large systemic vein in nature.

The pulmonary circulation normally contains about 10 per cent of the total blood volume, but this amount is easily altered by as much as 50 per cent. A rise in pulmonary blood volume is seen in negative pressure breathing, the supine position when compared to the upright position, systemic vasoconstriction from any cause, over-transfusion, and left ventricular failure. A fall in pulmonary blood volume occurs during positive pressure breathing, on assuming the upright posture, during Valsalva's manoeuvre, after haemorrhage, or as a result of systemic vasodilation from any cause. Thus it is a simple matter to shift blood from the pulmonary circulation to the systemic circulation, and vice versa.

Although on histological examination the pulmonary blood vessels can be seen to contain smooth muscle, control of the distribution of the blood flow within the vessels, and of the resistance offered to flow, appears to be largely passive. Although more than a dozen active reflexes have been described, none of them is as yet generally accepted. The one exception to this is the response of the pulmonary circulation to alveolar hypoxia. If alveolar hypoxia occurs for any reason, either generally or locally within the lung, the result is *vaso-constriction* and a reduction in blood flow in those vessels supplying the hypoxic area, so that the blood is diverted to oxygenated parts of the lung. This response to hypoxia is the opposite to that which occurs in the systemic circulation. In man 50 per cent of the final shift in blood flow has occurred within 2 minutes of the onset of alveolar hypoxia, and it is complete after 7 minutes. The reflex is accentuated by a local rise in H^+ ion concentration. The mechanism of this reflex is as yet unknown although its purpose is more readily apparent. For example, if pulmonary collapse occurs in a portion of the lung, ventilation will be reduced in the collapsed area, and oxygenation of the venous blood flowing to that area will be less effective. The blood is therefore diverted to parts of the lung where it can become adequately oxygenated, thus tending to maintain a normal arterial oxygen saturation.

Pulmonary Hypertension

Pulmonary hypertension is said to be present when the systolic pressure rises above 30 mm. Hg. It can be due either to an increase in flow, in pulmonary vascular resistance, or in left atrial pressure. An increase in pulmonary blood flow occurs when a left-to-right shunt is present, such as is found in atrial or ventricular defects or in the presence of a patent ductus arteriosus. In these conditions the blood flow through the lungs may be as much as three times the systemic cardiac output. If this state of affairs is allowed to persist, after some years the pulmonary vascular resistance begins to rise due to structural changes in the vessels and the pulmonary artery pressure rises even further. Eventually the pressure on the right side of the heart may exceed that in the left side, and a right-to-left shunt with central cyanosis then appears. The combination of a ventricular septal defect, pulmonary hypertension and a reversed shunt is called Eisenmenger's syndrome.

A rise in left atrial and pulmonary venous pressures causes pulmonary arterial hypertension by back-pressure, and may be secondary to aortic or mitral valve disease, or to left ventricular failure from any cause. A rise in pulmonary vascular resistance occurs in such conditions as massive or multiple pulmonary emboli and in some lung diseases, notably advanced chronic bronchitis. Pulmonary hypertension in the latter condition is thought to be due to a combination of chronic hypoxia and obliteration of the pulmonary vascular bed by the disease process.

Pulmonary Oedema

Normally the pressure in the pulmonary capillaries is low and is exceeded by the colloidal osmotic pressure of the plasma which tends to retain fluid within the circulation. If for any reason the pulmonary capillary pressure rises above the osmotic pressure, fluid passes across the alveolar-capillary membrane and pulmonary oedema results. This can occur in any disease in which the pulmonary venous pressure is high, such as those listed above, or as a result of over-transfusion, of brain damage, or following chemical damage to the pulmonary capillaries.

Measurement of Pulmonary Blood Flow

There are four principal methods. First, use of radio-active gases. Second, the direct Fick method requiring the measurement of the oxygen uptake per minute in the pulmonary circulation. Third, the dye-dilution method; and fourth, the body plethysmograph. The last method is a recent development and has the advantage that it measures blood flow instantaneously. The patient, enclosed in the body plethysmograph, sits in an air tight chamber, the interior pressure of which can be sensitively monitored. At the desired moment he inhales deeply from a bag inside the chamber containing a mixture of 80 per cent nitrous oxide and 20 per cent oxygen. The nitrous oxide rapidly leaves the bag and becomes dissolved in the pulmonary circulation. The bag empties and the interior pressure of the chamber decreases. The rate of pulmonary blood flow can then be calculated from a knowledge of the pressure of nitrous oxide in the patient's alveoli, the solubility of nitrous oxide in blood, and the volume of the alveoli.

Pulmonary Haemodynamics during General Anaesthesia

The haemodynamics of the pulmonary circulation in fit young volunteers during general anaesthesia have recently been described by Price and his colleagues (1969). They found that cyclopropane caused a rise in mean pulmonary artery pressure and wedge pressure, and that pulmonary vascular resistance was doubled. About 40 per cent of the rise in pulmonary artery pressure was estimated to be secondary to the increased vascular resistance, and about 60 per cent due to actions distal to the pulmonary capillaries. No significant change in these measurements was found during halothane anaesthesia, with or without nitrous oxide. A nitrous oxide/oxygen/*d*-tubocurarine sequence has no effect on the pulmonary artery pressure or vascular resistance, although both are elevated during ether anaesthesia (Wyant *et al.*, 1962).

Distribution of Pulmonary Blood Flow

Many years ago it was suggested that in the erect posture the simple factor of the weight of a column of blood in the lung would cause the upper part of the lung to receive less blood than the lower part. In recent years great advances have been made in the study of the amount and distribution of both air and blood in the lungs with the aid of radio-active techniques. Radio-active oxygen with a half-life of two minutes (West, 1963 *a* and *b*) or radio-active xenon with a half-life of 5·3 days are available (Ball *et al.*, 1962). So also is oxygen-15 labelled carbon dioxide. The principle of the method of measurement is simple. The patient's chest is surrounded with multiple counters which can detect radio-activity in a particular area of the lung. The subject then takes a single breath of radio-active gas. The distribution of this gas in the lung will reveal the regional ventilation per unit of lung volume. Alternatively, if the value of the pulmonary blood flow is required, then the technique differs according to which gas is used. In the case of oxygen (or oxygen-labelled carbon dioxide) the patient takes a breath and then holds it: the rate of the removal of this gas from the

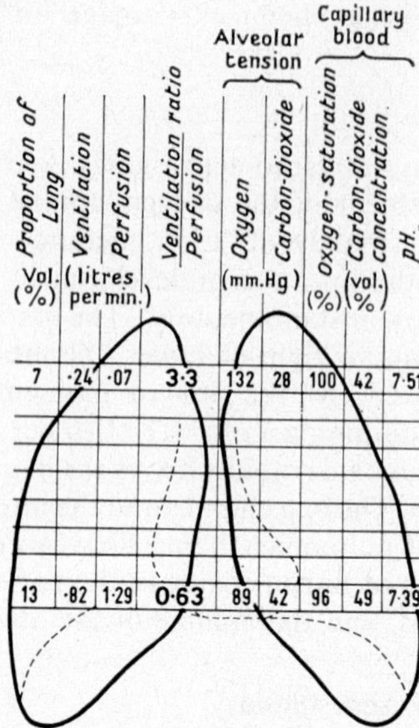

4/FIG. 7(*a*).—Differences in ventilation, blood flow and gas exchange in the normal upright lung.

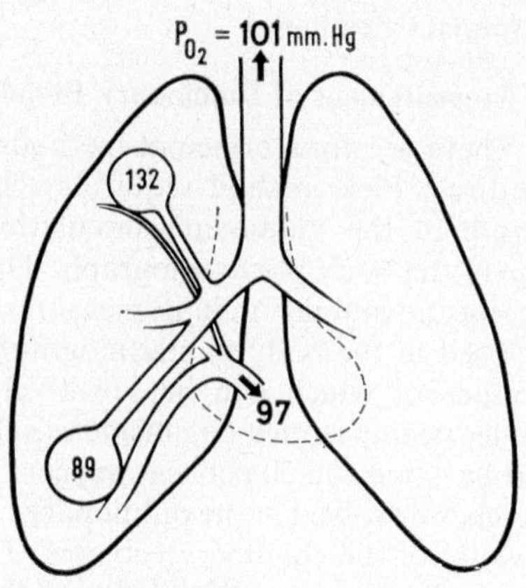

4/FIG. 7(*b*).—Diagram showing how normal alveolar-arterial oxygen difference arises. The P_{O_2} values in alveoli at the top and bottom of the lungs, in alveolar air (average value) and in mixed blood leaving the lungs are shown. Alveolar-arterial oxygen difference= 101−97 = 4mm. Hg.

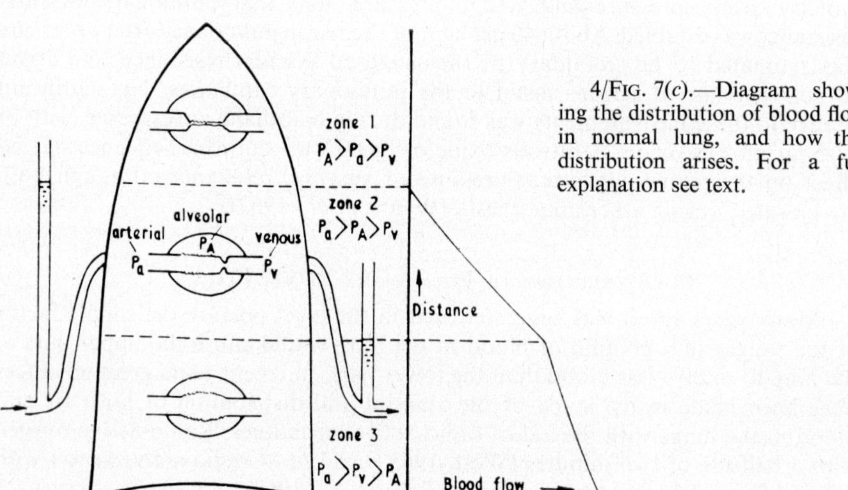

4/FIG. 7(*c*).—Diagram showing the distribution of blood flow in normal lung, and how this distribution arises. For a full explanation see text.

different areas of the lung signifies the pulmonary blood flow. In contrast, xenon is a relatively insoluble gas and is injected into an arm vein as a solution in saline: the xenon passes to the pulmonary capillaries and out into the alveoli. The precise areas in which this takes place are revealed by the counters.

In the normal conscious subject West (1962) found that, in the upright position, there was a nine-fold difference in the pulmonary blood flow between the first and fifth intercostal spaces, with almost no blood flow at the apex of the lung.

From Fig. 7*a* it will be observed that in passing from the apex to the base of the lung, the volume of the organ only increases from 7 to 13 per cent, yet the blood flow alters from 0·07 l./minute at the apex, to 1·29 l./minute at the base. In the *supine* position the blood flow at the apex increases considerably, so that its distribution becomes uniform from apex to base, although now perfusion anteriorly is less than that posteriorly. It appears, therefore, that gravity plays a dominating role in determining the distribution of blood flow within the lungs. The mechanisms through which gravity controls the distribution of blood in the upright lung are shown in Fig. 7*c*. The lung has been divided into three zones by considering the relationships between the alveolar pressure (PA), the pulmonary artery pressure (Pa) and the pulmonary venous pressure (Pv), and the effects these pressures have upon the collapsible pulmonary vessels. In zone 1, at the top of the lung, the alveolar pressure exceeds both the pulmonary artery and pulmonary venous pressures. The result is collapse of the local pulmonary vessels, and little or no blood flow. In zone 2 the pulmonary artery pressure exceeds the alveolar and pulmonary venous pressures. The pulmonary vessels are now held partly open, and blood flow begins to occur at the top of the zone, increasing rather rapidly down its length. In zone 3 the pulmonary artery pressure exceeds the pulmonary venous pressure, which itself is greater than the alveolar pressure. Blood flow continues to increase as we pass down zone 3, but at a slower rate than in zone 2. There is another important difference between zone 2 and zone 3. In zone 2, the blood flow depends mainly on the difference between the *alveolar* and *pulmonary artery* pressures, whereas in zone 3, it is the difference between the *pulmonary arterial* and *pulmonary venous* pressures which is important, the alveolar pressure having little influence.

The scheme outlined above satisfactorily explains most of the observed findings (e.g. the effect of lying supine). For instance, during exercise the perfusion of the lung becomes more evenly distributed, and this is probably due to the increase in pulmonary artery pressure which is observed under these conditions so that zone 1 becomes much smaller or disappears altogether.

In the normal lung at lung volumes below total lung capacity, the interstitial pressure at the lung base is raised because the lung parenchyma is less well expanded than at the lung apex. Perivascular oedema isolates the vessel from the normal expanding action of the lung parenchyma, with the result that the vessel closes by virtue of the inherent tension in its wall. A modification of the three zone model to take account of the reduction of blood flow in the most dependent regions of the lung has been proposed by Hughes and his colleagues (1968). Under pathological conditions, interstitial oedema may further raise the interstitial pressure, thus further reducing the basal blood flow (West *et al.*, 1965).

Distribution of Ventilation

In the normal upright lung the ventilation per unit lung volume is greater at the base than it is at the apex. The change in ventilation decreases approximately linearly with the distance up the lung, being about twice as great at the base than at the apex. It is an interesting fact that these differences disappear in the supine position, the ventilation becoming almost even from apex to base. Also, the differences in regional ventilation become less during exercise, and are reversed in the inverted position. The mechanism by which ventilation within the normal lung is controlled is not known for certain, although it appears that gravity plays a part, and it may be related to the different pleural pressures which exist at the top and bottom of the lungs. The local tension of carbon dioxide may also have a part to play. Severinghaus *et al.* (1961), found that a fall in alveolar CO_2 in one lung after occlusion of its pulmonary artery was accompanied by a fall in ventilation to the lung of about 25 per cent.

In diseased lung the two main factors controlling the distribution of ventilation are the patency of the airways, and local changes in compliance within the lungs. Any factor which reduces the airway calibre, and therefore raises the resistance to airflow, will result in a fall in ventilation to the affected region. Similarly, any area in which the local compliance has decreased will be less well ventilated than the surrounding more expandable normal lung tissue.

The Relationships Between Ventilation and Perfusion in Normal and Abnormal Lungs

The normal alveolar ventilation ($\dot{V}A$) in an adult is approximately 4 l./minute, and the total perfusion ($\dot{Q}$) about 5 l./minute. Therefore the proportion of ventilation to perfusion is $\frac{4}{5} = 0{\cdot}8$. This ratio is known as the VENTILATION/PERFUSION RATIO ($\dot{V}A/\dot{Q}$). The ventilation/perfusion ratio for a whole lung is a composite of the ratios for each individual alveolus, and in an "ideal" lung the ratio for each alveolus should be the same as that for the whole lung (namely 0·8), so that ventilation and blood flow are distributed absolutely evenly to each individual alveolus. As is apparent from the fore-going discussions on the distribution of blood flow and ventilation within the normal lung, this is far from the case (West, 1963 *a* and *b*).

The differences in ventilation and perfusion at the top and bottom of the upright lung, together with their effects on gas exchange, are shown in Fig. 7*a*. At the bottom of the lung ventilation is exceeded by blood flow, so that $\dot{V}A/\dot{Q}$ is low, namely 0·63. Because ventilation is proportionally low, the rate of supply of oxygen to these alveoli is less than the maximum rate at which it could be removed by the blood flow. This results in a low P_{O_2} in these over-perfused alveoli (i.e. 89 mm. Hg), and therefore, a low P_{O_2} in the blood leaving this portion of the lung. However, owing to the shape of the oxygen dissociation curve, a P_{O_2} of 89 mm. Hg only results in a small fall in oxygen saturation (to 96 per cent), as we are still working well on the flat upper portion of the curve. Similarly, the excretion of carbon dioxide is impaired, because the ventilation is not sufficient to wash out all the carbon dioxide passing into the alveoli from venous blood without a small rise in its alveolar concentration ($PA_{CO_2} = 42$ mm. Hg). The result is that blood leaving the base of the lungs is slightly hypoxic and hypercapnic.

Passing up the lungs, both ventilation and perfusion decrease, but perfusion decreases at about three times the rate at which ventilation does. By the time the top of the lung is reached, perfusion is almost nil, so that ventilation at the apices is proportionally far greater than perfusion, and the ratio of the two becomes very high ($\dot{V}A/\dot{Q} = 3{\cdot}3$). Therefore oxygen is supplied to the upper alveoli at a greater rate than it is removed, with the result that a new equilibrium is established, and the alveolar P_{O_2} is high ($PA_{O_2} = 132$ mm. Hg). The blood leaving these areas has a similar P_{O_2} and the saturation rises to nearly 100 per cent. The alveolar carbon dioxide pressure is lower than at the bases ($PA_{CO_2} =$

38 mm. Hg) owing to excessive wash out. Thus blood leaving the apices is almost 100 per cent saturated with a slightly low carbon dioxide content. It is clear that at the top of the lung much of the ventilation is "wasted", as it does not have the opportunity to partake in gas exchange owing to the very low blood flow. This wasted ventilation therefore, becomes part of the physiological dead space, by definition. Any further increase in the proportion of alveoli which are over-ventilated (i.e. with a *high* $\dot{V}_A/\dot{Q}$ ratio) will result in an increase in physiological dead space. This may be secondary to either an increase in relative ventilation in parts of the lung, or to a reduction in relative perfusion, because in both instances a rise in $\dot{V}_A/\dot{Q}$ will occur.

Blood leaving these parts of the lungs with different $\dot{V}_A/\dot{Q}$ ratios will become mixed in the left atrium and left ventricle, so that the arterial tensions of oxygen and carbon dioxide will be somewhere in between the extreme values found at the top and bottom of the lungs. In normal young people the arterial P_{O_2} is about 97 mm. Hg, and P_{CO_2} about 40 mm. Hg. As the normal average alveolar P_{O_2} is about 101 mm. Hg, there is, therefore, a difference of about 4 mm. Hg between the alveolar and arterial P_{O_2} values. This difference is known as the ALVEOLAR-ARTERIAL OXYGEN DIFFERENCE ($P_{A_{O_2}} - P_{a_{O_2}}$) (see Fig. 7*b*). The normal value for $P_{A_{O_2}} - P_{a_{O_2}}$ when breathing 21 per cent oxygen ranges from 5 to 25 mm. Hg, increasing with age (Raine and Bishop, 1963), and also becoming much greater when breathing high oxygen concentrations. Thus when interpreting figures for alveolar-arterial oxygen differences, the inspired oxygen concentration must be taken into account. The alveolar-arterial difference for carbon dioxide is less than 1 mm. Hg.

As has been explained the final value for arterial P_{O_2} and saturation is due to the mixing of fully saturated blood with blood from the relatively underventilated parts of the lung which is less fully saturated. This phenomenon is known as VENOUS ADMIXTURE. The venous admixture can be calculated from the following equation:

$$\frac{\dot{Q}s}{\dot{Q}t} = \frac{Cc' - Ca}{Cc' - C\bar{v}}$$

where $\dot{Q}s/\dot{Q}t$ is the venous admixture, expressed as a percentage of the cardiac output; Cc' is the oxygen content in pulmonary end-capillary blood; Ca is the oxygen content of arterial blood; and $C\bar{v}$ is the oxygen content of mixed venous blood. Cc' is calculated from the "ideal" alveolar P_{O_2}, itself calculated from the Alveolar Air Equation (Comroe, *et al.*, 1962), the haemoglobin content of the blood, and the relationship between P_{O_2} and saturation of haemoglobin (the oxygen dissociation curve). Full details of the methods and calculation are given by Finley *et al.* (1960). In man the normal venous admixture is 1 to 5 per cent of the cardiac output (Cole and Bishop, 1963).

It should be pointed out here that the figures obtained for venous admixture give that percentage of the cardiac output which appears *never to have come into contact with oxygen at all.* In other words, the effect of ventilation/perfusion maldistribution (see below), which results in blood of various oxygen contents being mixed together, is actually represented as an anatomical shunt of mixed systemic venous blood bypassing the lungs, as though the lung could be artificially divided into ideally ventilated and totally unventilated compartments.

Blood passing through the latter compartment does not come into contact with oxygen, and therefore appears as an anatomical right-to-left shunt. A figure of, say, 10 per cent venous admixture means that the lungs are behaving *as though an anatomical shunt of this value were present*. Nevertheless, the venous admixture and the alveolar-arterial oxygen difference are indispensible in quantitating the effectiveness of oxygen transfer within the lungs. The advantage of measuring $\dot{Q}s/\dot{Q}t$ rather than $P_{A_{O_2}} - Pa_{O_2}$ is that the latter can be increased in the presence of a low cardiac output (an extra-pulmonary factor), whereas this is accounted for in venous admixture figures. This is because the mixed venous oxygen content in a blood sample taken from the right ventricle or pulmonary artery must be known in order to calculate venous admixture. The assumption of an arterio-venous oxygen content difference can lead to error.

The various subdivisions and some causes of the venous admixture are shown in Table 4. *Physiological shunt* is the term used to describe the blood which passes through the thebesian and bronchial vascular systems to nourish the heart and lungs respectively. This blood is not oxygenated yet it finally arrives on the left side of the heart to dilute the oxygenated blood which has come from the lungs.

4/TABLE 4

A CLASSIFICATION OF SOURCES OF VENOUS ADMIXTURE

		OCCURRENCE		
		In the normal conscious subject	In the anaesthetised subject	In pathological states
Anatomical	Transfer of mixed venous blood from right heart to left heart	NIL	NIL	Septal defects, patent ductus arteriosus, pulmonary haemangioma
Physiological	Drainage of venous blood into left heart	1–2 per cent of cardiac output from bronchial and thebesian veins	Probably the same as in the conscious subject	Bronchial blood flow greatly increased in bronchial disease, e.g. bronchiectasis
Atelectatic Shunt	Pulmonary blood flow through *totally* unventilated lung	NIL	10–15 per cent of cardiac output depending on ventilatory history and other factors	Collapse or consolidation of lung—especially in lobar pneumonia
Ventilation/ perfusion Maldistribution	Pulmonary blood flow through *relatively* under-ventilated lung	Normal degree of maldistribution is responsible for reduction of arterial P_{O_2} by 2–10 mm.Hg	Increased during anaesthesia	Greatly increased in diseases such as emphysema in which it is the major cause of desaturation

Anatomical (or Pathological) *Shunt* describes blood which bypasses the lungs, passing from right to left through a septal defect or patent ductus arteriosus in the presence of pulmonary hypertension, or occasionally through communications within the lungs themselves. *Ventilation/Perfusion Maldistribution* is the term used to describe that portion of the pulmonary blood flow which has passed through relatively underventilated lung, whereas *Atelectatic Shunt* is used to describe blood which has passed through totally unventilated lung. The normal value for venous admixture—1 to 5 per cent—is made up partly by physiological shunt (1 to 2 per cent), and partly from the results of ventilation/perfusion maldistribution.

Considering the magnitude of the variations in ventilation/perfusion relationships within the normal upright lung, it is remarkable how efficient the lungs are at oxygenating venous blood when compared to the "ideal" lung. As mentioned above, the normal alveolar-arterial oxygen difference is only about 4 mm. Hg, with a venous admixture of less than 5 per cent of the cardiac output. This is due to the shape of the oxygen dissociation curve since, for blood leaving the over- or under-ventilated regions of normal lungs, only the flat upper portion of the curve is involved. In blood leaving the lung bases, therefore, a P_{O_2} of 89 mm. Hg corresponds to a saturation of 96 per cent, not far below full saturation. Because the upper portion of the oxygen dissociation curve is almost a straight line, this small fall in saturation can be compensated for by blood leaving the over-ventilated regions of the lung. In these regions at the top of the lung the P_{O_2} in the blood is 132 mm. Hg, corresponding to a saturation of nearly 100 per cent. The result is that when the two are mixed together the final P_{O_2} is 97 mm. Hg with a saturation of 97 per cent. However, arterial oxygenation is much less satisfactory when, for blood leaving the under-ventilated regions, the point of equilibration lies well down on the steep part of the dissociation curve. Under these circumstances the slightly higher oxygen content found in the over-ventilated regions is now unable to compensate for the rather lower saturations in blood leaving the under-ventilated areas. Significant desaturation therefore occurs in the final blood mixture leaving the left ventricle. This saturation occurs frequently in pathological states. For instance, if a region of atelectasis is present, in which no ventilation occurs, the blood leaving this part of the lung has an oxygen saturation equal to that in venous blood arriving at the lungs (i.e. $P_{O_2} = 40$ mm. Hg; saturation $= 75$ per cent), as no oxygen has been added to the blood. Here we have a saturation which is considerably lower than that found in the under-ventilated areas of normal lung. The small rise in saturation in the over-ventilated regions is now unable to compensate for the low saturation in the blood which has passed through the atelectatic lung, and arterial desaturation inevitably follows. Clearly, compensation becomes even more difficult in the presence of a low cardiac output, when systemic venous saturation may fall to 50 per cent or less. The relation between cardiac output, venous admixture and arterial oxygenation is shown in Fig. 8. As can be seen, for a given venous admixture arterial oxygenation falls considerably at low cardiac outputs. This accounts for the very low arterial P_{O_2} values found in patients with cardio-respiratory failure.

Ventilation/perfusion relationships can be quantified by making the following measurements: (1) The physiological dead space. This gives an estimate of

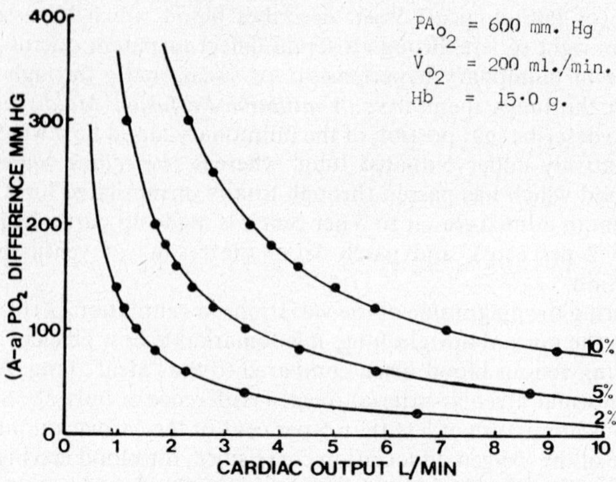

4/FIG. 8.—Graph showing the effect of venous admixture and cardiac output on the alveolar-arterial oxygen difference while breathing oxygen. As can be seen, for a given venous admixture, the alveolar-arterial oxygen difference rises steeply at low cardiac outputs. Also, a change in venous admixture causes a greater change in alveolar-arterial oxygen difference when the cardiac output is low.

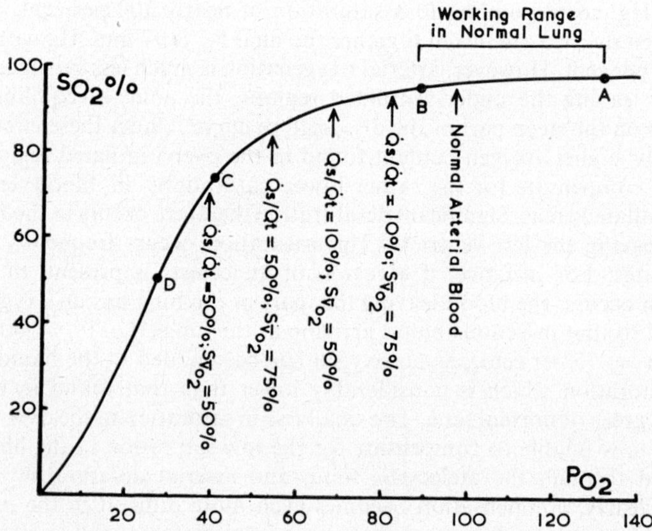

4/FIG. 9.—Diagram showing the approximate effects of various situations on arterial oxygenation in relation to the oxygen dissociation curve when breathing air. Blood which has come from relatively over-ventilated areas of normal lung is at point A, and that from relatively underventilated areas is at point B. Point C represents mixed venous blood in the presence of a normal cardiac output and point D mixed venous blood with a low cardiac output. The arterial oxygen saturation is above 90 per cent (P_{O_2} = 64 mm. Hg) unless the venous admixture rises above about 30 per cent with a normal cardiac output, or above 15 per cent when the mixed venous saturation is 50 per cent. $\dot{Q}s/\dot{Q}t$ per cent = venous admixture: $S\bar{v}_{O_2}$ = saturation of mixed venous blood.

the amount of wasted ventilation, and therefore of the amount of the lung which is being relatively over-ventilated. (2) The alveolar-arterial oxygen difference or venous admixture. The larger the value of either of these figures, the greater is the amount of lung which is relatively under-ventilated or non-ventilated. An increase in $\dot{Q}s/\dot{Q}t$ or $P_{A_{O_2}} - Pa_{O_2}$ can be due to the following pulmonary causes (a) a diffusion defect, (b) ventilation/perfusion maldistribution; or (3) atelectatic shunt. The effects of the first two can be abolished by breathing 100 per cent oxygen, whereas the effects of the atelectatic shunt are still present. Therefore, the relative contribution of atelectasis as compared to the other two causes can be estimated by calculating venous admixture firstly when breathing air, and then during oxygen breathing. While breathing air all three factors contribute to venous admixture; during oxygen breathing only atelectatic shunt is demonstrated.

4/TABLE 5

THE PULMONARY CAUSES OF ARTERIAL HYPOXAEMIA

<table>
<tr><td>(1) Hypoventilation.</td><td colspan="2">Excluded or confirmed by arterial P_{CO_2}. Hypoxaemia abolished by oxygen breathing.</td></tr>
<tr><td>(2) Diffusion Defect.</td><td rowspan="2">Effects abolished by oxygen breathing.</td><td rowspan="3">Relative over-ventilation appears as as high VD phys.
Relative under-ventilation appears as high $\frac{\dot{Q}s}{\dot{Q}t}$ or high $P_{A_{O_2}} - Pa_{O_2}$.</td></tr>
<tr><td>(3) Maldistribution.</td></tr>
<tr><td>(4) Atelectatic Shunt.</td><td>Unaffected by oxygen breathing.</td></tr>
</table>

Although most of the previous discussion has been concerned with the normal lung, in the presence of pulmonary disease exactly the same principles apply. The final result in terms of physiological dead space and arterial hypoxaemia depends on the balance of many factors. The extent, type and location of diseased areas, the relative amounts of lung which have a high or low $\dot{V}A/\dot{Q}$ ratio, the tidal volume, the physiological dead space, the cardiac output and the age of the patient. Each one of these factors contributes its quota to the overall function of the lungs as reflected in the arterial blood. However, the dominant influence on arterial oxygenation is usually the relationship between ventilation and perfusion.

The Ventilation/Perfusion Ratio and Carbon Dioxide Excretion

Variations in the relationship between ventilation and perfusion have a smaller effect on the excretion of carbon dioxide than upon the uptake of oxygen. This is because the physiological dissociation curve for carbon dioxide is almost a straight line (see 3/Fig. 11). The result is that it is possible for over-ventilated areas of the lung to compensate fairly easily for the high carbon dioxide tension found in blood which has passed through under-ventilated regions, in much the same way as has been described for the upper portion of the oxygen dissociation curve. Essentially the adequacy of carbon dioxide excretion depends mainly on the total alveolar ventilation, rather than upon its distribution. A potential rise in arterial P_{CO_2} due to ventilation-perfusion abnormalities can be compensated for by an increase in total ventilation. This is not so for a fall in P_{O_2}, unless it is secondary to hypercapnia. It is only when lung disease is very severe, with large variations in ventilation/perfusion relationships, coupled with an inability to increase total ventilation any further, that the arterial P_{CO_2} begins to rise. This explains the finding that the arterial P_{O_2} is a much more sensitive index of pulmonary disease than is the arterial P_{CO_2}.

SOME FACTORS AFFECTING PULMONARY FUNCTION
with special reference to anaesthesia

Advancing Age

The results obtained from almost any lung function test must be interpreted with the subject's age in mind. For the tests of ventilation increasing age is associated with a fall in maximum breathing capacity, forced expiratory volume, peak expiratory flow rate, vital capacity and total lung capacity. A progressive rise is seen in the ratios functional residual capacity/total lung volume and residual volume/total lung capacity. The physiological dead space rises, but the arterial P_{CO_2} remains constant. The alveolar-arterial oxygen difference rises, and may be as high as 25 mm. Hg in old age. The arterial P_{O_2} therefore falls progressively, and in an old person with clinically normal lungs may be as low as 75 mm. Hg.

Posture

Compared with the upright position, in a subject lying supine the distribution of both blood flow and ventilation becomes even from top to bottom of the lung. However, an anterior to posterior gradient now appears. In the inverted position ventilation is greater at the apex that at the base, the reverse of that found in the normal upright position.

When an anaesthetised patient, breathing spontaneously, is turned on his side, perfusion of the lowermost lung is encouraged at the expense of the upper. The proportion of the ventilation going to the lower lung is also increased because the diaphragm is able to contract more efficiently. This is due to the weight of the abdominal contents pushing the muscle higher up into the thorax and so permitting a greater range of movement on contraction. Thus, during spontaneous respiration both perfusion and ventilation of the lower lung are increased. Once the patient is paralysed and artificially ventilated, the upper lung now becomes preferentially ventilated, as its compliance is greater due partly to there being less pressure from the abdominal contents and diaphragm to be overcome, and partly because its vascular bed is less distended. If thoracotomy is now performed the amount of lung tissue which is ventilated but not perfused rises, and the fraction which is perfused but not ventilated (atelectatic shunt) also increases, but to a lesser extent (Virtue *et al.*, 1966).

Effect of Artificial Ventilation

It is now widely accepted that anaesthesia with artificial ventilation results in an increased physiological dead space, sometimes up to 50 per cent or more of the tidal volume. This means that parts of the lungs have become relatively over-ventilated. The precise effects of artificial ventilation on the regional distribution of ventilation are at present unknown although Bergman (1963) has suggested that there is no alteration from that found during spontaneous ventilation. The essential change is that the alveolar pressure is increased. It is, therefore, possible to predict some of the effects of positive pressure ventilation on the distribution of blood flow. An increase in alveolar pressure will result in an enlargement of zone 1, with the other two zones dropping down the lung. The amount of lung with a high $\dot{V}_A/\dot{Q}$ ratio is therefore greater, and an increased physiological dead space results. This effect was found by Campbell *et al.* (1958) who reported a rise in physiological dead space following a change from spontaneous to controlled ventilation, with no change in alveolar-arterial oxygen difference. For a further discussion of the effects of ventilation on the arterial oxygenation see the section on Anaesthesia (p. 167).

Effect of Duration of Inspiration

In the normal supine subject breathing spontaneously, the elastic resistance of the lung is only about 6 cm. water/litre (Attinger *et al.*, 1956; Howell and Peckett, 1957). This is largely because the chest wall is moving actively so that it provides no resistance. In a paralysed patient, however, the elastic resistance rises on average to about 19 cm. water/litre (Smith and Spalding, 1959), i.e. over three times as great as in a patient breathing spontaneously. Watson (1962*a*) has shown that this rise in resistance occurs very rapidly after the change from spontaneous to controlled respiration. It cannot, therefore, adequately be explained on a basis of atelectasis or blocked bronchi, because sufficient time is not allowed for this to occur. Apparently the most significant factor is the duration of inspiration. Thus, if inspiration during intermittent positive-pressure ventilation lasts more than 1·5 seconds, the physiological dead space and elastic resistance are within normal limits. On the other hand, if inspiration is shortened to only 0·5 second, then there is a steep rise in elastic resistance and physiological dead space. The most probable explanation of these findings is that very rapid inspiration leads to an abnormal distribution of air in the lungs so that again the ventilation-perfusion ratio is altered. With a very rapid inflation there is an abnormal distribution of air in the lungs, so that some alveoli are overventilated but relatively underperfused whilst others are underventilated and overperfused (Spalding and Crampton Smith, 1963).

Effect of Total Blood Volume and its Distribution

Freeman and Nunn (1963) working with anaesthetised dogs, found an increase in physiological dead space in the presence of haemorrhage. In fact under these conditions it could be increased to nearly 80 per cent of the tidal volume. Askrog *et al.* (1964) found similar changes during controlled hypotension in man, especially if the patient was tipped head up. Both experimental findings can be explained by a fall in pulmonary arterial and venous pressures, in one case secondary to a fall in total blood volume, in the other because of a shift of blood from the pulmonary to the systemic circulation. From Fig. 7*c* it can be seen that this will result in an increase in zone 1, with the other two zones dropping down the lung. Therefore, an increase in dead space results, the amount depending on the fall in pulmonary arterial and venous pressures.

Premedication

The work of Tomlin and his associates (1964) has suggested that when arterial hypoxaemia is observed during and after general anaesthesia it may in part be due to the pulmonary effects of subcutaneous atropine. They found that the mean oxygen saturation in a group of patients premedicated with atropine (93·4 per cent) was significantly lower than in a second unpremedicated group (96·0 per cent). In a second study they observed a significant fall in arterial P_{O_2} following atropine given subcutaneously (from a mean of 95·4 mm. Hg to 86·4 mm. Hg), and that post-operative hypoxaemia occurred in those patients premedicated with atropine but not in a group of unpremedicated patients. On the other hand, Nunn and Bergman (1964), in a study on conscious volunteers, agreed with the findings of Daly *et al.* (1963), who observed that arterial oxygenation was unchanged in conscious subjects even after the administration of up to 2 mg. of atropine intravenously. Similarly, Taylor and his colleagues (1964) found no change in the oxygen saturations of arterial blood in anaesthetised patients, and nor did Gardiner and Palmer (1964) after premedication with atropine. Conway (1964) has produced evidence that the route of administration may be important, hypoxaemia being most likely to appear after subcutaneous administration of the drug. Although the effect of atropine, if any, on arterial oxygenation has not yet finally been settled, there is general agreement that it increases both anatomical and physiological dead space. Nunn and Bergman (1964) found an increase in V_D/V_T ratio of 26·5 to 34·3 per cent. A similar increase in anatomical dead space has been reported by Smith *et al.* (1967) after both atropine (+ 22 per cent) and hyoscine (+ 25 per cent). The precise mechanism of this effect is not known, but it is probably related either to an action on the bronchial musculature or to an action on the lining membrane.

In 1965 Pierce and Garofalo found that arterial P_{O_2} was significantly lower in a group of patients awaiting open heart surgery after being given a mixture of pethidine, promethazine and pentobarbitone, although no change occurred in a second group given pentobarbitone alone. Arterial P_{CO_2} was unchanged in both groups. Egbert and Bendixen (1964) noted an alteration in the pattern of breathing after the administration of morphine, the main change being a large decrease in the frequency of spontaneous "sighing". They suggested that this might result in alveolar collapse, and therefore in arterial hypoxaemia. Fletcher and Barber (1966) agreed with this finding, but could detect no change in arterial P_{O_2}, $P_{A_{O_2}} - Pa_{O_2}$, or in lung compliance, in spite of the absence of "sighing" after morphine for up to one and a half hours. A transient increase in compliance followed a voluntary maximum inspiration, but did not occur after spontaneous sighing. Recently Martinez *et al.* (1967) have investigated the pulmonary effects of various premedications in patients with pulmonary or cardiovascular disease, but who were well compensated at the time. They studied the effects of intramuscular morphine (1·3 mg./10kg.), pentobarbitone (15 mg./10 kg.) and atropine (0·07 mg./10 kg.), morphine and hyoscine (0·07 mg./10 kg.), hyoscine alone and a placebo. Both arterial P_{O_2} and P_{CO_2} were unchanged in all groups after the drugs had been given, except for a small rise in Pa_{O_2} after morphine alone and after pentobarbitone and atropine. The most significant finding was a fall in alveolar ventilation, ranging between 5·4 per cent and 12·7 per cent of control values, following each drug combination except the placebo. They considered that the arterial P_{CO_2} remained constant despite a fall in ventilation because this was accompanied by a reduction in CO_2 production. The study is remarkable for the lack of effects demonstrated. Gardiner and Palmer (1964), investigating healthy patients awaiting surgery, also found no change in arterial P_{O_2} or P_{CO_2} thirty minutes after premedication with either atropine alone or with papaveretum and hyoscine.

In spite of these studies it is well known that opiates, given in sufficient dosage, cause a reduction in alveolar ventilation and a rise in arterial P_{CO_2}, and depress the ventilatory response to carbon dioxide (Smith *et al.*, 1967). They also cause systemic venodilatation, with a small shift of blood out of the pulmonary circulation (the likely mechanism through which they are effective in pulmonary oedema).

Anaesthesia

Although it had been suggested previously (Stark and Smith, 1960), the possibility that clinically unrecognised arterial hypoxaemia might occur during routine anaesthesia in healthy patients was first seriously considered following the publication of a paper by Bendixen and his colleagues in 1963. They reported that during anaesthesia with controlled respiration a progressive fall occurred in arterial P_{O_2} and total compliance, both of which could be reversed by passive hyperinflation. Pa_{O_2} fell most rapidly in those patients who were ventilated at the lowest tidal volumes. In 1964 Bendixen *et al.* published similar findings during spontaneous respirations with ether/oxygen anaesthesia, and Egbert *et al.* (1963), measuring total compliance under a variety of anaesthetics, found that in the absence of deep breaths a fall in compliance could be demonstrated after 5 to 10 minutes, and that passive hyperinflation returned compliance to control levels. Gold and Helrich (1965) also found a decrease in lung compliance to below pre-anaesthetic levels during nitrous oxide/oxygen/halothane anaesthesia with spontaneous respiration, and noted that the decrease was related to the magnitude of the decrease in tidal volume. At this time Nunn (1964) also published a study showing abnormally high alveolar-arterial oxygen differences during anaesthesia with spontaneous respirations, and recommended an inspired oxygen concentration of at least 35 per cent to maintain normal oxygenation during surgery. In a second study, this time during controlled ventilation, Nunn *et al.* (1965) again found abnormally low arterial P_{O_2} values and noted that they fell progressively in their older patients. Passive hyperinflation was not always successful in reversing these changes. Slater *et al.* (1965), in a study of nitrous oxide/oxygen/curare anaesthesia, suggested that a minimum oxygen concentration of 33 per cent was necessary to maintain a Pa_{O_2} of 80 mm. Hg or more in the majority of patients, and Sykes *et al.* (1965) found that high alveolar-arterial oxygen differences could be reduced by ventilating paralysed patients at high tidal volumes. At this time, therefore, it appeared that atelectasis, as shown by high alveolar-arterial oxygen differences and low compliance, was an inevitable accompaniment of general anaesthesia. The atelectasis appeared to be progressive although Askrog and his colleagues (1964) could find no evidence of this during either halothane, cyclopropane or nitrous oxide anaesthesia, and in some cases could be substantially reversed by passive hyperinflations. However up to this time few workers had measured arterial oxygen tensions immediately preceding the induction of anaesthesia, although many had examined changes in Pa_{O_2} during its course. Then Marshall (1966) reported that he could find no change in alveolar-arterial oxygen difference between blood samples taken before and during anaesthesia with halothane and oxygen, although he was able to detect a rise during the administration of ether and air compared to pre-operative values (Marshall and Grange, 1966). In an investigation into the effects of halothane and oxygen on functional residual capacity, compliance and alveolar-arterial oxygen differences, Colgan and Whang (1968) were unable to find any alteration from pre-operative values either during or after anaesthesia, and stated that "progressive atelectasis was not a predictable consequence of unassisted ventilation during anaesthesia in healthy dogs and man". However it is evident from their figures in man that some alveolar collapse may have been present in their patients after premedication but before the induction of anaesthesia, as they found abnormally high alveolar-arterial oxygen differences at this time (mean $P_{A_{O_2}} - Pa_{O_2} = 164$ mm. Hg; mean $Pa_{O_2} = 414$ mm. Hg, breathing 100 per cent oxygen). Recently an excellent investigation has been reported by Marshall *et al.* (1969) covering the periods before, during and after halothane and oxygen anaesthesia in man. Before the induction of anaesthesia they found the following data; breathing 100 per cent oxygen, mean $Pa_{O_2} = 572$ mm. Hg; mean $P_{A_{O_2}} - Pa_{O_2} = 70$ mm. Hg; mean shunt = 4·4 per cent of the cardiac output. Soon after induction evidence of an increase in intrapulmonary shunting had appeared (mean $Pa_{O_2} = 466$ mm. Hg; mean $P_{A_{O_2}} - Pa_{O_2} = 170$ mm. Hg; mean shunt = 12·1 per cent) which had increased at the end of operation (mean $Pa_{O_2} = 427$ mm. Hg; mean $P_{A_{O_2}} - Pa_{O_2} = 218$ mm. Hg; mean shunt = 14·8 per cent). These changes had all returned to pre-operative levels three hours after operation (Fig. 10).

At the present time the bulk of the evidence indicates that general anaesthesia is associated with the development of an intrapulmonary shunt, although its nature is not certain. The actual value of this shunt is remarkably constant at about 10–15 per cent of the cardiac output with a large variety of anaesthetic agents and from investigator to investigator. It seems likely that the appearance of intrapulmonary shunting is related to the state of anaesthesia rather than to the actions of individual agents (Webb and Nunn, 1967; Price *et al.*, 1969). Some workers have found little difference in venous admixture measurements made when breathing inspired oxygen concentrations of 21 per cent and 100 per cent, suggesting that ventilation/perfusion maldistribution plays little part in its aetiology (Nunn *et al.*, 1965; Bergman, 1967), and no changes have been reported in the distribution of either ventilation or perfusion following the induction of anaesthesia with or without controlled ventilation (Bergman, 1963; Hulands *et al.*, 1969). Low tidal volumes appear to predispose to greater shunting effects than high tidal volumes, although the ratio of inspiratory to expiratory time is not important (Lumley *et al.*, 1969). Many workers have not found the changes to be progressive with time (Askrog *et al.*, 1964; Sykes *et al.*, 1965; Panday and Nunn, 1968; Lumley *et al.*, 1969). However the volume history of the lungs immediately before taking blood for analysis is probably of great importance in determining the values found (Mead and Collier, 1959), and it is possible that

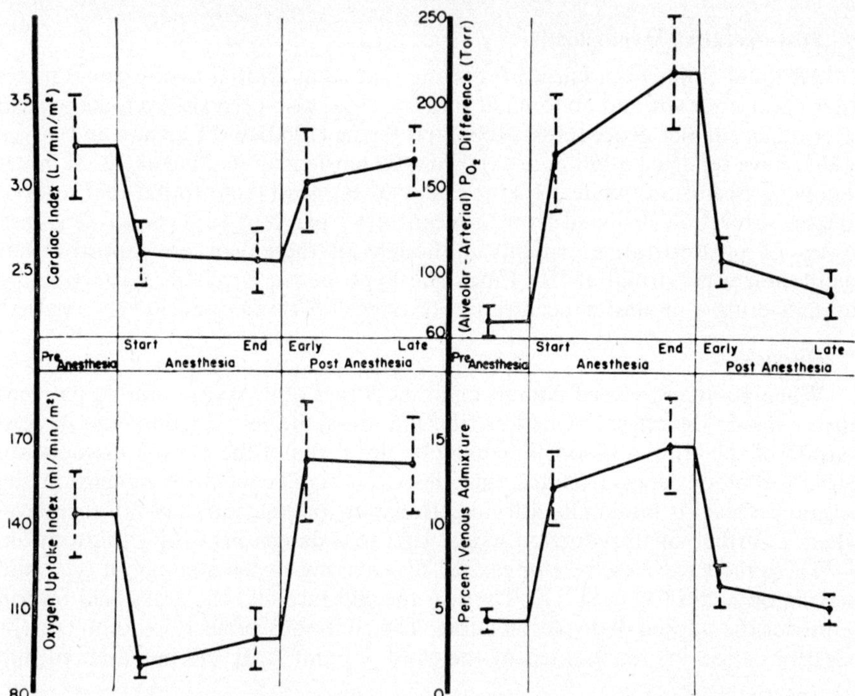

4/FIG. 10.—Changes in cardiac index, oxygen uptake, alveolar-arterial oxygen difference and venous admixture during and after halothane/oxygen anaesthesia with spontaneous respiration. The post-anaesthetic measurements were made 30 minutes ("early") and 3 hours ("late") after discontinuing the halothane. Mean data from 10 patients, ± S.E.

during controlled ventilation small differences in techniques could explain the contradictory results of different workers.

One incontrovertible fact arises out of these experiments, namely that during general anaesthesia the transport of oxygen through the lungs is often impaired, and that to ensure adequate arterial oxygenation during an anaesthetic at least 33 per cent oxygen should be administered in the inspired gas mixture. A substantial part of these changes is in all probability due to complete alveolar collapse and can sometimes be partially reversed by passive hyperinflation.

As well as affecting oxygen transfer within the lungs, anaesthesia also impairs the efficiency of carbon dioxide excretion. The most important adverse effect is due to a reduction in alveolar ventilation, brought about by (1) direct depression of the respiratory centres; (2) decreased ventilatory response to a rise in arterial P_{CO_2}; (3) the addition of apparatus dead space; and (4) an increase in physiological dead space. Another factor which has to be taken into account is that the arterio-alveolar CO_2 difference (normal = less than 1 mm. Hg) rises during anaesthesia. Nunn and Hill (1960) found an average value of 4·5 (S.D. = ± 2·5) mm. Hg during spontaneous respiration, and 4·7 (S.D. = ± 2·5) mm. Hg during controlled ventilation. It has been suggested that these findings might be secondary to a fall in pulmonary artery pressure.

Post-operative Hypoxaemia

Although it has been known for many years that arterial hypoxaemia occurs after major thoracic and abdominal surgery, it has also been shown to be present after much simpler procedures. Nunn and Payne (1962) and Conway and Payne (1963) have reported a fall in arterial oxygen tension for as long as 12–24 hours following operation, while Buckley and Van Bergen (1960) found that arterial oxygen saturation dropped from a mean of 97 per cent to 93·8 per cent in a group of post-operative patients, although all these workers reported that ventilation was normal at this time. The hypoxaemia is readily correctible by administering a modest concentration of oxygen (Conway and Payne, 1963).

Discussion

When an anaesthetised patient breathes 20 per cent oxygen and 80 per cent nitrous oxide the effects of maldistribution are sufficient to reduce the oxygen tension of the arterial blood. Fortunately, the shape of the oxygen dissociation curve for blood is so arranged that despite a significant drop in tension the saturation level is minimally affected. However, the tension may fall to a level where a further small reduction would lead to a dangerous drop in saturation.

These facts can best be emphasised by referring to the analogy of the child playing on a cliff top (Fig. 11). The sea, the cliff face and the grass field on top represent the oxygen dissociation curve. The conscious subject breathing air (21 per cent oxygen) is represented by the child at point A. It will be observed that

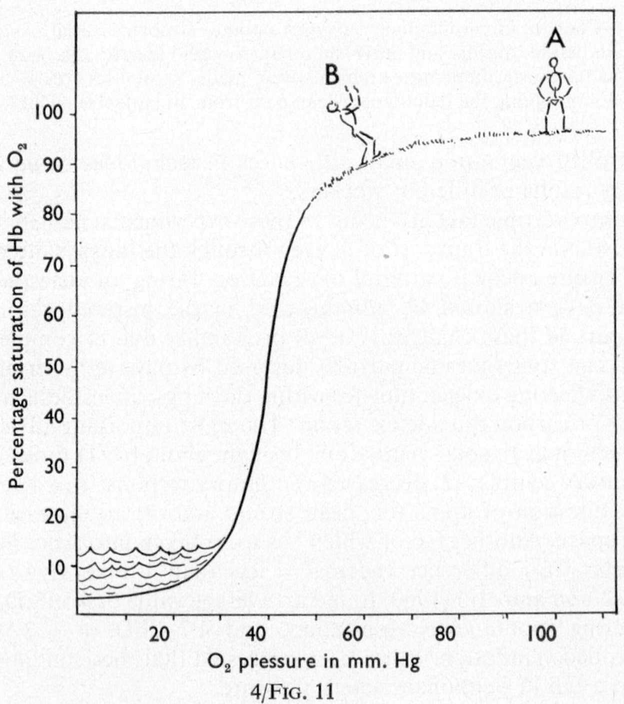

4/Fig. 11

fairly wide movements to the right or left will lead to only a very small change in oxygen saturation. The anaesthetised patient, or those in the immediate post-operative period under analgesic drugs, are quite different. Now the child has moved to point B. Any movement to the left (as, for example, with atelectasis or mild respiratory obstruction) can lead to a perilous descent towards desaturation. If, however, such patients are given extra oxygen, they are rapidly transported to the safety zone (point A) enjoyed by the conscious subject.

It is recommended, therefore, that at least *33 per cent* oxygen should be the *minimum* inspired concentration for the anaesthetised patient breathing spontaneously and also that a periodic hyperinflation should be used to simulate the "sigh" of the conscious subject. This work also underlines the value of oxygen therapy in the post-operative period, although in most instances good physiotherapy with encouragement of deep breathing is sufficient.

A simple assessment of respiratory function must always be made before operation and anaesthesia. Observation of the patient at rest and at light exercise, such as walking in the ward, together with a clinical examination, are likely to prove just as satisfactory as more complicated tests in the majority of cases. The breath-holding test of Sebrasez is a useful but rough method for estimating cardio-respiratory reserve. It consists of taking a maximum inspiration while at rest and then holding the breath for as long as possible. Failure to hold the breath for less than 25 seconds is abnormal.

Properly chosen and adequately given anaesthesia need not necessarily hamper respiratory function during the time of its administration if a mixture containing at least 33 per cent oxygen is breathed. Assisted or controlled respiration will compensate for most types of decreased ventilatory capacity, though there are occasions when even intermittent positive-pressure may be better avoided, e.g. cases of obstructive emphysema. The general reduction of metabolism and rest associated with a carefully chosen anaesthetic is a therapeutic factor of importance. In the immediate post-operative period and for some time after, however, unaided respiratory function must be sufficient to maintain a normal oxygen and carbon dioxide tension in the blood. Pain, the increased metabolism of the body which follows an operation, and occasionally the central respiratory effects of depressant doses of opiates and the like, all tend in differing ways to reduce respiratory function; furthermore, the results of surgery on the lungs, and of post-operative complications in them, may be decisive factors leading to decompensation. It is the ability of the patient to withstand the immediate post-anaesthetic period as well as the period of operation that anaesthetists ought to try to assess pre-operatively.

Dyspnoea is the most obvious clinical symptom and sign of this incapacity; it is an index of the relation between ventilatory capacity and ventilatory volume. Subjects with a normal capacity may show dyspnoea on heavy exercise. In the presence of lung disease, however, the capacity is limited and a slight increase in ventilatory volume leads to difficulty in breathing. It is because so many thoracic operations are considered against a background of disease in the lungs that specialised tests may have to be carried out to determine the function of that portion which will remain.

The value of these tests to the anaesthetist is very limited, and it is doubtful whether, at the moment, they offer much more information in cases of disease than can be obtained by simple observation of the patient's dyspnoea and cyanosis. In so far as the special tests substantiate clinical investigation they may be helpful in the choice of practical anaesthesia. Thus emphysema or bronchial spasm may necessitate special techniques or special treatment. One of the difficulties in assessing the results of the tests is the differentiation between normal and abnormal, and in deciding from the results of respiratory function tests what the chances are of post-operative complications. Nevertheless, they do enable an objective assessment to be made of the severity of dyspnoea, and hence of true impairment of ventilatory function. This may be of value not only in evaluating the results of surgical treatment, but also in preparing patients for operation when the results of treatment could with advantage be measured and compared with previous figures. Broncho-spirometry, despite its many disadvantages, may occasionally give valuable information concerning the adequacy of the lung which is to be left after pneumonectomy.

The geriatric patient who is physically handicapped by pulmonary disease is increasingly frequently submitted to surgery and therefore to anaesthesia. Although gross in its practical implications, the basic advantages of properly chosen and administered anaesthesia, and the relative tolerance to it of even diseased patients, enables most operations to be performed with a limited mortality and morbidity. If, however, any improvement is to be made on the present best, and the occasional patient is to be saved from a major complication, objective measurements of the pulmonary state of patients of this type before, during and after operation and anaesthetic, and following pre-operative treatment, must be carried out. Only by such means can progress eventually be made towards a reasoned pre-operative assessment of what a patient can be expected to tolerate during and after an operation.

THE ACID-BASE STATUS OF THE BLOOD

Terminology

The relationship between acids and bases can be described by the following equation:

$$\text{Acid} \rightleftarrows \text{H}^+ + \text{Base}^-$$

An acid is a hydrogen ion donor. A strong acid is almost completely dissociated when in an aqueous solution. A weak acid is less completely dissociated. *A base* is a hydrogen ion acceptor. A strong base is one for which the above equilibrium is displaced almost completely to the left, and a weak base is one for which it is displaced only partly to the left. *Buffers* are substances which by their presence in solution increase the amount of acid or alkali which must be added to cause a unit shift in pH. The combination in solution of a weak acid and its strong base (as a salt) is called a *buffer pair*. The weak acid is the *buffer acid* and the strong base is the *buffer base*. A buffer system obeys the Law of Mass Action, so that

$$\text{K [Acid]} = [\text{H}^+] + [\text{Base}^-]$$

where K is a constant. Rearranging this formula

$$[H^+] = K \frac{[Acid]}{[Base^-]}$$

and converting to negative logarithms to the base 10, this equation becomes:

$$pH = pK' + \log \frac{[Base^-]}{[Acid]}$$

For the bicarbonate buffer system the equation becomes:

$$pH = pK' + \log \frac{[HCO_3^-]}{[H_2CO_3]}$$

This is the Henderson-Hasselbach equation. $[HCO_3^-]$ represents the plasma bicarbonate, and $[H_2CO_3]$ represents the sum of the dissolved carbon dioxide and carbonic acid, according to the equation

$$CO_2 + H_2O \rightleftharpoons H_2CO_3$$

For plasma at 38°C, pK′ = 6·1 (the dissociation constant). Numerous graphic representations of the Henderson-Hasselbach equation have been suggested, the best known being the pH-bicarbonate plot (Davenport, 1958), and the pH-log P_{CO_2} plot (Siggaard-Andersen, 1966).

The acidity of a solution depends on the concentration of hydrogen ions contained in it, and is most often expressed in pH units. pH is the negative logarithm of the molar hydrogen ion concentration (or, more correctly, the hydrogen ion activity). The normal pH of whole blood is 7·4 units, equivalent to a hydrogen ion concentration of 40 nano-equivalents/litre. A nano-equivalent is an equivalent $\times 10^{-9}$, or one millionth of a milli-equivalent. The relationship between pH and the hydrogen ion concentration is shown in Table 6.

4/Table 6

Equivalent values of pH and Hydrogen Ion concentration

$[H^+]$ nano Eq/1.	pH.
100	7·0
63	7·2
40	7·4
25	7·6
16	7·8
10	8·0

P_{CO_2} is the partial pressure of carbon dioxide in a gas mixture, and at 37°C is given by the equation:

$$P_{CO_2} = (F_{CO_2}) \text{ (B.P.} - 47\text{), mm. Hg}$$

where F_{CO_2} is the fractional concentration of carbon dioxide in the mixture, B.P. (mm. Hg) is the barometric pressure, and 47 mm. Hg is the saturated vapour pressure of water at 37°C. The P_{CO_2} of a solution of carbon dioxide in a liquid such as plasma is best understood by considering a gas-liquid system in equilibrium. The carbon dioxide tension of the liquid phase is equal to the P_{CO_2} in the gas phase when no net exchange of CO_2 occurs between the two phases. At any given equilibrium the carbon dioxide content of the liquid is a reflection of the P_{CO_2} of the gas phase, and therefore the CO_2 content of the liquid can be described by stating the P_{CO_2} of the gas phase. The P_{CO_2} of blood is thus defined as that P_{CO_2} in a gas mixture which, when in contact with the blood, results in no net exchange of CO_2 between the two phases.

An *acidosis* is said to be present when the hydrogen ion concentration in blood is higher than normal (low pH), or would be if no compensation had occurred. An *alkalosis* (baseosis) is present when the hydrogen ion concentration is lower than normal (high pH), or would be if compensation had not occurred. These definitions enable combinations of changes to be described, e.g. a respiratory acidosis and a metabolic alkalosis present at the same time, although the pH may lie within the normal range. A *respiratory acidosis* or *alkalosis* is a change, or potential change, in pH resulting from alterations in the P_{CO_2}. A *metabolic acidosis* or *alkalosis* is a change, or potential change, in pH resulting from alterations in the non-volatile acids in the blood, e.g. lactic acid.

Buffer base is the sum of the buffer anions in the blood. It includes bicarbonate, haemoglobin, proteins and phosphates, and therefore alters with changes in the haemoglobin. The total buffer base does not alter with respiratory changes in the blood, but does alter as a result of non-respiratory (metabolic) changes. The total buffer base can therefore be used to quantitate a metabolic acidosis or alkalosis. Instead of measuring total buffer base, which is difficult, metabolic factors can be described in terms of the change in buffer base from its normal

4/TABLE 7

THE NORMAL VALUES AND CHANGES FOUND IN THE BLOOD RESULTING FROM UNCOMPENSATED CHANGES IN ACID-BASE STATUS

	pH	P_{CO_2}	*Plasma bicarbonate*	*Total buffer base*	*Base excess*	*Standard bicarbonate*
Normal values	7·35–7·44	36–46 mm.Hg	23–28 mEq/litre	44–48 mEq/litre	0 ± 3 mEq/litre	22–26 mEq/litre
Respiratory acidosis	Low	High	High	Normal	Normal	Normal
Respiratory alkalosis	High	Low	Low	Normal	Normal	Normal
Metabolic acidosis	Low	Normal	Low	Low	Negative	Low
Metabolic alkalosis	High	Normal	High	High	Positive	High

value. This change is termed the *base excess*, and is defined as the amount of titratable base on titration to normal pH at normal P_{CO_2} and temperature (i.e. to pH = 7·4, at P_{CO_2} = 40 mm. Hg and 38°C). A positive value for the base excess indicates a metabolic alkalosis, and a negative value a metabolic acidosis (sometimes termed a *Base Deficit*). The base excess as read from Astrup charts is independent of the haemoglobin level. *Standard bicarbonate* is the plasma bicarbonate concentration of fully oxygenated blood at 38°C when the P_{CO_2} has been adjusted to 40 mm. Hg. By adjusting the P_{CO_2} to 40 mm. Hg, alterations in the plasma bicarbonate in whole blood secondary to changes in P_{CO_2} disappear, and the standard bicarbonate, like base excess, therefore describes metabolic acid-base changes.

The normal values and changes found in the blood resulting from uncompensated alterations in acid-base status are shown in Table 7.

Buffering Systems in the Body

About three-quarters of the chemical buffering power in the body lies within the cells, and is due to the high concentration of intra-cellular proteins, phosphate and other inorganic compounds. The remainder is due to the buffering power of the extracellular fluids. The buffering power of a system depends on the pH at which it is working and on the concentrations of the buffer elements.

The bicarbonate buffer system.—As previously explained this sytem consists of a mixture of H_2CO_3 (the weak acid) and $NaHCO_3$ (the strong base). The relationship between their concentrations and the pH is described by the Henderson-Hasselbach equation:

$$pH = pK' + \log \frac{[HCO_3^-]}{[H_2CO_3]}$$

so that the pH is determined by the ratio $\frac{[HCO_3^-]}{[H_2CO_3]}$. In Fig. 12 the relation

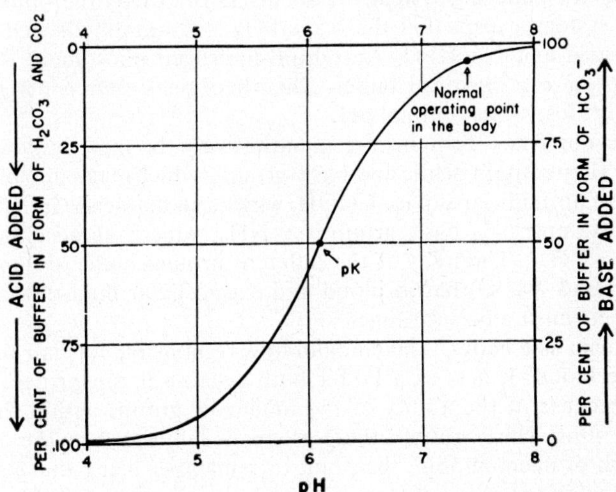

4/Fig. 12.—The reaction curve for the bicarbonate buffer system.

between the relative concentrations of the two and the pH is shown. This S-shaped curve is typical of many buffers. The following points should be noted: (1) The buffering power of the system is greatest when the slope of the curve is steepest so that, for the addition of a given amount of acid or base the smallest change in pH occurs around this part of the curve. (2) The buffer system is most efficient when the concentrations of HCO_3^- and H_2CO_3 are equal, or when pH = pK (under these conditions $\log \frac{[HCO_3^-]}{[H_2CO_3]} = 0$). Once the relative concentrations of bicarbonate and carbonic acid exceed about 8:1 in either direction the buffering power of the system falls off rapidly. Normally the system functions at a pH of around 7·4, when the ratio of bicarbonate to carbonic acid is 20:1, well outside its optimal working range.

From these considerations it is evident that the *chemical* buffering power of the bicarbonate system in the body is poor. However, its efficiency is vastly improved by the fact that both the carbonic acid and bicarbonate concentrations can be regulated by the body, the former by the lungs and the latter by the kidneys. Herein lies the importance of the bicarbonate buffer in the regulation of the acid-base state of the body. It is the only buffer which can be physiologically adjusted to maintain a normal pH. For instance, if a strong acid is added to the blood the following reactions occur:

$$HCl + NaHCO_3 = H_2CO_3 + NaCl$$

$$H_2CO_3 \rightleftarrows H_2O + \boxed{CO_2} \rightarrow \text{Excreted by the lungs}$$

In the first instance the strong acid is "swapped" for a weak acid (chemical buffering). The carbonic acid dissociates into water and CO_2, and the latter is excreted by the lungs (physiological buffering).

The phosphate buffering system.—This works in exactly the same way as the bicarbonate system, except that the NaH_2PO_4 (sodium dihydrogen phosphate) is the weak acid and Na_2HPO_4 (disodium hydrogen phosphate) is the strong base. The system is a chemical buffer. The pK of the system is 6·8, so that it is working fairly close to its optimal pH.

Proteins as buffers.—Proteins are quantitatively the most important buffers in the body. They contain acidic and basic groups, which make up "buffer pairs". An example of an acidic group is –COOH, which can dissociate into $-COO^- + H^+$, and an example of a basic group is $-NH_2$, which can accept a hydrogen ion to form $-NH_3^+$. The pK's of the different protein buffer systems vary, but many are around 7·4, so that in blood and extracellular fluid they are working at or near their most efficient ranges.

Haemoglobin as a buffer.—Haemoglobin is responsible for half the buffering power of the blood. It acts as a buffer both because it is a protein and, more important, because of the ability of the imidazole groups within the molecule to accept H^+ ions. The acidity of these groups is influenced by the oxygenation and reduction of haemoglobin, the point to remember being that haemoglobin is a weaker acid in the reduced form than when it is oxygenated (Fig. 13). When oxygenated haemoglobin gives up oxygen to the tissues it becomes reduced and

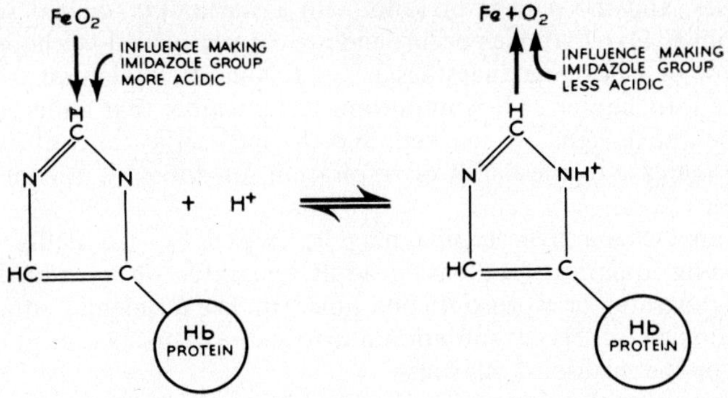

4/FIG. 13.—The effect of the oxygen saturation of haemoglobin upon the buffering power of the imidazole group.

is therefore more able to accept H^+ ions and CO_2. In the lungs the reverse effect occurs.

The buffers in the blood, in order of importance, are haemoglobin, bicarbonate and plasma proteins, and phosphate. In interstitial fluid the main buffers are bicarbonate, phosphate, and interstitial proteins. In the cells the main buffers are proteins, phosphate, and other inorganic substances.

Respiratory Acidosis (Hypercapnia, hypercarbia)

In a healthy conscious subject a reduction in the alveolar ventilation immediately leads to a rise in the arterial P_{CO_2}. This in turn results in an attempt to increase the ventilation again and to return the P_{CO_2} to normal. For a discussion of the carriage of CO_2 in the blood see page 99. If for any reason the patient is unable to increase his ventilation, a respiratory acidosis develops. The P_{CO_2} rises, plasma bicarbonate rises and the pH falls. The kidney compensates for these changes by excreting H^+ ions and retaining bicarbonate. This secondary response is slow to develop, and it may take many days for full compensation to occur. The response to a chronic respiratory acidosis is therefore a metabolic alkalosis which tends to, and often succeeds in, returning the pH to normal. A fully compensated respiratory acidosis is then said to be present. In the presence of acute hypercarbia, such as happens during general anaesthesia, there is no time for any appreciable renal compensation to occur. During apnoea the arterial P_{CO_2} rises about 3 mm. Hg per minute and H^+ ions accumulate at a rate of 10 mEq/minute. This is some 20 times faster than the kidney can excrete them.

The systemic effects of hypercapnia are widespread. The central nervous effects include impairment of mental activity and loss of consciousness, a rise in cerebral blood flow and C.S.F. pressure and the stimulation of respiration, followed by depression if the P_{CO_2} rises further. General sympathetic overactivity occurs. If a high inspired oxygen tension is not delivered to the patient hypoxaemia follows hypercapnia (see p. 142). Profound effects are seen in the circulation. The heart muscle is depressed, although this effect is offset by the increased sympathetic activity, and a rise in cardiac output follows, accompanied by peripheral dilatation. Increased bleeding is seen in surgical wounds. The blood pressure rises, and the patient presents with a warm skin, dilated veins and a bounding pulse. Dysrhythmias occur, and are especially likely to happen during cyclopropane or halothane anaesthesia. For further discussion on the effects of hypercarbia see Chapter 5. It is important to remember that under anaesthesia many of the above signs are masked, and the only indications of hypercapnia may be an increase in the depth of respiration, or difficulty in controlling the ventilation.

Under anaesthesia hypercapnia may be caused by: (a) Badly chosen or malfunctioning apparatus, e.g. using adult apparatus on a child, incorrectly assembled apparatus or worn out soda lime. (b) The accidental administration of carbon dioxide. (c) Hypoventilation due to such factors as central respiratory depression or the misuse of relaxants.

This treatment of hypercarbia due to apparatus faults or the accidental administration of carbon dioxide is self-evident. But a word of warning: the P_{CO_2} should be returned to normal values slowly or serious cardiac dysrhythmias and/or hypotension may be preciptitated. Hypoventilation should be treated by assisting or controlling the respirations until the patient is himself once more able to maintain adequate ventilation. If hypercapnia is suspected a generous concentration of oxygen should be given in the inspired gas mixture.

Hypoventilation during anaesthesia.—Under anaesthesia the function of the lungs is often impeded. For example, most sedative and anaesthetic agents depress the activity of the respiratory centres. Thus, many patients breathing spontaneously through any anaesthetic system show a rise in the carbon dioxide tension of the blood. In some cases the degree of hypoventilation may be greater than realised and the P_{CO_2} then rapidly reaches very high levels. It is, therefore, important to emphasise that during anaesthesia the anaesthetist (not the patient) is largely responsible for controlling the carbon dioxide tension at about the normal level. Sometimes the patient's spontaneous respiration may be adequate, but often assistance to ventilation will be required. The principal difficulty for the anaethetist is to recognise minor degrees of hypoventilation; the time-honoured custom of looking at the reservoir bag and thinking that ventilation is "adequate" is often grossly erroneous. Fluctuations in arterial P_{CO_2} from 40–60 mm. Hg are probably of little consequence in the normal, healthy patient but values in excess of 80 mm. Hg denote severe and dangerous hypoventilation. When the level rises to 110 mm. Hg, carbon dioxide narcosis occurs and the patient will not recover consciouness when the anaesthetic drugs are withdrawn. If, at this moment, the patient is allowed to breathe room air simply because the operation is finished, he will not only have to contend with the disadvantages of alveoli filled with anaesthetic gases escaping from the circulation (Diffusion hypoxia, see p. 222) and the uneven ventilation-perfusion ratio which normally follows anaesthesia (see p. 164 *et al.*), but also with a reduced quantity of available oxygen from the lungs due to the high carbon dioxide tension. Hypoxia will occur.

For example: see table opposite.

Fluctuations—both up and down—in the carbon dioxide content of the plasma are not always due to respiratory complications but may equally be the result of changes in tissue metabolism. Both respiratory acidosis and metabolic acidosis sometimes occur in a patient at the same time under conditions of

PARTIAL PRESSURE OF GASES IN ALVEOLI, BREATHING AIR

	Normal ventilation (arterial P_{CO_2} = 40 mm. Hg)	*Hypoventilation (arterial P_{CO_2} = 100 mm. Hg)*
Oxygen	95 mm. Hg	35 mm. Hg
Nitrogen	578 ,, ,,	578 ,, ,,
Carbon dioxide	40 ,, ,,	100 ,, ,,
Water vapour	47 ,, ,,	47 ,, ,,
Total	760 mm. Hg	760 mm. Hg

anaesthesia. The reasons for this are not yet clear but may be related to pre-operative starvation, the reaction of the body to surgical trauma and to the effects of the various anaesthetic agents.

During controlled respiration in the presence of severe chronic bronchitis the ventilation required to maintain a normal or low P_{CO_2} may have to be much greater than in a patient with normal lungs. Tidal volumes of up to one litre may be necessary to produce a large enough alveolar ventilation to keep the P_{CO_2} from rising. Unless this point is borne in mind the patient may suffer from the effects of hypercapnia while the anaesthetist is happy in the mistaken belief that ventilation is adequate.

Respiratory Alkalosis (Hypocapnia, hypocarbia)

This state of affairs commonly occurs during controlled respiration. Excessive ventilation leads to a reduction in the P_{CO_2}. The kidney compensates for a rise in pH by excreting more HCO_3^- ions and reabsorbing more H^+ ions, thus producing an alkaline urine. The secondary response to a respiratory alkalosis is therefore a metabolic acidosis, but in an anaesthetised patient this secondary response is reduced by the fall in renal blood flow caused by the anaesthetic agents. However, it is not uncommon to find a mild metabolic acidosis in the anaesthetised and hyperventilated patient. An uncompensated respiratory alkalosis leads to the following changes in the blood: a low P_{CO_2}, a low plasma bicarbonate, a high pH and a normal base excess and standard bicarbonate.

The principal theoretical danger of a respiratory alkalosis under anaesthesia is cerebral vasoconstriction, as it is known that the P_{CO_2} of the blood reaching the brain largely controls the diameter of these vessels. Thus, a severe alkalosis may produce intense cerebral vasoconstriction. Cerebral effects of hyperventilation, such as euphoria and analgesia, have been demonstrated but whether they are due to cerebral vasoconstriction or to a direct action of a low CO_2 tension on the cells is not definitely known, although the latter seems to be much more likely. Satisfactory evidence that long periods of even severe respiratory alkalosis lead to cerebral damage is still lacking and most clinicians believe that a mild respiratory alkalosis is more beneficial for the patient than a mild respiratory acidosis. Furthermore, severe vasoconstriction is probably prevented by the reaction of the cerebral vessels to the change of oxygen tension, because a reduced oxygen tension leads to cerebral vasodilatation (Severinghaus, 1964).

During anaesthesia with controlled ventilation a low P_{CO_2} causes the cardiac output to fall. In fact one of the main determinants of the cardiac output during anaesthesia is the P_{CO_2} level (Prys-Roberts, 1968). As the P_{CO_2} rises from low, through normal to high values the cardiac output increases, at first due only to increases in the stroke volume, and then to increases in both stroke volume and in heart rate. These changes are accompanied by a rise in mean arterial pressure and in left ventricular stroke work, and by a fall in peripheral resistance.

Metabolic Acidosis

A metabolic acidosis follows the accumulation in the body of non-volatile acids, e.g. lactic acid, or aceto-acetic and α-keto-glutaric acids in uncontrolled diabetes mellitus. Uncompensated, the changes seen in blood are as follows: a low pH, low plasma bicarbonate, normal P_{CO_2}, a negative base excess and a low standard bicarbonate. These changes are usually followed by a secondary hyperventilation with a fall in the P_{CO_2}, so that the pH tends to return towards normal.

The effects of a metabolic acidosis are severe. The heart muscle is depressed and the cardiac output falls. Intense peripheral vasoconstriction may occur. These changes tend to perpetuate the acidosis so that a vicious circle is set up. The cardiovascular responses to sympathetic activity and sympathomimetic drugs are reduced so that the natural protective mechanisms are interfered with. Metabolic acidosis stimulates the peripheral chemoreceptors. If these are inactive and provided the acidosis is sufficiently intense, then H^+ ions may leak into the brain and stimulate the respiratory centre directly (Severinghaus, 1964). There is no evidence available to support the clinical suggestion (Brooks and Feldman, 1962) that metabolic acidosis is capable of depressing the activity of the respiratory centre.

A mild metabolic acidosis sometimes occurs in patients undergoing general anaesthesia (see below). It is commonly observed after a period of extracorporeal perfusion, after circulatory arrest and hypothermia, and immediately following the temporary occlusion of a major vessel such as the aorta. Other causes are massive blood transfusion, respiratory distress of the newborn, renal failure and diabetic coma.

Treatment should be directed towards immediate correction of the acidosis with sodium bicarbonate or T.H.A.M., and treatment of the precipitating cause. The dose of bicarbonate can be calculated from the base excess, assuming that equilibration throughout the extracellular fluid will occur (about 20 per cent of the body weight).

$$\text{Dose (mEq.)} = \frac{\text{Base excess} \times \text{Body weight (kg.)}}{5}$$

This dose should be given intravenously over about twenty minutes. The results of administering the dose of bicarbonate as suggested above are not always predictable due to the possible development of further acidosis since the original blood sample was taken, and because of altered equilibration with the extracellular fluid in a deranged circulation. For these reasons it is essential to reassess the acid-base status of the arterial blood after the bicarbonate has been given, and to correct further if necessary. Sodium bicarbonate is a poor buffer in its own right, as explained previously, and acts mainly by combining with H^+ ions to form CO_2 and water:

$$H^+ + HCO_3^- \rightleftharpoons H_2CO_3 \rightleftharpoons CO_2 + H_2O$$

The administration of bicarbonate to correct a metabolic acidosis therefore presents a carbon dioxide load for the lungs to excrete, and efficient buffering of a metabolic acidosis depends on adequate pulmonary ventilation. One disadvantage of using bicarbonate as a buffer is that its use necessitates loading with sodium a circulation that may already be in failure. If this is considered to be undesirable then T.H.A.M. may be used instead, as it is virtually sodium free.

Metabolic acidosis and anaesthesia.—During uncomplicated anaesthesia in normal man metabolic acidosis is rarely encountered (Bunker, 1962). In dogs, however, it is commonly observed during ether anaesthesia and this perhaps has tempted some authors to assume the same is true in man. The reason for this discrepancy is that ether anaesthesia causes equal amounts of adrenaline and noradrenaline to be liberated in the dog but principally noradrenaline in man. Noradrenaline is largely free of metabolic effects (Bearn *et al.*, 1951), whereas adrenaline stimulates the release of lactic acid from the tissues in dogs.

There are, however, a few exceptions to this rule. Small children who possess increased sympathetic nervous activity tend to produce a moderate metabolic acidosis during ether anaesthesia. Furthermore, adult patients who are suffering from metabolic diseases in which lactic acid utilisation is impaired (i.e. Cushing's disease, cirrhosis of the liver) also tend to develop severe metabolic acidosis during ether anaesthesia (Bunker, 1962). This state of affairs is peculiar to ether anaesthesia and it is not observed after cyclopropane or thiopentone-nitrous oxide-oxygen anaesthesia.

4/TABLE 8

THE MECHANISMS BY WHICH PRIMARY ACID-BASE CHANGES ARE COMPENSATED. If the pH has been fully returned to normal the primary change is said to be FULLY COMPENSATED. If the pH has not been completely returned to normal the primary change is said to be PARTIALLY COMPENSATED.

Original acid-base change	*Compensatory Mechanism*	*Compensating Organ*
Respiratory Acidosis	Metabolic alkalosis, with a further rise in plasma $[HCO_3^-]$.	Kidney
Respiratory Alkalosis	Metabolic acidosis, with a further fall in plasma $[HCO_3^-]$	Kidney
Metabolic Acidosis	Respiratory alkalosis, with a further fall in plasma $[HCO_3^-]$	Lungs
Metabolic Alkalosis	Respiratory acidosis, with a further rise in plasma $[HCO_3^-]$	Lungs

Metabolic Alkalosis

Under normal circumstances this is rarely observed in the anaesthetised patient. Two uncommon situations in which an alkalosis may be seen are (1) Excessive administration of base to correct a metabolic acidosis, and (2) In the presence of severe pyloric stenosis. In the latter situation hyperventilation may be dangerous, as the combination of both a respiratory and a metabolic alkalosis will lead to a very high pH. A mild metabolic alkalosis is often observed post-operatively, especially in association with potassium depletion.

Measurement of Acid-base Status

(1) Respiratory Acidosis and Alkalosis

Such measurements are in effect an assessment of the efficiency of ventilation. There are three principal methods:

1. *Tidal volume measurement.*—This is the simplest, yet least accurate, method available. The amount of air or gases expired with each breath by the patient can easily be measured by a suitable respirometer (e.g. Wright, Dräger or Monaghan). Most of these instruments add a small amount of resistance to respiration and are least accurate over low flow rates—the circumstances where they are most needed. Once the tidal volume and the number of respirations per minute have been assessed the minute volume can easily be calculated. This figure must then be related to the patient's metabolic requirements. The latter will depend on the age, body-weight, surface area and metabolic state of the patient. The correct requirements for each individual subject can best be calculated either with the aid of the Radford nomogram or the Nunn slide rule.

2. *Measurement of alveolar carbon dioxide tension.*—There are two principal ways in which this can be achieved—an end-tidal sampling method or a re-breathing technique. The *end-tidal sample* is taken at the close of expiration and provided there is a sufficient volume of ventilation it represents the contents of the alveolar air. The sample is then analysed for carbon dioxide content. One of the principal disadvantages of this technique is uneven ventilation, as is found in some patients with emphysema, for air-trapping will lead to consistently low readings. However, even in normal subjects the end-tidal CO_2 differs from arterial blood during anaesthesia by as much as 10 mm. Hg for reasons which are not yet explained. *The rebreathing technique* (Campbell and Howell, 1960; Collier, 1956) is based on the principle of equilibrating the air in the patient's lungs with oxygen in a rebreathing bag. First the patient breathes oxygen (spontaneously or by controlled respiration) for two minutes in and out of the bag, which is attached by a mask to the face or directly on to the end of an endotracheal tube. During this period the carbon dioxide content within the re-breathing bag gradually rises until it approximates the mixed venous carbon dioxide concentration. At this stage the method aims at obtaining a rough equilibration between the carbon dioxide tension in the bag and the mixed venous blood in the pulmonary artery. The contents of the bag are then temporarily sealed whilst the patient breathes room air or anaesthetic gases again for a few minutes. At the end of this period the mask is again applied and the patient

re-breathes the contents in the bag for a further 45 seconds, which represents approximately the time taken for blood leaving the lungs at the beginning to recirculate. If the patient is unconscious or hypoventilating, then gentle assistance can be given to the bag to ensure that a true alveolar sample is obtained. At the end of the period the carbon dioxide content of the bag is analysed in a modified Haldane apparatus (Fig. 14). Now the CO_2 per cent is converted to partial pressure (multiply by $\frac{BP - 47^*}{100}$), and the figure obtained represents the P_{CO_2} of mixed venous blood. The arterial P_{CO_2} is obtained by subtracting 8 mm. Hg. The main technical error arises from having leaks around the face-piece during rebreathing. The method is not affected by the presence of nitrous oxide or halothane provided 70 per cent potassium hydroxide is used for the absorption of the carbon dioxide. The principal advantage of this technique lies in its simplicity, the relative cheapness of the apparatus, and the rapidity with which successive estimations can be made. However, in cases with a very high alveolar carbon dioxide tension (i.e. 80 mm. Hg or above) the values obtained are consistently lower than those measured by a direct arterial technique. The reason for this

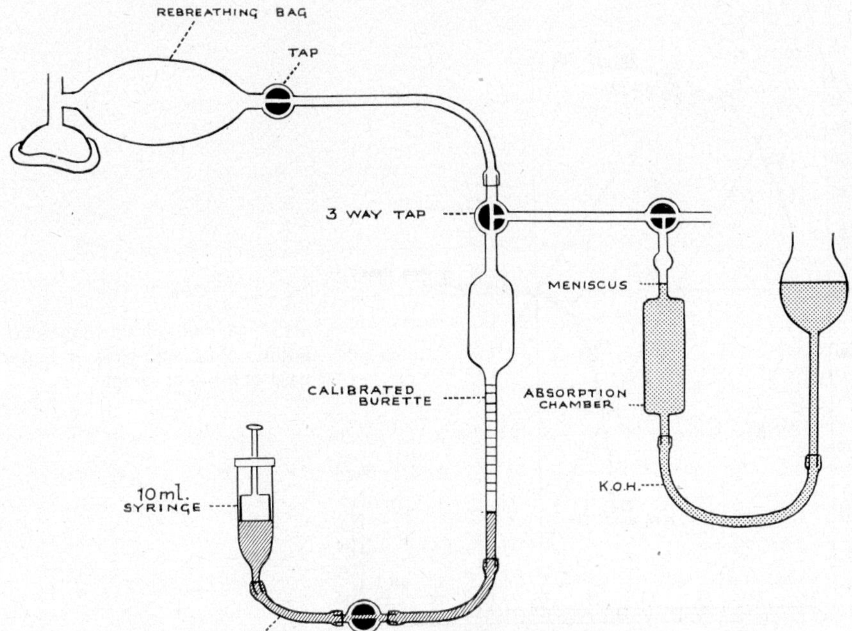

4/Fig.14.—Modified Haldane Apparatus.

The calibrated burette is filled with mercury from the 10 ml. syringe and after levelling the potassium hydroxide solution to the meniscus the tap above the meniscus is turned to position ⊥. The rebreathed sample is blown through and this tap is then closed. The sample is drawn into the burette. The tap above the calibrated burette is turned to position T and the first tap to position ⊣. The sample is then pushed into the absorption chamber fifteen times. The meniscus is levelled and the volume change due to carbon dioxide absorption is read from the burette.

* BP = Barometric pressure; 47 = water vapour pressure in mm. Hg. at 37C°.

anomaly is that in the rebreathing technique originally the bag contents are without CO_2 and insufficient time is available for equilibration. If one were to start with a higher value of CO_2 in the bag the correct answer could be obtained.
3. *Measurement of arterial carbon dioxide tension* (P_{CO_2}).—The most commonly used methods are the interpolation micro-method (Astrup, 1959) or the carbon dioxide electrode (Severinghaus, 1959).

(*a*) *The interpolation micro-method* has the advantage that a sample of capillary blood is sufficient for each measurement.* The method is based on the principle that the relation between the logarithm of P_{CO_2} and pH is always a straight line. If this line can be constructed for a particular sample of blood then merely knowing the pH will enable the P_{CO_2} to be predicted. The interpolation method, therefore, measures only the pH. Thus, a sample of blood is first taken from the patient and the pH measured; it is then exposed to a known high level of P_{CO_2} (e.g. 60 mm. Hg = Point A on Fig. 15) and a known low level of P_{CO_2} (e.g. 30 mm. Hg = Point B on Fig. 15) and the pH measured on each occasion. A straight line can now be drawn connecting points A and B. The actual pH of the sample is then located on this line. The pH of the blood sample is found to be 7·1 and this corresponds with a P_{CO_2}, or 50 mm. Hg.

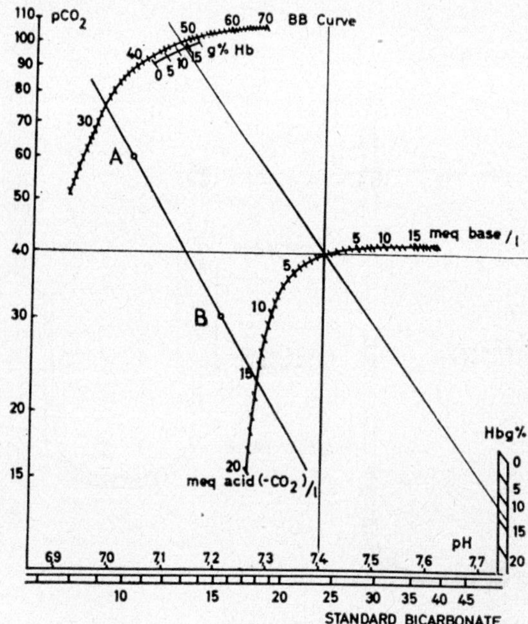

4/FIG. 15.—Graph showing calculations of Δ acid-base or buffer base of a blood sample.

* *Note on collection of blood for P_{CO_2} estimations.*
The best sample is one taken anaerobically into a sealed heparinised syringe from a large artery, stored in an ice-cold container for transport and then analysed without contact with the atmosphere. If venous or capillary blood is used, in addition to the foregoing precaution an attempt should be made to stimulate the peripheral circulation by warmth so that the errors associated with stagnation are minimised.

(*b*) *The principle of the carbon dioxide electrode* (Smith and Hahn, 1969) is that it produces an electrical signal directly proportional to the logarithm of the P_{CO_2} of a sample of either a liquid or a gas. It consists of a pH electrode separated from the sample by a teflon membrane which is permeable to CO_2 but not to ions in the sample. CO_2 diffuses through the membrane into a thin layer of dilute sodium bicarbonate solution controlling the pH of this solution. The electrode has the advantage that the partial pressure of CO_2 may be read directly from a meter in one to two minutes.

(II) Metabolic Acidosis and Alkalosis

The best way to quantitate the metabolic component of acid-base equilibrium has long been a matter for debate. However at present the most convenient and practical methods are to measure either the base excess/deficit or the standard bicarbonate. There are two principal ways of estimating the base excess:

(a) *By measuring the pH, P_{CO_2} and haemoglobin.*

Measurement of pH.—The glass electrode.

This instrument is based on the characteristics of special glass which is selectively permeable to H^+ ions. This glass has the property that if each side of the glass is bathed in a solution of different pH, an e.m.f. is generated across it. This e.m.f. is directly and linearly proportional to the difference between the pH's of the two solutions. If the pH on one side of the glass is stabilised, and a solution of unknown pH is introduced onto the other side of the glass, the e.m.f. thus generated gives an indication of the unknown pH. The e.m.f. across the pH sensitive glass can be measured by placing metal electrodes in the solutions on either side of it. But a problem arises here, because at any metal-electrolyte interface an e.m.f. is developed and this can obscure that across the glass. For this reason the electrodes on either side must be electrically very stable, so that little or no variation in potential occurs at their surfaces. If variations do occur it is impossible to separate these from alterations across the pH glass, which is what we are trying to measure. Suitably stable electrodes are (1) silver, coated with a layer of silver chloride, and immersed in a solution containing chloride ions; and (2) calomel coated mercury, in contact with saturated KCl. The general arrangement of a pH electrode is shown in Fig. 16. On one side of the glass is a solution of 0·1M HCl (stable pH) into which is dipped a silver:silver chloride electrode. On the other side of the glass is the test solution.

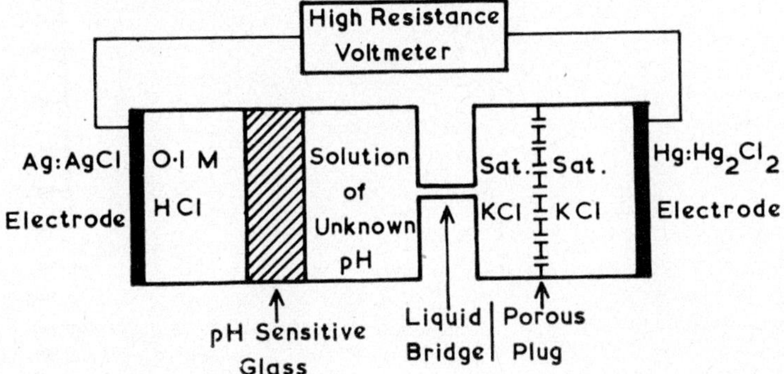

4/Fig. 16.—Schematic diagram of a pH electrode. See text for full details.

This is connected electrically via a liquid bridge to a saturated solution of KCl, which is itself in contact with a mercury: calomel electrode. A porous plug is inserted in the KCl to prevent contamination of the calomel electrode by the test solution. The e.m.f. across the whole assembly can now be measured by connecting the silver and calomel electrodes through a sensitive high resistance voltmeter. The instrument is calibrated by setting it up against solutions of known pH, and the pH of an unknown solution can then be measured by comparing the e.m.f. it generates with that produced by the solutions of known pH. Although for each measurement the potential across the whole apparatus is read, the stability of the system is that such changes in e.m.f. across the whole are due to changes across the pH sensitive glass.

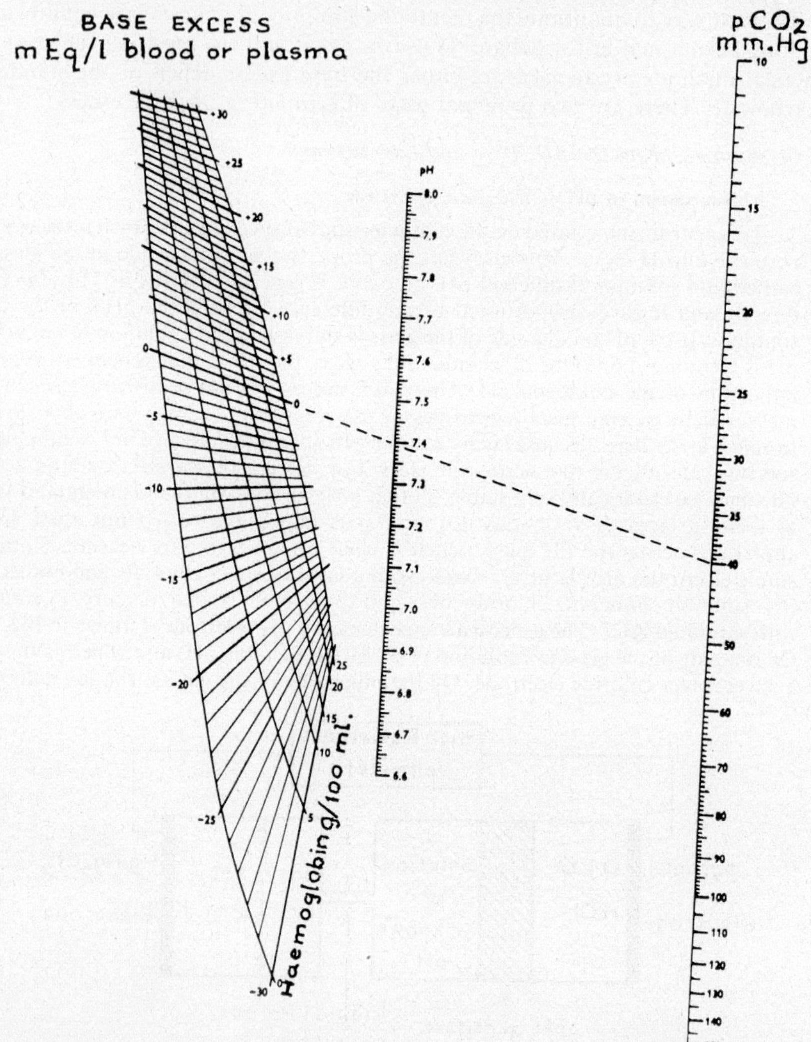

4/FIG. 17.—Nomogram for blood acid-base calculation (Siggaard-Andersen, 1963).

If the pH, P_{CO_2} and haemoglobin content of a sample of blood are known, the base excess can be read from a special slide rule, such as that designed by Severinghaus, or from a nomogram such as that of Siggaard-Andersen (1963) (Fig. 17). To use this nomogram, place a ruler against the value for the blood P_{CO_2}, and then bring it into line with the value for the pH. The ruler will now cross the large column for base excess. The lattice-work is due to various values of the haemoglobin. The base excess can now be read off directly from the appropriate haemoglobin column.

(*b*) *By the interpolation method* (Astrup, 1959).

This method is the same as that previously described for measuring the P_{CO_2} (p. 184), and the example shown in Fig. 15 can be used again. The lower curved line gives values for base excess. The point at which the straight line constructed for the sample of blood under examination cuts this curve gives the base excess value. In the example the line AB cuts the base excess line at the point marked −15 mEq/litre, indicating a severe metabolic acidosis.

The standard bicarbonate can also be measured by dropping a perpendicular from the point at which the line AB cuts the $P_{CO_2} = 40$ mm. Hg line, and reading off its value from the point at which the perpendicular meets the standard bicarbonate scale. In this example the standard bircarbonate is equal to 14 mEq/litre, a very low value (normal = 22–26 mEq/litre).

If we now had to decide how much bicarbonate would be required to correct such a metabolic acidosis, the dose can be calculated from the equation on page 180. Assuming that the patient weighs 60 kg., the dose of bicarbonate works out at $\frac{15 \times 60}{5} = 180$ mEq. After this dose has been administered, another sample of arterial blood must be analysed, and a further dose given if necessary.

4/TABLE 9

CAUSES OF VARIATIONS IN P_{O_2}, P_{CO_2} AND pH AND THEIR EFFECT ON ACID-BASE BALANCE.

	P_{O_2} (*in mm.Hg*)	P_{CO_2} (*in mm. Hg*)	*pH*	*Base excess or deficit (in mEq/litre)*
Normal values	100	40	7·4	0
Raised	(a) Oxygen inhalation (b) Hyper-ventilation	(a) Hypo-ventilation (b) Carbon dioxide inhalation	Alkalosis (a) Respiratory (b) Metabolic	+ 3 or more (a) Excessive bicarbonate administration (b) Pre-existing metabolic alkalosis
Lowered	(a) Intrapulmon-ary factors (b) Lowered alveolar concentration 1. Low inspired conc. 2. Hypo-ventilation	Hyperventilation	Acidosis (a) Respiratory (b) Metabolic	− 3 or less (a) Tissue ischaemia or hypoxia (b) Pre-existing metabolic acidosis

Interpretation of blood gas analysis.—The impact of the glass electrode system and development of this technique has made sweeping changes in the anaesthetist's requirements for the interpretation of laboratory data. Now that it is possible for the relatively uninitiated to make measurements of P_{O_2}, P_{CO_2}, and pH, the whole problem of the control of patients undergoing anaesthesia or in the post-operative period has been greatly simplified. If suitable apparatus is available, then a knowledge of P_{O_2}, P_{CO_2}, and pH is sufficient to diagnose the majority of problems of ventilation and acid-base balance.

The value of these measurements is emphasised in Table 9.

A few simple examples will illustrate the value of this table, e.g.

(a) *The patient's blood (whilst breathing air) reveals the following data:*

P_{O_2} 60 mm. Hg
P_{CO_2} 42 mm. Hg
pH 7·4
Base excess/deficit = 0 mEq/litre

Interpretation.—The P_{O_2} is low yet the P_{CO_2}, pH and base excess/deficit are normal. The normal P_{CO_2} signifies that ventilation is adequate whereas the low P_{O_2} indicates that there is some interference with the transfer of oxygen from the alveoli to the pulmonary circulation. The commonest cause of this situation is an alteration of the ventilation-perfusion ratio.

Diagnosis.—This situation is observed in patients with scattered areas of pulmonary collapse. It could also be present if the patient was inspiring a mixture with a low percentage of oxygen: however, the normal P_{CO_2} rules out the possibility of hypoventilation.

Treatment.—In the past it was often assumed that all areas of pulmonary collapse were secondary to blockage of the bronchiole by mucous secretions or "plugs". A number of investigators have found that under anaesthesia and in the post-operative period under sedation the normal control of the ventilation-perfusion ratio is altered (see p. 167). The patient should be given oxygen to breath, and re-expansion of the lungs should be encouraged with coughing and deep breathing. Conway and Payne (1963) have shown that this type of hypoxaemia occurring in the early post-operative period can readily be corrected by giving oxygen. An oxygen flow of 2 litres/minute into a plastic oxygen mask is perfectly satisfactory.

(b) *The patient's blood (whilst breathing air) reveals the following data:*

P_{O_2} 45 mm. Hg
P_{CO_2} 80 mm. Hg
pH 7·2
Base excess/deficit = 0

Interpretation.—The raised P_{CO_2} suggests under-ventilation and this could also account for the lowered P_{O_2}. A pH on the acid side without any change in the base excess confirms a respiratory rather than a metabolic problem.

Diagnosis.—Hypoventilation is the cause of the respiratory acidosis. Measuring the minute volume with a Wright respirometer will confirm this finding. If the patient was breathing 100 per cent oxygen rather than air when the test samples were taken then the P_{O_2} would rise to 550 mm. Hg (if no increased shunt were present), yet the other figures would remain the same.

Treatment.—Improved ventilation. This can be achieved by applying intermittent positive-pressure ventilation, but careful monitoring of the P_{CO_2} level will be required before normal spontaneous respiration can be allowed to resume.

(c) *The patient's blood (whilst breathing air) reveals the following data:*

P_{O_2} 100 mm. Hg
P_{CO_2} 40 mm. Hg
pH 7·1
Base excess = − 17·5 mEq/litre

Interpretation.—Normal values for P_{O_2} and P_{CO_2} suggest that ventilation and oxygen transfer within the lungs are normal. A pH on the acid side with a large base deficit indicates a metabolic acidosis probably due to poor peripheral blood flow.

Diagnosis.—Metabolic acidosis due to poor peripheral perfusion.

Treatment.—Sodium bicarbonate, in the requisite amount, should be given on the basis of the patient's extracellular fluid volume to correct the metabolic acidosis. For example, if the patient has a weight of 70 kg. and a base excess of − 17·5 mEq/litre then he requires an intravenous injection of $\frac{70 \times 17{\cdot}5}{5} =$ 245 mEq/litre to correct the metabolic acidosis.

Hyperventilation

Geddes and Gray (1959) have stressed the value of hyperventilation in association with complete muscular paralysis for providing ideal conditions for surgery. Using a mixture of nitrous oxide/oxygen (70:30 per cent) for ventilation together with electro-encephalographic recordings they found a state indistinguishable from that obtained with anaesthetic agents such as ether or halothane. On the other hand Bridge and Eger (1966) found that, during halothane anaesthesia, hyperventilation *per se* had no effect on the depth of anaesthesia.

The precise role of carbon dioxide in brain function is not yet clear but Bonvallet *et al.* (1956) found a low P_{CO_2} reduced activity in the reticular formation; Morrice (1956) suggested an adequate carbon dioxide tension was essential for the Krebs tricarboxylic acid cycle.

In the past it was often believed that when patients were hyperventilated the carbon dioxide level had to rise back to normal again before spontaneous respiration was resumed. Utting and Gray (1962) have emphasised the fallacy of this conception. In a study of twelve patients they found that spontaneous breathing recommenced even when a severe degree of respiratory alkalosis was present (Fig. 18). They concluded that provided the respiratory centre was not depressed by an anaesthetic or analgesic agent then respiration could be resumed with a peripheral stimulus.

Apnoea

Literally, apnoea means "without breathing". Its importance in relation to anaesthesia has waxed and waned. Before the days of controlled respiration, the

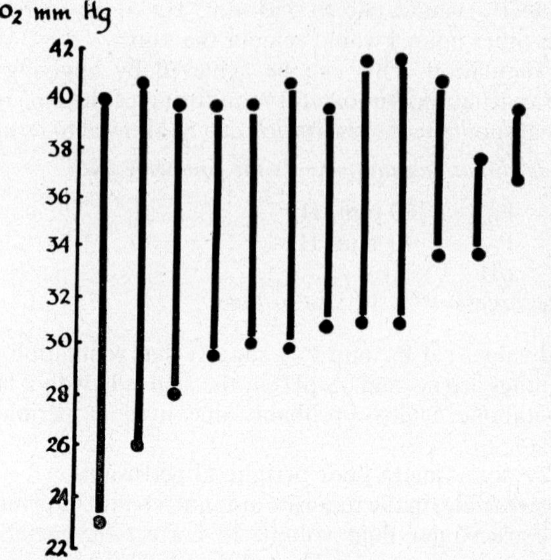

4/Fig. 18.—The results of P_{CO_2} estimations in twelve patients. The top dot represents the value of P_{CO_2} pre-operatively and the bottom dot signifies the level of P_{CO_2} as respiration recommenced after a period of hyperventilation.

cessation of breathing was regarded almost with horror as a sign of possible death. The realisation that respiration could easily be maintained by manual inflation of a rebreathing bag was instrumental in the popularisation of carbon dioxide absorption techniques and controlled respiration. However, although apnoea is frequently and deliberately produced during anaesthesia, a prolonged cessation of respiration in the post-operative period is most undesirable. In recent years, however, a number of these prolonged apnoeas, particularly following the use of muscle relaxants, have been reported. Indeed, their occurrence, and a fear of the potential dangers of inadequately "controlled" respiration, has led some authorities to suggest that it is wiser to use assisted rather than controlled respiration. The respective merits of these two types of respiration have already been discussed (p. 59).

Prolonged apnoea in anaesthesia.—The causes of prolonged apnoea in clinical anaesthesia are various. The factors concerned fall naturally into two groups, namely those affecting the brain and spinal cord (central causes) and those impairing respiration at the neuromuscular junction (peripheral causes). The differentiation between these two main causes can only be satisfactorily achieved by the use of a peripheral nerve-stimulator. If the muscles show evidence of paresis, then clearly a peripheral cause is suspect, whereas if there is no obvious peripheral weakness, then a central depression of the respiratory centre must be sought.

A. *Central causes of apnoea.*—One of the commonest reasons why a patient fails to resume respiratory activity after a long period of controlled respiration is *central depression* of the respiratory centre by hypnotic, analgesic, or anaesthetic drugs. The cause can frequently be traced back to the use of heavy premedication, followed by a large dose of a thiobarbiturate for the induction of anaesthesia. Often pethidine has been given intermittently throughout the operation, so that an accumulation of it may play one of the principal parts in suppressing the onset of spontaneous respiration. Some anaesthetic agents, such as halothane and cyclopropane, have a particularly marked central depressant effect and therefore are best used sparingly in the completely paralysed patient. However, they possess an advantage over the analgesic group of drugs in that they can be rapidly withdrawn at the end of the anaesthetic. The analgesic drugs are difficult to administer to the completely paralysed patient during anaesthesia, because in the absence of spontaneous respiration it is difficult to estimate the effect of a particular dose on respiratory centre activity. In a few patients (especially those with a heavy premedication) even a small intravenous dose of an analgesic drug may lead to apnoea. For this reason it is unwise to combine the use of the muscle relaxants with large doses of analgesic drugs.

It has been suggested that *d*-tubocurarine may in some circumstances cross the blood-brain barrier and depress the respiratory centre directly. This matter is discussed elsewhere (Chapter 31), but at the present time there is very little evidence to support this hypothesis.

The use of controlled respiration may mask a cerebrovascular accident or the effects of surgical interference with the medulla in neurosurgery. Either of these may cause prolonged apnoea in the post-operative period.

B. *Peripheral causes.*—These are mostly concerned with the use of muscle relaxants and the causes are discussed in detail elsewhere (Chapter 31), but some of the principal reasons are listed in Table 10.

4/TABLE 10

PRINCIPAL CAUSES OF PROLONGED APNOEA ASSOCIATED WITH ANAESTHESIA

Central	*Peripheral*
1. Depression of the respiratory centre by analgesics, hypnotics and anaesthetics	1. Overdose of the muscle relaxant
	2. Inadequate anti-cholinesterase therapy
2. Excessive alteration in level of P_{CO_2} of blood Over-ventilation++→Apnoea	3. Inadequate hydrolysis of suxamethonium by plasma cholinesterase
	4. Pathological disease of the respiratory muscles, e.g. myasthenia gravis.
	5. Impaired renal excretion of the relaxant

RESISTANCE TO RESPIRATION

Under normal conditions of breathing the respiratory resistance comprises the force required to drive air to and fro' along the bronchial tree from the mouth to the alveoli. The resistance to the flow of air in a tube is the pressure difference between the two ends. If a subject breathes through an anaesthetic apparatus then the resistance of the extra breathing pathway must be taken into account, because the respiratory muscles will have to do more work. A simple test can be made by asking a conscious subject to breathe through a small endotracheal tube (Magill No. 4 or 6) held between his lips, when the extra effort required soon becomes apparent. Expiration is affected most, because there is a rise in intrapulmonary pressure with inadequate emptying of the alveoli. This leads to an increase in carbon dioxide and, therefore, an increase in the depth of respiration in an attempt to wash out more carbon dioxide. The abdominal muscles soon come into action during expiration in an endeavour to drive air out of the lungs.

Nearly every piece of anaesthetic apparatus increases in varying degree the respiratory resistance. One of the most important factors is the type of flow of the gases. This largely depends upon the diameter and shape of the breathing tubes and connection pieces, the number, style and setting of valves in the system, and the size and packing of the soda-lime canister.

Gas flows.—When the flow of gas along a tube is smooth and regular it is called laminar, but as the rate of flow increases a critical velocity is reached at which the flow becomes turbulent (Fig. 19). The flow of air in the respiratory tract of a normal patient is laminar, and the flow of gases during inspiration in anaesthetic practice does not reach sufficiently high rates to produce turbulent flow. The internal diameter of the tubes along which the gases flow and the presence of obstruction in them may, however, affect the critical velocity and

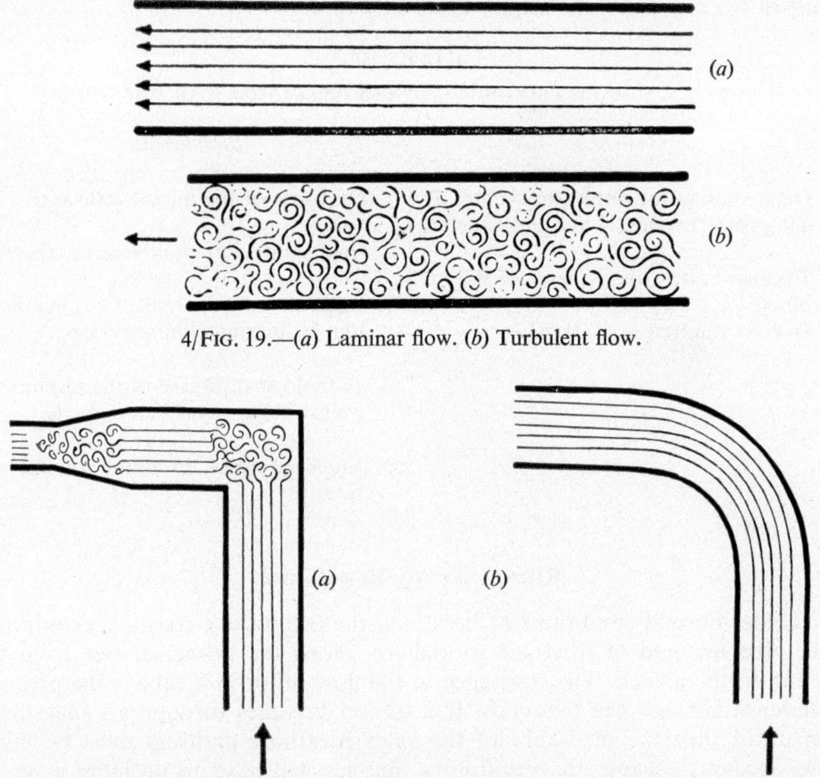

4/FIG. 19.—(*a*) Laminar flow. (*b*) Turbulent flow.

4/FIG. 20.—(*a*) Mixed laminar and turbulent flow. (*b*) Laminar flow in a curved tube.

hence produce turbulent flow. It is important, therefore, that the anaesthetist should use the largest sized tube that will pass easily through the glottic aperture, since in the adult this is the narrowest portion of the respiratory tract between the lips and the carina. In children the cricoid is the limiting factor. Furthermore, the endotracheal connections should be of a wide bore, and curved rather than sharply angled (Fig. 20). Macintosh and Mushin (1946) have described and illustrated the different effects of a No. 10 and No. 6 endotracheal tube on intrapleural pressure (Fig. 21).

Valves.—The number and the types of unidirectional valve used in the different pieces of anaesthetic apparatus vary, but the majority are of the disc type which is lifted by the flow of gases either against its own weight (simple disc type) or against the resistance of a spring (spring-loaded type). The latter offer too great a resistance to the flow of gases and, where possible, should be

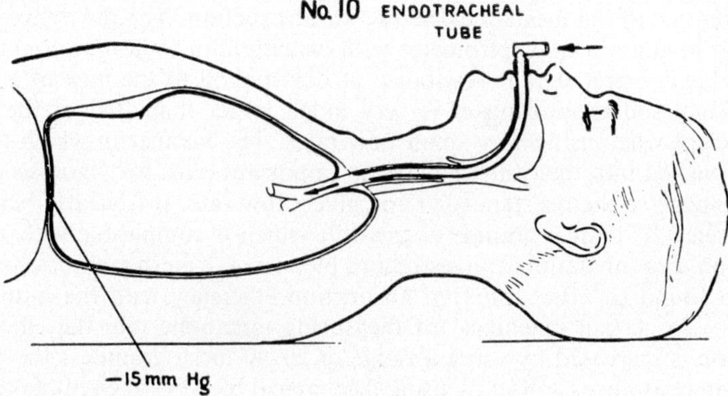

(*a*) Large bore endotracheal tube means less resistance to respiration and therefore a lower intrapleural pressure.

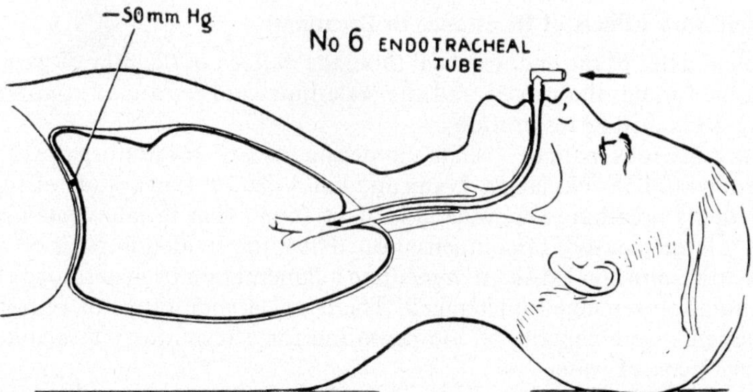

(*b*) Small bore endotracheal tube means a greater resistance to respiration and therefore a high intrapleural pressure.

4/Fig. 21.—Diagrams to Show the Effect of Endotracheal Tube Size on Intrapleural Pressure, and therefore on Inspiratory Effort

eliminated. Hunt (1955) has described the optimum design of disc valves. They should be made to have approximately equal cross-sectional flow areas for air at all the constricted portions and these areas should be approximately equal to that of the main duct. The disc should be as light as practicable and should have a lift approaching one quarter of the diameter of the duct. If a disc becomes wet from the moisture of the expired gases a slight increase in respiratory resistance will occur, not only from the greater weight of the disc but from the surface tension of the water between the disc edges and its seating. For paediatric anaesthesia not only is resistance of great importance but also the quantity of air contained in the valve, since this may markedly increase deadspace in a small infant (see p. 205). The effects of various pieces of anaesthetic apparatus in the external resistance to respiration in infants has been extensively reviewed by Smith (1961).

Soda-lime canister.—The insertion of a soda-lime canister into a respiratory system is, in the mechanical sense, an obstruction. The difference between breathing in and out of a spirometer with or without a soda-lime container can be easily demonstrated. The resistance or obstruction to the flow of gases of a conventional soda-lime canister is very much larger than that of the average valve, except when using very small flow rates. The manner in which the granules are packed into the canister plays an important part, for vigorous compaction will increase the resistance for any given flow rate. It is clearly best, therefore, to select as large a granule as possible which is compatible with adequate absorption. For inhalational anaesthesia a blend of 4–8 mesh granules (see p. 202) has been found to offer optimum absorption efficiency with the minimum of resistance. In certain machines for measuring metabolic rate the efficiency of absorption is increased by using a range of 20–40 mesh granules; the resulting increase in resistance is offset by using mechanical blowers to circulate the gases. A wide, short canister (as used in circle absorbers) offers less resistance than the long narrow (Waters) canister, because the gases travel at a lower velocity between the granules and also have a shorter over-all passage through the canister.

Respiratory Effects of Resistance to Breathing

The diameter of the endotracheal tube, the pattern of the flow of gases along the flexible tubing, the valves, and the soda-lime canister are all capable of increasing resistance to respiration.

In a conscious patient even a moderate rise in respiratory resistance is followed by a fall in ventilation. Nunn and Ezi-Ashi (1961) in a study of anaesthetised patients breathing spontaneously have found that in many such patients there is a large measure of compensation. Thus, the sudden imposition of a resistance to respiration led to an immediate augmentation of inspiratory effort so that ventilation remained unchanged. There was a wide range of response but some patients were capable of compensating for a respiratory resistance of as much as 17 cm. of water.

A further finding of interest was the difference in the effect of a 5 kilogram weight placed first on the chest and then on the epigastrium. The anaesthetised patient showed almost no change in ventilation following pressure on the chest, whereas there was a 20 per cent reduction in ventilation if the same weight was placed on the upper abdomen (Table 11).

4/TABLE 11

EFFECT OF EXTERNAL INTERFERENCE WITH RESPIRATION ON VENTILATION

	Change in Lung volume (ml.)	*Change in tidal volume (%)*	*Change in respiratory rate (%)*	*Change in minute volume (%)*
5 kg. on sternum	– 70	– 4·1	+ 2·8	– 1·7
5 kg. on epigastrium	– 45	– 19·2	+ 2·0	– 17·8

The reason for this discrepancy is that the diaphragm is the principle muscle of respiration and any pressure in the epigastric region will seriously impede its function. These figures help to emphasise the importance of intermittent positive-pressure respiration in patients undergoing upper abdominal surgery, particularly where firm retraction on liver or bowel is used to gain exposure.

The endotracheal tube is always considered an important source of resistance to respiration. It is known that the resistance presented by a tube is proportional to the flow of gases and the diameter of the tube. Munson and his colleagues (1963) have shown in a group of patients that whereas the mean peak flow rate in the conscious state was 21 litres/min., it rose to 28–43 litres/min. when anaesthesia was induced. A glance at Fig. 22 shows how the peak flow rate is high

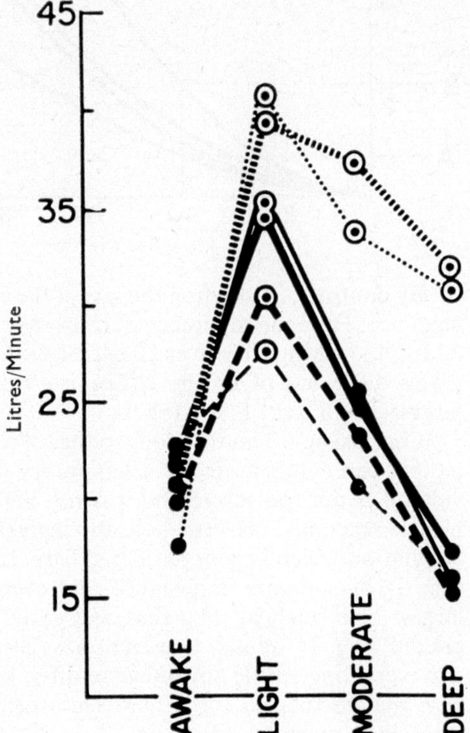

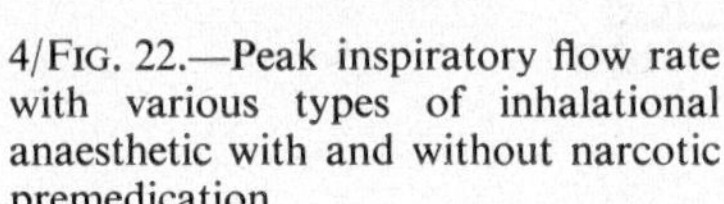
4/FIG. 22.—Peak inspiratory flow rate with various types of inhalational anaesthetic with and without narcotic premedication.

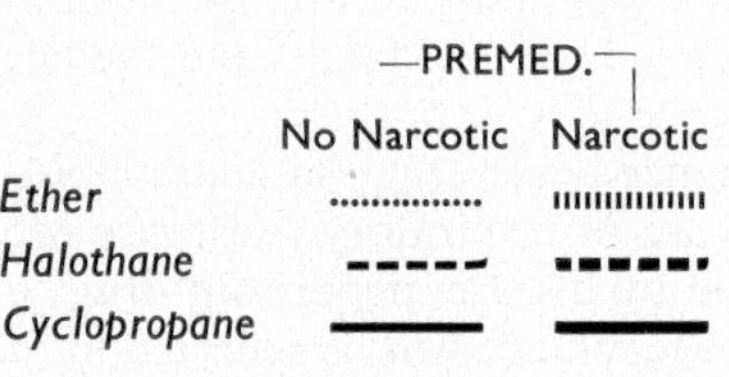

during light anaesthesia with most anaesthetic agents but drops down again when moderate or deep levels of anaesthesia are reached. With ether anaesthesia high peak flow rates are maintained at most levels of anaesthesia.

Interpretation of these flows in relation to the various sizes of endotracheal tube available reveals some interesting data. In adults, the difference in resistance encountered between a 42 F (No. 10 Magill) and a 32 F (No. 7 Magill) with a common peak flow rate of 40 litres/min. is only 1 cm. H_2O (Fig. 23). Thus under anaesthesia there is a very small increase in resistance over a wide range of endotracheal tube sizes in adults. This discrepancy may in part be due to the large bore of the trachea being required for fight or flight rather than the more tranquil event of anaesthesia where only relatively low flow rates are present.

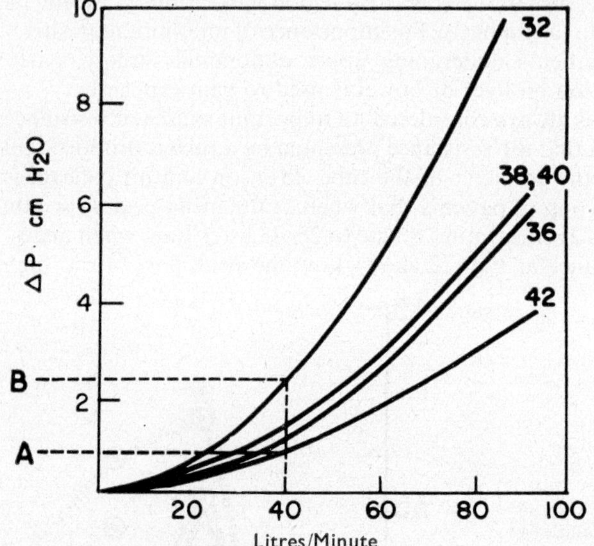

4/FIG. 23.—Resistance through endotracheal tubes.

By contrast, in children the size of the endotracheal tube is of paramount importance. Here the difference in resistance between a 12 F (No. O Magill) and a 22 F (No. 3 Magill) is over 80 cm. H_2O. Close observation of Fig. 24 will show that a difference of 60 cm. H_2O exists between a 12 F (O Magill) and the next largest size, i.e. 14 F (1 Magill).

Conclusion.—These various studies of resistance suggest that the anaesthetised patient can compensate for a temporary increase of respiratory resistance provided it is not too severe and it is not impeded by disease, depressant drugs or muscle relaxants. Nevertheless, any increase in resistance will be reflected in the circulation which is not considered here. In children the size of the endotracheal tube is of supreme importance and every effort should be made to pass the largest endotracheal tube that will easily traverse the narrow opening at the cricoid ring. In adults, however, sizes larger than 36 F or No. 8 Magill have correspondingly little advantage to offer, but for good anaesthetic practice it is a wise maxim to pass the largest endotracheal tube that will comfortably pass through the vocal cords.

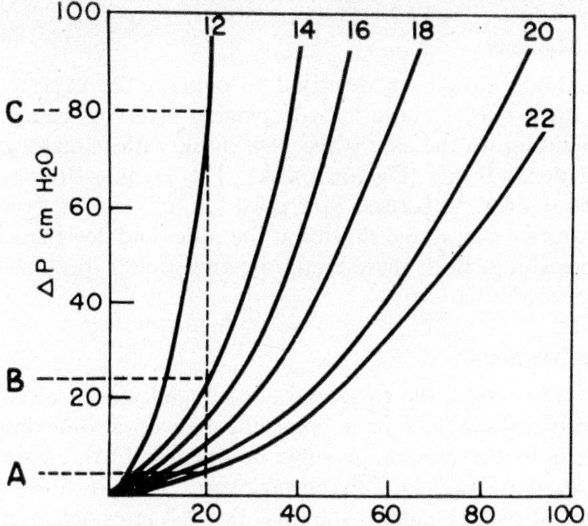

4/Fig. 24.—Resistance through endotracheal tubes.

ANAESTHETIC BREATHING SYSTEMS

A badly designed or improperly used anaesthetic breathing system adversely affects the respiratory function of the patient. At the extremes of age, and in ill patients, such a disturbance may have serious consequences. The principles of good practice must be recognised when selecting and administering anaesthesia with any particular system, and the advantages and disadvantages peculiar to it appreciated. No one of the schemes to be described is perfect in itself, but some are of greater value for special types of case or anaesthesia than for routine use whatever the condition. When making a final choice, and after consideration of all the basic facts, the preference and experience of the anaesthetist concerned must be decisive.

Open Mask

Volatile liquid anaesthetics can be administered by a "drop" technique with an open mask. The open mask is widely used for anaesthetising infants and small children since it is safe, simple, and satisfactory for short surgical procedures when the advantages of a complicated method would be lost, while the disadvantages might be accentuated. Needless to say, the open mask still has a place in adult anaesthesia in situations where apparatus is unavailable or impracticable. Usually on the open mask the patient inspires an anaesthetic-air mixture which is at about 0° C: evidence for this during ether anaesthesia can be seen in the snow which forms on the mask. The respiratory tree is called upon to raise the temperature of the inspired gases to 37° C and also to saturate them with water vapour. It is estimated that, using the open method, there is a heat loss of about 300 calories per minute (Macintosh and Mushin, 1946).

Semi-open Methods

Various methods have been designed to contain the vapour in the direct vicinity of an open mask. These include placing layers of gamgee gauze over the mask or building up the side walls of a mask with gamgee gauze or linen stretched on a metal frame (Ogston mask). The Dennis Browne inhaler is a cylindrical tube with a rubberised face mask at one end, a gauze diaphragm in the middle, and an adjustable shutter at the other end designed to control the amount of rebreathing. Both these methods, and similar modifications, lead to carbon dioxide accumulation.

Semi-closed Methods

In a semi-closed system the gases and vapours delivered from an anaesthetic machine accumulate and mix in a breathing bag or a wide bore tube from whence they pass to the patient. A valve or opening in the system allows the patient's expiration to pass into the atmosphere. The position of the bag—if one is incorporated in the system—the total flow of gases delivered into it from the machine, their site of entry into the system, and the placing of the expiratory aperture, are all of importance. So also is the pressure at which a valve is set to allow gases to pass through it.

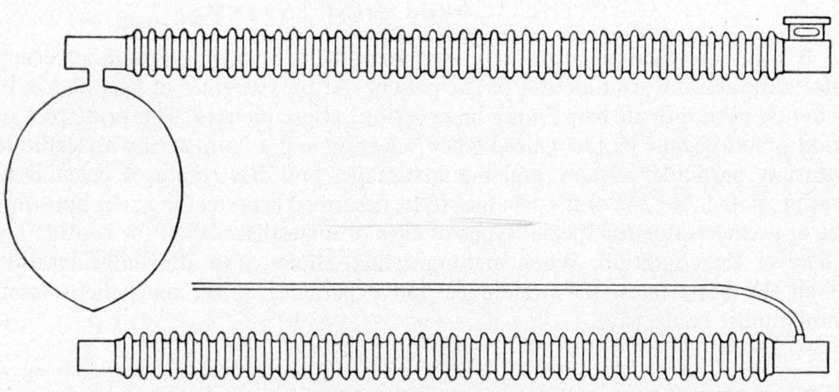

4/Fig. 25.—Semi-closed systems.

The two semi-closed systems in common use are the original Magill attachment and the modified Ayre's "T" piece (Fig. 25), but there are modifications of each. Both systems have been extensively investigated to assess the degree of rebreathing in relation to certain flows of fresh gases (Woolmer and Lind, 1954; Mapleson, 1954; Davies *et al.*, 1956; Inkster, 1956; Ayre, 1956). For economy in total gas flow with virtual elimination of rebreathing the original Magill attachment is still the best for an adult. The fresh gas flows into the Magill attachment have recently been investigated by Kain and Nunn (1967). These workers, measuring minute volume and end-tidal CO_2 while reducing the fresh gas flow in steps, found that significant rebreathing (as indicated by a rise in minute volume and end-tidal CO_2) did not occur until the gas inflow was reduced to between 2 and

4 litres/minute, or about equal to the patient's alveolar ventilation (Fig. 26). Previously it had been considered that a gas inflow equal to the patient's minute volume was necessary to prevent rebreathing. This state of affairs only holds when the patient is breathing spontaneously, but not if such a system is used for

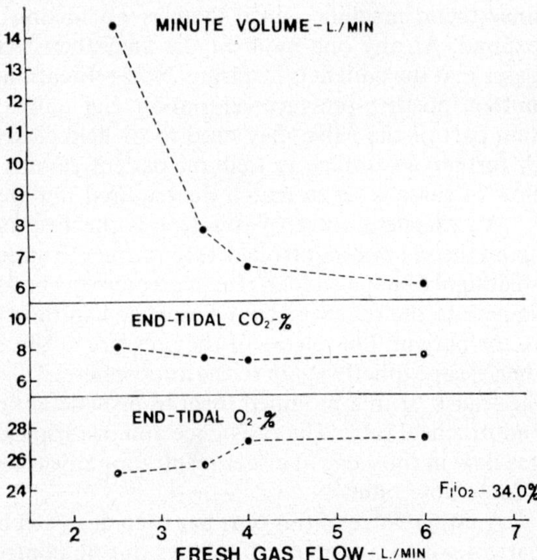

4/Fig. 26.—Diagram showing the changes in minute volume, end-tidal CO_2 and end-tidal O_2 with step-wise reductions in fresh gas flow into a Magill anaesthetic circuit.

intermittent positive-pressure respiration. Then a far greater flow of gases must be used to prevent carbon dioxide accumulation.

With a "T" piece the dead space gases pass down the open end of the tube first, while the alveolar gases, leaving last, may be reinspired. A high flow of gases (approximately twice the respiratory minute volume of the patient) is needed to prevent rebreathing with a "T" piece if the capacity of the expiratory limb of the system is to be ignored. Rebreathing can be eliminated with a small expiratory limb provided that the volume of the gases that can be held in it is no greater than the volume of fresh gases that can enter it during an expiratory pause (Mapleson, 1954). With a small expiratory limb some mixing with the atmospheric air may occur.

In a semi-closed system the resistance that the expiratory valve offers to expiration must be set against the far greater flow of gases needed with a "T" piece. This resistance may be a matter of some importance in very small children since even a specially designed valve will offer more resistance than the expiratory limb of a wide-bore "T" piece.

In all these systems the temperature of the inspired gases is raised to that of the room by the time they have traversed the breathing tubes to reach the patient. However, as the anaesthetic gases are specially prepared without water vapour the respiratory tract is called upon to saturate them fully. The estimated heat loss for the semi-closed method is 250 calories per minute (Macintosh and Mushin, 1946).

Non-rebreathing Valves

The non-rebreathing valve may be considered as a modification of the semi-closed system. Designed primarily to prevent rebreathing by ensuring unidirectional flow of all expired gases, such valves have therefore the additional advantage of enabling the patient to inspire a constant proportion of gases from the anaesthetic machine, since there is no mixing of these with those which are expired. At any one moment the anaesthetist can tell the exact proportion of gases that the patient is inspiring. Non-rebreathing valves are also useful for intermittent positive-pressure ventilation, but unless specially designed, the exhalation part of the valve may need to be held closed when the pressure is applied. A further advantage is that the patient cannot be hyperventilated if the total flow of gases is set to match the required minute volume of the patient.

An excellent valve of this type is the Frumin, which can be used for both spontaneous and controlled respiration (Frumin, Lee and Papper, 1959). It is so designed that a sudden rise in pressure (as produced by the anaesthetist's hand squeezing the reservoir bag) closes the expiratory leak so that all the gases pass to the patient. On release of the pressure at the end of inspiration the gases can then escape quietly again to the atmosphere. This valve can be used either with a face-mask or in a modified form to provide an 'in-line' gas flow for use with an endotracheal tube. The resistance and dead space are minimal. The resistance to gas flow in the valve at either inspiration or expiration is 1·5 mm. Hg at 60 litres/minute flow rates.

Another valve of this type has been designed by Ruben (1955), the exhalation part of which automatically closes during controlled or assisted respiration. It has a possible disadvantage in that it is "noisy". The dead space measures 9 ml. and the resistance at a flow of 25 litres per minute is only 0·8 cm. of water during inspiration and 1 cm. of water during expiration. Other recently introduced one-way valves include the Ambu "E" valve, and the Laerdal valve.

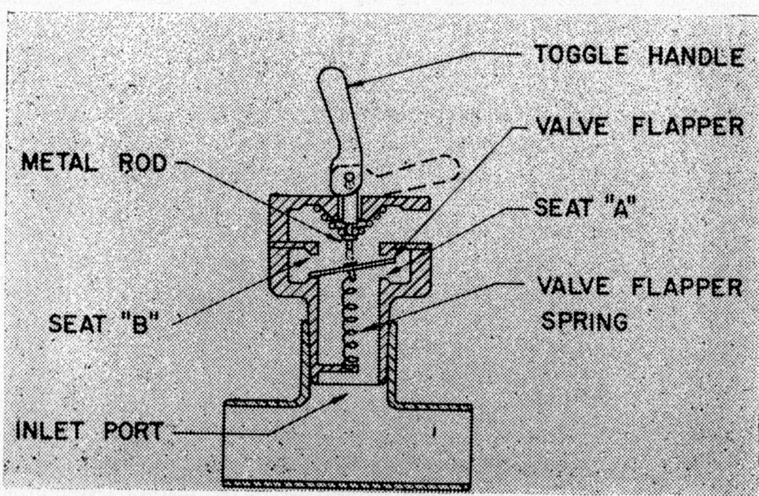

4/FIG. 27.—Pressure equalising valve.

When using a non-rebreathing valve, a pressure-equalising valve should be included in the system (Fig. 27) (Steen and Lee, 1960). Such a device prevents the build-up of excess gases in the reservoir bag, and without it it is necessary to admit to the system only the same amount that the patient will remove. This valve is fitted with a device which permits a leak of gases at a low pressure, and also allows the anaesthetist to stop the leak by squeezing the reservoir bag sharply.

Carbon Dioxide Absorption Techniques

John Snow in 1850 was one of the first to realise the potentialities of carbon dioxide absorption, but it was not until the work of Dennis Jackson on animals (1915) and Waters' application of this work to man (Waters, 1924) that the method came to be widely adopted. The principle is that if sufficient oxygen is added to the anaesthetic system to supply the patient's basic metabolic requirements and the carbon dioxide is removed from the exhalation, then the same mixture of gases or vapours can be breathed over and over again.

The primary justification for absorption techniques in anaesthesia is economy. Heat preservation and moistening of the inspired gases are secondary and minor advantages. It must, however, be borne in mind that the ability of the anaesthetist to reduce the level of carbon dioxide to below normal levels in a patient by means of such a system was, and still is, one of the basic factors in inducing controlled respiration. The risk of an explosion with an inflammable anaesthetic can be minimised by using it in a closed system.

Soda lime.—This is a mixture of about 94 per cent calcium hydroxide, 5 per cent sodium hydroxide, and recently 1 per cent potassium hydroxide has been added to some preparations to enhance absorption. Small amounts of silica are sometimes added as this reacts with calcium and sodium hydroxide to form calcium and sodium silicate. The silicate of calcium is extremely hard and brittle, whereas sodium silicate is gelatinous. The more silica that is added, the harder the soda lime becomes, and therefore the less dust that is formed. As a general rule, however, the efficiency of absorption of soda lime varies inversely with its hardness: for this reason silicates are omitted altogether in many present-day preparations of soda lime.

Sodium hydroxide, present in a 5 per cent proportion, plays the role of catalyst. Increasing this amount will improve absorption but unfortunately leads to excessive heating and "caking". Calcium hydroxide, on the other hand, represents the main bulk of soda lime and absorbs well, but it forms dust easily and is hygroscopic. The optimum moisture content of the mixture is from 14–19 per cent and such soda lime is described as "non-hygroscopic" because it does not readily absorb moisture from the surrounding atmosphere.

In preparation, the whole mass is fused into sheets and then allowed to harden. After this it is fragmented and then graded according to the size of the granules. For this purpose a wire mesh screen is used as a sieve. A 4-mesh screen means that there are four quarter-inch square openings per inch (approximately four 6·2 mm. square openings per 25 mm.); an 8-mesh screen signifies eight eighth-inch openings per inch (approximately eight 3·1 mm. openings per 25 mm.), and so on. In general anaesthesia the granules should be in the 4–8 mesh range, as this size represents the optimum surface area of absorption with the minimum resistance.

Hardness is measured by placing the granules in a standard steel pan together with 15 steel balls of fixed diameter. The whole is then shaken for thirty minutes, after which the granules are placed on a 40-mesh sieve and again shaken for a further three minutes. The amount retained on the screen should be not less than 75 per cent of the original and is described as the hardness number.

4/TABLE 12

SPECIFICATIONS FOR SODA LIME
(*Based on B.P. and U.S.P. standards*)

Colour:	White
Content:	Calcium hydroxide 94 per cent Sodium hydroxide 5 per cent Potassium hydroxide 1 per cent
Moisture content:	Not less than 14 per cent Not more than 19 per cent
Granule size:	4–8 mesh
Hardness number:	75 or more

Baralyme.—This comprises 80 per cent calcium hydroxide and 20 per cent barium hydroxide. This mixture is sufficiently hard not to require the addition of silica. Barium hydroxide (like sodium hydroxide in soda lime) plays the role of activator so that barium carbonate, calcium carbonate and water are formed. Heat is produced in a similar manner, but as both barium and calcium carbonate are insoluble, no interaction can take place. For this reason baralyme has no powers of regeneration like soda lime, where any sodium carbonate (soluble) formed can combine with any unneutralised calcium hydroxide available. Recent studies by Adriani (1963) suggest that modern soda lime is nearly 50 per cent more efficient than baralyme.

Indicators in soda lime.—Many dyes will change colour as hydroxides are neutralised and converted to carbonates.

Ethyl violet is an example of a colourless base indicator which can be impregnated into soda lime. The base of the indicator reacts with carbonic acid to form a soluble carbonate which is purple in colour. When all the sodium hydroxide is converted to sodium and calcium carbonate, a purple colour develops. Examples of other dyes are given in Table 13.

Too much reliance should never be placed on any indicator for soda lime as hypercarbia can always develop before signs of soda lime exhaustion are evident. Furthermore, complete reliance on a colour change may lead to a dangerous situation if a soda lime without any indicator is suddenly used. Such findings as the presence of channelling along the sides of a canister may prove misleading in judging the time of exhaustion of soda lime. Nevertheless, the presence of an indicator in soda lime is a useful guide, particularly if a double canister system is being used, in that it allows one chamber to be replaced. The final proof of the efficacy of a particular soda-lime canister's contents can only lie in the periodic testing of the gases flowing through it for the possible presence of carbon dioxide. This can be achieved by using a simple analyser.

4/TABLE 13

Indicators	Soda lime	
	Fresh	*Exhausted*
Methyl orange	Orange	Yellow
Phenolphthalein	Colourless	Pink
Ethyl violet	Colourless	Purple
Clayton yellow	Pink	Yellow

Mechanism of absorption.—When the patient's exhalations are passed through the canister containing the soda-lime granules the carbon dioxide combines with the hydroxides to form carbonates and water. This chemical change requires the presence of some moisture, which is provided by the patient's expiration, and at the same time it produces heat. There is also an overall increase in the weight of the canister contents which amounts to about 33 per cent when they are worn out.

$$(1)\ CO_2 + 2NaOH \rightarrow H_2O + Na_2CO_3 + \text{heat.}$$
$$(2)\ Na_2CO_3 + Ca(OH)_2 \rightarrow 2NaOH + CaCO_3.$$

A small quantity is also absorbed thus:

$$CO_2 + Ca(OH)_2 \rightarrow H_2O + CaCO_3 + \text{heat.}$$

The heat produced is known as the heat of neutralisation. Temperatures up to 60° C have been recorded inside canisters. The production of some heat is a sign that the soda lime is functioning efficiently.

Regeneration of soda lime.—The surface of the soda-lime granule rapidly becomes exhausted. There are pores, however, which penetrate into the interior and allow carbon dioxide to diffuse inwards to find a fresh hydroxide surface. Clinically it has been observed in the past that if soda lime was taken out of the system and rested when apparently exhausted, then after a few hours it was again able to absorb carbon dioxide efficiently. This observation led to the suggestion of having two canisters and interchanging them every hour to allow one to have a rest period.

The explanation of this regeneration is complex but is clearly concerned with the pores in the granule. The sodium hydroxide in the moisture on the surface of the granule is more soluble than calcium hydroxide, so it combines with the carbon dioxide in the usual manner to form sodium carbonate. Now this substance is very soluble, so it passes into the interior of the granule through one of the pores to react with the less soluble calcium hydroxide lying in the inner sanctum. Here calcium carbonate, which is insoluble, is formed along with sodium hydroxide. The sodium hydroxide then diffuses out to the surface and the process is repeated.

Due to improved soda lime, regeneration is rarely seen today. There are three main reasons (Adriani, 1963). First, less silica is now used. The granule is not so hard but is capable of better absorption. Second, the moisture content is better controlled and more uniform. Third, small quantities (1 per cent) of potassium hydroxide have been added to improve absorption. Furthermore, experiments using a tidal volume of 500 ml. containing 200 ml. of carbon dioxide have shown that the modern circle absorber will remove virtually all the carbon dioxide for the first three hours, but after that the content of carbon dioxide escaping from the canister rises rapidly to reach about 0·5 per cent after five hours. There was no evidence of regeneration.

The to and fro'.—The canister is placed between the breathing bag and face-piece or endotracheal tube. Fresh gases are introduced near the face-piece so that any alteration in the gas concentration is immediately transmitted to the patient. The presence of a warm canister so close to the patient's respiratory tract ensures that the heat and humidity loss is negligible, but the system has largely fallen into disfavour because of the inadequacy of the carbon dioxide absorption, the awkwardness of the apparatus so close to the patient's head, and the possibility of inhalation of dust particles.

A standard adult to and fro' canister is cylindrical and measures 8 by 13 cm. Ideally the air space should equal the patient's tidal volume. When filled with soda lime the air capacity lies between 375 and 425 ml. As the patient breathes in and out of the canister, so the soda lime nearest the mouth becomes exhausted. The respirations usually travel along the sides of the canister because in this region the flow of gases apparently encounters least resistance. With this system, as the soda lime becomes exhausted, so the entrapped air around it becomes dead space because this air can now be rebreathed without first having the carbon dioxide removed. For the first 1½ hours the standard canister appears to be capable of absorbing almost all the carbon dioxide but after that there is a progressive rise up to 0·5 per cent after 5½ hours (Adriani, 1963). In clinical practice, where the tidal volume may be high due to controlled or assisted respiration and the carbon dioxide output may be in excess of 200 ml. per minute, it is clear that the efficiency of this canister would be much shorter.

A neat and simple method of obtaining a well-packed canister is to place a nylon pot scourer between the soda lime and the cap (Robson and Pask, 1954). This also helps to prevent channelling of gases in the canister.

The circle.—In this system the gases have to pass great distances along flexible tubing so that the rate of flow is lower than in a to and fro' apparatus. The presence of unidirectional valves also offers an increase in resistance, though if these are properly constructed with a wide surface area this is reduced to a minimum.

The canister itself requires a number of comments. First, it is immaterial whether it is placed vertically or horizontally though, in the latter case, there is a greater tendency to leave a gap along the upper surface in the packing or settling of the granules. The gases may enter from the top or the bottom of the canister. The capacity of the absorber should be at least equal to the patient's tidal volume; if the tidal volume is greater then some of the expired gases will pass directly through the canister without coming to rest in the interior, thus impeding efficient absorption. The total air space normally available in an absorber lies between 40–60 per cent of the total volume of the unit, but this volume can be varied by changing the size of the granules and also the firmness of the packing.

In recent years large canisters have become more popular because they ensure better absorption, in that their capacity far exceeds any predictable tidal volume and all expired gases are in contact with a large number of granules during their passage through the absorber. The ideal capacity has not yet been determined, but the greater this is the longer becomes the period of uninterrupted use before renewal is required. These units are often constructed of transparent plastic material so that a change in the colour of the indicator in the soda lime can be seen. Nevertheless, the heat and alkali needed in absorption techniques tend to destroy rubber and plastic materials.

In some cases these large absorbers are made in two interchangeable sections so that one half can be replaced when exhausted. An alternative method to having one large canister in the circuit is to use two absorbers mounted in series. However, these large-size canisters should be used solely for the purpose of more efficient absorption rather than as an economy measure, for it is known that inadequate absorption commences before the indicator has changed completely.

Although soda lime is believed to act as a bactericidal filter and the heat and presence of alkali possibly do have a germicidal effect, for a known infected patient it is advisable to use a "to and fro'" system since the soda lime can be discarded and the apparatus can be thoroughly and efficiently sterilised at the end of the anaesthetic. If economy of anaesthetic gases or vapour is the primary consideration then very low flows can be used with the closed circle system provided the concentration of oxygen and anaesthetic agent in the inspired mixture is carefully monitored.

PAEDIATRIC ANAESTHETIC SYSTEMS

Elimination of apparatus dead space and minimal resistance to respiration are the most important factors to be considered. Any addition to the normal dead space of a small child can seriously hamper the adequacy of pulmonary exchange. This becomes evident when one considers that the tidal volume of a full-term normal neonate is about 20 ml., and that the physiological dead space is half this amount (Strang, 1961), alveolar ventilation therefore amounting only to some 10 ml. (see Table 14). The addition of only a few ml. of apparatus dead space therefore represents a large proportionate increase in the newborn baby.

4/TABLE 14

THE RESPIRATION OF NEWBORN AND ADULT SUBJECTS

(*From C. A. Smith in Mitchell-Nelson's* Textbook of Pediatrics. *Saunders*, 1950)

	Rate	*Tidal Volume*	*Minute volume*	*Vital capacity*
Newborn infant (3·5 kg.)	44	19·0 ml.	838 ml.	170 ml.
Premature baby (1·7 kg.)	58	12·3 ml.	713 ml.	—
Adult	18	450·0 ml.	7100 ml.	3500 ml.

Masks.—Even a small mask adds to the dead space of the anaesthetic system, and in proportion to the small tidal and alveolar ventilation of a child becomes a factor of importance. A good mask for small babies must be designed to reduce apparatus dead space to a minimum and also to suit the flat contour of the face which is normal at the start of life. The most suitable mask at present available is that described by Rendall-Baker and Soucek (1962). The nominal dead space in the size intended for mature neonates is 4 ml.

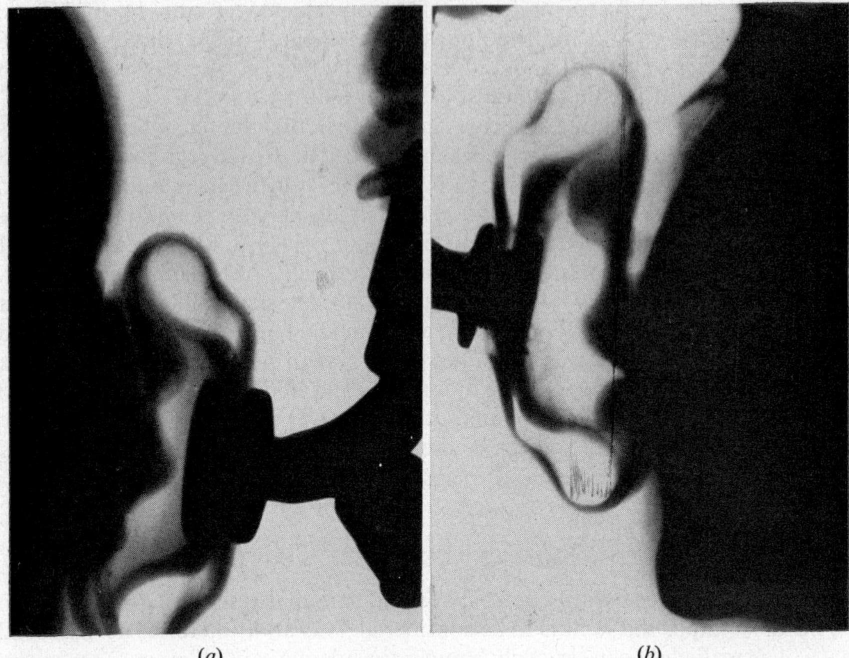

(*a*) (*b*)

4/Fig. 28.—X-ray pictures showing the difference in contour of the face of an infant (*a*), and a 4-year old child (*b*). This illustrates the need for a special type of mask for the infant.

Apparatus.—Paediatric anaesthetic equipment should offer the least possible dead space and resistance to respiration for the child to contend with. It should also be light and easily managed. In this country two systems are most commonly used.

(1) *The Rendall-Baker apparatus.*—This equipment is excellent for mask anaesthesia with spontaneous respiration, and can be adapted for use during controlled ventilation (Fig. 29). It consists of a partitioned mask adaptor fitted with an inlet tube and a light expiratory valve on one side of the partition, and a large port on the other side onto which an open-ended bag can be attached. Fresh gases are directed by the partition so that they flow over the child's face, and therefore the apparatus dead space is almost nil. The apparatus can be assembled in two ways. Fresh gases can be introduced into the side-arm on the partitioned adaptor, passing down over the child's face and out of the large port into the open-ended bag. Used like this it acts as a type of Ayre's T-piece. Alternatively gases can be led in through the open-ended bag, expiration taking place via the expiratory valve. Fresh gas flows should exceed twice the minute volume of the child.

(2) *Ayre's T-piece.*—This equipment is used for endotracheal anaesthesia with either controlled or spontaneous respiration. Ayre (1965) has summarised the approximate gas flow rates and sizes for the expiratory limb of a T-piece.

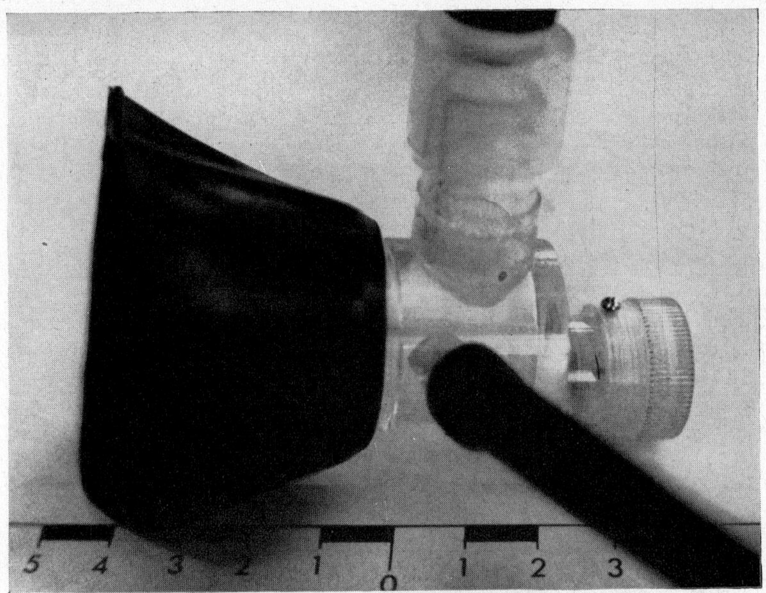

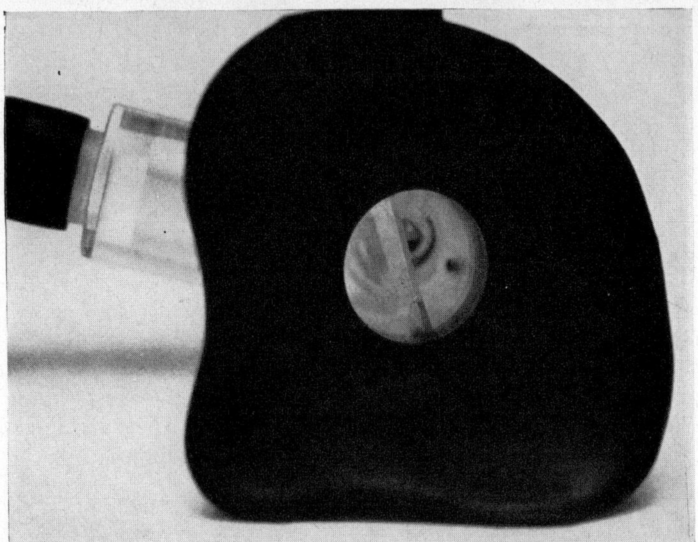

4/Fig. 29 (*a*) and (*b*).—The Rendall-Baker paediatric anaesthetic apparatus. See text for details. The scale is in centimetres.

At present it is customary to deliver a generous gas flow to the side-arm of the T-piece (at least twice the minute volume of the child) and to use only one size for the expiratory limb. An open-ended bag may be attached to the expiratory limb in order to monitor spontaneous respiration, or to manually control ventilation, as suggested by Jackson Rees.

Age	*Rate of flow of fresh gases (litres/minute)*	*Capacity of expiratory limb (ml.)*
0–3 months	3–4	6–12
3–6 months	4–5	12–18
6–12 months	5–6	18–24
1–2 years	6–7	24–42
2–4 years	7–8	42–60
4–8 years	8–9	60–72

Other types of apparatus (one-way valves, and both to and fro' and circle absorber systems) have been designed for paediatric use, but have not achieved

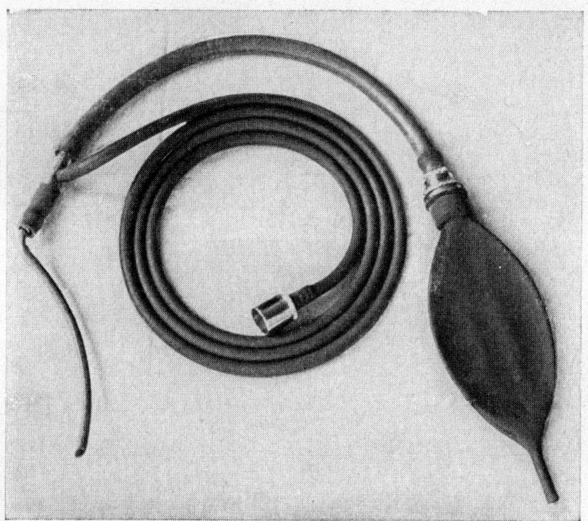

4/Fig. 30.—T-piece system for paediatric anaesthesia.

popularity in this country. When used for neonatal anaesthesia they often have too large a dead space, present too high a resistance to respiration, or are difficult to fix alongside the small head of a baby. They are unnecessarily complicated where simple equipment is extremely satisfactory.

REFERENCES

Adriani, J. (1963). *Chemistry and Physics of Anesthesia.* Springfield, Ill.: Charles C. Thomas.

Askrog, V. F., Pender, J. W., and Eckenhoff, J. E. (1964). Changes in physiological deadspace during deliberate hypotension. *Anesthesiology*, **25,** 744.

Askrog, V. F., Pender, J. W., Smith, T. C., and Eckenhoff, J. E. (1964). Changes in respiratory deadspace during halothane, cyclopropane and nitrous oxide anesthesia. *Anesthesiology*, **25,** 342.

ASTRUP, P. (1959). "Ultra-micro methods for determining pH, pCO_2 and standard bicarbonate in capillary blood". In: *A Symposium on pH and Blood Gas Measurement*, pp. 81–92. Ed. R. F. Woolmer. London: J. & A. Churchill.

ATTINGER, E. O., MONROE, R. G., and SEGAL, M. S. (1956). The mechanics of breathing in different body positions. I. In normal subjects. *J. clin. Invest.*, **35,** 904.

AYRE, P. (1956). The T-piece technique. *Brit. J. Anaesth.*, **28,** 520.

BALL, W. C., STEWART, P. B., NEWSHAM, L. G. S., and BATES, D. V. (1962). Regional pulmonary function studied with Xenon^{133}. *J. clin. Invest.*, **41,** 519.

BEARN, A. G., BILLING, B., and SHERLOCK, S. (1951). Effect of adrenaline and noradrenaline on hepatic blood flow and splanchnic carbohydrate metabolism in man. *J. Physiol. (Lond.)*, **115,** 430.

BENDIXEN, H. H., BULLWINKEL, B., HEDLEY-WHITE, J., and LAVER, M. B. (1964). Atelectasis and shunting during spontaneous ventilation in anesthetised patients. *Anesthesiology*, **25,** 297.

BENDIXEN, H. H., HEDLEY-WHYTE, J., and LAVER, M. B. (1963). Impaired oxygenation in surgical patients during general anesthesia with controlled ventilation. A concept of atelectasis. *New Engl. J. Med.*, **269,** 991.

BERGMAN, N. A. (1963). Distribution of inspired gas during anesthesia and artificial ventilation. *J. appl. Physiol.*, **18,** 1085.

BERGMAN, N. A. (1967). Components of alveolar-arterial oxygen tension difference in anesthetised man. *Anesthesiology*, **28,** 517.

BONVALLET, M., HUGELIN, A., and DELL, P. (1956). Milieu intérieur et activité automatique des cellules réticulaires mésencéphaliques. *J. Physiol. (Paris)*, **48,** 403.

BRIDGE, B. E., Jr., and EGER, E. I. (II) (1966). The effect of hypocapnia on the level of halothane anesthesia in man. *Anesthesiology*, **27,** 634.

BROOKS, D. K., and FELDMAN, S. A. (1962). Metabolic acidosis: a new approach to "neostigmine-resistant curarisation". *Anaesthesia*, **17,** 161.

BUCKLEY, J. J., and VAN BERGEN, F. H. (1960). Assessment of respiratory efficiency in the post-operative patient. *Anesthesiology*, **21,** 93.

BUNKER, J. P. (1962). Metabolic acidosis during anesthesia and surgery. *Anesthesiology*, **23,** 107.

CAMPBELL, E. J. M., and HOWELL, J. B. L. (1960). Simple rapid methods of estimating arterial and mixed venous pCO_2. *Brit. med. J.*, **1,** 458.

CAMPBELL, E. J. M., and HOWELL, J. B. L. (1963). Sensation of breathlessness. *Brit. med. Bull.*, **19,** 36.

CAMPBELL, E. J. M., NUNN, J. F., and PECKETT, B. W. (1958). A comparison of artificial ventilation and spontaneous respiration with particular reference to ventilation-blood flow relationships. *Brit. J. Anaesth.*, **30,** 166.

CARLENS, E. (1949). A new flexible double-lumen catheter for broncho-spirometry. *J. thorac. Surg.*, **18,** 742.

CASE, E. H., and STILES, J. A. (1946). The effect of various surgical positions on vital capacity. *Anesthesiology*, **7,** 29.

CHURCHILL, E. D. (1925). Pulmonary atelectasis, with especial reference to massive collapse of the lung. *Arch. Surg. (Chicago)*, **11,** 489.

COLE, R. B., and BISHOP, J. M. (1963). Effect of varying inspired oxygen tension on alveolar-arterial oxygen tension difference in man. *J. appl. Physiol.*, **18,** 1043.

COLGAN, F. J., and WHANG, T. B. (1968). Anesthesia and atelectasis. *Anesthesiology*, **29,** 917.

COLLIER, C. R. (1956). Determination of mixed venous carbon dioxide tension by rebreathing. *J. appl. Physiol.*, **9,** 25.

COMROE, J. H., FORSTER, R. E., DUBOIS, A. B., BRISCOE, W. A., and CARLSEN, E. (1962). *The Lung. Clinical Physiology and Pulmonary Function Tests*, p. 103, 2nd edit. Chicago: Year Book Medical Publishers.

NUNN, J. F., and HILL, D. W. (1960). Respiratory deadspace and arterial to end-tidal CO_2 tension difference in anesthetized man. *J. appl. Physiol.*, **15,** 383.

NUNN, J. F., CAMPBELL, E. J. M., and PECKETT, B. W. (1959). Anatomical subdivisions of the volume of respiratory dead space and effect of position of the jaw. *J. appl. Physiol.*, **14,** 174.

NUNN, J. F., and EZI-ASHI, T. I. (1961). The respiratory effects of resistance to breathing in anesthetized man. *Anesthesiology*, **22,** 174.

NUNN, J. F., and EZI-ASHI, T. I. (1962). The accuracy of the respirometer and ventigrator. *Brit. J. Anaesth.*, **34,** 422.

NUNN, J. F., and PAYNE, J. P. (1962). Hypoxaemia after general anaesthesia. *Lancet*, **2,** 631.

PANDAY, J., and NUNN, J. F. (1968). Failure to demonstrate progressive falls of arterial P_{O_2} during anaesthesia. *Anaesthesia*, **23,** 38.

PAPPENHEIMER, J. (1950). Standardisation of definitions and symbols in respiratory physiology. *Fed. Proc.*, **9,** 602.

PIERCE, J. A., and GAROFALO, M. L. (1965). Preoperative medication and its effect on blood gases. *J. Amer. med. Ass.*, **194,** 487.

POOLER, H. E. (1949). Relief of post-operative pain and its influence on vital capacity. *Brit. med. J.*, **2,** 1200.

PRICE, H. L., COOPERMAN, L. H., WARDEN, J. C., MORRIS, J. J., and SMITH, T. C. (1969). Pulmonary haemodynamics during general anesthesia in man. *Anesthesiology*, **30,** 629.

PRYS-ROBERTS, C. (1968). Ph.D. Thesis, Univ. of Leeds.

RAINE, J. M., and BISHOP, J. M. (1963). A—a difference in O_2 tension and physiological deadspace in normal man. *J. appl. Physiol.*, **18,** 284.

RENDALL-BAKER, L., and SOUCEK, D. H. (1962). New paediatric face-masks and anaesthetic equipment. *Brit. med. J.*, **1,** 1960.

ROBSON, J. G., and PASK, E. A. (1954). Some data on the performance of Waters' canister. *Brit. J. Anaesth.*, **26,** 333.

RUBEN, H. (1955). A new non-rebreathing valve. *Anesthesiology*, **16,** 643.

SEVERINGHAUS, J. W. (1959). Recent developments in blood O_2 and CO_2 electrodes: In: *A Symposium on pH and Blood Gas Measurement*, pp. 126–142. Ed. R. F. Woolmer. London: J. & A. Churchill.

SEVERINGHAUS, J. W. (1964). Personal communication.

SEVERINGHAUS, J. W., SWENSON, E. W., FINLEY, T. N., LATEGOLA, M. T., and WILLIAMS, J. (1961). Unilateral hypoventilation produced in dogs by occluding one pulmonary artery. *J. appl. Physiol.*, **16,** 53.

SIGGAARD-ANDERSEN, O. (1963). Blood acid-base alignment nomogram. *Scand. J. Clin. Lab. Invest.*, **15,** 211.

SIMPSON, B. R., PARKHOUSE, J., MARSHALL, R., and LAMBRECHTS, W. (1961). Extradural analgesia and the prevention of post-operative respiratory complications. *Brit. J. Anaesth.*, **33,** 628.

SLATER, E. M., NILSSON, S. E., LEAKE, D. L., PARRY W. L., LAVER, M. B., HEDLEY-WHITE, J., and BENDIXEN, H. H. (1965). Arterial oxygen tension measurements during nitrous oxide/oxygen anesthesia. *Anesthesiology*, **26,** 642.

SMITH, A. C., and HAHN, C. E. W. (1969). Electrodes for the measurement of oxygen and carbon dioxide tensions. *Brit. J. Anaesth.*, **41,** 731.

SMITH, A. C., and SPALDING, J. M. K. (1959). Intermittent positive-pressure respiration. Some physiological observations. *Proc. roy. Soc. Med.*, **52,** 661.

SMITH, C. A. (1950). In Mitchell-Nelson's *Textbook of Pediatrics*, 5th edit. Philadelphia: W. B. Saunders.

SMITH, T. C., STEPHEN, G. W., ZEIGER, L., and WOLLMAN, H. (1967). Effects of premedicant drugs on respiration and gas exchange in man. *Anesthesiology*, **28,** 883.

SMITH, W. D. A. (1961). The effects of external resistance on respiration. Part I. General review. *Brit. J. Anaesth.*, **33,** 549.

SPALDING, J. M. K., and CRAMPTON SMITH, A. (1963). *Clinical Practice and Physiology of Artificial Respiration.* Oxford: Blackwell Scientific Publications.

STARK, D. C. C., and SMITH, H. (1960). Pulmonary vascular changes during anaesthesia. *Brit. J. Anaesth.*, **32,** 460.

STEEN, S. N., and LEE, A. S. J. (1960). Prevention of inadvertent excess pressure in closed systems. *Curr. Res. Anesth.*, **39,** 264.

STRANG, L. B. (1961). Alveolar gas and anatomical deadspace measurements in normal newborn infants. *Clin. Sci.*, **21,** 107.

SYKES, M. K., YOUNG, W. E., and ROBINSON, B. E. (1965). Oxygenation during anaesthesia with controlled ventilation. *Brit. J. Anaesth.*, **37,** 314.

TAYLOR, S. H., SCOTT, D. B., and DONALD, K. W. (1964). Respiratory effects of general anaesthesia. *Lancet*, **1,** 841.

TOMLIN, P. J., CONWAY, C. M., and PAYNE, J. P. (1964). Hypoxaemia due to atropine. *Lancet*, **1,** 14.

UTTING, J. E., and GRAY, T. C. (1962). The initiation of respiration after anaesthesia accompanied by passive pulmonary hyperventilation. *Brit. J. Anaesth.*, **34,** 785.

VIRTUE, R. W., PERMUTT, S., TANAKA, R., PEARCY, C., BANE, H., BROMBERGER-BARNEA, B. (1966). Ventilation-perfusion and changes during thoracotomy. *Anesthesiology*, **27,** 132.

WAKAI, I. (1963). Human oxygenation by air during anaesthesia. The relation o ventilatory volume and arterial oxygen saturation. *Brit. J. Anaesth.*, **35,** 414.

WATERS, R. M. (1924). Clinical scope and utility of carbon dioxide filtration in inhalation anesthesia. *Curr. Res. Anesth.*, **3,** 20.

WATSON, W. E. (1962*a*). Some observations on dynamic lung compliance during intermittent positive pressure respiration. *Brit. J. Anaesth.*, **34,** 502.

WATSON, W. E. (1962*b*). Observations on dynamic lung compliance of patients with respiratory weakness receiving intermittent positive pressure respiration. *Brit. J. Anaesth.*, **34,** 690.

WEBB, S. J. S., and NUNN, J. F. (1967). A comparison between the effects of nitrous oxide and nitrogen on arterial P_{O_2}. *Anaesthesia*, **22,** 69.

WEST, J. B. (1962). Regional differences in gas exchange in the lung of erect man. *J. appl. Physiol.*, **17,** 893.

WEST, J. B. (1963*a*). Blood-flow, ventilation and gas exchange in the lung. *Lancet*, **2,** 1055.

WEST, J. B. (1963*b*). Distribution of gas and blood in normal lungs. *Brit. med. Bull.*, **19,** 53.

WEST, J. B., DOLLERY, C. T., and HEARD, B. E. (1965). Increased pulmonary vascular resistance in the dependant zone of the isolated dog lung caused by perivascular oedema. *Circulat. Res.*, **12,** 301.

WOOLMER, R., and LIND, B. (1954). Rebreathing with a semi-closed system. *Brit. J. Anaesth.*, **26,** 316.

WYANT, G. M., CHANG, Chung Ai, and MERRIMAN, J. E. (1962). The effect of anesthesia upon pulmonary circulation. *Curr. Res. Anesth.*, **41,** 338.

FURTHER READING

CHERNIACK, R. M., and CHERNIACK, L. (1961). *Respiration in Health and Disease.* Philadelphia: W. B. Saunders Co.

COMROE, J. H., FORSTER, R. E., DUBOIS, A. B., BRISCOE, W. A., and CARLSEN, E., (1962). *The Lung*, 2nd edit. Chicago: Year Book Medical Publishers.

Davenport, H. W. (1958). *The ABC of Acid-Base Chemistry*. Chicago: Univ. of Chicago Press.

Nunn, J. F. (1969). *Applied Respiratory Physiology*. London: Butterworth & Co.

Siggaard-Andersen, O. (1966). *The Acid-Base Status of the Blood*. Copenhagen: Munksgaard.

West, J. B. (1965). *Ventilation/Blood Flow and Gas Exchange*. Oxford: Blackwell Scientific Publications.

Wilton, T. N. P. and Wilson, F. (1965). *Neonatal Anaesthesia*. Oxford: Blackwell Scientific Publications.

Chapter 5

OXYGEN AND ASSOCIATED GASES

OXYGEN (O_2)

History

Although Stephen Hale prepared oxygen along with many other gases in 1727, the full credit for its discovery and the realisation of the importance of this gas as a normal constituent of air must go to Priestley (1777). Following upon this discovery Lavoisier and his colleagues (1780 and 1789) demonstrated that it was absorbed by the lungs and, after metabolism in the body, eliminated as carbon dioxide and water. Since that time its value as a therapeutic agent has gradually increased with improved methods of administration.

Preparation

In the laboratory. Numerous methods are available, though they serve no practical purpose. Amongst the commonest is to heat potassium chlorate in the presence of a catalyst such as manganese dioxide:

$$\underset{\text{potassium chlorate}}{2KClO_3} \xrightarrow[\text{manganese dioxide}]{\text{Heat and}} \underset{\text{potassium chloride}}{2KCl} + \underset{\text{oxygen}}{3O_2}$$

Commercially. Fractional distillation of liquid air is the method now almost universally adopted. Before liquefaction of the air carbon dioxide is removed, and afterwards the nitrogen and oxygen are separated by making use of the difference in their boiling points (oxygen = − 182·5° C: nitrogen = − 195·8° C) The gaseous oxygen is then collected and stored in cylinders, coloured black with white shoulders, at a pressure of approximately 120 atmospheres, or roughly 1800 lb./sq. inch.

Presentation

Cylinders up to 48 cu. ft. capacity for anaesthetic use are supplied with pin index valves. Cylinders larger than 48 cu. ft. are supplied with bull-nosed threads.

Large volume users may consider piped oxygen supplies to be justified. The oxygen may be supplied to piped systems in large compressed gas cylinders attached to a manifold in banks of two or more cylinders. Various devices are employed to ensure a continuity of gas supply, one bank of cylinders "running" whilst the other is held in reserve, with facilities for automatic opening of the reserve when the "running" bank nears exhaustion and with the simultaneous activation of a warning device.

Another form of oxygen supply is from liquid oxygen. In general, users in excess of 5,000 cubic feet of oxygen per week will find the liquid oxygen source economical. In one type of installation the liquid oxygen is boiled in a vacuum insulated evaporator (V.I.E.) and supplied to the pipeline at 60 lb. per sq. inch. No compressor is necessary with such an installation.

Physical Properties

Oxygen is a tasteless, colourless and odourless gas; with a specific gravity of 1·105 (air = 1) and a molecular weight of 32. At normal atmospheric pressure it liquefies at − 183° C, but on increasing the pressure to 50 atmospheres, the temperature at which liquefaction occurs rises to − 119° C. The liquid may be cooled to a solid which melts at − 218° C. The solubility in water is 2·4 volumes per cent at 37° C and 4·9 volumes per cent at 0° C.

Inflammability

Oxygen cannot be ignited, but its presence aids combustion. Fires which occur during oxygen therapy are due to the rapid conflagration favoured by the high concentration of oxygen, though oxidisable substances such as cloth, wool or rubber must be present. With oil or grease, oxygen under pressure may cause an explosion, and this type of fire was particularly liable to happen when the old type of Endurance reducing valve was used. As the cylinder was turned on, a sudden jet of gas through this valve might come in contact with extraneous grease and result in an explosion. Combustion was favoured by the rubber diaphragm in the valve and enhanced by the continual flow of oxygen. The present-day Adams valve is less susceptible to this risk, but nevertheless grease should always be avoided in the presence of oxygen.

Pharmacological Actions

Oxygen is a normal constituent of air, and in order to appreciate the importance of an oxygen-rich atmosphere it is necessary to recall a few fundamental facts concerning respiration. About one-fifth (20·9 per cent) of the air we inhale at each breath consists of oxygen. Thus, in the inspired air, oxygen has a partial pressure of one-fifth of the atmospheric pressure, i.e. 20·9 per cent of 760 mm. Hg = 159 mm. Hg. As the air passes down the bronchial tree it becomes mixed with expired gases which are partially depleted of their oxygen so that the partial pressure of oxygen in the alveoli is about 100 mm. Hg. This is the force that drives the oxygen across the pulmonary membrane, because the tension of oxygen in the venous blood is only 40 mm. Hg.

1. *Oxygen Content*

The oxygen content of the blood is the amount of oxygen that can be extracted from 100 ml. of blood. It is expressed in ml. of dry gas at standard temperature and pressure (S.T.P.D.).

2. *Oxygen Capacity*

The oxygen capacity is the volume of oxygen at S.T.P.D. carried by 100 volumes of blood after saturation with room air.

The oxygen capacity of blood includes oxygen in combination with haemoglobin (1·39 ml. O_2 per gram Hb) and oxygen in solution in the plasma (0·3 ml. O_2 per 100 ml. blood).

3. *Oxygen Saturation*

Oxygen saturation is the oxygen content of a sample compared with the oxygen capacity of that sample expressed as a percentage.

More exactly, it is the

$$\frac{O_2 \text{ combined with Hb}}{O_2 \text{ combined with Hb after equilibration with air}} \times 100$$

$$= \frac{O_2 \text{ content} - \text{dissolved } O_2}{O_2 \text{ capacity} - \text{dissolved } O_2} \times 100$$

The oxygen saturation may be obtained by spectrophotometric methods but it should be noted that actual oxygen content may not be obtained in this manner.

Oxygen content is traditionally measured by the manometric method of Peters and Van Slyke which was first described in 1924, but the modern micro-manometric technique of Natelson (1951) is presently favoured. More recently an excellent correlation with such techniques has been obtained by Davies (1970) using a gas chromatograph.

In the arterial circulation, 100 ml. of blood carries about 19·8 ml. of oxygen combined with haemoglobin, while a small amount (0·3 ml.) of oxygen is also carried in solution in the plasma. Although this latter quantity is not large its importance is great, because it is via this pathway that the oxygen passes to and from the haemoglobin and so reaches the tissues.

The percentage saturation of haemoglobin with oxygen depends largely on the tension of oxygen in the blood. An increase in oxygen tension results in a rise in the amount of oxygen carried by the haemoglobin, but the relationship is not linear as it is with the oxygen in solution in the plasma. The graph obtained is expressed as the *oxygen dissociation curve* (Fig. 1). This dissociation curve of

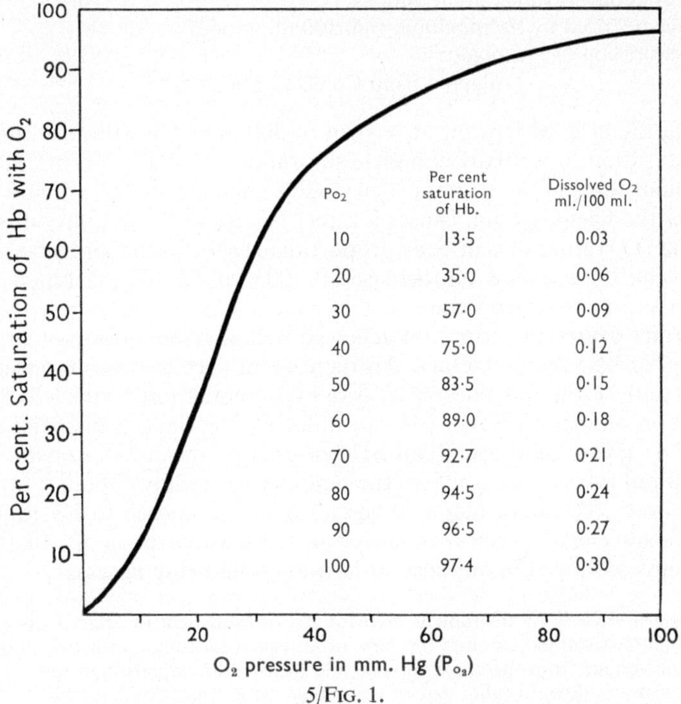

5/Fig. 1.

haemoglobin is of particular importance to anaesthetists because it is possible to vary the percentage of oxygen in the inspired mixtures of gases (thus altering the tension of oxygen, i.e. P_{O_2}) and so determining the oxygen saturation of the patient's blood. The peculiar S-shape of the curve has certain advantages for the patient. First, the tension of oxygen (P_{O_2}) in the arterial blood can fall from 95 mm. Hg to 80 mm. Hg, as may happen with slight respiratory obstruction, yet the haemoglobin of arterial blood remains virtually fully saturated (i.e. 97·0 per cent). In fact, the P_{O_2} has to fall to about 60 mm. Hg before cyanosis is visible and even then the arterial oxygen saturation is around 85 per cent. Secondly, at the beginning of the curve when the P_{O_2} is low in the tissues the haemoglobin readily gives up its oxygen content.

The small, but vital amount of oxygen (0·3 ml./100 ml. blood) which is dissolved in the plasma does not have any such dissociation curve, for the oxygen content of plasma bears a direct linear relationship to the tension to which it is exposed. Thus, a patient breathing air will have an alveolar partial pressure of oxygen of 100 mm. Hg, and this will give a 95–97 per cent saturation of the haemoglobin. The total oxygen content of 100 ml. of blood is about 20·3 ml. of which only 0·3 ml. is carried by the plasma (Table 1).

5/Table 1

Mean Values for Oxygen in Blood

	Arterial	*Venous*
Oxygen tension (Po_2) in mm. Hg	95	40
Oxygen dissolved in plasma (ml./100 ml. blood)	0·3	0·12
Total oxygen content (ml./100 ml. blood)	20·3	15·5
Total oxygen carried by haemoglobin (ml./100 ml. blood)	20	15·4
Per cent saturation of haemoglobin	97·0	75

(Adapted from Comroe *et al.*, 1962)

Increasing the arterial tension of oxygen to 300 mm. Hg will raise the haemoglobin saturation to virtually complete saturation (i.e. 100 per cent). Such a tension, though leading to an almost negligible increase in the amount actually carried by the haemoglobin, causes a threefold rise in the quantity dissolved in the plasma. This amount is directly proportional to the partial pressure no matter how high the P_{O_2} rises, i.e. an increase of 0·003 ml. O_2/100 ml. blood for each mm. Hg rise in partial pressure.

The exact degree of saturation achieved with a given tension of oxygen can be influenced by various factors. An increase in carbon dioxide tension shifts the curve to the right and a decrease, as in hyperventilation, to the left. Similarly, variations in temperature and pH can influence the oxygen dissociation curve (see p. 97). Oxygen saturation can be measured by means of an oximeter.*

At normal rates of metabolism the body tissues remove about 5 ml. of oxygen from every 100 ml. of blood. When a subject is exposed to 2·3 atmospheres of oxygen, sufficient oxygen is dissolved in the plasma to supply all the tissue requirements without the presence of haemoglobin being necessary.

* *Oximeter.*—This is an instrument used for the measurement of arterial oxygen saturation. The light transmitted through the lobe of an ear is measured with two photo-electric cells, and the voltage from these is combined and measured by a galvanometer. The scale of the galvanometer is directly calibrated in percentage saturation (Millikan, 1942).

The inhalation of 100 per cent oxygen at atmospheric pressure may slightly interfere with the transport of carbon dioxide from the tissues to the lungs. The reason is that larger quantities of carbon dioxide are taken up by reduced haemoglobin than by oxyhaemoglobin, so that the whole transport of carbon dioxide is very dependant on the amount of reduced haemoglobin available. If a subject breathes a high percentage of oxygen, the increased quantity dissolved in the plasma will then lead to less dissociation of oxyhaemoglobin and, therefore, a diminution in the amount of reduced haemoglobin available for carbon dioxide transport. The possible effects of an increase in carbon dioxide in the tissues are discussed later.

Physiological Results of Oxygen Excess

Recent work has been directed to the design of a safe environment for astronauts in space capsules for prolonged periods.

Studies performed on volunteers enclosed in controlled environments have shown that the critical factor involved in the causation of the toxic effects of oxygen is not the percentage of oxygen within the atmosphere but the absolute tension of oxygen within that environment. Provided the oxygen tension is kept below 418 mm. Hg, toxic effects do not become apparent (Michael, 1960). The oxygen tension decided upon for the Apollo flights was 247 mm. Hg. The safety of man in an atmosphere of pure oxygen has been proven by Bartek (1967) and by successful Apollo missions. It should be noted that though the cabin atmosphere on these missions from the third day onwards was pure oxygen, the cabin pressure was approximately one-third of normal atmospheric pressure.

The inhalation of 100 per cent oxygen as opposed to room air leads to certain physiological changes, namely:

Respiratory system.—Fowler and Comroe (1948) studied 32 subjects breathing 100 per cent oxygen and found that the minute volume became decreased by about 3 per cent after one to two minutes. This they explained on the basis that normal air—with its lower oxygen tension—leads to a continuous tonic stimulation of respiration via the chemoreceptors in the carotid and aortic bodies. The inhalation of a high oxygen mixture results in abolition of this reflex stimulation and thus in a fall in the minute volume. This observation suggests that in most subjects there is some slight regulation of breathing through these reflexes.

After a number of minutes have passed respiratory depression gives way to stimulation. In the 32 subjects mentioned above there was an increase over normal of 7·6 per cent in the minute volume at the end of 6–8 minutes. There are many possible explanations of this phenomenon, but the most likely is either stimulation of the lower respiratory passages by the oxygen acting as an irritant or dilatation of the pulmonary capillaries by oxygen with the production of reflex respiratory stimulation from mild pulmonary congestion.

Circulatory system.—In studies in volunteers breathing pure oxygen (Eggers *et al.*, 1962) it has been shown that there is a slight fall in both heart rate and cardiac output during the inhalation. The most striking feature was the generalised increase in peripheral resistance and systemic pressure. The effects of oxygen inhalation on the general circulation have been likened to the effects of administering a peripheral vasoconstrictor, for the blood pressure goes up and the heart rate goes down. On this basis it is suggested that the slowing of the heart rate may be a reflex action following upon stimulation of the baroreceptors rather than any direct action on the chemoreceptors.

Blood.—Inhalation of 100 per cent oxygen for as long as three days has not been found to affect significantly the number of red or white cells, or the amount of haemoglobin (Comroe *et al.*, 1945). Nevertheless, using the shorter life span of the red blood cell in sickle cell anaemia and chronic haemolytic anaemia, Reinhard *et al.* (1944) and Tinsley *et al.* (1949) have clearly demonstrated that inhalations of a high concentration of oxygen will, within the safe period of administration, lower the red blood cell count in the peripheral blood. A decline in reticulocytes (young red cells) appears about the fourth or fifth day of oxygen therapy and is followed on the sixth or seventh day by the start of a fall in the number of red cells. In these patients a rise in the red cell count began about 48 hours after the cessation of oxygen therapy.

Elimination of nitrogen.—The inhalation of 100 per cent oxygen leads to a rapid fall in the nitrogen content of the arterial circulation so that the blood is almost completely cleared in a few minutes, but the loss from other tissues is more gradual. The brain takes 15–20 minutes before it is largely free of nitrogen. The cerebrospinal fluid clears relatively slowly, only 50 per cent leaving in the first hour, while fat tissues—with their poor blood supply—may take many hours before denitrogenation is complete. Oxygen inhalation may also be used to remove air from body cavities such as the gastro-intestinal tract and cerebral ventricles.

Clinical Results of Oxygen Excess

Under ordinary conditions the inhalation of concentrations of 50–60 per cent oxygen does not cause any harm in man and the breathing of 100 per cent oxygen cannot subjectively be distinguished from air by trained pilots (Bartlett and Hertz, 1962).

Patients with heart failure secondary to chronic lung disease (cor pulmonale) do not tolerate oxygen therapy well, however, and may lose consciousness when it is given. The type of lung disease most often associated with cor pulmonale is emphysema, in which the blood carbon dioxide tension is already high. The administration of oxygen to patients with this disease will only aggravate the situation, since it not only temporarily diminishes pulmonary ventilation by removing the stimulus of hypoxia from the chemoreceptors, but it also decreases the amount of reduced haemoglobin available for the transport of carbon dioxide. Concentrations of 50–100 per cent oxygen given to this type of patient may also cause a sudden increase in cerebrospinal fluid pressure (Davies and MacKinnon, 1949). During chronic hypoxaemia mental confusion, delirium and restlessness are not uncommon and are probably due to cerebral stimulation. Comroe and Dripps (1950) consider that relief of the hypoxaemia by the use of oxygen removes this stimulus, with resulting loss of consciousness. Storstein (1952) has shown that continued administration of oxygen to cases with cor pulmonale leads to an undesirable increase in cardiac work. It would seem that oxygen should be given to this type of patient only in company with some mechanical means of ventilation, such as an I.P.P.R. (intermittent positive-pressure respiration) ventilator with a negative suck phase, in order to ensure that the carbon dioxide concentration does not rise.

Using an oxygen tent, nasal catheter, or loose-fitting mask, oxygen tensions in excess of 50 per cent in the inspired air are rarely attained. If a carefully adjusted face-mask is used with a high flow of oxygen, however, high concentrations may be achieved and then toxic manifestations encountered. In the conscious subject they may take several forms:

(*a*) *Substernal pain.*—On breathing oxygen, pain may come on as early as the fourth hour, but usually not until the twelfth or sixteenth. It is a sharp burning pain which may become very severe; it is worse on inspiration, and the pain is accentuated by deep breathing or cold air. The causation is unknown but may be associated with drying of the mucous membrane of the trachea and the development of tracheo-bronchitis.

(*b*) *Diminution of vital capacity.*—The average fall is about 400 ml. after 24 hours on 100 per cent oxygen. Again the causation is unknown, but alveolar damage, dilatation of the pulmonary vessels by the high concentration of oxygen, or changes due to the alteration in carbon dioxide transport may play a part. At pressures greater than 0·6 Atm. pulmonary atelectasis may occur if the inert gas concentration is less than 15 per cent (Ernsting, 1965).

(*c*) *Other effects.*—The administration of concentrations of 50 per cent or more to premature children may lead to blindness (see Retrolental fibroplasia, p. 126). In animals damage to the alveolar walls has been reported from prolonged inhalation of high concentrations of oxygen and is probably caused by high arterial oxygen tensions rather than by high alveolar oxygen concentrations (Gupta, 1969). Certain patients receiving ventilator treatment have developed pulmonary lesions and these have been shown to be associated with high oxygen tensions (Nash *et al.*, 1967).

Oxygen Lack

The failure of the tissues to receive adequate quantities of oxygen is variously described as anoxia, hypoxia, or oxygen lack, but strictly interpreted anoxia means *total* lack of oxygen. The lack of oxygen represents a severe hazard to the tissues and has been aptly described by Haldane as causing "not only stoppage of the machine, but also total ruin of the supposed machinery." Under ordinary conditions the body has certain regulatory mechanisms which prevent the tissues from suffering oxygen deprivation, but during the course of anaesthesia oxygen lack may become a factor of prime importance. There are four main types of hypoxia that may occur, viz. (1) Anoxic, (2) Anaemic, (3) Stagnant, (4) Histotoxic.

1. **Anoxic Hypoxia**

The haemoglobin is insufficiently oxygenated in the lungs. During anaesthesia the simplest cause of anoxic hypoxia is a failure to administer a sufficient percentage of oxygen in the inspired air. Usually it is inadvisable to use less than 25 per cent oxygen from the anaesthetic machine, since the actual concentration inspired by the patient after mixing with expired gases may be much less. Hypoxia is frequently caused by mechanical factors, such as laryngeal spasm, simple obstruction to the airway by the tongue, or the presence of foreign material like blood, vomit, mucus and sputum, and partial respiratory paralysis. Shallow breathing or periods of apnoea also influence the oxygen saturation of blood. Moreover, collapse of part of a lung may lead to oxygen lack. In all these instances prevention is the best form of cure, and no amount of oxygen therapy is likely to cure the hypoxia until the primary cause has been removed.

Another common cause of anoxic hypoxia is the administration of a "gas", or nitrous oxide anaesthesia. Opinion is sharply divided as to how much of the unconsciousness produced is simply due to hypoxia and how much to the anaesthetic properties of nitrous oxide. During a rapid induction in an unpremedicated patient it would seem highly probable that the speed at which unconsciousness is reached is closely related to the degree of oxygen deprivation (see Nitrous Oxide).

During thoracic anaesthesia it is often necessary to place a "blocker" or balloon in one of the main bronchi to prevent secretions leaking out and flowing over to the other side. It should be remembered that whilst the balloon is in position, and until the affected lung has been allowed to collapse fully by opening the pleural cavity, about half the cardiac output is passing through that lung. A period of half to one hour may pass during which it is found to be increasingly difficult to keep the patient well oxygenated unless the percentage inspired is increased. On opening the pleural cavity the lung collapses readily on handling and a rapid improvement in the patient's oxygenation is often noted. The exact mechanism of the transfer of gases in a lung shut off from the atmosphere by a blocker is not sufficiently understood, but this cause of hypoxia can be largely offset by filling the patient's lungs with a high percentage of oxygen before the blocker is placed in position.

Diffusion hypoxia.—Fink (1955) has drawn attention to a mild condition of anoxic hypoxia that may occur in the immediate period following a long anaesthesia with nitrous oxide and oxygen and which is due to the outward diffusion of nitrous oxide from the pulmonary blood lowering the alveolar partial pressure of oxygen in the inhaled air. He has measured the arterial oxygen saturation on such occasions and finds that it may fall 5 to 10 per cent, often reaching values below 90 per cent. Although this type of hypoxia is rarely severe and can be simply prevented by administering oxygen to a patient for five to ten minutes from the time that anaesthesia ceases, its clinical significance may well be important, since it could account for occasional mishaps in ill patients.

2. Anaemic Hypoxia

When there is a reduction in the oxygen-carrying power of the blood, then anaemic hypoxia may result. It occurs either because there is insufficient haemoglobin in the blood or because some of the haemoglobin has been modified so that it can no longer transport oxygen. Lack of haemoglobin occurs in many chronic disease states, and particularly in the presence of infections, haemorrhage, and carcinomata, but during surgery the primary cause is blood loss. Anaemic hypoxia is characterised by a fall in the oxygen-capacity of arterial blood.

Methaemoglobinaemia and sulphaemoglobinaemia.—Clinically, these conditions are so similar that they are best considered together. They can be defined as diseases characterised by chronic cyanosis, unaccompanied by polycythaemia or dyspnoea, due to the presence of methaemoglobin or sulphaemoglobin in the blood (Whitby and Britton, 1957).

Sulphaemoglobinaemia produces a cyanotic tinge which is sometimes described as leaden-blue or mauve-lavender. Methaemoglobinaemia gives a chocolate-brown appearance. The two conditions can be identified separately in the laboratory by studying the different wavelengths of their respective absorption spectra.

The causative factors are essentially the same. A large number of coal-tar derivatives, such as phenacetin, acetanilide, sulphonal, sulphonilamide and some nitrates may produce either condition. The presence of some foreign substance in the blood is believed to favour the combination of sulphur and haemoglobin or a reduction in haemoglobin. Nevertheless, idiopathic cases also occur.

The only useful purpose achieved by distinguishing between these two conditions is that one can be treated and the other cannot. Apart from withdrawing the causative agent, methaemoglobinaemia can be cured by the injection of a 1 per cent solution of methylene blue (0·1–0·2 ml./kg. of body weight). As this treatment is relatively harmless it can also be used as a diagnostic test when the cyanosis of the methaemoglobinaemia will rapidly disappear, but the dark tinge of sulphaemoglobinaemia remains. Large doses of vitamin C (200 mg./diem) are also effective in the treatment of methaemoglobinaemia.

Carbon monoxide.—A further possible cause of anaemic hypoxia is the great affinity of haemoglobin for carbon monoxide, resulting in the formation of carboxyhaemoglobin. Although it is unlikely that a patient would require surgical intervention whilst suffering from acute carbon monoxide poisoning, it should be remembered that haemoglobin has about 300 times greater affinity for carbon monoxide than for oxygen.

3. Stagnant Hypoxia

When both the cardiac output and the peripheral blood flow fall to a low level, the circulation through the tissues becomes too slow to meet the requirements of the cells for oxygen: the result is stagnant or ischaemic hypoxia. This type of hypoxia is most commonly seen in states of shock, trauma, and haemorrhage. It may be local or generalised. For example, during anaesthesia the lobe of an ear or the bed of the finger nail may be seen to look dusky or cyanosed, yet if they are squeezed and rubbed briskly, fresh oxygenated blood enters, giving a bright tinge to the colour of the skin. This local phenomenon is particularly well seen in cases with poor peripheral vasomotor control, and is also seen as a more generalised state in association with intense vasoconstriction at the end of a long and perhaps haemorrhagic operation, or as a compensatory measure in cases with a low cardiac output due to heart disease. The state of the peripheral circulation may be used as an index of the onset or degree of "shock".

In hypotensive anaesthesia combined with posture there is widespread vasodilatation with pooling of the blood in the most deyendant parts. The large veins become distended with blood and these parts usually show some signs of stagnant hypoxia due to local pooling of the blood. In itself, this is not necessarily detrimental to the patient, but when the venous return is handicapped, the cardiac output falls.

4. Histotoxic Hypoxia

It is commonly believed that the production of unconsciousness by most anaesthetic drugs is due to depression of tissue-oxidation by interference with the denydrogenase systems (see Central Nervous System section). This has been considered as a form of histotoxic hypoxia, which is classically and most grossly typified by the effect of cyanide on the body. It also occurs in alcohol poisoning. In histotoxic hypoxia the blood does not unload oxygen during its passage through the tissues, since the cells are unable to utilise it. This condition, therefore, is characterised by a venous oxygen saturation higher than normal.

Cyanosis

The term indicates a bluish colour of the skin or mucous membranes which becomes evident when the absolute amount of reduced haemoglobin present in the blood is greater than 5 g. per cent. In almost every case its onset is closely associated with that of hypoxia and in considering the possible causes the two conditions are best taken together (see Table 2). Cyanosis and hypoxia are not necessarily synonymous, however, and either condition can occur independently of the other, particularly during anaesthesia.

In polycythaemia, there may be a great increase in the number of red cells and consequently also in the total amount of reduced haemoglobin. When the level rises above 5 g. per cent, cyanosis is present yet there is no hypoxia. Alternatively, in severe anaemia, hypoxia may be present without any cyanosis, because there is less than a total of 5·0 g. per cent of reduced haemoglobin in the circulation. In patients with Fallot's tetralogy the chronic hypoxia leads to a compensatory polycythaemia, so that hypoxia and cyanosis are both present.

5/Table 2

Hypoxia and Cyanosis

Possible Causes likely to be met by the Anaesthetist

1. Factors present before operation:
    a. Lesions involving the respiratory tract
        Oedema of the glottis, e.g. Ludwig's angina, bilateral quinsy.
        Carcinoma of the larynx.
        Tracheal compression and stenosis.
        Foreign bodies in bronchus.
        Neoplasms in bronchial tree.
        Asthma and severe bronchitis.
        Pulmonary disease, e.g. tuberculosis, emphysema, fibrosis, etc.
        Space-occupying lesions of the chest wall.
        Air or fluid in the pleural space.
        Paresis of the muscles of respiration, e.g. poliomyelitis, myasthenia gravis, etc.
    b. Lesions involving the circulation
        Cyanotic heart disease.
        Pulmonary oedema (e.g. mitral stenosis).
        Congestive cardiac failure.
        "Shock" states (e.g. blood loss; coronary thrombosis).
        Polycythaemia.

N.B. Methaemoglobin, sulphaemoglobin, and the injection of blue dyes give the appearance of cyanosis.

2. Factors developing during operation:
   a. Lesions of the respiratory tract
      Inhalation of blood or vomit.
      Mucus or sputum.
      Laryngeal spasm.
      Insufficient oxygen in respired mixture.
      Inadequate ventilation due to paresis of respiratory muscles.
      Central respiratory depression.
      Collapse of trachea and bronchial bronchiolar spasm.
      Insertion of bronchial blocker.
   b. Lesions of the circulation
      Stagnation of the peripheral circulation.
      Cardiac failure and pulmonary oedema.
      Injection of blue dye.
3. Factors developing after operation:
   a. Lesions of the respiratory tract
      Tongue falling back and obstructing glottis.
      Inhalation of blood or vomit.
      Mucus or sputum.
      Laryngeal spasm.
      Inadequate ventilation.
      Pulmonary collapse.
      Tracheal collapse.
   b. Lesions of the circulation
      Cardiac failure and pulmonary oedema.
      Peripheral circulatory failure.
      Excessive transfusion therapy.

Effect of Oxygen Lack

During conscious respiration, if the subject hypoventilates then a reduction in the oxygen saturation of the blood is accompanied by a corresponding increase in the concentration of carbon dioxide. Under the conditions of anaesthesia, however, the use of carbon dioxide absorption techniques and alteration of the concentrations of the respired gases allows both oxygen lack and carbon dioxide excess to become separate entities. The possible causes of oxygen lack are intimately connected with those already described for hypoxia and cyanosis. The effects will vary according to their severity and rapidity of onset.

Acute oxygen lack.—A subject breathing nitrous oxide alone through a non-return valve rapidly suffers from severe anoxia. Carbon dioxide does not accumulate because, apart from the slight increase in dead space due to the mask etc., there is no rebreathing. The absence of oxygen in the inspired mixture means that the oxygen in the alveoli is rapidly washed out. Ultimately the pressure of oxygen in the venous blood coming to the lungs is greater than that in the alveoli, so that instead of taking up oxygen in the lungs, the blood actually gives up oxygen. Unconsciousness is rapidly produced. It must be remembered, however, that although nitrous oxide possesses anaesthetic properties, when it is administered with a subnormal concentration of oxygen such a rapid loss of consciousness is much more likely to have been brought about by the acute hypoxia than the anaesthetic properties of the nitrous oxide (see Nitrous Oxide). Acute hypoxia leads first to stimulation of the chemoreceptors and then to direct depression of the respiratory centre, resulting in weak respiratory movements which—in turn—increase the degree of hypoxia and create a vicious circle. Finally, breathing ceases from failure of the respiratory centre and convulsions or jactitations occur.

Subacute oxygen lack.—Small changes in the oxygen content of the inspired mixture often produce little change in respiratory activity. The reason for this is that the response of the chemoreceptors and the respiratory centre to changes in oxygen concentration are relatively sluggish when compared with those of the centre to carbon dioxide. For example, in some subjects there is no increase in respiratory rate until the oxygen content of the inspired gases falls to 16 per cent, whereas in others it has to be as low as 14 per cent. Below 12 per cent there is, in every case, an increase in pulmonary ventilation.

The hyperpnoea that results from the hypoxia compensates in part for the reduced oxygen content by making better use of such oxygen as is available in the inspired gases. The extra work of breathing may at first slightly increase the amount of carbon dioxide produced, but very soon the tension of this gas in the blood falls, leading to a direct depression of the respiratory centre.

Oxygen lack
↓
Increased rate of breathing
↓
Increased pulmonary ventilation
↓
Lowering alveolar CO_2 tension
↓
Alkalaemia (lowered arterial CO_2 tension)
↓
Depression of respiration

Chronic oxygen lack.—A gradual decline in the oxygen tension of inspired air occurs most commonly on flying to high altitudes; this matter therefore is more naturally concerned with aviation medicine. As the altitude increases so the total atmospheric pressure is reduced and the partial pressure of oxygen declines proportionately. Thus:

At sea level—partial pressure of O_2 in air	=	159 mm. Hg
At 10,000 ft. „ „ „ „	=	110 mm. Hg
At 20,000 ft. „ „ „ „	=	73 mm. Hg
At 50,000 ft. „ „ „ „	=	18 mm. Hg

The tension of oxygen in arterial blood (P_{O_2}) is nearly identical with that in the alveoli. Unfortunately, the concentration of oxygen in the alveoli is not the same as that in air. The reasons for this are simple: oxygen is removed from the alveolar gases and carbon dioxide enters. All the air entering is fully saturated with water and under quiet ventilation only 14 per cent of the composition of the alveolar air comes directly from the atmosphere. The difference in the partial pressure of oxygen in air and in the alveoli is best seen in the example below:

	Air	*Alveolar air*
Partial pressure of	O_2 = 159 mm. Hg	O_2 = 103 mm. Hg
		CO_2 = 40 mm. Hg
,, ,,	N_2 = 601 mm. Hg	N_2 = 570 mm. Hg
		Water = 47 mm. Hg
	Total = 760 mm. Hg	Total = 760 mm. Hg

The higher the altitude, therefore, the lower the partial pressure of oxygen in the alveoli and consequently the lower the arterial saturation of blood. At sea level the $P_{A_{O_2}}$ is 100 mm. Hg and the arterial saturation 95 per cent: on rising to 10,000 feet the $P_{A_{O_2}}$ is 67 mm. Hg and the arterial saturation has dropped to 90 per cent, whereas at 30,000 feet the $P_{A_{O_2}}$ is 21 mm. Hg and the arterial oxygen saturation is only 20 per cent. Mountaineers and people who live at high altitudes can partially compensate for this lower arterial oxygen saturation by increasing the number of red blood cells in the circulation (compensatory polycythaemia).

A normal person loses consciousness when the arterial oxygen saturation falls to 50 per cent or below. Breathing air, this gives an upper ceiling of 23,000 feet, but if oxygen is substituted for air a height of 47,000 feet may be reached before unconsciousness ensues.

The various physiological changes that can be noted in a patient suffering from chronic hypoxia are:

(*a*) Decreased mental efficiency.
(*b*) Sleepiness, headache, lassitude and fatigue.
(*c*) Euphoria.
(*d*) Increased ventilation. Above 8,000 feet the arterial saturation falls to 93 per cent or less and this is sufficient to stimulate the chemoreceptors into activity leading to increased ventilation.

The persistent increase in pulmonary ventilation results in a reduction in the alveolar carbon dioxide tension. This alkalaemia is compensated for by changes in renal excretion: the kidneys excrete more base and the urine becomes less acid.

The most significant instances of chronic oxygen lack are to be found in patients with severe lung or heart disease when there is interference with the oxygen transport mechanism.

Other Effects of Oxygen Lack

The inhalation of mixtures with a low oxygen tension produces a rise in the pulmonary artery systolic pressure which is independent of changes in the systemic blood pressure (Motley *et al.*, 1947). Similarly, it has been shown in cats that a rise in oxygen tension results in a fall in pulmonary arterial pressure (von Euler and Liljestrand, 1946). These findings have led to the suggestion that oxygen tension may produce a local mechanism for regulating the blood flow through various parts of the lung. Thus, if an area of the lung is poorly ventilated or collapsed this region of pulmonary tissue leads to local hypoxia, which, in turn brings about a constriction of the vessels in that area. Such constriction would tend to prevent blood passing into the collapsed area and becoming inadequately oxygenated. Conversely, an area of the lung may be well ventilated yet not receiving sufficient pulmonary blood flow. The increased oxygenation resulting from the ventilation leads to local dilatation of the vessels and a rise in the pulmonary blood flow (Comroe and Dripps, 1950). Ross and his co-workers (1962) studied the effect of varying concentrations of oxygen saturation (from 10–100 per cent) on the forelimb of the dog. They noted that a decrease in oxygen saturation led to an increase in blood flow through the limb. At the maximum level the flow was three times greater than normal and was unaffected by spinal analgesia. These experiments tend to confirm the suggestion that local tissues can autoregulate their blood flow in an attempt to maintain an adequate supply of oxygen. This may be by a direct action of the oxygen saturation level or through the medium of a vasodilator substance.

Hypoxia causes an increase in coronary blood flow (Eckenhoff *et al.*, 1947). The effects of oxygen lack on the central nervous system are discussed in Chapter 45.

Indications for Oxygen Therapy

Oxygen therapy is clearly indicated in the presence of acute cyanosis, yet it is well-known that the oxygen tension of arterial blood can fall to dangerously low levels without there being obvious changes in the colour of the skin. Nevertheless, during surgery observation of the shade of red exhibited by arterial blood will usually give a rough but valuable guide to the state of oxygenation of the patient.

It is often falsely assumed that the anaesthetised patient requires only the same percentage of oxygen as is present in air to maintain a normal arterial oxygen saturation. Recent work has shown that for a variety of reasons the anaesthetised patient requires *more* oxygen than the conscious patient breathing air (see Chapter 4).

Principally, there are three factors responsible for carrying sufficient oxygen to the tissues:

1. Haemoglobin value of the blood.
2. The blood flow (indirectly related to the cardiac output).
3. Oxygen saturation of the blood (as reflected by the oxygen dissociation curve). The concept of available oxygen is useful in this context. It is the amount of oxygen that is readily available to the tissues (Freeman, 1966).

$$\text{AVAILABLE OXYGEN} = \dot{Q} \times SaO_2 \times Hb \times 1{\cdot}34$$

where $\dot{Q}$ is the blood flow and SaO_2 is the oxygen saturation of arterial blood.

Any of these factors can be reduced by as much as one-third without causing any harm to the patient, yet if all three are depressed by this amount the effect will be lethal!

Anaesthesia appears to increase the difficulty of maintaining the tissue oxygen tension for a number of reasons. First, the shunt in the pulmonary vessels is increased, so that a larger quantity than usual of the blood passing down the pulmonary arteries by-passes the alveoli and thus passes directly to the left side of the heart. Secondly, variations in the ventilation-perfusion ratio lead to an increasing degree of maldistribution of the blood and gas in the lungs so that they become less efficient as an oxygenator. It seems that anaesthesia in some way interferes with the careful mechanism which normally ensures that the pulmonary blood flow passes to alveoli that are functioning, and vice versa. Thus, whereas in the normal conscious state only about 1–5 per cent of the blood entering the pulmonary arteries fails to be exposed to the alveolar gases, in the anaesthetised patient this figure may rise to as much as 10–15 per cent. To these two must be added the effect of hypoventilation due to respiratory depressant drugs. In these circumstances, the tissue oxygen tension can fall to very low levels.

Anaesthesia, however, does offer the patient some advantages as far as oxygen requirements are concerned. On the credit side the induction of unconsciousness depresses metabolism and this may lower the total body oxygen consumption by as much as 15–20 per cent. In certain rare instances hypothermia can increase this figure. Furthermore, if the patient breathes a mixture of nitrous oxide and oxygen the "diffusion effect" (see p. 222) *increases* the oxygen saturation of the blood during the period of uptake of the gas. Finally, if hyperventilation is used this can raise the amount of the alveolar oxygen tension just as hypoventilation can lower it.

The various factors influencing the tissue oxygen tension of the anaesthetised patient breathing an inhalational anaesthetic with 21 per cent oxygen (same as air) are summarised below (Table 3).

5/TABLE 3

SUMMARY OF FACTORS INFLUENCING OXYGEN TENSION OF TISSUES IN ANAESTHETISED PATIENT

(A) Factors lowering oxygen tension.
  (1) Pulmonary SHUNT.
  (2) Maldistribution, i.e. alteration in the ventilation-perfusion ratio.
  (3) Hypoventilation (if present).

(B) Factors raising oxygen tension.
  (1) Depression of metabolism.
  (2) Diffusion effect.
  (3) Hyperventilation.

The practical significance of all these various factors is best exemplified by referring to studies of the arterial oxygen saturation of a patient *spontaneously* breathing anaesthetic concentrations of halothane and air. It is found that the oxygen saturation in the arterial blood often falls below normal. For this reason the optimum concentration of oxygen in the inspired mixture for a patient under general anaesthesia is nearer 30 per cent than 20 per cent. A concentration of 33 per cent oxygen in the inspired gases will compensate for the detrimental effects of anaesthesia except in the presence of hypoventilation, severe anaemia, or a reduced cardiac output (see also Chapter 4).

So far only the anaesthetised patient has been considered, but it must be remembered that many of these factors persist for a number of hours after the anaesthetic has been withdrawn and the patient is in the recovery room. During anaesthesia suboxygenation is unlikely to occur in skilled hands, but it can commonly be observed in the post-operative period. Nunn and Payne (1962) have demonstrated that nearly all patients undergoing general anaesthesia have a period of reduced oxygen saturation lasting for many hours after operation. In this period hypoventilation (see p. 140) is liable to play a much more important role and for the first quarter of an hour or so diffusion hypoxia (see pp. 222 and 275) will also work to the patient's disadvantage if nitrous oxide has been used.

Just how important changes in oxygen saturation of the blood are in the post-operative patient is not yet clear. Fortunately, owing to the shape of the oxygen dissociation curve, a large fall in the oxygen saturation of the blood is only reflected in a relatively small reduction in tissue oxygen tension (see Fig. 11, p. 170). Nevertheless, this dissociation curve has been likened to a precipice and once over the cliff edge it will be seen that both saturation and tension fall fast. Clearly it is better for the patient to be kept on the plateau, well away from the dangerous cliff edge.

The importance of the oxygen saturation of the blood can be emphasised with a few simple examples. Assuming a cardiac output of 5 litres per minute and a tissue oxygen consumption of 250 ml. per minute, then with an arterial oxygen saturation of 100 per cent there is 1,000 ml. of oxygen available to the tissues (100 ml. of blood at 100 per cent saturation carries about 20 ml. of oxygen). Thus, the tissues' oxygen requirements are covered fourfold. Even under conditions of hypoxia, when the arterial saturation may drop to 40 per cent, there will still be enough oxygen available for the tissues (e.g. 400 ml.) But, if the hypoxia is combined with anaemia then the oxygen carrying capacity of the blood is reduced below that needed for tissue survival. Nevertheless, even in these adverse circumstances the inhalation of 100 per cent oxygen will immediately raise the amount of oxygen available to the tissues above the danger level. These situations are illustrated below:

	Arterial saturation %	*Hb %*	*O_2 consumption ml./min.*	*O_2 available ml./min.*
Normal	100	100	250	1,000
Hypoxia	40	100	250	400
Hypoxia + Anaemia	40	50	250	200
Hypoxia + Anaemia + Oxygen Therapy	100	50	250	400

Effects of Oxygen Therapy

1. **Oxygen saturation of the blood.**—With the inhalation of air in a normal subject at sea level the tension of oxygen in the alveoli is about 104 mm. Hg and 100 mm. Hg in the arterial blood, giving a saturation of 95–97 per cent. If 100 per cent pure oxygen is now breathed the alveolar oxygen tension rises to 673 and the arterial tension to 640 with a saturation of 100 per cent. Thus, breathing:

	Air	100 *per cent oxygen*
Alveolar P_{O_2} (mm. Hg)	104	673
Arterial P_{O_2} (mm. Hg)	100	640
Arterial O_2 per cent saturation	97	100

A study of these figures reveals a point of importance. Oxygen tension gives a far wider range and therefore a better indication of the state of oxygenation of the patient's blood than oxygen saturation.

2. **Carbon dioxide tension of the blood.**—Theoretically, breathing pure oxygen can interfere with the transport of carbon dioxide because reduced haemoglobin is a stronger base than oxyhaemoglobin, and therefore carries more carbon dioxide. This only becomes of practical importance when oxygen is breathed at high pressures. Nevertheless, in patients with diseased lung tissue in whom chronic hypoxia and a raised P_{CO_2} are present, then the sudden inhalation of oxygen may lead to hypoventilation and a rise in carbon dioxide tension of the blood.

3. **Ventilation.**—The clinical effects of breathing excess of oxygen have already been considered (p. 220). The immediate result of the inhalation of oxygen in normal man is a slight decrease in minute volume, lasting for a few minutes only. This is presumably due to the temporary reduction of stimuli reaching the respiratory centre from the carotid and aortic bodies. Following this slight reduction in ventilation there is an increase of approximately 10 per cent minute volume during the period of inhalation. The cause of this increase is unknown but it may be due either to oxygen acting as an irritant to the lower respiratory tract or to a local increase in the P_{CO_2} of cells in the respiratory centre, due either to vasoconstriction from the raised P_{O_2} or to the diminished amount of reduced haemoglobin available for the removal of carbon dioxide (Comroe *et al.*, 1962).

In any consideration of oxygen therapy it is important to stress that occasionally it is possible to do more harm than good. This is most likely to occur in two principal situations. First, the patient with severe chronic bronchitis and emphysema who is admitted to hospital with cyanosis and respiratory failure. Secondly, the post-operative patient who has received large doses of respiratory depressant drugs. In both these instances respiration is probably largely maintained by the "anoxic drive" of the chemoreceptors of the carotid and aortic bodies. The sudden inhalation of a high concentration of oxygen leads to diminished ventilation with an increase in P_{CO_2} and a fall in P_{O_2}. However, if a careful watch is undertaken to prevent underventilation, oxygen therapy can do no harm and may certainly do a lot of good, provided the concentration does not exceed 50 per cent.

4. **Blood volume and haemorrhage.**—The role of oxygen in the treatment of haemorrhage has been controversial (Wood *et al.*, 1940; Frank and Fine, 1943). Freeman and Nunn (1963) suggest that it may have a more important part to play than has hitherto been supposed. Under conditions of haemorrhage and a reduced blood volume the fall in cardiac output leads to a drop in peripheral

blood flow. In turn, this leads to stagnant anoxia in the tissues and a metabolic acidosis develops. The increased acidity of the blood stimulates the respiratory centre and hyperventilation or "air hunger" develops.

Studies on dogs undergoing haemorrhage have revealed that raising the inspired oxygen from 21 per cent (air) to 30 per cent nearly halves the mortality (Freeman, 1962). One of the most remarkable features is that the physiological dead space in the haemorrhagic animal rises from a normal value of 30 per cent of the tidal volume to nearly 80 per cent. This must, of course, seriously reduce the effective alveolar ventilation. There is no comparable data available in man but Cournand *et al.* (1943) demonstrated a similar but smaller rise in physiological dead space in patients suffering from haemorrhage.

The explanation of this reduction in effective alveolar ventilation probably lies in a fall in cardiac output and therefore of pulmonary blood flow. Under these conditions, it is possible to visualise that "only a thin trickle of blood passes through certain favoured alveoli leaving the rest ventilated but unperfused—a state which accords closely with the necropsy appearances" (Freeman and Nunn, 1963).

Anaesthesia or heavy sedation in the post-operative period may not only depress the activity of the respiratory centre and thus reduce the compensatory hyperventilation, but it may also lead to an increase in peripheral vasodilation and a further reduction in cardiac output. For these reasons, there now seems to be good evidence for the administration of an increased percentage of oxygen to the patient with a reduced blood volume, though clearly adequate blood transfusion is most important. Furthermore, these findings support the clinical observation that patients undergoing vascular surgery with severe haemorrhage are best anaesthetised without halothane, which is known to produce marked peripheral vasodilatation.

The value of artificial ventilation with the possible disadvantage of a further reduction in cardiac output due to increased positive intrathoracic pressure, as opposed to the advantage of improved ventilation, still remains to be elucidated.

Methods of Oxygen Therapy

Selection of equipment.—There are three principal types of apparatus available for oxygen therapy: face-masks, nasal catheters including spectacles, and oxygen tents. The selection of a particular piece of apparatus will depend on several factors. First, the concentration of oxygen required for the patient. In an emergency the only satisfactory way to give 100 per cent oxygen is to use intermittent positive-pressure ventilation with a mask, valve and a bag. Secondly, the equipment must be reliable. Many of the earlier models of plastic disposable masks did not mould accurately to the contours of the patient's face so that the concentration of oxygen varied greatly. Finally, comfort is an important factor in the conscious or semi-conscious patient. Humidity and flow rate influence the comfort of a particular mask.

General considerations.—During recent years great strides have been made in the design of equipment for oxygen therapy. The B.L.B. mask, the nasal catheter, and the oxygen tent are gradually being superseded in many cases by new and more accurate equipment. The need for this accuracy arose from the treatment of patients with chronic respiratory failure (e.g. severe bronchitis and emphysema). The sudden administration of a high inspired oxygen concentration removes the respiratory drive created largely by the low oxygen tension, ventilation becomes reduced and acute acidosis and carbon dioxide narcosis may follow (see Clinical Results of Oxygen Excess, p. 220). On the other hand, if these patients are given a gradually increasing concentration of oxygen the ventilation is not affected as the oxygen tension rises. In the past many physicians attempted to use intermittent oxygen therapy but Haldane likened this technique to "occasionally bringing a drowning man to the surface"!

Oxygen Masks.—There are a great many available and only a number of those in use are listed here.

B.L.B. and nasal masks.—These are fitted with a small reservoir bag of about 500 ml. capacity into which the supply of oxygen is led. There is no expiratory valve, only a hole placed in the middle of the mask. Some rebreathing and accumulation of water vapour occurs in the bag, though unless the mask fits exceptionally well a carbon dioxide concentration of clinical importance is unlikely to occur. At a flow rate of 8 litres/minute the inspired concentration may reach 90 per cent and the carbon dioxide concentration in the bag rise to about 0·4 per cent (air = 0·03 per cent). These masks are rarely used nowadays, and have no advantages over disposable masks of the types described below.

Disposable oxygen inhaler ("Polymask") (Fig. 2).—The mask is made of polyvinyl chloride and is divided into two communicating compartments. The mask can easily be shaped to conform to the patient's face since it is fitted with a malleable wire. Values as high as 50–60 per cent inspired oxygen have been reported (Burns and Hall, 1953), though lower concentrations are often encountered due to leakage of air around the mask.

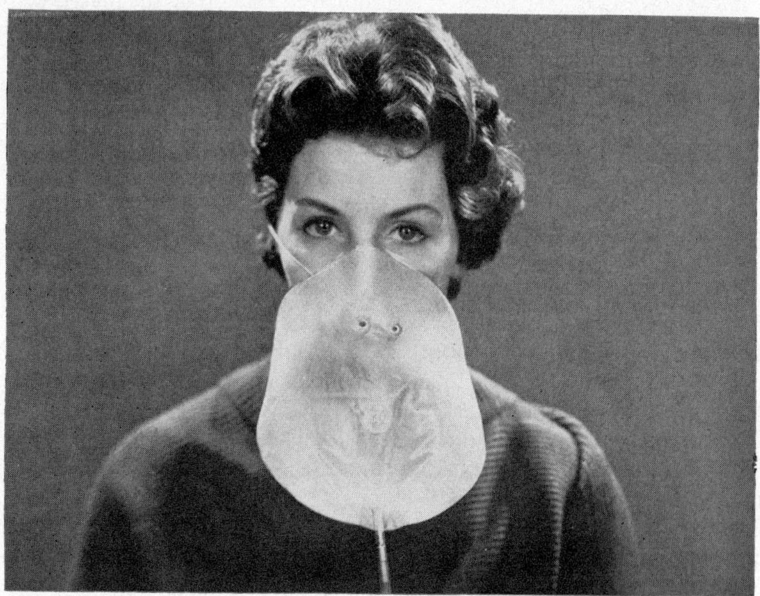

5/Fig.2 .—Disposable oxygen mask.

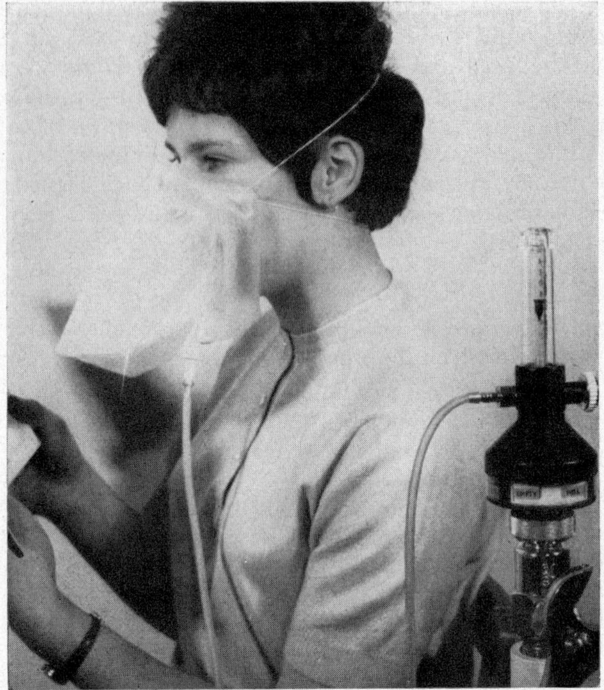

5/Fig. 3.—The "Pneumask".

"*Pneumask*" (Fig. 3).—This is an improved version of the plastic disposable mask which is particularly suitable for use in the unconscious patient. The oxygen supply is first routed through the inflatable cuff surrounding the perimeter of the mask before finally flowing into the interior. The advantage of this arrangement is that should the oxygen supply fail then the cuff will deflate and the mask will fall away from the patient's face. Inspired concentrations of about 40–45 per cent oxygen can be obtained with gas flows of 4 litres.

"*MC*" *mask* (Fig. 4).—This is a disposable mask that is very suitable for patients in recovery areas. At gas flows of 4 litres an inspired concentration of approximately 45 per cent oxygen can be obtained.

"*Ventimask*" (Fig. 5).—This mask uses the Venturi principle so that a low flow of oxygen can be used to draw in large quantities of air. The advantage of this principle is that it is not only economical with oxygen but it also permits accuracy in the concentration of oxygen delivered to the patient, even in the presence of a poorly fitting mask.

The mask is disposable and contains a single inlet tube. There are two types designed to give an under-mask concentration of either 28 per cent oxygen in air or 35 per cent oxygen in air.

Nasal catheters.—A size 9 rubber Jacques catheter, with two or three side holes cut in the terminal part to prevent all the flow of oxygen impinging on the same area of pharyngeal mucosa, is satisfactory for adults. It should be well-lubricated before use and inserted so that the tip lies in the oropharynx. Too deep insertion leads to gastric dilatation. Flows up to 3 litres/minute are well tolerated and give an inspired oxygen concentration of 27 per cent. Higher flows of 4–6 litres are often possible and give a concentration of between 30–40 per cent inspired oxygen (Miller, 1962).

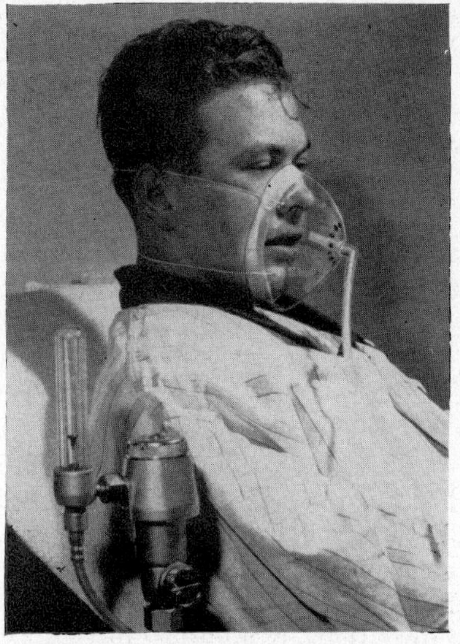

5/FIG. 4.—The "MC" mask.

Comment

The performance of these devices for oxygen therapy has been assessed on "patient-model" devices (Bethune and Collis, 1967) and on patients (Leigh, 1970). The results emphasise the irregular performance of high flow devices with regard to carbon dioxide accumulation, whilst the low flow venturi devices provide inspired oxygen tensions close to the specification.

Oxygen tents.—A tent must be used when other methods of oxygen administration are impracticable. Such occasions arise when the patient is very young or incapable of tolerating a mask or catheter.

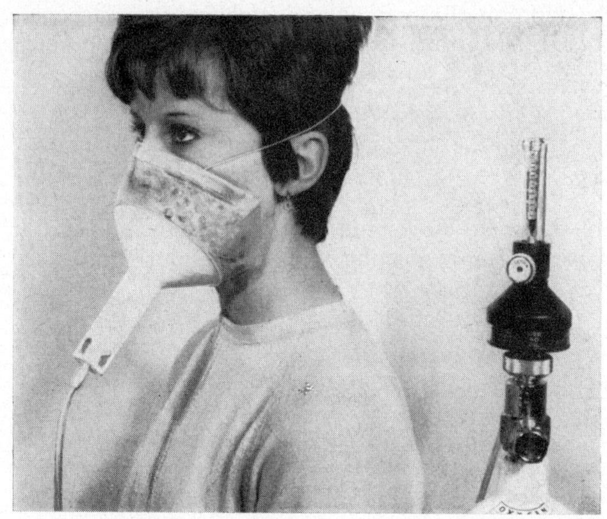

5/FIG. 5.—The "Venti-mask".

Hewer and Less (1957) have listed the essential components of a modern oxygen tent:

1. Positive ventilation of the atmosphere in the tent must be secured.
2. The temperature and humidity of the atmosphere in the tent must be amenable to regulation.

3. Carbon dioxide must not be allowed to accumulate within the tent.
4. Adequate provision must be made for nursing, flushing the tent, and sampling the internal atmosphere.
5. The materials from which the tent is made must be non-inflammable.
6. It must be possible to sterilise the interior of the tent.

The established design of an oxygen tent has been re-examined by Wayne and Chamney (1967) who describe an economical, efficient model which enables an oxygen concentration of 47 per cent to be achieved within the tent.

CARBON DIOXIDE (CO_2)

History

Carbon dioxide was first isolated by Black in 1757. The physiological significance of this gas was not fully appreciated until the work of Yandell Henderson in the United States (1925) and J. S. Haldane in England (1926). It soon gained widespread popularity amongst anaesthetists as a stimulus to respiration, but in more recent years the emphasis has been on its elimination rather than its addition in view of the high figures for carbon dioxide tensions in the blood that have been recorded with certain anaesthetic systems and techniques.

Preparation

In the laboratory.—The addition of any strong mineral acid to a carbonate or bicarbonate frees carbonic acid, which is an unstable, volatile substance. Thus it liberates its anhydride—carbon dioxide.

$NaHCO_3$	$+ HCl$	$\rightarrow NaCl$	$+ H_2O$	$+ CO_2$
Sodium bicarbonate	Hydrochloric acid	Sodium chloride	Water	Carbon dioxide

Commercially.—Carbon dioxide is a common by-product in the preparation of the alkaline earth oxides, notably calcium and magnesium, from their respective carbonates:

$CaCO_3$	$\xrightarrow{\text{Heat}}$	CaO	$+ CO_2$
Calcium carbonate		Calcium oxide	Carbon dioxide

Physical Properties

Carbon dioxide is a very stable substance, representing a minute proportion of the atmosphere—namely 0·03 per cent. It combines readily with water to form carbonic acid, the solubility diminishing as the temperature increases. The gas has a pungent odour which in high concentrations may be irritating to mucous membranes. The molecular weight is 44. On compression by a pressure of 50 atmospheres at 20° C it forms a colourless liquid and as such is stored in cylinders for medical use. The cylinders are coloured grey.

Inflammability

Carbon dioxide—in a concentration of 5 per cent—is very effective in reducing the range of inflammability of any mixtures of gases, because it possesses a high molar heat capacity. Charges of static electricity are more easily dissipated when the concentration of carbon dioxide in the atmosphere is 0·5 per cent or greater.

Pharmacological Actions

Carbon dioxide is a waste product of tissue metabolism. It is carried in the blood in three forms, namely in physical solution, combined with the protein in the red cell and plasma as carbamino-protein, and as bicarbonate in the plasma (see transport of carbon dioxide, p. 99).

Carbon Dioxide Excess

A high concentration of carbon dioxide can produce unconsciousness. After a few breaths of 40 per cent carbon dioxide with oxygen a patient will show many of the signs of anaesthesia. In psychiatric practice, a mixture of 50 per cent carbon dioxide with oxygen is sometimes used to produce a convulsion, as an alternative to electric shock treatment. It may well be that a high carbon dioxide tension in the blood is the reason why some patients with a "prolonged apnoea" do not recover consciousness during a period of inadequate artificial respiration without an anaesthetic mixture.

Respiratory effects.—When the concentration of carbon dioxide in the body is allowed to rise slowly (as in partial respiratory obstruction) the depth, and later the rate, of respiration is increased. The respiratory centre is stimulated both by a direct action of the gas and by changes in the pH of the blood. This latter mechanism can also activate the centre reflexly through the medium of the chemoreceptors in the carotid and aortic bodies and the central chemoreceptor on the ventro-lateral surface of the medulla (see Chapter 3). High concentrations of carbon dioxide depress respiration.

The carbon dioxide tension of arterial blood (40 mm. Hg) is controlled so finely that a rise of 1·5 mm. Hg leads to an increase in tidal exchange of 100 per cent in an attempt to "blow off" the excess and return the tension to normal. Conversely, a fall of 1·5 mm. Hg, in the absence of other stimuli, may lead to apnoea.

Circulatory effects.—A rise in carbon dioxide tension leads to a rise in the systolic blood pressure with a complementary bradycardia, and an increase in the cardiac output and the blood flow through the brain and skin capillaries. The mechanism of the pressor response is believed to be both direct and reflex (chemoreceptor) stimulation of the vasomotor centre. High concentrations of carbon dioxide depress nervous conduction in the heart, particularly in the bundle of His, so that heart block and a slow ventricular rhythm are commonly observed with an increased myocardial irritability. A rise in the carbon dioxide level of the blood increases the excretion of catechol amines (principally noradrenaline) by the sympathetic nerve-endings within the myocardium. Thus, with most anaesthetic agents—principally cyclopropane and halothane—the higher the carbon dioxide level of the blood the greater is the chance of arrhythmias. As both these agents are respiratory depressants hypoventilation bears a close correlation with the onset of ventricular arrhythmia. Furthermore, both these agents "sensitise" the myocardium to this increased catechol amine excretion so that clinically both improving ventilation and reducing the depth of anaesthesia will help to restore normal rhythm.

In dogs, dramatic changes in cardiac rhythm can be produced by a sudden termination of a period of hypercarbia. Severe arrhythmias are observed if a vigorous attempt to lower the P_{CO_2} is made. Under the conditions of clinical anaesthesia in man there is no satisfactory evidence to support the view that a similar situation arises. In fact, it appears to be quite the contrary (Price, 1960) and it would appear to be both safe and advisable to remove the excess CO_2 from the body at a rapid rate. Capillary dilatation in the tissues, together with hypertension, is the cause of increased oozing from excess carbon dioxide during an operation.

In a patient who is slowly recovering consciousness after an anaesthetic, the presence of partial respiratory obstruction or inadequate ventilation, with a consequent rise in the tension of carbon dioxide in the blood, may cause many of the signs just mentioned. To the untrained observer, the circulatory state of such a patient will seem satisfactory, as exemplified by a normal blood pressure and pulse rate. As time passes, however, the effects of the anaesthetic finally wear off and ventilation improves. The excess carbon dioxide is now rapidly removed and this stimulus to the vasomotor centre is no longer present. At this moment the patient may well pass into a state of apparent circulatory collapse, as the blood pressure falls to a low level. The heart rate may reflexly increase. Before the dangers of inadequate ventilation were fully appreciated, this form of post-operative circulatory collapse occurred relatively frequently. It was also sometimes associated with deep cyclopropane anaesthesia, when it certainly accounted for many cases of "cyclopropane shock" (see p. 293).

Use of Carbon Dioxide in Anaesthesia

For anaesthetic purposes a concentration of 5 per cent is usually sufficient to produce a temporary increase in the depth of respiration during induction with an irritant volatile agent such as ether. The mechanisms regulating the concentration of carbon dioxide in the blood are extremely sensitive, however, and the administration of anaesthetic and analgesic drugs can so depress the respiratory centre that it may no longer respond to even gross changes in the tension of the gas, and only be reflexly stimulated by the chemoreceptors. Morphine, pethidine and the barbiturates are most commonly responsible.

In the presence of respiratory depression, concentrations of carbon dioxide which are themselves depressant to the respiratory centre may accumulate. The opportunity for such an occurrence is very much increased in anaesthetic practice when patients are inadequately ventilated after the use of muscle relaxants or anaesthetised with unphysiological techniques. Pask (1955) has drawn attention to the potential danger of this combination of circumstances, and the culminating effect during the early post-operative period of slight respiratory obstruction—due perhaps to loss of tone in the muscles of the jaw and tongue—with a further rise in carbon dioxide. Tensions as high as 160 mm. Hg have been reported in partially paralysed patients during anaesthesia. On the other hand, with excessive hyperventilation and the use of carbon dioxide absorption techniques the tension of carbon dioxide may fall as low as 15–20 mm. Hg.

Clinical Use

For resuscitative purposes carbon dioxide is no longer recommended unless ample facilities are available for determining either alveolar or blood tensions of the gas. In nearly all cases of respiratory failure or marked depression the concentration in the body is already high enough to provide ample stimulation of the centres and may have reached concentrations which are actively depressant.

The most reasonable indication for the use of carbon dioxide occurs at the end of operation when it is desired to restart spontaneous respiration after a period of properly controlled respiration, which is normally maintained in part by moderate hyperventilation with temporary hypocapnia. A patient with emphysema is especially likely to need carbon dioxide at this stage, as his respiratory centre is normally accustomed to a high tension of the gas.

The intermittent inhalation of carbon dioxide may be beneficial in the treatment of post-operative hiccup.

The inhalation of 5 per cent carbon dioxide has been used to produce cerebral vasodilatation during anaesthesia for carotid artery surgery.

HELIUM (He)

History

Helium was first noted by Lockyer and Eden in 1867 when examining the spectrum of the sun. It was isolated by Ramsay and Lockyer in 1895.

Preparation

The main source is from the abundant supplies of natural gas found in the United States, chiefly in Texas and Kansas. The other gases present are removed by absorption, liquefaction or scrubbing with water and sodium hydroxide. Helium is difficult to liquefy, so that when the temperature is lowered to −195° C the other gases can easily be removed and helium remains as a gaseous residue.

Physical Properties

Helium is an inert, colourless, odourless gas. It is one of the "rare gases" present in air, the others being radon, argon, xenon and krypton. Apart from hydrogen, helium is the lightest known gas, with a molecular weight of 4 and specific gravity of 0·178 (air = 1). The oil/water solubility ratio is 0·187 at 37° C. It diffuses through skin and rubber.

Clinical Use

The therapeutic value of helium lies in its capacity to lower the specific gravity of any mixture of gases of which it forms a part. Thus in the presence of respiratory obstruction a helium-oxygen mixture may be of greater benefit than oxygen alone. Dean and Visscher (1941) have shown that other factors than density must be taken into account, such as the type of gas flow in the respiratory tract. In normal circumstances this is streamlined but if the speed of flow is increased, as is the case with any incomplete obstruction in the upper respiratory tract, a velocity is reached at which the flow becomes turbulent. The pressure required to move a streamlined gas flow is proportional to the rate of flow and the *viscosity* of the mixture. The viscosity of air is 1·00 compared with 1·11 for a mixture of 80 per cent helium and 20 per cent oxygen, so that air is best under such conditions. The pressure required to move a turbulent flow is proportional to the square of the rate of flow and to the *density* of the mixture. A mixture of 80 per cent helium and 20 per cent oxygen with a density of 0·33 is under these conditions better than air with a density of 1·00. Doll (1946) reviewing the therapeutic value of helium in the light of these facts, recommends this gas when respiratory obstruction exists in the larger air passages but presents evidence to show that in asthma—a disease of the smallest passages where air flow is not turbulent—it is unlikely to be of value.

The inhalation of a helium-oxygen mixture for a short period prior to the induction of anaesthesia in cases with upper respiratory obstruction, will considerably improve the arterial oxygen saturation and may enable a rapid intubation to be performed with safety. For such a purpose cylinders are available containing 79 per cent helium and 21 per cent oxygen. Alternatively, helium can with advantage be added to a mixture of inhalational gases to decrease the specific gravity of the anaesthetic mixture and increase the speed of induction for the patient when there is some obstruction in the upper respiratory tract. A mixture of 25 per cent oxygen, 15 per cent cyclopropane and 60 per cent helium has a specific gravity of 0·50, or half that of air.

PRINCIPLES OF GAS ANALYSIS

In anaesthetic practice a knowledge of the concentration of a gas such as oxygen, carbon dioxide, or nitrous oxide is often required for the satisfactory management of the patient. This information can be obtained in a variety of ways depending on the apparatus available. In general the methods available can be classified in three groups—first, those based on *chemical* analysis; second, those requiring *physical* measurement; and third, the use of a *specific electrode.*

Chemical Analysis

The principal methods require the absorption of a gas by a particular reagent. After the gas has been removed from the sample the volume change is measured. Under these conditions both the temperature and the pressure must be kept constant. Examples of this type of apparatus are the Haldane, Orsat-Henderson and Van Slyke (see Rebreathing Technique, p. 182). The Scholander micropipette analyser is based on the same principle but has the advantage that very small quantities of gas are required, yet accurate determinations of oxygen and carbon dioxide can be obtained (Adriani, 1962).

A variation of this system is the manometric technique, where both the volume and the temperature are kept constant and variations in pressure can be measured by an apparatus such as that of Van Slyke and Niell. This type has the advantage of great accuracy and permits the determination of the pressure of gases in blood. Oxygen, for example, is absorbed by sodium hydrosulphite and carbon dioxide by sodium hydroxide. Nitrous oxide interferes with the estimation but allowance can be made for its presence. A micro-manometric modification of the Van Slyke method of analysis has been described by Natelson (1951).

Physical Analysis

In recent years such techniques have become more popular because of the introduction of electronics in medicine and also because the very small quantities required permit continuous gas analysis.

The principal methods employed are:

Magnetic.—Oxygen is a paramagnetic gas and will thus alter the magnetic flux existing between the poles of a permanent magnet. A small dumb-bell shaped vessel containing nitrogen—a weakly, diamagnetic gas—is suspended between the poles of the magnet. This dumb-bell will rotate in the presence of a paramagnetic gas such as oxygen to a degree proportional to the concentration of oxygen present. A mirror attached to the dumb-bell reflects a light beam which is displayed on a calibrated ground-glass screen.

A high degree of accuracy is obtainable.

Infra-red Analyser.—A sample gas is compared continuously with a reference gas—usually carbon dioxide—for absorption of infra-red radiation. An infra-red radiator is "shone" through the sample and the reference cell alternately by means of a rotating shutter which "chops" the infra-red beam. The difference in the signal obtained from the detector when the beam is transmitted through the sample and the reference is a measure of the concentration of gas in the sample. The speed of rotation of the "chopper" determines the response time of the system. The response of the analyser should be sufficiently rapid to enable end-tidal analysis of each expiration to be seen.

Mass spectrograph.—The gas mixture to be analysed is drawn into a vacuum chamber where the individual molecules are ionised. The ionised particles are then subjected to a strong electromagnetic field which causes the ionised particles to move in an arc, the radius of which is determined by the mass of the particular ion. The response of the apparatus is extremely fast and accurate, and enables the uptake of gases to be measured on a breath-to-breath basis.

When tracer gases such as xenon or krypton are used, small changes in uptake, dependant upon alteration in pulmonary blood flow, may be estimated, and when coupled to a digital computer can give an indication of the cardiac output from beat to beat (Bushman, personal communication).

Gas chromatography.—The measurement of gases and vapours by the gas chromatograph has advanced considerably, but the basic technique remains the same in principle. Measurement of blood oxygen and carbon dioxide content may now be performed rapidly using this technique (Davies, 1970).

A column consisting of crushed firebrick or Celite (or Kieselguhr, a diatomaceous earth) is usually heated to 70°–100° C. A carrier gas, being hydrogen, nitrogen, helium, argon or carbon dioxide, is used to carry the constituents to be distinguished. Each constituent then separates in the column and arrives at the detector as a separate entity and is revealed as an individual response. The various substances are distinguished by the time taken following injection for the response to appear. The record is usually displayed on a pen recorder and the amount of each constituent represented as a peak height. More exactly, it is proportional to the area under the peak, and the output of the detector may be fed directly to an integrating amplifier and the result obtained as a digital print out.

The detectors in gas chromatographs are of three main types:

1. Hot wire (katharometer) which detects changes in the thermal conductivity of the carrier gas.

2. Gas density.

3. Ionisation

(i) Micro-argon using Sr^{90} as a radioactive source of β rays.
(ii) Electron capture, using Ni_{63} as a source of free electrons.
(iii) Flame ionisation. A hydrogen flame is the means whereby ions are formed. This type of detector is extremely sensitive to organic compounds.

Specific Electrodes

During recent years great progress has been made in the development of gas electrode systems so that these are now commercially available for oxygen, carbon dioxide and pH. They have been so simplified that the anaesthetist can personally operate them and obtain vital information on the blood gas tension of the patient. In the future, it seems likely that these techniques will replace all others for blood gas analysis in clinical practice. Several manufacturers now produce complete electrode systems for blood gas analysis.

1. **Oxygen electrode.**—The principle is that a platinum electrode is polarised from a mercury cell battery to about 650 mV. Oxygen molecules in the vicinity of the electrode (cathode) become polarised thus:

$$O_2 + 4e \rightarrow 2\,O^{--}$$

The ionised molecules may thus carry a current to a silver/silver chloride electrode of the opposite polarity (anode), the resulting current being proportional to the concentration of oxygen in the solution. The electrodes are separated from the blood sample by a semi-permeable membrane of polypropylene, and immersed in a solution of potassium chloride and phosphate buffer to minimise the effect of gases other than oxygen. Basically, the present-day model is a development of the original Clark electrode.

2. **Carbon dioxide electrode.**—The design and principle of this electrode has already been described (see Hypoventilation, p. 185). Modifications have included a special glass electrode with a nearly flat surface, a calomel reference electrode and a special butyl rubber seal (relatively insoluble to CO_2) to hold the electrode in the cuvette. The original "Cellophane" spacer was found to be responsible for the slow response and this has now been obviated by using a nylon stocking covering. Fibres of glass wool are also included, because this increases the speed of the response.

3. **pH electrode.**—Developments in this type of electrode have included the return to the use of capillary glass electrodes, with the sample inside the capillary to ensure anaerobic measurement.

REFERENCES

BARTEK, M. J. (1967). A study of man during prolonged exposure to oxygen. *Aerospace Med.*, **38,** 1037.

BARTLETT, R. G., and HERTZ, R. A. (1962). Differentiation between air and oxygen. *Aerospace Med.*, **33,** 552.

BETHUNE, D. W., and COLLIS, J. M. (1967). The evaluation of oxygen masks: a mechanical method. *Anaesthesia*, **22,** 43.

BURNS, T. H. S., and HALL, J. M. (1953). A disposable oxygen mask. *Brit. med. J.*, **2,** 672.

BUSHMAN, J. (1970). Personal communication.

COMROE, J. H., Jr., and DRIPPS, R. D. (1950). *Physiological Basis for Oxygen Therapy.* Springfield, Ill.: Charles C. Thomas.

COMROE, J. H., Jr., DRIPPS, R. D., DUMKE, P. R., and DEMING, M. (1945). Oxygen toxicity. *J. Amer. med. Ass.*, **128,** 710.

COMROE, J. H., FORSTER, R. E., DUBOIS, A. B., BRISCOE, W. A., and CARLSEN, E. (1962). *The Lung. Clinical Physiology and Pulmonary Function Tests*, 2nd edit. Chicago: Year Book Medical Publishers.

COURNAND, A., RILEY, R. L., BRADLEY, S. E., BREED, E. S., NOBLE, R. P., LAWSON, M. D., GREGERSON, M. I., and RICHARDS, D. W. (1943). Studies of the circulation in clinical shock. *Surgery*, **13,** 964.

DAVIES, C. E., and MACKINNON, J. (1949). Neurological effects of oxygen in chronic cor pulmonale. *Lancet*, **2,** 883.

DAVIES, D. D. (1970). A method of gas chromatography for quantitative analysis of blood gases. *Brit. J. Anaesth.*, **42,** 19.

DEAN, R. B., and VISSCHER, M. B. (1941). The kinetics of lung ventilation. An evaluation of the viscous and elastic resistance to lung ventilation with particular reference to the effects of turbulence and the therapeutic use of helium. *Amer. J. Physiol.*, **134,** 450.

DOLL, R. (1946). Helium in the treatment of asthma. *Thorax*, **1,** 30.

ECKENHOFF, J. E., HAFKENSHIEL, J. H., and LANDMESSER, C. M. (1947). Coronary circulation of the dog. *Amer. J. Physiol.*, **148,** 582.

EGGERS, G. W. N., Jr., PALEY, H. W., LEONARD, J. J., and WARREN, J. V. (1962). Haemodynamic responses to oxygen breathing in man. *J. appl. Physiol.*, **17,** 75.

ERNSTING, J. (1965). The influence of alveolar nitrogen and environmental pressure on rate of gas absorption from non-ventilated lung. *Aerospace Med.*, **36,** 948.

FINK, R. B. (1955). Diffusion anoxia. *Anesthesiology*, **16,** 511.

FOWLER, W. S., and COMROE, J. H., Jr. (1948). Lung function studies. Rate of increase of arterial oxygen saturation during inhalation of 100 per cent. oxygen. *J. clin. Invest.*, **27,** 327.

FRANK, H. A., and FINE, J. (1943). Traumatic shock. V. A study of the effects of oxygen on haemorrhagic shock. *J. clin. Invest.*, **22,** 305.

FREEMAN, J. (1962). Survival of bled dogs after halothane and ether anaesthesia. *Brit. J. Anaesth.*, **34,** 832.

FREEMAN, J. (1966). *Oxygen Measurements in Shock. Symposium on Oxygen Measurement in Blood and Tissues*, pp. 221–243. London: Churchill.

FREEMAN, J., and NUNN, J. F. (1963). Ventilation-perfusion relationships after haemorrhage. *Clin. Sci.*, **24,** 135.

GUPTA, R. K. (1969). Histochemical studies in pulmonary oxygen toxicity. *Aerospace Med.*, **40,** 500.

HALDANE, J. S. (1926). Some bearings of the physiology of respiration on the administration of anaesthetics. *Proc. roy. Soc. Med.*, **19,** Sect. of Anaesth., p. 33.

HENDERSON, Y. (1925). Physiological regulation of the acid-base balance of the blood and some related functions. *Physiol. Rev.*, **5,** 131.

HEWER, C. L., and LEE, J. A. (1957). *Recent Advances in Anaesthesia and Analgesia,* 8th edit. London: J. & A. Churchill.

LAVOISIER, A. L., and DE LA PLACE, P. S. (1780). Mémoire sur la chaleur. *Mém. prés Acad. Sci. (Paris)*, **94,** 355.

LEIGH, J. M. (1970). Variation in performance of oxygen therapy devices. *Anaesthesia,* **25,** 210.

MICHAEL, E. L. (1960). Exposure to oxygen tension of 418 mm. Hg for 168 hours. *Aerospace Med.*, **31,** 138.

MILLER, W. F. (1962). Oxygen therapy catheter, mask, hood and tent. *Anesthesiology,* **23,** 445.

MILLIKAN, G. A. (1942). Oximeter, instrument for measuring continuously oxygen saturation of arterial blood in man. *Rev. sci. Instrum.*, **13,** 434.

MOTLEY, H. L., COURNAND, A., WERKO, L., HIMMELSTEIN, A., and DRESDALE, D. (1947). The influence of short periods of induced acute anoxia upon pulmonary artery pressures in man. *Amer. J. Physiol.*, **150,** 315.

NASH, G., BLENNERHASSETT, J. B., and PONTOPPIDAN, H. (1967). Pulmonary lesions associated with oxygen therapy and artificial ventilation. *New Engl. J. Med.*, **276,** 368.

NATELSON, S. (1951). Routine use of ultra micro methods in the clinical laboratory. *Amer. J. clin. Path.*, **21,** 1153.

NUNN, J. F., and PAYNE, J. P. (1962). Hypoxaemia after general anaesthesia. *Lancet,* **2,** 631.

PASK, E. A. (1955). Committee on deaths associated with anaesthesia. Review of cases where post-operative care was inadequate to meet the circumstances which arose. *Anaesthesia*, **10,** 4.

PRICE, H. L. (1960). Effects of carbon dioxide on the cardiovascular system. *Anesthesiology*, **21,** 652.

PRIESTLEY, J. (1777). *Experiments and Observations on Different Kinds of Air*. London.

RAMSAY, —., and LOCKYER, J. N. (1895). L'hélium, élément terrestre. (Abstr.) *Rev. sci.*, **3,** 654.

REINHARD, E. H., MOORE, C. V., DUBACH, R., and WADE, L. J. (1944). Depressant effects of high concentrations of inspired oxygen in erythrocytogenesis. *J. clin. Invest.*, **23,** 682.

ROSS, J. M., FAIRCHILD, H. M., WELDY, J., and GUYTON, A. C. (1962). Autoregulation of blood flow by oxygen lack. *Amer. J. Physiol.*, **202,** 21.

SÉGUIN, A., and LAVOISIER, A. L. (1789). Premier mémoire sur la respiration des animaux. *Mém. prés. Acad. Sci. (Paris)*, **103,** 566.

STORSTEIN, O. (1952). Effect of pure oxygen breathing on circulation in anoxaemia in patients with lung and heart diseases and normal individuals subjected to experimental anoxaemia. *Acta med. scand.*, **143,** Suppl. 1, p. 269.

TINSLEY, J. C., Jr., MOORE, C. V., DUBACK, R., MINNICH, V., and GRINSTEIN, M. (1949). The role of oxygen in the regulation of erythropoesis. Depression of the rate of delivery of new red cells to the blood by high concentrations of inspired oxygen. *J. clin. Invest.*, **28,** 1544.

VON EULER, U. S., and LILJESTRAND, G. (1946). Observations on the pulmonary arterial blood pressure in the cat. *Acta physiol. scand.*, **12,** 301.

WAYNE, D. J. and CHAMNEY, A. R. (1967). A new oxygen tent. *Lancet*, **2,** 344.

WHITBY, L. E. H., and BRITTON, C. J. C. (1957). *Disorders of the Blood*, 8th edit. London: J. & A. Churchill.

WOOD, G. O., MASON, M. F., and BLALOCK, A. (1940). Studies on effects of inhalation of high concentrations of oxygen in experimental shock. *Surgery*, **8,** 247.

Chapter 6

HYPERBARIC AIR AND OXYGEN

THE normal atmosphere contains approximately 20 per cent oxygen and under normal circumstances this is sufficient for the body's requirements. However, in the presence of acute or chronic hypoxia this percentage must be increased if tissue damage is to be avoided. Furthermore, in the presence of circulatory disturbances the uptake of oxygen by the body may be satisfactory yet the blood-flow to the tissues is inadequate. Increasing the tension of oxygen in the blood not only raises the amount physically dissolved in the plasma but also improves the gradient of oxygen tension available to the stagnant area.

At sea level arterial blood is about 95 per cent saturated with oxygen and the tension of this gas in the trachea during inspiration is 149 mm. Hg (i.e. 21 per cent of 760 mm. Hg less the tension of water vapour at 37° C = 47 mm. Hg). Breathing 100 per cent oxygen displaces the nitrogen and the tension of oxygen now rises to 713 mm. Hg (i.e. 760–47 mm. Hg).

The oxygen dissociation curve permits a wide latitude of oxygen tension for man breathing air. Thus, climbing in an aircraft reduces the atmospheric pressure but the oxygen tension can fall to as low as 40 mm. Hg before the saturation is reduced to a level where cyanosis and symptoms occur. The partial pressures at various altitudes of both air and oxygen are illustrated in Table 1 with the equivalent conditions to be expected, but these take no account of the physical fitness and acclimatisation of the individual. In this respect it will be recalled that in 1952 Sir Edmund Hilary was able to remove his oxygen mask on the summit of Everest for a period of ten minutes without becoming acutely hypoxic.

Diving under the sea produces the reverse effect. Here, the tension of oxygen steadily increases. Thus the pressure is raised 1 atmosphere or 760 mm. Hg for every 33 feet of sea water or 30 feet of salt-free water descended. For example, at a depth of 33 feet under the surface of the sea the tension of air is 2 atmospheres or $760 \times 2 = 1520$ mm. Hg. The proportion of oxygen remains the same but the tension of this gas will be doubled. If pure oxygen is breathed at this depth then the tension will be raised accordingly.

In any description of hyperbaric therapy it is most important that the terminology for the actual pressure the patient is receiving should be completely understood. Thus when a patient is described as being exposed to 2 atmospheres (absolute) of either air or oxygen it means that these gases are being delivered at atmospheric pressure plus one extra atmosphere. Thus, the situation is most easily denoted as 2 atmospheres absolute or 2 AT.A.

Atmospheric Pressure + 1 atmosphere = 2 AT.A.
Atmospheric Pressure + 2 atmospheres = 3 AT.A.
Atmospheric Pressure + 3 atmospheres = 4 AT.A.

In recent years attention has centred on the possibility of using a high tension of oxygen in clinical practice to increase the amount of oxygen available to tissue cells in need.

6/TABLE 1

EFFECT OF ALTITUDE ON THE BAROMETRIC PRESSURE OF OXYGEN

Altitude	Conditions	Barometric pressure: Total air pressure in mm. Hg	Barometric pressure: Oxygen tension in mm. Hg
100,000 ft.	On towards space!	7	1·15
63,000 ft.	Body fluids boil at 98·6 F.	47	10
40,000 ft.	Severe oxygen lack in spite of breathing 100 per cent O_2	141	30
29,028 ft.	Summit of Everest	235	49
18,000 ft.	Highest permanent human habitation	379	79
12,000 ft.	Definite signs of oxygen lack	483	101
8,000 ft.	Safety zone	564	118
5,000 ft.	Slight or no effects of oxygen lack	632	132
Sea level		760	159

(After Lambertsen, 1961)

Haemoglobin is the principal carrier of oxygen and as has already been stated it is normally 95-97 per cent saturated so that there is little room for further improvement. However, the amount carried in the plasma bears a direct relationship with the tension of oxygen in the air breathed. Thus, at a tension of 3·5 atmospheres* (2660 mm. Hg) the amount of oxgyen carried in the plasma is greater than the normal arterio-venous oxygen difference so that haemoglobin is no longer required.

Thus:	*Oxygen content of Plasma*
Breathing Room Air	0·3 ml./100 ml. Blood
Breathing 100 per cent O_2	2·0 ml./100 ml. Blood
Breathing 100 per cent O_2 at 2 Atmos.	3·8 ml./100 ml. Blood
Breathing 100 per cent O_2 at 3 Atmos.	5·3 ml./100 ml. Blood
Breathing 100 per cent O_2 at 3·5 Atmos.	6·5 ml./100 ml. Blood

In brief: For every rise of 100 mm. Hg in tension there is an approximate increase of 0·3 ml. of oxygen for every 100 ml. of plasma.

This increased oxygen content and to a lesser extent the improved pressure

* 1 atmosphere = 14·7 pounds per square inch (P.S.I.)

gradient available to the tissues are the basis of the theoretical advantage of the use of hyperbaric oxygen. It still remains to be proved whether this advantage will be borne out in clinical practice.

The only method of increasing the pressure of inspired oxygen above atmospheric requires the use of a specially constructed pressure chamber. Such a chamber may be small (for the patient only) or it may be large and capable of containing not only a patient but also a number of attendants. The problems involved in the use of these two types of chambers are different. In the small single-person chamber the interior is filled with pure oxygen and therefore the problems are centred around the toxicity of oxygen under pressure. In the larger chamber the atmosphere is air-under-pressure which the attendants can breathe whilst the patient receives either pure oxygen or an anaesthetic mixture; in the latter case whatever gases are employed the total tension of the mixture will be the same as the interior of the chamber. The advantage of the attendants breathing air as opposed to oxygen lies in the greater safety margin of hyperbaric air, not only to the individual but also with regard to the risk of explosion.

In considering the various problems raised by the use of a pressure chamber these can be conveniently grouped under first the effects of hyperbaric oxygen and secondly the limitations and dangers of hyperbaric air.

Hyperbaric Oxygen

If man breathes oxygen under pressure, then sooner or later he will develop the signs of oxygen toxicity. The time interval or latent period depends both on the tension of oxygen and the time for which the gas is breathed. The response also varies between different individuals, and the same individual at different exposures (Donald, 1947). The symptoms and signs of oxygen toxicity are almost all concerned with the central nervous system. Animal experiments suggest that if it is ever found necessary for man to breathe oxygen at high pressures for a long time then pulmonary symptoms will also develop. It has also been shown that pulmonary abnormalities can appear in normal subjects after prolonged exposure to hyperbaric oxygen (Fisher, 1968). Finally, if premature babies are exposed to high atmospheric oxygen then the risk of retrolental fibroplasia must be considered to be greatly increased.

Oxygen Toxicity

Aetiology.—Unfortunately the cause of this condition is unknown, but it is generally believed that high oxygen pressures interfere with oxidative reactions. It is possible that the oxygen inactivates a specific enzyme—the dehydrogenases including the sulphydryl group—which are essential for activity. This matter will be considered in greater detail below.

Symptoms and signs.—Among the most prominent prodromal features are nausea and dizziness with ringing in the ears and tingling of the hands. Anxiety is also a common symptom. Twitching of the lips, eyelids or small muscles of the hand may develop and the respiration becomes "cogwheel" in character as the diaphragm undergoes spasmodic contractions. Convulsions, which are the essential feature of oxygen toxicity, often develop suddenly without warning or the patient may show increasing myoclonic movements over several minutes.

Nevertheless, clarity of consciousness is retained until just after the onset of the convulsions.

Diagnosis.—The suddenness of onset of convulsions make the detection of the pre-convulsive state difficult. However, the pattern of the electro-encephalogram will reveal hyper-irritability prior to their onset and an electromyogram of the lip muscles has been used to detect the earliest signs of muscle-twitching.

Treatment.—Provided the high pressure of oxygen is immediately withdrawn and the patient allowed to breathe air (either at atmospheric pressure or above) the convulsions will cease and no permanent cerebral damage will result. The danger of oxygen convulsions *per se* lies in the possible injury to the individual during a spasm in a small chamber.

However, if the patient is lying in a small single chamber then rapid decompression is not always advisable because in the conscious state laryngeal spasm may develop during the convulsions and close the glottis. In this case, a sudden drop of environmental pressure would lead to a dangerously high pressure trapped within the lungs thus increasing the possible risk of rupture. If the patient continues to breathe spontaneously (denoting an open glottis) or there is an endotracheal tube *in situ* (as in the anaesthetised subject), then the dangers of rapid decompression under hyperbaric oxygen are minimal.

Factors Influencing Onset of Toxicity

(*a*) *Duration and pressure.*—The duration of time that a patient is exposed to a high pressure of oxygen, and the height of the atmospheric pressure, are the principal factors concerned in the onset of oxygen toxicity. There is a wide variation in man. For example, during diving operations (similar to a pressure chamber) at a pressure of 2 and 2·5 atmospheres (absolute) some subjects develop symptoms of oxygen toxicity (though not necessarily convulsions) in less than thirty minutes of oxygen breathing. Most fit young males can withstand 2 atmospheres (absolute) of oxygen for thirty minutes without symptoms. Yarborough *et al.* (1947) in a study of servicemen under diving conditions, found that about one half could withstand 4 atmospheres (absolute) for 30 minutes.

It must be emphasised, however, that most of the data available is based on studies in servicemen, who are usually described as "fit, young and healthy." This group is not typical of the usual hospital patient. However, Foster and Churchill-Davidson (1970—personal communication) have had experience with a large number of patients who have been exposed to high pressures of oxygen in combination with radiotherapy treatment for cancer. In a group of 410 conscious patients (mostly over 50 years of age) who were exposed to 3 atmospheres (absolute) for periods lasting 20–66 (av. 35) minutes, there were four cases of convulsions. These figures are even more impressive when it is remembered that each patient was given this treatment on a number of occasions, so that the figure could be interpreted as 4 cases developing convulsions out of 2,278 exposures to 3 atmospheres absolute. In another series, 73 patients were anaesthetised and then exposed to 4 atmospheres absolute for 21–75 (av. 36) minutes, and only one case developed convulsions.

The wide variation in the response of man to high pressures of oxygen makes it difficult to predict an exact safe limit, but it is now clear that most patients can withstand 3 atmospheres (absolute) for at least 30 minutes.

(*b*) *Carbon dioxide.*—Lambertsen (1961) has shown conclusively that raising the percentage of inspired carbon dioxide concentration will increase the risk of convulsions. Under normal conditions of breathing oxygen under pressure no gross accumulation of CO_2 occurs in the brain and the small amount that is retained is not directly responsible for oxygen convulsions. However, if 2 per cent CO_2 is added to the inhaled mixture there is a pronounced reduction in the time the patient can breathe oxygen-under-pressure without developing signs of toxicity. A possible cause of this increased toxicity is the consequent dilatation of the cerebral blood vessels brought about by the carbon dioxide which, in turn, leads to a greatly increased cerebral blood-flow. This would result in an enormous increase in the cerebral venous oxygen tension. As only 3 ml. of oxygen per 100 ml. of blood is removed from the arterial blood perfusing the brain, the cerebral venous blood is still virtually 100 per cent saturated and this may influence the onset of convulsions.

(*c*) *Exercise.*—Although unlikely to be a factor in clinical oxygen therapy, exercise is also known to reduce the time interval before the onset of convulsions.

Prevention of Oxygen Toxicity

Clearly, reducing either the height of the atmospheric pressure or the duration of exposure will reduce the possibility of oxygen toxicity. However, one of the principal factors in prevention—if a high tension is required—lies in anaesthetising the patient. Both narcotic drugs and anaesthetic agents possess the ability to partially protect the patient. There is evidence from animal experiments that halothane at 4 AT.A. of oxygen delays the onset of convulsive E.E.G. activity, but there is no information available for other drugs (Harp, 1966). The fact that patients can withstand higher pressures for longer periods when anaesthetised (Foster and Churchill-Davidson, 1963) suggests that anaesthetics —particularly the barbiturates—exert some protective influence on the brain. Periodic interruption of oxygen breathing, as would be possible in a large chamber filled with air, has also been found to greatly extend the tolerance of oxygen in small animals (Kaufman and Morgarger, 1956). Finally, the use of muscle relaxants can prevent the motor activity of convulsions.

Mechanism of Toxicity

A study of tissue slices (rat) has revealed that all tissues are not equally susceptible to *in vitro* poisoning so that the effect on the central nervous system is far greater than that on kidney or muscle. As animals killed by high pressure oxygen show no general reduction of their oxidative metabolism it must be assumed that a generalised depression of metabolism can be excluded. However, it is now commonly accepted that some specific enzyme systems, particularly those dependent on the sulphydryl group for their catalytic potency, can be inhibited by oxygen. This inactivation is thought to be specific because many other enzymes including cytochrome oxidase are not affected. Prominent amongst those inhibited are enzymes involved in the tricarboxylic acid cycle, particularly in the oxidation of pyruvate, succinate, α-ketoglutarate and maleate (see p. 250).

Other workers consider that the observed enzyme inhibition is caused by the oxidation of sulphydryl containing co-enzymes (Haugaard, *et. al.*, 1959). One of the attractions of this concept is that mammalian tissues possess enzymic mechanisms for the regeneration of sulphydryl co-enzymes; this could explain the complete recovery from the acute phase of oxygen toxicity.

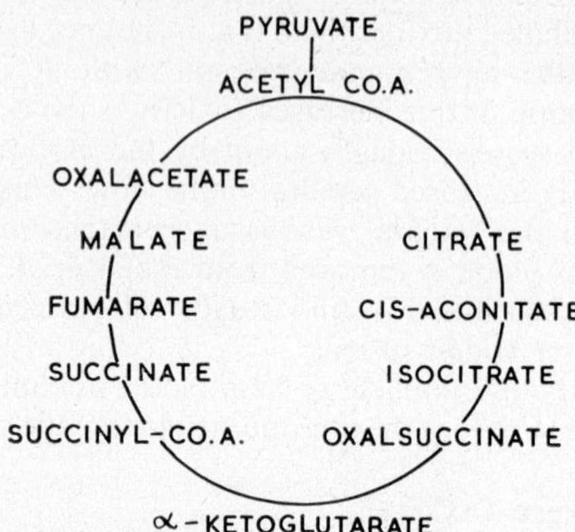

Effects of Oxygen on the Respiratory Tract

At atmospheric pressure, the inhalation of 80 per cent oxygen or more for longer than twelve hours leads to symptoms of irritation of the respiratory tract with substernal soreness, coughing and sore throat. The inhalation of 100 per cent oxygen for longer than twenty-four hours may give rise to bronchopneumonia. These symptoms following the inhalation of a high percentage of oxygen can be prevented merely by reducing the concentration inspired; thus up to 50 per cent oxygen can be breathed for up to 8 days without risk.

If the pressure is raised above atmospheric then experiments in animals have shown that the symptoms of pulmonary damage develop. For example, rats subjected to 5 atmospheres of oxygen show signs of pulmonary congestion and alveolar exudates within 20–40 mins. and an atelectatic appearance within the hour (Smith, 1899).

In man lung damage is rarely seen (Fuson, 1964—personal communication) perhaps because to date exposures have not been sufficiently prolonged. However, in six normal subjects exposed to pure oxygen at 2 AT.A. for 6–11 hours, all showed a decrease in the vital capacity of approximately 15 per cent and changes in dynamic pulmonary compliance. The subjects all returned to normal in 14–22 hours (Fisher, 1968). It is thought that a high oxygen tension possibly causes an alteration of the surfactant layer of the lungs and a temporary alteration in the pulmonary elastic element.

Effect of Oxygen on Cerebral Blood Vessels

At atmospheric pressure the inhalation of a high concentration of oxygen leads to cerebral vasoconstriction. This is rarely sufficient to be of any significance except in the premature and newborn infant, where this constriction may be sufficient to produce permanent damage i.e. retrolental fibroplasia. Saltzman and his colleagues (1964) have studied the vascular response of the retinal vessels to hyperbaric oxygenation in adults. They found no evidence of damage to the eye or visual fields following short periods of exposure; they concluded that the increased oxygenation of the blood more than compensated for the intense vasoconstriction. It remains to be seen whether prolonged periods of hyperbaric oxygenation will lead to cerebrovascular damage. Henkind (1964) in a study of retinal vessels states that "there is little or no evidence to suggest that oxygen can cause obliteration of vessels other than immature retinal vessels."

HYPERBARIC AIR

Apart from the use of compressed air for diving operations, one of the earliest reports of the use of air under increased atmospheric pressure came from Cunningham in 1927. In Kansas City he constructed two large chambers (11 feet wide and 100 feet long) in which patients with cancer, diabetes and syphilis were treated for periods of time varying from a few hours up to four weeks at pressures of 1·6 to 4 atmospheres. A huge chamber, constructed as a gigantic sphere measuring 64 feet in diameter, and the equivalent height of a 5 storey building, was also used in Cleveland. Though the value of these chambers was never proven at least they established that man could live at pressures of 3 atmospheres of air for periods of a week or longer.

However, hyperbaric air is not without dangers. As the pressure is increased so does the likelihood that nitrogen narcosis will occur. Similarly, after breathing air under pressure for a long time the possibility of decompression sickness or "bends" is present. Finally, a rapid return to normal atmospheric pressure may cause lung damage and air embolus in certain individuals.

Nitrogen Narcosis

It appears that all the inert gases are capable of exerting a depressant effect upon the peripheral and central nervous systems. Although these gases cannot be called anaesthetics it is believed that their mode of action is very similar. Thus, it has been suggested that if nitrogen and oxygen (in a 4:1 ratio) are breathed at 38 atmospheres, the depth of unconsciousness produced would be similar to that produced by nitrous oxide and oxygen (4:1) at 1 atmosphere pressure. However, nitrogen narcosis is routinely observed at pressures between 3·5 and 6·0 atmospheres and severely curtails any logical thought at a pressure above 8 atmospheres.

Symptoms.—Nearly all subjects show symptoms of nitrogen narcosis on their first exposures to pressure above 2 AT.A, these tending to diminish on subsequent exposures (Ledingham, 1969). It has also been shown that there is some deterioration in mental performance at 2 AT.A (Poulton *et al.*, 1963). The earliest sign of nitrogen narcosis is euphoria. The subsequent sequence of events somewhat resembles the symptoms of chronic hypoxia and is similar to those of increasing alcoholic intoxication. This condition is so serious that it is highly improbable that surgery could be attempted in a chamber above 6 atmospheres with air breathing alone. For this reason it is vitally important that the pressure within the chamber be controlled from outside lest the occupants get too euphoric!

Mechanism.—This is not clearly understood but it is believed to be similar to the mechanism of action of anaesthetic gases. The greater the lipid solubility of an inert gas the more likelihood there is that it will produce narcosis. Thus xenon, krypton and argon, which have a greater solubility in olive oil than nitrogen, would all be expected (under standard conditions) to produce signs of narcosis at a lower atmospheric pressure. Helium and hydrogen, however, are relatively insoluble in olive oil. No narcotic effects have been reported in diving experiments when helium and oxygen or hydrogen and oxygen mixtures are breathed at 30 atmospheres pressure (1,000 ft. sea water). The narcotic property of an inert gas also appears to decrease as the molecular weight of the gas grows smaller. Carpenter (1955) has proposed that any inert substance present in sufficient concentration in the cell lipids can exert a depressant effect on metabolism. He has been able to show that nitrous oxide at high partial pressures can depress pyruvate oxidation by enzymatic reaction in the citric acid cycle.

Prevention.—It appears from the above data that the only satisfactory method of avoiding nitrogen narcosis is to breath air at a pressure not greater than 3 atmospheres. If, in clinical practice, higher pressures are required in the chamber and skilled work is necessary, then it is probable that a helium and oxygen mixture should be breathed. Such a mixture is non-explosive, non-toxic, but expensive and it will make vocal communication difficult because of the alteration in viscosity that it causes in the inhaled gases.

Decompression Sickness ("Bends" or Caisson Disease)

Aetiology.—Under normal conditions the nitrogen in the atmosphere is in equilibrium with the gaseous nitrogen in the tissues. On entering a pressure chamber additional nitrogen will become dissolved in the tissues in direct proportion to the rise in atmospheric pressure. Those tissues with a large blood supply e.g. brain, liver, kidney and heart, will rapidly receive the increased tension of nitrogen. Poorly perfused tissues such as fat take some time before they reach equilibrium with the arterial blood. Thus, if the period of the pressurisation is short, on returning rapidly to atmospheric pressure the tissues with a rich blood supply (i.e. brain, etc.) can give up their increased tension just as fast as they were able to take it up; the extra amount dissolved in the poorly perfused tissues (e.g. fat) is minimal so no ill-effects are observed.

On the other hand, if the subject is exposed to a high pressure for a long period of time, the poorly perfused tissues are able to take up large quantities of nitrogen. The fact that nitrogen is some five times more soluble in fat than in water also aids the build-up. Due to the poor vascularity of fatty tissues it may take as long as 12 hours for equilibrium to be reached between the partial pressure of nitrogen in these tissues and that within the chamber. In contrast, the kidney (a high blood flow organ) requires only about one hour for equilibration.

On sudden decompression after a prolonged exposure to a high pressure, the high blood flow tissues are cleared rapidly, but the tension remains high in the poorly perfused tissues merely because it cannot dispose quickly of its contents. If the decompression is very slow then the high tension of nitrogen can gradually diffuse out into the passing circulation without difficulty. On the other hand, if decompression is rapid the nitrogen in the tissues will still be at a relatively high tension whilst that in the circulation has returned to atmospheric pressure. The tissue gas, therefore, comes out of solution, expands, and then gives rise to symptoms and signs in various parts of the body.

Symptoms and signs.—The commonest symptom is pain in the muscles and joints (usually shoulder or knees). The periarticular tissues become distended by gas bubbles so that severe arthralgia develops. Similarly small gas emboli form in the peripheral nerve sheathes leading first to sensory disturbances (formication, pruritus, tingling and thermal sensations) and then to motor weakness (Table 2). In the skin and subcutaneous tissue the bubble formation causes eruptions of an urticarial and herpetic type. In the central nervous system, vertigo, deafness, vomiting, dyspnoea and finally convulsions and coma may develop.

In a severe case the symptoms of pain in the joints are followed rapidly by motor paralysis and the subject falls to the floor. Respiration becomes laboured, cyanosis develops and the pulse becomes weak. Coma and convulsions can ensue at any time if the pressure is not immediately increased again and the patient decompressed slowly. In the event of a fatal outcome, the post-mortem findings show intense congestion of the viscera with small haemorrhagic areas in the brain, spinal cord, pleura, and pericardium. The subcutaneous tissue reveals the presence of gas bubbles (subcutaneous emphysema). Despite popular belief to the contrary, gas emboli only rarely appear in the circulation; such instances are usually only observed in very rapid decompression of animals from a very high atmospheric pressure.

6/Table 2

Symptoms and Signs of Decompression Sickness

Mild symptoms	— Pain in muscle and joints (shoulder and knees) — Sensory disturbances (tingling, pruritis, etc.) — Skin eruptions of urticarial or herpetic type — Vertigo, deafness and vomiting
Moderate	— Motor paralysis — Dyspnoea and laboured respirations — Tachycardia and hypotension — Dyspnoea
Severe	— Coma — Convulsions

Prevention.—Fortunately, if strict rules for work in a pressure chamber are obeyed decompression sickness is completely avoidable. Provided these conditions are fulfilled then breathing air under pressure is a safe procedure. The following factors are of importance:

(*a*) *Limitation of pressure in chamber.*—Since tissues can be moderately saturated with an inert gas without formation of bubbles, it is possible to spend unlimited time in a chamber at 2 atmospheres without the need for slow decompression.

(*b*) *Limitation of duration in chamber.*—Experience with deep-sea diving has shown that if the time spent at a given atmospheric pressure is limited then no decompression is necessary (Table 3). However, if the chamber is re-entered within a specific time interval then allowance must be made for the small amount of nitrogen that is still present in the tissues and the subsequent exposures must be shorter.

(c) *Limitation of rate of decompression.*—It is safe to decompress to half the original pressure rapidly but if the pressure is then still above atmospheric, a suitable pause must be made at this new pressure before further decompression is undertaken.

(d) *Use of helium/oxygen mixtures.*—Substitution of helium for nitrogen as the inert gas eliminates the dangers of narcosis but not of decompression sickness. However, helium reduces the time required for decompression because it is only about one-half as soluble as nitrogen in the body tissues and also it diffuses twice as fast through living membranes. Thus, the amount of helium absorbed in a given time would be considerably less than nitrogen under the same conditions, and the rate of elimination will also be much faster. The fact that helium has less density as a gas than nitrogen means that less effort is required to breathe it at high atmospheric pressures and this may prove to be important in maintaining good alveolar ventilation if great pressures are used in the chamber.

6/TABLE 3

Atmospheres	*Maximum time in chamber without decompression in mins.*
2	—
2·25	320
2·5	200
3·0	60
3·5	40
4·0	25
5·0	10
6·0	5

Figures based on U.S. Navy Diving Manual (1958)

(e) *Use of oxygen decompression.*—It has already been stated that decompression to half the original pressure can be achieved rapidly. On reaching this stage the time interval required at this new level can be shortened if the subject then breathes oxygen. The lungs will now fill with oxygen and therefore the maximum possible gradient between the pressure of nitrogen (P_{N_2}) in the tissues and the zero level in the alveoli will be established. This will speed the elimination of nitrogen and decompression time will be shortened. The large P_{N_2} gradient does not result in bubble formation because the total pressure still remains high. This technique is used in decompressing patients from pressure above 2 AT.A. A special mask system may be used for the purpose (McDowall, 1965) and has led to a decrease in the time necessary for decompression (Ledingham, 1968).

In civil engineering contracts involving tunnel work, the tunnel workers may be frequently exposed to pressures in excess of 3 AT.A. for periods of up to 8-hour shifts. Rigid adherence to a decompression schedule is clearly here of great importance.

Air Embolism

If one of the personnel selected for working in a high pressure chamber has an undetected lung cyst or any other volume of trapped gas, which is not in communication with the respiratory tract, then exposure to a high atmospheric pressure results in a similar pressure within the cyst. A sudden reduction in the extrathoracic pressure will cause expansion of the gas in the cyst, so that the cyst may rupture into the pleural cavity, or stretch and lacerate the lung, resulting in interstitial emphysema or air embolism if the gas enters the circulation. A similar set of circumstances can arise in the presence of emphysema. This emphasises the need for careful selection of personnel working in a pressure chamber.

Bone Necrosis

Avascular necrosis of bone, commonly the head of the femur, proximal or distal ends of the humerus and the proximal end of the tibia, has been reported. It may occur many months or even years after exposure to compressed air or it may occur after only one exposure (Davidson, 1964: Walder, 1966). When the lesion invades the articular surface of a joint it may be severely disabling. It is believed to be related to decompression sickness in that small gas bubbles enter and block the main vessels of the bone. A study of 241 tunnel workers on the Clyde tunnel showed that 19 per cent of workers had bone lesions from this cause (McCallum, 1968).

It seems likely that this complication can be avoided if the code for duration of compression and the ritual of decompression times are closely followed.

Otitic Barotrauma

The middle ear communicates with the pharynx via the Eustachian tube and an equalisation of pressure is achieved when the subject swallows. However it is much easier to equalise pressure during decompression than during compression. If the Eustachian tube is blocked for any reason it may not be easy to equalise the pressure and the tympanic membrane may be retracted. This will give rise to severe earache and a possible rupture of the tympanic membrane. The situation is worse if pure oxygen is used for decompression as this is more rapidly absorbed from the middle ear. In a small number of people compression may have to be abandoned because of this problem, and anaesthetised or unconscious patients should have a preliminary myringotomy before decompression.

Indications for Hyperbaric Oxygen Therapy

At the present time many of the indications for hyperbaric oxygen are only theoretical, because there have been insufficient controlled studies to prove the value of this type of therapy. Nevertheless, the results so far achieved permit an optimistic outlook for the future. The indications for hyperbaric oxygen may be classified in two groups according to their clinical application—Present and Possible:

Present Clinical Application

1. **Infections.**—Anaerobic infections, in particular those due to clostridial

organisms, respond dramatically to this type of therapy (Brummelkamp *et al.*, 1963; Slack *et al.*, 1969). This is because the environment created is unfavourable to the continued growth of the organism and consequent production of toxins with a subsequent dramatic decrease in the toxicity of the patient.

Laboratory studies have also shown that hyperbaric oxygen has a bacteriostatic action on coagulase positive staphylococci and *Pseudomonas pyocyanea* (Shreiner, 1964; Irvin, 1966).

2. **Poisoning.**—Hyperbaric oxygen therapy is the method of choice in the treatment of carbon monoxide poisoning (Lawson *et al.*, 1961). It has been known for many years that the inhalation of pure oxygen in cases of carbon monoxide poisoning speeds the elimination of this gas from the body. The process is greatly enhanced if hyperbaric oxygen is used and tissue hypoxia is halted. To achieve the optimum results this type of therapy should be applied at the earliest possible moment. It is therefore necessary to carry a portable chamber in the ambulance sent to the patient.

3. **Acute arterial insufficiency.**—Tissues that are deprived of their blood supply either by trauma, embolism or thrombosis can be supported during the critical period in an attempt to diminish the area of anoxaemia and permit the improvement of collateral flow (Sharp *et al.*, 1962). Hyperbaric oxygen has been used in plastic surgery for the treatment of ischaemic pedicle grafts (Perrin, 1966).

4. **In combination with radiotherapy and chemotherapeutic agents.**—Gray and his colleagues (1953) working with animals found that all cells become highly resistant to radiotherapy when exposed to low tensions of oxygen. This resistance disappeared if a normal oxygen tension was restored. Churchill-Davidson and his colleagues (1955) conceived that some cancer cells in a tumour must be living in a region of low oxygen tension and therefore would be very resistant to radiotherapy. They reasoned that if the oxygen tension in these cells could be raised then the results of radiotherapy should be improved. On this basis a number of patients with various types of malignant disease were treated in a chamber filled with oxygen at 3 atmospheres absolute. This work has now been extended and similar encouraging results have been obtained at other centres, particularly in Melbourne (Van den Brenk *et al.*, 1962). It is possible that the use of hyperbaric oxygen may improve the results obtained by treatment with chemotherapeutic agents.

Possible Clinical Applications

1. **Cardiac surgery.**—The surgery of congenital heart disease in children may be aided when conducted in a hyperbaric environment possibly combined with hypothermia (Smith *et al.*, 1963). There is some evidence that at 3 atmospheres pressure the peripheral blood flow is increased due to a probable reduction in effective viscosity in the peripheral vascular bed. This will permit a greater artificial perfusion rate than is normal when a pump oxygenator is used. Another factor of significance is that the myocardium becomes less sensitive to external manipulation under hyperbaric oxygen so that the incidence of ventricular fibrillation is reduced. Furthermore, hypothermia increases the solubility of oxygen in blood so that at 20° C the amount is increased by 50 per cent (Severinghaus, 1959). As the excitability of nervous tissue is also reduced by cold it can be

anticipated that the danger of oxygen toxicity under these conditions will be reduced.

2. **Myocardial infarction.**—It has been suggested that hyperbaric oxygen may be useful in the treatment of myocardial infarction by decreasing the incidence of arrhythmias and ventricular fibrillation and perhaps by increasing the viability of the tissue immediately surrounding the infarcted area. Clear evidence of the value of hyperbaric oxygen therapy in myocardial infarction is still lacking.

3. **Storage of organs.**—Hyperbaric conditions may prove to be useful in the storage of organs before transplantation (Ackerman and Barnard, 1966).

4. **Resuscitation of the newborn.**—Hutchison and his colleagues (1966) suggest from a controlled trial that the resuscitation of apnoeic newborn babies by the use of hyperbaric oxygen in a chamber is as effective as tracheal intubation and intermittent positive pressure respiration. These results are not, however, accepted by all workers in this field and the use of hyperbaric oxygen for the treatment of asphyxia neonatorum is not recommended.

Anaesthesia for a Patient in a Hyperbaric Chamber

One of the effects of raising the pressure is to increase the density and viscosity of the gases so that the effects of any obstruction to respiration are more serious, as is any added resistance to respiration in the anaesthetic apparatus.

Since it is the partial pressure of anaesthetic vapour in the brain which determines the depth of anaesthesia, the percentage concentration of the vapour in the inspired air should be reduced corresponding to the working pressure of the chamber.

When anaesthetising a patient in a large chamber the anaesthetist is in direct contact with the patient and can exercise moment-to-moment control. Since the object of the procedure is to raise the oxygen tension in the body as much as possible, oxygen will be the vehicle used for an anaesthetic vapour. Because of the explosion risk ether and cyclopropane must be excluded. Halothane may be ignited in clinical concentrations at 4 AT.A. and above in the presence of diathermy. It is safe below these pressures provided that it is vaporised in 100 per cent oxygen and not in a mixture of nitrous oxide and oxygen because these gases together widen the inflammability gap of halothane under hyperbaric conditions. Intravenous agents can be used, as can the muscle relaxants. Great care is necessary to prevent respiratory depression, because any increase in the carbon dioxide content of the blood leads to an increased need for anaesthetics and shortens the latent period before the development of oxygen toxicity. All the expired vapour should be led away to the exhaust from the chamber, so that there is no risk of accumulation in the chamber to affect the team.

The problems of anaesthesia in a pressure chamber have been described by McDowall (1964). Many concern anaesthetic apparatus. Cylinders containing the gases used in anaesthesia are usually at a pressure high enough to function normally in a hyperbaric environment. Reducing valves work normally provided the supply pressure is sufficiently high, and this means that any gas piped to them in the chamber from an extraneous source must have a higher pressure than the usual pipeline pressure of 60 lbs/sq. inch. Rotameters depend on the density of the gas flowing through them, which will be raised in a hyperbaric environment, It has been shown experimentally that at 2 AT.A. they read high by about 30 per cent (McDowall, 1964). In practice, flow meters should be calibrated against a spirometer at the appropriate pressure. Vaporisers of the "Fluotec" type should deliver the set concentration because the partial pressure of a vapour in equilibrium with its liquid is proportional to absolute temperature and is not affected by total ambient pressure. Experimentally this has been shown to be true of a "Fluotec" in concentrations above 2 per cent but below this value the readings are high. Ventilators may be used provided—because of the explosion hazard—they are not electrically operated.

Several practical points should be borne in mind. If a cuffed endotracheal tube is used, the cuff should be filled with water or saline, in order to prevent large changes in volume, and the same applies to the balloons of Foley and similar urethral catheters. Pleural drainage tubes should be left unclamped at all times to avoid a build-up of pressure in the pleural cavity. Vaporisers should be left open during compression and decompression to prevent implosion or explosion. Intravenous drips may run more rapidly following decompression if the pressures are not equalised by a suitable air inlet thus increasing the risk of air embolism.

The fire hazard in a hyperbaric chamber, especially when oxygen is used, is greatly increased and the consequences of any spark etc. are very much more serious than at normal pressures.

Anaesthesia for a patient in a small chamber is complicated, since when it is used with radiotherapy no attendants can be in the room. Some system of remote monitoring is therefore required. The essentials for this are an electrocardiograph and a microphone to monitor respiration. A pneumotachygraph and electroencephalograph are useful but more elaborate devices. The latter is better than an electromyograph from the lip. The use of gaseous anaesthetics lowers the oxygen tension available and the control of vapour concentration and elimination of the expired vapour from the chamber present problems, so that a single-dose basal anaesthetic is the most suitable. The barbiturates have the special advantage of being anti-convulsants. The technique originally described by Sanger *et al.* (1955) has now been modified. A myringotomy is still performed in each ear and a long segment of a hypodermic needle is inserted through the hole in the drum. This remains *in situ* for the time required to complete the course of treatments.

Premedication consists of phenobarbitone 90 mg. given the night before and the morning of the day of treatment. One and a half hours before the treatment, atropine 1 mg., pethidine 100 mg. and promethazine 50 mg. are injected intramuscularly. Anaesthesia is induced by the slow intravenous injection of from 0·3 to 1·0 g. of pentobarbitone sodium with from 75 to 200 mg. of pethidine. A dose of suxamethonium is given and after oxygenation the larynx and trachea are sprayed with 3 ml. of 4 per cent cocaine and a plain endotracheal tube, well-lubricated with lignocaine ointment, is passed. At this stage of the first treatment the myringotomy needles are inserted. The electrodes are then attached to the patient and he is positioned on the couch ready for the radiotherapy (Fig. 1*a* and *b*). The couch is then slid into the chamber, and whilst the patient is being positioned so that the tumour is exactly in the right position, the correct functioning of the monitoring apparatus is checked and the washout of air from the chamber begun. Originally, the patient's expirations were passed through a soda-lime canister via a one-way circle system. Experience has now been gained with the deliberate addition of 2 per cent carbon dioxide to the oxygen in the chamber for patients with cerebral tumours (where the cerebral vasoconstriction produced by high pressure oxygen would tend to undo the benefits), and with conscious patients in the chamber. As a result the use of the canister has been stopped without any ill effects occurring.

Design of High Pressure Chambers (Figs. 1*a–e*)

Essentially there are three types of chamber available:

(*a*) *Portable.*—These require maximum lightness and portability. The presently available commercial models weigh less than 300 pounds and can be folded to a length of three feet for transportation.

(*b*) *Small personal chamber.*—These are eminently suitable for treatment of a single patient with attendants outside as in radiotherapy (Fig. 1*b*).

(*c*) *Large multiple chamber.*—At present the most promising design is the triple chamber incorporating a large central container with facilities for surgery, together with two smaller associated chambers. This system provides maximum efficiency and adaptability of use. The patient and attendants first enter one of the smaller chambers where air compression is achieved. If necessary the team can then move to the larger chamber for specific therapy or surgery. Finally the team can pass to the second small chamber for decompression. In this manner it is possible to treat three different patients at any one time with the greatest possible flexibility. Though all three chambers are filled with air the patient can receive oxygen or an anaesthetic mixture as soon as the required atmospheric pressure has been achieved.

Requirements of a Pressure Chamber

The following control systems are of principal importance in the satisfactory maintainance of a hyperbaric chamber.

(*a*) *Compressed air pump.*—Ideally there should be two. One large pump for rapid compression and a smaller one for maintaining adequate ventilation of the chamber once the requisite pressure has been reached. Experience has shown that these compressors must be oil free i.e. the pistons are sealed for lubrication or do not require oil for lubrication. A steady increase in pressure is necessary to reduce the painful effects of pressure changes on such semi-closed air cavities as the various sinuses in the skull and the middle ear. However, recent investigations have shown that there is a large personal element in this matter and a steady rise of pressure *per se* is not capable of eliminating the incidence (Foster and Churchill-Davidson, 1963).

(*b*) *Climate control.*—Provision must be made for heating, cooling and humidification of the air in the chamber. There is a rise in temperature within the chamber on compression and a fall on decompression.

(*c*) *Electrical equipment* must be spark-proof.

(*d*) *Anaesthetic gases and oxygen* are best administered from cylinders stored within the chamber with facilities for the spent gases to be vented.

(*e*) *Sterile instruments etc.* should be available through a subsidiary compartment.

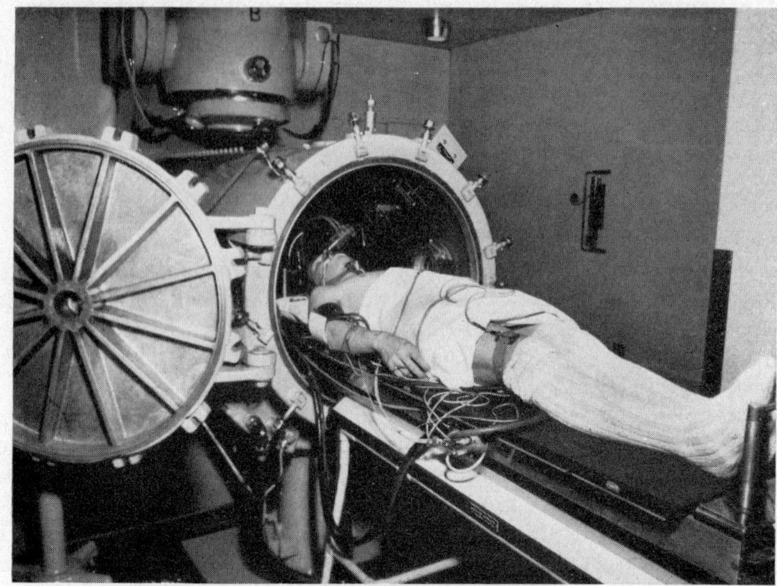

6/Fig. 1(*a*).

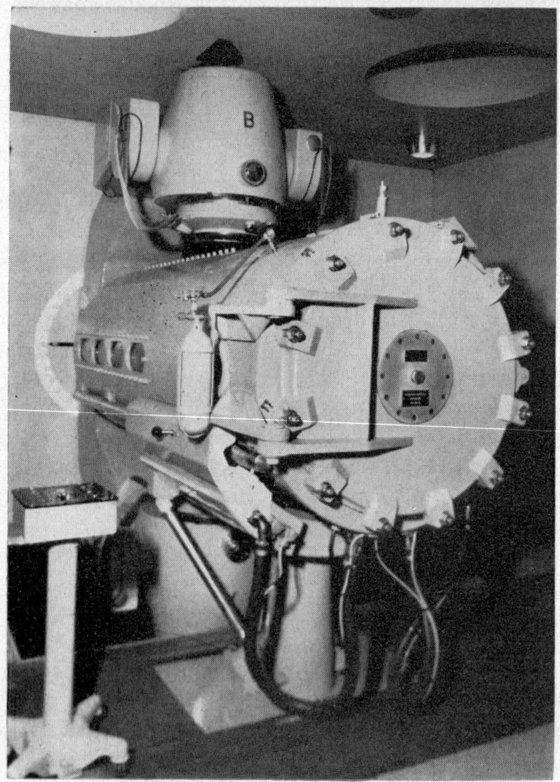

6/Fig. 1(*b*).

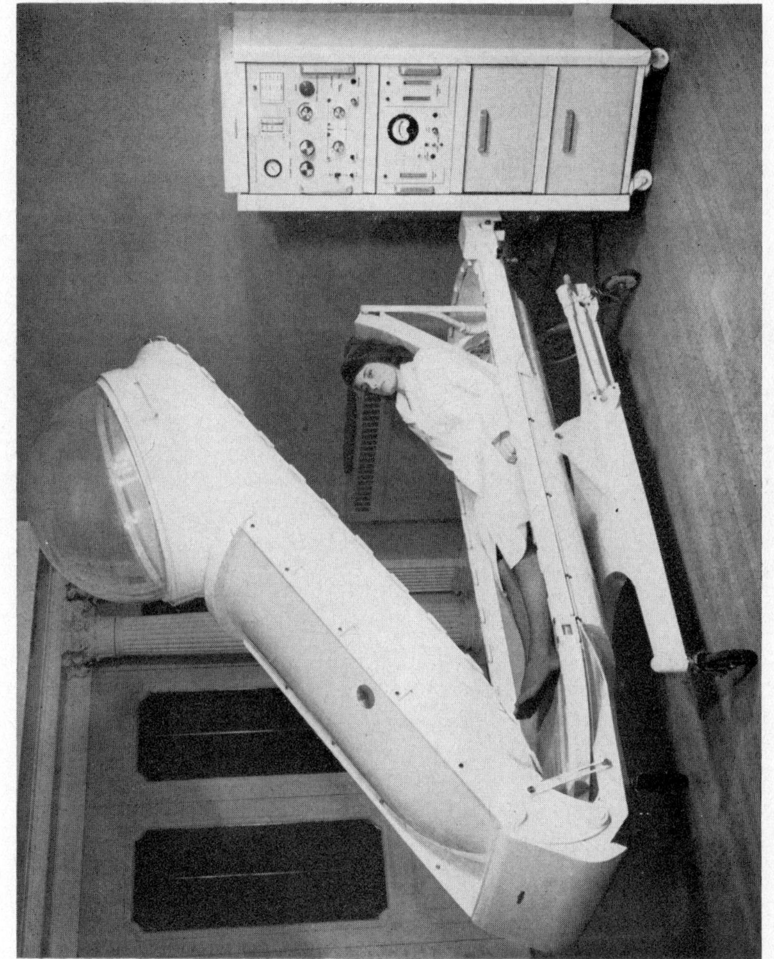

6/Fig. 1(*c*).

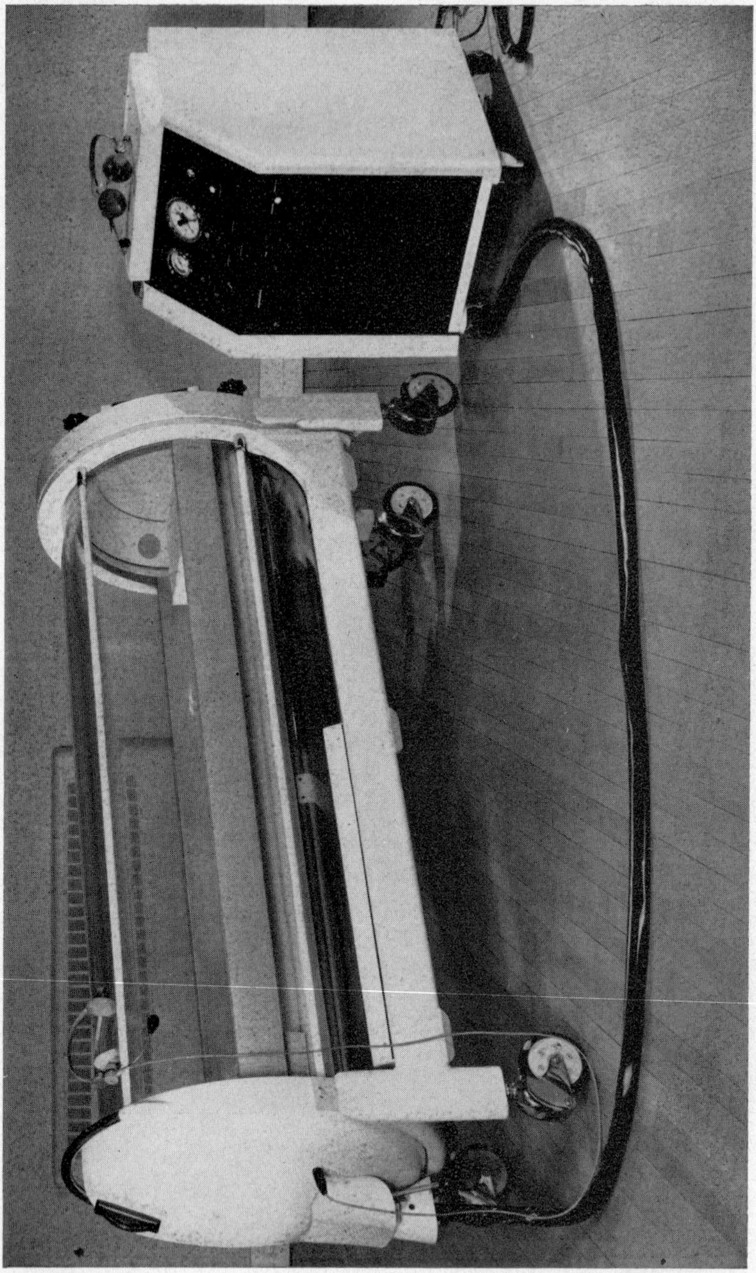

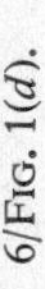

6/FIG. 1(*d*).

6/FIG. 1(*e*).

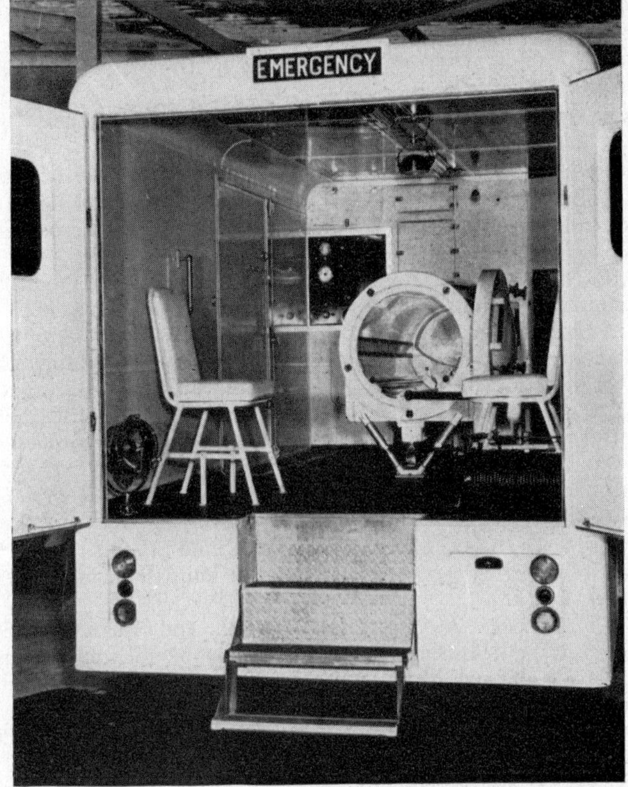

6/FIG. 1.—CHAMBERS FOR HYPERBARIC OXYGEN THERAPY

(*a*) and (*b*) General anaesthesia for radiotherapy with hyperbaric oxygenation.

(*c*) Reclining pressure chamber for patients requiring hyperbaric oxygen therapy in the sitting position. The oxygen is re-circulated through a semi-closed system with carbon dioxide absorption. Maximum working pressure is 2 atmospheres absolute.

(*d*) Horizontal chamber. The model designed for radiotherapy uses fresh oxygen supply to keep down the carbon dioxide level of the chamber and has a maximum working pressure of 4 atmospheres. The general purpose model uses re-circulation and carbon dioxide absorption; it has a maximum working pressure of 3 atmospheres absolute.

(*e*) Mobile emergency chamber. This is used for resuscitation, as in carbon monoxide poisoning, and has a maximum working pressure of 3 atmospheres absolute.

REFERENCES

ACKERMAN, J. W. R., and BARNARD, D. N. (1966). Successful storage of kidneys. *Brit. J. Surg.*, **53**, 525.

BRUMMELKAMP, W. H., BOEREMA, I., and HOOGENDYK, L. (1963). Treatment of clostridial infections with hyperbaric oxygen drenching. (A report of 26 cases). *Lancet*, **1**, 235.

CARPENTER, P. G. (1955). "Inert gas narcosis". In *Proceedings of the Underwater Physiology Symposium*, p. 377. (Ed. C. G. Goff). (Nat. Research Counc. Publ.). Washington, D.C.: Nat. Acad. of Sciences.

CHURCHILL-DAVIDSON, I., SANGER, C., and THOMLINSON, R. H. (1955). High-pressure oxygen and radiotherapy. *Lancet*, **1**, 1091.

CUNNINGHAM, O. J. (1927). Oxygen therapy by compressed air. *Curr. Res. Anesth.*, **6**, 64.

DAVIDSON, J. K. (1964). Radiology in decompression sickness: the Clyde tunnel. *Scot. med. J.*, **9**, 1.

DONALD, K. W. (1947). Oxygen poisoning in man. *Brit. med. J.*, **1**, 667–712.

FISHER, A. B., HYDE, R. W., PUY, R. J. M., CLARK, J. M., and LAMBERTSEN, C. J. (1968). Effect of oxygen at 2 atmospheres on the pulmonary mechanics of normal man. *J. appl. Physiol.*, **24**, 529.

FOSTER, C. A., and CHURCHILL-DAVIDSON, I. (1963). Response to high pressure oxygen of conscious volunteers and patients. *J. appl. Physiol.*, **18**, 492.

GRAY, L. H., CONGER, A. D., EBERT, M., HORNSEY, S., and SCOTT, O. C. A. (1953). The concentration of oxygen dissolved in tissues at the time of irradiation as a factor in radiotherapy. *Brit. J. Radiol.*, **26**, 638.

HARP, J. R., GUTSCHE, B. B., and STEPHEN, C. R. (1966). Effect of anaesthetics on central nervous system toxicity of hyperbaric oxygen. *Anesthesiology*, **27**, 608.

HAUGAARD, N., NESS, M. E., and ITSLEVITS, H. (1959). The toxic action of oxygen on glucose and pyruvate oxidation in heart homogenates. *J. biol. Chem.*, **227**, 605.

HENKIND, P. (1964). Hyperbaric oxygen and corneal revascularisation. *Lancet*, **2**, 836.

HUTCHISON, J. H., KERR, M. M., INALL, J. A., and SHANKS, R. A. (1966). Controlled trials of hyperbaric oxygen and tracheal intubation in asphyxia neonatorum. *Lancet*, **1**, 935.

IRVIN, T. T., NORMAN, J. N., SUGWANAGUL, A., and SMITH, G. (1966). Hyperbaric oxygen in the treatment of infections by aerobic microorganisms. *Lancet*, **1**, 392.

KAUFMAN, W. C., and MORGARGER, J. P. (1956). Pressure breathing: functional circulatory changes in dogs. *J. appl. Physiol.*, **9**, 33.

LAMBERTSEN, C. J. (1961). "Harmful effects of oxygen". In: *Medical Physiology*, p. 710, 11th edit. (Ed. P. Bard). St. Louis: C. V. Mosby Co.

LAWSON, D. D., MCALLISTER, R. A., and SMITH, G. (1961). Treatment of acute experimental carbon monoxide poisoning with oxygen under pressure. *Lancet*, **1**, 800.

LEDINGHAM, I. MCA., and DAVIDSON, J. A. (1968). Hazards in hyperbaric medicine. *Brit. J. Anaesth.*, **41**, 324.

MCCALLUM, R. I. (1968). Decompression sickness: a review. *Brit. J. industr. Med.*, **25**, 4.

MCDOWELL, D. G., LEDINGHAM, I. MCA., JACOBSON, I., and NORMAN, J. M. (1965). Oxygen administration by mask in a pressure chamber. *Anesthesiology*, **26**, 720.

PERRIN, D. J. D. (1966). Hyperbaric oxygenation of skin flaps. *Brit. J. plast. Surg.*, **19**, 110.

POULTON, E. C., CARPENTER, A., and COTTON, M. J. (1963). Mild nitrogen narcosis. *Brit. med. J.*, **2**, 1450.

SALTZMAN, H. A., HART, L., SIEKER, H. O., and DUFFY, E. J. (1964). Retinal vascular response to hyperbaric oxygenation. *J. Amer. med. Ass.*, **188**, 450.

SANGER, C., CHURCHILL-DAVIDSON, I., and THOMLINSON, R. H. (1955). Anaesthesia for radiotherapy under high-pressure oxygen. *Brit. J. Anaesth.*, **27**, 436.

SEVERINGHAUS, J. W. (1959). "Respiration and hypothermia". In: *Hypothermia*, p. 384–94. *Ann. N.Y. Acad. Sci.*, **80**, Art 2. pp. 285–550.

SHARP, G. R., LEDINGHAM, I. MCA., and NORMAN, J. N. (1962). The application of oxygen at two atmospheres pressure in the treatment of acute anoxia. *Anaesthesia*, **17**, 136.

SLACK, W. K., HANSON, G. C., and CHEW, H. E. R. (1969). Hyperbaric oxygen in the treatment of gas gangrene and clostridial infection. *Brit. J. Surg.*, **56**, 505.

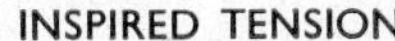

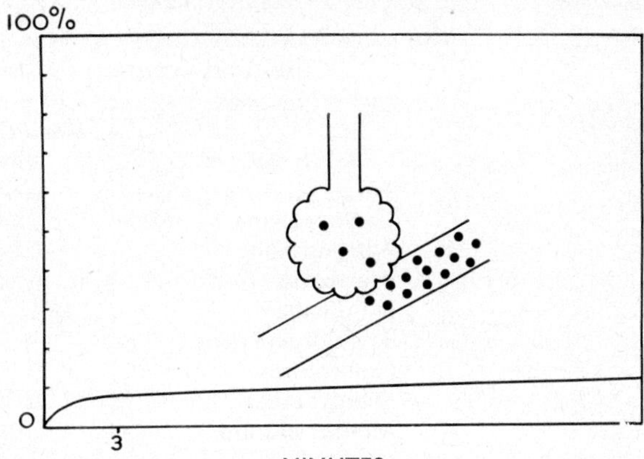

7/Fig. 3.—Alveolar tension curve of a gas which has a high solubility in blood, i.e. ether.

solubility only a small quantity is absorbed, the alveolar concentration therefore rises rapidly so that the tension of the gas is also quickly increased (Fig. 2*b*). As the brain has a rich blood supply the cerebral tension mounts equally rapidly, so that unconsciousness soon supervenes. On withdrawal of the anaesthetic agent the reverse process takes place and recovery is rapid.

Conversely, if a gas or vapour has a *high* blood solubility, then large amounts can be absorbed just as though the blood were like a piece of blotting paper, so that it is difficult for the alveolar concentration to rise (Fig. 3). As the concentration in the alveolus remains low, the tension in the blood also is low so that induction of anaesthesia is slow. The anaesthetist learns to partially compensate for this difficulty by giving a very high inspired concentration on induction, which if continued indefinitely would rapidly prove lethal. Ether is an example of an anaesthetic agent with a high blood solubility. Clinically, it is administered in high concentration at the outset of anaesthesia and then gradually reduced once a satisfactory level of surgical anaesthesia has been achieved. However, if this latter concentration was used from the start it would take many hours to anaesthetise the patient! Unfortunately, there is no such clinical dodge that can be used to speed recovery, because it is impossible to reduce the alveolar concentration below zero.

The solubility coefficients for a variety of anaesthetic gases are listed in detail in Table 1. A knowledge of these figures will immediately reveal to the reader whether a particular agent produces a rapid or slow induction and, furthermore, whether recovery would be fast or prolonged.

Another practical implication of the blood solubility coefficient values is that an agent in which the blood tension—and hence the brain and myocardial tension—can only rise slowly (i.e. one with a high blood solubility, like ether) has clearly the greatest safety margin in the hands of the inexperienced.

3. **Blood flow.**—The greater the flow of blood through the lungs, the more anaesthetic agent it will be able to remove from the alveolus. Thus, an increase in cardiac output means a greater amount of anaesthetic vapour is removed from the alveolus and there is, therefore, a *fall* in the alveolar concentration. This

7/Table 1

Values of Partition Coefficients in Blood of the Common Anaesthetic Agents

Agent	*Blood/Gas solubility Coefficient*
Cyclopropane	0·42
Nitrous oxide	0·47
Fluroxene	1·37
Halothane	2·36
Trichloroethylene	9·15
Chloroform	10·3
Diethyl ether	12·1
Methoxyflurane	13·0

(Eger and Larsen, 1964)

means that the blood and tissue tension also fall, so that the plane of anaesthesia will lighten or induction will take longer. Conversely, if the cardiac output is *reduced* the alveolar tension will rise, so that there is an increase in the depth of anaesthesia.

(D). **The Tissues**

The uptake of an anaesthetic agent by the tissues depends on virtually the same factors as those already described for blood, namely—the tension gradient between the circulation and the tissues, the solubility of the agent in a particular organ and finally the blood flow.

1. **Tissue tension gradient.**—This depends primarily on the tension of the agent in the arterial blood and therefore directly on the alveolar concentration. Once equilibrium in tension between the blood and the tissues has been reached (i.e. the point of saturation) then no further uptake can occur in these organs.

2. **Tissue/blood solubility.**—Another factor of importance is the solubility of the agent in the tissues themselves. Fortunately most inhalational anaesthetic agents have approximately the same solubility in the principal tissues as they do in blood; thus, for most of them the coefficient of tissue/blood solubility is in the region of 1·0 (see Table 2). There is, however, one principal exception—halothane. With this agent the solubility in brain and muscle is some three times greater than that in blood. This means that these organs have a remarkable capacity for removing halothane from the circulation.

Fatty tissue.—A mass of tissue of particular importance is the adipose depots throughout the body. Although these areas receive only a small percentage of the cardiac output, fatty tissue has a special affinity for most inhalational agents because they are all extremely lipid soluble. It will be observed that the solubility coefficient of halothane in human fat is 60 (see Table 2), as opposed to only 1·6 for kidney tissue. This remarkable capacity of fat to remove anaesthetic agents from the circulation means that this tissue comprises a vast storage potential. Unfortunately, though there is abundant data available on the solubility of the

7/TABLE 2

PARTITION COEFFICIENTS OF SOME INHALATIONAL ANAESTHETICS AT 37° C ± 0·5° C

Agent	*Blood/Gas*	*Tissue/Blood*
Cyclopropane	0·42	1·34 (brain) 0·81 (muscle)
Nitrous oxide	0·47	1·0 (lung) 1·06 (brain) 1·13 (heart)
Fluroxene	1·37	1·44 (brain)
Halothane	2·36	1·6 (kidney) 2·6 (brain) 2·6 (liver) 3·5 (muscle) 60·0 (fat)
Chloroform	10·3	1·0 (heart) 1·0 (brain)
Diethyl ether	12·1	1·2 (lung) 1·14 (brain)
Methoxyflurane	13·0	1·34 (muscle) 1·70 (brain—grey) 2·34 (brain—white)

(After Eger and Larsen, 1964)

various anaesthetic agents in olive oil, there is little information available for human fat.

3. **Blood flow.**—This represents one of the most important factors in determining the uptake of a particular anaesthetic agent by the tissues. For this reason, Eger (1964) has divided the various tissues into four groups depending principally on their blood supply. The *vessel-rich* group (VRG) comprises the principal organs of the body such as the brain, heart, liver and kidney. These organs receive some 70–75 per cent of the total cardiac output and therefore the tension of the anaesthetic agent will rise rapidly in these structures. The *intermediate* group is represented mainly by skeletal muscle and skin. The *fat* group comprises the adipose tissue throughout the body. And finally the *vessel-poor* group is made up of such relatively non-vascular structures as ligaments, tendons, and cancellous bone. To all intents and purposes these structures play no part in the uptake of anaesthetic agents. An example of the average percentage of the total cardiac output received by the various tissues is shown in Table 3.

7/TABLE 3

Group	*Region*	*Mass in kg.*	*Per cent Cardiac output*
Vessel-rich	Brain	1·4	14
	Liver (splanchnic)	2·6	28
	Heart	0·3	5
	Kidney	0·3	23
Intermediate	Muscle	31·0	16
	Skin	3·6	8
Fat	Adipose tissue	12·5	6
Vessel-poor	Residual tissue	11·3	Nil
Total	—	63·0	100

(After Bard, 1961)

A study of the uptake of a relatively insoluble agent may help to emphasise the importance of blood flow. For example, with nitrous oxide (Fig. 4) the bulk of the initial uptake is undertaken by those organs with a large blood supply (VRG). Equilibrium between the tension in the alveolus and in the vessel-rich

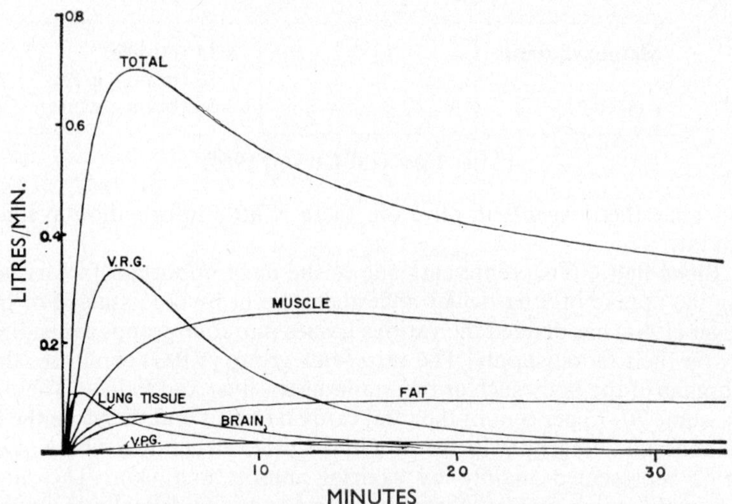

7/FIG. 4.—Tissue uptake of an insoluble anaesthetic—nitrous oxide.

group (e.g. brain) is achieved in about ten minutes. After this the importance of the intermediate group (e.g. muscle) becomes obvious and these structures soon are responsible for a large proportion of the total anaesthetic uptake in the succeeding minutes. In time, even these organs come to reach equilibrium with the alveolar concentration so that finally the task of further uptake falls on the fatty tissues. The fat depots, owing to their high lipoid content have a special affinity for anaesthetic agents so that they can continue to remove the molecules from the circulation for many hours. In fact, with an agent such as halothane it may be a matter of days before complete saturation of these tissues is finally reached. Even then, minute losses would still occur through organs such as the skin, so that the venous blood tension would always be slightly lower than the alveolar tension and a steady but minimal uptake would continue.

The whole process of uptake of any anaesthetic agent is most often expressed as a simple diagram based on the original curve described by Kety (1950) (Fig. 5).

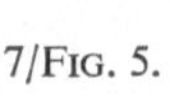

7/Fig. 5.

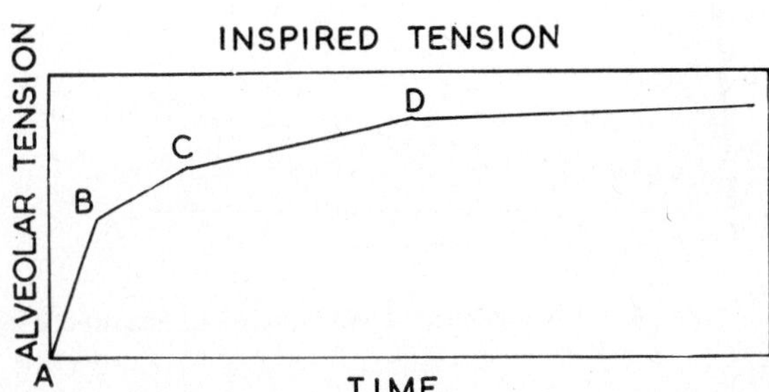

During the time of AB, ventilation is bringing fresh anaesthetic gas or vapour into the alveoli faster than it is being removed by the circulation. Point B represents the moment at which input due to ventilation is balanced by output due to absorption into blood. The period BC then represents the time taken for equilibrium between alveolar and tissue tension to be reached in the vessel-rich group. At point C this is finally achieved. The period CD then illustrates the continually decreasing uptake by muscle until finally from point D onwards the uptake by fat is the only consideration. Occasionally points B, C, and D are referred to as "knees" of the curve.

Additional Factors

1. **Variation in solubility of the agents.**—The fact that some agents are more soluble in blood than others has already been discussed. This will have an important bearing on the alveolar concentration so that the curve will vary considerably with the individual agent. The influence of solubility is illustrated in Fig. 6. For example, cyclopropane with a blood/gas solubility coefficient of 0·42 rises to a higher alveolar concentration far more rapidly than halothane with a solubility coefficient of 2·36. Similarly, ether with a coefficient of 12·1 rises more slowly than halothane. Clinically, anaesthetics with a high solubility in blood give a slow induction and a slow recovery, whereas the reverse is true for those agents with a low solubility.

2. **The concentration effect.**—It has already been pointed out that nitrous oxide and cyclopropane have approximately the same solubility coefficient in blood (e.g. cyclopropane = 0·42; nitrous oxide = 0·47). From this it might be

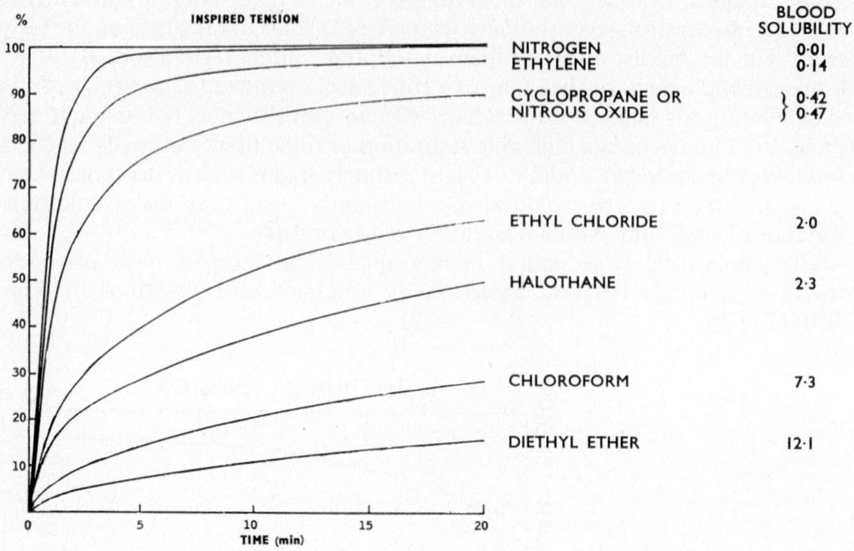

7/FIG. 6.—The influence of solubility of an anaesthetic agent on alveolar concentration.

anticipated that these two agents would have almost identical alveolar concentration curves. This is not the case. The reason for this difference is that nitrous oxide is administered at a much higher *concentration* than cyclopropane. This is the concentration effect (Eger, 1963).

The importance of the concentration effect is that if an anaesthetic is administered in a high concentration then the alveolar concentration will rise much more rapidly (towards the inspired concentration) than it would if it were given in a low concentration (Fig. 7). Hence there is a different curve for each concentration. This can perhaps be understood best by considering a mythical closed lung filled with 100 per cent of an anaesthetic agent. Under these conditions the alveolar concentration curves are the same for all agents. No matter how much or how little gas is removed by the circulation the concentration in the lung must remain at 100 per cent even though the lung gets smaller. If, however, this lung is filled with only 80 per cent of the anaesthetic gas and the remaining 20 per cent is a diluent gas, then as the anaesthetic agent is absorbed so the proportion must be altered as the concentration of the diluent gas remains the same. In other words, the diluent gas comes to represent a greater proportion of the whole and the concentration of the anaesthetic gas will fall. The rate and amount of this fall will depend largely on how soluble the particular anaesthetic agent is in blood.

Clinically, the concentration effect is best seen in anaesthetic gases with a high blood solubility when they are used over a wide range of concentration. Fluroxene and ether are highly soluble agents and therefore the concentration effect can easily be observed. Nitrous oxide and cyclopropane are relatively insoluble but can be used over a wide range of concentrations so that this effect is observed to a lesser degree. Halothane and methoxyflurane, on the other hand, which are

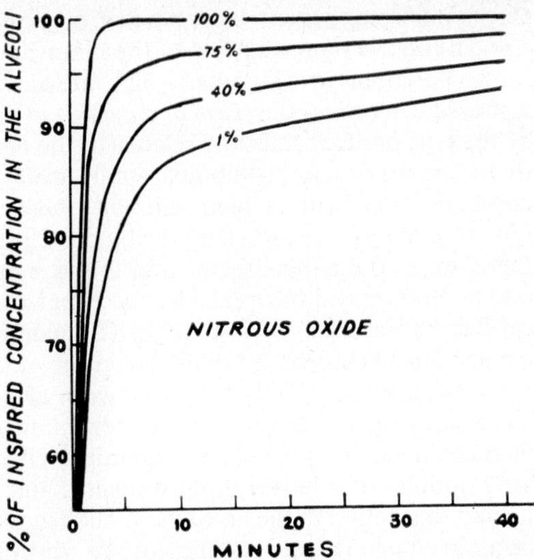

7/Fig. 7.—The Concentration Effect.

This diagram illustrates that the higher the concentration of an anaesthetic agent the more rapidly the alveolar concentration approaches to that inspired.

seldom used in high concentrations, do not exhibit this phenomenon to any marked degree.

3. **Diffusion hypoxia** (also called the Fink phenomenon) in essence is the reverse of the concentration effect. At the end of an anaesthetic when the mask is withdrawn the patient breathes room air. The alveoli will soon become filled with a mixture of nitrogen, oxygen, carbon dioxide and water vapour. Nevertheless, there is still an appreciable quantity of nitrous oxide dissolved in the circulation and tissues. Though nitrous oxide is always referred to as an insoluble anaesthetic agent it is some 34 more times soluble than nitrogen. This means that blood can carry that much more nitrous oxide than it can nitrogen. Thus during the first few minutes of breathing room air large quantities of nitrous oxide leave the body. In fact breathing a 75:25 per cent mixture of nitrous oxide and oxygen as much as 1500 ml. of nitrous oxide may be expired in the first minute, 1200 ml. in the second and 1000 ml. during the third. The net result of this exodus is that the volume of expiration exceeds that of inspiration, so that more carbon dioxide is carried out than usual. This lowers the carbon dioxide tension of the blood, reduces the stimulus to respiration and brings about a depression of ventilation.

The other and even more important effect of this mass movement of nitrous oxide into the alveoli is that it dilutes the concentration of oxygen present. Normally in the alveoli there is approximately 14 per cent oxygen, but under these conditions the oxygen content may drop to as low as 10 per cent, with the result that some hypoxia may ensue.

Clinically, diffusion hypoxia is only significant when nitrous oxide is employed as the anaesthetic agent, because this is the only anaesthetic agent that is commonly used in high concentrations. The effect is only likely to persist in a rapidly diminishing manner for the first ten minutes after the end of a nitrous oxide anaesthetic. In the presence of normal ventilation at the close of an anaesthetic then diffusion hypoxia is of little significance, but in the presence of depressed ventilation it develops an increasing importance. The adverse effects of this hypoxia can largely be prevented by permitting the patient to breathe pure oxygen for five minutes prior to the removal of the anaesthetic face-piece.

4. **Variations in ventilation.**—The rate at which a high tension in the blood is achieved determines the *speed of induction* of anaesthesia, whereas it is the height of the tension itself which is related to the *depth* of the anaesthesia. An anaesthetic agent with a low solubility rapidly achieves a high tension in the blood, and conversely one with a high solubility takes a long time even though large quantities may be absorbed by the blood. The alveolar tension or concentration, therefore, is the critical factor and this is a balance between input from ventilation and removal or uptake by the circulation. If ventilation is increased and cardiac output remains unchanged (Yamamura *et al.*, 1963) then the alveolar tension must be raised. With nitrous oxide or cyclopropane, which are relatively insoluble agents, a high tension between alveolus and the circulating blood is established rapidly during the first few minutes of induction, so that any later increase in ventilation will have a minimal effect. Ether and halothane, however, are examples of relatively soluble agents and the tension in the blood lags far behind that found in the alveolus. A sudden increase in ventilation, such as may occur in changing from spontaneous to controlled respiration, will lead to a rise in both alveolar and arterial blood tension. Figure 8*a* demonstrates the different effect of ventilation at 2, 4 and 8 litres per minute (Eger, 1964). Thus, with ether anaesthesia an increase in ventilation from 2 litres/min. to 8 litres/min. will lead to a three-fold increase in alveolar tension and with halothane under similar circumstances to a two-fold increase. This emphasises that with a soluble anaesthetic agent a sudden *increase* in ventilation may create a profound and potentially dangerous increase in depth of anaesthesia (Eger, 1964).

5. **Variations in cardiac output.**—The more soluble the anaesthetic gas or vapour the greater will be the effect of changes in cardiac output on alveolar concentration. The alveolar tension (less the venous blood tension) tends to drive the anaesthetic vapour into the circulation. Thus an *increase* in cardiac output means a greater amount of anaesthetic vapour is removed from the alveolus and there is a *fall* in alveolar tension. Conversely, if the cardiac output is *reduced* there is a rise in alveolar tension and this will lead to an increase in depth of anaesthesia. Figure 8*b* demonstrates the effect of different cardiac outputs of 2, 6 and 18 litres/min. with nitrous oxide, ether and halothane (Eger, 1964).

Decreasing the cardiac output from 18 to 2 litres per minute produces little change with an insoluble anaesthetic agent such as nitrous oxide or cyclopropane. However, a similar decrease under ether or halothane anaesthesia may lead to a three-fold and a two-fold increase respectively in alveolar concentration. Clinically, in a patient with a high cardiac output, as, for example, an extremely nervous or a thyrotoxic patient, the induction of anaesthesia will take longer than usual if a soluble anaesthetic such as ether is used. Conversely, if there is a low cardiac output, as in haemorrhage or mitral stenosis, the rate of induction of anaesthesia may be greatly increased.

To summarise:

INCREASE IN VENTILATION }
DECREASE IN CARDIAC OUTPUT } . . . INCREASE in Depth of Anaesthesia

Thus, if a patient is breathing spontaneously under halothane anaesthesia and the anaesthetist suddenly decides to institute controlled respiration, there may be a rapid increase in the depth of anaesthesia. This will be caused by increased ventilation and a reduction in cardiac output, the last possibly being accentuated by a fall in arterial $P_{\bar{C}O_2}$ (Prys-Roberts *et al.*, 1967).

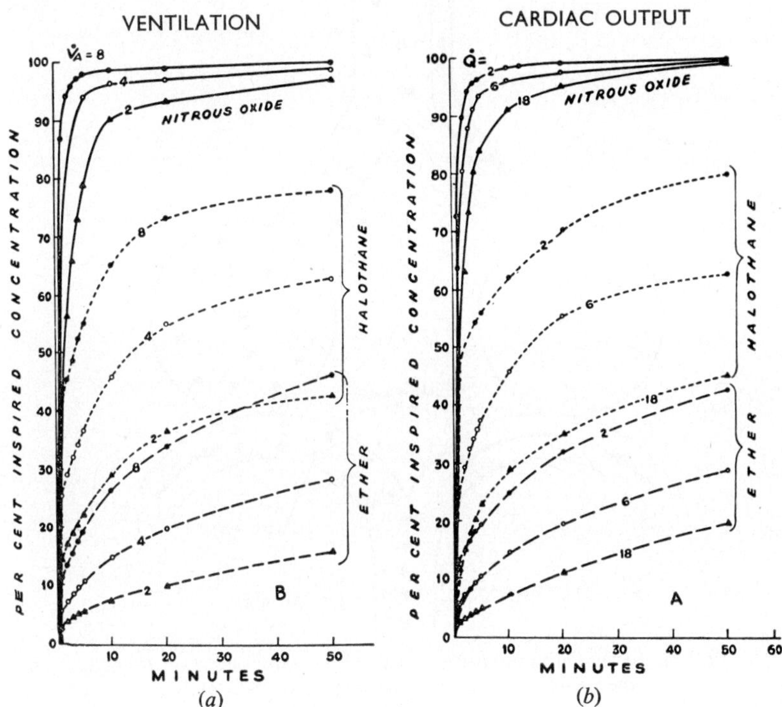

7/FIG. 8.—Effect of variations in cardiac output and ventilation on uptake and distribution of anaesthetic agents.

(*a*) Changes in alveolar concentration in relation to alteration of ventilation (2, 4, 8 litres per minute).

(*b*) Effect of variations of cardiac output on alveolar concentration (2, 6 and 18 litres per minute).

6. **Right to left shunts and variations in ventilation-perfusion ratio.**—Any right to left shunt due to a heart defect means that a proportion of the cardiac output does not go through the lungs. The same situation occurs in an emphysematous patient with large numbers of alveoli which are perfused but not ventilated, whilst others may be ventilated but not perfused. There is therefore an alteration in the ventilation-perfusion ratio. This situation also occurs to some extent in normal patients undergoing general anaesthesia (see p. 166 *et seq.*).

Another example of the effects of an alteration in ventilation-perfusion ratio can be seen when the anaesthetist places an endobronchial blocker in the main bronchus of one lung during thoracic anaesthesia. The remaining lung will receive double its normal ventilation, whilst the affected lung will be perfused yet will receive no anaesthetic vapour from the alveoli (Fig. 9).

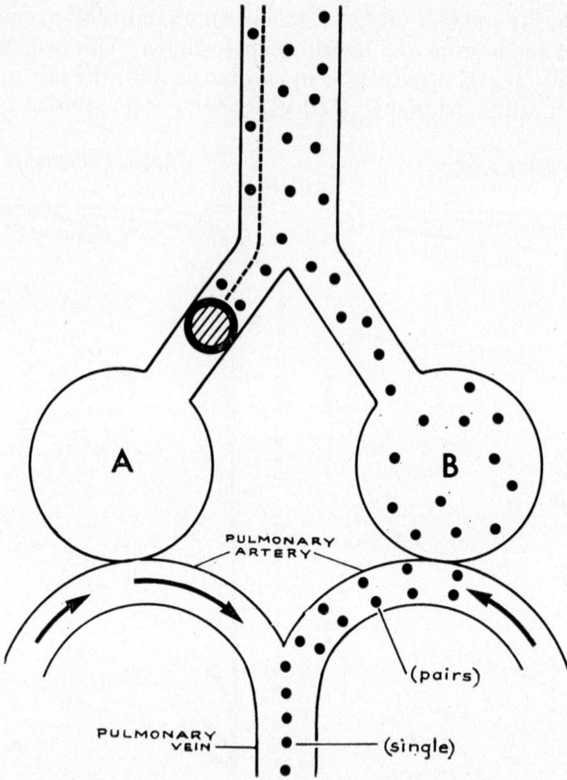

7/FIG. 9.—Effect on the ventilation/perfusion ratio of blocking one main bronchus. The dots represent molecules of anaesthetic gas. (See text).

Blood passing along the pulmonary artery to Lung B will pick up molecules of the anaesthetic vapour in the capillaries, but on draining into the pulmonary vein the tension of the anaesthetic vapour in this blood is *diluted* to half by blood coming from the non-ventilated Lung A. This dilution effect is much more significant when an insoluble anaesthetic agent is used. To appreciate this point it is necessary to consider the tensions of anaesthetic agents in both alveoli and the circulation when (*a*) a *soluble* and (*b*) an *insoluble* agent is used (Fig. 10).

Before one main bronchus is obstructed the assumption is made that equilibrium exists between alveolar and blood tension so that the pulmonary vein contains blood with a tension of 10 mm. Hg. When the bronchus is blocked, then the ventilation to the remaining lung is doubled. If a soluble anaesthetic agent is used then the increased ventilation will lead to a doubling of the alveolar tension to 20 mm. Hg. This increased tension is reflected in the blood in the pulmonary capillaries but on reaching the pulmonary vein it comes in contact with blood without any anaesthetic tension, so that the dilution effect reduces the tension to the original 10 mm. Hg. In fact, blocking the bronchus has made no change in the tension of the anaesthetic agent in the mixed blood of the pulmonary vein. On the other hand, if an insoluble anaesthetic agent is used then doubling the

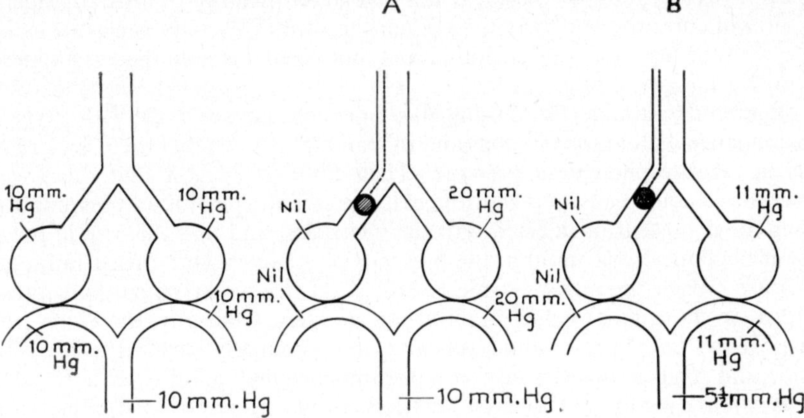

7/FIG. 10.—**Diagram** to show different anaesthetic tensions with (*A*) soluble agent, (*B*) insoluble agent.

ventilation to one lung does not appreciably alter the tension (see Variations in ventilation, p. 276), so that only a small rise results. In this case, therefore, the dilution effect produces a profound reduction of the anaesthetic tension.

7. **Variations in body temperature.**—As a general rule the solubility of a gas in blood increases as the temperature falls (Fig. 11).

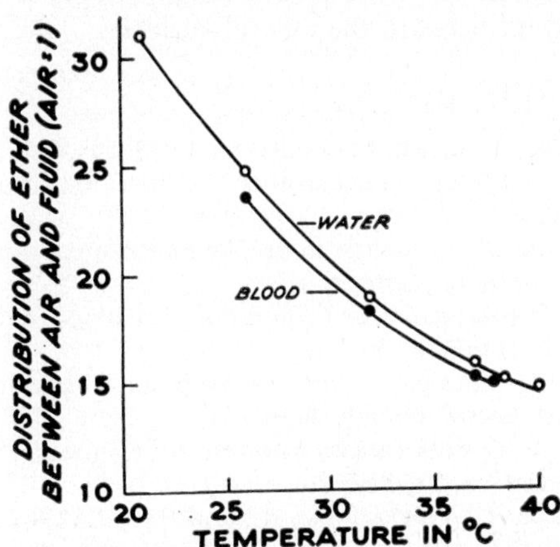

7/FIG. 11.—The effect of temperature change on the solubility of ether in blood and water.

It might quite naturally be assumed, therefore, that as the body temperature falls during hypothermia so more anaesthetic agent would be taken up by the body and the depth of anaesthesia increased. This is borne out in clinical practice because the lower the body temperature falls, the less anaesthetic the patient requires.

Effect of Anaesthetic Agents on Air in Closed Body Cavities

Under normal circumstances, with the exception of the lungs, the sinuses and the intestines, there is no air in the various body cavities. However, during a pneumoencephalogram air is introduced into the ventricles of the brain, in a pneumothorax it is placed in the pleural cavity, and in acute intestinal obstruction it accumulates in the lumen of the intestine. If such patients are anaesthetised with nitrous oxide and oxygen (75:25 per cent) then the gas will rapidly enter the enclosed space and the volume will increase. The reason for this is that nitrous oxide is thirty-four times more soluble than nitrogen in blood. Thus because the partial pressure of a gas in the blood and in a body cavity must be the same, a much larger quantity of nitrous oxide than of air will enter the body cavities. When the wall of a cavity is elastic, as is the case with the intestines, distension occurs, but when it is rigid there is an increase in pressure (Eger, 1965).

Eger and Saidman (1965) using 70–75 per cent nitrous oxide with oxygen for pneumoencephalography in dogs and in man have shown that there is a dramatic rise in cerebrospinal fluid pressure. Their findings suggest that this form of anaesthesia could cause a serious increase in cerebrospinal fluid pressure if used when air is present or injected into the ventricles, and that this rise in pressure might be clinically harmful in the presence of a pre-existing raised intracranial pressure. When the nitrous oxide is turned off the cerebrospinal fluid pressure returns to its original value in about ten minutes. Clinically, therefore, on the basis of this evidence it would appear to be potentially harmful to use nitrous oxide and oxygen anaesthesia for a pneumoencephalogram if air is to be used as the filling medium. However, this risk would be removed if either nitrous oxide or oxygen were used to outline the ventricles. Similarly, in artificially induced intestinal obstruction in dogs the same process occurs, but the changes are slower. The volume doubles in two hours and triples in four hours. This increase in volume may contribute to the surgeon's difficulty in closing the peritoneal cavity in the presence of distended bowel. Similar problems occur when a pneumothorax, pneumoperitoneum or pneumopericardium are present, or when air is trapped in the respiratory tract, e.g. in an isolated air cyst or bulla. The rate at which pleural gas expands is fifteen times more rapid than that of gas in the bowel, a fact which may be due to the good pleural blood supply and the direct diffusion of gas from the alveoli beneath the pleural surfaces.

REFERENCES

BARD, P. (1961). *Medical Physiology*, p. 240, 11th edit. St. Louis: C. V. Mosby Co.

EGER, E. I. (II) (1963). Effect of inspired anaesthetic concentration on the rate of rise of alveolar concentration. *Anesthesiology*, **24**, 153.

EGER, E. I. (II) (1964). Respiratory and circulatory factors in uptake and distribution of volatile anaesthetic agents. *Brit. J. Anaesth.*, **36**, 155.

EGER, E. I. (II), and LARSON, C. P., Jr. (1964). Anaesthetic solubility in blood and tissues: values and significance. *Brit. J. Anaesth.*, **36**, 140.

EGER, E. I. (II), and SAIDMAN, L. J. (1965). Hazards of nitrous oxide anesthesia in bowel obstruction and pneumothorax. *Anesthesiology*, **26**, 61.

KETY, S. S. (1950). The physiological and physical factors governing the uptake of anesthetic gases by the body. *Anesthesiology*, **11**, 517.

PRYS-ROBERTS, C., KELMAN, G. R., KAIN, M. L., GREENBAUM, R., and BAY, J. (1967). Cardiac output and blood carbon dioxide levels during halothane anaesthesia in man. *Brit. J. Anaesth.*, **39**, 687.

YAMAMURA, H., WAKASUGI, B., OKUMA, Y., and MAKI, K. (1963). The effects of ventilation on the absorption and elimination of inhalational anaesthetics. *Anaesthesia*, **18**, 427.

FURTHER READING

Symposium on Pharmacokinetics of Inhalation Anaesthetic Agents (1964). *Brit. J. Anaesth.* (No. 3), **36.**

PAPPER, E. M., and KITZ, R. J., Eds. (1962). *Uptake and Distribution of Anesthetic Agents.* New York: McGraw-Hill.

Chapter 8

THE ANAESTHETIC GASES

NITROUS OXIDE (N_2O)

NITROUS oxide was first prepared by Priestley in 1772, and its anaesthetic properties were first demonstrated by Sir Humphrey Davy in 1800. It was not until 1844, however, that it came to be used in clinical practice. In that year Gardner Quincy Colton, a lecturer in chemistry, gave a demonstration of the effects of inhaling nitrous oxide at Hartford, Connecticut. Amongst his audience was Horace Wells, a local dentist, who was so impressed that he persuaded Colton to give him some nitrous oxide the following day for extraction of a tooth. The procedure was completely painless. Later that year Wells gave a demonstration of the technique at Harvard Medical School, but the patient complained of pain and Wells was dubbed a fraud. The introduction of ether soon afterwards delayed a full appreciation of nitrous oxide until nearly twenty years later, when Colton reintroduced it for use in dental practice.

Preparation

In the laboratory.—Small amounts may be prepared by reacting iron with nitric acid. Nitric oxide (NO) is first produced, but this is reduced to nitrous oxide since an excess of iron is present:

$$2NO + Fe \rightarrow FeO + N_2O$$

Commercially.—Nitrous oxide is produced by heating ammonium nitrate to between 245 and 270° C.

$$NH_4NO_3 \xrightarrow[245\text{–}270^\circ\ C]{Heat} N_2O + 2H_2O$$

The processes involved in drying and purifying the gas may vary but that used by the British Oxygen Company in the United Kingdom is briefly as follows (British Oxygen Co., 1967). A strong solution of ammonium nitrate when heated produces nitrous oxide with ammonia, nitric acid, nitrogen and traces of nitric oxide (NO) and nitrogen dioxide (NO_2). Cooling of the emerging gases results in reconstitution of the ammonia and nitric acid to ammonium nitrate and this is returned to the reactor. The gases are now passed through water scrubbers which remove any residual ammonia and nitric acid, and then through caustic permanganate scrubbers which remove the higher oxides of nitrogen to leave a residuum of 1 Vpm (volume per million) of nitric acid and nitrogen dioxide with the purified nitrous oxide and some nitrogen. Acid scrubbers now remove any final traces of ammonia and the gases are then compressed and dried in an aluminium drier. As the gases leave the drier continuous sampling takes place by passing a small stream of them through a visual bubbler. This consists of two solutions in series, the first containing acid potassium permanganate which converts any nitric oxide to nitrogen dioxide. The second consists of a colourless solution of Saltzman reagent in which any nitrogen dioxide present dissolves causing a chemical reaction which produces a magenta colour. The compressed and dried gases are now expanded into a liquefier with resultant liquefaction of the nitrous oxide and escape of the gaseous nitrogen. The pure nitrous oxide is now evaporated, compressed to a liquid, and passed through a second aluminium drier to the cylinder filling line. At this stage visual and electronic checks are carried out on samples leaving the drier to ensure that the nitrogen dioxide content does not exceed 1 Vpm.

About nine tenths of the contents of a full nitrous oxide cylinder are in liquid form. Great care is taken during manufacture to prevent moisture being included in the cylinder contents, since water vapour tends to freeze as it passes through a reducing valve and leads to a drop in the flow of gas.

When a nitrous oxide cylinder is turned on, the gaseous tension within it is first reduced and then immediately built up again as some of the liquid vaporises. Thus a pressure manometer attached to such a cylinder will show a steady reading until all the liquid nitrous oxide is used up, when a rapid fall is registered as the remaining gas escapes. Latent heat is required for the vaporisation of liquid nitrous oxide and this is obtained from the casing of the metal cylinder, which, as a result, rapidly cools. This in turn leads to freezing of the water vapour in the air immediately surrounding the cylinder, and to the formation of a layer of ice on the cylinder.

Nitrous oxide cylinders are marketed in various sizes, and coloured blue. In the United Kingdom 100 and 200 gallon cylinders are the most commonly used.*

Physical Properties

Nitrous oxide is non-irritating, sweet-smelling and colourless, and is the only inorganic gas used to produce anaesthesia in man. The molecular weight is 44·01 and the specific gravity is 1·527 (air = 1). It is readily compressible under 50 atmospheres pressure at 28° C to a clear and colourless fluid with a boiling point of −89° C. It is stable in the presence of soda lime. The oil/water solubility ratio is 3·2. The blood/gas solubility coefficient is 0·47.

Impurities

The main impurities which may occur have already been mentioned, and to them carbon monoxide should be added. This may be produced from burning particles of the sacks in which ammonium nitrate is delivered. The consequences of inhaling higher oxides of nitrogen, especially nitrogen dioxide, in concentrations over 50 Vpm are reflex inhibition of breathing with laryngospasm, and the rapid onset of intense cyanosis (Prys-Roberts, 1967). The last is due to both the formation of methaemoglobin and to altered pulmonary gas exchange. Pulmonary oedema may occur in the acute phase, but with concentrations lower than 50 Vpm it may not appear for some hours. If the patient does not die quickly, chronic chemical pneumonitis may follow, with resultant pulmonary fibrosis.

* 100 gallons of nitrous oxide weigh 30 oz.: 1 U.S. gallon is 5/6th Imperial gallon.

Respiratory acidosis, from associated ventilatory failure, and metabolic acidosis, from production of nitric and nitrous oxide formed from solution of the gases in the body fluids, may occur. Hypotension may be marked and results from the effect of nitrate and nitrite ions on vascular smooth muscle. The cases of poisoning described by Clutton-Brock (1967) illustrate vividly the clinical consequences.

The detection of higher oxides of nitrogen has been reviewed by Kain *et al.* (1967). In clinical practice the best method involves the use of a starch iodide paper. The moistened paper is placed in a 20 ml. syringe and 15 ml. of oxygen are drawn up, followed, by 5 ml. of the sample gas. Any nitric oxide will be oxidised by the oxygen to nitrogen dioxide, and the latter by oxidising iodide to iodine will turn the starch from a faint purple to a bright blue, depending on the amount of iodine present. The sensitivity of this test is 300 Vpm.

The principles of treatment of poisoning by the higher oxides of nitrogen have been discussed by Prys-Roberts (1967). He stresses that the advice he gives, although based on current concepts for the correction of the physiological disturbances that occur, is only a conjectural suggestion for those faced with the problem. Oxygen, either by spontaneous or assisted ventilation, and methylene blue, 2 mg./kg. of body weight intravenously, will be required initially to overcome the intense cyanosis resulting from methaemoglobinaemia. Further increments of methylene blue may be required, but excessive amounts can result in the production of methaemoglobin and also haemolytic anaemia.

Bronchial lavage and suction, together with endobronchial and parenteral steroids, have been suggested for the treatment of the chemical pneumonitis, whilst the metabolic acidosis will require intravenous sodium bicarbonate for its correction. The severe systemic hypotension from vasodilation can be improved by intravenous fluid and minimal doses of a vasopressor. The use of dimercaprol is suggested for severe cases since it has a protective action against the higher oxides of nitrogen.

Inflammability

It is neither inflammable nor explosive but will support combustion of other agents, even in the absence of oxygen, because at temperatures above 450°C it does decompose to nitrogen and oxygen.

Pharmacological Actions

Nitrous oxide is rapidly absorbed from the alveoli. 100 ml. of blood will carry 45 ml. of nitrous oxide in its plasma. It does not combine with haemoglobin nor does it undergo any chemical combination within the body, so that elimination is as speedy as absorption.

Anaesthetic action.—Nitrous oxide is a weak anaesthetic. At one time it was thought that any anaesthetic action that followed its use was produced solely by the exclusion of oxygen from the brain cells, since it is 15 times more soluble in plasma than nitrogen, and 100 times more so than oxygen.

Some patients can be rendered unconscious by the inhalation of mixtures containing at least 20 per cent oxygen—indeed a few subjects lose consciousness with mixtures containing equal parts of nitrous oxide and oxygen. If nitrogen is substituted for nitrous oxide in such a mixture anaesthesia rapidly ceases, and even if the oxygen is reduced to 10 per cent—with 90 per cent nitrogen—no anaesthesia occurs (Goodman and Gilman, 1955). Faulconer and Pender (1949) showed that a 50:50 mixture of nitrous oxide and oxygen at 2 atmospheres pressure rapidly produces surgical anaesthesia with complete oxygen saturation of the arterial blood, whereas the same concentration at atmospheric pressure in their patients did not produce loss of consciousness.

There is nowadays, therefore, no doubt that nitrous oxide is a weak anaesthetic agent, but the problem still remains as to how much of the anaesthesia produced (when it is used without supplement) is due to the potency of the gas and how much to the hypoxia which so frequently accompanies its use in these circumstances. The fact that these two features are intimately connected is emphasised by the following statement of Clement (1951): ". . . control of anaesthesia is synonymous with control of oxygen". From time to time a case of anoxic damage to the brain, or even of death, is reported following the use of nitrous oxide for a short period. If such gross manifestations of hypoxia can occur, it may well be that minor damage to the brain tissue arises more frequently and passes unnoticed at the time, but is reflected later in altered mental performance. Faulconer *et al.* (1949) showed that to produce in man surgical anaesthesia (stage III) with nitrous oxide a partial pressure of 760 mm. Hg is required if full oxygenation is maintained. Since an 80 per cent mixture of nitrous oxide in oxygen at normal atmospheric pressure results in a partial pressure of nitrous oxide of only about 600 mm. Hg, surgical anaesthesia cannot be achieved without some hypoxia. The use of a mixture of nitrous oxide and oxygen in the proportion 85:15 for induction causes a marked fall in arterial saturation in approximately two minutes, even when previous preoxygenation is carried out for three minutes. When pure nitrous oxide is used to induce anaesthesia, loss of consciousness is rapid enough—about 60 seconds—to suggest that this is primarily caused by displacement of oxygen from the brain rather than by saturation with nitrous oxide to a degree sufficient to cause anaesthesia without hypoxia (Bourne, 1954). The amount of saturation needed to produce unconsciousness is not known—partial rather than complete saturation may be sufficient—but whatever it is it takes time, and clinical observations have suggested seven to fifteen minutes (Mushin, 1952; Kaye, 1951). Bourne believes that a rapid induction with pure nitrous oxide is achieved by a sudden reduction in cerebral oxygen content, and that once unconsciousness is achieved, oxygenation can be increased and compensated for by the accumulating quantities of nitrous oxide in the central nervous system. Even from then on anaesthesia can be maintained with adequate oxygenation in only a proportion of people, while in many, if conditions satisfactory for the surgeon are to be maintained, sub-oxygenation must be continued.

Resistance to nitrous oxide.—Bourne (1954) has described two types of resistance to nitrous oxide, namely "false" and "true". "False" resistance is seen in those patients who are not minded to taking it lying down. Usually this indicates an inadequate mental approach to the patient on the part of the anaesthetist. Moreover, once these patients' circulation has become saturated with nitrous oxide they can be kept anaesthetised without hypoxia ."True" resistance, on the other hand, is seen in a patient who is barely unconscious even when saturated with 80 or 90 per cent nitrous oxide. Thus, whereas "false" resistance is a product of temperament and training, "true" resistance seems to develop from habituation to alcohol or narcotic drugs.

Contra-indications to nitrous oxide anaesthesia.—There are no contra-indications to the use of nitrous oxide in combination with an adequate percentage of oxygen. But present practice suggests that there are no occasions when this combination alone is justified. It is always preferable either to precede the inhalation by an intravenous induction of anaesthesia or to supplement it with a more potent inhalational agent, thereby ensuring a satisfactory level of oxygenation in the inspired mixture at all times. Indeed, a minimum concentration of 30 per cent oxygen is recommended when nitrous oxide is used for anaesthetic purposes.

Methods of Administration

Nitrous oxide can be administered by intermittent or continuous flow machines.

Intermittent flow.—This is an economical method as gas only flows during inspiration, and it is based upon two different techniques.

The first technique depends upon nitrous oxide and oxygen flowing into a mixing bag from which the patient inspires via corrugated tubing and a mask. As the bag empties, so it is refilled from the cylinders, and when it is full the flow of gases is automatically cut off until the next inspiratory effort starts the process once more. This type of apparatus is used almost entirely in midwifery and dental practice. The percentage of gas and oxygen in the mixture breathed can be readily adjusted by setting the dial to the required figure, and a simple device enables the intermittent flow to be replaced by continuous flow at various pressures—a factor which may be particularly useful in dental anaesthesia. Many machines incorporate a small trichloroethylene or halothane inhaler and a reservoir bag between the patient and the machine.

The second technique makes use of a premixed cylinder of nitrous oxide and oxygen under pressure with a demand valve to allow a high flow of gas to the patient on inspiration. The premixing of these two gases in the same cylinder was first suggested by Barach and Rovenstine (1945). At room temperature and at a pressure of 2,000 pounds per square inch certain proportions of nitrous oxide in oxygen exist as a single phase gas, due to the solvent action (Poynting effect) of the oxygen at this pressure. Tunstall (1961) described this phenomenon, making the point that up to 75 per cent nitrous oxide-oxygen remains in the gas phase under these conditions. He also reported the clinical use of a mixture of 50 per cent nitrous oxide and 50 per cent oxygen contained in one cylinder for the relief of pain in childbirth. Cooling such a mixture produces liquid nitrous oxide at the bottom of the cylinder, and this remains even when the cylinder is rewarmed (Cole, 1964). In these circumstances, if the cylinder is used it will first deliver a mixture with an oxygen content that is higher than intended, and then one that is lower. Delivery of a constant mixture from the cylinder can be assured either by preventing cooling or, should cooling occur, by briskly inverting the cylinder several times after rewarming (Tunstall, 1963; Cole, 1964). A detailed study of premixed nitrous oxide and oxygen (50:50) has been described by Gale *et al.* (1964). (See also Chapter 52.)

Continuous flow.—A continuous flow of gases is supplied from the anaesthetic machine, and a semi-closed system is most frequently used, with almost all the expired mixtures passing into the atmosphere through the expiratory valve. A closed system with absorption of carbon dioxide is not indicated when nitrous oxide is used, since it is extremely difficult to adjust the patients' oxygen requirements accurately and to maintain anaesthesia with this weak agent in such circumstances. Semi-closed anaesthesia is, however, frequently practised with a carbon dioxide absorber in place so that a more economical flow of gases can be used (see below).

Clinical Uses of Nitrous Oxide

For the reasons already stated, there is no place for the use of nitrous oxide as the sole anaesthetic.

Nitrous Oxide Analgesia

The introduction of premixed cylinders of 50:50 nitrous oxide and oxygen has revolutionised the use of nitrous oxide for analgesia. Parbrook (1968) has reviewed the possible indications, which include obstetric analgesia, the relief of pain in acute trauma and for cardiac ischaemia—particularly when a high oxygen content of the inspired gases is required—and other more traditional situations such as burns and painful dressings. Parbrook (1967) has also outlined four zones of analgesia, which are essentially subdivisions of Stage I of anaesthesia, and he believes that the first of these is the most useful, because in it the patient remains in full contact with his surroundings. This zone is generally achieved with concentrations of 6–25 per cent of nitrous oxide.

Nitrous Oxide in Dental Surgery (see Chapter 12)

Nitrous Oxide with Supplements

Though lacking in potency nitrous oxide is the least toxic of all the various anaesthetic agents available and has come to occupy an important role in anaesthetic technique. It is often used in conjunction with oxygen as the vehicle for delivering an anaesthetic vapour such as halothane or ether to the patient. In this respect as a weak anaesthetic agent it reduces the amount of the inhalational agent required for the same level of anaesthesia. It is also used extensively, sometimes with supplements of thiopentone, pethidine or other narcotic analgesics in conjunction with the muscle relaxants in major surgery.

It is frequently administered in a ratio of 75:25 per cent nitrous oxide and oxygen. The 25 per cent oxygen in the normal patient is sufficient to maintain adequate saturation of arterial blood, but under anaesthesia the effect of increased shunting and maldistribution (see p. 167) are such that in some cases an inspired concentration of 33 per cent must be used to maintain the same oxygen *tension* as before the onset of anaesthesia. Though the arterial saturation is virtually unaffected by this drop in tension owing to the oxygen dissociation curve (see p. 170), the fall alone must signify some reduction in reserve. In seriously ill patients requiring a high oxygen intake then nitrous oxide is not the most suitable agent.

Significance of uptake.—The high cost of some inhalational anaesthetic agents has increased the interest in using a low flow technique. As nitrous oxide is the principal carrier gas it is important to emphasise a few points in relation to its uptake by the blood. Nitrous oxide is relatively insoluble in blood, therefore the tension rises rapidly on induction and falls equally fast at the end of anaesthesia (see Chapter 7). The brain, an organ with a rich blood supply, has a similar solubility to that of blood so the brain tension also rises fast. Equilibrium between alveolar, blood and brain concentrations is achieved in a few minutes, but this must not be interpreted as meaning that a state of complete saturation has been achieved. Other tissues such as muscle and fat with a relatively low blood supply will gradually extract nitrous oxide from the blood, so that even after many hours some gas is still leaving the circulation. For example, with a patient breathing 75:25 per cent nitrous oxide/oxygen the uptake by the body (mostly muscle and fat) is about 175 ml./minute at the end of one hour, and at two hours it is still around 100 ml./minute. After about thirty hours complete saturation could theoretically be achieved but this is thwarted by the constant loss of 5–10 ml./minute of nitrous oxide through the skin.

Low flow technique.—The flow rate of nitrous oxide is important for two reasons. First, if it is the sole induction agent (in combination with oxygen) and it is used in a circle system (i.e. rebreathing allowed but carbon dioxide absorbed), then a 1 litre flow of 75:25 N_2O/O_2 will not render the patient unconscious even after 10 minutes of breathing this mixture. The reason for this is that the capacity of air in the lungs and in the anaesthetic apparatus is so great that they dilute the nitrous oxide to a level below which unconsciousness can be produced. On the other hand, if an 8 litre flow of the same mixture is used then unconsciousness is lost within two minutes because the apparatus is rapidly flushed out (Eger, 1960). Therefore, if a low flow nitrous oxide technique is to be used it should always start with a high flow for a few minutes before reducing to smaller flows.

Once on a low flow technique it must not be assumed that because the inspired concentration of oxygen is 25 per cent the alveolar concentration is at this level. Assuming for a moment that the input flow is 1·0 litre per minute and the oxygen consumption is 250 ml./minute and also that "complete saturation" with nitrous oxide has been achieved, then after one breath all the oxygen in the alveoli (i.e. 25 per cent of 1 litre = 250 ml.) will be taken up by the blood and the alveoli will then contain pure nitrous oxide. This will remain to dilute the next breath containing the inspired concentration of 75:25 N_2O/O_2. Consequently the oxygen content in the alveoli is considerably below the 25 per cent in the inspired concentration. This example emphasises the paramount importance of using an oxygen analyser in the circle system when low flows of nitrous oxide are being administered. Provided the concentration of oxygen in the inspired mixture does not fall below 25 per cent and total minute volume is adequate then this technique can safely be used, but for reasons described in Chapter 4, p. 167 *et seq.*, it is best not to use an inspired mixture of less than 33 per cent oxygen.

Finally, it is interesting to consider the question of what happens to the patient with abdominal distension or a closed pneumothorax who also breathes a mixture of N_2O/O_2. Nitrous oxide, though relatively insoluble in blood, is still much more soluble than nitrogen. Therefore more molecules will present themselves at the cavity site and for every one molecule of nitrogen leaving, at least ten molecules of nitrous oxide will be available. On this basis the induction of nitrous oxide and oxygen anaesthesia might be predicted to increase abdominal distension. (See p. 279.)

ETHYLENE (C_2H_4)

There is a wide discrepancy in the anaesthetic literature as to the origin of the hydrocarbon, ethylene. In 1779 Priestley gave the credit to Ingenhousz, but the exact date of preparation remains obscure. Other authorities claim that Becher, in 1669, was the first person to prepare the gas. In 1923 Brown, whilst working in the Henderson Laboratory at Toronto, published some observations on the anaesthetic properties of this gas in animals. That same year Luckhardt and Carter of Chicago reported their findings on the use of this drug in human subjects. The evidence available suggests that the credit for its introduction as an anaesthetic should go to Luckhardt, since he had observed its anaesthetic and analgesic properties in animals years before.

Preparation

In the laboratory: Ethyl bromide is reacted with alcoholic potassium hydroxide to form ethylene, potassium bromide, and water.

$$C_2H_5Br + KOH \rightarrow C_2H_4 + KBr + H_2O$$

Ethyl bromide + potassium hydroxide (alcoholic) → Ethylene + potassium bromide + water

Commercially: by dehydration of ethyl alcohol with either sulphuric (H_2SO_4) or phosphoric (H_2PO_4) acid.

$$C_2H_5OH + H_2SO_4 \xrightarrow{150^\circ C +} C_2H_4 + H_2O$$

Ethyl alcohol + Sulphuric acid Ethylene + Water

At temperatures below 150° C ethyl ether may be formed when sulphuric acid is used.

Natural gas can be used to produce ethylene by a process of breakdown or "cracking" with heat. Propane is formed as an intermediate process.

Physical Properties

Ethylene is a colourless, non-irritating gas with a slightly sweetish and unpleasant odour. It is lighter than air, having a specific gravity of 0·97 (air = 1). Molecular weight is 28·03. It liquefies at 10° C under 60 atmospheres pressure and the boiling point of this liquid is—104° C. It is the least soluble in blood of the commonly used anaesthetic agents having an Ostwald blood-gas solubility coefficient of 0·140 (*cf.* nitrous oxide = 0·468). The oil/gas coefficient is 1·28 and the solubility in blood and tissue (e.g. heart and brain) is about equal, i.e. 1·0 and 1·2 respectively (Marshall and Grollman, 1928; Meyer and Hopff, 1923; Kety, 1951). It is not altered by soda lime but diffuses through rubber.

Impurities

These are either contaminants from the manufacturing process or from decomposition. Alcohol, aldehydes, ether, oxides of sulphur or phosphorus, carbon dioxide, carbon monoxide, olefins or acetylenes may be present.

Inflammability

Ethylene is highly combustible, when mixed with oxygen or air, and exposed to sparks or flames. Thus in air 3·1–32·0 per cent ethylene is explosive, while in oxygen the range is from 3·0–80·0 per cent. The risk of explosion is increased on account of its low density which allows it to rise in the atmosphere.

The addition of nitrous oxide (40 per cent) to a mixture of ethylene (50 per cent) and oxygen (10 per cent) does not prevent an explosion, but helium and nitrogen, when used as diluents, reduce the explosive range.

Pharmacological Actions

Ethylene is rapidly absorbed from the alveoli and, when given in a concentration of 100 per cent, it brings about unconsciousness slightly more rapidly than nitrous oxide. Ethylene in mixtures of 20–40 per cent with oxygen is said to produce analgesia, but 80–90 per cent is required for anaesthesia. The main advantages over nitrous oxide are a more rapid induction, greater muscular relaxation, and the ability to use a slightly higher percentage of oxygen. Against these must be set the disadvantage of a highly explosive agent with an unpleasant odour.

In a report from the United States of nearly 200,000 cases of ethylene-oxygen anaesthesia, there were five deaths in the operating room and three in the post-operative period attributed to this agent. There were three non-fatal explosions in this series.

Ethylene is rapidly eliminated through the lungs, although a very small percentage may be excreted through the skin. The incidence of post-operative nausea and vomiting is greater than that with nitrous oxide.

Method of Administration

This is similar to that already described for nitrous oxide.

CYCLOPROPANE (C_3H_6)

Cyclopropane, or trimethylene, was first prepared by the chemist Freund in 1882. Nearly fifty years later, in 1929, Lucas and Henderson of Toronto noted that it possessed better anaesthetic properties than propylene, in which they were primarily interested. In 1933 Waters and his colleagues, at Madison, Wisconsin, introduced cyclopropane into clinical anaesthesia.

Preparation

Cyclopropane can be prepared from the natural gas found in the United States, or from trimethylene glycol. This substance is produced during the fermentation of molasses to obtain glycol. In the first stage trimethylene glycol is reacted with hydrobromic acid to form trimethylene dibromide, and in the second stage this latter substance is treated with zinc which brings about the production of cyclopropane and zinc dibromide.

$$\begin{array}{ccccc} CH_2OH & & & & CH_2Br & \\ | & & & & | & \\ CH_2 & + & 2HBr & \rightarrow & CH_2 & + 2H_2O \\ | & & & & | & \\ CH_2OH & & & & CH_2Br & \end{array}$$

Trimethylene glycol — Hydrobromic acid — Trimethylene dibromide

$$\downarrow \quad + Zn$$

$$\text{cyclo-}(CH_2)_3 \text{ (}CH_2\text{ above } H_2C - CH_2\text{)} + ZnBr_2$$

Cyclopropane — Zinc dibromide

Physical Properties

Cyclopropane is a pleasant, sweet-smelling gas, which is irritating to the respiratory tract when inhaled in concentrations over 40 per cent. The molecular weight is 42·08 and the vapour density 1·42 (air = 1), and because it is heavier than air it tends to gravitate towards the floor. When subjected to pressures of five atmospheres or more, it liquefies. It is stored as a liquid at a pressure of 75 lb. per square inch in light metal cylinders which are coloured orange. Because of this relatively low pressure no reducing valves are required, the flow being regulated through a simple fine-adjustment pin. One ounce of the liquid gives 3·5 U.K. gallons or 4·29 U.S. gallons of gas. The boiling point is −33° C and freezing point −127° C. It has a solubility coefficient in blood of 0·415 (*cf.* nitrous oxide 0·468) and therefore it is relatively insoluble in blood. This accounts for the rapid induction and recovery that can be achieved with this agent. The solubility coefficient in human fat is 6·8 (Eger, 1963—personal communication) and the solubility in the tissues is about the same as in blood. Cyclopropane is not altered or decomposed by alkalis, and so undergoes no change in the presence of soda lime, but diffuses through rubber.

Impurities

Propylene, allene, cyclohexane, carbon dioxide, various halides such as brom- or chlor-propane and, finally, nitrogen, are possible impurities. Concentrations of propylene above 3 per cent may prove dangerous.

Inflammability

Cyclopropane, when mixed with air, oxygen or nitrous oxide, becomes explosive over a variable range. In air 2·4–10·4 per cent cyclopropane is explosive, in oxygen 2·5–60·0 per cent, and in nitrous oxide 3–30 per cent.

Pharmacological Actions

Uptake.—Cyclopropane, when inhaled, is absorbed from the alveoli and carried in the circulation attached principally to the red cells by virtue of their high protein and lipoprotein content. Some is attached to the serum protein but as the water solubility of cyclopropane is relatively low (0·204 as opposed to 15·61 for ether) only a small portion is physically dissolved in the plasma.

Elimination.—Cyclopropane is excreted almost entirely by the lungs, although a small quantity is lost through the skin. Approximately 50 per cent of cyclopropane in the body is removed within ten minutes of discontinuing its administration.

Concentration for anaesthesia.—The amount of cyclopropane required for induction must necessarily be higher than that used for maintenance because of the dilution caused by the contents of the lungs and the anaesthetic apparatus. For a rapid induction of anaesthesia the reservoir bag of the apparatus should be filled with 50:50 cyclopropane and oxygen. The patient is asked to take five or six deep breaths of this mixture. Unconsciousness sets in within thirty seconds and this is rapidly followed by a period of apnoea in most cases. Sometimes uncoordinated twitching movements may be observed throughout the body lasting for about half a minute.

Inhalation of a concentration of 4 per cent cyclopropane in oxygen produces analgesia, 6 per cent abolishes consciousness, 8 per cent light anaesthesia and 20–30 per cent deep anaesthesia. These figures, however, are of limited value since the concentration of cyclopropane inhaled and its effect vary widely, depending on the response of the patient and the duration of the inhalation.

Action on the respiratory system.—Cyclopropane given with oxygen to the unpremedicated patient produces a progressive decrease in alveolar ventilation as the depth of anaesthesia increases (Jones *et al.*, 1960). The depression of ventilation is due to a fall in tidal volume, for the respiratory rate increases as anaesthesia deepens. This increase in rate was at one time thought to result from a sensitisation by cyclopropane of the pulmonary stretch receptors in the respiratory tract, but there is strong evidence that anaesthetics abolish this reflex (Paskin, 1968). If morphine or pethidine are used as part of the premedication then there is a progressive decrease in tidal volume without any change in respiratory rate. This leads to profound hypoventilation at a much lighter level of anaesthesia than would be experienced in the unpremedicated patient. From a clinical standpoint heavy premedication with analgesics before cyclopropane anaesthesia invariably leads to apnoea long before a sufficient concentration is given for adequate muscular relaxation. Munson and his colleagues (1966) suggest that at equipotent anaesthetic concentrations cyclopropane is less depressant to respiration than halothane.

In the experimental animal cyclopropane produces bronchial constriction and though such a response is not commonly seen in clinical practice, it should be remembered when considering this agent for anaesthesia for a patient liable to bronchospasm.

Action on the circulatory system.—*General response.* Much work has been done on the study of the effects of cyclopropane on the circulation (Price, 1961). In the past, most of the data concerning the effects of this anaesthetic have been based on studies involving premedication of the patient, intermittent positive-pressure ventilation, endotracheal intubation and the trauma of surgery. All of these are believed to influence the action of cyclopropane on the circulation and therefore the actions quoted below are those reported as being due solely to cyclopropane anaesthesia.

Effect on the heart.—Cyclopropane when administered to the heart-lung preparation causes a depression of cardiac contractility which is directly related to the concentration used. In direct contrast, in anaesthetised man cyclopropane brings about an increase in cardiac output with a rise in right ventricular stroke volume, stroke work and end-diastolic pressure. This increase in cardiac output is only seen under light anaesthesia, for the output falls to normal or below as depth is increased. These findings in intact man suggest that the increase in cardiac output under light anaesthesia is related to the stimulation of the sympathetic nerves supplying the heart. It is known that the noradrenaline concentration in the myocardium increases proportionately with the concentration of cyclopropane. The adrenaline concentration is not affected. Thus, the increase in cardiac output in light anaesthesia may be due to increased noradrenaline production and as anaesthesia deepens so the direct depressant effect of cyclopropane on the myocardium becomes manifest. If, however, cyclopropane is administered to a patient with sympathetic blockade then only the depressant action on the myocardium could be anticipated.

Effect on the heart rate.—It is widely believed by all users of cyclopropane that this anaesthetic agent produces a slowing of the pulse rate. Yet, if the patient is not premedicated with a narcotic, the effect of cyclopropane on the heart rate is negligible. As the anaesthetic depth is increased no obvious change in pulse rate is observed. If, however, some premedication is given in the form of morphine, then a bradycardia may be observed with cyclopropane anaesthesia (Li and Etsten, 1957).

In the absence of any premedicant drugs concentrations of cyclopropane as high as 14–18 vols. per cent can be inspired without any observable change in pulse rate (Price, 1961). Furthermore, if a large dose of atropine (1·0—2·0 mg.) is then given, a very dramatic increase in pulse rate takes place (i.e. an average increase of 70 beats/minute). This increase is far greater than that produced by the same dose of atropine without cyclopropane anaesthesia. The inference is made, therefore, that cyclopropane may increase vagal activity and this effects cardiac impulse generation, conduction and improved atrial contractility. At the time it increases vagal activity it also stimulates sympathetic activity within the heart. In the unpremedicated patient these two forces balance each other out and there is little change of pulse rate. When atropine is given not only is vagal activity blocked but sympathetic activity is allowed to proceed unheeded. Hence the dramatic tachycardia. However, atropine administration during cyclopropane anaesthesia leads to a high incidence of arrhythmias, and might lead to ventricular fibrillation (Eger, 1962).

Arrhythmias.—An increase in the alveolar carbon dioxide tension precipitated the onset of arrhythmias in every one of a series of twenty-eight patients anaesthetised with cyclopropane (Price *et al.*, 1958). It is known that both hypercarbia and cyclopropane increase the rate of noradrenaline liberation from sympathetic nerves terminating in the myocardium. Catecholamines liberated from other areas of the body are relatively ineffective. It would appear, therefore, that the combination of a raised carbon dioxide tension of the blood and cyclopropane lead to an excessive noradrenaline excretion in the myocardium. Nevertheless, Price *et al.* (1968) demonstrated that cyclopropane itself has a direct effect on the myocardium. Thus, during sympathetic nerve stimulation there is an increased chronotropic response and this is not directly related to the amount of transmitter substance released. Clinically, therefore arrhythmias under cyclopropane anaesthesia can largely be prevented if particular attention is paid to the prevention of hypoventilation. In fact Price and his colleagues (1960) concluded that "in persons anaesthetised with cyclopropane the most reliable circulatory indication of hypercarbia was the presence of cardiac arrhythmias."

"*Cyclopropane shock*".—This term became popular during the era of cyclopropane to explain the sudden cardiovascular collapse that was sometimes observed at the end of a long anaesthetic under deep cyclopropane. At first it was believed to be solely due to the accumulation of carbon dioxide brought about by the respiratory depression of the deep cyclopropane. Now it would seem that it is a combination of both cyclopropane and carbon dioxide causing a period of intense sympathetic nervous activity. The hypotension and collapse that occurs at the end of the anaesthesia is believed to be due to the sudden withdrawal of this activity. The whole process is akin to the rapid withdrawal of an intravenous infusion of adrenaline or noradrenaline, resulting in a period of hypotension which is believed to be due to ganglionic blockade (Price, 1960).

Action on the peripheral circulation.—Cyclopropane, unlike most other anaesthetic agents, produces peripheral vasoconstriction in both skin and muscle even under light general anaesthesia. The magnitude of this vasoconstriction is directly related to the depth of anaesthesia. The mechanism of this constriction is interesting. It would appear to be due either to a direct action of cyclopropane on the vessel wall itself or to some humoral substance such as noradrenaline. The evidence to support this hypothesis is that the vasoconstriction occurs even after the nerve supply to that area has been blocked (Fig. 1) (McArdle and Black, 1963).

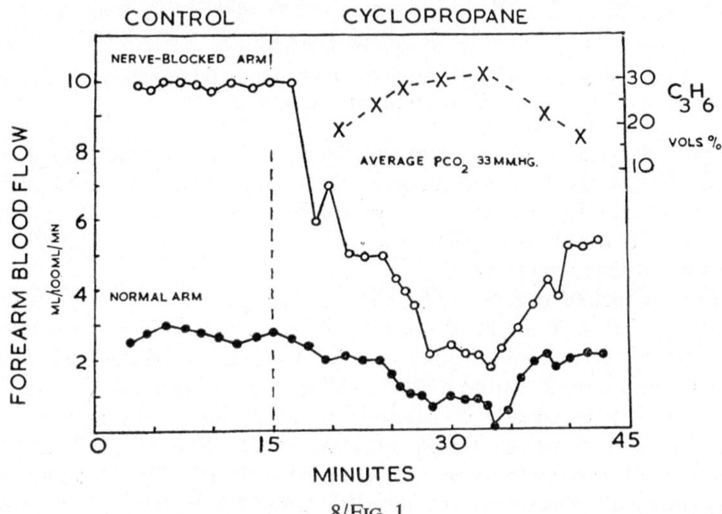

8/FIG. 1.

Cristoforo and Brody (1968), using a dog muscle preparation, found no evidence of either activation of the sympathetic nervous system or sensitisation of vascular smooth muscle to noradrenaline by cyclopropane. They concluded, therefore, that the maintenance or slight elevation of blood pressure during cyclopropane anaesthesia was due to a direct stimulating effect on smooth muscle by the anaesthetic agent itself. These findings are at variance with those of other workers (Gravenstein *et al.*, 1960; Price and Price, 1962). It is possible, therefore, that in man the maintenance of systemic pressure is brought about by a variety of mechanisms—liberation of noradrenaline, sensitisation of the vessel wall to the effect of the catecholamines and also a direct effect of the cyclopropane on the smooth muscle of the vessel wall.

Surgical stimulation also appears to influence the effect of cyclopropane on the vessel wall. Under light cyclopropane anaesthesia the normally observed vasoconstriction gives way to vasodilatation (Fig. 2). This response is not

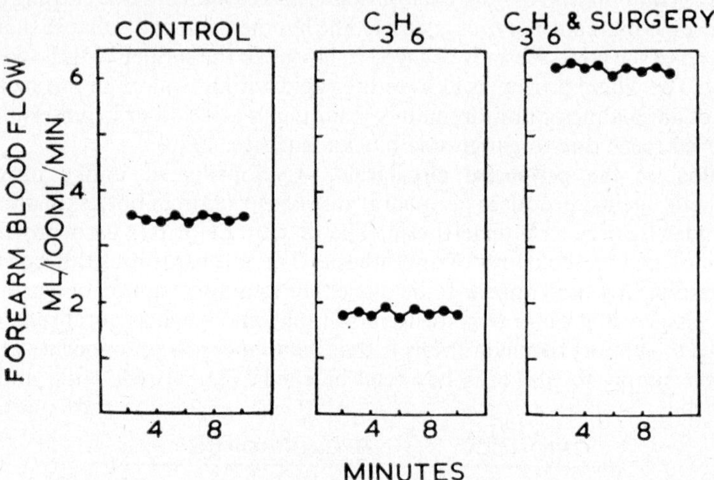

8/FIG. 2.—Effect of cyclopropane anaesthesia alone and cyclopropane with surgery on the forearm blood flow in man.

observed under deep cyclopropane anaesthesia but the mechanism is not understood. Nevertheless, this observation may explain some of the contradictory results obtained with studies of the peripheral circulation under cyclopropane anaesthesia. It would also explain the increased "oozing" sometimes seen under light cyclopropane anaesthesia.

Action on various organs.—*The kidney.* Cyclopropane produces a reduction of renal blood flow in direct proportion to the concentration. Thus under light anaesthesia there is about a 30 per cent fall in renal blood flow, whereas under deep anaesthesia it may fall to as low as 80 per cent of normal. This fall in renal blood flow with increasing concentrations of cyclopropane signifies that the agent produces a constriction of the renal vessels (Miles *et al.*, 1952). Deutsch and his co-workers (1967), studying normal unpremedicated human subjects, found that cyclopropane anaesthesia produced a dramatic reduction in both glomerular filtration and renal plasma flow (about 40 per cent). They concluded that their findings could be explained on the basis of increased sympathetic nervous system activity during cyclopropane anaesthesia. At the same time they observed that cyclopropane anaesthesia was associated with an anti-diuresis which was probably brought about by increased production of anti-diuretic hormone (ADH), and they also noted an increase in plasma renin levels. The latter finding is particularly interesting as the renin-angiotensin system has been considered to be responsible for the autoregulation of renal blood flow, so it is theoretically possible that cyclopropane may act on the renal blood flow through the mechanism of this system.

The liver.—Cyclopropane reduces liver blood flow in direct relation with the depth of anaesthesia (Shackman *et al.*, 1953). This finding has been corroborated by the work of Price and his colleagues (1965) who found that cyclopropane reduced splanchnic blood flow to both the gut and the liver. They concluded that this effect was brought about not only by increased sympathetic activity in the vasoconstrictor fibres to the liver and intestine but also by sensitisation of the vascular smooth muscle to the action of noradrenaline.

The uterus.—Cyclopropane depresses the contractions of the gravid uterus again in direct relation to the concentration used. It passes quickly through the placental barrier and equilibrium between maternal and foetal blood is rapidly established. For this reason high concentrations of cyclopropane are rarely used for Caesarian section or forceps delivery in obstetrical anaesthesia, though if cyclopropane is used as an induction agent only the respiratory depression of the foetus is eliminated within a few minutes of the withdrawal of the agent.

The lungs.—Cyclopropane increases central venous pressure. This may be due to stimulating vagal activity but it results in the right heart and great veins becoming firmer with increased tone. Thus, when the lungs are inflated with positive pressure the veins (and indirectly the cardiac output) are less susceptible to this compression. This may explain why the blood pressure does not usually fall under cyclopropane anaesthesia even in the seriously ill patient. Nevertheless, hypotension and diminished cardiac output do sometimes occur on induction with cyclopropane anaesthesia, particularly if a narcotic agent has been used. As time progresses this depression is usually offset and the blood pressure returns to normal, suggesting that some homeostatic mechanism is at work. This may be due to stimulation of baroreceptor reflex activity. Price and Widdicombe (1962) have demonstrated in dogs and cats that cyclopropane anaesthesia acts by a direct stimulant effect on the baroreceptors in the carotid sinus. Another possible explanation, supported by some evidence in animal experiments, is that cyclopropane diminishes the sensitivity of the medullary vasomotor centre to afferent inhibitory impulses thus allowing the centre free rein to send out efferent constrictor reactions.

Central nervous system.—Price and his colleagues (1969), working with cats, have confirmed that cyclopropane increases sympathetic nervous activity and they conclude that this effect is brought about by a selective depression of certain neurones in the medulla oblongata. Thus, cyclopropane inhibited the "depressor" neurones whilst stimulating the "pressor" ones. An additional excitatory action on the spinal cord neurones could not be excluded but appeared relatively unimportant.

Cyclopropane and adrenaline.—Price and his co-workers (1958) studied the different blood levels of adrenaline required to produce ventricular arrhythmias with either a simple infusion technique or that produced by a raised carbon dioxide level of the blood. They found that hypercarbia was far more effective in producing arrhythmias than adrenaline infusion. In fact the catecholamine level under hypercarbia was only one-tenth as high as in the infusion series yet the incidence of arrhythmias was high, suggesting that endogenous adrenaline is far more effective than the exogenous material.

Matteo and his associates (1963), however, found that the subcutaneous injection of a 1:60,000 solution of adrenaline during cyclopropane anaesthesia with adequate ventilation (i.e. normal CO_2 level) led to a 30 per cent incidence of ventricular arrhythmias. From data available it would seem that the use of a subcutaneous infiltration with even a weak solution of adrenaline (i.e. 1:200,000) is contra-indicated during cyclopropane anaesthesia in man.

Clinical Use

Owing to the risk of an explosion, the popularity of cyclopropane as an anaesthetic has gradually faded with the introduction of newer and non-inflammable anaesthetics. Cyclopropane may, however, be the agent of choice for the induction of anaesthesia when a rapid loss of consciousness is necessary, coupled with a high concentration of oxygen and maintenance of the systemic blood pressure. This type of induction is most commonly required in obstetric practice, but the need also arises for some patients with acute intestinal obstruction. In such circumstances cyclopropane is best administered as a 50:50 mixture with oxygen (Bourne, 1954). The patient breathes from a six-litre bag filled with the mixture. Five to six breaths are sufficient to produce loss of consciousness. Some motor excitement (tonic or clonic contractions) may be observed at this point, and its onset is usually associated with a momentary period of breath-holding which lasts for a few seconds.

Summary

Cyclopropane anaesthesia is particularly suitable as an anaesthetic agent for the seriously-ill patient because it is accompanied by a high oxygen concentration and a rise of cardiac output (under light anaesthesia only), peripheral vasoconstriction, and virtually no change in heart rate. The result is that the blood pressure is well maintained even when intermittent positive-pressure respiration is introduced. The latter procedure is often necessary because cyclopropane diminishes tidal volume. Most of the beneficial effects of cyclopropane on the myocardium are abolished if a narcotic is given as part of the premedication. Barbiturates, phenothiazine derivatives and atropine do not have this adverse effect. Morphine and pethidine also reduce ventilation in their own right so that when combined with cyclopropane there is a serious risk of hypoventilation; both the increased carbon dioxide level of the blood and cyclopropane combine to raise the amount of noradrenaline excreted in the myocardium so that the risk of arrhythmias is increased. The presence of these arrhythmias under cyclopropane anaesthesia should suggest inadequate ventilation or too deep anaesthesia; in either case it has often been observed that the inhalation of a low concentration of ether vapour will bring about a return of normal rhythm.

Disease, trauma and narcotic agents appear to influence both the sympathetic and the parasympathetic responses to cyclopropane. Atropine tends to remove the effect of increased vagal stimulation whereas ganglion blocking drugs will remove the sympathetic response and may cause cyclopropane to produce a profound hypotension through direct myocardial depression.

REFERENCES

BARACH, A. L., and ROVENSTINE. E. A. (1945). The hazards of anoxia during nitrous oxide anesthesia. *Anesthesiology*, **6,** 449.

BOURNE, J. G. (1954). General anaesthesia for out-patients with special reference to dental extraction. *Proc. roy. Soc. Med.*, **47,** 416.

BOURNE, J. G. (1957*a*). Fainting and cerebral damage. A danger in patients kept upright during dental gas anaesthesia and after surgical operations. *Lancet*, **2,** 499.

BRITISH OXYGEN CO. LTD. (1967). Current methods of commercial production of nitrous oxide. *Brit. J. Anaesth.*, **39,** 440.

BROWN, W. E. (1923). Preliminary report on experiments with ethylene as a general anaesthetic. *Canad. med. Ass. J.*, **13,** 210.

CLEMENT, F. W. (1951). *Nitrous Oxide-Oxygen Anesthesia*, 3rd edit. Philadelphia: Lea & Febiger.

CLUTTON-BROCK, J. (1967). Two cases of poisoning by contamination of nitrous oxide with higher oxides of nitrogen during anaesthesia. *Brit. J. Anaesth.*, **39,** 388.

COLE, P. V. (1964). Nitrous oxide and oxygen from a single cylinder. *Anaesthesia*, **19,** 3.

CRISTOFORO, M. F., and BRODY, M. J. (1968). The effect of halothane and cyclopropane on skeletal muscle vessels and baroreceptor reflexes. *Anesthesiology*, **29,** 36.

DAVY, H. (1800). *Researches, Chemical and Philosophical, chiefly concerning Nitrous Oxide*. London.

DEUTSCH, S. PIERCE, E. C., and VANDAM, L. D. (1967). Cyclopropane effects on renal function in normal man. *Anesthesiology*, **28,** 547.

EGER, E. I. (1960). Factors affecting the rapidity of alteration of nitrous oxide concentration in a circle system. *Anesthesiology*, **21,** 348–358.

EGER, E. I. (II) (1962). Atropine, scopolamine, and related compounds. *Anesthesiology*, **23,** 365.

FAULCONER, A., and PENDER, J. W. (1949). The influence of partial pressure of nitrous oxide on the depth of anesthesia and the electroencephalogram in man. *Anesthesiology*, **10,** 601.

FAULCONER, A., PENDER, J. W., and BICKFORD, R. G. (1949). The influence of partial pressure of nitrous oxide on the depth of anesthesia and the electro-encephalogram in man. *Anesthesiology*, **10,** 601.

FREUND, A. (1882). Über Trimethylene. *Mschr. Chemie.*, **3,** 625.

GALE, C. W., TUNSTALL, M. E., and WILTON-DAVIES, C. C. (1964). Premixed gas and oxygen for midwives. *Brit. med. J.*, **1,** 732.

GOODMAN, L. S., and GILMAN, A. (1955). *The Pharmacological Basis of Therapeutics*, 2nd edit. New York: The Macmillan Company.

GRAVENSTEIN, J. S., SHERMAN, E. T., and ANDERSEN, T. W. (1960). Cyclopropane epinephrine interaction on the nictitating membrane of the spinal cat. *J. Pharmacol. exp. Ther.*, **129,** 428.

JONES, R. E., GULDMANN, N., LINDE, H. W., DRIPPS, R. D., and PRICE, H. L. (1960). Cyclopropane Anesthesia III. Effects of cyclopropane on respiration and circulation in normal man. *Anesthesiology*, **21,** 380.

KAIN, M. L., COMMINS, B. T., DIXON-LEWIS, G., and NUNN, J. F. (1967). Detection and determination of higher oxides of nitrogen. *Brit. J. Anaesth.*, **39,** 425.

KAYE, G. (1951). Note on hypoxia during nitrous oxide anaesthesia in dentistry. *Med. J. Aust.*, **1,** 577.

KETY, S. S. (1951). Theory and application of exchange of inert gas at the lungs and tissues. *Pharmacol. Rev.*, **3,** 1.

LI, T. H., and ETSTEN, B. (1957). Effect of cyclopropane anesthesia on cardiac output and related hemodynamics in man. *Anesthesiology*, **18,** 15.

LUCAS, G. H. W., and HENDERSON, V. E. (1929). A new anaesthetic gas: cyclopropane. A preliminary report. *Canad. med. Ass. J.*, **21,** 173.

LUCKHARDT, A. B., and CARTER, J. B. (1923). Ethylene as a gas anesthetic: preliminary communication. Clinical experience in 106 surgical operations. *J. Amer. med. Ass.*, **80,** 1440.

MCARDLE, L., and BLACK, G. W. (1963). Effects of cyclopropane on peripheral circulation. *Brit. J. Anaesth.*, **35,** 352.

MARSHALL, E. K., and GROLLMAN, A. (1928). Method for determination of the circulatory minute volume in man. *Amer. J. Physiol.*, **86,** 117.

MATTEO, R. S., KATZ, R. L., and PAPPER, E. M. (1963). The injection of epinephrine during general anesthesia with halogenated hydrocarbons and cyclopropane in man. *Anesthesiology*, **24,** 327.

MEYER, K. H., and HOPFF, H. (1923). Theorieder Narkose durch Inhalationoanesthetika. *Hoppe-Seylers Z. physiol. Chem.*, **126,** 281.

MILES, B. E., DE WARDENER, H. E., CHURCHILL-DAVIDSON, H. C., and WYLIE, W. D. (1952). The effect on the renal circulation of pentamethonium bromide during anaesthesia. *Clin. Sci.*, **11,** 73.

MUNSON, E. S., LARSON, C. P., Jr., BABAD, A. A., REGAN, M. J., BUECHEL, D. R., and EGER, E. I. (II) (1966). The effects of halothane, fluroxene and cyclopropane on ventilation. A comparative study in man. *Anesthesiology*, **27,** 716.

MUSHIN, W. W. (1952). Anaesthesia for minor procedures. *Brit. med. J.*, **1,** 431.

PARBROOK, G. D. (1967). The levels of nitrous oxide analgesia. *Brit. J. Anaesth.*, **39,** 974.

PARBROOK, G. D. (1968). Therapeutic uses of nitrous oxide. *Brit. J. Anaesth.*, **40,** 365.

PASKIN, S. SKOVSTED, P., and SMITH, T. C. (1968). Failure of the Hering-Breuer reflex to account for tachypnea in anesthetized man. *Anesthesiology*, **29,** 550.

PRICE, H. L. (1960). General anaesthesia and circulatory homeostasis. *Physiol. Rev.*, **40,** 187.

PRICE, H. L. (1961). Circulatory actions of general anesthetic agents and the homeostatic roles of epinephrine and norepinephrine in man. *Clin. Pharmacol. Ther.*, **2,** 163.

PRICE, H. L., DEUTSCH, S., COOPERMAN, L. H., CLEMENT, A. J., and EPSTEIN, R. M (1965). Splanchnic circulation during cyclopropane anesthesia in normal man. *Anesthesiology*, **26,** 312.

PRICE, H. L., LURIE, A. A., BLACK, G. W., SECHZER, P. H., LINDE, H. W., and PRICE, M. L. (1960). Modifications by general anesthetics (cyclopropane and halothane) of circulatory and sympathoadrenal responses to respiratory acidosis. *Ann. Surg.*, **152,** 1071.

PRICE, H. L., LURIE, A. A., JONES, F. E., PRICE, M. L., and LINDE, H. W. (1958). Cyclopropane anesthesia. *Anesthesiology*, **19,** 619.

PRICE, M. L., and PRICE, H. L. (1962). Effects of general anesthetics on contractile responses of rabbit aorta strips. *Anesthesiology*, **23,** 16.

PRICE, H. L., WARDEN, J. C., COOPERMAN, L. H., and MILLAR, R. A. (1969). Central sympathetic excitation caused by cyclopropane. *Anesthesiology*, **30,** 426.

PRICE, H. L., WARDEN, J. C., COOPERMAN, L. H., and PRICE, Mary L. (1968). Enhancement by cyclopropane and halothane of heart rate responses to sympathetic stimulation. *Anesthesiology*, **29,** 478.

PRICE, H. L., and WIDDICOMBE, J. (1962). Actions of cyclopropane on carotid sinus baroreceptors and carotid body chemoreceptors. *J. Pharmacol. exp. Ther.*, **135,** 233.

PRIESTLEY, J. (1779). *Experiments in Natural Philosophy, with continuation of the Observations on Air*. Vol. I.

PRIESTLEY, J. (1774). *Experiments and observations on different kinds of Air*. London.

PRYS-ROBERTS, C. (1967). Principles of treatment of poisoning by higher oxides of nitrogen. *Brit. J. Anaesth.*, **39,** 432.

SHACKMAN, R., GRABER, I. G., and MELROSE, D. G. (1953). Liver blood flow and general anaesthesia. *Clin. Sci.*, **12,** 307.

TUNSTALL, M. E. (1961). Obstetric analgesia. The use of fixed nitrous oxide and oxygen mixture from one cylinder. *Lancet*, **2,** 964.

TUNSTALL, M. E. (1963). Effect of cooling on premixed gas mixtures for obstetric analgesia. *Brit. med. J.*, **2,** 915.

WATERS, R. M., ROVENSTINE, E. A., and GUEDEL, A. E. (1933). Endotracheal anesthesia and its historical development. *Curr. Res. Anesth.*, **12,** 196.

Chapter 9

VOLATILE ANAESTHETICS

DIETHYL ETHER $(C_2H_5)_2O$

ETHER was first described by Valerius Cordus in 1540. In 1841, Crawford Long used ether in his own home in Jefferson, Georgia, and, in the following year, he used it during three surgical operations. Unfortunately these events were not published until after William Morton's famous demonstration of the potentialities of ether as an anaesthetic at the Massachusetts General Hospital in 1846 (Morton, 1847). After this, ether became widely publicised and the news spread to London, where Drs. Boot and Squires soon used it on surgical cases at University College Hospital.

Preparation.—Dehydration of alcohol by sulphuric acid at a temperature below 140° C.

$$C_2H_5OH + H_2SO_4 \rightarrow C_2H_5HSO_4 + H_2O$$

Ethyl alcohol + Sulphuric acid

$$C_2H_5HSO_4 + C_2H_5OH \rightarrow H_2SO_4 + C_2H_5OC_2H_5$$

Ethyl alcohol — Diethyl ether

Physical properties.—Ether is a colourless, volatile liquid (boiling point 36·5° C) with a characteristic pungent smell. At room temperature (20° C) it has a vapour pressure of approximately 425 mm. Hg.

Significance of vapour pressure.—A knowledge of the vapour pressure of a volatile anaesthetic agent enables the anaesthetist quickly to calculate the inspired concentration being delivered to the patient by a "bubble-through" type of vaporiser e.g. copper kettle or "Vernitrol". It is of very little value if only a portion of the stream of gases are exposed to the liquid as in a "blow-over" type of vaporiser e.g. Boyle's bottle. Even when the latter type of vaporiser is converted to "bubbling" then the constantly changing temperature of the liquid make a calculation difficult unless this temperature is known.

The principle of the copper kettle (Fig. 1) is that the vaporiser is constructed of a highly conductive metal and when attached directly to an anaesthetic table-top of similar material it has a large heat reservoir available which will prevent the temperature in the vaporiser from falling. A known flow of oxygen is then bubbled through the liquid anaesthetic agent at room temperature.

Taking ether as an example, at a room temperature of 20° C the vapour pressure is 425 mm. Hg. With flow rates of up to 500 ml. of oxygen per minute passed through this instrument the temperature does not alter appreciably. Above this figure it falls in proportion to the flow rate. However, if the temperature of the liquid is known then the concentration of the ether vapour emitted can still be accurately predicted. For example, at a room temperature of 20° C the vapour pressure is 425 mm. Hg (Fig. 2) and the ether concentration is 52 vols. per cent;

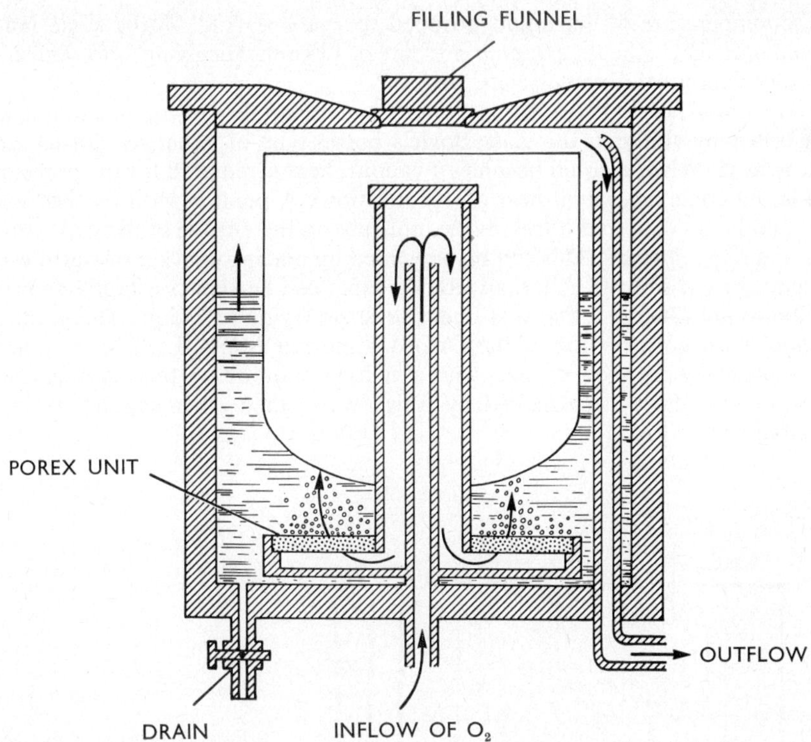

9/FIG. 1.—Diagram of flow of gases through a copper kettle. (After Morris).

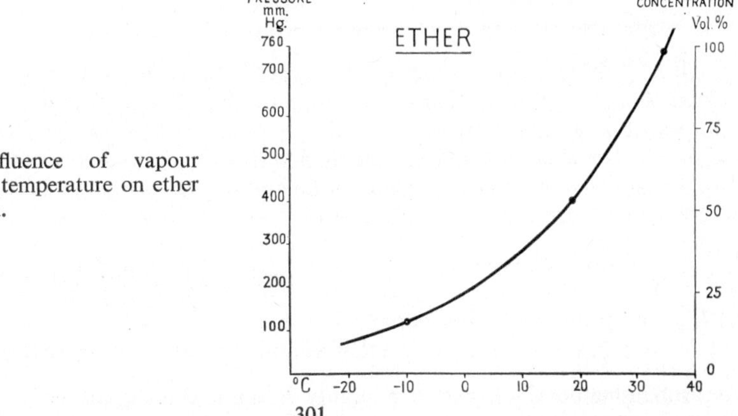

9/FIG. 2.—Influence of vapour pressure and temperature on ether concentration.

if the temperature of the liquid dropped to $-10°$ C (Fig. 2) the same inflow would only meet ether at a vapour pressure of 120 mm. Hg giving a concentration of ether vapour of about 14 vols. per cent.

The important part played by a changing temperature in vaporisation is well illustrated by studying the glass Boyle's bottle type of vaporiser during ether anaesthesia. When a liquid becomes a vapour, heat is required for the process so the liquid cools (i.e. latent heat of vaporisation). A point is soon reached when the liquid is so cool that it freezes the moisture on the outside of the glass vaporiser and frost appears. This can be prevented by placing a jacket of warm water around the glass bottle. Alternatively, the ether can be kept constantly above its boiling-point (36·5), so that it is under pressure trying to escape. This principle is used in the construction of the Oxford Vaporiser Mark II where the ether is surrounded by chemical crystals with a melting point above that of ether. Once these crystals have been melted by warm water then ether vapour will issue spontaneously (Fig. 3).

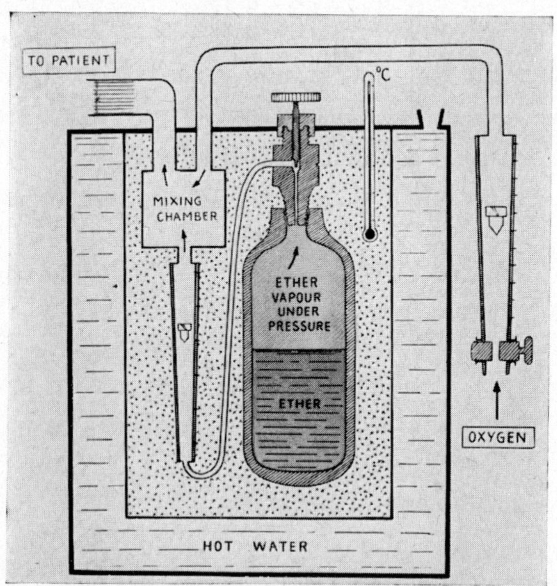

9/Fig.3.—Oxford Vaporiser Mark II.

If a "bubble-through" vaporiser (copper kettle) is used at a room temperature of 20° C then a flow of 500 ml. of oxygen through this instrument will give an output of 1000 ml. of 50 per cent ether vapour. Except for the total volume involved it is easier to think of this as 500 ml. of pure ether vapour. When this total is added to 4 litres of nitrous oxide and oxygen the patient will then receive a 10 per cent ether concentration, viz.

$$\left.\begin{array}{c}\text{4 litres of } N_2O/O_2 \\ + \\ \text{1 litre of 50 per cent ether vapour}\end{array}\right\} \text{5 litres total gas flow with 500 ml. of ether vapour.}$$

= 5 litres of 10 per cent ether vapour in nitrous oxide/oxygen.

Inflammability.—Ether is a highly inflammable liquid which ignites at a temperature of 154° C (the presence of peroxides may lower the ignition point to 100° C). Provided sufficient oxygen is present, low concentrations of ether burn with a clear blue flame, whereas high concentrations explode. In air, the range of inflammability of ether is 1·9–48·0 per cent, but with the addition of more oxygen this is increased to 2·0–82·0 per cent. Since ether vapour is two and a half times heavier than air, the vapour collects like an invisible blanket over the floor. A spark from an electric motor or a switch can ignite this, causing a characteristic "cold blue" flame to spread slowly across the floor. In daylight this flame may be invisible. The chief danger is that it may reach a richer source of oxygen than the air, thus causing an explosion of devastating consequences.

Stability.—The two important impurities caused by decomposition of ether are acetic aldehyde and ether peroxide, the former can be detected by Nessler's solution (complex mercuric iodide solution), and the latter by potassium iodide solution—both of which are turned yellow. Decomposition is favoured by air, light and heat but prevented by copper and hydroquinone. Ether should, therefore, be kept in sealed, dark bottles in a cool cupboard.

Other impurities are alcohol, sulphuric acid, sulphur dioxide, mercaptans, and ethyl esters.

Some doubt has been expressed about the toxicity of these impurities of ether in man. An investigation in animals revealed that aldehyde (0·5 per cent) was without significant effect, whereas mercaptans (1·0 per cent) and peroxide (0·5 per cent) could cause gastric irritation but had no other obvious deleterious action. During anaesthesia the presence of mercaptans in the ether should be suspected if the patient's expirations have a peculiar "fishy" odour; in such cases tachycardia and an unexplained hypotension may also occur.

Pharmacological Actions

Uptake and distribution.—Ether has a blood/gas solubility coefficient of 12·1 (Eger *et al.*, 1963). This signifies that blood has a tremendous capacity for absorbing ether so that it is constantly being removed from the alveoli. Consequently it takes a long time for the alveolar tension to rise to the same height as the inspired tension. As alveolar tension is virtually synonymous with brain tension then induction of anaesthesia will be slow and equally recovery will be affected in the reverse manner. This combined with the fact that it is irritant to the respiratory tract means that it will take 15–25 minutes to achieve deep anaesthesia.

The solubility of ether in the various tissues is similar to that of blood (Table 1).

9/TABLE 1

THE TISSUE/BLOOD COEFFICIENT FOR ETHER

1·14	in Brain tissue
1·2	in Lung tissue
3·3	in Fat tissue

(Eger *et al.*, 1963).

Significance of oil/gas solubility.—The value for ether is 65; this signifies a relatively low lipoid solubility when compared with other agents, e.g. 224 for halothane and 960 for trichloroethylene. The oil/gas solubility coefficient is another way of indicating anaesthetic potency. For example, to produce the 1st plane of surgical anaesthesia with ether an alveolar concentration of 2·5 vols. per cent is required, whereas with trichloroethylene only 0·17 vols. per cent is needed (Eger, personal communication).

Estimation of ether concentration.—In the past the concentration of ether in the blood was measured by complex chemical analysis of the level in blood (Andrews *et al.*, 1940). Newer methods such as gas chromatography or infra-red analysis are now available and these indicate the alveolar concentration of ether in vols. per cent (Table 2).

9/TABLE 2

APPROXIMATE BLOOD AND ALVEOLAR LEVELS OF ETHER IN RELATION TO DEPTH OF ANAESTHESIA

	Blood level in mg. per cent	*Alveolar concentration in vols. per cent*
Stage I	10– 40	0·284–1·14
Stage II	40– 80	1·14 –2·27
Stage III, Plane I	80–110	2·27 –3·12
„ II	110–120	3·12 –3·41
„ III	120–130	3·41 –3·69
„ IV	130–140	3·69 –3·98
Stage IV	140–180	3·98 –5·11

Excretion.—Ether is not broken down in the body. The majority (85–90 per cent) is excreted unchanged through the lungs and the remainder is eliminated via the skin, body secretions and urine.

Action on the respiratory system.—Ether, in anaesthetic concentrations, is an irritant to the mucosa of the respiratory tract. It increases the amount of bronchial secretions but at the same time it also increases the internal diameter of the bronchi and bronchioles. For this reason, it is an extremely useful anaesthetic agent for patients with asthma or bronchiolar spasm. Ether does not affect the action of surfactant in reducing surface tension in the alveoli (Miller and Thomas, 1967).

Ether is believed to stimulate the nerve endings in the bronchial tree and thus reflexly excite the respiratory centre. It may also sensitise the baroreceptors. The ultimate effect is to increase the *rate* of respiration. At a later stage, as the paralysant action of ether manifests itself in deep anaesthesia, the minute volume steadily declines until apnoea finally supervenes. Larson and his colleagues (1969) have shown that in healthy unpremedicated patients, the resting preinduction arterial carbon dioxide tension does not rise until deep levels of ether anaesthesia (alveolar ether concentrations of 6 per cent) are reached. They doubt the need for controlled or assisted ventilation to maintain a satisfactory arterial carbon dioxide tension during anaesthesia.

Action on the cardiovascular system.—There is still a wide margin of discrepancy in the reported findings of the action of ether on the cardiovascular system in man. This is because countless studies have been made but each has varied the technique or the quantity or quality of premedicant and other drugs used. As most patients undergoing ether anaesthesia require premedication, it has been argued that studies made on patients without premedication are only academic, yet it is only through such studies that it is possible to determine the precise effect of ether anaesthesia in man.

If ether vapour is added to the circulation in a heart-lung preparation there is a dramatic depression of myocardial activity. Brewster and his colleagues (1953) working with adrenalectomised dogs have convincingly shown that ether can depress the myocardium. Jones and his co-workers (1962) have demonstrated that ether produces increased sympathetic nervous activity, mainly in the form of liberation of noradrenaline. The plasma level of noradrenaline rises with increasing depth of ether anaesthesia (Black *et al.*, 1969) (Fig. 4).

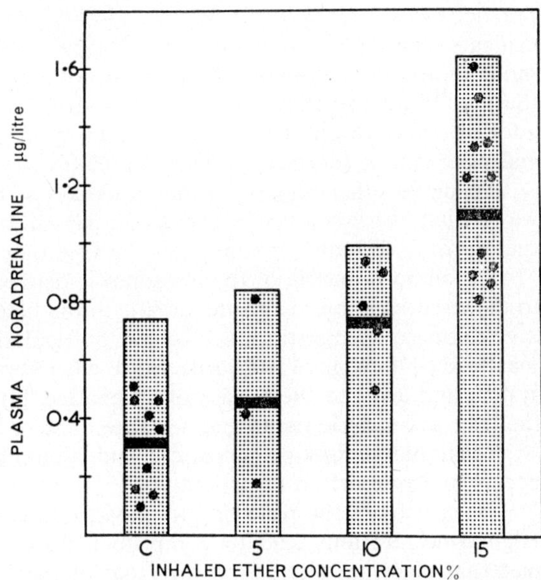

9/FIG. 4—Plasma noradrenaline levels in relation to increasing concentration of inhaled ether. The horizontal black lines indicate mean values (Black *et al.*, 1969).

Ether anaesthesia produces remarkably small alterations in blood pressure and pulse rate. It rarely leads to cardiac irregularities and does not sensitise the myocardium (like cyclopropane) to the action of noradrenaline and adrenaline. In fact, in the past, small concentrations of ether were often given to stop irregularities produced by cyclopropane anaesthesia. The evidence of tachycardia when ether is given without atropine premedication is taken as an indication of the parasympathetic blocking action of ether. To summarise, ether appears to increase sympathetic nervous activity and block parasympathetic activity in normal man (Price, 1961). The increase in noradrenaline liberation under ether anaesthesia partially offsets the direct myocardial depressant action of ether seen in the isolated heart preparation. Deep ether anaesthesia, therefore, should be used with caution in those patients with reduced catecholamine secretion or in the presence of ganglion blockade. β blocking agents, such as propranolol, are particularly dangerous during ether anaesthesia (Jorfeldt *et al.*, 1967).

Action on the peripheral circulation.—McArdle and his colleagues (1968) have measured the effects on forearm blood flow and conclude that increasing concentration leads to a reduction in flow. There is no change in flow with inspired concentrations of 5 per cent ether, a slight fall with 10 per cent and a significant reduction with 15 per cent. When the sympathetic nerve supply to one forearm is blocked by local analgesia, the reduction in blood flow to that side still equals the fall on the unblocked side as increasing concentrations of ether are inspired, thus suggesting that the vasoconstriction is not nervously mediated. Black *et al* (1969) suggest that there is a close relationship between the increase in vascular resistance and a rising plasma noradrenaline concentration.

Action on skeletal muscle.—Ether causes skeletal muscle relaxation by depressing the central nervous system (Ngai *et al.*, 1965), and by affecting the nerve, the motor end-plate and the muscle itself. Concentrations used in clinical practice cause a block at the motor end-plate (Secher, 1951*a*), and there is some evidence that the post-junctional membrane is affected (Karis *et al.*, 1966). The mode of action is probably similar (but not identical) to that of *d*-tubocurarine (Secher, 1951*b*), so that when these two drugs are used in the same patient an additive effect results from their synergism. The effect of ether at the motor end-plate can be reversed by neostigmine (Gross and Cullen, 1943).

Action on other organs.—Ether provokes sickness (see Chapter 47) in two ways. First, it is absorbed in saliva and passed to the stomach where it irritates the mucosa. Secondly, it stimulates the vomiting centre in the medulla.

The smooth muscle of the intestines is depressed by ether in direct relation to the concentration of the anaesthetic in the blood.

Prolonged administration of ether, particularly in the presence of hypoxia, may lead to damage of liver cells. Since ether stimulates the autonomic nervous system and leads to the release of adrenaline, glycogen is mobilised from both the liver and muscle tissue and a marked rise in blood sugar follows.

Renal blood flow is depressed, and albuminuria from tubular irritation, occurs in a proportion of patients.

Ether reduces the tone of the gravid uterus even in slight concentrations. High concentrations lead to complete relaxation. It rapidly passes from the maternal placental circulation into that of the foetus, so that equilibrium between the two is soon achieved.

Clinical Use

The objective in the administration of any anaesthetic is not only to produce unconsciousness but also to suppress the reflex activity of the patient to just a sufficient degree to enable the surgeon to perform a particular operation. Modern anaesthetic techniques often go far beyond this maxim, but ether still remains the safest and most effective means of gradually producing reflex suppression.

In the conscious state, if the skin of a patient's hand is incised with a knife, the hand is rapidly withdrawn unless the patient deliberately brings other muscles into force which overcome this withdrawal reflex. The moment unconsciousness is produced, the central controlling force is removed, and the patient responds to stimuli in a reflex manner. Now, if the skin is cut, not only is the limb withdrawn but, owing to "facilitation" produced by the reflex, there is a spread to many other pathways, so that the larynx may close, the abdominal muscles may contract, and the other limbs move across in an unco-ordinated effort to ward off the stimulus. As the depth of anaesthesia increases so, one by one, the reflex pathways become blocked, until finally all are suppressed. The exact position in which the reflex arc is broken differs with the various anaesthetic agents. Ether not only has a direct suppressant action on the central nervous system but also raises the excitation threshold of the motor end-plate, in a similar manner to *d*-tubocurarine chloride, thus producing a neuro-muscular block.

Even in minimal concentrations ether irritates the bronchial tree, stimulating the vagal afferent fibres leading to an increase in depth and rate of respiration together with an outpouring of mucous secretions. The latter reflex is successfully depressed by adequate doses of atropine or hyoscine. As the depth of anaesthesia increases the respiratory pattern changes, more reflexes become suppressed, and characteristic changes in the size of the pupil can be seen. This slow progression of change has made it possible to divide up the various alterations in reflex activity into stages of ether anaesthesia. First described by Guedel after an exhaustive study of open ether anaesthetics, these stages remain today amongst the basic requirements for the student of anaesthesia. They are given in Table 3.

The pre-operative use of even small doses of the opiates prevents the correct interpretation of the pupil signs. The changes are best seen in children premedicated with barbiturates. During rapid lightening of ether anaesthesia the changes in pupillary diameter (together with all the other reflexes) tend to lag behind the more accurate respiratory-pattern changes. Sometimes even the respiratory patterns of deep anaesthesia may persist until the patient is practically awake.

Guedel's classification refashioned.—Many authors have attempted to refashion Guedel's classification to embrace the changes seen with such anaesthetic drugs as cyclopropane and with the muscle relaxants. With ether, a relatively slow process of events underlines the stages and enhances the intrinsic safety of the drug. Newer agents do not respect such an orderly sequence; amongst others, the capacity of the intravenous thiobarbiturates to depress respiration in light anaesthesia, and of muscle relaxants to simulate most of the signs of anaesthesia yet produce no anaesthesia, are well known. The idea of anaesthetic depth is outmoded when combinations of drugs are used, but the need for a guide to the assessment of anaesthesia remains. Mushin (1948) and Laycock (1953) have restated the orthodox stages in modern terms. Analgesia, characterised by consciousness and disorientation, is an essential feature of the first stage, and merges into the second, when unconsciousness supervenes, often with marked reflex activity. Both these stages may be lost, however, when the induction of anaesthesia is rapid. It is in the third stage that surgery is performed when the reflexes are depressed. The fourth stage represents overdosage.

Each or all of these stages of general anaesthesia can usually be assessed from the specific and objective signs that surgical stimuli produce. Thus modern polypharmacy in anaesthesia is devised to select a combination of drugs, each with a more or less distinct action, and to avoid the unnecessary depression of other parts of the body that must occur occasionally when a single agent is used.

9/TABLE 3. THE STAGES AND SIGNS OF ETHER ANAESTHESIA

	Respiration			Pupils		Reflex Depression
	Rhythm	Volume	Pattern	Size	Position	
Stage I (Analgesia) Analgesia to loss of consciousness	Irregular	Small	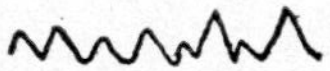	Small	Divergent	Nil
Stage II (Excitement) Loss of consciousness to rhythmical respiration	Irregular	Large	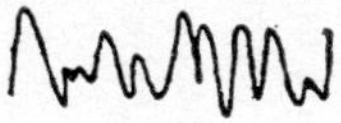	Large	Divergent	Eyelash Eyelid
Stage III (Surgical anaesthesia)						
Plane I Rhythmical respiration to cessation of eye movement	Regular	Large	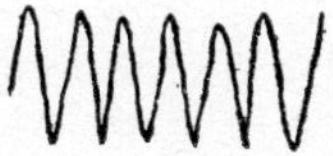	Small	Divergent	Skin Vomiting Conjunctival Pharyngeal Stretch from limb-muscles
Plane II Cessation of eye movement to start of respiratory muscle paresis (excl. diaphragm)	Regular	Medium	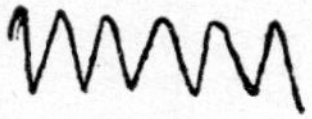 *	$\frac{1}{2}$ dilated	Fixed centrally	Corneal
Plane III Respiratory muscle paresis to paralysis	Regular Pause after expiration	Small	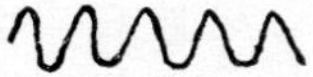	$\frac{3}{4}$ dilated	Fixed centrally	Laryngeal Peritoneal
Plane IV Diaphragmatic paresis to paralysis	Jerky Irregular Quick inspiration Prolonged expiration, i.e. "see-saw"	Small	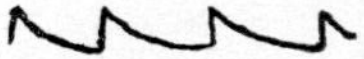	Fully dilated	Fixed centrally	Anal sphincter Carinal
Stage IV Apnoea						

* If the respiration rate is slow, an expiratory pause may be seen in Plane II.

Gray (1957) has summarised this type of technique in the single word "control". Others have termed it "balanced anaesthesia", but this idea of utilising more than one agent to offset the disadvantages of a single one, was suggested long before anaesthesia reached its present state (Lundy, 1926).

The anaesthetist chooses a drug or mixture of drugs that best fits the anticipated needs of the operation, and as Laycock (1953) has written, reflexes are his essential guides in this matter. He must understand them, look out for them, nurse them, leave them alone, depress or abolish them.

Methods of Administration

A patient can be anaesthetised with ether by any one of the five standard methods (see p. 197), namely open, semi-open, semi-closed and closed with carbon dioxide absorption.

For an open technique the Schimmelbusch mask is commonly used. This consists of a wire frame covered with a layer or two of gauze or a single layer of lint. The ether is dropped on to it from a suitable bottle, the aim being to supply the maximum concentration that the patient will tolerate without coughing or breath-holding. The mask should be kept moist over its whole surface since this will provide the maximum vapour concentration, bearing in mind that the liquid vaporises very rapidly. It is helpful during open ether administration to allow a slow trickle of oxygen under the margin of the mask, and during the induction of anaesthesia to add a little carbon dioxide to increase the depth of respiration. An alternative to the addition of carbon dioxide is to allow some of this gas to accumulate from the patient's exhalations by covering the mask with gamgee gauze so that the system becomes semi-open. Such an arrangement also helps to contain the ether vapour.

The chief disadvantage of these techniques is the unpleasant induction, but this can be mitigated by the use of ethyl chloride prior to ether. Very high vapour concentrations are seldom achieved—indeed the concentration may be insufficient for some adults. Under experimental conditions, using an external method of warming, concentrations of 40 per cent or more have been obtained, but in clinical practice the rapid evaporation of ether results in a corresponding fall in temperature and therefore in the volume concentration of the inspired vapour.

In the semi-closed method the ether is vaporised in a glass container by a flow of anaesthetic gases and oxygen. One of the factors adding to the safety of ether as an anaesthetic agent, when used in this way, is that as vaporisation increases, so the temperature of the liquid ether falls which in turn slows the rate of vaporisation. If, therefore, the control is set to deliver a strong concentration of ether vapour, the depth of anaesthesia increases, but after a time, with the control still in the same position, there is a reduction in the vapour concentration. It is inadvisable to warm the outside of the glass container unless a strong concentration is required during the induction of anaesthesia. Even then this practice is generally considered too dangerous and it is safer to surround the bottle with cold water to prevent icing.

The vaporisation of ether in a closed system depends upon the particular type of apparatus. When it is to and fro', vaporisation is exactly as in a semi-closed system, but owing to the small basal flow of gases, only slight concentrations of ether can be obtained. In a circular system the whole volume of ventilation can be passed through an ether bottle, so that high concentrations of ether can be relatively quickly built up. Moreover, vaporisation is assisted both by heat from the patient and by heat produced in the canister.

The E.M.O. inhaler.—This "draw-over" inhaler was designed by Epstein and Macintosh (1956) to deliver a required concentration of anaesthetic vapour irrespective of variations in the temperature of the liquid anaesthetic throughout the range likely to be met in clinical practice. The apparatus incorporates a water bath which surrounds the vaporising chamber and, by acting as a heat buffer, prevents sudden, marked changes in the temperature of the liquid anaesthetic. A bellows type thermostat automatically ensures that a constant vapour concentration of anaesthetic leaves the inhaler. The E.M.O. inhaler must be calibrated to suit the particular volatile anaesthetic used in it.

Convulsions occurring during ether anaesthesia (see Chapter 45).

DIVINYL ETHER $(C_2H_3)_2O$

In 1887 Semmler described a substance which he believed to be divinyl ether. The anaesthetic properties of divinyl ether were first described by Leake and Chen in 1930, and three years later Gelfan and Bell (1933) published the first report on its use in clinical anaesthesia.

Preparation.—This is a complicated and costly process. Ether is first chlorinated to prepare $\beta\beta$-dichlor-ether which is then fused with molten potassium hydroxide to produce divinyl ether, potassium chloride and water.

$(C_2H_4Cl)_2O$ +	2KOH →	$(C_2H_3)_2O$ +	2KCl +	$2H_2O$
$\beta\beta$-dichlor-ether +	Potassium hydroxide →	Divinyl ether +	Potassium chloride +	Water

Physical properties.—Divinyl ether is a colourless, non-irritating liquid with a sweet odour. The molecular weight is 70, the specific gravity of the liquid is 0·77 and of the vapour 2·2 (air = 1). The boiling point is 28·3° C. Divinyl ether is believed to be less soluble in water than ethyl ether, but the oil/water solubility ratio is a matter of disagreement. Adriani (1952) claims it is 41·3, whereas Kochmann (1936) states it is similar to that of diethyl ether, or 3·2. The very rapid recovery from anaesthesia with this agent favours Adriani's figure.

Stability.—Divinyl ether has a relatively low stability, which is made worse by acids and improved by alkalis. When it is chemically pure it is so volatile that moisture tends to freeze on the anaesthetic face-piece. For this reason 3·5 per cent absolute alcohol is added to diminish volatility. A non-volatile organic base—phenyl-alpha-naphthylamine—in a concentration of 0·01 per cent is also added to improve the stability. The commercial product is known as "Vinesthene" in the United Kingdom. The liquid decomposes on exposure to air, light and heat to form formaldehyde, acetaldehyde, formic and acetic acid. It is, therefore, best kept in dark, well-stoppered bottles in a cool place. The manufacturers do not recommend use two years after production and it is inadvisable to use the contents of a bottle that has been opened for more than two weeks. It is not affected by soda lime even when the heat in the canister reaches temperatures as high as 70° C.

Inflammability.—Divinyl ether is explosive when mixed with air in concentrations between 1·7 and 27·0 per cent, and with oxygen between 1·8 and 85·0 per cent.

Pharmacological Actions

Divinyl ether is absorbed and eliminated almost entirely through the lungs, but a small percentage is excreted through the skin. A vapour, with a concentration of 4 per cent, will give a light plane of anaesthesia with a blood concentration of 20–30 mg. per cent, whereas a vapour with 10 per cent divinyl ether may lead to a blood level of 70 mg. per cent and respiratory arrest. Induction is more rapid and pleasant than with ether owing to the increased potency and the absence of irritation of the bronchial tree. Recovery is also more rapid than after ether.

Action on the cardiovascular system.—Divinyl ether has similar effects to diethyl ether. The pacemaker may be displaced, leading to auricular extrasystoles, but the adrenergic stimulation leads to improvement in myocardial contraction.

Action on the respiratory system.—Bronchial dilatation is produced, and in light anaesthesia respiration is increased in rate. An overdose leads to failure of the respiratory centre before the heart finally stops beating.

Action on the alimentary system.—Divinyl ether can cause toxic damage to the liver if used in high concentration for prolonged periods. Central lobular necrosis is produced, and though this complication is rare it is inadvisable to use the agent for more than 30 minutes at one administration. As with chloroform, the incidence of this complication can be greatly reduced by pre-operative treatment with glucose, protein and amino-acids in order to protect the liver, and also by a high percentage of oxygen with a low carbon dioxide tension during anaesthesia.

Other actions.—Salivation is apt to be produced by divinyl ether, particularly if premedication has been omitted. It has few side effects and causes little or no nausea and vomiting after short administrations. It depresses uterine tone in labour and quickly crosses the placenta into the foetus.

Clinical Use

Divinyl ether is both volatile and expensive, so that its clinical use is restricted; although it has some value for the induction of anaesthesia, divinyl ether alone is generally used in a special closed inhaler as a single dose method. A quantity of the agent is evaporated in the bag of an inhaler which has previously been filled with oxygen. About 3–5 ml. of divinyl ether will produce anaesthesia in about six breaths and give approximately 2–3 minutes of unconsciousness, depending upon the size of the patient. The method is particularly suitable for guillotine tonsillectomy, and sometimes for dental extractions, in children.

A mixture of 75 per cent diethyl ether and 25 per cent divinyl ether marketed under the trade name of "Vinesthene Anaesthetic Mixture" (V.A.M.) has a wider application, however, since it gives a rapid induction of anaesthesia with less irritation of the bronchial tract than does diethyl ether alone. V.A.M. may be vaporised by any of the methods described for ether.

ETHYL CHLORIDE (C_2H_5Cl)

Ethyl chloride was first prepared by Basil Valentine during the early part of the seventeenth century. Flourens in 1847 (Flourens 1847 *a* and *b*) and Heyfelder in 1848 described its general anaesthetic properties, but it continued to be used solely for local refrigeration analgesia until in 1894 Carlson inadvertently produced unconsciousness in a patient whilst spraying the gum for a dental extraction. Since that time it has been used extensively in anaesthesia.

Preparation.—There are two common methods of preparation:

By reacting ethylene with hydrochloric acid:

$$C_2H_4 + HCl \rightarrow C_2H_5Cl.$$

By treating ethyl alcohol with hydrochloric acid:

$$C_2H_5OH + HCl \rightarrow C_2H_5Cl + H_2O.$$

Physical properties.—Ethyl chloride is a clear fluid with an ethereal odour which is not irritating to the respiratory tract. Frequently this is masked by the addition of eau-de-Cologne. The molecular weight is 64·5. The specific gravity of the liquid is 0·921 at 20° C and of the vapour 2·28 (air = 1). The boiling point is 12·5° C, so that at ordinary room temperatures it is a vapour. Nevertheless, it is easily compressed to form a highly volatile liquid which can be stored in glass or metal tubes. It has a high lipoid solubility, for at 38° C five volumes of vapour dissolves in one volume of blood.

Impurities.—It may contain traces of alcohol, aldehydes, chlorides or polyhalogenated ethanes.

Inflammability.—The vapour is heavier than air and is capable of explosion when mixed with air in concentrations between 3·8–15·4 per cent and with oxygen between 4·0 and 67·0 per cent.

Pharmacological Actions

Ethyl chloride is non-irritant to the respiratory mucosa. Concentrations of 3–4·5 per cent in the inspired air produce anaesthesia and a blood concentration of 20–30 mg. per cent leads to the signs of surgical anaesthesia. Forty mg. per cent leads to respiratory arrest.

Action on the cardiovascular system.—There is very little evidence that ethyl chloride produces an irritable myocardium, and arrhythmias are rare during induction. The pulse rate may be slowed from stimulation of the vagal centre and there is widespread vaso-dilatation due to vasomotor depression. As anaesthesia progresses the heart dilates slightly, owing to the effect on the myocardium. Although both the cardiac output and peripheral vascular tone are depressed in deep anaesthesia, there is no evidence that myocardial failure will occur before respiratory arrest—most cases of sudden circulatory failure during the induction of anaesthesia can be traced to relative overdosage at the time rather than to peculiar side-effects. Overdosage easily and quickly results on account of the physical properties of the drug.

Other actions.—Ethyl chloride anaesthesia is frequently followed by headache, nausea and vomiting. It depresses uterine tone in labour and quickly crosses the placenta into the foetus.

Clinical Use

Local analgesia.—A fine spray is allowed to fall on the operation area. The liquid vaporises and the skin cools to $-20°$ C, and the surrounding water vapour freezes and deposits fine snowy crystals over the wound. The incision is painless but as the thaw sets in the pain may become excruciating.

General anaesthesia.—Ethyl chloride is an extremely potent and simple anaesthetic to administer—so much so that the greatest possible care should be exercised in its use. It is particularly suitable for induction in children, but once a rhythmical respiratory exchange has commenced it should be abandoned: if necessary, the anaesthesia can be maintained by the much safer agent—diethyl ether.

It is inadvisable to spray more than 5 ml. of the ethyl chloride on to an open mask for the induction of anaesthesia; subsequent doses should be much smaller. Great care should be taken to prevent a child holding its breath for a prolonged period and then taking a large inspiration of a highly-concentrated vapour, which can lead to circulatory collapse.

Ethyl chloride may be used with oxygen in a closed inhaler in a manner similar to that described for divinyl ether. A dose of 3–5 ml. is sufficient for a single administration.

TRICHLOROETHYLENE (CCl_2CHCl)

Originally described by E. Fischer, a German chemist, in 1864, it was first used as a anaesthetic agent in animals by Lehmann in 1911 whilst working at Wurzburg University.

The finding that trichloroethylene was a powerful grease solvent led to its wide application in industry for the removal of grease from metal and machinery. This led to toxic symptoms in some of the factory workers, however, and in 1915 Plessner described the syndrome of acute trichloroethylene poisoning—one of the main features of which is sensory paralysis of the fifth cranial nerve. Such symptoms were almost certainly due to the impurities associated with trichloroethylene. In the same year Oppenheim described twelve cases of trigeminal neuralgia that were successfully treated by inhalations of trichloroethylene vapour.

In 1934, Dennis Jackson of Cincinnati University redescribed its anaesthetic properties and one year later, at the same University, Striker and his colleagues published the first report of the successful administration of trichloroethylene to 304 patients for dental extractions or minor operative procedures. Hewer and Hadfield (1941) popularised it in the United Kingdom.

Preparation.—Acetylene when treated with chlorine forms tetrachlorethane; this is reacted with calcium hydroxide in a "lime slurry" to form trichloroethylene, which is purified by distillation.

$$\underset{\text{Acetylene}}{C_2H_2} + \underset{\text{Chlorine}}{2Cl_2} \rightarrow \underset{\text{Tetrachlorethane}}{C_2H_2Cl_4}$$

$$\underset{\text{Tetrachlorethane}}{2C_2H_2Cl_4} + \underset{\text{Calcium hydroxide}}{Ca(OH)_2} \rightarrow \underset{\text{Trichloroethylene}}{2C_2HCl_3} + \underset{\text{Calcium chloride}}{CaCl_2} + \underset{\text{Water}}{2H_2O}$$

Physical properties.—Trichloroethylene is a heavy colourless liquid with a low volatility (boiling point 87·5° C) and has a smell similar to that of chloroform but not so sweet. The vapour pressure at 20° C is about 57 mm. Hg. Thus with a high boiling point and low vapour pressure it is relatively difficult to vaporise high concentrations.

However, it has an oil/gas solubility coefficient of 960; on this basis it is the most potent of all known anaesthetic agents and it is calculated that a concentration as low as 0·17 vols. per cent will achieve the 1st plane of surgical anaesthesia (or minimal anaesthetic concentration).

"Trilene", the trade name for the preparation which is used in anaesthesia in Great Britain, consists of purified trichloroethylene, thymol (stabilising agent) 1:10,000 and waxoline blue (dye) 1:200,000. The dye is added to distinguish it from chloroform.

In the United States the trade name is "Trimar". It consists of 99–99·5 per cent purified trichloroethylene with the remainder alcohol. Ammonium carbonate is added as a preservative.

Stability.—Trichloroethylene is decomposed by strong light or by contact with hot surfaces into phosgene and hydrochloric acid. It is, therefore, best kept in metal containers.

It is contra-indicated in the presence of soda lime for two reasons—first, it decomposes to phosgene and hydrochloric acid when in contact with a hot surface. Secondly, in the presence of an alkali and heat it may be broken down to hydrochloric acid and dichloracetylene, a substance which is both inflammable and toxic. Dichloracetylene may itself decompose to phosgene and carbon monoxide. Thus:

1.
$$\begin{matrix} CHCl \\ \| \\ CCl_2 \end{matrix} \xrightarrow{NaOH} \begin{matrix} CCl \\ ||| \\ CCl \end{matrix} + HCl \text{ (absorbed by NaOH)}$$

Trichloroethylene + Heat → Dichloracetylene + Hydrochloric acid

2.
$$\begin{matrix} CCl \\ ||| \\ CCl \end{matrix} + O_2 \longrightarrow COCl_2 + CO$$

Dichloracetylene + Oxygen → Phosgene + Carbon monoxide

The rate of decomposition of trichloroethylene in the presence of soda lime depends largely on the temperature. At 15° C it is slow, but over 60° C the rate rises sharply (Fig. 5). It has been suggested that decomposition can be inhibited by the addition of 10 per cent silica.

Some of the early cases of cranial nerve palsy following the use of trichloroethylene in the presence of soda lime are believed to have been due to the high percentage of sodium hydroxide present in the absorbents used. Soda lime of this type was five times more hygroscopic and also generated more heat than that available today. It has also been shown that the temperature of modern soda lime rarely rises above 40° C during clinical anaesthesia, nevertheless at this temperature small amounts of dichloracetylene can be formed.

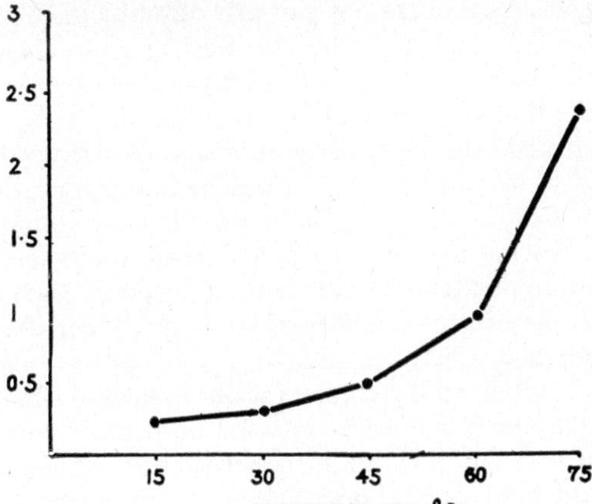

9/FIG. 5.—Chart to show how the rate of decomposition of trichloroethylene to dichloracetylene rises rapidly with temperature.

It is inadvisable to use cautery or diathermy in the immediate presence of trichloroethylene vapour, such as during an oral operation, because at temperatures above 125° C phosgene and hydrochloric acid may be rapidly formed, particularly if a high percentage of oxygen is present (Carney and Gillespie, 1945; Firth and Stuckey, 1945).

Toxicity.—Cranial nerve lesions are amongst the commonest toxic manifestations of impure trichloroethylene or its degradation products, such as dichloracetylene. The fifth nerve is the most commonly involved but lesions of all the nerves except the first, ninth and eleventh have been reported.

The onset of toxic symptoms and signs is usually characterised by a complaint of numbness or coldness around the lips starting about twenty-four to forty-eight hours after the anaesthetic ceased. During the next few days the area of sensory loss spreads to involve the whole field supplied by the trigeminal nerve. There is no motor involvement. Recovery usually begins between the fifth and tenth days and may be complete in a fortnight.

Inflammability.—Trichloroethylene vapour is non-inflammable and non-explosive in the concentrations used in anaesthesia (see also Chapter 18).

Pharmacological Actions

Uptake and distribution.—Trichloroethylene has a blood/gas solubility coefficient of 9·15, which indicates that it is relatively soluble in blood. In other words blood has a great capacity for taking up trichloroethylene. A long time will elapse, therefore, before alveolar tension reaches equilibrium with the inspired concentration. Clayton and Parkhouse (1962) found that the administration of a 1 per cent v/v trichloroethylene concentration resulted in an arterial concentration in the blood of 12·17 mg./100 ml. Furthermore, in slim subjects the concentration in venous blood approximated to that of arterial blood after about 30 minutes, whereas in fat subjects it took twice as long. This is because trichloroethylene is extremely soluble in human fat due to its high oil/gas solubility; in fact, it is probably 100 times more soluble in fat than in muscle.

To summarise, this agent has a low volatility and a high blood solubility.

The slow induction is partially offset by the high degree of potency due to the remarkable oil/gas solubility. Recovery, however, is prolonged.

Trichloroethylene is partly excreted unchanged by the lungs and partly metabolised. Depending upon the duration of time for which the vapour is inhaled, the percentage recovery of trichloroethylene in expired gases varies from 67 to 83 per cent (Malchy and Parkhouse, 1969). Metabolic degradation is slow, and the metabolic products are found in the urine from 10 to 18 days following a single period of trichloroethylene administration. Assuming that approximately 20 per cent of inspired trichloroethylene is metabolised, then 10 per cent of trichloroethanol and 10 per cent of trichloracetic acid will result (Greene, 1968).

Action on the cardiovascular system.—Almost every known form of cardiac arrhythmia has been reported during trichloroethylene anaesthesia, but always in association with high concentrations of the inhaled vapour. Sinus tachycardia and bradycardia, nodal rhythm and partial heart block are usually associated with light anaesthesia, whereas ventricular extrasystoles may occur in deep anaesthesia.

The incidence of cardiac arrhythmias is likely to be increased if adrenaline is used during anaesthesia. Opinion is divided on the incidence of primary cardiac failure due to trichloroethylene, though it appears that this condition may very rarely occur (Edwards *et al.*, 1956).

Trichloroethylene produces no significant alteration in forearm blood flow, heart rate or mean arterial blood pressure (McArdle *et al.*, 1968).

Action on the respiratory system.—Trichloroethylene in moderate concentrations (1–3 per cent) is non-irritant to the respiratory tract; in high concentrations, however, it may cause tachypnoea. This is believed to be due to simultaneous paralysis of the stretch receptors in the lung and a concomitant stimulation of the deflation receptors, resulting in a rapid shallow respiration (see lung receptors, p. 93). The increased respiratory rate leads to a diminished tidal volume and in severe cases this may be so reduced that hypoxia occurs.

Other actions.—Post-operative vomiting and headache occasionally follow trichloroethylene anaesthesia, while circumoral herpes has been reported.

Trichloroethylene causes a rise in intracranial pressure. Jennett and his associates (1969) report that such an increase occurs even when the arterial carbon dioxide is low, and that it is associated with cerebral vasodilation and an increased cerebral blood flow.

Trichloroethylene will depress the contractions of the uterus during labour. Analgesic concentrations—0·5 per cent v./v. in air or less—have little effect on uterine muscle unless inhaled for periods approaching 4 hours, when accumulation of the drug in the body occurs. At this stage both the rate and tone of uterine contraction may be decreased. Trichloroethylene rapidly crosses the placenta into the foetal circulation, and animal experiments (sheep) show that within sixteen minutes the foetal concentration is higher than that in the maternal circulation (Helliwell and Hutton, 1950).

The effect of trichloroethylene on the liver has been studied by determining concentrations of glutamic acid, pyruvic acid, transaminase and lactic dehydrogenase in the blood of patients undergoing anaesthesia. Elevated values were not found in any case (Bløndal and Fagerlund, 1963).

Clinical Use

The fact that trichloroethylene is non-inflammable, relatively non-irritant and with minimal post-operative side-effects, has made it popular as a supplement to the sequence thiopentone, nitrous oxide and oxygen for the maintenance of light anaesthesia. The chief disadvantage in general surgery is that it is unsuitable for the production of muscular relaxation, since when this is attempted tachypnoea and cardiac arrhythmias are quickly encountered. Nevertheless, within the safe limits of its application it is a useful agent. For the production of analgesia it is widely used in both obstetrics and dentistry. It is also useful for post-operative analgesia, particularly during physiotherapy (Ellis and Bryce-Smith, 1965; Hovell *et al.*, 1967).

Administration.—The low volatility makes trichloroethylene barely suitable for administration on an open mask, but as it is over four times as heavy as air this route can be used to produce analgesia if no apparatus is available. The drug is most commonly used in a semi-closed system using a Tritec vaporiser or, for analgesia, in a "draw-over" type of apparatus (see Chapter 51). It can also be given in an accurate concentration by volume in air from an E.M.O. inhaler after suitable calibration of the apparatus.

CHLOROFORM ($CHCl_3$)

Chloroform was independently discovered by Soubeiran, Liebig and Guthrie in 1831. Its chemical and physical properties were first described by Alexandre Dumas in 1835, and twelve years later, in 1847, Flourens reported on its anaesthetic properties (Flourens, 1847 *a* and *b*). That same year James Simpson, acting on a suggestion from a Liverpool chemist David Waldie, experimented upon himself and his colleagues, and finally gave it to patients with great success. Soon after its introduction into clinical practice chloroform largely replaced ether in popularity, but since then its popularity has gradually waned.

Preparation.—Chloroform may be prepared in a number of ways, but those most commonly encountered are:

In the laboratory: acetone or ethyl alcohol is heated with bleaching powder and the mixture is then submitted to steam distillation.

$$\underset{\text{Acetone}}{2CH_3.CO.CH_3} + \underset{\text{Bleaching powder}}{Ca(OCl)_2} \rightarrow \underset{\text{Trichlor-acetone}}{CH_3COCCl_3} + \underset{\text{Chloroform}}{CHCl_3} + \underset{\text{Calcium acetate}}{Ca(CH_3.COO)_2}$$

Commercially: carbon tetrachloride and hydrogen are allowed to react in the presence of iron.

$$\underset{\text{Carbon tetrachloride}}{\begin{array}{c} Cl \\ | \\ Cl-C\ \ Cl \\ | \\ Cl \end{array}} + \underset{\text{Hydrogen}}{2H} \xrightarrow[\text{Iron}]{Fe} \underset{\text{Chloroform}}{\begin{array}{c} Cl \\ | \\ Cl-C-H \\ | \\ Cl \end{array}} + \underset{\text{Hydrochloric acid}}{HCl}$$

frequently than not (Hill, 1932). Waters (1951) studied fifty-two patients, and in this small series noted four cases of temporary cardiac arrest, and only seven cases in which no cardiac irregularities occurred. In all induction deaths with chloroform the heart stops before respiration ceases.

During the inhalation of moderate concentrations of chloroform (1·5–2 per cent) the cardiac output and peripheral resistance are progressively decreased, together with a continuous fall in blood pressure. It is incorrect to assume, however, that maintenance of light anaesthesia with low constant concentrations of chloroform leads to a steady fall in blood pressure. In fact perfectly reasonable pressures can be maintained.

Action on the respiratory system.—Chloroform depresses respiration both by a direct effect on the respiratory centre and by the production of progressive depression of the respiratory muscles.

Action on the liver.—It is generally accepted that central hepatic necrosis occurs in some degree after chloroform anaesthesia or analgesia irrespective of the concentration used or the length of administration. But Rollason (1964) using serum glutamic pyruvic transaminase (SGPT) activity in patients with good nutrition could find no evidence of liver damage following chloroform anaesthesia, provided the concentration did not exceed 2·25 per cent in an oxygen-rich mixture and there was no carbon dioxide retention. Repeated short administrations may sensitise the liver, and certainly increase the risk of a bad attack. In severe cases, leading to death, section of the liver will show necrosis with fatty degeneration of the cells surrounding the vein in the centre of the lobule. Signs and symptoms of poisoning are produced only by severe necrosis.

Delayed chloroform poisoning was originally described by Casper in 1850. The first symptoms may occur as early as six hours after the operation, although more commonly they present themselves twenty-four to forty-eight hours later. Nausea and vomiting start early and progressively increase in severity. The diagnosis becomes certain with the development of jaundice, and death, preceded by coma, may occur at any time during the first ten days. Delayed chloroform poisoning is not restricted in its symptomatology to the liver, the heart and kidneys also being affected. Fatty degeneration of the heart and necrosis of the tubular epithelium of the kidneys take place and result in incipient cardiac and renal failure.

A poor nutritional state increases the risk of this complication, whereas the pre-operative use of carbohydrates, proteins and amino-acids helps to protect the liver. Moreover, the avoidance of hypoxia and carbon dioxide retention is of practical help. Waters (1951) has shown that if chloroform is given in the presence of a high percentage of oxygen, and if steps are taken to avoid carbon dioxide accumulation, hepatic and renal function tests in a group of patients show no significant difference from those of controls.

The treatment of delayed chloroform poisoning consists primarily of the administration of intravenous fluids, together with carbohydrates, protein and amino-acids. Of the various amino-acids methionine is the most useful because it plays an important part in building up the reserves of glycogen in the liver.

Action on the kidneys.—The toxic effects of chloroform are mainly on the renal tubules, which at microscopy can be seen to be swollen with the lumina filled with fat globules and coagulated serum. After chloroform anaesthesia transient albuminuria is a common occurrence, while prolonged administration often leads to glycosuria. In cases of delayed poisoning as described above ketonuria also occurs.

Other actions.—Toxic effects may be found in other organs. In severe cases fatty degeneration occurs in the pancreas and spleen, while nausea and vomiting in some degree usually follow all but the briefest anaesthetic. Chloroform depresses uterine contractions during labour and quickly crosses the placenta to reach the foetus.

Clinical Use

The main advantages of chloroform are a sweet-smelling, non-irritant vapour, portability, potency, and non-inflammability. It permits a rapid, smooth induction, while the decreased bleeding which results from circulatory depression was the forerunner of the "hypotensive" technique. Low volatility and a high potency make it particularly valuable in hot and humid countries, while the fact that an experienced administrator can produce such excellent conditions for surgery from a small bottle and simple mask has undoubtedly done much to recommend it in the past. It is interesting to recall in this respect that John Snow is believed to have given 4,000 chloroform anaesthetics without any mortality.

Nevertheless, despite all these advantages, chloroform is not nowadays commonly used. As long ago as 1912 the Committee on Anesthesia of the American Medical Association went so far as to say that in their opinion the use of chloroform for major surgical operations was no longer justifiable. The reason for its elimination from major anaesthetic practice is to be found in the toxic effects it produces on the various parts of the body, and the fact that most, if not all, of its advantages can be obtained with a combination of other agents and with less risk to the patient. Only on an occasion where there is no suitable alternative, such as may occur for instance in certain circumstances in domiciliary midwifery, should chloroform now be used.

Administration

Chloroform may be dropped on to an open mask. One drop weighing 20 mg., if vaporised in 500 ml. of air, forms a 1 per cent concentration of the vapour. At the start of induction 20 drops a minute is adequate, increasing later to 30 drops a minute. Great care should be taken to prevent the sudden inspiration of a high concentration, which is most likely with a struggling patient, and to avoid liquid chloroform reaching the skin, since it may cause a burn. Sometimes patients breathe shallowly during induction and then suddenly take a deep inspiration just before the second stage is reached. Nosworthy (1958) found that this could be avoided by adding a little carbon dioxide to the inspired mixture so that the depth of respiration could be regulated from the onset of unconsciousness. Once rhythmical and regular respiration has become established it is advisable to change over to ether or a chloroform-ether mixture (1 part chloroform to 4 parts diethyl ether). The safety of chloroform is at all times increased by the addition of oxygen to the inhaled mixture.

Administration in a semi-closed system has the advantage that it can be combined with an adequate oxygen flow and a more accurate increase in vapour concentration, but both in this type of system, and particularly in a closed system, the danger of accumulation cannot be over-emphasised.

THE FLUORINATED HYDROCARBONS

The introduction of halothane into clinical practice provides one of the great landmarks in the development of anaesthesia. In an attempt to find an agent that was basically as "safe" as ether yet non-inflammable, Suckling (1957) examined a number of fluorinated hydrocarbons. This group was known to be highly stable, volatile and non-inflammable (under clinical conditions).

In these compounds the fluorine atoms have a strong chemical bond with the carbon atoms. The result is that the fluorine atom is quite unreactive, particularly when the compound contains a CF_2 or CF_3 grouping. Such agents would be unlikely to interfere with body metabolism because of their high chemical stability, and therefore would tend to have a low toxicity (Sadove and Wallace, 1962).

Robbins (1946) in a study of many of the fluorinated hydrocarbons found that those with low boiling points produced convulsive movements; that the potency increased as the boiling point rose, yet recovery time became more prolonged, and that substitution of a bromine atom in the fluorohydrocarbon not only increased potency but also appeared to improve the safety margin.

The inclusion of several halogen atoms in a compound confers inflammability in the clinical range. If the halogen selected is a fluorine atom then there is no decrease in volatility, but the presence of at least one hydrogen atom is necessary for anaesthetic potency.

A large number of fluorinated hydrocarbons have been synthesised but only three have to date received extensive clinical trials. These are halothane, methoxyflurane and fluroxene:

```
   F  Br         Cl  F       H        F  H       H       H
   |  |          |   |       |        |  |       |      /
F—C—C—H      H—C—C—O—C—H     F—C—C—O—C = C
   |  |          |   |       |        |  |              \
   F  Cl         Cl  F       H        F  H               H
 Halothane     Methoxyflurane             Fluroxene
(B.P. 50·2° C) (B.P. 104·65° C)          (B.P. 43·2° C)
```

Of these three compounds halothane has received the widest clinical acclaim. One of the principal features of these fluorohydrocarbons is that they have relatively low boiling points (with the exception of methoxyflurane) when compared with similar agents containing only chlorine or bromine. For example, if all of the five halogens in halothane were chlorine then the boiling point would be 162° C. In fact, the boiling point of halothane is 50·2° C at atmospheric pressure.

A fourth compound that has had limited clinical trials during recent years is teflurane, or 1,1,1,2-tetrafluoro-bromethane, which is similar in structure to halothane. The incidence of cardiac arrhythmias during light surgical anaesthesia with this agent is so high that it cannot be considered as a potentially useful addition to the existing fluorinated hydrocarbons of proven safety.

HALOTHANE ("FLUOTHANE")

Halothane was prepared and examined by Raventós (1956). It was introduced into clinical anaesthesia by Johnstone (1956) and Bryce-Smith and O'Brien (1956).

Physical properties.—Halothane is a heavy, colourless liquid with a sweet smell somewhat resembling chloroform. It contains 0·01 per cent of thymol for stability. The formula is:

```
   F  Br
   |  |
F—C—C—H
   |  |
   F  Cl
```

Halothane

It has a molecular weight of 197·39 and a boiling point of 50·2° C (at 760 mm. Hg). It does not react with soda lime. One of the contaminants is butene in a concentration of 0·001 per cent. When exposed to light for several days it will decompose to various halide acids such as HCl, HBr, free chlorine, bromine radicles and phosgene. The presence of thymol helps to prevent the liberation of free bromine.

The vapour pressure of halothane is 241 mm. Hg at 20° C. It is, therefore, very suitable for vaporisation in a bubble-through (e.g. copper kettle) or temperature and flow-controlled vaporiser (e.g. "Fluotec"). If a flow of 100 ml. of oxygen is passed through the copper kettle (or "Vernitrol") vaporiser then as the vapour pressure is $\frac{240}{760}$ mm. Hg or approximately $\frac{1}{3}$ of an atmosphere 100 ml. of oxygen will pick up 50 ml. of halothane (i.e. a total of 150 ml. of $33\frac{1}{3}$ per cent halothane or 50 ml. of pure halothane vapour). If this quantity (i.e. 50 ml. of halothane vapour) is added to 5 litres of nitrous oxide and oxygen then the patient will receive an inspired concentration of 1 per cent halothane. Similarly, if 200 ml. is put through the vaporiser and this is again added to 5 litres of nitrous oxide and oxygen the patient will receive a 2 per cent halothane vapour.

In the absence of water vapour halothane does not attack most metals. However, if water vapour is present it will attack aluminium, brass and lead. Copper and fault-free chromium are not attacked.

Halothane is readily soluble in rubber (coefficient 121·1 at 760 mm. and 24° C) and less so in polyethylene (coefficient 26·3). This significant rubber solubility together with the large amount of this material used in an anaesthetic system means that the uptake of halothane by rubber could be significant if a low-flow circle absorption technique is used. High flows eliminate this problem (Eger *et al.*, 1962).

Analysis.—Halothane can be estimated by gas chromatography (Dyjverman and Sjövall, 1962) or by infra-red (Robson *et al.*, 1959) or ultra-violet light analysis.

Pharmacology

Uptake and distribution.—Halothane has a blood solubility coefficient of 2·3 (*cf.* nitrous oxide 0·46 and ether 12·1) and might be described as being in the medium range of solubility. Because it is relatively insoluble in blood it is not taken up very rapidly from the alveoli. This means that the alveolar concentration or tension can soon approach the inspired concentration. Now alveolar *tension* is virtually synonymous with brain *tension*, so a high tension is rapidly achieved in the brain. This means induction of anaesthesia is relatively rapid. On withdrawal of the anaesthetic the same process is reversed so that recovery is rapid.

Mapleson (1962) has shown that though the rate of uptake is high at the start, after twenty minutes, for every 1 per cent of halothane vapour in the inspired mixture, the patient has an uptake of 10 ml. of halothane vapour per minute. This first goes to the organs with a rich blood supply such as the heart and brain. Resting muscle and fat have a much poorer blood supply so that they receive their quota of halothane long after the tension in the alveoli and brain have reached equilibrium. Thus, in the first few minutes of halothane anaesthesia most goes to the heart, brain, liver and kidneys. After ten or twenty minutes the muscles are tending to remove their quota from the circulation so that 10 ml. of halothane vapour is removed from the lungs every minute. In time even the poorly perfused fat receives its share. In this manner the body continues almost indefinitely to keep removing halothane vapour from the lungs. If, therefore, a 1 per cent inspired concentration is given to a patient it is estimated that it will take 5 days or more for the concentration in the alveoli to rise to this level. In fact, equilibrium between inspired and alveolar concentrations is probably never reached because a small amount is lost through the skin.

One of the principal reasons for the prolonged uptake of halothane by the body is the remarkable capacity of human fat to absorb it. So great is this affinity—the solubility coefficient of halothane in fat is 60·0 (*cf*, nitrous oxide = 1·0)—that it is capable of removing almost all the halothane it receives in the circulation.

Other tissues also show a slightly greater affinity for halothane than blood, e.g.

9/TABLE 4

TISSUE/BLOOD SOLUBILITY COEFFICIENT OF HALOTHANE

2·6 in Brain
2·6 in Lung
1·6 in Kidney
3·5 in Muscle
60 in Fat

Metabolism.—Isotope labelling techniques have now established that about 12 per cent of inspired halothane is metabolised by the liver microsomes and the resulting products are excreted in the urine (Van Dyke and Chenoweth, 1965). Halothane undergoes both oxidation and dehalogenation to form trifluoracetic acid, as well as bromide and chloride radicals (Rehder *et al.*, 1967). This metabolism may be stimulated by barbiturates and also by further doses of halothane itself (Cascorbi *et al.*, 1970).

Work with mice has shown that the metabolites of halothane may persist in the liver for as long as twelve days after administration (Cohen, 1969). Chronic exposure to halothane can impair liver cell function in small mammals and this may be due to the accumulation of metabolites. A matter of some concern to all anaesthetists, as well as those working in operating theatres, is whether such small concentrations of expired halothane from patients could have any harmful effects on the attendant staff.

Action on respiration.—Halothane is a respiratory depressant. This is more marked in the presence of narcotic premedication. Increasing the inspired concentration of halothane leads to a progressive diminution of volume rather than rate of respiration. In fact, surgical stimulation under light anaesthesia decreases basal metabolism in direct proportion to the depth of anaesthesia; in surgical anaesthesia the oxygen consumption is reduced about 20 per cent (Severinghaus and Cullen, 1958; Nunn and Matthews, 1959).

In view of the respiratory depressant action of halothane it is advisable occasionally to assist the ventilation whenever spontaneous respiration is present. At least 30 per cent oxygen should always be present in the inspired mixture.

The action of sufactant in the lungs is not affected by halothane anaesthesia (Miller and Thomas, 1967).

Halothane may be accidentally injected intravenously, in which case severe pulmonary lesions may occur, leading to death. Sandison and his colleagues (1970), in an experimental study of intravenous halothane in dogs, found that the predominant lesions produced in the lungs were generalised oedema and patchy alveolar haemorrhages, and that pathological changes occurred in other organs and in the blood. They note that in the dog, a dose equivalent to 3–5 ml. for an adult human can cause severe lung damage.

Action on the heart.—One of the principal problems in the study of the action of halothane on the cardiovascular system is the wealth of contradictory evidence. This appears to be largely due to the multiplicity of premedicant and intravenous drugs used in the study. Price (1960), however, administered halothane and oxygen alone to a group of unpremedicated patients and observed the results. The cardiac contractile force was diminished; stroke volume and cardiac output were reduced despite an increased venous pressure. The heart rate and arterial pressure were also reduced, but the total systemic peripheral resistance was only slightly affected. Atropine reversed the bradycardia but failed to correct the arterial hypotension or to improve the cardiac output. Prys-Roberts and his colleagues (1967) found no significant change in calculated systemic peripheral resistance during oxygen-halothane anaesthesia with spontaneous respiration.

There appears to be unanimity of opinion amongst most authors that myocardial depression is directly related to the depth of halothane anaesthesia (Mahaffey *et al.*, 1961; Morrow and Morrow, 1961; Severinghaus and Cullen, 1958; Wenthe *et al.*, 1962), and animal experiments suggest that this is due to inhibition of enzyme activity in the muscle (Brodkin *et al.*, 1967). Nevertheless, an overall picture of the action of halothane is more complex. For example, the ability of atropine to reverse the bradycardia suggests that halothane has a parasympathetic stimulant action as well as producing myocardial depression.

An interesting hypothesis that might explain most of the actions of halothane throughout the body is that in increasing concentration it gradually blocks the action of noradrenaline at the effector sites in the heart, central nervous system and peripheral tissues (Price, 1960). Two important findings support this suggestion. First, unlike most other anaesthetic agents, halothane does not produce an increase in the plasma catechol amine level of blood. Secondly, halothane partially blocks the constrictor action of noradrenaline on the skin vessels (Black and McArdle, 1962). On this basis the effect of halothane on the heart would be to reduce the secretion and activity of noradrenaline at the sympathetic nerve endings in the myocardium and at the same time to sensitise the parasympathetic nerve endings leading to bradycardia. There is experimental evidence from dogs to show that halothane can inhibit and, in adequate concentration, completely block stellate ganglion transmission (Price and Price, 1967).

Arrhythmias occurring during halothane anaesthesia bear a direct relationship to hypercarbia from respiratory depression. Adrenaline can be safely used in the presence of halothane provided the concentration and total dose used are within acceptable limits and the patient is neither hypercarbic nor hypoxic. Katz and Katz (1966) suggest concentrations of 1 in 100,000 to 1 in 200,000 and a total dose of the former of not more than 10 ml. in any one ten-minute period. Whenever an infiltration of adrenaline is used during anaesthesia it is important to remember that the adrenaline itself is the most dangerous factor, and that this danger is enhanced when the injection is made in a vascular part of the body. The prophylactic administration of propranolol intravenously before infiltrating with adrenaline has been recommended (Ikezon *et al.*, 1969), but there are inherent dangers in using propranolol during general anaesthesia, particularly with halothane, and these may well be greater than those of the controlled use of adrenaline.

Action on the peripheral circulation.—Despite a wealth of studies on the action of halothane on the myocardium, there are singularly few available on the action of this drug on the peripheral circulation. Black and McArdle (1962) investigated a group of unpremedicated patients inhaling 1–4 per cent halothane (with thiopentone induction and nitrous oxide/oxygen maintenance). They found a persistant vasodilatation of the skin and muscle vessels along with a fall in both the arterial pressure and the vascular resistance (Fig. 6).

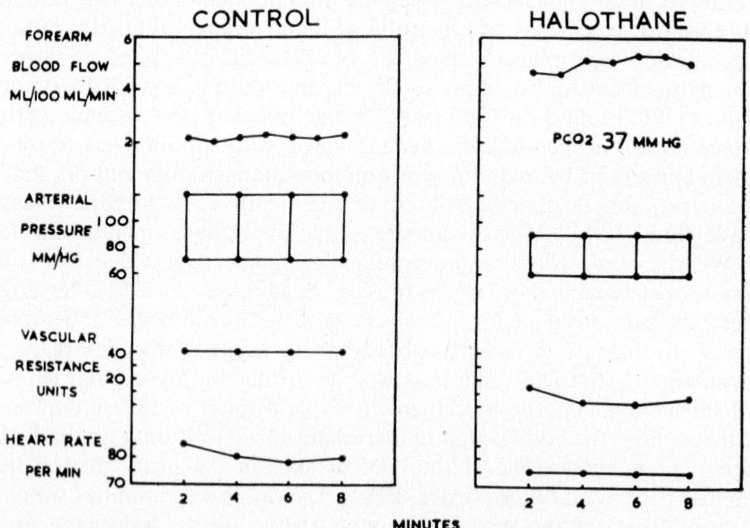

9/Fig. 6.—The effects of halothane on the circulation.

In an attempt to explain the mechanism of the vasodilatation produced by halothane they infused a solution of noradrenaline into the brachial artery of a series of patients (Fig. 7). In the absence of halothane anaesthesia, noradrenaline promptly produced severe vasoconstriction, but when halothane was inhaled this constrictor action of noradrenaline was partially blocked.

In another study they found that if a nerve block was produced in one arm then halothane anaesthesia had no effect on the blood flow through this arm, yet it produced an increase in the normal arm (Fig. 8).

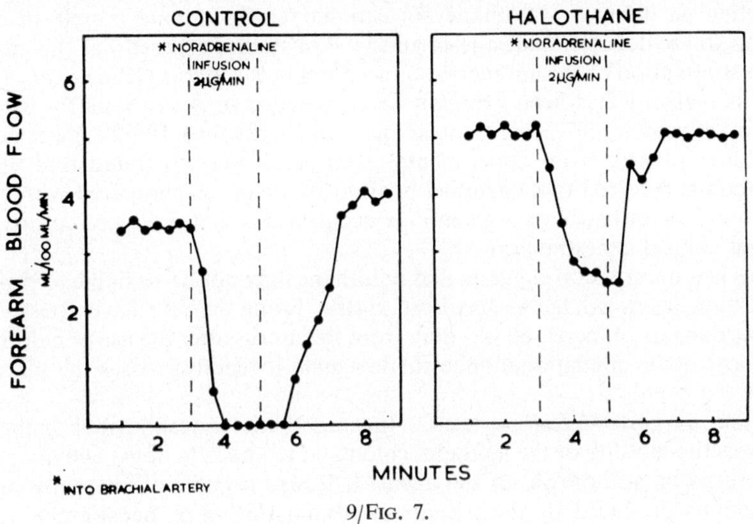

9/FIG. 7.

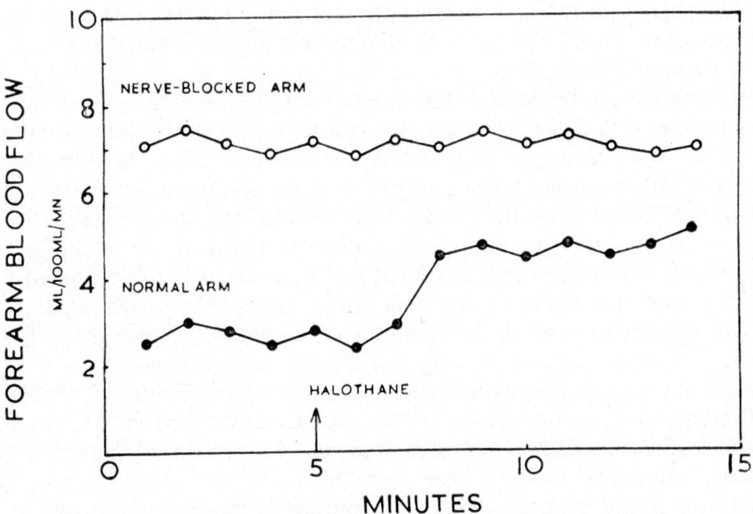

9/FIG. 8.—Effect of halothane on forearm blood flow.

These results suggest that halothane does not have a direct action on the vessel wall itself but acts rather by blocking the action of noradrenaline. This concept fits well with the possible action of halothane on the myocardium mentioned above.

Action on kidney and liver.—Halothane causes a decrease in renal flow probably related to a fall in glomerular filtration rate and a reduction in ADH release (Deutsch *et al.*, 1966). It also leads to a fall in hepatic blood flow (Epstein *et al.*, 1966). The possible association of halothane and liver damage is considered below.

Action on uterus.—Halothane anaesthesia relaxes uterine muscle in direct relation to the depth of anaesthesia and *in vitro* studies suggest that this may be due to stimulation of the adrenergic β receptors in the uterus (Klide *et al.*, 1969). For this reason it has been expressly recommended in anaesthesia for external version, manual removal or contraction ring (Crawford, 1962). Vasicka and Kretchmer (1961), from experimental studies in women, found that uterine contractions recurred twice as quickly after halothane as compared with ether, when these anaesthetics were given in concentrations that produced comparable levels of clinical anaesthesia.

This last observation suggests that halothane may not be so liable to produce postpartum haemorrhage as has been stated. Some authors have stressed the possible dangers of increased bleeding from the uterus after the use of halothane. Like most other inhalational anaesthetic agents it readily crosses the placental barrier.

Action on gastro-intestinal tract.—In anaesthetic concentrations halothane depresses the motility of the jejunum, colon and stomach in dogs; activity promptly returns on withdrawal of the agent. It is also capable of antagonising the contractions produced by the parenteral administration of neostigmine (Marshall *et al.*, 1961).

Action on skeletal muscle.—Halothane has minimal neuromuscular blocking action but potentiates the action of the non-depolarising agents, whilst antagonising the effect of drugs which act by depolarisation (Graham, 1958; Hanquet, 1961; Katz and Gissen, 1967).

Action on the cerebral blood flow and intracranial contents.—Cerebral blood flow is increased and cerebral vascular resistance decreased during halothane anaesthesia. These changes occur when the arterial carbon dioxide tension is maintained within normal limits and provided there is not a considerable fall in mean arterial blood pressure (McDowall, 1967; Christensen *et al.*, 1967). At normal arterial carbon dioxide tension halothane causes a rise in cerebrospinal fluid pressure, but this can be prevented if the patient is hyperventilated before the addition of halothane to the anaesthetic gases (McDowall *et al.*, 1966). Intracranial pressure rises during halothane anaesthesia, especially so in those patients who have space-occupying intracranial lesions (Jennett *et al.*, 1969). Headache may follow halothane anaesthesia (Tyrell and Feldman, 1968).

Shivering.—Intense muscle spasms are occasionally observed in the early part of the post-operative period. These movements are sometimes jocularly referred to as the "halothane shakes". Moir and Doyle (1963) studied a large group of patients and found that the body temperature in those who "shivered" after operation was 0·5 °C lower than those who did not shiver, and Jones and

McLaren (1965) noted a close relationship between falls in central body temperature and shivering following halothane anaesthesia. Bay and his colleagues (1968) studied arterial oxygen and carbon dioxide tensions and cardiac output during post-operative shivering. They found that both ventilation and cardiac output were adequate for the increased demands imposed by shivering, but that there is a potential danger of hypoxaemia in patients who have ventilatory embarrassment or a fixed low cardiac output. The high incidence of shivering after halothane anaesthesia is probably related to the vasodilatory action of the drug and the environmental temperature.

Action on cells.—Experimental work by Nunn *et al.* (1969) has shown that halothane interferes with mitosis in cells.

Clinical Use

There is little doubt that halothane has proved one of the most useful agents in the whole history of clinical anaesthesia. It is non-inflammable, potent and non-irritating to the respiratory tract in anaesthetic concentrations. Furthermore, it has a low post-operative incidence of nausea and vomiting. In abdominal surgery it is often combined with a muscle relaxant in order to achieve good relaxation without resorting to high concentrations of halothane that would depress the systemic pressure. It is widely used in anaesthesia for all types of surgery including neurosurgery, ear, nose and throat, orthopaedic and paediatric cases. A reduction in blood pressure, which at one time was regarded as an undesirable side-effect, is now often used to advantage in major surgery to reduce the blood loss.

Methods of vaporisation.—Halothane can be vaporised in a number of ways but its high cost demands that reasonable economy be used. For this reason it is unsuitable for open-mask application. When placed in a bubble-through vaporiser (copper kettle, see Fig. 1) (Morris, 1952), a flow rate of 100 ml. of oxygen through the apparatus (at room temperature) when added to 5 litres of nitrous oxide and oxygen will give an inspired concentration of 1 per cent. Similarly 200 ml. of oxygen will give a concentration of 2 per cent.

On the other hand, the "Fluotec" vaporiser (Fig. 9*a*) receives all the inspired gas en route to the patient and adds a predicted amount of halothane to the mixture of gases. This apparatus is both temperature- and flow-controlled (Fig. 9*b*) and it is a satisfactory vaporiser for routine clinical use (Paterson *et al.*, 1969).

Vaporiser inside or outside circle system.—Various authorities have argued for and against the policy of whether the vaporiser should be always placed outside the circle system or whether it is safe to incorporate it inside the system to permit rebreathing and thereby exercise economy.

Halothane with a relatively high vapour pressure, low boiling point and low blood solubility can be regarded as a potent anaesthetic in which low concentrations (i.e. 0·4 per cent with nitrous oxide/oxygen) are capable of maintaining unconsciousness. The only justification, therefore, for using a vaporiser within the circle system is on the grounds of economy.

Vaporiser inside the circle system.—One of the principal fears of using a halothane vaporiser within the circle system has been the possibility that the concentration of halothane would rapidly rise to a fatal level; in fact this does not occur if the patient is breathing spontaneously because not only does the patient continue to remove halothane from the system but as soon as the anaesthetic concentration rises the respiratory minute volume becomes depressed. In this manner the patient will then vaporise less halothane and this acts to prevent a rapid build up of halothane within the system. The patient, at this point, will

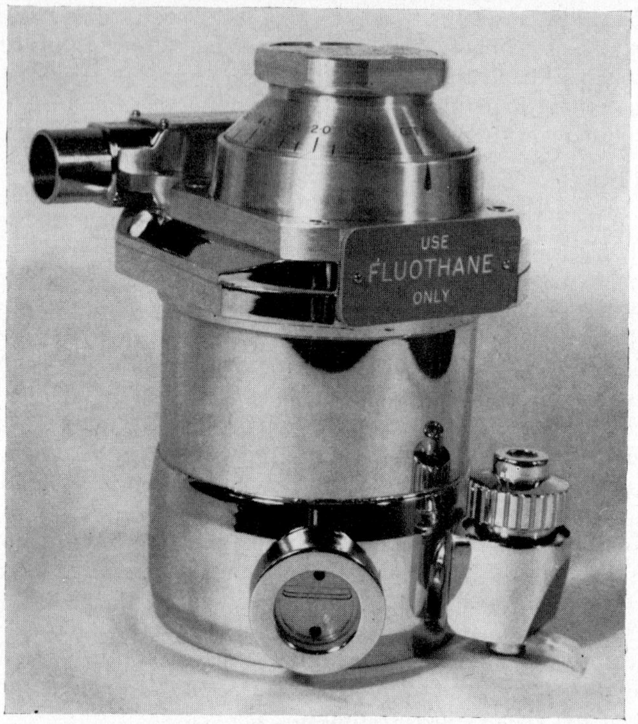

9/Fig. 9(*a*).—The "Fluotec" Mark III vaporiser.

show all the clinical signs of deep halothane anaesthesia, i.e. depressed ventilation, slow pulse rate and hypotension. Provided the anaesthetist uses these signs and reduces (or turns off) the concentration delivered by the vaporiser then this method can be used. However, to achieve a satisfactory level of anaesthesia, in some cases it is necessary to depress ventilation below normal. If the anaesthetist then institutes assisted or controlled respiration without modifying the vaporiser setting a rapid and fatal concentration of halothane may develop. In short, the vaporiser should only be used within the circle system in the presence of spontaneous respiration. If assisted respiration is required then great care must be exercised to see that the concentration of halothane does not rise unexpectedly.

Vaporiser outside the circuit.—If the vaporiser is placed outside the circle system then the concentration within the system cannot rise above that entering it. In fact, due to the constant uptake of halothane by the body it takes many hours or even days for the alveolar concentration to reach equilibrium with the inspired concentration. A vaporiser outside the circle system, therefore, is

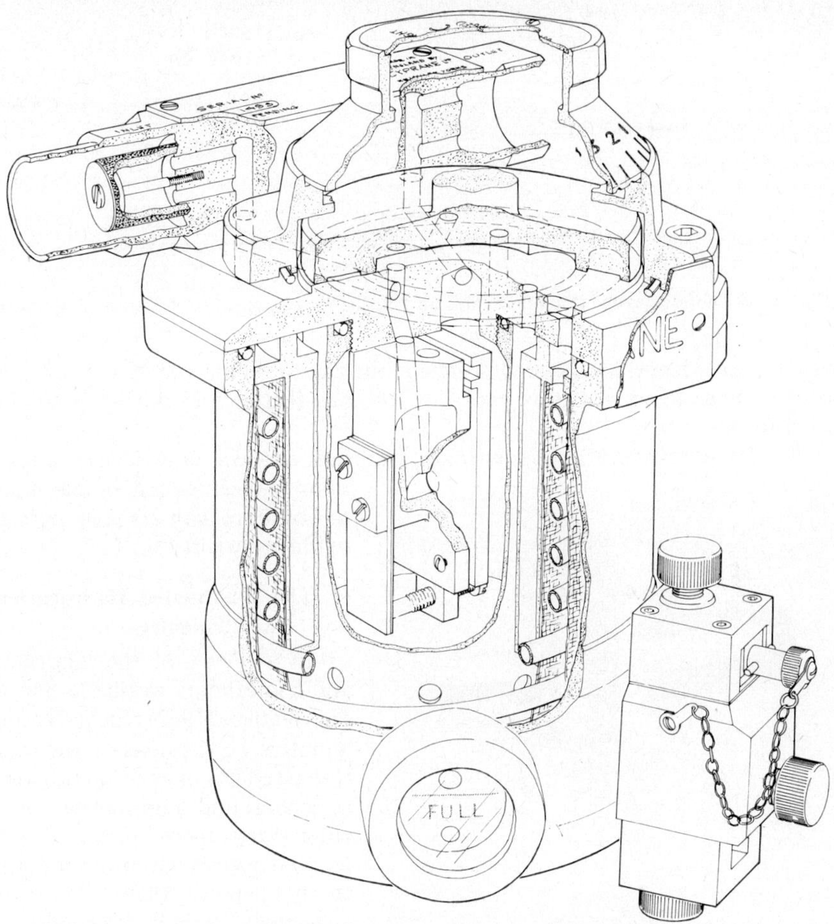

9/Fig. 9(*b*).—Diagram to illustrate the interior of the "Fluotec" Mark III.

relatively safe provided an excessive concentration is not used and the patient is carefully observed for the signs of increasing depth of anaesthesia.

It is often not fully realised that even though the vaporiser is placed outside the circle system, fluctuations in concentration can occur when assisted or controlled respiration is used (Hill and Lowe, 1962). On squeezing the bag the back-pressure in the anaesthetic apparatus rises to 15–20 cm. of water. This forces more gases into the interior of the vaporiser and this increased volume of gases collects additional vapour. The exact increase in the vapour concentration delivered to the patient will depend on the flow of gases used. If a high flow of gases is used then the extra 50 ml. or so that can be compressed into the vaporiser does not pick up enough vapour to seriously increase the concentration. On the other hand, if a low flow is used then it is possible the concentration received by the patient may actually be double that indicated by the vaporiser. For this reason a flow of gases of at least 4 litres/minute is recommended for use on the circle

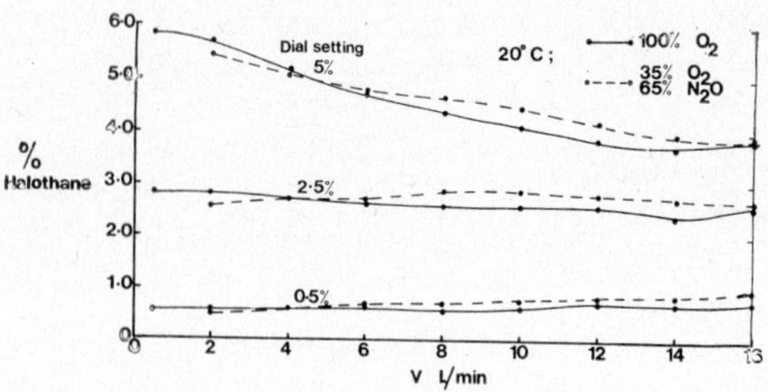

9/Fig. 10.—The effects of varying flow rates on halothane concentration ("Fluotec" Mark III).

system even when the vaporiser is outside the circuit. Some vaporisers contain a special device to prevent this back-flow of anaesthetic gases during controlled respiration.

A small, convenient and inexpensive vaporiser that will only develop a maximum concentration of halothane of not more than 2·3 vols. per cent is illustrated in Fig. 11.

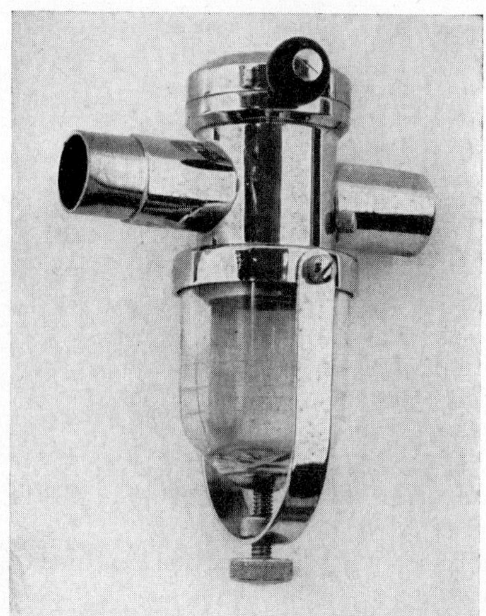

9/Fig. 11.—The Goldman vaporiser.

The Fluorinated Hydrocarbons and Jaundice

In a review of the laboratory and clinical data available Sadove and Wallace (1962) reached certain tentative conclusions on the hepatotoxic effects of anaesthetic agents in general and halothane in particular. First, there appears to be a marked species variation in regard to the hepatotoxicity of various anaesthetic agents. Secondly, in man halothane is probably no more or less hepatotoxic than other commonly used anaesthetic agents, excluding chloroform. Thirdly, many other factors will accentuate the toxic potentiality of anaesthetic agents, particularly the pre-operative nutritional state of the patient, blood transfusions, and the occurrence of hypoxia, hypercarbia or hypotension during or after anaesthesia (Morris and Feldman, 1963).

Since that time a number of reports have appeared in the literature linking both halothane and methoxyflurane with liver damage. Prior to 1963 there were only a handful of cases giving a possible link between halothane and toxic hepatitis (Burnap *et al.*, 1958; Virtue and Payne, 1958; Barton, 1959; Vourc'h *et al.*, 1960; Temple *et al.*, 1962). In 1963 two reports appeared in the *New England Journal of Medicine* which attracted particular attention. The first entitled "Liver necrosis after halothane anaesthesia" (Bunker and Blumenfeld, 1963) reviewed two cases with a fatal outcome. One of these cases was a young girl (*aet.* 16) who had a lacerated wrist repaired under halothane anaesthesia lasting 4½ hours. The anaesthesia and post-operative course were uneventful, but the patient developed signs of a hepato-renal syndrome on the 10th post-operative day and died three days later. Post-mortem examination showed profound central lobular necrosis of the liver.

In the second report (Lindenbaum and Leifer, 1963) the association between recurrent fever and hepatic dysfunction after repeated use of halothane anaesthesia was noted. A retrospective study revealed eight similar cases and these authors concluded that there was a relationship between halothane or methoxyflurane anaesthesia and hepatic dysfunction.

Since this time a number of reports attempting to link halothane anaesthesia and hepatic disturbance have appeared in the world literature (Tornetla and Tamaki, 1963; Gordon, 1963; Brody and Sweet, 1963; etc.).

Although no definite cause and effect relationship has yet been established it is important to consider every possibility, such as blood transfusion, viral hepatitis, antibiotics and other therapeutic agents. (See also Chapter 48.)

Laboratory studies.—Studies *in vitro* of the effects of halothane on cultures of human liver cells show little or no detectable alterations in cell morphology, unless the period of exposure is very prolonged (2 days) and the concentration of halothane equivalent to that which would be required to produce deep surgical anaesthesia. Even at these extremes, the cell vacuolation which is produced is partially reversible on withdrawal of the halothane (Corssen *et al.*, 1966; Rees and Zuckerman, 1967).

A number of impurities are known to be present in halothane in minute quantities. One of these compounds—dichlorohexafluorobutene—has a higher boiling point than halothane and is said to increase twofold or more during the clinical use of halothane in a vaporiser (Cohen *et al.*, 1963). Albin *et al.* (1964) cannot substantiate this finding, and state that the impurity is *not* increased when the copper kettle is used with halothane. Preliminary animal studies have suggested the possible toxicity of this compound in man.

The presence of copper appears to accelerate the formation of this butene compound and a possible pathway has been suggested (Cohen *et al.*, 1963) as follows:

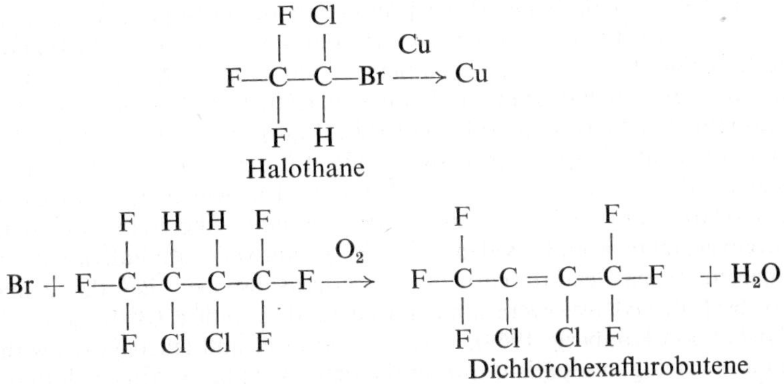

```
     F  Cl
     |  |       Cu
  F—C—C—Br ——→ Cu
     |  |
     F  H
   Halothane
```

```
          F  H  H  F                  F             F
          |  |  |  |     O2           |             |
Br + F—C—C—C—C—F ——→   F—C—C = C—C—F   + H2O
          |  |  |  |                  |   |   |   |
          F  Cl Cl F                  F  Cl  Cl  F
                                   Dichlorohexaflurobutene
```

cation). This high anaesthetic potency, together with the absence of irritation of the respiratory tract, helps to reduce the time taken for induction of anaesthesia.

With the exception of the fatty tissues, methoxyflurane is only a little more soluble in other tissues than it is in blood (Table 5).

9/TABLE 5

TISSUE/BLOOD SOLUBILITY COEFFICIENT OF METHOXYFLURANE

Coefficient	Tissue
2·34	Brain tissue/White matter
1·70	Brain tissue/Grey matter
1·34	Muscle
38·5	Fat

Action on the respiratory system.—Methoxyflurane depresses respiration in direct relationship with the depth of anaesthesia. The tidal volume is affected more than the rate of respiration. This agent does not appear to stimulate salivation or bronchial secretions and is relatively free from irritant effects on the respiratory mucosa.

Action on the cardiovascular system.—Walker and his colleagues (1962) have measured the effects of methoxyflurane in unpremedicated patients. They observed a decrease in cardiac output, systemic vascular resistance and stroke volume. There was an increase in heart rate. The cardiovascular effects of methoxyflurane resembled halothane rather than ether, and they concluded that the hypotension produced by methoxyflurane was primarily due to a fall in cardiac output. Bagwell and Woods (1962) working with dogs found that methoxyflurane produced a progressive depression of ventricular contractile force, aortic pressure and total aortic flow with increasing concentration of the anaesthetic agent. Miller and Morris (1961) demonstrated that methoxyflurane does not increase the concentration of plasma catecholamines in the dog.

Action on skeletal muscle.—The basis for the profound muscular relaxation during methoxyflurane anaesthesia has been studied in man (Ngai *et al.*, 1962). It was found that even when anaesthesia was deepened to a stage where electromyographic activity in the diaphragm was abolished, the twitch response to ulnar nerve stimulation remained unaffected. This suggests that the principle cause of muscle paralysis in methoxyflurane anaesthesia is an action on the central nervous system (probably the spinal cord).

Action on other organs.—As with all the halogenated hydrocarbon anaesthetic agents there is no positive evidence definitely proving that these drugs produce toxic reactions in the liver and kidney. Such damage, however, has been reported in patients who have received these agents, yet there is no evidence at present definitely connecting the two events. Moricca and his co-workers (1962) studied liver function in normal dogs and found a consistant modification of cellular function after methoxyflurane anaesthesia.

Clinical use

Methoxyflurane can be used as the principal anaesthetic agent for most surgical procedures (Boisvert and Hudon, 1962; Denton and Torda, 1963; McCaffrey and Mate, 1963). It has a relatively slow induction time (Thomason *et al.*, 1962) and some patients may complain about the unpleasant odour. In abdominal surgery the relaxation obtained is not as profound as that with a muscle relaxant

DEUTSCH, S., GOLDBERG, M., STEPHEN, G. W., and WEN-HSIEN, W. U. (1966). Effect of halothane on renal function in normal man. *Anesthesiology*, **27**, 793.

DRAGON, A., and GOLDSTEIN, I. (1967). Methoxyflurane: preliminary report on analgesic and mood-modifying properties in dentistry. *J. Amer. dent. Ass.*, **75**, 1176.

DYJVERMAN, A., and SJÖVALL, J. (1962). Estimation of Fluothane by gas chromotography. *Acta anaesth. scand.*, **6**, 171.

EDWARDS, G., MORTON, H. J. V., PASK, E. A., and WYLIE, W. D. (1956). Deaths associated with anaesthesia. A report on 1,000 cases. *Anaesthesia*, **11**, 194.

EGER, E. I. (II), and BRANDSTATER, B. (1963). Solubility of methoxyflurane in rubber. *Anesthesiology*, **24**, 679.

EGER, E. I. (II), LARSON, P., and SEVERINGHAUS, J. (1962). The solubility of halothane in rubber, soda lime and various plastics. *Anesthesiology*, **23**, 356.

EGER, E. I. (II), SHARGEL, R., and MERKEL, G. (1963). Solubility of diethyl ether in water, blood and oil. *Anesthesiology*, **24**, 676.

ELLIS, M. W., and BRYCE-SMITH, R. (1965). Use of trichloroethylene inhalation during physiotherapy. *Brit. med. J.*, **2**, 1412.

EPSTEIN, H. G., and MACINTOSH, Sir R. (1956). An anaesthetic inhaler with automatic thermo-compensation. *Anaesthesia*, **11**, 83.

EPSTEIN, R. M., DEUTSCH, S., COOPERMAN, L. H., CLEMENT, A. J., and PRICE, H. L. (1966). Splanchnic circulation during halothane anaesthesia and hypercapnia in normal man. *Anesthesiology*, **27**, 654.

FIRTH, J. B., and STUCKEY, R. E. (1945). Decomposition of Trilene in closed circuit anaesthesia. *Lancet*, **1**, 814.

FISCHER, E. (1864). Ueber die Einwirkung von Wasserstoff aus Einfach-Chlorkohlenstoff. *Jena. Z. Med. Naturw.*, **1**, 123.

FLOURENS, M. J. P. (1847*a*). Note touchant l'action de l'éther sur les centres nerveux. *C. R. Acad. Sci. (Paris)*, **24**, 340.

FLOURENS, M. J. P. (1847*b*). Note touchant l'action de l'éther injecte dans les artères. *C. R. Acad. Sci. (Paris)*, **24**, 482.

GELFAN, S., and BELL, I. R. (1933). The anesthetic action of divinyl oxide on humans. *J. Pharmacol. exp. Ther.*, **47**, 1.

GORDON, J. (1963). Jaundice associated with halothane anaesthesia. *Anaesthesia*, **18**, **299**.

GOTTLIEB, S. F., FEGAN, F. J., and TIESLINK, J. (1966). Flammability of halothane, methoxyflurane and fluroxene under hyperbaric conditions. *Anesthesiology*, **27**, 195.

GRAHAM, J. D. P. (1958). The myoneural blocking action of anaesthetic drugs. *Brit. med. Bull.*, **14**, 15.

GRAY, T. C. (1957). Reflections on circulatory control. *Lancet*, **1**, 383.

GREENE, N. M. (1968). The metabolism of drugs employed in anesthesia. Part II. *Anesthesiology*, **29**, 327.

GROSS, E. G., and CULLEN, S. C. (1943). The effect of anesthetic agents on muscular contraction. *J. Pharmacol. exp. Ther.*, **78**, 358.

GUEDEL, A. E. (1951). *Inhalation Anesthesia*, 2nd edit. New York: The Macmillan Co.

HANQUET, M. (1961). The action of halothane on inhibitors of neuromuscular transmission (observations carried out in humans). *Anesth. et Analg.*, **18**, 461.

HELLIWELL, P. J., and HUTTON, A. M. (1950). Trichlorethylene anaesthesia. *Anaesthesia*, **5**, 4.

HEWER, C. L., and HADFIELD, C. F. (1941). Trichlorethylene as an inhalation anaesthetic. *Brit. med. J.*, **1**, 924.

HEYFELDER, F. (1848). *Die Versuche mit dem Schwefeläther, Salzäther und Chloroform, und die daraus gewonnenen Resultate in der chirurgischen Klinik zu Erlangen.* Erlangen.

HILL, D. W., and LOWE, H. J. (1962). Comparison of concentration o ı halothane in closed and semiclosed circuits during controlled ventilation. *Anesthesiology*, **23**, 291.

HILL, I. G. W. (1932). The human heart in anaesthesia. An electrocardiographic study. *Edinb. med. J.*, **39,** 533.

HOVELL, B. C., MASSON, A. H. B., and WILSON, J. (1967). Trichloroethylene for postoperative analgesia. *Anaesthesia,* **22,** 284.

IKEZONO, E., YASUDO, K., and HATTORI, Y. (1969). Effects of propranolol on epinephrine-induced arrhythmias during halothane anesthesia in man and cats. *Curr. Res. Anesth.*, **48,** 598.

JACKSON, D. E. (1934). A study of analgesia and anesthesia with special reference to such substances as trichlorethylene and vinesthene (divinyl ether), together with apparatus for their administration. *Curr. Res. Anesth.*, **13,** 198.

JARMAN, R., and EDGHILL, H. B. (1963). Methoxyflurane (Penthrane): a clinical investigation. *Anaesthesia,* **18,** 265.

JENNETT, W. B., BARKER, J., FITCH, W., and MCDOWALL, D. G. (1969). Effect of anaesthesia on intracranial pressure in patients with space occupying lesions. *Lancet,* **1,** 61.

JOHNSTONE, M. (1955). Some mechanisms of cardiac arrest during anaesthesia. *Brit. J. Anaesth.*, **27,** 566.

JOHNSTONE, M. (1956). The human cardiovascular response to Fluothane anaesthesia. *Brit. J. Anaesth.*, **28,** 392.

JONES, H. D., and MCLAREN, A. B. (1965). Postoperative shivering and hypoxaemia after halothane, nitrous oxide, oxygen anaesthesia. *Brit. J. Anaesth.*, **37,** 35.

JORFELDT, L., LÖFSTRÖM, B., MÖLLER, J. and ROSEN, A. (1967). Propranolol in ether anesthesia. Cardiovascular studies in man. *Acta anaesth. scand.*, **11,** 159.

KARIS, J. H., GISSEN, A. J. and NASTUK, W. L. (1966). Mode of action of diethyl ether in blocking neuromuscular transmission. *Anesthesiology*, **27,** 42.

KATZ, R. L. and GISSEN, A. J. (1967). Neuromuscular and electromyographic effects of halothane and its interaction with *d*-tubocurarine in man. *Anesthesiology*, **28,** 564.

KATZ, R. L., and KATZ, G. J. (1966). Surgical infiltration of pressor drugs and their interaction with volatile anaesthetics. *Brit. J. Anaesth.*, **38,** 712.

KLATSKIN, G., and KIMBERG, D. V. (1969). Recurrent hepatitis attributable to halothane sensitization in an anaesthetist. *New Engl. J. Med.*, **280,** 515.

KLIDE, A. M., PENNA, M., and AVIADO, D. M. (1969). Stimulation of adrenergic beta receptors by halothane and its antagonism by two new drugs. *Curr. Res. Anesth.*, **48,** 58.

KOCHMANN, M. (1936). Narkotica der Fettreihe. *In* Heffter's *Handbuch der experimentellen Pharmakologie.* Berlin: Ergünzungswerk, Vol. 2.

KRANTZ, J. C., CARR, C., LU, G., and BELL, F. K. (1953). The anesthetic action of trifluorethyl vinyl ether. *J. Pharmacol. exp. Ther.*, **108,** 488.

KUBOTA, Y., SCHWEIZER, H. J., and VANDAM, L. D. (1962). Haemodynamic effects of diethyl ether in man. *Anesthesiology*, **23,** 306.

LARSON, C. B., Jr., EGER, E. I. (II), MUALLEM, M., BUECHEL, D. R., MUNSON, E. S., and EISELE, J. H. (1969). The effects of diethyl ether and methoxyflurane on ventilation: II. A comparative study in man. *Anesthesiology*, **30,** 174.

LAYCOCK, J. D. (1953). Signs and stages of anaesthesia. A restatement. *Anaesthesia*, **8,** 15.

LEAKE, C. D., and CHEN, M. Y. (1930). Anesthetic properties of certain unsaturated ethers. *Proc. Soc. exp. Biol.* (*N.Y.*), **28,** 151.

LEHMANN, K. B. (1911). Experimentelle Studien über den Einfluss technisch und hygienisch wichtiger Gase und Dämpfe auf den Organismus. Die gechlorten Kohlenwasserstoffe der Fettreihe nebst Betrachtungen über die einphasische und zweiphasische Giftigkeit ötherischer Körper. *Arch. Hyg.* (*Berl.*), **74,** 1.

LEVY, A. G. (1913). The exciting causes of ventricular fibrillation in animals under chloroform anaesthesia. *Heart*, **4,** 319.

LINDENBAUM, J., and LEIFER, E. (1963). Hepatic necrosis associated with halothane anesthesia. *New Engl. J. Med.*, **268**, 525.

LU, G., JOHNSON, S. L., LING, M. S., and KRANTZ, J. C., Jr. (1953). Anesthesia XLI: The anesthetic properties of certain fluorinated hydrocarbons and ethers. *Anesthesiology*, **14**, 466.

LUNDY, J. S. (1926). Balanced anesthesia. *Minn. Med.*, **9**, 399.

MCARDLE, L., BLACK, G. W., and UNNI, V. K. N. (1968). Peripheral vascular changes during diethyl ether anaesthesia. *Anaesthesia*, **23**, 203.

MCARDLE, L., UNNI, V. K. N., and BLACK, G. W. (1968). The effects of trichloroethylene on limb blood flow in man. *Brit. J. Anaesth.*, **40**, 767.

MCCAFFREY, F. W., and MATE, M. J. (1963). Methoxyflurane. A report of 1,200 cases. *Canad. Anaesth. Soc. J.*, **10**, 103.

MCDOWELL, D. G. (1967). Effects of clinical concentrations of halothane on the blood flow and oxygen uptake of the cerebral cortex. *Brit. J. Anaesth.*, **39**, 186.

MCDOWALL, D. G., BARKER, J., and JENNETT, W. B. (1966). Cerebrospinal fluid pressure measurements during anaesthesia. *Anaesthesia*, **21**, 189.

MACINTOSH, R. R., MUSHIN, W. W., and EPSTEIN, H. G. (1963). *Physics for the Anaesthetist.* 3rd Edit. Oxford: Blackwell Scientific Publications.

MAHAFFEY, J. E., ALDINGER, E. E. SPROUSE, J. H. DARBY, T. D., and THROWER, W. B. (1961). The cardiovascular effects of halothane. *Anesthesiology*, **22**, 982.

MAJOR, V., ROSEN, M., and MUSHIN, W. W. (1967). Concentration of methoxyflurane for obstetric analgesia by self-administered intermittent inhalation. *Brit. med. J.*, **4**, 767.

MALCHY, H., and PARKHOUSE, J. (1968). Respiratory studies with trichloroethylene. *Canad. Anaesth. Soc. J.*, **16**, 119.

MAPLESON, W. W. (1962). The rate of uptake of halothane vapour in man. *Brit. J. Anaesth.*, **34**, 11.

MARSHALL, F. N., PITTINGER, C. B., and LONG, J. P. (1961). Effects of halothane on gastro-intestinal motility. *Anesthesiology*, **22**, 363.

MILLER, R. A., and MORRIS, M. E. (1961). A study of methoxyflurane anaesthesia. *Canad. Anaesth. Soc. J.*, **8**, 210.

MILLER, R. N., and THOMAS, P. A. (1967). Determination from lung extracts of patients receiving diethyl ether or halothane. *Anesthesiology*, **28**, 1089.

MOIR, D. D., and DOYLE, P. M. (1963). Halothane and post-operative shivering. *Curr. Res. Anesth.*, **42**, 423.

MORRICA, G., CAVALIERE, R., MANNI, C., and MASSONI, P. (1962). Effects of methoxyflurane on the liver. *Gazz. int. Med. Chir.*, **67**, 1293.

MORRIS, L. E. (1952). A new vaporiser for liquid anesthetics. *Anesthesiology*, **13**, 586,

MORRIS, L. E., and FELDMAN, S. A. (1963). Influence of hypercarbia and hypotension upon liver damage during halothane anaesthesia. *Anaesthesia*, **18**, 32.

MORROW, D. H., and MORROW, A. G. (1961). The effects of halothane on myocardial contractile force and vascular resistance. *Anesthesiology*, **22**, 537.

MORTON, W. T. G. (1847). *A memoir to the Academy of Sciences at Paris on a new use of sulphuric ether.* Reprinted by Henry Schuman, New York, 1946.

MUSHIN, W. W. (1948). The signs of anaesthesia. *Anaesthesia*, **3**, 154.

MUSHIN, W. W., ROSEN, M., BOWEN, D. J., and CAMPBELL, H. (1964). Halothane and liver dysfunction: a retrospective study. *Brit. med. J.*, **2**, 329.

MUSHIN, W. W., ROSEN, M., and JONES, F. V. (1971). Post-halothane jaundice in relation to previous administrations of halothane. *Brit. med. J.*, **2**, 18.

NAGEL, E. L. (1965). Personal communication.

NGAI, S. H., HANKS, E. C., and BRODY, D. C. (1962). Effect of methoxyflurane on electromyogram, neuromuscular transmission and spinal reflexes. *Anesthesiology*, **23**, 158.

NGAI, S. H., HANKS, E. C., and FARHIE, S. E. (1965). Effects of anesthetics on neuromuscular transmission and somatic reflexes. *Anesthesiology*, **26,** 162.

NOSWORTHY, M. D. (1958). Personal communication.

NUNN, J. F., DIXON, K. L., and LOUIS, J. D. (1969). Effects of halothane on mitosis. *Anesthesiology*, **30,** 348.

NUNN, J. F., and MATTHEWS, R. L. (1959). Gaseous exchange during halothane anaesthesia: the steady respiratory state. *Brit. J. Anaesth.*, **31,** 330.

OPPENHEIM, H. (1915). Über Trigeminuserkrankung infolge von Trichloräthylenvergiftung (Discussion). *Neurol. Zbl.*, **34,** 918.

OSTLERE, G. (1953). *Trichlorethylene Anaesthesia.* Edinburgh: E. & S. Livingstone.

PACKER, K. J., and TITEL, J. H. (1969). Methoxyflurane analgesia for burns dressings: experience with the Analgizer. *Brit. J. Anaesth.*, **41,** 1080.

PATERSON, G. M., HULANDS, G. H., and NUNN, J. F. (1969). Evaluation of a new halothane vaporiser. The Cyprane Fluotec Mark 3. *Brit. J. Anaesth.*, **41,** 109.

PITTINGER, C. B. (1966). *Hyperbaric Oxygenation*, p. 74. Springfield, Ill.: Charles C. Thomas.

PLESSNER, W. (1915). Über Trigeminuserkrankung infolge von Trichloräthylenvergiftung. *Neurol. Zbl.*, **34,** 916.

PRICE, H. L. (1960). General anaesthesia and circulatory homeostasis. *Physiol. Rev.*, **40,** 187.

PRICE, H. L. (1961). Circulatory actions of general anesthetic agents. *Clin. Pharmacol. Ther.*, **2,** 163.

PRICE, H. L., and PRICE, M. L. (1967). Relative ganglionic blocking potencies of cyclopropane, halothane, nitrous oxide and the interaction of nitrous oxide with halothane. *Anesthesiology*, **28,** 349.

PRYS-ROBERTS, C., KALMAN, G. R., KAIN, M. L., and GREENBAUM, R. (1967). Cardiac output—blood carbon dioxide levels during halothane anaesthesia in man. *Brit. J. Anaesth.*, **39,** 687.

RAVENTÓS, J. (1956). The action of Fluothane—a new volatile anaesthetic. *Brit. J. Pharmacol.*, **11,** 394.

REES, K. R., and ZUCKERMAN, A. J. (1967). Lack of toxicity of halothane on differentiated liver cell cultures. *Brit., J. Anaesth.*, **39,** 851.

REHDER, K., FORBES, J., ALTER, H., HESSLER, O., and STIER, A. (1969). Biotransformation in man; a quantitive study. *Anesthesiology*, **31,** 560.

ROBBINS, B. H. (1946). Preliminary studies of the anaesthetic activity of fluorinated hydrocarbons. *J. Pharmacol. exp. Ther.*, **86,** 197.

ROBSON, G., GILLIES, D. M., CULLEN, W. G., and GRIFFITH, H. R. (1959). Fluothane (Halothane) in closed circuit anesthesia. *Anesthesiology*, **20,** 251.

ROLLASON, W. N. (1964). Chloroform, halothane and hepatotoxicity. *Proc. roy. Soc. Med.*, **57,** 307.

SADOVE, M. S., BALAGOT, R. C., and LINDE, H. W. (1957). The effect of Fluoromar on certain organ functions. *Curr. Res. Anesth.*, **36,** 47.

SADOVE, M. S., and WALLACE, V. E. (1962). *Halothane.* Philadelphia: F. A. Davis Co.

SAIDMAN, L. J., and EGER, E. I. (II) (1965). Effect of nitrous oxide and of narcotic premedication on the alveolar concentration of halothane required for anesthesia. *Anesthesiology*, **26,** 67.

SANDISON, J. W., SIVAPRAGASAM, S., HAYES, J. A., and WOO-MING, M. O. (1970). An experimental study of pulmonary damage associated with intravenous injection of halothane in dogs. *Brit. J. Anaesth.*, **42,** 419.

SECHER, O. (1951*a*). The peripheral action of ether estimated on isolated nerve-muscle preparation. (IV.) Measurement of action potentials in nerve. *Acta pharmacol. (Kbh.)*, **7,** 119.

SECHER, O. (1951*b*). The peripheral action of ether estimated on isolated nerve-muscle preparation. (III.) Antagonistic and synergistic action of ether and neostigmine. *Acta pharmacol.* (*Kbh.*), **7,** 103.

SEVERINGHAUS, J., and CULLEN, S. C. (1958). Depression of myocardium and body oxygen consumption with Fluothane in man. *Anesthesiology*, **19,** 165.

SIMPSON, J. Y. (1847). *Account of a new anaesthetic agent as a substitute for sulphuric ether in surgery and midwifery*. Edinburgh.

SLATER, E. M., GIBSON, J. M., DYKES, H. M. H., and WALZER, S. G. (1964). Post-operative hepatic necrosis. Its incidence and diagnostic value in association with the administration of halothane. *New Engl. J. Med.*, **270,** 983.

STRIKER, C., GOLDBLATT, S., WARM, I. S., and JACKSON, D. E. (1935). Clinical experiences with the use of trichlorethylene in the production of over 300 analgesias and anesthesias. *Curr. Res. Anesth.*, **14,** 68.

SUCKLING, C. W. (1957). Some chemical and physical features in the development of Fluothane. *Brit. J. Anaesth.*, **29,** 466.

TEMPLE, R. L., COTE, R. A., and GORENS, S. W. (1962). Massive hepatic necrosis following general anesthesia. *Curr. Res. Anesth.*, **41,** 586.

THOMASON, R., LIGHT, G., and HOLADAY, D. A. (1962). Methoxyflurane anesthesia. *Curr. Res. Anesth.*, **41,** 225.

TORNETLA, F. J., and TAMAKI, H. T. (1963). Halothane jaundice and hepatotoxicity. *J. Amer. med. Ass.*, **184,** 658.

TYRELL, M. F., and FELDMAN, S. (1968). Headache following halothane anaesthesia. *Brit. J. Anaesth.*, **40,** 99.

VAN DYKE, R. A., and CHENOWETH, M. B. (1965). Metabolism of volatile anaesthetics II. *Biochem. Pharmacol.*, **14,** 603.

VAN POZNAK, A., and ARTUSIO, J. F. (1960). Anaesthetic properties of a series of fluorinated compounds. *Toxicol. appl. Pharmacol.*, **2,** 374.

VASICKA, A., and KRETCHMER, H. (1961). Effect of conduction and inhalation anesthesia on uterine contraction. *Amer. J. Obstet. Gynec.*, **82,** 600.

VIRTUE, R. W., and PAYNE, K. W. (1958). Post-operative death after Fluothane. *Anesthesiology*, **19,** 562.

VOURC'H, G., SCHNOEBELEN, E., BUCK, F., and FRUHLING, L. (1960). Hepatonéphrite aiguë mortelle après anesthésie comportant de l'halothane (Fluothane). *Anesth. et Analg.*, **17,** 466.

WALKER, J. A., EGGERS, G. W. N., and ALLEN, C. R. (1962). Cardiovascular effects of methoxyflurane anesthesia in man. *Anesthesiology*, **23,** 639.

WATERS, R. M. (1951). *Chloroform. A Study after* 100 *years*. Madison: Univ. Wisconsin Press.

WENTHE, F. M., PATRICK, R. T., and WOOD, E. H. (1962). Effects of anesthesia with halothane on the human circulation. *Curr. Res. Anesth.*, **41,** 381.

Chapter 10

EXAMINATION OF THE RESPIRATORY TRACT AND TRACHEAL INTUBATION

A GENERAL clinical examination of the patient is a valuable aid to the diagnosis of most ailments of the respiratory tract, and an essential preliminary for assessment of any patient's fitness to undergo operation and anaesthesia. Particularly in diseases affecting the lungs and bronchi, specific investigations may be necessary to establish a precise diagnosis before operation is undertaken, and some of these may need anaesthesia for their successful accomplishment. The three commonest special investigations in thoracic disease are examination of the sputum, radiography of the chest, and direct examination of the respiratory tract by laryngoscopy and bronchoscopy. From the anaesthetist's point of view, the importance of sputum examination lies not only in any possible contamination of the anaesthetic apparatus* but in the theoretical and practical possibilities that follow upon the presence of considerable quantities in the respiratory tract during anaesthesia. A great deal of practical information—which may be of value in choosing a particular anaesthetic or technique—can be gleaned from macroscopical examination of the sputum, and from a knowledge of the quantity expectorated during the course of 24 hours.

RADIOGRAPHIC INVESTIGATIONS

The interpretation of X-rays of the chest in the standard posterior-anterior, oblique and lateral views, particularly in relationship to the normal anatomy of the lungs, is important and in most instances is sufficient for accurate diagnosis. The lungs and their normal sub-divisions are illustrated in Figs. 1 to 6 inclusive. Bronchography (see below) is a method of determining the state of the bronchial tree and is nowadays infrequently used in the United Kingdom. Good standard X-rays of the lungs provide almost as much, and usually sufficient, information for accurate diagnosis, while there are fewer and fewer patients with diseases such as bronchiectasis for whom bronchographic investigation may be essential. Bronchography has, too, its own morbidity which may result from plugging of the bronchi and bronchioles or from reactions to the substances used for the investigation.

Bronchography

The bronchial tree can be outlined either by instillation of a radio-opaque liquid or by insufflation of a radio-opaque powder.

Radio-opaque liquids.—An aqueous, rather than an oily, suspension of contrast medium is preferred because it is less irritating to the bronchial tree, does not require much reflex suppression during instillation and mixes with bronchial secretions.

* Sterilisation of anaesthetic equipment is discussed in Appendix 3.

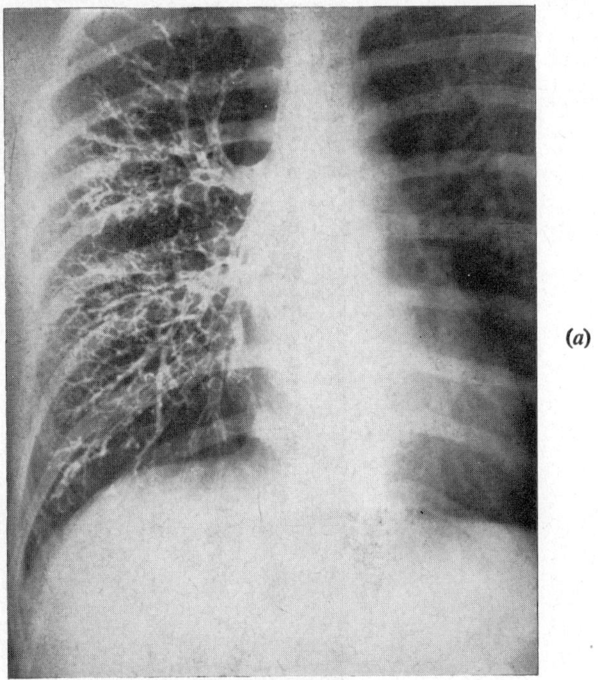

(a)

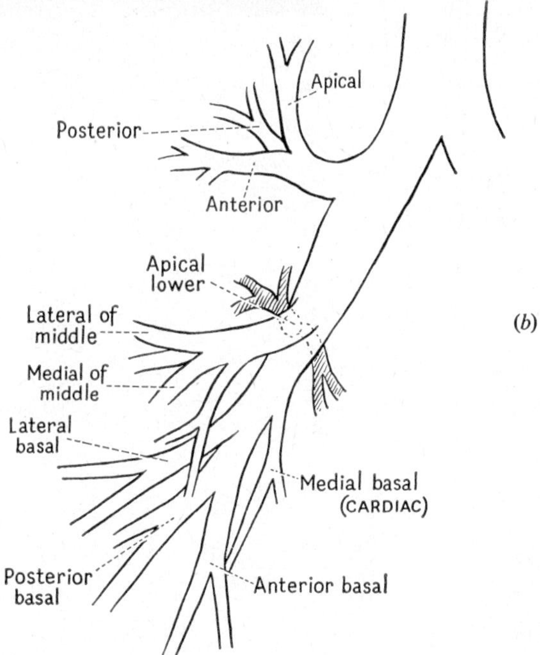

(b)

10/Fig. 1.—Normal right bronchogram—anterior-posterior.

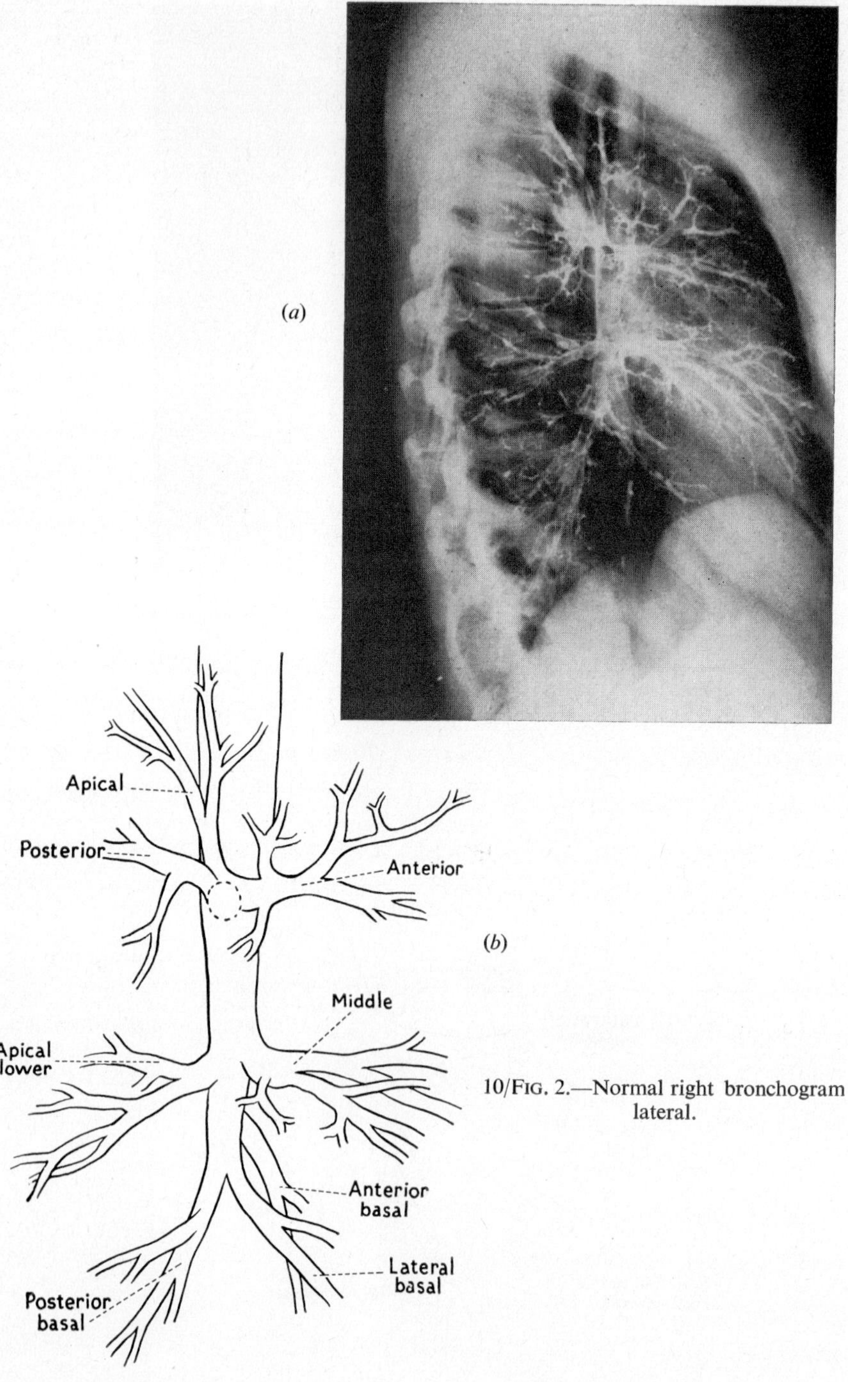

10/FIG. 2.—Normal right bronchogram lateral.

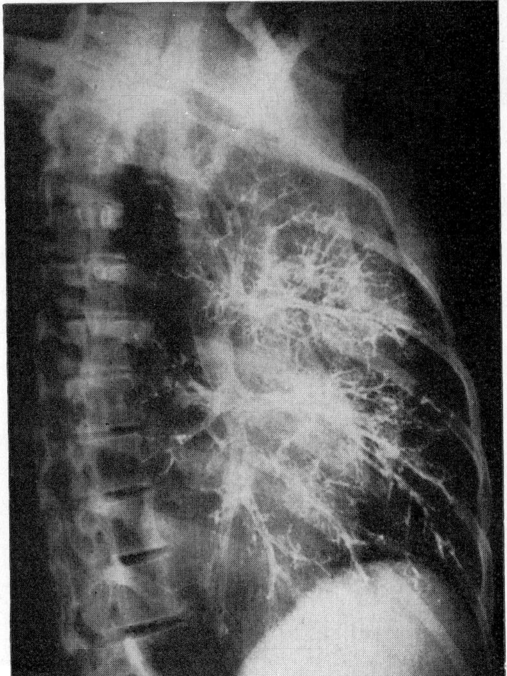

(*a*)

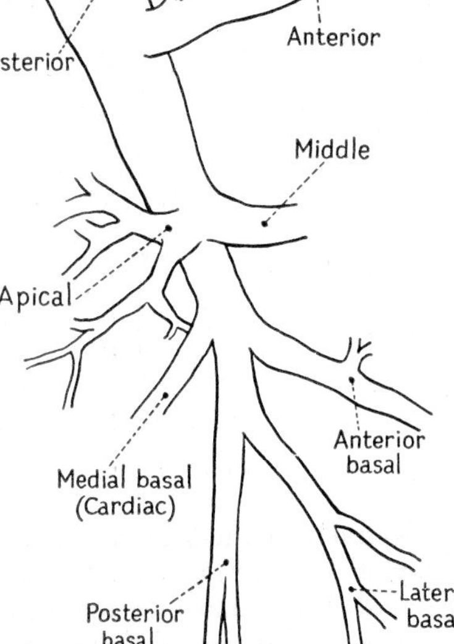

(*b*)

10/Fig. 3.—Normal right bronchogram—oblique.

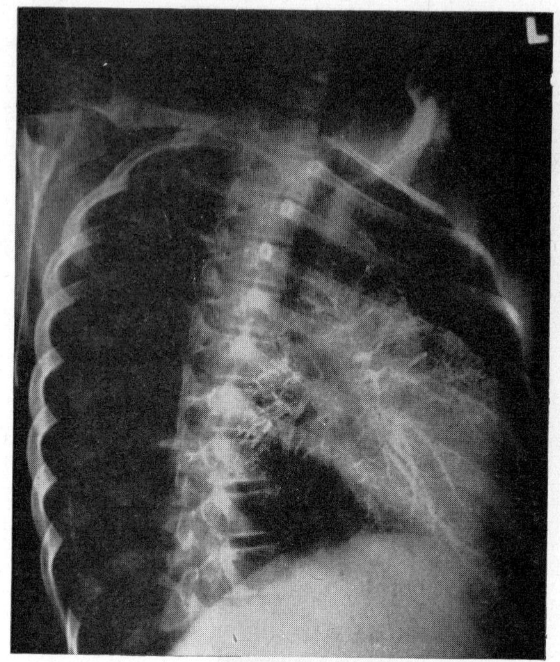

(*a*)

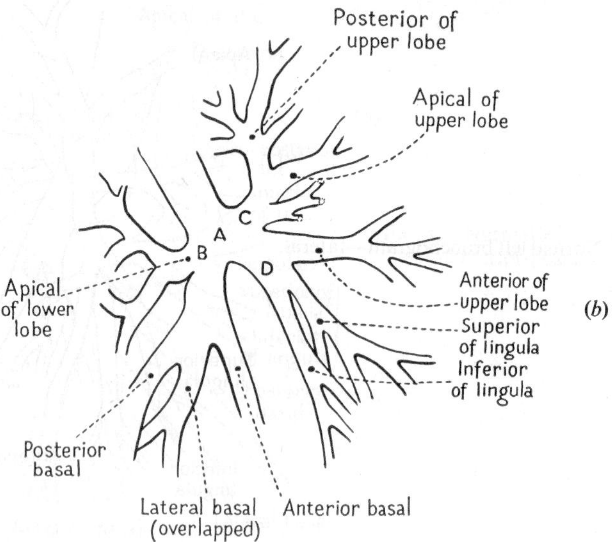

(*b*)

10/Fig. 6.—Normal Left Bronchogram—Oblique

A = Upper lobe bronchus.
B = Lower lobe bronchus.
C = Apico-posterior bronchus (of upper lobe).
D = Lingular bronchus.

considerably more may be required for adequate filling in cases of marked bronchiectasis. A child takes about 6–8 ml. for a single side.

Alternatives to "Hytrast".—Propyliodone ("Dionosil") or the n'propyl ester of 3:5 diodo-4-pyridone n-acetic acid is sometimes used. Propyliodone may be suspended in water with the aid of sodium carboxymethyl-cellulose but it has the disadvantage of being hydrolysed and is in part excreted from the body through the kidneys. Iodism may therefore follow its use. An acute disadvantage of some alternatives to "Hytrast" and propyliodone is that they may inter-react with volatile inhalational anaesthetic agents, particularly halothane, to produce toxic fatal reactions in the patient. Such reactions have not been seen with "Hytrast" or propyliodone.

Iodism.—Reactions to iodine during or following bronchography are extremely uncommon. An acute reaction is most likely to be anaphylactic in type and will require immediate emergency treatment including the use of adrenaline and hydrocortisone. However, in the early stages of a reaction it is almost impossible to forecast its probable extent. Thus treatment must be undertaken in all suggestive cases, and should consist of attempts to remove any residual contrast medium by posturing with encouragement to cough, and by aspiration from the stomach. Next the patient may usefully be given sodium chloride to enable the free iodine to attach itself to a sodium ion, thereby assisting renal excretion. An oral dose of 0·7 g. of sodium chloride in a capsule four hourly is usually tolerated, and may be supplemented by half a litre of 0·9 per cent sodium chloride intravenously every three days.

Radio-opaque powders.—The bronchial tract can be outlined by the insufflation of particles of a heavy metal in the form of a powder. Tantalum oxide has been used for this purpose (Nedel *et al.*, 1968). It has a particle size of 3–4μ. The technique requires manipulation of a catheter into a major bronchus with the aid of fluoroscopy. A few squeezes of an insufflator distribute the powder, which is non-irritant, down to secondary bronchi and because of the high density of the metal particles, low concentrations of tantalum oxide contrast well on the X-rays. This method does not block the smaller bronchi, but it does require fluoroscopy and probably general anaesthesia.

Technique for bronchography with a radio-opaque liquid.—Adequate postural drainage should be carried out for some time before bronchography in wet cases, in order to reduce the sputum as much as possible; this not only makes for safety, but also gives the contrast medium a chance to reach the smaller bronchi. The contrast medium is introduced into the bronchial tree either through a rubber catheter passed via the nose or over the back of the tongue, or by direct injection through the cricothyroid membrane. A third method, now used as a rule only under general anaesthesia, is to pass an endotracheal tube, down which a small rubber catheter is introduced. In adults and co-operative children local analgesia is perfectly satisfactory for bronchography, which is at the most an uncomfortable procedure. In the young, up to about the age of 6 years, and in older children who are unco-operative, general anaesthesia may be necessary, and this permits good pictures being taken with safety. Indeed, from the practical point of view, general anaesthesia for all children may save a lot of time and lead to better overall results, since a slight movement or a bout of coughing can easily spoil the final result.

Adults.—Premedication is unnecessary unless the patient is particularly nervous, when a barbiturate such as pentobarbitone (100 to 200 mg.) is helpful. Surprisingly little surface analgesia is needed, since it is not essential to anaesthetise the tracheal or bronchial mucosa, the contrast medium usually running smoothly without producing any marked irritation.

When the catheter is to be passed over the back of the tongue some surface analgesia of this area and perhaps of the glottis itself may be helpful—although if the operator is skilled the whole procedure can be done without it. Effective analgesia can be quickly produced by spraying the area with 4 per cent lignocaine a minute or two beforehand. The patient then sits up in a chair with his neck extended, and grasping his tongue with a piece of gauze between finger and thumb holds it firmly forward. He is told to breathe deeply and the appropriate amount of contrast medium to outline the particular lobe is then injected over the back of the tongue. A similar technique is used for the nasal route.

When a needle of the requisite bore is to be inserted through the cricothyroid membrane, local analgesia of the skin and tissues down to the membrane is necessary. The patient lies on his back with his head extended on a pillow, and when the membrane has been located by palpation a skin weal is raised over it and the deeper tissues also infiltrated with 2 per cent lignocaine. After the patient has been warned that it will make him cough, 1 ml. of 2 per cent lignocaine is squirted through the membrane during inspiration, and the needle immediately withdrawn to avoid breakage. When the coughing has subsided a special flanged needle of 12 or 14 gauge is pushed through the same track into the trachea, and attached by its bayonet fitting to the syringe already charged with contrast medium. The careful aspiration of a little air to show that the trachea has been entered is essential before making the injection. Dangers are the production of a haematoma, intravascular injection, and breakage of the needle. The subcutaneous injection of "Hytrast" is not dangerous. The suspension is non-irritant to the tissues, but it will remain *in situ* for up to eight weeks. The cricothyroid route is potentially a hazardous and complicated method but it gives great control of the instillation and enables a more deliberate positioning of the patient between the intermittent injections, and therefore more accurate localisation of the contrast medium. An alternative to direct injection is to thread a fine catheter through the needle and then with the aid of fluoroscopy to manipulate the tip of it into the desired bronchus.

Positioning for bronchography.—Three distinct positions are necessary to fill the lower lobe, middle (or lingular) lobe and upper lobe respectively (Fig. 7). It is preferable to fill each in turn and to instil into the trachea a small quantity of contrast medium—3 to 5 ml.—on each occasion. For the lower lobe the patient is partially sitting, inclined about 20° posteriorly and to the side to be filled, and a minute is allowed for the contrast medium to reach the branches of the lower lobe bronchus. The patient then lies on the side to be filled in the horizontal plane, and if an X-ray shows no reflux of contrast medium from the lower lobe bronchus to the upper lobe, a further 5 ml. are added with the head raised during the injection.

The upper lobe bronchus may be filled by alternative methods. First, after the instillation of 5 ml. of contrast medium in the lateral, horizontal position, the patient is turned almost into the prone position and the table tilted head-

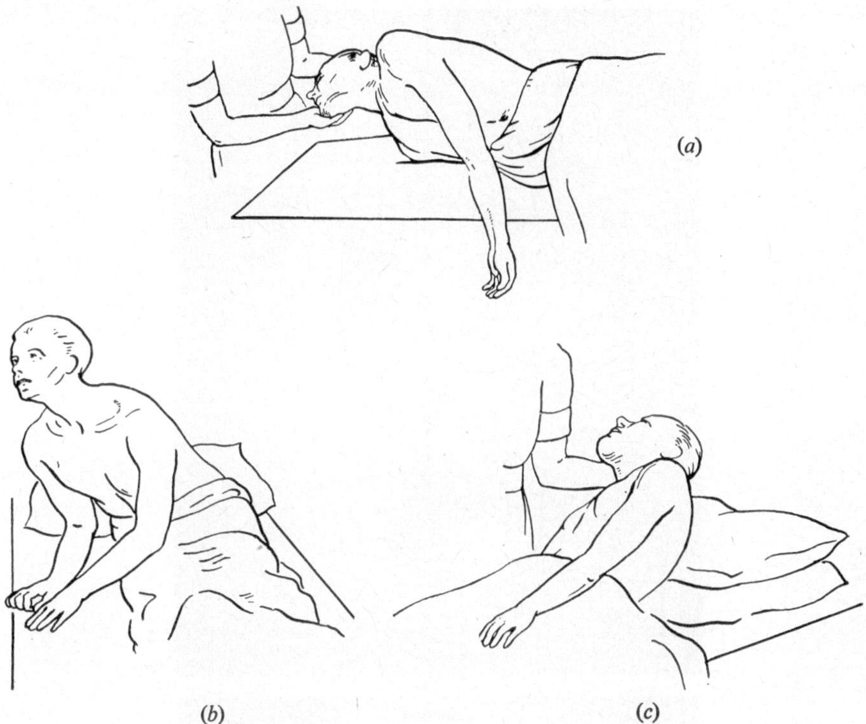

10/FIG. 7.—THE THREE POSITIONS FOR BRONCHOGRAPHY
(*a*) Upper lobe; (*b*) Middle lobe; (*c*) Lower lobe.

down. Secondly, provided a catheter lies in the trachea, the patient is placed in the Trendelenburg position on the side to be filled and 5 ml. of contrast medium is injected. In this method, if the lower and middle lobes have just been filled, it is worth waiting a minute and then taking an X-ray, before adding more contrast medium, to see whether the upper lobe will fill by reflux from the lower.

Pictures of each lobe should be taken in postero-anterior, lateral and oblique views. It is generally better to restrict a bronchogram to one side at a time in order to avoid overlap of structures in lateral views. If localisation of disease is unimportant, and the bronchogram is being performed for purely diagnostic reasons (Fig. 8), both sides can be done at the same performance since a good oblique will often show all branches of the bronchi in both lungs. Bronchography should be restricted to one lung at a session when the patient has a very reduced pulmonary function.

Children.—If the child is co-operative, any of the techniques described for adults can be used, though the nasal route is the least satisfactory owing to the smallness of the passage and the likely presence of adenoid tissue. Careful training is a wise precaution, not only to gain the confidence of the child but to accustom him to the X-ray department, the various procedures, and the positions needed. This may take a week or longer, and should be carried out along with postural drainage and breathing exercises. The quantity of local analgesic

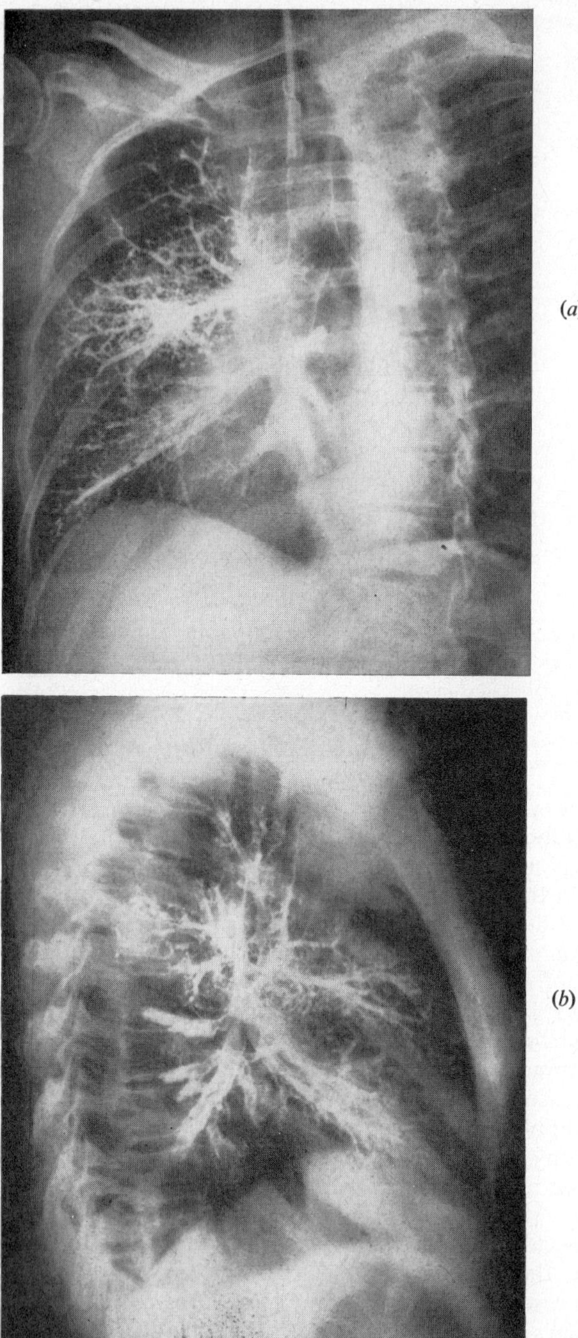

10/FIG. 8.—Bronchiectasis of right lung.

and contrast medium must be proportionate to the size of the child. The dose of lignocaine should not exceed 2·6 mg./kg. Bronchography under topical analgesia in children is not always successful, particularly when they are unco-operative, and it can be dangerous. The hazard of too much local analgesic drug has been referred to, but there is also a danger of respiratory obstruction (Atwood, 1965). It is best to limit bronchography under topical analgesia in children to one lung at a session.

General anaesthesia.—Preparation designed to drain as much of the secretions away prior to the bronchogram is just as important before general anaesthesia as local analgesia. Premedication depends upon the size and age of the child, but in general basal anaesthesia to ensure that the child arrives in the X-ray department asleep is our preference. This can be achieved in several ways (see Chapter 11, p. 375) and should be followed by atropine sulphate 0·6 mg. subcutaneously.

If the child has a considerable quantity of sputum such preliminary sedation may introduce the dangers of respiratory obstruction, both in the pre-investigation period and during post-investigation recovery. For such cases kindness must give way to safety, and either atropine only be ordered, or a combination of opiate and atropine suited to the child's size.

The child is brought to the radiological department in his cot and anaesthesia induced. When a barbiturate or phenothiazine has been given for premedication, nitrous oxide and oxygen followed by halothane is the best, but after atropine alone, or atropine with an opiate, a small dose of thiopentone may be used. Relaxation is procured by intermittent injections of suxamethonium or by a single injection of gallamine triethiodide, the object being complete control of respiration during the whole procedure. After intubation with an endotracheal tube attached to a Cobb's suction connection piece, as much sputum as possible is sucked out of the lungs. It is undesirable to inflate the lungs by intermittent positive-pressure before suction when a fair quantity of sputum is present; when this is the case, after induction and before the muscle relaxant is given, the child must be allowed to breathe a high concentration of oxygen for a minute or so in order to prevent hypoxia occurring during suction. Anaesthesia is maintained for this period by the combined effects of any sedative premedication and the residue of halothane or thiopentone left over from the induction.

After the sputum has been removed, the child is inflated with oxygen and the contrast medium is injected through a separate rubber catheter passed down the endotracheal tube. The child is then placed in the required positions for filling the various lobes on one side, but only kept in each position for a few seconds since the contrast medium flows more quickly under general anaesthesia. The pictures are taken while the child is still apnoeic, and if oxygenation has been properly performed before the injection of the contrast medium, cyanosis will not occur. After the completion of one side, as much contrast medium as possible is quickly aspirated and then the child is ventilated.

Positioning of an anaesthetised child is basically the same as that for the adult, but the whole of the contrast medium for one side should be injected into the trachea at once, with the child held in the sitting position but inclined 40° to that side. Immediately after the injection the child, while inclined laterally, is moved backwards and forwards so that the middle (or lingular) and lower lobe bronchi are entered by the contrast medium, and after a few seconds it is held on its side head-down over the end of the table so that the upper lobe bronchus can be filled. X-ray pictures are then taken as soon as the child has been returned to the horizontal.

If both lungs are to be outlined at the same session the views should be restricted, and taken in the following order:

1. *Right lung.* Right lateral followed by an antero-posterior view.
2. *Left lung.* Right antero-oblique followed by antero-posterior view.

Atwood (1965) strongly recommends that bilateral bronchography at the same session should be avoided in a child under 18 months of age. For such an infant, airway obstruction is a particular hazard, bearing in mind the relative sizes of the bronchial tree, the endotracheal tube and the catheter for the contrast medium. Removal of the contrast medium by suction is difficult, and an infant has a relatively poor power of coughing (Freifeld *et al.*, 1964; Atwood, 1965).

Respiration should be spontaneous at the end of the whole procedure, but after using gallamine, neostigmine preceded by atropine may be needed. The child should be nursed on one or other side and with his head and thorax tilted downwards until fully conscious to facilitate some lung drainage.

The essential requirements of any general anaesthetic technique for bronchography are control of the airway with adequate oxygenation at all times and a brief suppression of the cough reflex. The return of reflex activity must be rapid at the end of the procedure. There must be no explosion hazard. Although individual drugs, depending upon personal preference, are used to procure the necessary conditions, a clear distinction can be made between methods entailing the use of an endotracheal tube, and those in which the glottic reflexes are depressed by general anaesthesia and opaque oil poured into the trachea over the back of the tongue. Complete safety and control of secretions can only be achieved by intubation of the trachea and the use of suction, but these procedures and the associated depression of reflexes by relaxants or deep anaesthesia complicate the anaesthetist's work. A further advantage of endotracheal intubation is that the whole examination can be carried out deliberately and smoothly without undue haste, while the use of explosive and inflammable agents is easily excluded. Good team work between radiologist, anaesthetist and nurse is an essential prerequisite for safety and perfect pictures.

LARYNGOSCOPY AND BRONCHOSCOPY

Indirect Laryngoscopy

Indirect inspection of the glottis, even though performed by someone other than the anaesthetist, may provide information valuable to the anaesthetist concerning the type and extent of any laryngeal lesions, the degree of obstruction present, if any, and how the vocal cords move. These facts are of considerable importance when choosing an anaesthetic sequence for any form of operation, but more particularly when an operation in the neighbourhood of the glottis is contemplated, or intubation of the trachea intended.

Method.—A small circular laryngeal mirror set at an angle on the end of a metal stem is used. The mirror must be warmed by dipping in hot water just before use to prevent steaming up when the larynx is visualised. The patient sits opposite the operator with his mouth wide open and pulls his tongue well forward between a piece of gauze with his right hand. The back of the mirror is gently pushed up against the soft palate while a light is shone on the glass so that an inverted vision of the glottis is shown. In sensitive patients who tend to gag during the procedure, it is helpful to spray the soft palate and back of the tongue with a little 4 per cent lignocaine a few minutes before starting.

Direct Laryngoscopy

All anaesthetists are familiar with the two principal types of laryngoscope—the straight and the curved (Macintosh) blade. The straight blade exposes the

LARYNGOSCOPE BLADES

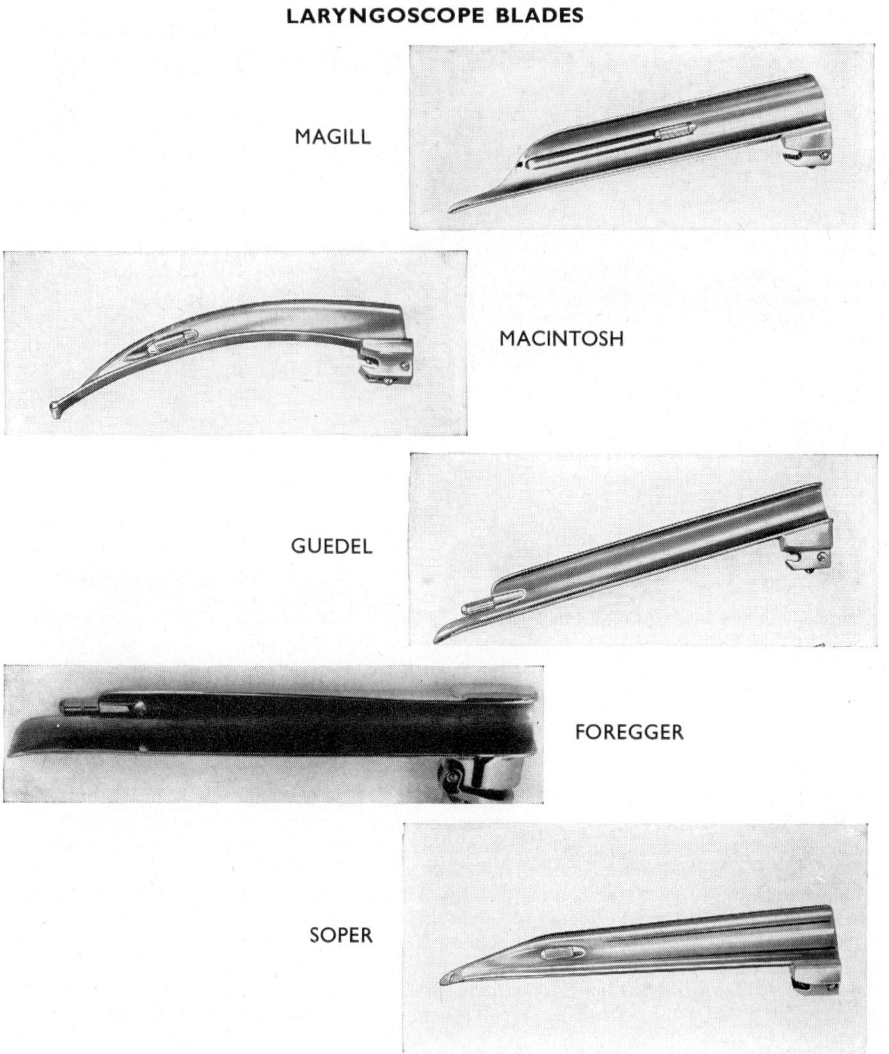

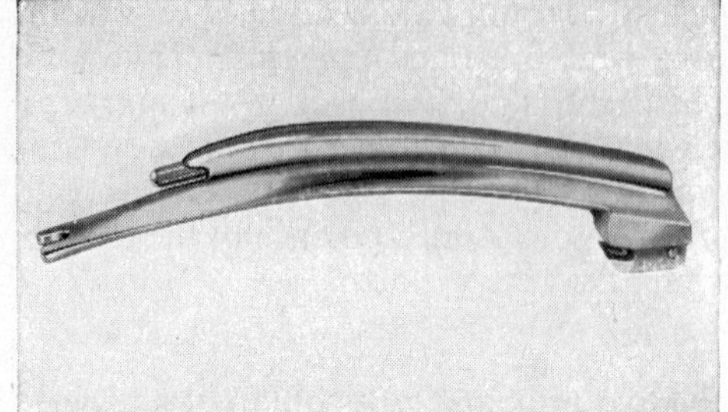

B-J (Bowen-Jackson)

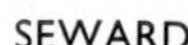

SEWARD

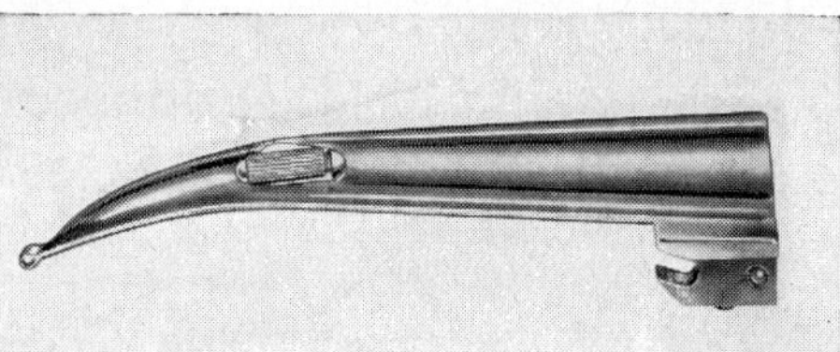

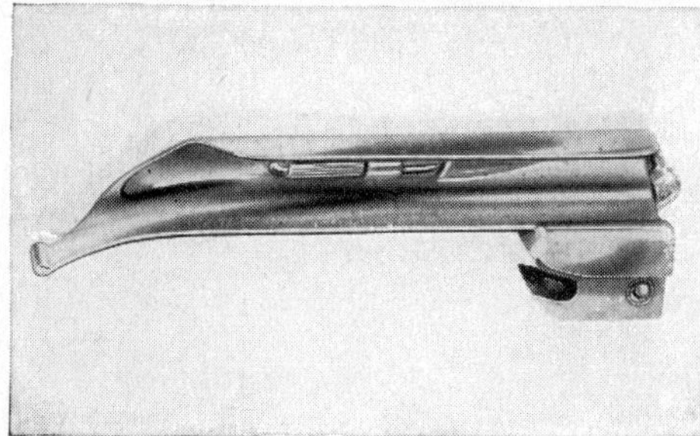

OXFORD INFANT

ROBERTSHAW

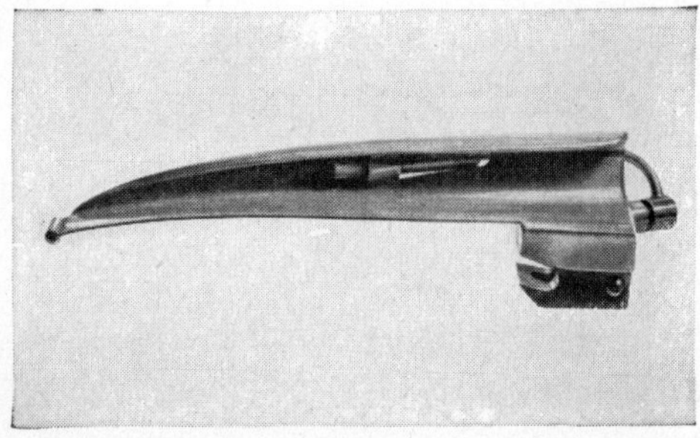

10/Fig. 9.—Some Styles of Laryngoscope Blades.

The Magill, Macintosh, Guedel, Foregger and Soper blades were designed primarily for adults, though each is available in a size suitable for children. The Soper blade combines the "Z" part of the Macintosh design with a straight blade. The B-J (Bowen-Jackson) is a compromise, and can be used for children and adults. The blade has a cleft at the end which enables it to straddle the glosso-epiglottic fold and enter the depths of the vallecula. It also has a marked curve at the distal end, while its depth is shallow so that it can be easily inserted between large teeth. The Seward, Oxford Infant and Robertshaw blades were all produced for infants and children. The Oxford Infant has an overhang on the open side to prevent the lips obscuring vision, and a broad, flat lower surface which is helpful for a child with a marked degree of cleft palate.

vocal cords by lifting the epiglottis itself; whereas the curved blade, which was designed to avoid stimulation of this sensitive structure, indirectly raises the epiglottis and brings the larynx into view by pressing upon the base of the tongue. Several variations of these two styles are described. Some of those that are commonly used by anaesthetists are illustrated in Fig. 9. For diagnostic purposes, particularly when biopsy is necessary, the straight bladed type is essential, not only to fix a particular cord, but also to evert it so that its inferior surface can be inspected. For anaesthetic purposes individual preference and practice is more important than theoretical argument, but most anaesthetists accept the curved blade as offering a broader view of the glottic area with greater room for passing an endotracheal tube, while seeing the cords until the last moment. The curved blade is also easier to use in a patient with a full set of teeth, and there is some evidence that it is less liable to produce bruising in the soft tissues of the pharynx and around the glottis and epiglottis (Wylie, 1950).

Bronchoscopy

Bronchoscopy may be performed for diagnostic reasons, for purposes of treatment when it is necessary to remove excessive or troublesome secretions from the respiratory tract, or as an essential part of an anaesthetic technique when it is desirable to block off the whole or part of a lung for a particular pulmonary operation.

Apparatus.—For diagnostic purposes and for the introduction of blockers the Negus bronchoscope is most satisfactory (Fig. 10). The lighting is distal and supplied by a battery separate from the instrument; the lumen is unobstructed, and various sizes are made. The smallest Negus bronchoscope has a circumference of 15·0 mm. with an internal diameter of 3·2 mm. at the distal, and 4·1 mm. at the proximal end. This size is used for babies up to about 1 year of age while the infant's bronchoscope has a circumference of 19·5 mm., a length of 27·5 cm. and an internal diameter of 4·1 mm. and 5·4 mm. respectively. The sizes gradually increase up to a maximum of 25 mm. circumference, 40 cm. in length and internal diameters of 8·7 mm. at the distal and 10 mm. at the proximal end. In general an instrument with the greatest circumference at the distal end compatible with the size of the patient is preferable for most anaesthetic purposes. On the rare occasion nowadays when an endobronchial blocker is required, it must be remembered that the distal end of the bronchoscope may restrict its passage. Moreover, the greater the circumference the better the view obtained.

Many other bronchoscopes have been designed, but it is proposed to mention only two. First the Magill intubating bronchoscope, built to carry around it an endobronchial tube and, therefore, of relatively small circumference itself. Secondly, a bronchoscope of the Negus style, but designed with the battery in the handle, for portability. Wherever bronchoscopy is carried out it is essential to have suction available, and a special metal suction catheter which will pass down the bronchoscope used.

Method.—The patient should be flat on the table with the head extended at the atlanto-occipital joint and slightly raised on a pillow or special support by flexion of the neck, with the object of getting the mouth and trachea in a straight line (Fig. 11). This enables the rigid straight bronchoscope to be passed

by the introduction of the short-acting muscle relaxants such as suxamethonium, and it is possible to have a patient fully conscious with complete reflex activity within a minute or two of the investigation ending. This rapid return of full reflex activity makes the use of suxamethonium, with brief general anaesthesia, the technique of choice when some bleeding is likely to follow a laryngoscopy or bronchoscopy. Furthermore, such patients can go home about two hours later, so long as they are accompanied.

The use of a muscle relaxant does introduce the hazards associated with respiratory paralysis which are here complicated by the presence of the bronchoscope, and may be further accentuated by any blood or pus that lies in the respiratory tract. In practice a fair division of the use of the bronchoscope between the endoscopist and the anaesthetist, the one for purposes of diagnosis and, if necessary, suction, and the other for inflation of the lungs, works well. There are, moreover, alternative methods of ensuring adequate ventilation of the patient (see below). Certain relatively uncommon conditions, such as a broncho-pleural fistula or a tension cyst in the lung, may contra-indicate general anaesthesia with intermittent positive-pressure respiration (see p. 428).

With local analgesia cord movements are usually unaffected, but even under general anaesthesia these can be observed as the relaxant wears off at the termination of either laryngoscopy or bronchoscopy. General anaesthesia with respiratory paralysis drastically limits the duration of direct laryngoscopy; if a small nasal endotracheal tube is placed through the glottis for the insufflation of oxygen the examination can take a little longer, as for micro-laryngoscopy.

Technique of general anaesthesia.—Premedication must be chosen to suit the physical and mental state of the patient, but sedation is not essential unless the patient is agitated. Bronchoscopy is likely to be carried out because of pulmonary disease, so that drugs of the phenothiazine class may have a special value in preventing bronchiolar spasm and avoiding respiratory depression. But unless such drugs are particularly indicated, papaveretum 10 mg. and hyoscine 0·4 mg. are effective between the ages of 15 and 60 years. Atropine sulphate 0·6 mg. should be substituted for hyoscine for patients over 60 years.

Anaesthesia is induced with 0·2–0·3 g. thiopentone, depending on the physical build and state of the patient, and complete relaxation obtained with 30–50 mg. of suxamethonium. Ventilation is then carried out with oxygen for a minute or two. It may now be desirable to spray the mucous membranes of the trachea and vocal cords with 3 ml. of 4 per cent lignocaine using a Macintosh spray. Topical analgesia helps to prevent laryngeal spasm on withdrawal of the bronchoscope should the effect of the relaxant then be wearing off. On the other hand, this practice leaves the patient with some depression of reflex activity.

When a local spray is used, this must be followed by ventilation with oxygen until the endoscopist is ready to start. Oxygenation can be continued throughout the investigation through a 4 mm. Ryle's tube, the tip of which is placed at the level of the carina before the bronchoscope is passed. Additional doses of suxamethonium and thiopentone are given as necessary. If bleeding is present at the end of a bronchoscopy, the instrument should be left in place until it has been controlled or the cough reflex has returned.

The principle of the technique of general anaesthesia for bronchoscopy is to fill the lungs with a high concentration of oxygen and to maintain this through a catheter in the trachea. Then even if the patient is apnoeic, the arterial oxygen saturation will not fall to a low level for some time. Nevertheless, without some ventilation of the lungs the carbon dioxide tension of the arterial blood must rise steadily. The rate of rise in these circumstances is about 3·4 mm. Hg/min. without ventilation of the lungs, and about 2·7 mm. Hg/min. with intermittent ventilation, but in both situations the arterial oxygen tension remains pretty constant (Jenkins and Sammons, 1968; Pender *et al.*, 1968). Thus the technique of *apnoeic oxygenation* can be safely maintained for about ten minutes and is limited by the rate of rise of the arterial carbon dioxide tension. It has not been proven that the rising arterial carbon dioxide tension plays a part in causing cardiac arrhythmias during bronchoscopy under general anaesthesia of the type outlined; indeed about one-third of all patients undergoing bronchoscopy get electrocardiographic changes irrespective of the technique of anaesthesia or the level of the arterial carbon dioxide tension (Jenkins, 1966; Jenkins and Sammons, 1968; Kostel and Neilsen, 1968).

Pulmonary ventilation during the examination can be ensured by periodic inflation with high gas flows through an endotracheal tube plugged into the end of the bronchoscope or via a special endpiece with a glass window and side aperture. Every opportunity must be taken for this inflation between the surgeon's activities, or, if necessary, his examination must be momentarily interrupted.

For laryngoscopy lasting for about two minutes, an initial inflation with oxygen will usually be sufficient, and if spontaneous respiration has not returned when the laryngoscope is removed, further inflation with a face mask can then be carried out.

Technique of local analgesia.—The nerve supply to these regions is principally derived from the glossopharyngeal and vagus—the 9th and 10th—cranial nerves. The glossopharyngeal, through its pharyngeal, tonsillar and lingual branches, supplies the sensory innervation of the pharynx, tonsils and posterior third of the tongue, while the vagus, through the internal laryngeal branch of the superior laryngeal nerve, innervates both surfaces of the epiglottis, the aryepiglottic folds and the mucous membrane of the larynx down to the false cords, and through the recurrent laryngeal nerves the rest of the mucous membrane of the larynx and the upper part of the trachea.

The patient is premedicated and given an analgesic lozenge containing lignocaine 150 mg. to suck about 10 minutes prior to the procedure. Excessive drying of the mucosa from hyoscine and atropine must be avoided or the local analgesic action of the lozenge will not be widespread, but some drying of secretions, particularly if they are plentiful, is needed to enable the subsequent topical analgesia to reach the surface before being washed away. If the lozenge has been effective it is a comparatively simple matter to spray the whole of the pharynx over the back of the tongue and right down to the epiglottis and glottis with 2 ml. of 4 per cent lignocaine either with a simple spray or by means of a curved canula attached to a syringe. Some analgesic will enter the larynx by this method. Alternatively, after less complete spraying, the tongue is held forward with a piece of gauze and a swab dipped in 4 per cent lignocaine and held in a pair of curved Krause forceps (Fig. 12) is passed over it. When Krause's forceps are not available a cholecystectomy forceps makes a good substitute. The swab is then pressed firmly into each pyriform fossa region in turn. By this method some analgesic may penetrate the mucosa in the pyriform fossa and block the internal laryngeal nerve which runs superficially at this point. It is more probable, however, that all the mucous membrane in the vicinity, including that of the aryepiglottic folds, larynx and epiglottis, is made analgesic by direct contact as the swab is later moved backwards and forwards in the fossa. The mucous membrane on the inferior surface of the vocal cords and that in the larynx and upper

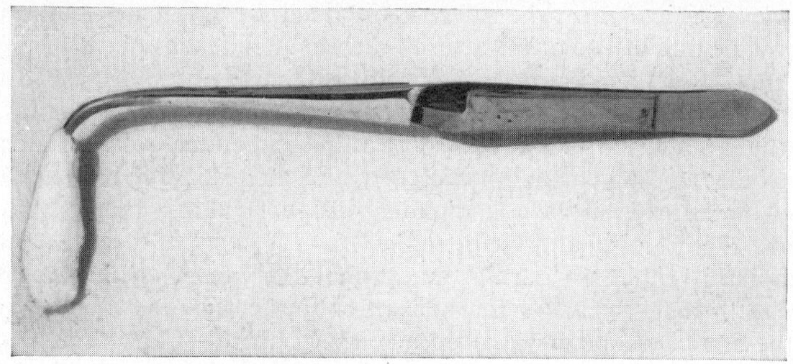

10/FIG. 12.—Krause's forceps with cotton wool swab.

part of the trachea can only be reached by spraying between the vocal cords or by injecting 1 ml. of 4 per cent lignocaine through the cricothyroid membrane as previously described for bronchography. If the lower part of the bronchial tree is still sensitive, more spraying can be done down the bronchoscope as it is advanced.

Following topical analgesia an occasional patient may develop a gruff voice due to some of the solution reaching the external laryngeal nerve (see Chapter I, p. 16).

The whole paint-up can be made more pleasant for the patient if it is immediately preceded by the slow, intravenous injection of a 1 per cent solution of 50 to 100 mg. of pethidine, or 5 mg. of diazepam.

Anaesthesia for Direct Laryngoscopy and Bronchoscopy in Children

There is no intrinsic reason why children should not be dealt with in a similar manner to adults, but it is unlikely that they will tolerate any form of local analgesia. In very young infants up to about three to four weeks of age no anaesthesia is required, and for those up to approximately three years the difficulties and hazards of a muscle relaxant technique may be sufficiently great to make a purely inhalational method preferable. Then the safest and most effective agent is open ether to a deep level of anaesthesia, so that the examination can be carried out while the anaesthesia wears off. Provided oxygen is not insufflated during the examination there is no risk of an explosion, and respiration is spontaneous the whole time. An alternative method is to use halothane with oxygen. This provides a pleasant induction to anaesthesia, but necessitates a quick bronchoscopy since halothane is eliminated from the child more rapidly than ether.

INTUBATION OF THE TRACHEA

The principal reasons for passing an endotracheal tube may be broadly summarised in two groups:—

1. Maintenance of an efficient airway.
2. Intermittent positive-pressure respiration.

1. Maintenance of an Efficient Airway

In many operations about the head and neck the maintenance of a clear airway without an endotracheal tube may be impossible, and any tendency to obstruction will be the more serious because access to the lower jaw is difficult for the anaesthetist once the surgeon has commenced. Even in these situations, however, intubation—though frequently a wise precaution—is not invariably essential. In fact, provided the anaesthetist is experienced and both the head and jaw are correctly positioned, then in many cases of lower abdominal surgery a very satisfactory airway can be obtained without the use of an endotracheal tube. The ideal position for opening up the pharynx and carrying the tongue forward is to place the head and neck in extension. However, it is advisable to use an endotracheal tube routinely for all upper abdominal surgery. Factors which strongly indicate the passage of a tube into the trachea, whatever the site of operation, are an awkward anatomical build of the patient, any tendency to laryngeal irritability either before or developing during the induction of anaesthesia, operations of long duration, and surgical procedures upon patients in poor physical health—a state which makes the sure provision of adequate ventilation at all times a vital necessity. The production of induced hypotension should be added to the last category since this technique leaves a very small margin of safety should any possible upset cause respiratory obstruction. The presence of material such as pus, blood or excessive mucus in the respiratory tract is also an indication for intubation so that intermittent suction can be carried out.

Simple intubation will not prevent vomit, pus or blood from entering the trachea, and may even assist aspiration by allowing fluid to track down the side of the tube. An essential precaution is either to use a cuffed endotracheal tube or pack off the glottis round the tube. A pack is unsatisfactory should vomiting be likely, as straining loosens it and the vomit may then push it up and enter the trachea. A cuffed tube is not ideal when blood or pus is in the oropharynx, as they may track down its side and collect below the level of the cords and above the cuff.

The oral route is always preferable to the nasal, provided it is compatible with the surgical procedure, as it allows a large-bore tube to be introduced into the trachea.

2. Intermittent Positive-Pressure Respiration

If it is intended to use either controlled or assisted respiration for more than short periods of time, then the indications for an endotracheal tube will outweigh any disadvantages. In modern anaesthesia the use of relaxant drugs invariably affects respiration, so that their continued addition during operations of more than brief duration is better combined with the passage of a tube. Artificial respiration is then not only more efficient, but the risk of inflation of the stomach is decreased. When the patient is totally paralysed and unintubated, gentle inflation by pressure on the anaesthetic bag causes air to enter the glottis, provided the tongue is well forward. Pressures above 25 cm. of water are likely to lead to some air entering the oesophagus and hence the stomach through the relaxed cricopharyngeal sphincter, but in cases of incomplete muscle paralysis or when there is partial or complete obstruction to the glottis, the oesophagus is more likely to be inflated than the lungs, even at low pressures, since the air will take the route of least resistance. This is a point of some practical importance where muscle relaxants have produced only partial paralysis since the glottis, being reflexly very active, will partially close in the presence of a stimulus at a stage when the less sensitive cricopharyngeus is well relaxed.

Distension of the stomach may be an undesirable—and post-operatively an unpleasant—accompaniment of intermittent positive-pressure respiration. Such a factor may also account for the occurrence of hiccup on inflation after partial paralysis with a muscle relaxant, the assumption being that each forced inspiration sends some air into the stomach with consequent slight distension of this organ and indirect stimulation of the diaphragm.

Contra-indications and Disadvantages

There are no absolute contra-indications to intubation when there are sufficient reasons for believing that an endotracheal tube is essential, but on occasion it may be inexpedient to intubate—or indeed frankly unnecessary. Those complications of intubation which are discussed below do not of themselves outweigh the advantages in essential cases, although the probability of some occurring more frequently than others suggests that alternative methods of maintaining a satisfactory airway may, on occasion, be preferable. Difficulty in intubating may, on certain specific occasions, make an alternative imperative, especially in the case of inexperienced practitioners, when the hazards so induced of laryngoscopy and intubation may be greater than those of an uncontrolled airway. Cass and his colleagues (1956) have summarised the six common anatomical causes of difficult oral intubation. They are:—

1. A short muscular neck with a full set of teeth.
2. A receding lower jaw with obtuse mandibular angles.
3. Protruding upper incisor teeth associated with relative overgrowth of the premaxilla.
4. Poor mobility of the mandible.
5. A long high-arched palate associated with a long narrow mouth.
6. Increased alveolar-mental distance which necessitates wide opening of the mandible for laryngoscopy.

Even in the presence of these difficulties, oral intubation can frequently be accomplished with the help of a curved introducer made to lie inside the tube but without protruding past the end.

Children present special problems. The size of the cricoid ring—which is the narrowest part of the laryngeal cavity until puberty—and not the glottic aperture, determines the diameter of the endotracheal tube. A comparison of the epiglottis in an adult and a young child will demonstrate the flat spade shape in the one and the curled form in the other, and illustrate the advantages of a straight-bladed laryngoscope in small children. Congenital abnormalities, such as micrognathia, may also add to the difficulties of intubation.

Complications

The introduction of muscle relaxants into anaesthesia not only widened the indications for intubation but also very much simplified and quickened the procedure. Thus there is a tendency to intubate for convenience, and to forget that even a straightforward and generally easy procedure has a morbidity rate. Minor disabilities and occasionally major disasters do occur, however, although it would be untrue to suggest that the worst of these constitute any more than a very small percentage of the total number of intubations performed.

General.—The gross traumatic manifestations of intubation are those most frequently associated with inexperience on the part of the anaesthetist; even so there is little excuse for broken teeth, torn lips and abraded gums if reasonable conditions of anaesthesia are produced and care is taken (Rosenberg and Borga, 1968). Trauma to the nasal passages is more difficult to avoid if this route is chosen, even when a careful pre-operative examination is made beforehand. The passage of a tube through the nasopharynx frequently leads to abrasion of the mucous membrane whether haemorrhage occurs or not, though this risk can be lessened by pre-operative shrinking of the mucosa with cocaine. There is a chance of infection being introduced into the lower air passages from this area and withdrawal of the tube may carry infection from a septic oropharynx into the neighbourhood of the sinuses. In actual practice infection either of the lower air passages or of the sinuses following nasal intubation rarely occurs, and the greatest disadvantages of this route are the production of haemorrhage on some occasions and the limitations to the size of the endotracheal tube which it imposes. The oral route is therefore the one of choice.

Sore throat or pharyngitis is undoubtedly the commonest complication of intubation, and probably occurs in something like 60 per cent of all cases, irrespective of the way in which laryngoscopy and the passage of the tube are carried out. It can be quite severe, and symptomatically sufficient to upset the patient, particularly when the operative procedure is elsewhere on the body and of a relatively minor type. Drugs of the atropine class, post-operative medication and any essential limitation of post-operative oral fluid, all increase the severity of the symptoms, which, however, rarely extend into the second post-operative day. Although considerably less troublesome, sore throat following intubation has become almost as common a complication of modern anaesthesia as vomiting was after ether anaesthesia in years gone by. This fact alone should encourage anaesthetists to practise endotracheal anaesthesia only when a good reason is apparent, rather than as a near-routine procedure for every type of surgery, anaesthesia and patient!

Complications may occasionally arise from the endotracheal tube itself. An endotracheal tube may be obstructed by its own inflated cuff overlapping its distal end, or in the case of some armoured tubes by an expansion of the tube lining into its own lumen. Gilston (1969) has described how accumulation of secretions in an endotracheal tube may cause obstruction during prolonged intubation, and Dickson and Harrison (1969) have reported a neonatal emergency following the gastric aspiration of a neonatal endotracheal tube. The position of an intubated patient during anaesthesia may lead to narrowing or total obstruction of its lumen (Heinonen *et al.*, 1969).

The larynx.—Laryngitis occurs in about 2 per cent of cases intubated, particularly when wide bore tubes—such as the use of an inflated cuff in the trachea necessitates—hold the cords in abduction for a considerable period. It is characterised by loss of power in the voice or by complete, but temporary, aphonia on the return of consciousness.

An even rarer complication is granuloma formation, and this, when organised, may result in a polyp. Young and Stewart (1953) record their findings in twelve patients, and summarise the sequence of events as probably being abrasion or haematoma, infection, ulceration and granulation, with finally organisation to a nodule or web-cicatrix. In most recorded cases a granuloma has followed the presence of an endotracheal tube for a prolonged period, suggesting that continued pressure and friction, as the tube moves with respiration, are the essential causative factors. Tonkin and Harrison (1966) have recorded the sequence of events that follows prolonged intubation of the trachea. Coughing and straining are likely to accentuate this state of affairs, and during both intubation and extubation increase the risk of trauma. Direct trauma from the point or bevel of an endotracheal tube may occasionally occur, particularly during blind nasal intubation, when the vocal process of one or other arytenoid cartilage is most likely to be prodded (Wylie, 1950).

Although granulomata with such an aetiology are undoubtedly rare, there is at least a possibility that cases may go unrecognised until the connection with anaesthesia is forgotten. Many affected patients are symptomless and have been found to have a lesion at routine laryngeal examination on the follow-up after thyroidectomy, although most have had minimal but persistent hoarseness or occasional weakness of voice. Treatment by complete voice rest may allow the ulcer to heal without much granulation formation so that spontaneous cure results, but usually piecemeal removal by direct laryngoscopy is needed. This should be carried out if improvement is not apparent on indirect laryngoscopy after a week or so, and even this treatment may need repeating.

In very small children traumatic intubation or the presence of a tightly fitting tube between the vocal cords for a long time may be potential causes (either singly or together) of glottic oedema with obstruction. The former factor is the more important and careful technique has led to the virtual disappearance of this complication. Subglottic stenosis has followed intubation in children (Taylor *et al.*, 1966). Instrumentation in the region of the glottis of a small infant quickly leads to bruising and oedema, with consequent narrowing of an already minute orifice. It is the relative size which makes this very rare complication of anaesthesia almost entirely limited to children. Oedema of the glottis, both in children and adults, may also be caused by sensitivity or overdosage of a local analgesic incorporated in the lubricant used on the tube, and in general it is preferable to avoid anything but a simple unmedicated base in children under about one year of age. If oedema should follow endotracheal anaesthesia in a child, a temporary tracheostomy may have to be done as a life-saving measure, but the early use of a moist atmosphere in an oxygen tent often tides over partial obstruction.

The trachea and bronchi.—Tracheitis characterised by retrosternal soreness may occur as part and parcel of a post-operative sore throat, but rarely, except in the case of infection from contaminated apparatus, as a definite entity. There is, however, evidence that cuffed endotracheal and endobronchial tubes sometimes lead to actual sloughing of localised areas of mucosa, or produce a membranous tracheobronchitis (Turner, 1949; Dark and Jewsbury, 1955). A variety of factors is responsible, principal amongst which are local pressure producing anaemia of the mucous membrane, most commonly in an ill, debilitated patient, trauma from local movement and the effect of irritants such as local analgesic pastes. The slough or membrane usually comes away within the first 48 hours after operation, and may cause partial or complete obstruction to the airway until coughed up or removed by suction. Such a causal factor is unlikely to be diagnosed except after the event and only then when the offending tissue can be seen, but it has been shown to be a possible factor to be remembered when faced with a post-operative episode bordering on acute asphyxia.

Intubation and post-operative pulmonary complications.—There is no worthwhile evidence to suggest that endotracheal anaesthesia materially affects the incidence of post-operative chest complications after any form of surgery (Tomlin *et al.*, 1968).

REFERENCES

ATWOOD, J. M. (1965). Respiratory obstruction during bronchography. *Anesthesiology*, **26,** 234.

CASS, N. M., JAMES, N. R., and LINES, V. (1956). Difficult direct laryngoscopy complicating intubation for anaesthesia. *Brit. med. J.*, **1,** 488.

DARK, J., and JEWSBURY, P. (1955). Post-operative membranous tracheobronchitis. *Lancet*, **1,** 430.

DICKSON, J. A. S., and FRASER, G. C. (1967). "Swallowed" endotracheal tube: a new neonatal emergency. *Brit. med. J.*, **2,** 811.

FREIFELD, S., and ZALVENDO, P. (1964). A technic for anesthesia in pediatric bronchography. *Curr. Res. Anesth.*, **43,** 45.

GILSTON, A. (1969). Obstruction of endotracheal tube. *Anaesthesia*, **24,** 256.

HEINONEN, J., TAKKI, S., and TAMMISTA, T. (1969). Effect of the Trendelenburg tilt and other procedures on the position of endotracheal tubes. *Lancet*, **1,** 850.

JENKINS, A. V. (1966). Electrocardiographic findings during bronchoscopy. *Anaesthesia*, **21,** 449.

JENKINS, A. V., and SAMMONS, H. G. (1968). Carbon dioxide elimination during bronchoscopy. *Brit. J. Anaesth.*, **40,** 533.

KOSTER, N., and NIELSEN, S. E. (1968). Electrocardiographic findings during bronchoscopy. *Anaesthesia*, **23,** 27.

NEDEL, J. R., WOLFE, W. G., and GRAF, P. D. (1968). Tantalum oxide. *Invest. Radiol.*, **3,** 229.

PALMER, P. E. S., BARNARD, P. J., CUSHMAN, R. P., and CRAWSHAW, G. R. (1967). Bronchography with Hytrast. *Clin. Radiol.*, **18,** 94.

PENDER, J. W., WINCHESTER, L. W., JAMPLIS, R. W., LILLINGTON. G. A., and MCCLENAHAN, J. B. (1968). Effects of anesthesia on ventilation during bronchoscopy. *Curr. Res. Anesth.*, **47,** 415.

ROSENBERG, N., and BORGA, J. (1968). Protection of teeth and gums during endotracheal intubation. *Curr. Res. Anesth.*, **47**, 34.

TAYLOR, T. H., NIGHTINGALE, D. A., and SIMPSON, B. R. (1966). Subglottic atenosis after nasal endotracheal intubation. *Brit. med. J.*, **2**, 451.

TOMLIN, P. J., HOWARTH, F. H., and ROBINSON, J. S. (1968). Postoperative atelectasis and laryngeal incompetence. *Lancet*, **1**, 1402.

TONKIN, J. P., and HARRISON, G. A. (1966). Sequence of events from prolonged intubation up to 72 hours, including post-mortem findings. *Med. J. Aust.*, **11**, 581.

TURNER, F. L. (1949). Sloughs of the tracheal mucosa. *Lancet*, **2**, 237.

WYLIE, W. D. (1950). Hazards of intubation. *Anaesthesia*, **5**, 143.

YOUNG, N., and STEWART, S. (1953). Laryngeal lesions following endotracheal anaesthesia: A report of twelve adult cases. *Brit. J. Anaesth.*, **25**, 32.

FURTHER READING

LINDOHOLM, C. C. (1969). Prolonged endotracheal intubation. *Acta anaesth. scand.*, Suppl. 33.

PROCTOR, D. F. (1968). Anesthesia for peroral endoscopy and bronchography. *Anesthesiology*, **29**, 1025.

Chapter 11

ANAESTHESIA FOR SURGERY OF THE EARS, NOSE, THROAT AND MOUTH

General Principles

Surgery in this region of the body is rarely complicated by factors such as great haemorrhage or trauma of the type which leads to circulatory failure. In many cases the operations are elective and the mortality, or even morbidity, are as often attributable to anaesthesia as to the operation. The main concern of the anaesthetist must be to provide with safety a quiet patient and an uncongested operating field—assets which are almost entirely dependent on complete control of the airway. A rapid return of reflex activity is also essential after many of the common operations.

An endotracheal method is usually indicated, although individual procedures, and indeed some patients—particularly children—may be more conveniently dealt with unintubated, especially when the operating time is short. Oral intubation is preferable to the nasal route when the site of the operation permits, since it is less traumatic, certainly cleaner, and allows the use of a wider bored tube which makes for freer breathing.

Prevention of Aspiration

With endotracheal anaesthesia the tracheobronchial tract can be adequately sealed off by either a pack or an inflated cuff on the tube, so that the risk of aspiration of blood or pus during the operation is removed. In this respect a pack is better than a cuff. The latter may easily leak and must lie below the vocal cords, with the result that fluid can accumulate in the larynx just above it. A pack, unless very firmly placed, is unlikely to be so efficient as a cuff, yet does in practice act as a perfectly good seal to fluids, since it tends to absorb them. This is illustrated by the effectiveness of two vaginal tampons, placed one on either side of the tube deep in the pharynx. As an alternative an ordinary bandage soaked in water and then squeezed out is satisfactory if it is placed well down on both sides of the endotracheal tube above the glottis. The use of any pack increases post-operative pharyngitis, particularly if it becomes dry and remains in place for a very long time. For this reason a greasy pack may be better for long operations. The use of sterile paraffin as the lubricant is best avoided since it introduces a very remote risk of an irritant pneumonia should any of this substance get into the lungs. Whatever method is used care must be taken to ensure that the pack is removed at the end of the procedure. Total laryngeal obstruction may quickly result if the pack is left in the pharynx after removal of the endotracheal tube.

Control of blood or foreign material does not cease at the end of the operation, since the risk of aspiration or obstruction is considerable in the immediate post-operative period. Adequate reflex activity is essential after all operations in the mouth or nasal cavities before the endotracheal tube is removed.

Before the tube or pack is removed, the patient must be placed in the semi-prone position, preferably over a pillow, so that the head and neck are at a lower level than the glottis, and all blood sucked out of the oropharynx.

Choice of Technique

There is little to be gained from controlled or assisted respiration unless an adequate tidal volume cannot be maintained spontaneously.

Excessive bleeding, which particularly hampers the surgeon's vision into the nasal cavities, is the principal reason for some practitioners' preferring local analgesia. A slight reaction by the patient upon an endotracheal tube leads to a very marked increase in the vascularity of the operation site, while the use of sufficient muscle relaxant to correct this will depress spontaneous respiration enough to cause a rise in the carbon dioxide tension of the blood. Bleeding can in practice be usually kept within normal limits by a combination of adequate anaesthesia, local vasoconstriction of the mucous membranes, freedom of expiratory or inspiratory obstruction to respiration, normal ventilation, and simple posturing of the patient. However, some patients are likely to strain unless specific steps are taken to reduce the irritation of the tube in the trachea—even though this is apparently contra-indicated by the need for active reflexes at once post-operatively. When a patient reacts it takes quite a long time for the venous engorgement to subside, so that straining and coughing are best avoided.

It is perhaps more skilful to attend to these details of technique in advance, either by deepening the level of anaesthesia or by a judicious use of an intravenous analgesic such as pethidine, rather than by the less refined but effective therapy of partial paralysis, if freedom from excessive haemorrhage is essential. It is also probable that the potential danger of specific depression of protective glottic reflexes in the immediate post-operative period has been exaggerated. If the patient is only semi-conscious then such a state of affairs is obviously most undesirable, but a return to full consciousness can be ensured so easily and so rapidly nowadays that the danger need be no greater than that produced by the use of a post-operative dose of morphine. Moreover a local analgesic effect can be produced with a drug of short duration. Bourne (1954) considers that the tracheal mucosa adapts itself to the continuous presence of the endotracheal tube, even if the surface analgesia is transient, and that coughing is usually due to movement caused by the surgeon's manipulations, which make the tube touch a fresh piece of mucosa. He controls coughing by the intravenous addition of suxamethonium and the use of artificial respiration, arguing that by the time spontaneous respiration returns the tracheal mucosa will have adapted itself to the tube once more. This, however, results in an uneven form of anaesthesia and encourages venous congestion, and it is better to deepen anaesthesia by inhalational methods if moderate doses of pethidine do not succeed. Halothane is particularly valuable for brief nasal and oral operations where it is desirable to have more control and yet provide a rapid return of consciousness.

Individual experience of agents must condition the eventual choice for various operations, although some drugs appear more suitable for certain procedures than others. These are mentioned specifically later, when the particular operations are discussed. For general purposes, ever since Bourne (1947) described the use of thiopentone-curare-nitrous oxide-oxygen anaesthesia for head and neck surgery, increasing use has been made of the muscle relaxants to facilitate intubation and reduce the total quantity of anaesthetic. Suxamethonium is nowadays frequently substituted for curare, but its short action with the rapid return to full muscular activity can be a disadvantage. Moreover, because the sequelae of most operations for ear, nose, throat and oral disease are minimal, those of anaesthesia, especially the muscle pains produced by suxamethonium, are more likely to be noticed by the patient. These several factors suggest that there are occasions when the use of other relaxants, more particularly gallamine which has a shorter action and a less prolonged effect on respiration than *d*-tubocurarine, may be advisable.

In practice general anaesthesia for many nasal and aural operations is combined with the use of locally applied or injected vasoconstricting solutions such as cocaine or adrenaline. It is important to remember the potential dangers of adrenaline in relation to halothane (see also Chapter 9, page 326). Induced hypotension must never be used as a cover for excessive bleeding due to bad anaesthesia.

These several points concerning anaesthesia need not be limited to adults, provided the dose of each agent is related to the weight and physical condition of the child. However, in small children it is often more convenient and simpler to rely upon one principal inhalational agent like ether, rather than to use a combination of many drugs.

Many operations in this region of the body are eminently suitable for local analgesia. For some, the production of good analgesia may be time-consuming and take longer than the induction of general anaesthesia, but, in an area which is notable for its vascularity, the time is often justified by the better end-results. Yet general anaesthesia is most commonly used for every type of operation, with the exception of dental, in this country. The reader is referred to more specialised works for descriptions of the various local techniques in this part of the body.

Anaesthesia for Specific Operations

Tonsils and Adenoids in Children

Tonsils are removed in the vast majority of cases by dissection, removal by guillotine now being rarely performed.

Dissection tonsillectomy in children.—The principles of this method are completeness and full control of bleeding. Time should not be a major consideration. A controlled level of adequate anaesthesia with return of reflex activity at the end of the operation is required.

Two controversial points need amplification—first premedication, and secondly choice of anaesthetic technique.

Premedication with barbiturate, with reasonable timing, will guarantee that a child arrives in the anaesthetic room asleep. Oral barbiturates may be unpleasant to take and may in a few cases lead to some post-operative depression. Increased restlessness may also occur when the anaesthetic wears off and pain is felt. Properly used it has the advantage of ensuring that a child had no knowledge of leaving the ward, let alone of the induction of anaesthesia—two points of some importance for the very young or unco-operative children. Provided competent nursing staff are available, post-operative difficulties do not in practice commonly occur, and post-operative restlessness may be lessened by the prolonged analgesic effect of ether if this agent is used during the procedure. Oral phenothiazines such as trimeprazine tartrate ("Vallergan") are of equal value. They are more pleasant to take than barbiturates. Most children are well sedated and in those who arrive restless and tearful in the anaesthetic room there appears to be a high incidence of amnesia of the event. Post-operative restlessness is less common, though a fast pulse rate is often observed and the children may remain drowsy for some time post-operatively. In the older child, papaveretum and hyoscine in a dose suited to the weight, will usually enable him to be brought to the anaesthetic room in a quiet and co-operative frame of mind. Frequently the induction of anaesthesia is forgotten at a later date in a general amnesia for the whole immediate pre-operative period. Correct management of the child should aim to ensure that even if he remembers the induction of anaesthesia it should not be resented.

The choice of an anaesthetic technique largely depends upon the decision whether or not to intubate. Doughty (1957*a*) advocates a similar sequence of drugs as would generally be selected for an adult—thiopentone: relaxant: nitrous oxide: oxygen—with doses scaled down to suit the child, and an oral endotracheal tube. By means of a modified tongue-plate on the standard Boyle-Davis gag (Doughty, 1957*b*), the oral tube can be accommodated between the tongue and the gag without infringing on the surgeons operation field. The advantages of intubation by this method are a speedy induction of anaesthesia, control of the airway, protection of the trachea and bronchi from aspiration of blood. Also after an adequate depth of anaesthesia initially to allow full opening of the gag, a light level of anaesthesia ensures a rapid return of consciousness. The surgeon, incidentally, is protected from the inhalation of anaesthetic vapours associated with an open technique, Care should be taken that the endotracheal tube is not compressed by the tip of a Doughty blade or by the blade against the lower incisor teeth. Webster (1963) found the degree of compression at the tip of the blade varies with extension of the neck and was more liable to occur when the blade was too short. Compression against the lower incisor teeth was common if a standard curved Magill endotracheal tube was used. The Worcester Connector (Steel and Needs, 1963) and modifications (Ozorio and Cohen, 1964) are designed to overcome this problem. Whatever connection is used the endotracheal tube should not be soft thus making compression more likely. The alternative to intubation is insufflation down a tube on the side of the tongue spatula of the Boyle-Davis gag, and this demands an adequate depth of anaesthesia, particularly at the moment when the gag is placed in the mouth and the operation commenced. Without an endotracheal tube safety is best achieved by a depth of anaesthesia sufficient to prevent any gagging or reflex glottic irritation during the operation, and maintenance of a free airway by the surgeon. An anaesthetic sequence based on ether or halothane as the main agent is the most satisfactory in these circumstances. Deep anaesthesia is only necessary to suppress reflex activity during positioning of the gag at the start of the operation. A competent surgeon and anaesthetist are unlikely to have any operative difficulties despite the absence of an endotracheal tube, and a speedy return of reflex activity can be assured, but recovery of full consciousness will depend on the type of premedication. As in so many other situations, results depend more upon the individual concerned than upon the agents and techniques. For tonsillectomy, however, simple anaesthesia is not necessarily synonymous with increased safety in the hands of an inexperienced anaesthetist. Here indeed are the ingredients of disaster—an uncontrolled airway, blood in its immediate vicinity and, all too often, an equally inexperienced surgeon. The answer to this problem does not lie in the selection of more complicated techniques for junior anaesthetists, but rather in adequate supervision during elementary methods or, more simply, personal administration by the experienced. Trouble may also develop if the surgeon makes over-zealous use of suction as this lowers the concentration of the anaesthetic agent in the pharynx and may lead to gagging and coughing.

Whatever the technique of anaesthesia, the operation is most safely carried out with the patient in the supine position and the shoulders raised on a sandbag or pillows, so that the head and neck lie at a lower level. Bleeding must be adequately controlled by the surgeon at all times.

Guillotine tonsillectomy in children.—The two most important needs for this type of operation are good relaxation and an immediate return of reflex activity as soon as the operation is over. Adequate sedative premedication is precluded, atropine sulphate alone being given. The insufflation technique using a Boyle-Davis gag already described is the standard method of anaesthesia. Adequate depth of anaesthesia is required for introduction of the gag. Once this is achieved satisfactorily oxygen only should be given so that adequate return of reflex activity is ensured by the end of the procedure. Care should be taken during the operation to prevent aspiration and preserve the airway.

Adenoidectomy follows guillotine tonsillectomy and the child should be placed on his side as soon as the curetting is completed. He should not leave the theatre until fully conscious.

Tonsillectomy in Adults

Proper control of general anaesthesia for an adult with the surgeon operating in the mouth cannot be maintained without the use of an endotracheal tube. As this is almost always passed through the nose, the pre-anaesthetic use of a cocaine spray to enlarge the cavities by mucosal shrinkage is a useful preliminary.

Although a rare procedure in this country, the tonsils can be removed under local analgesia in adults provided they are not grossly fibrotic from repeated infections. An advantage of a local technique is diminished bleeding, but the risk of post-operative sepsis and reactionary haemorrhage may be increased. The technique of analgesia (Macintosh and Ostlere, 1955) principally consists of topical analgesia, followed by the injection of a local analgesic solution into the posterior pillar of the tonsillar fossa from top to bottom, and then injection into the anterior pillar. The patient should be sitting comfortably in a chair facing the operator.

Post-Tonsillectomy Bleeding

Post-operative haemorrhage after removal of tonsils and adenoids is not uncommon and is severe enough to require surgical ligation in about 1–2 per cent of cases (Gorham, 1964). It is the chief cause of death from the operation. Severe shock or even death, though rare, usually result from failure to judge the severity of blood loss. Assessment of this may be difficult. There may be continuous slow loss over many hours. Although bleeding from the tonsillar fossa can be seen by looking into the mouth, bleeding from the adenoid bed cannot be observed in this way. The patient may be constantly swallowing blood and there may be more blood in the stomach than on the pillow (Tate, 1963). Restlessness may be attributed to pain rather than blood loss and opiates wrongly given, the central depression produced masking the important signs and resulting in collapse. There is the additional hazard of vomiting or regurgitation, blood being aspirated into the lungs.

Such post-operative blood loss is especially dangerous in small children who may have lost a higher proportion of their blood volume at the time of operation (usually unmeasured). It is vital that haemostasis is secured under general anaesthesia as quickly as possible before the patient becomes dangerously shocked.

As soon as the decision has been taken to return the patient to theatre an intravenous infusion should be set up and blood cross-matched. The patient should be placed head down on his side so that if vomiting or regurgitation occur blood will not enter the larynx. Pre-operative sedation is unnecessary and should never be given. Induction of anaesthesia should be performed on a tipping table with a sucker in good working order close at hand. Intravenous barbiturates are contra-indicated as further hypotension may result. A gaseous induction using cyclopropane and oxygen or halothane and oxygen is much safer. A cuffed endotracheal tube is passed via the mouth using ether or halothane to provide the necessary relaxation for this manoeuvre. Suxamethonium may be preferred as this provides better conditions for intubation but may also lead to regurgitation of blood from the stomach. Once the airway is protected the patient can be turned onto his back, anaesthesia being continued in a light plane using halothane or ether. Blood should be sucked out of the stomach using a wide bore tube. This will often produce an improvement in the patient's general condition and blood can be transfused whilst the source of bleeding is located and dealt with. An alternative to intubation in children is to insufflate ether via a Boyle-Davis gag, full extension of the head ensuring that though blood may accumulate in the pharynx it will not enter the trachea (Gorham, 1964).

At the end of the procedure the patient should be extubated on his side and remain in the tonsil position closely observed until full recovery has taken place.

Aural Operations

The potential dangers associated with some depression of glottic activity in the presence of blood or pus do not arise, so that a combination of light anaesthesia and specific depression of respiratory tract reflexes can be successfully and safely used while the patient breathes spontaneously. (For a fuller description of techniques of this type the reader is referred to Chapter 39.) Bleeding can thus be kept within normal limits, but even so it may be troublesome for the surgeon; a very small amount of blood quickly obscures the view should a microscope be in use. There is, however, very little substantiation for the opinion, sometimes expressed, that the success of an operation in this area of the body can only be assured by the use of hypotension to produce a completely dry operating field. Induced hypotension is not essential, but as an ancillary to the basic anaesthetic technique it will make the surgical procedure simpler and possibly quicker. It certainly should not be used to circumvent the difficulties of inexperienced surgeons. Many operations on the ear, especially those involving mobilisation, or removal of the stapes and replacement by a prosthesis, lend themselves to simple local analgesia. Despite this, general anaesthesia is most commonly favoured in this country.

Saidman (1965) and Eger (1965) have shown that nitrous oxide anaesthesia influences the pressures and volumes in closed gas-filled cavities. Nitrous oxide is about thirty times more soluble than nitrogen in blood and therefore nitrous oxide molecules will collect in the air spaces quicker than nitrogen molecules leave, causing a temporary increase in the size of the non-rigid air space. Thomsen (1965) observing bulging of a graft during myringoplasty under nitrous oxide anaesthesia showed that there was a marked increase in pressure in the middle ear cavity, the rate of increase in pressure being related to the percentage of nitrous oxide inhaled. Matz (1967) experimenting with 60 per cent nitrous oxide in oxygen in cats showed that there was a slow rise in pressure, in the middle ear over 10–15 minutes until a peak pressure was reached at which stage the Eustachian tube opened and a temporary pressure drop occurred. Both Thomsen and Matz considered it possible that nitrous oxide inhalation, with its resultant rise in middle ear pressure, might be responsible for tympanic perforation, otitis media and other aural sequelae of general anaesthesia, particularly in patients with any interference of normal Eustachian tube function. It is probably best, therefore, in such patients either to use a halothane-oxygen mixture and avoid the use of nitrous oxide altogether, or simply to turn the nitrous oxide off about 10 minutes prior to final closure of the middle ear cavity.

One other factor is worthy of comment when choosing an anaesthetic sequence for surgery of the ear. Many operations, including fenestration, stapedectomy, destruction or removal of the labyrinth, and some mastoidectomies, are followed in the post-operative period by intense vestibular disturbances, so that even raising the head from the pillow may cause sickness. This can often be offset by the post-operative use for two or three days of a phenothiazine drug by mouth—chlorpromazine 25 mg. b.d. or prochlorperazine 25 mg. b.d.—and to some extent prevented by their use intramuscularly during the operation, so that the patients come round with specific central sedation in this respect.

Laryngofissure

The presence of a relatively small endotracheal tube does not obstruct the surgical field during laryngofissure and removal of a vocal cord or its mucous membrane. Intubation ensures an adequate airway, makes the maintenance of anaesthesia simple, and with an inflated cuff or small pack—placed by the surgeon as soon as the larynx is opened—prevents the aspiration of blood. It is most important to have full reflex activity present at the end of operation. With light anaesthesia alone there is a tendency for the patient to cough when the sensitive mucous membrane of the larynx and cords is touched, unless conditions are just right. Occasionally it may be better to control the patient fully with a relaxant and to use intermittent positive-pressure respiration rather than give more anaesthetic drugs, the choice of which is frequently restricted by use of the diathermy. When controlled respiration is carried out, a cuffed tube is essential or the surgeon's pack may be blown out during inflation.

Some surgeons start the operation by making a temporary tracheostomy. The anaesthesia can then be started in the way described, but once the trachea is opened the endotracheal tube must be removed and a special short cuffed and sterilised tube of the requisite size inserted into the tracheostomy opening by the surgeon. The anaesthesia is continued through this. Montando's tube (Fig. 1) is particularly useful, as it is curved to avoid the need for a connection piece very near to the operation site. If this is unavailable a cut endotracheal tube will be of value.

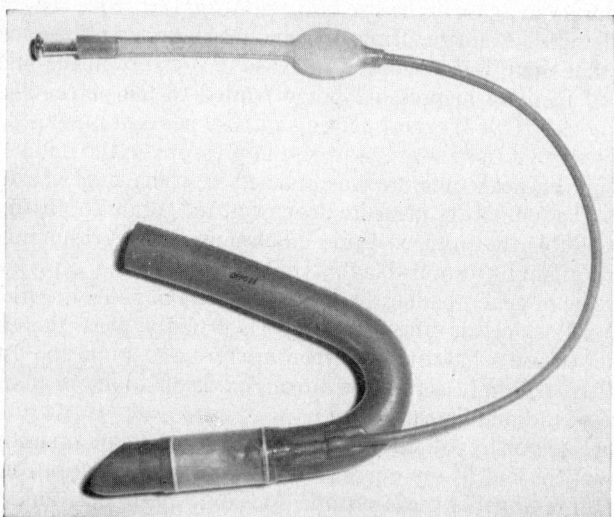

11/Fig. 1.—Montando's tube.

Laryngectomy

In this operation the anaesthetic sequence is largely conditioned by the surgical technique, and whether or not a tracheostomy has already been performed. If there is a tracheostomy, a suitable plastic tracheostomy tube should be inserted into which an adaptor can secure an airtight fit between tracheostomy tube and catheter mount. Alternatively, simple intubation with a short cuffed tube, as described above, may be used.

In cases where there is no tracheostomy the more usual procedure is for the surgeon to dissect out the larynx completely before dividing the lower end from the top of the trachea preparatory to removing the whole organ. In this event pre-operative assessment of the degree of respiratory obstruction is essential. If the patient is slightly obstructed and stridor is present, respiratory depressant drugs should be omitted and atropine only be given for premedication. Special precautions (see below) will be needed for induction. Anaesthesia is maintained with the aid of a cuffed oral endotracheal tube placed in position with considerable care considering the presence of the new growth and the risk of causing bleeding. Distortion of the normal anatomy by tumour or oedema may make intubation difficult and it may only be possible to get a small size tube into the trachea. As the trachea is divided this tube is removed and the surgeon introduces a sterile, short, cuffed tube fitted with an angled connection into the trachea direct. This is then attached to the anaesthetic apparatus. This tube can remain in position until the very end of the operation, when it will have to be removed so that a permanent tracheostomy can be formed by sewing the skin to the edges of the trachea. It is therefore essential that the patient be breathing spontaneously by then and that the surgeon prevent any risk of aspiration by suction.

The alternative surgical procedure consists of dissecting the larynx from the pharynx in the first place. At this stage the disconnected endotracheal tube has to be delivered from the mouth through the surgical incision and reconnected to the anaesthetic system below the chin. At a later stage the larynx is severed from the trachea, when the procedure follows that described above.

In practice, whatever the approach, there is a time during a laryngectomy when continuous inhalational anaesthesia is no longer practicable. Deepening of the level of anaesthesia using halothane prior to this may avoid the patient waking during this time. The use of trichloroethylene or methoxyflurane in the early stages of the operation may be a help, as they tend to delay recovery of full consciousness. Intermittent injection of thiopentone may be necessary to supplement the residue of inhalational drugs but great care must be taken not to depress the respiration.

Oesophagoscopy

Oesophagoscopy is at best an unpleasant investigation under any form of local analgesia, and may be difficult, if not impossible, to perform in the presence of inadequate conditions. Consideration must be given to the disease for which it is being performed before any anaesthetic is commenced, since there may be a considerable danger of aspiration of oesophageal or stomach contents. Special precautions (see Chapter 47) will be needed to avoid this. Suxamethonium should be used for intubation and to maintain perfect surgical conditions throughout the procedure, which is considerably simplified by full relaxation of the jaw muscles and the cricopharyngeal sphincter. Some surgeons prefer spontaneous ventilation while advancing the instrument as the oesophagus dilates during expiration, thus avoiding damage. Better assessment can also be made of the state of the cardio-oesophageal junction. Where this is preferred, halothane provides adequate relaxation. Care should be taken that the endotracheal tube is not compressed by the oesophagoscope at any time during the procedure.

Anaesthesia in the Presence of Upper Respiratory Obstruction

There are many potential causes of respiratory obstruction, varying from swellings in or near the trachea and glottis, to the simple obstructive effects of

in the body. It may then be necessary to administer carbon dioxide for a spell, gradually weaning the patient back to air over a period of time, or to perform intermittent positive-pressure ventilation until the patient once more breathes spontaneously.

Further relief will result from adequate suction removing retained secretions which may have accumulated in large quantities whilst the upper respiratory obstruction progressed.

Hare-Lip and Cleft Palate

An operation for repair of hare-lip is carried out when the child is about three months old. When the abnormality is bilateral a bone graft can be inserted in a stage one procedure or, each side is repaired separately with an interval of from 2 to 3 weeks between the operations. A cleft palate is treated when the child is between 12 and 15 months old, preferably before the child starts to talk.

To avoid feeding difficulties an operation for hare-lip is best carried out at an hour of the day least likely to upset the child's normal routine, bearing in mind that 4 hours' pre-operative starvation is essential. Anaesthetic requirements should consist of premedication with 0·3 mg. atropine sulphate and endotracheal nitrous oxide, oxygen and halothane, spontaneous ventilation and a T-piece system. Induction can be conveniently performed with cyclopropane and oxygen, a litre of each administered for a period of from 3 to 4 minutes being excellent for this purpose. Suxamethonium 1·0 mg./kg. injected into a vein in the front of the wrist provides the best conditions for intubation; however, an inhalation method without relaxant should be used if extreme difficulty is anticipated with intubation. An Oxford tube avoids kinking during the operation and is connected to the T-piece system below the centre of the lower lip. A latex rubber tube incorporating a coil of nylon will also avoid kinking.

Most of the anaesthetic problems are associated with intubation and the endotracheal tube, and immediately following extubation. Both laryngoscopy and the passage of the tube may be troublesome to the inexperienced anaesthetist. The hare-lip tends to obscure the field of vision and the laryngoscope blade may slip into a cleft palate if this is present as well as the hare-lip. Additional malformations may also make intubation difficult. The Pierre Robin syndrome combines micrognathia, a large tongue and a posterior cleft palate. In micrognathia the underdeveloped lower jaw tends to hold the tongue against the posterior pharyngeal wall. Intubation is made easier by using an introducer with the Oxford tube and a pliable urethral bougie of suitable size is ideal for this purpose. This protrudes an inch beyond the distal end of the Oxford tube and is introduced into the larynx, the endotracheal tube being threaded into the trachea. When subglottic stenosis is present this may not be recognised until intubation is attempted and, of course, necessitates a tube of smaller size than average for the child's age group. The length of the tube must be carefully assessed to avoid intubation of the right bronchus and avoid stimulation of the carina with subsequent coughing or extubation during surgical manoeuvres in the mouth. A Boyle-Davis gag is used to provide surgical access for the repair of a cleft palate and care should be taken that this does not compress the endotracheal tube but presses on the metal connector from the tube to the T-piece system.

For either lesion the level of anaesthesia should be as light as possible to ensure that the child will cry immediately the operation is completed; yet care must be taken to avoid vomiting before the gag is removed. Light halothane provides adequate respiratory activity, which can be conveniently gauged by fitting a stethoscope attachment over the outlet tube of the T-piece. Alternatively a stethoscope can be placed over the precordium so that both respiration and heart beat can be heard.

The operations are performed with the infant supine in the tonsillectomy position, a sandbag being placed under the shoulders and the head tilted downwards towards the surgeon's lap as he sits at the head of the table. Blood loss is rarely excessive but it is usual to lose between 5 and 10 per cent of the infant's blood volume. Over 10 per cent of the blood volume may be lost if a bone graft is being used in the repair of a bilateral hare-lip and transfusion in such cases will be necessary.

Extubation should be performed with the lungs expanded with the infant on its side. A tongue stitch pulling the tongue forward may help provide a good airway. Laryngeal spasm should be avoided as administration of oxygen via a mask or reintubation in such circumstances may damage the repair of the hare-lip. The child should not leave the anaesthetist's care until full consciousness has been recovered and a clear airway established.

REFERENCES

ABERDEEN, E. (1960). *A Classification of Neonatal Risk in Oesophageal Atresia: Tracheo-Oesophageal Fistula.* 7th Internat. Conf. of the British Assn. of Paediatric Surgeons, London 1960.

BOURNE, J. G. (1947). Thiopentone – nitrous oxide – oxygen anaesthesia with curare for head and neck surgury. *Brit. med. J.*, **2,** 654.

BOURNE, J. G. (1954). Anaesthesia for ear, nose and throat operations. *Med. ill.* (*Lond.*), **8,** 110.

DOUGHTY, A. G. (1957*a*). Anaesthesia for adenotonsillectomy, a critical approach. *Brit. J. Anaesth.*, **29,** 407.

DOUGHTY, A. G. (1957*b*). A modification of the tongue-plate of the Boyle-Davis gag. *Lancet*, **1,** 1074.

EGER, E. I. (1965). Hazard of nitrous-oxide anaesthesia in bowel obstruction and pneumothorax. *Anesthesiology*, **26,** 61.

GORHAM, A. P. (1964). The role of the anaesthetist in the management of post-tonsillectomy haemorrhage in children. *Anaesthesia*, **19,** 565.

MACINTOSH, R. R., and OSTLERE, M. (1955). *Local Analgesia; Head and Neck.* Edinburgh: E. & S. Livingstone.

MATZ, G. J., RATTENBORG, C. G., HOLADAY, D. A. (1967). Effects of nitrous-oxide on middle ear pressure. *Anesthesiology*, **28,** 948.

OZORIO, H. P. L., and COHEN, M. (1964). An anaesthetic technique for adenotonsillectomy in children. *Brit. J. Anaesth.*, **36,** 432.

SAIDMAN, J. L. (1965). Change in C.S.F. pressure during pneumoencephalogram under nitrous-oxide and oxygen. *Anesthesiology*, **26,** 67.

STEEL, W. D., and NEEDS, R. E. (1963). Cuffed orotracheal intubation for removal of tonsils and adenoids. *Brit. J. Anaesth.*, **35,** 43.

STIRLING, J. B. (1964). Anaesthesia for tonsilectomy. *Brit. J. Anaesth.*, **26,** 411.

TATE, N. (1963). Deaths from tonsillectomy. *Lancet*, **2,** 1090.

Thomsen, K. A. (1965). Middle ear pressure during anaesthesia. *Arch. Otolaryng.*, **82,** 609.

Webster, A. C. (1963). Endotracheal anaesthesia for adenotonsillectomy: A modification of Doughty's technique. *Canad. Anaesth. Soc. J.*, **10,** 66.

Waterston, D. J., Bonham Carter, R. E., and Aberdeen, E. (1963). Congenital tracheo-oesophageal fistula in association with oesophageal atresia. *Lancet*, **2,** 55.

Chapter 12

ANAESTHESIA FOR DENTAL SURGERY

INTRODUCTION

History

GARDNER QUINCY COLTON first administered nitrous oxide to Horace Wells for the extraction of a tooth in 1844. It is just over 100 years since anaesthesia for dental extractions was introduced into England by Thomas Evans, an American dental surgeon, in 1868. A brief period of unconsciousness was induced using nitrous oxide delivered via a face-mask, allowing enough time for the painless removal of one or two teeth. The method was not associated with fatalities nor, as far as is established, with cerebral complications (Goldman, 1968). The invention of the nosepiece about 1899 allowed a longer period of unconsciousness, and hence more surgical time. This greatly increased the dangers to the patient as it allowed protracted periods of hypoxia. The introduction of the demand-flow apparatus by McKesson in 1910 and the technique of secondary saturation in which nitrogen and oxygen were "washed out" of the lungs by nitrous oxide, further added to the hazards of dental surgery. Even though a very large number of anaesthetics were given safely, fatalities and cerebral complications were far from rare. This era of "anoxic unconsciousness" (Goldman, 1968) to provide pain-free dental extraction continued until recent years. Klock (1955) and Tom (1956) demonstrated that oxygen restriction at any stage was unnecessary, but even after the dangers of hypoxia were well established, 31 patients died undergoing dental treatment under anaesthesia in the dental chair between the years 1961–1965 (Editorial *Brit. J. Anaesth.*, 1968).

General anaesthesia in dentistry is, however, an expanding field. There are now about 2 million dental anaesthetics given each year in the United Kingdom, a number exceeding the sum total of anaesthetics given for all other branches of surgery. The vast majority of these are given to healthy individuals for the extraction of teeth or conservative dentistry as out-patients either in dental surgeries, clinics, or dental hospital out-patient departments. A much smaller number are given to hospital in-patients for oral and maxillo-facial surgery.

Problems in Dental Surgery

Dental operations are rarely life-saving. The problems encountered by the anaesthetist are similar to those described in the chapter on anaesthesia for ear, nose and throat surgery. The airway is shared with the surgeon and as it lies in close proximity to the operation site, must be protected from inhalation of blood, saliva and operation debris. Further, dental burrs, whether used for surgery or conservation, are irrigated with water. Careful packing of the oropharynx is therefore essential and facilities for adequate suction should always be available and in perfect working order. The surgeon requires a wide open unobstructed mouth, the anaesthetist a clear unobstructed airway.

For out-patient surgery there is a combination of problems not encountered in any other surgical field. Firstly, the average person regards dental treatment as a minor event, arriving in the dental surgery relatively unassessed and unprepared, and expecting to return to the normal routine of life shortly after the procedure is completed; secondly, the majority of patients are seated upright during the anaesthetic. The upright position is used in certain neurosurgical and neuroradiological procedures, but both are carried out under careful anaesthetic control and monitoring. By comparison, the relatively unprepared and unassessed patient is also met for minor procedures in the casualty department, but these are performed with the patient in the supine position.

The combination of these two factors makes anaesthesia for out-patient dentistry unique. The safety of the individual in such circumstances must depend to a great extent on the brevity of surgery, most patients having only one or two teeth extracted, and the youth and fitness of the majority treated. Dental extraction technique was originally developed to cope with quick removal of a tooth causing unbearable pain. The sitting position became so entrenched in the extraction technique that it was carried on into the age of multiple extractions undertaken to remove sepsis rather than alleviate severe pain (Love, 1963), and in recent years is still practised for conservative dentistry. The supine position for out-patient dental treatment under general anaesthesia has been advocated for many years (Scott, 1952; Bourne, 1957; Love, 1963), the erect posture for such treatment being considered reckless as long ago as 1873 (Morrison). It requires a different surgical approach, to which most operators adapt easily, and its use appears to be becoming more widespread in dental surgeries.

Whatever position is adopted the dental surgeon requires certain things of his anaesthetist in order that a large number of cases can be treated with skill and safety (Moore, 1968). Induction of anaesthesia must be smooth and swift. During the operation the patient should be still and quiet, breathing spontaneously without obstruction, retching or coughing, especially if instruments such as dental drills and chisels are used in the mouth. There should be sufficient relaxation of jaw muscles to allow the mouth to be opened by gentle pressure of a gag and to allow insertion and changing of dental props and packs without difficulty. The surgeon will require free access to the mouth unobstructed by masks, tubes or supporting fingers on the jaw. Recovery has been divided into waking time, walking time and the time it takes before the patient is able to leave the surgery or recovery room (Young and Whitwam, 1964). This period should be as short as possible. There should be no straining or fighting as this may encourage post-operative bleeding or cause damage to oral wounds or appliances. Post-operative nausea and vomiting should also be avoided.

Finally, the anaesthetist should be aware of, and be able to deal with, any complication that may arise.

THE UPRIGHT POSITION

Traditionally, out-patient dental treatment under general anaesthesia is performed with the patient seated upright in the dental chair (Love, 1963). Man spends most of his waking life in the upright position. It is essential, therefore, that those mechanisms which ensure adequate brain cell oxygen in this position in everyday life are not lost under general anaesthesia. The oxygen tension of the brain depends on two factors; firstly, the arterial tension of oxygen reaching the brain and secondly, the rate of cerebral blood flow.

Cerebral Arterial Oxygen Tension

The arterial oxygen tension reaching the brain depends on the partial pressure of inspired oxygen, on adequate respiratory activity, alveolar-capillary gas exchange and on an adequate haemoglobin content of the blood. This last factor being of no greater importance in the upright than in any other position.

Respiratory activity and ventilation perfusion are better in the upright position than if the patient is lying flat, so long as the patient is allowed to breathe without the restriction of tight clothing. Blood drains by gravity to the lung bases where there is a much larger area for gas exchange than in other parts of the lung. The lung bases are also better ventilated by unimpeded diaphragmatic excursion.

The most important factor in determining the arterial oxygen tension under dental anaesthesia is the partial pressure of oxygen in the inspired gases. Until recent years this has been reduced to dangerously low levels by deliberate exclusion of oxygen from the inspired mixture during the induction period. This method relied on the use of 100 per cent nitrous oxide to induce a state of hypoxic unconsciousness rather than true surgical anaesthesia. The safety of this method depended on the fact that the period of total hypoxia was very short. Smith (1964) found that the average duration of administration of not more than 5 per cent oxygen was about 50 seconds, although over 10 per cent of his series were deprived of oxygen for longer than this time and the onset of jactitations, indicating that hypoxia had been taken too far, occurred in at least 5 per cent of cases. Although jactitations could not necessarily be associated with damage to central neurones, it was impossible to be sure that no damage had been done. Patient susceptibility to hypoxia obviously varies and of course, cannot be anticipated.

Bourne (1967) considers that in the traditional hypoxic method of anaesthesia, in which anoxic anoxia is deliberately introduced, severe anoxia of the brain only develops after a certain time lag, the body's entire oxygen reserve intervening to delay the effect on the cerebral cells. The real danger is the effect on the cerebral blood flow. When the flow rate begins to slow down to a critical level (450 ml./min.) stagnant anoxia is produced in the brain, and irreversible brain damage may rapidly occur without the characteristic cyanosis seen in anoxic anoxia.

Cerebral Blood Flow

The rate of cerebral blood flow is normally about 750 ml./min. It depends on the mean arterial blood pressure and the cerebrovascular resistance. In the sitting position cerebrovascular resistance is minimal and the blood flow varies directly with variations in the mean arterial blood pressure. Normally, this pressure is kept higher in the sitting than in the recumbent position due to overcompensation for the effect of gravity by the carotid sinus and aortic stretch mechanisms. These mechanisms will probably remain intact during nitrous oxide anaesthesia (Coplans, 1962), but may be depressed if adjuvants such as halothane are used.

During anaesthesia in the dental chair certain situations may alter the cerebral blood flow. Hypoxia is known to lead to an increased flow, a 35 per cent increase being produced breathing a mixture containing only 10 per cent oxygen (Keele and Neil, 1966). While hypoxia develops during the induction period using 100 per cent nitrous oxide the circulation is in a hyperdynamic state, cerebral blood vessels are fully dilated, there is a rise in mean blood pressure (Goldman *et al.*, 1958), and the cerebral blood flow is increased to the maximum possible limit. This is probably the vital safety factor which has allowed millions of dental extractions to be performed under hypoxic conditions with remarkably few disasters.

Diminished cerebral blood flow occurs if the arterial blood pressure is reduced in any way. It is also diminished as a result of cerebral arteriolar constriction, following either reduction in carbon dioxide tension or inhalation of high percentages of oxygen.

A fall in arterial pressure occurs in two situations in the dental chair. It may occur because of direct stimulation of the carotid sinus. This usually results from incorrect support of the patient's jaw by the anaesthetist and it is important that pressure should only be applied to the mandible itself to support the jaw. Pressure on the soft tissues below the mandible should be avoided at all costs as this may lead to carotid sinus stimulation. A fall in arterial pressure may also result from fainting in the dental chair.

Fainting

Bourne (1960, 1966) considers that nearly all the catastrophies with nitrous oxide in the dental chair are due to the common fainting attack and that this danger will continue until the traditional upright position of the patient is abandoned in favour of the supine position during anaesthesia. Fainting in the conscious patient is characterised by a sudden decrease in blood pressure and heart rate, with pallor and sweating preceding loss of consciousness and muscle tone.

Initially, there is a gradual decrease in right atrial filling pressure and therefore cardiac output, the arterial pressure being maintained by vasoreceptor reflexes. Massive parasympathetic discharge from the vasomotor centres occurs resulting in sweating, decrease in the heart rate and active vasodilatation. The fall in total peripheral resistance affects principally the muscle and splanchnic vessels. The associated cutaneous vasoconstriction and pallor is due to outpouring of posterior pituitary hormone. The resultant massive (muscle) vasodilatation effectively withdraws a considerable amount of blood from the active circulation and simulates haemorrhage (Bourne, 1965).

There are many predisposing factors to fainting in the dental chair. Important ones include anxiety and emotional stress, fatigue, fasting prior to the anaesthetic and poor health. The young are more likely to faint than the old, but any healthy person can be made to faint, and it is impossible to predict which individual will faint under a given stimulus. Fear, pain, the upright position with the weight off the feet, nausea and the inhalation of mixtures poor in oxygen all lead to simulated haemorrhage. Thus the not uncommon situation in the dental surgery where an unprepared, nervous individual is anaesthetised in a frightening way in the sitting position, by a mixture containing little or no oxygen, seems an ideal precipitant to fainting.

The onset of fainting may be so abrupt that there is little warning. It may occur prior to induction of anaesthesia, during anaesthesia, or during the recovery period. Whilst the patient is conscious there are always observable signs such as yawning, pallor and sweating. Under anaesthesia, however, such signs are absent and the loss of muscle tone from fainting may be thought to be due to the onset of surgical anaesthesia. Under an anaesthetic the pallor associated with fainting is usual, but of greater importance is bradycardia. Careful monitoring of the pulse throughout the procedure is therefore vital. If the blood pressure falls precipitously, cerebral blood flow is diminished below the critical level and the resultant stagnant anoxia leads to fatal brain damage very rapidly unless the situation is relieved. An individual who faints falls into the horizontal position and this quickly restores the blood pressure to normal. In the dental chair the patient may be actively prevented from falling and if the faint is not recognised soon enough severe brain damage and even death will result. Once recognised, the patient should be removed from the chair with all haste and laid on the floor, if possible with the feet raised to increase the venous return. Modern dental chairs have been designed to tilt the patient into the horizontal position and thus save valuable time. After initial recovery of consciousness it is important that the patient is kept lying flat until complete recovery has taken place. It should be remembered that the tendency to faint may persist for many hours after the initial episode and recurrence will occur if attempt is made to stand up again too soon.

Latham (1951) noticed that fainting occasionally occurred very shortly after administration of oxygen following a period of hypoxia. He termed this "oxygen paradox" and considered that the sudden re-oxygenation increased the size of the pulmonary vascular bed and muscle blood flow and so gave rise to fainting. A fall in blood pressure following administration of oxygen at the end of a dental anaesthetic has also been noted by Goldman *et al.* (1958), whilst Bourne (1960) studying reports of deaths in the dental chair observed that two such patients "went pale when oxygen was delivered" during the recovery period.

To summarise, fainting in the dental chair is not uncommon, the dental anaesthetist must carefully watch for pallor and change in pulse rate at all stages of the procedure and once recognised, simple treatment should be started as quickly as possible. Such accidents appear to have occurred even in the safest hands. It is therefore difficult to justify the single operator-anaesthetist who cannot monitor the pulse and observe the patient's condition with such care and who will almost certainly miss the earliest signs of fainting in the upright position.

Other Aspects of Posture

There are other problems met in out-patient dentistry that are associated with the position of the patient, be he supine or upright. These include regurgitation of stomach contents, inhalation of blood and debris, and airway maintenance.

Regurgitation of Stomach Contents

Silent regurgitation or active vomiting of stomach contents is a hazard during anaesthesia in any unprepared patient. Silent regurgitation is especially likely if an undiagnosed hiatus hernia or similar condition is present. The upright position protects against this problem and the complication is rarely if ever encountered in the sitting position (Coplans, 1962). It is, however, often encountered in unprepared patients in the supine position. Active vomiting may occur under anaesthesia if the patient has a full stomach. Although this should not occur in adults requiring treatment, fear of dental treatment may keep undigested food in the stomach for many hours. It may also be a hazard in anaesthesia for children, who may have been given sweets to pacify them on the way to the dental surgery. The upright position gives no protection against active vomiting, indeed the position is ideal for overwhelming invasion of the trachea. This is a situation made more difficult by the time involved in getting the patient out of the chair into a head down position and can only be avoided by stress laid on the importance of pre-operative fasting, and by ensuring that a careful smooth induction of anaesthesia is obtained. Premature insertion of the pack invariably leads to retching, and vomiting may follow. The supine position does not protect against active vomiting but makes immediate treatment such as turning the patient on the side much easier and is especially valuable if the head of the table or dental chair can quickly be tipped down.

Inhalation of Blood and Debris

Inhalation of blood and debris may occur as readily in the upright position as in the supine despite appearances to the contrary. Love (1963) states that the patient in the sitting position is safer from inhalation of material spilled in the mouth only when the floor of the mouth is horizontal or tilted forwards. In this position it is difficult to maintain a clear airway and surgical access is difficult. In fact there is usually a change in the patient's position after induction of anaesthesia, either because the patient slips down in the chair or the dentist actually tilts the chair backwards prior to surgery to gain better access to the upper teeth. The head will also tilt backwards if the anaesthetist does not apply adequate counter-pressure to the patient's head or if he is trying to maintain a good airway. Head retraction will occur if the patient is too lightly anaesthetised. These effects will produce a situation similar to that found with the supine position in which blood and debris will pool in the pharynx and are very liable to be inhaled. This is especially the case if back teeth are extracted. Correct placing of the pack therefore is just as vital in the upright position as in the supine to absorb blood as it gravitates to the back of the tongue. There should be adequate packing of the back of the mouth from retromolar triangle to retromolar triangle. The pack should be placed and maintained by the dentist to guard the glottic area without encroaching on the airway. Careful watch should be kept on the area where the pack touches the buccal walls as there is often a space here through which blood and debris can pass (Love, 1963). Further points recommended by Love to avoid inhalation include tranquil anaesthesia, unhurried surgery, reliable suction and careful positioning of the patient in the immediate post-operative period. Respiratory obstruction, coughing, struggling, vomiting and heavy bleeding all make the likelihood of inhalation greater, whatever the position of the patient and these factors are mostly under the anaesthetist's control.

Airway Control

Once anaesthesia has been induced with the patient in the supine position, the tongue falls backwards by gravity and leads to varying degrees of airway obstruction. In dental surgery the operator often displaces the mandible and the tongue backwards. This displacement is easier to counteract in the upright than in the supine position. It is thus much easier for obstruction and resultant hypoxia to occur in the supine position than in the upright (Coplans, 1962). Danziger (1962) suggested intubation in the dental chair to overcome these problems but this seems impractical for most out-patient procedures. However, a nasopharyngeal airway may be of value in this situation.

OUT-PATIENT DENTAL SURGERY

Indications for General Anaesthesia

The majority of out-patient dental procedures, either extractions or conservation work, can be performed under local analgesia, and this will provide adequate operating conditions. There are, however, certain groups of patients in whom general anaesthesia is either definitely indicated or is of great value (Ministry of Health, 1967; Goldman, 1968).

1. Young children do not like local techniques.
2. Acute infective conditions, except where there is oedema of the floor of the mouth or Ludwig's angina, and in whom acute sepsis has not lead to trismus with limitations of the opening of the mouth. Due to the low pH of infected tissues local analgesia will not relieve pain. When severe infection is present treatment is best carried out as an in-patient.
3. Uncooperative patients, either those who are mentally subnormal or who have physical infirmity enough to become uncontrollable under local analgesia, e.g. spastics.
4. Multiple extractions, in more than one quadrant of the mouth.
5. Those individuals who are sensitive or allergic to local analgesic drugs.
6. A large number of people, often very intelligent who are extremely nervous of all forms of dental treatment and to whom general anaesthesia for conservative dentistry as well as extractions is a great benefit.

Preparation of the Patient

It is important to stress at the outset that in no other form of anaesthesia is the "psychological approach" more important than when giving an anaesthetic to a patient in the dental chair. The administrator is often required to assess the clinical state of an out-patient, whom he has never seen before, without causing any unnecessary alarm, and at the same time allay any apprehension. Commonsense and a few simple questions are what is needed. Indeed, even if there were time to do a full clinical examination (which is rarely the case), it is doubtful whether the information gained in most patients would be worth the apprehension produced.

Some simple instruction should be given to the patients before they come up for treatment. They should take no food or drink for at least four hours prior to the time of anaesthesia. Special precautions should be taken with children as they and/or their parents, may have differing ideas as to what is meant by food. Beware of the child who has been given sweets to pacify him on the way to the dental surgery. The bladder should be emptied to avoid micturition during anaesthesia. Patients should be instructed to wear clothing which is not tight round the neck or waist and have sleeves that are easily drawn up above the elbow in case intravenous agents are used. False teeth should be removed as they may cause obstruction when the patient becomes unconscious.

On meeting a patient for the first time much can be learnt by a quick study of the general condition and features to decide whether the patient is dyspnoeic, cyanotic, flushed, anaemic or plethoric. The age, muscular build and degree of mental apprehension of the patient should also be assessed. As Thompson (1964) notes: is the patient pale, palsied, panicky, panting, plethoric, porcine, pregnant or purple? Certain questions should be asked (Bourne, 1967):

1. Have you ever had any serious illness?
2. Have you, during the last year or so, been taking any pills, capsules or other medicines?
3. When did you last have anything to eat or drink?

While these are being asked a finger on the patient's pulse and careful observation will detect any obvious signs of disability. In general, if a patient can climb stairs or run for a bus without becoming unduly breathless or developing pain in the chest he may be regarded as fit for anaesthesia for a brief period in the dental chair. Absolute contra-indications to general anaesthesia as an out-patient include recent food or fluid, coronary disease, respiratory obstruction especially if there is oedema of the floor of the mouth or swelling of the neck, limited opening of the jaw from trismus, and cerebrovascular disease. There are many relative contra-indications to general anaesthesia. They include diabetes, pregnancy, congenital and acquired heart disease, respiratory disease and anaemia including sickle-cell anaemia. The urgency and importance of dental treatment may also be factors influencing the decision to give an anaesthetic in the dental surgery.

Drugs used in the treatment of disease may modify the patient's response to dental anaesthesia. Hypoglycaemic agents, antidepressants, tranquillisers, anti-hypertensives and anticoagulants are but a few examples of the multiplicity of drugs that may be met. It is important that the anaesthetist should know exactly the nature of the patient's treatment for concurrent disease. Whilst some drugs will have little effect on the patient's response to anaesthesia in the dental chair, others, for example the monoamine oxidase inhibitors and the corticosteroids, may have a profound effect. If necessary the patient should be referred to hospital for treatment and if thought advisable have his dental treatment as an in-patient.

Premedication is unnecessary for most patients and is a disadvantage for the ambulant as the recovery period may be increased and the time of departure delayed. Most patients can be calmed by a proper approach to their fears. The promise of an intravenous induction will allay the fears of most nervous individuals.

Methods of Administration

Dental anaesthetic machines are designed to deliver accurate mixtures of nitrous oxide and oxygen either by intermittent or continuous flow. A suitable vaporiser, able to deliver accurate concentrations of an adjuvant should be included.

Intermittent flow.—Intermittent or demand-flow apparatus must give reasonably accurate percentages of nitrous oxide and oxygen administered to the patient under all conditions of tidal volume and respiratory rate. The method is economical—gases flow only during inspiration into a mixing bag from which the patient inspires via corrugated tubing and a mask. As the bag empties, so it is refilled from the cylinders, and when it is full of gases is automatically cut off until the next inspiratory effort starts the process once more. The "Walton" (Fig. 1) and the "A.E." machines (Fig. 2) are the most commonly used demand-flow machines used in dental anaesthesia in the United Kingdom. There are two controls (Fig. 3). The percentage of gas and oxygen in the mixture breathed can be readily adjusted by setting the dial to the required figure. A pressure control can be adjusted to provide either demand or continuous flow. A vaporiser and the reservoir bag are incorporated between the patient and the machine. The reservoir bag is actually not necessary in a demand-flow situation as variations in the patient's tidal volume are compensated by the patient's own inspiratory effort (Goldman, 1968).

Continuous flow.—A continuous flow of gases is supplied from the machine, almost all the expired gases passing into the atmosphere through the expiratory valve. A standard Boyle machine can be perfectly satisfactory for dental anaes-

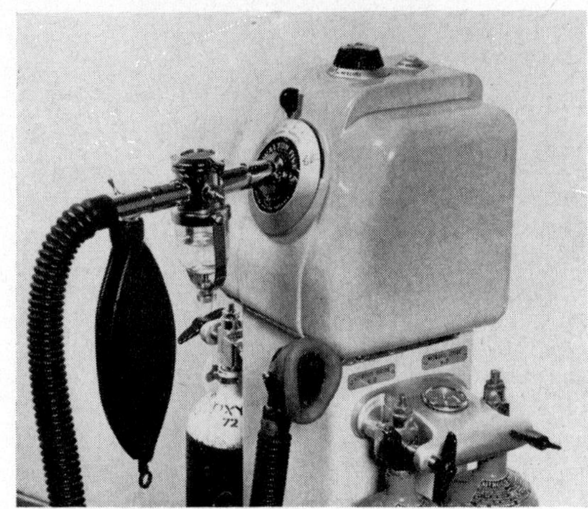

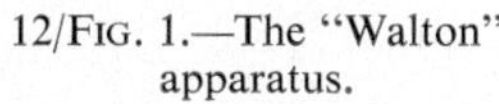

12/FIG. 1.—The "Walton" apparatus.

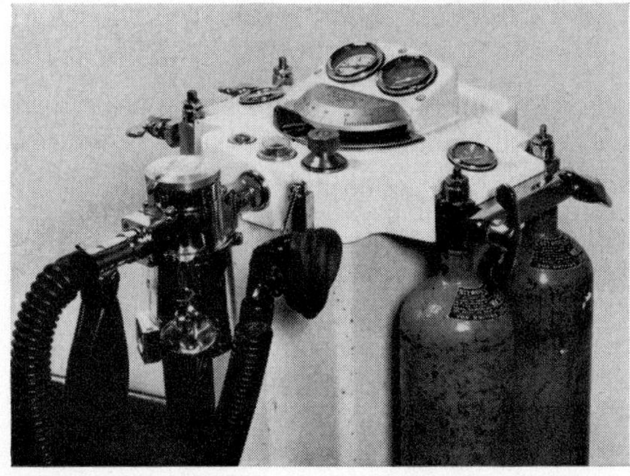

12/FIG. 2.—The "A.E." apparatus.

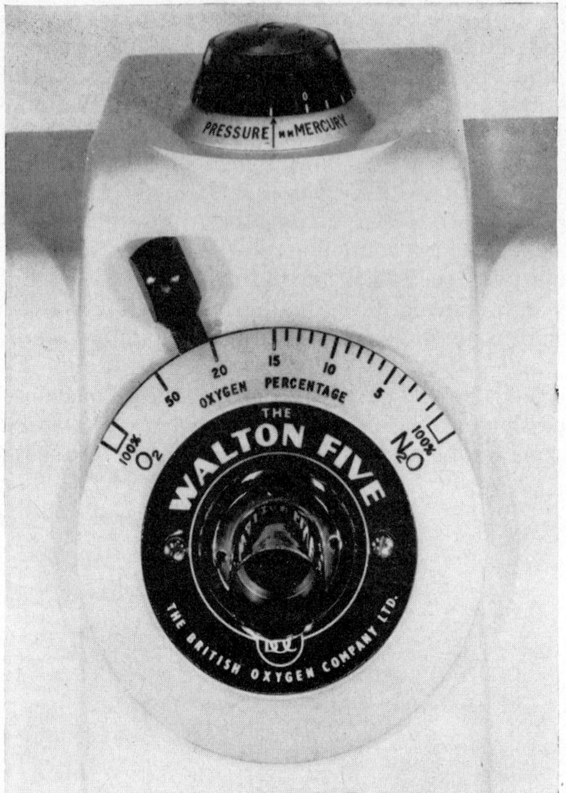

12/Fig. 3.—The "Walton" head, showing mixture control.

thesia and simplified versions of the apparatus, such as the "Salisbury" machine (Fig. 4), have been introduced for this purpose. In the continuous flow method, a reservoir bag must be included in the system. A high flow is needed to ensure an adequate volume during induction when the mask or nose piece is not applied to the face but is held some distance away (Goldman, 1968), a situation desirable especially when inducing children.

Position in the Dental Chair

The patient should sit comfortably with the seat of the dental chair tilted slightly backwards (Fig. 5). The occiput should rest on a head rest which is adjusted to bring the head into a more upright position or that of "sniffing the morning air." The hands rest across the abdomen, the knees are bent at right angles and the feet brought together. Small shildren are more easily controlled in a special seat attached to the back of the dental chair. Care should be taken to prevent powerful lamps shining in the patient's face. A bib is placed round the neck to prevent any soiling of the clothes. A mouth prop is often inserted prior to induction in adults but with the methods of anaesthesia now available this can easily be inserted when the patient is asleep. In children the prop should not be inserted until they are fully anaesthetised.

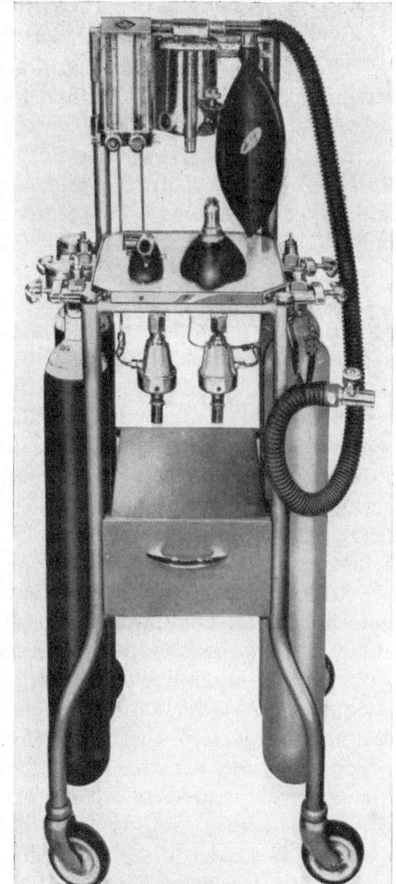

12/FIG. 4.—The "Salisbury" apparatus.

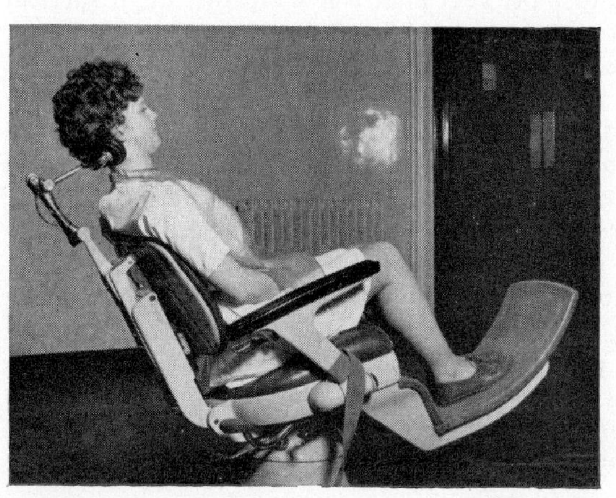

12/FIG. 5.—Posture for dental anaesthesia.

Anaesthesia for Dental Extractions

There is now no place for the induction of anaesthesia with 100 per cent nitrous oxide. If an inhalational technique is chosen not less than 20 per cent oxygen should be delivered with the nitrous oxide and this can rapidly be increased to 25 per cent if an adjuvant such as halothane is used. Latham and Parbrook (1966) go further and suggest the use of premixed 50:50 nitrous oxide and oxygen as this is a constantly accurate mixture and therefore safer, and incidentally, more economical than using separate cylinders of the two gases.

Adults and older children can be encouraged to breath the gases through a nose piece. A high flow should be used but the gases should not be delivered at a pressure which is unpleasant for the patient. If the nose breathing is found difficult or impossible a mouth attachment or a pack held over the mouth may be of value. An alternative would be to use a standard face mask which is gradually lowered to cover both nose and mouth during induction. The mask should initially be held away from the face especially in children. In small children a nose piece may be used to cover both mouth and nose for induction, being reapplied to cover the nose only when surgical anaesthesia has been achieved.

Although trichloroethylene and divinyl ether ("Vinesthene") are still used, halothane is the commonest adjuvant to nitrous oxide at present in use in dental anaesthesia in this country. It has many desirable features for out-patient dental treatment. It is relatively non-irritant, provides a smooth quick induction, and adequate muscle relaxation so that the mouth can be opened without force. It is non-explosive and therefore safe to use in the presence of dental instruments which sometimes produce sparks from friction with the teeth. The patient recovers quickly and post-operative nausea and vomiting are uncommon. It can be vaporised from a Goldman vaporiser or some modification if a demand flow machine is used, or from a Fluotec or similar compensated vaporiser if a continuous flow machine is used.

Halothane can be added at the start of induction allowing 25 per cent oxygen to be given with the nitrous oxide. 1 per cent halothane vapour is given initially and this is gradually increased to 2 per cent after a few breaths. Light surgical anaesthesia is achieved in about 1–1½ minutes so long as there is no breath holding or obstruction to breathing. Resistant cases require longer to achieve this state.

Light surgical anaesthesia can be recognised by the onset of regular rhythmical ventilation, expiration being about twice as long as inspiration. The eyelash reflex, i.e. contraction of the eyelid in response to touching the eyelash goes at the same time and adequate muscle relaxation will have been achieved to allow the mouth to be easily opened. At this stage, the dental prop is inserted and a small pack placed at the back of the tongue to prevent blood and tooth fragments being aspirated. Whilst the teeth are being extracted the anaesthetist should support the head and jaw and also be prepared to introduce a mouth gag to allow the dental prop to be switched over to the other side. Once light surgical anaesthesia has been achieved the halothane vaporiser can be turned down to deliver about 1 per cent, and 25 per cent oxygen with nitrous oxide should be administered.

For the simple extraction of one or two teeth the halothane can be turned off altogether once the prop and pack have been inserted.

Consciousness normally returns within a few seconds to a minute, depending on the duration of anaesthesia. During the phase of returning consciousness the prop is removed and the pack either removed or replaced. At this stage the head should be held well forward with the jaw supported allowing any blood to drain forwards. If the anaesthetic is being given in the supine position the patient should be turned on his side for the recovery phase to prevent blood going back onto the glottis. Whatever the technique of anaesthesia employed, it is important that there are adequate facilities for recovery—a couch or trolley where those patients who take longer than a few seconds to wake up can be recovered on their sides, in good lighting conditions with adequate suction facilities.

Intravenous induction.—An intravenous induction may be preferable to inhalational methods. It is the method of choice for nervous individuals. Two agents, methohexitone and propanidid, are in common use.

Methohexitone produces a more rapid return of consciousness compared with equipotent doses of thiopentone. Full recovery time, however, is similar to thiopentone and a hypnotic effect with reduced mental altertness may persist for up to 24 hours after a single dose. Propanidid has a significantly shorter duration of action. It is completely broken down in the body within 30 minutes. There is therefore no hangover effect as is found after methohexitone and there is complete mental awareness.

Both cause excitatory movements during induction with involuntary arm movements and hiccup if larger doses are given. Both produce cardiovascular depression. Whereas methohexitone causes respiratory depression if too large an induction dose is given, propanidid has a biphasic respiratory effect with initial hyperventilation leading to transient apnoea. Methohexitone is antanalgesic. Propanidid was originally thought to have general analgesic properties but the feature is not clinically very noticeable (Howells, 1968). Propanidid, being produced in viscous solution is more difficult to inject, especially through small needles used in children. It can be diluted satisfactorily with water or normal saline. Extravascular injection is not painful using propanidid, but venous thrombosis has been reported though this is more likely to occur after multiple injection rather than after a single dose. Methohexitone can be given as a 1 or 2 per cent solution in a dose of 1 mg/kg., propanidid in a 2·5 per cent solution, the initial dose being 5–10 mg./kg.

Whichever intravenous agent is used for induction, as soon as the patient is asleep a nose piece is placed directly on the face, the expiratory valve partially closed and anaesthesia continued using 50 per cent nitrous oxide and oxygen. This mixture may be quite adequate for the removal of a few teeth. If a longer period of operating time is required or if it is found difficult to open the mouth it may be necessary to add 1 per cent halothane to the mixture.

There is an increased incidence of nausea and vomiting after a propanidid/ nitrous oxide/oxygen sequence as compared with inhalation anaesthesia preceded by barbiturates (Dundee, 1965). Swerdlow (1965) showed an incidence of over 80 per cent of patients developing nausea and vomiting after propanidid, nitrous oxide and oxygen.

As patients expect to return to a full normal ambulatory state as soon as possible, propanidid would seem to be the drug of choice as an intravenous induction agent prior to maintenance by inhalational methods. It ensures that the patients will have full mental activity on leaving the dental surgery though some may feel sick.

Anaesthesia for Conservative Dentistry

Traditionally, conservative dentistry or "fillings" (as opposed to "extractions") has been carried out under local analgesia, either by local infiltration or nerve block techniques. There is a great problem of fear of pain in dental treatment of this type, indeed fear of pain is probably the greatest deterrent to proper dental care (Monheim, 1957). Despite the improvement in local analgesic agents, the use of local sprays and analgesic jellies, and the use of sharp disposable needles, there has been little change in this inherent fear of the discomfort involved. Wide individual variation exists in the pain threshold and the degree of discomfort may to some extent depend on the patient's past experience. Conservative dental treatment means not only physical pain, but great mental stress. This is especially the case when a long period of time is necessary for treatment or when multiple nerve blocks are required. To deal with this problem local analgesia can be supplemented by sedation or dispensed with altogether, treatment being performed under a state of "ultra-light" anaesthesia. These allow the dentist to complete treatment, if necessary in more than one quadrant of the mouth, at a single sitting rather than subject the patient to the mental stress of several visits to the surgery. With all these methods the same care must be taken to assess the patient's general condition as if he were to undergo a full general anaesthetic. It should be stressed that whether supplements are added to the local block or ultralight anaesthesia is employed this is an additional hazard to the patient's welfare and should only be justified after careful consideration of all factors. It should not be given just because the patient demands this service.

Supplements to Local Analgesia (sedation)

Although sedation helps minimise the discomfort of treatment, recovery time is undoubtedly prolonged. There must be facilities therefore to allow patients to recover slowly and in safety. Sedatives can be given orally. This route of administration, though comparatively safe, is unpredictable both in timing and effectiveness. Hypnotics (barbiturates), tranquillisers (chlordiazepoxide), analgesics and even alcohol have all been tried with variable results. They may be of value in helping the moderately anxious. For the very nervous patient, the intravenous route is more certain of producing the ideal tranquil situation as the dose can be finely adjusted to suit the individual requirements. At the same time, care ensures that a relative overdose, through individual variation, leading to respiratory or cardiovascular depression does not occur.

One of the best known methods of intravenous sedation was introduced by Jorgensen and Leffingwell (1961) and was designed to make dentistry acceptable to the very nervous, and prolonged operations endurable to all. Consciousness is not abolished. Pentobarbitone ("Nembutal"), pethidine and hyoscine are used to provide sedation, amnesia and additional analgesia. Pentobarbitone is injected first, 5 mg. being given intravenously and a couple of minutes' pause allowed to see if any unusual sensitivity to the drug should appear. Further doses of 10 mg. are then given at half minute intervals until the patient seems relaxed and at ease. Up to 100 mg. can be given. At this stage a mixture of pethidine 25 mg. and hyoscine 0·2 mg. diluted in 5 ml. of water is given slowly, 2–5 ml. of the mixture being given. The patient is now in a state of "light sedation" and the local block can be injected without much discomfort. Although good results will be achieved in expert hands it may be difficult to judge correct doses. There is always a "hangover" effect and there may be nausea post-operatively. It is probably best to operate with the patient lying in the supine position to avoid the risk of fainting.

Modified Jorgensen techniques have been tried using smaller doses of pento-barbitone and using intermittent methohexitone rather than pethidine/hyoscine. It is worth remembering with such a method that the potential convulsive properties of methohexitone may summate with those of lignocaine.

Diazepam ("Valium") is an excellent tranquilliser prior to dental treatment. It provides a feeling of well-being, a shortening of the patient's time sense (even the most prolonged treatment appears to last only a few minutes), and amnesia of the event. Healy *et al.* (1970*b*) used an intravenous dose of up to 0·2 mg./kg. and found no untoward physiological disturbances other than incompetence of laryngeal closure during the first few minutes after drug administration. The patient should be supine. 10–20 mg. diazepam is given slowly intravenously over a period of about 2 minutes. Care should be taken to retain consciousness to avoid the danger of respiratory obstruction and inhalation of vomit. Injection should be made into a large vein because injections into small veins may be painful and also lead to venous thrombosis. The local block can be started immediately after the diazepam has been given. The technique gives satisfactory operating conditions for the dentist even in the most anxious patient, and Healy *et al.* (1970*a*) consider it a real and practical advantage in the management of such patients. Recovery time is prolonged but most patients are clinically safe to leave the surgery accompanied by a responsible adult within 90 minutes of administration of the drug.

Ultra-light Anaesthesia (Methohexitone analgesia)

For many years Drummond Jackson (1952) has pioneered the use of an intravenous barbiturate, such as hexobarbitone or thiopentone, as the sole agent to provide pleasant yet safe conditions for out-patient dental surgery. More recently methohexitone and propanidid have been widely used for this purpose. A patient's response to dental pain differs from the response to cutaneous pain. Cutaneous pain, for example cutting the skin with a knife, evolves brisk reflex defensive movement prohibiting surgery unless full surgical anaesthesia is given. Dental pain evokes much less response, allowing treatment to continue under a level of narcosis short of full surgical anaesthesia. There are various ways of producing ultra-light anaesthesia with intravenous agents. A common technique is described here. After a dental prop has been inserted into the mouth, methohexitone or pro-panidid is given intravenously, the size of the initial and subsequent doses being titrated against the patient's response to the stimulus of surgery. The aim—to provide a steady semi-narcotised state throughout the procedure—is difficult to achieve and requires high skill on the part of the administrator in judgement of size and timing of each dose. As doses are given intermittently an even plane of narcosis cannot be achieved, periods of full surgical anaesthesia alternating with periods of partial environment detachment (Howells, 1968). There is also wide individual variation in response to the drug used. Too light a plane of narcosis will evoke a marked response from the patient, but even if he cries out there appears to be amnesia of the event. It must be stressed that at all times careful observation of the patient must be carried out so that overdose, leading to even the most minimal clinical respiratory obstruction or depression, does not occur. To avoid the possibility of hypotension developing with methohexitone or propanidid, treatment is best carried out in the horizontal position.

The patient should be settled comfortably with an arm fixed to a board. The apparatus consists of either a reservoir bottle containing 250 ml. of 1 per cent methohexitone or a 50 ml. reservoir syringe containing 2·5 per cent propanidid connected to a 3-way tap. On one limb of the tap is fitted a 10 ml. syringe for delivering each dose of solution, and this communicates via the tap to a length of disposable polythene tubing and a fine needle (No. 12 gauge). The system is cleared of air before use, the needle inserted, and the initial dose given from the syringe. Bourne (1967) recommends the following initial dosage scheme for methohexitone :

Patients under 20 years of age	2·2 mg./kg.	body weight
20–40 „ „	1·5 mg./kg.	„ „
40–60 „ „	1·1 mg./kg.	„ „
over 60 „ „	0·75 mg./kg.	„ „

Less should be given for the obese and for those in poor health. With all patients it is best to err on the side of caution. Increments vary with the individual's requirements but up to 20 mg./min. may be needed. Howells (1968) recommends the initial dose of propanidid to be 4–5 mg./kg., whilst Cadle *et al.* (1968) suggest a higher initial dose especially in young females. Increments of 100–200 mg. propanidid per minute may be necessary. Whichever drug is used, an increment is given if the patient reacts to surgical stimulus either by screwing up the eyes or by slight limb movement.

For a period of treatment lasting less than 20 minutes, propanidid would seem the drug of choice. Its rapid rate of metabolism, 50 per cent being metabolised in 20 minutes, ensures that recovery is swifter than from methohexitone. There is also no hangover effect after propanidid. Treatment for over 20 minutes, necessitating high doses of propanidid, has occasionally led to stiffening of the limbs, suggestive of extrapyramidal influences (Cadle *et al.*, 1968). Therefore, if a long period of treatment is anticipated methohexitone appears the better drug. It is essential if patients are receiving large doses of these drugs that adequate recovery facilities are available.

The advantages of such a method appear overwhelming, both to the patient and to the dentist. Induction is swift and certain and even in the most robust, management less complicated than with inhalational methods, recovery pleasant, the method cheap—a most important factor when large numbers of patients are involved. Drummond Jackson (1962) describes it as the era of pleasanter dentistry for both patient and dentist.

Certain cautionary facts must however be mentioned. It is vital that throughout the period of ultra-light anaesthesia, which incidentally may be over an hour in length, a perfect airway is maintained and at no stage is there clinical evidence of respiratory obstruction or depression, or hypotension. This requires even greater vigilance on the part of the anaesthetist than during a full general anaesthetic administration.

Recent work by Wise *et al.* (1969) suggests that under methohexitone for conservative dentistry, clinically undetectable respiratory obstruction and arterial hypoxaemia may be present, cyanosis being masked by pronounced peripheral vasodilatation. Methohexitone in cumulative doses above 200 mg. leads to widespread vasodilatation with a marked fall in peripheral resistance. In such a situation a normal blood pressure is maintained by virtue of a large increase in cardiac output. This increase should appear in response to hypoxaemia, but under methohexitone this normal circulatory response appeared obtruded. Wise and his colleagues suggest therefore that patient comfort is obtained at the expense of the integrity of the respiratory and cardiovascular systems—a potentially dangerous situation. They further showed that the laryngeal reflexes were depressed and that in some cases there was radiological evidence of aspiration of radio-opaque dye (placed on the back of the tongue) into the trachea. Although the validity of parts of this work has been challenged (Coplans, 1969), and clinical evidence based on many thousands of cases shows the method to be safe in expert hands, it is obvious that extremely careful management of such a situation is essential, especially as the method is unnecessary in most cases except for patient convenience.

Faced with such facts it should be stressed that the recent trend for the single-handed dentist to give his own ultra-light anaesthetic is to be deplored. Indeed, the Joint Sub-Committee of the Ministry of Health on dental anaesthesia (Ministry of Health, 1967) deprecated the practice. It was considered that the administration of the anaesthetic and the performance of dental surgery could only lead to a division of attention and therefore an increased risk to the patient.

ANAESTHESIA FOR IN-PATIENT DENTAL SURGERY

When more extensive surgery is required than can be dealt with in the dental surgery, or when the patient's general condition contra-indicates out-patient treatment, he should be admitted to hospital. Although the majority of patients treated on an in-patient surgical list are young healthy adults who require removal of impacted wisdom teeth, every list is likely to contain patients whose general condition demands a full general anaesthetic for their dental treatment. Amongst these are diabetics, patients with severe heart disease and chronic respiratory disease, mental defectives, spastics, mongols and those with some haemorrhagic disorder such as haemophilia or those individuals with a history of post-extractionl haemorrhage. Careful pre-operative assessment is therefore of the greatest importance. Local hazards should also be assessed. The patient may have loose teeth, prostheses, bridges and other dental work or a deviated nasal septum. Finally, it is valuable to know the extent to which the patient can open his mouth prior to surgery.

A nasal endotracheal tube is used except for certain procedures involving the maxilla. Nasal tubes are usually uncuffed, but special streamlined cuffed tubes can be used. In any patient a smaller diameter nasal tube has to be used than the equivalent oral tube. Resistance to breathing is therefore greater. Damage can easily be done to the nasal mucosa resulting in haemorrhage. Infection present in the nose may also be carried to the bronchial tree.

Packing of the pharynx is essential. Towels are usually wrapped firmly around the face, hence the eyes must be protected and connections safely secured. Although no sequence of anaesthesia is ideal, a nitrous oxide-oxygen-halothane sequence with spontaneous breathing is satisfatory. Bleeding is seldom severe.

At the end of the procedure the pharyngeal pack is removed, the pharynx cleared of any blood, gauze packs placed in the cheeks to stop oozing and an oral airway inserted. The nasal tube is best removed with the patient turned onto the side, recovery taking place in the post-tonsillectomy position. At this stage post-halothane shivering sometimes occurs, especially if the patient has been stimulated, and care must be taken that respiratory obstruction does not result.

MAJOR JAW SURGERY

Operations for the correction of jaw deformities are usually carried out in young healthy adults. Ostectomies and osteotomies of the mandible or maxilla vary in their complexity and sometimes require a bone graft. The problems during these procedures are as described in the previous section, but blood loss may be severe enough to require transfusion. At the end, the jaws are immobilised with either elastic bands or wire. Swelling of the soft tissues occurs up to 48 hours post-operatively and is especially common if an intra-oral approach has been employed. The second post-operative night is therefore often dangerous as swelling is then at its maximum. If a prognathic mandible has been reduced by an osteotomy on the angle or ascending ramus, the base of the tongue may be positioned more posteriorly into the pharynx with a danger of airway obstruction.

The pharyngeal pack is removed immediately prior to immobilisation. To help maintain the airway post-operatively the nasal tube is partially removed and left in place as a pharyngeal airway. A safety pin should be inserted into the proximal end of the tube which is cut close to the nose. This pharyngeal airway is left in position at least until full recovery from the anaesthetic has taken place, but if tolerated it is best left until the following day. Care should be taken to see that the tube does not become blocked with blood and mucous. A tongue stitch may also be valuable in the immediate post-anaesthetic period. These patients are best nursed in an intensive care unit for at least 24 hours post-operatively. The nursing staff should be provided with a diagram of the wiring and wire cutters must be beside the patient in case of emergency, so that the bands or wires may be cut if severe respiratory obstruction occurs and cannot quickly be relieved by simple measures. Post-operative vomiting may be avoided by using anti-emetics such as perphenazine. However, if vomiting does occur, the patient should be placed in the post-tonsillectomy position allowing the vomit to drain through the space between the molar teeth and cheek. Suction may be invaluable.

Diseases for which hemimandibulectomy, hemiglossectomy and maxillary resection, with or without block dissection of glands of the neck, are required may make endotracheal tube insertion difficult. Displacement of normal anatomy in these cases sometimes requires blind introduction of a nasal tube, this manoeuvre being best performed with the patient breathing spontaneously. These operations are usually long and high blood loss can be expected. Controlled hypotension may be indicated (Davies and Scott, 1968). Recovery in the intensive care unit will require vigilance similar to that described above for post-operative care after correction of jaw deformity.

Acute Trauma

Trauma may cause a wide variety of maxillo-facial injuries. These injuries range in severity from fracture of the nasal bones requiring simple reduction to complicated injuries involving facial bones, nose, maxilla and mandible. There may be considerable soft tissue damage. Concomitant injuries to the head with loss of consciousness, the chest and abdomen, and limb fractures may also be present. Many patients with maxillo-facial injuries sustain concussion. When the head injury is serious, treatment of the face may have to be delayed while an assessment of the head injury is made and priority of treatment given if it is considered the more dangerous to life (Ennis and Gilchrist, 1968). Maxillo-facial injuries seldom require immediate operation unless there is uncontrollable haemorrhage or an obstructed airway. Other injuries must be carefully assessed and hypovolaemia corrected.

An obstructed airway is frequently present as a result of blood, teeth and dentures (rarely radio-opaque) lying in the pharynx. There may be direct obstruction where a fractured maxilla has been displaced downwards and backwards on to the dorsum of the tongue, or by the tongue itself falling back when the anterior portion of the mandible has been severely comminuted.

Atropine only should be given for premedication and opiate drugs should be avoided as there may be bleeding in the mouth and pharynx, and the stomach may contain swallowed blood. In addition, in an acute emergency the patient may have had a recent meal.

Intubation is the first important step. If the mouth can be opened sufficiently it may be simpler to pre-oxygenate and then go on to a thiopentone-suxamethonium -cricoid pressure-rapid intubation sequence, especially as it may be difficult to induce anaesthesia by inhalation alone if a face mask cannot be properly applied. If an inhalational induction is considered safer this may be prolonged. A head-down position will allow blood to drain freely and be sucked out if necessary. If respiratory obstruction cannot be relieved, tracheostomy under local analgesia may be life-saving and induction can then take place via this route. Once the respiratory tract is protected blood and debris can be removed from the pharynx. A large bore oesophageal tube can be passed to remove blood and other contents from the stomach. The route of the endotracheal tube must be discussed between the anaesthetist and oral surgeon prior to induction, the nasal or oral routes depending on the extent and position of the injuries. The direction of the tube may be changed during the procedure. If cerebrospinal fluid is seen draining from the nose a nasal tube should not be used because of the danger of infection. Any anaesthetic sequence which allows quick post-operative recovery is satisfactory for maintenance.

Post-operative management is similar to that described for other major jaw surgery and will depend on whether or not there is immobilisation of the jaws. Severe head injury and concomitant injuries to the chest may make tracheostomy essential. Skilled nursing must always be available to ensure that the airway remains clear and that the patient's general condition does not deteriorate. Post-operative restlessness may be due to partial hypoxia and must be carefully assessed. Sedation should be avoided unless the patient actually complains of pain. Pain, in fact, is usually minimal post-operatively in these patients (Davies and Scott, 1968).

The treatment of facial injuries is rarely life-saving but the restoration of the normal contours of the facial skeleton and repair of soft tissues with minimal scarring are of the utmost importance to the patient. Correct management of such patients during the acute phase is therefore vital.

REFERENCES

Bourne, J. G. (1957). Fainting and cerebral damage. *Lancet*, **2**, 499.

Bourne, J. G. (1960). *Nitrous Oxide in Dentistry: Its Danger and Alternatives*. London: Lloyd-Luke.

Bourne, J. G. (1965). The common fainting attack. A danger in dental chair anaesthesia. *Brit. dent. J.*, **119**, 65.

Bourne, J. G. (1966). A dental anaesthetic death. *Lancet*, **1**, 879.

Bourne, J. G. (1967). *Studies in Anaesthetics: Including Intravenous Dental Anaesthesia*, pp. 56 and 103. London: Lloyd-Luke.

British Journal of Anaesthesia (1968). Editorial. **40**, 151.

Cadle, D. R., Boulton, T. B., and Spencer Swaine, M. (1968). Intermittent intravenous anaesthesia for out-patient dentistry. A study using propanidid. *Anaesthesia*, **23**, 65.

Coplans, M. P. (1962). An assessment of the safety of the 'sitting posture' and hypoxia in dental anaesthesia. *Brit. dent. J.*, **113**, 15.

Coplans, M. P. (1969). Letter. Intermittent methohexitone in dentistry. *Brit. med. J.*, **2**, 760.

Danziger, A. M. (1962). Tracheal intubation for anaesthesia in the dental chair. *Brit. dent. J.*, **113**, 426.

Davies, R. M., and Scott, J. G. (1968). Anaesthesia for major oral and maxillo-facial surgery. *Brit. J. Anaesth.*, **40**, 202.

Drummond Jackson, S. L. (1952). *Intravenous Anaesthesia in Dentistry*. London: Staples.

Drummond Jackson, S. L. (1962). A milestone in intravenous anaesthesia. *Brit. dent. J.*, **113**, 303.

Dundee, J. W. (1965). Comparison of side effects of methohexital and thipentone with propanidid. *Acta anaesth. scand.*, Suppl. 17, 77.

Ennis, G. E., and Gilchrist, D. T. (1968). In *Fractures of the Facial Skeleton*, p. 554. Eds. Rowe, N. L., and Killey, H. C. Edinburgh: E. & S. Livingstone.

Evans, T. W. (1869). Correspondence. *Amer. J. dent. Sci.*, 525.

Goldman, V. (1968). Inhalational anaesthesia for dentistry in the chair. *Brit. J. Anaesth.*, **40**, 155.

Goldman, V., Cornwall, W. B., and Lethbridge, V. R. E. (1958). Blood pressure under anaesthesia in the sitting position. *Lancet*, **1**, 1367.

Healy, T. E. J., Lautch, H., Hall, N., Tomlin, P. J., and Vickers, M. D. (1970*a*). Interdisciplinary study of diazepam sedation for outpatient dentistry. *Brit. med. J.*, **3**, 13.

Healy, T. E. J., Robinson, J. S., and Vickers, M. D. (1970*b*). Physiological responses to intravenous diazepam as a sedative for conservative dentistry. *Brit. med. J.*, **3**, 10.

Howells, T. H. (1968). Intravenous anaesthetic agents in dental anaesthesia. *Brit. J. Anaesth.*, **40**, 182.

JORGENSEN, N. B., and LEFFINGWELL, F. (1961). Premedication in dentistry. *Dent. Clin. N. Amer.*, July, 299.

KEELE, C. A., and NEIL, E. (1966). *Sampson Wright's Applied Physiology*, 11th edit., p. 141. London: Oxford Univ. Press.

KLOCK, J. H. (1955). New concepts of nitrous-oxide anesthetic. *Curr. Res. Anesth.*, **34,** 379.

LATHAM, F. (1951). The oxygen paradox. Experiments on the effects of oxygen in human anoxia. *Lancet*, **1,** 77.

LATHAM, J. and PARBROOK, G. D. (1966). The use of premixed nitrous-oxide and oxygen in dental anaesthesia. *Anaesthesia*, **21,** 472.

LOVE, S. H. S. (1963). The dangers of inhalation of debris during anaesthesia. *Brit. dent. J.*, **115,** 503.

MINISTRY OF HEALTH (1967). Dental anaesthesia. (Report of a joint sub-committee of the Standing Medical and Dental Advisory Committee). London: H.M.S.O.

MONHEIM, L. M. (1957). *Local Anesthesia and Pain Control in Dental Practice*, p. 218. St. Louis: V. Mosby.

MOORE, J. R. (1968). The surgeons requirements for intra-oral surgery. *Brit. J. Anaesth.*, **40,** 152.

MORRISON, E. M. (1873). *Brit. J. dent. Sci.*, **16,** 566.

SCOTT, G. W. (1952). Inhalation and chest infection following dental extraction. *Guy's Hosp. Rep.*, **101,** 77.

SMITH, W. D. A. (1964). 410 dental anaesthetics. Part 1. Introduction, methods, material and anaesthetic techniques. *Brit. J. Anaesth.*, **36,** 620.

SWERDLOW, M. (1965). A trial of propanidid (F.B.A. 1420): a new ultra-short-acting anaesthetic. *Brith. J. Anaesth.*, **37,** 785.

THOMPSON, P. W. (1964). Dental anaesthesia. *Ann. roy. Coll. Surg. Engl.*, **35,** 362.

TOM, A. (1956). An innovation in technique for dental gas. *Brit. med. J.*, **1,** 1085.

WISE, C. C., ROBINSON, J. S., HEATH, M. J., and TOMLIN, P. J. (1969). Physiological response to intermittent methohexitone for conservative dentistry. *Brit. med. J.*, **2,** 540.

YOUNG, D. S., and WHITWAM, J. G. (1964). Observation on dental anaesthesia introduced with methohexitone. 11: Maintenance and recovery. *Brit. J. Anaesth.*, **36,** 94.

Chapter 13

ANAESTHESIA FOR PULMONARY OPERATIONS

GENERAL CONSIDERATIONS

PATIENTS about to undergo a pulmonary operation need a careful explanation of what they are expected to do in the immediate post-operative period. Particular attention must be paid to the fitting and practical use of an oxygen mask or tent, and instruction must be given in breathing exercises and postural drainage, although the latter may not be necessary pre-operatively. When employed for these purposes a physiotherapist must have a clear understanding of the different operations which are likely to be performed and their individual requirements.

Breathing Exercises and Postural Drainage

These are described in detail in Chapter 14, but are here discussed in relationship to pulmonary disease. Ventilatory movement, even of sound areas, is often diminished in pulmonary disease, partly because these patients are often confined to bed for relatively long periods and partly because they find that shallow breathing reduces the tendency to cough. A further specific factor is the effect of retraction on the lung on the side of the operation; and following a thoracoplasty respiration may be further embarrassed by strapping to prevent paradoxical movement.

Breathing exercises are designed to increase the capacity of all areas of the lungs, including those affected by disease. Excessive or sudden movements may by harmful to an area of healing tuberculosis, but movement and increased capacity of the normal parts is important. With the exception of tuberculous patients, the aim should be good and equal movements on *both* sides of the thorax. The emphasis should be on the affected side to bring it up to the standard of the good. Even after pneumonectomy, bilateral chest movements help to prevent deformity and keep the mediastinum central.

In wet cases postural drainage must be continued until the sputum can be reduced no further in quantity. Amounts of 30 ml. or less, in a twenty-four hour period should be aimed at, and although such a result might be expected after a week of treatment, it may be necessary to persevere for a month in some patients.

Blood Gas Tensions

Impaired arterial gas tensions may be expected in patients with severe disease of the lungs. Generally, during pulmonary operations the arterial oxygen tension falls to a greater extent than the concurrent rise in carbon dioxide tension. When a patient with pre-existing impairment of gas exchange in the lungs undergoes a pulmonary operation there will be a further deterioration and some degree of consequential hypoxia unless positive steps are taken to avoid this. It has been suggested that in such circumstances the oxygen-fraction of the inspired gas mixture should not fall below 50 per cent (Nilsson *et al.*, 1965; Lunding and Fernandes, 1967).

Antibiotics

Although anaesthetists are most likely to be concerned with the administration of these drugs for respiratory tract infections, certain general principles determining the use of antibiotics are worthy of discussion. It must first be emphasised that when problems do exist they are best solved by close co-operation between the clinician and the bacteriologist. The need for this co-operation stems largely from the increasing number of bacterial strains hitherto sensitive, but now resistant, to certain antibiotics, and from the many new antibiotics that have been produced to cope with the resistant bacterial strains.

All specimens should whenever possible be obtained from the patient before treatment is started with any antibiotic. The choice of a particular antibiotic, or combination of antibiotics, may then be made on the basis of a clinical judgement, but it is preferable whenever possible to wait until *in vitro* sensitivity tests have been carried out in the laboratory. These, however, though normally reliable when translated to the patient are not always so. When there is an apparent discrepancy of this nature, other possible causes of failure—such as inadequate dosage, lack of absorption, organisms isolated in an abscess, and inactivation of the antibiotic—should be sought. Furthermore, it is important to be sure that sufficient time has elapsed for the antibiotic given to be effective, since the patient's response may be delayed. Changing from one antibiotic to another too rapidly is unhelpful.

Generally speaking, the penicillins, streptomycin and the cephalosporins are bactericidal, while the tetracyclines are notably bacteriostatic. The former group should always be used when it is important to kill organisms, rather than merely stop their multiplication and allow the patient's natural resistance to do the rest. An overwhelming infection—particularly in the very young or the very old—is the sort of absolute indication for a bactericidal drug. Although there are exceptions, it is best not to combine a bactericidal with a bacteriostatic antibiotic.

There is good evidence that the prophylactic use of antibiotics may cause a higher rather than a lower incidence of infection, although, of course, this risk may have to be taken in certain instances. It is important to remember that in hospital practice resistant bacteria stem from the previous use of antibiotics. To put a patient on an antibiotic (particularly one of the broad spectrum variety) will increase the risk of superinfection of that patient with resistant bacteria.

Non-tuberculous pulmonary infections.—As already outlined, antibiotics are best prescribed on the basis of bacterial sensitivity and there is good evidence that they are most valuable when started early in an infection (Malone *et al.*, 1968). When the occasion demands speedy action, such as an acute post-operative infection or a pre-operative acute bronchitis in a patient needing an operation urgently, then either ampicillin or tetracycline can be used. The adult dose of the former is from 250 mg. to 1 g. q.d.s. and of the latter 200 mg. q.d.s. Both are broad spectrum antibiotics, but tetracycline is less so than when it was originally introduced, due to the appearance of strains of bacteria resistant to it. A recent broad spectrum drug of value is trimethoprim sulphamethoxazole ("Bactrim").

Empyema, lung abscess and other infected cases will need a systemic cover of a specific antibiotic depending on the sensitivity of the particular organism. Such a drug may also be usefully given intrapleurally to a patient with an empyema, but this is not a substitute for drainage by rib resection once the pus is too thick for aspiration, or when the lung stops expanding before closing the infected space.

Tuberculous pulmonary infections.—Pulmonary tuberculosis is still a major infectious disease in many parts of the world. In the British Isles the main problems concerning its treatment arise from the side-effects of streptomycin and PAS (para-amino salicylic acid) and resistance to these and other anti-tuberculous drugs. The former inevitably cause some patients to default from treatment, while the latter is fortunately not increasing. New drugs available for the treatment of tuberculosis are "Rifampicin", which is relatively free from side-effects, "Ethambutol", which may cause a condition similar to retrobulbar neuritis, and "Capreomycin", an antibiotic which is potentially nephrotoxic. The first two of these can be taken orally but the third must be administered parenterally.

ANAESTHESIA

Controlled respiration is the most practicable method of ensuring adequate oxygenation and elimination of carbon dioxide in the presence of an open thorax (see p. 59). It also offers considerable advantages to the surgeon in terms of pulmonary and diaphragmatic movements suited to the practical procedure. Occasionally there are contra-indications to intermittent positive-pressure respiration for the whole or part of an anaesthetic, while some diseases, or the physical condition of the patient, may make a particular procedure or choice of drugs more valuable than the general routine. These points, as they arise, are mentioned in the pages that follow during the discussion of the specific conditions. The common routine—provided the sputum is not excessive—is suitable premedication, then an intravenous induction and intubation with the aid of suxamethonium or a longer acting muscle relaxant after ventilation with oxygen. Anaesthesia is maintained with nitrous oxide and oxygen and doses of a longer acting muscle relaxant, such as *d*-tubocurarine, are added when required. Pethidine and phenoperidine may be helpful to make up for the lessening effect of the premedication. They help the maintenance of controlled respiration by central depression so that the total dose of muscle relaxant need not be so great, and they also ensure that after a lengthy operation, some analgesia extends into the immediate post-operative period—an important point when the patient is fully conscious so soon after nitrous oxide. The principal disadvantage of pethidine and phenoperidine is the risk of overdosage, with inactive respiratory tract reflexes and respiratory depression during the early post-operative period.

Replacement of blood loss can be a very important factor in some pulmonary operations, particularly if there has been any chronic sepsis with the formation of adhesions in the pleural space. Even with minimal loss it is probable that an average thoracotomy requires at least some blood to cover the operation and immediate post-operative period.

Normally, spontaneous breathing is allowed to return as soon as the skin suturing is started. On occasions when the chest is closed without drainage, however, controlled respiration must be continued because the thorax cannot be considered airtight until after the skin has been sutured; were spontaneous breathing to start before this, there is the possibility that the lung might collapse and be difficult to re-expand.

Basal pleural drainage with an under-water seal is, overall, an asset to the anaesthetist and the patient—many surgeons use one routinely whenever the pleural cavity is opened. It has three advantages:

i. The anaesthetist can force air out of the pleural cavity after the skin of the operation wound is closed. Post-operatively, the patient does this when he coughs. Both these factors militate against pulmonary collapse.

ii. Blood will not accumulate in the pleural cavity, so that bleeding can be quickly and simply assessed by looking at the contents of the drainage bottle.

iii. After lobectomy or segmental lung operations, suction—at about minus 5 cm. H_2O—can be applied from a pump to the drain to encourage expansion of the remaining lung tissue. For such cases, basal and apical drains are normally used. Suction removes air from any leaks in the lung tissue, but may tend to keep such holes open. It should not be used after pneumonectomy, since it increases the risk of bronchial fistula and it may pull the mediastinum and its contents unduly into the thoracotomy cavity. In the latter instance the cardiac action can be hampered.

The disadvantage of pleural drainage is the increased risk of introducing sepsis into the operation site. Basal drains are normally removed after one or two days, depending on the amount of blood that is draining. Following a lobectomy or segmental removal, one or other of the drains should be left in place for at least four days.

Tracheobronchial suction down the endotracheal tube is a wise precaution at the end of operation. Bronchoscopy is rarely necessary and may do far more harm than good because the anaesthetic conditions for its performance at this stage are not ideal, and to produce them specially is rarely to the patient's advantage.

CONTROL OF SECRETIONS

With proper preparation few, if any, patients should come to operation with large quantities of infected sputum, although this may occasionally be loculated in the form of a lung abscess. The production of anaesthetic conditions adequate for thoracic surgery depresses all protective reflexes in the tracheo-bronchial tract so that secretions, squeezed by the manipulation of the surgeon, may easily spread to normal parts of the pulmonary tree during operation and are even likely to do so as soon as the patient is placed on the operating table in the lateral position. In this position (Fig. 1), the most commonly used for pulmonary

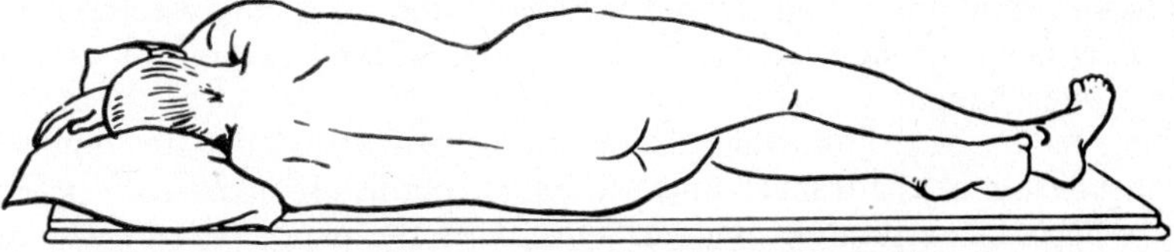

13/Fig. 1.—The lateral position for thoracic operations.

operations because of the excellent approach which it affords to the hilar vessels, the diseased lung is uppermost, and draining both towards the normal lung below and its own upper lobe which is also frequently normal. No amount of head-down tilt can prevent this risk of spread (see Fig. 2), though it is valuable as an aid towards some drainage down the trachea.

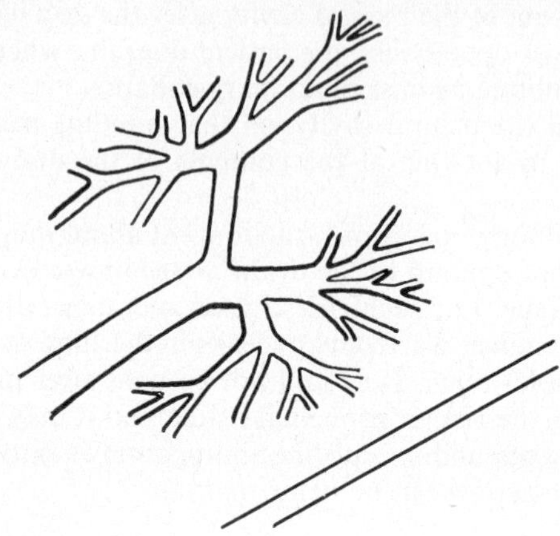

13/FIG. 2.—Diagram to illustrate how, in the right lateral position, the uppermost and diseased left lung may drain into its own upper lobe, despite a steep head-down tilt, and empty into the dependent right lung.

Obstruction to respiration with consequent hypoxia, lung collapse, and spread of infection is a likely complication, so that special precautions must be taken to deal with secretions from the moment that anaesthesia is induced.

Simple Suction

This is the mainstay in the control of secretions in the respiratory tract, whether excessive or normal in amount. It must be to hand at all times and used not only intermittently throughout the operation when there are suggestive signs of mucus being present, but also at more specific moments during both the production of anaesthesia and certain surgical manipulations when large quantities are most likely to be released from the diseased areas. The presence of secretions in the trachea or major bronchi is usually apparent from an increased resistance to positive-pressure respiration, or from audible râles transmitted to and amplified in the rebreathing bag. The use of a stethoscope attachment incorporated in the anaesthetic system just above the endotracheal tube helps in their early recognition. Nevertheless a considerable amount of material can collect without very obvious clinical evidence, so that suction must be carried out at regular intervals throughout the operation in wet cases.

Thin, watery sputum or blood may easily pass, or indeed be forced with positive-pressure respiration, into the small bronchioles and eventually into the alveoli of normal lung. Apart from the risk of pulmonary collapse and infection, fluid of either type may coat the alveoli and effectively prevent the normal gaseous interchange.

The specific occasions when suction must be carried out are immediately after intubation of the trachea and—when secretions are excessive—before any positive-pressure respiration is used, as soon as the patient is turned from the supine to the lateral position on the operating table, when the pleural cavity is opened, and whenever the surgeon manipulates the lung. Since suction may stimulate some reflex activity such as coughing, the surgeon must be warned before it is performed while surgery is in progress, but in the presence of large quantities of secretions there must be no delay.

Suction Combined with a Bronchus Clamp

A useful addition to suction is occlusion by the surgeon of the main bronchus of the affected side with a non-crushing clamp. This can only be carried out after the chest has been opened, but it is a valuable technique for producing not only control of secretions but also one lung anaesthesia (see also p. 420).

Bronchial Block

Secretions may be isolated in the affected area by blocking the bronchus concerned, or if it is impracticable to block the actual bronchus to a particular lobe, less specific control may be produced by blocking that which serves the whole lung. Block may be produced by placing in the bronchus a blocker of the Thompson, Magill or Macintosh-Leatherdale inflatable cuff type or by plugging this area with a strip of gauze (Fig. 3).

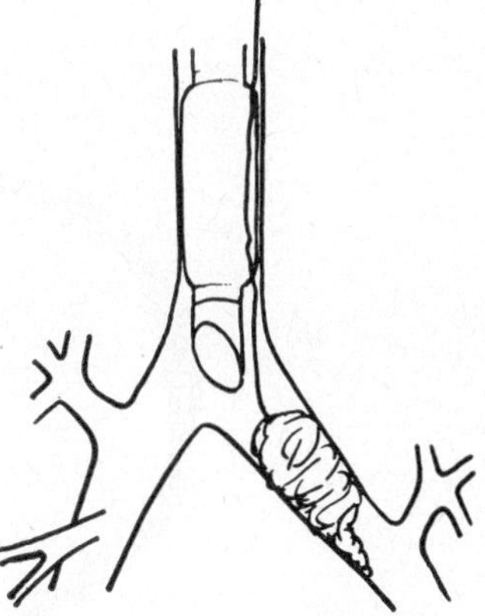

13/Fig. 3.—Crafoord's tampon.

Complete block is unsatisfactory because it shuts the lobe or lung off completely from the rest of the pulmonary tree and delays its collapse. In these circumstances not only does the lung tend to obscure the surgeon's field of vision, but a proportion of the pulmonary circulation passes through the non-functioning area without either elimination of carbon dioxide or uptake of oxygen. For this reason blockers consist of a drainage or central suction tube surrounded by an inflatable cuff. A further objection to tamponage of the bronchus is the difficulty in carrying it out accurately even under direct vision, particularly when the smaller bronchi are concerned. There is a risk of movement of the gauze during the operation even though it is held down by a wire stilette.

Bronchial block is not commonly practised nowadays, isolation of one or other bronchus generally being produced either by the use of an endobronchial tube or a double lumen tube.

Blockers (Figs. 4 and 5).—The Thompson blocker consists of a gauze-covered cuff which can be inflated through a narrow tube. This tube is fused with a larger tube running through the cuff to provide drainage from the blocked lung (Fig. 4 *a*). The gauze cover tends to keep the cuff securely fixed by friction against the bronchial mucous membrane and prevents over-inflation with the risk of rupture. The covered cuff, even when deflated, will only pass with ease down a large bronchoscope. The Magill blocker is designed on a similar principle but without a gauze cover, so that the deflated cuff is small and adaptable for passing down a small bronchoscope—minimum size 8 mm.—and placing in the small bronchi. However, the cuff ruptures easily and there is a danger of over-inflation with ballooning over the end of the drainage tube

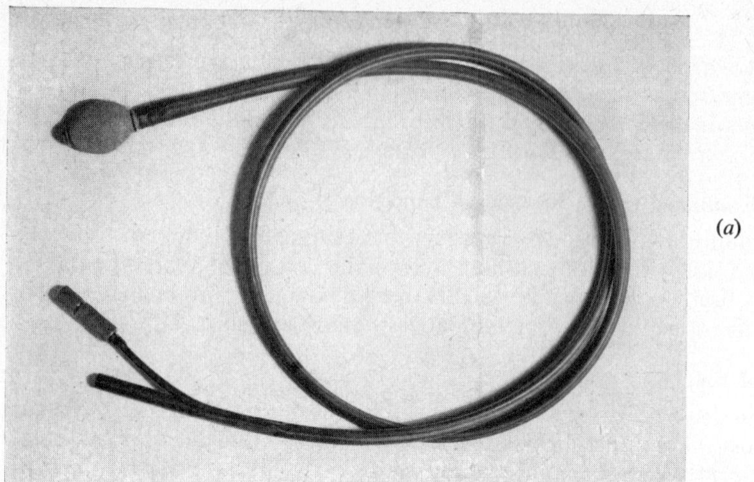

(*a*)

(*b*)

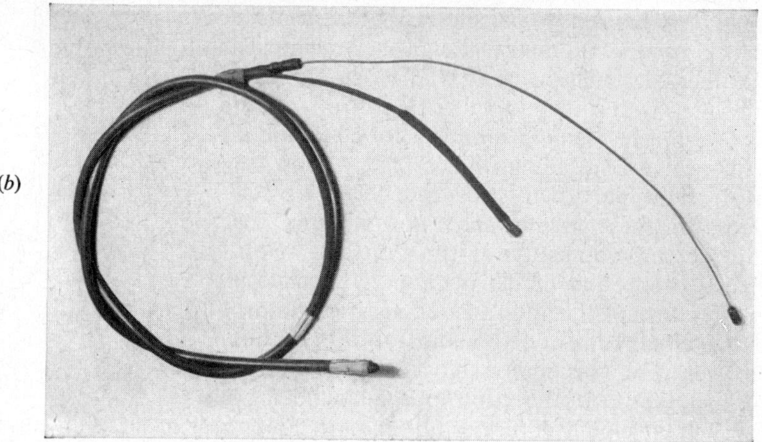

13/FIG. 4.—ENDOBRONCHIAL BLOCKERS
(*a*) Thompson's endobronchial blocker. (*b*) Magill's endobronchial blocker.

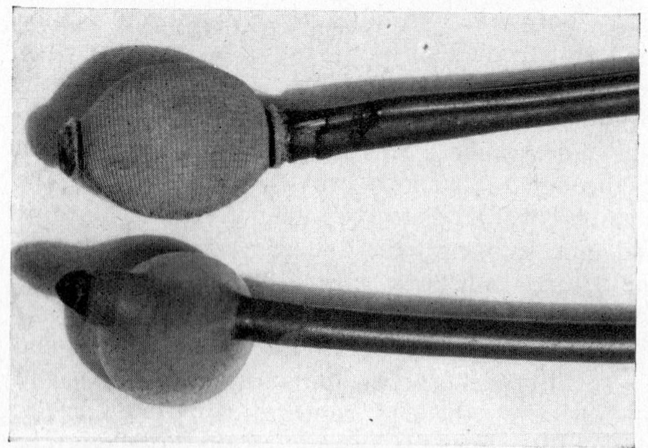

13/FIG. 5.—Comparison of inflated cuffs on the Thompson (above) and Magill blockers.

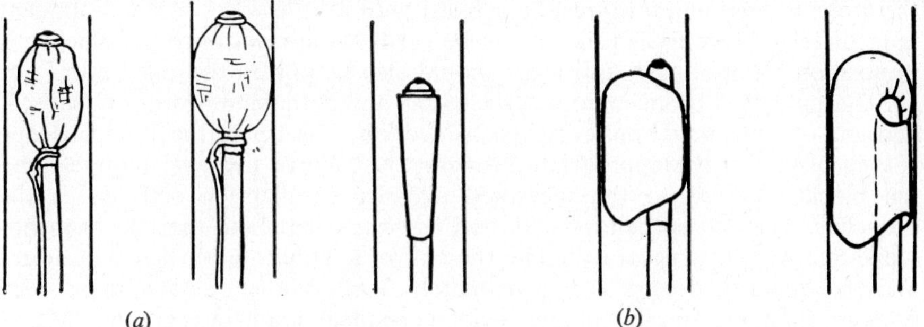

13/FIG. 6.—DIAGRAMMATIC ILLUSTRATION TO SHOW HOW A BLOCKER MAY LIE IN THE BRONCHUS

(a) Thompson. Uninflated and inflated.
(b) Magill. Note how over-inflation blocks the lumen of the tube.

(Fig. 6). For routine use the Thompson blocker is most favoured, but for upper lobes and children large enough for consideration of the technique the Magill, or modified Magill (see p. 417), being smaller, is more valuable. The Macintosh-Leatherdale bronchus blocker (Fig. 7) has two cuffs, one to lie in the trachea and the other in the left main bronchus. This tube is passed without the aid of a bronchoscope and combines the advantages of an endotracheal tube and a bronchus blocker.

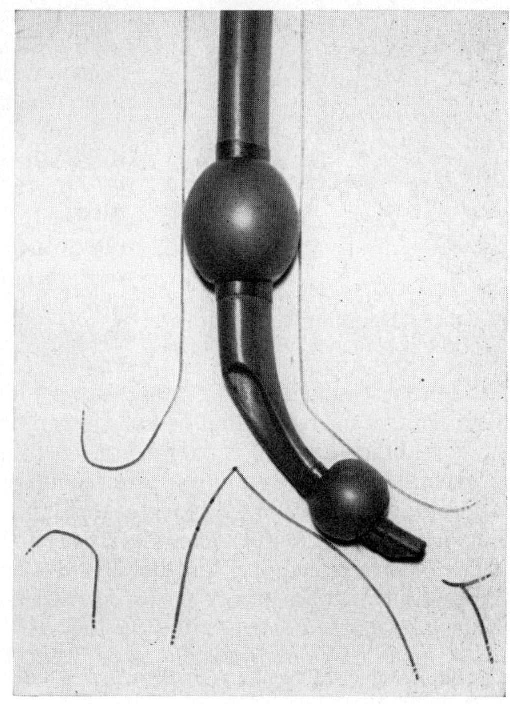

13/FIG. 7.—Macintosh-Leatherdale bronchus blocker.

Technique for passing blockers.—Prior to use the cuff must be tested for leaks and the blocker must be pushed down the bronchoscope until the deflated cuff is just beyond the distal end (with the Thompson blocker and a large bronchoscope this will be felt as a definite give). An ink mark is then made on the tubing at the level of the proximal end of the bronchoscope so that when the actual operation is performed there will be no doubt that the cuff has reached the bronchus. This is very important, since, although the place in the bronchus is first visualised down the bronchoscope, the actual positioning of a blocker cannot be done under direct vision. The blocker is fitted with a wire stilette which runs down the drainage tube and this must be greased with a little water-soluble lubricant immediately before use so that it can be easily withdrawn once the blocker is in position. A little pasta lubricans should also be put on the cuff.

The patient is bronchoscoped, the carina and both main bronchi visualised, and any obvious secretions removed by suction. The tip of the bronchoscope is then placed in the appropriate bronchus just above the level required and the blocker passed to the measured distance so that the cuff lies in the bronchus. The cuff is then inflated, and first the stilette and then the bronchoscope removed. It is usual to inflate the cuff of a Thomson blocker with water and the quantity needed is approximately 3 ml. Water offers a more even pressure than air, and its volume is not dependent upon temperature. Magill blockers are inflated with air, since they hold more and the risk of rupture and leakage of water into the lung is greater. At this stage the patient is intubated with a large endotracheal tube which can be most easily passed with the tubing of the blocker lying posteriorly in the glottis.

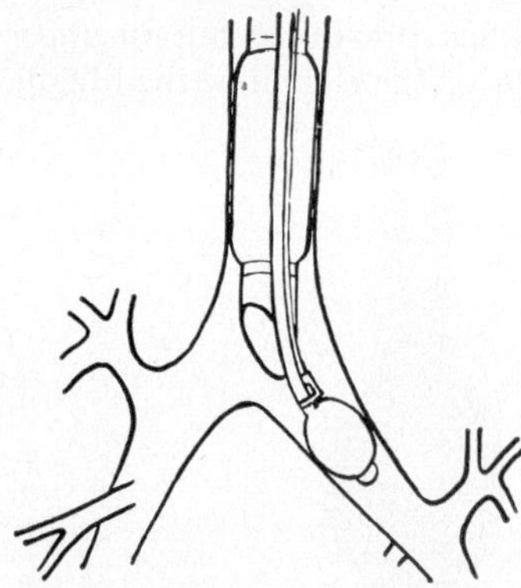

13/Fig. 8.—Diagram to show relationship of blocker to endotracheal tube.

A glance at Fig. 8 will show that this method of bronchial blocking is particularly useful for block of the left main bronchus just past the carina and of the left lower lobe or right middle and lower lobes. Upper lobe bronchus block is a more specialised technique which is described below. The distance of 5 cm. between the carina and the orifice of the left upper lobe bronchus leaves plenty of room for the cuff when it is desired to collapse the left lung, and block of the lower lobe bronchus on this side is no more difficult, since plenty of room is available below the opening of the upper lobe bronchus. However, on this side the lingula is frequently removed at the same time as the lower lobe, but since its bronchus arises from the upper lobe bronchus it cannot be blocked separately or in conjunction with the lower lobe. On the right side the problem is more difficult. There is only 2·5 cm. between the carina and the upper lobe bronchus, so that the cuff must be placed very accurately (Fig. 9). The principal difficulty is to avoid direct block of the upper lobe bronchus by the side of the cuff. This may be useful sometimes (Fig. 10), but not only prevents drainage of secretions from the upper lobe but also the escape of air, and leaves a partially inflated lobe in the surgeon's way. Furthermore, a ball valve may be produced leading to marked distension of the lobe as the anaesthetic progresses.

A much commoner mistake is to place the blocker too far down the right bronchus, leaving the upper lobe bronchus partially or completely open so that this lobe is not affected. Block of the middle and lower lobes is not difficult to accomplish, but attempted block of the lower lobe by pushing the blocker well down to avoid the middle lobe bronchus usually leaves the apical lower lobe bronchus open. These several practical disadvantages of the right bronchial tree will be discussed further in the comparison of contralateral bronchial block and endobronchial anaesthesia.

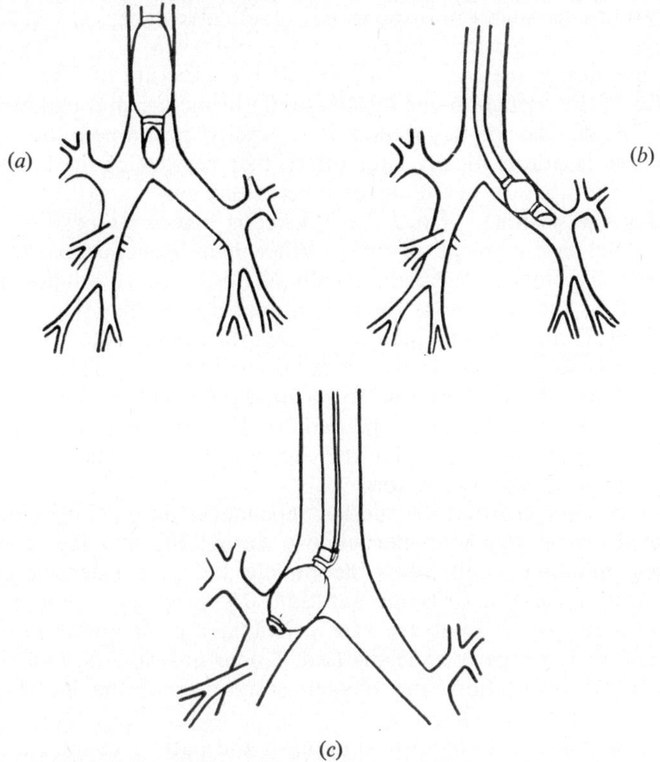

13/Fig. 9.—(*a*) Endotracheal cuffed tube. (*b*) Left endobronchial tube. (*c*) Right endobronchial blocker.

Upper lobe blocking (Stephen, 1952).—A special Magill blocker with a small cuff of approximately half the normal length is necessary for this procedure, since the upper lobe bronchus frequently sub-divides soon after leaving the main bronchus. This leaves very little room for insertion of a blocker, and the difficulty may be further accentuated by disease. Upper lobectomies are most often performed for tuberculosis, which more than other lesions is likely to lead to fibrosis with narrowing of the lumen and distortion of the angle formed between this bronchus and the parent stem. An acute angle makes the procedure difficult, if not impossible. With the stilette in position the cuff end of the blocker is slightly angulated so as to increase the ease of insertion, without preventing its free passage down the bronchoscope. When the bronchoscope is passed an attempt must be made to get it and the orifice of the particular upper lobe bronchus in a straight line by bending the patient's head as far as possible

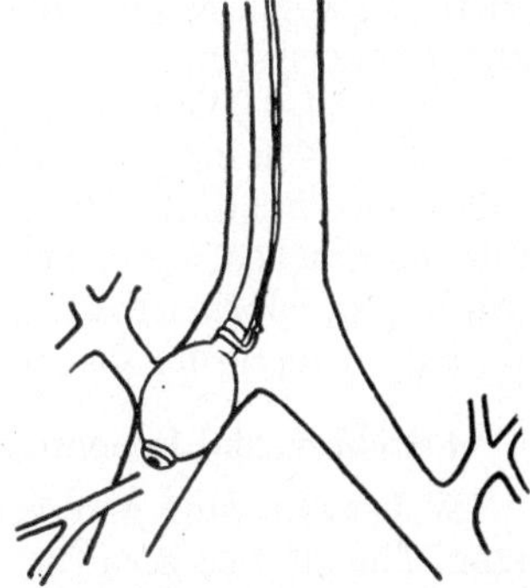

13/Fig. 10.—Diagram to show blocker placed to occlude right upper lobe bronchus completely.

to the opposite side. Such a position is only practicable under general anaesthesia. The chances of success are greater on the right side where the upper lobe bronchus lies nearer the carina. This avoids the necessity of introducing more than the tip of the bronchoscope into the main bronchus, and makes for greater flexibility. When the bronchoscope is correctly positioned the rest of the bronchial tree is automatically shut off so that passage of the blocker should lead easily to intubation of the upper lobe bronchus.

Checking the position.—Once the blocker is placed its position should be checked. In the case of block of one or other main bronchus, particularly after suction down the blocker, there are usually obvious signs of pulmonary collapse present, such as the absence of thoracic movement on that side and of breath sounds on auscultation during inflation. When the bronchus to a lobe is blocked these signs may be equivocal, due to aeration of the remaining lobes, but unless there are other reasons for doubting a good position this should not be taken as an indication for repeating the procedure. The true test of success can only be made when the thorax is open and movement of the lung can be watched during positive-pressure respiration.

It might be expected that the sudden dependence on one lung would lead to obvious evidence of hypoxia—particularly during the first few minutes after block when pulmonary collapse is incomplete and a considerable quantity of blood is still circulating without aeration. In practice, visible cyanosis or evidence of circulatory upset are rare provided the remaining lung is sound and the patient is properly anaesthetised. Under anaesthesia, and particularly with controlled respiration, the oxygen saturation of the blood should be normal.

There is a risk of the blocker slipping if the patient coughs, after sudden movement—such as might occur when positioning on the operating table—or when the surgeon handles the lung near it. In these circumstances the whole cuff may come back into the trachea and perhaps cause obstruction to respiration. If there is any difficulty in inflating a patient after inserting a blocker, particularly in the absence of other more obvious factors, the blocker must be deflated and removed at once. But a blocker may slip back into the trachea without causing complete obstruction and its dislodgement will only be appreciated when suction is applied to it. This will lead to rapid removal of gas from the lungs and anaesthetic system.

Removal.—The blocker must be removed just before the surgeon clamps the bronchus. The cuff is deflated by sucking out the water or air and the whole tube pulled out of the tracheo-bronchial tree. This can be done without removing the endotracheal tube, but its cuff must be momentarily let down. While removing the blocker the trachea and bronchus should be thoroughly sucked out through it to ensure that no secretions remain.

Endobronchial Intubation

A diseased lung may be isolated by intubating the bronchus of the normal lung. The affected area remains in communication with the atmosphere but not with the anaesthetic system, and as it is not ventilated pulmonary collapse follows. Secretions will drain from it with posture into the trachea and oropharynx. The endobronchial tube is normally placed in the main bronchus.

Endobronchial tubes are made in several sizes, the essential points being a narrow cuff and beyond this a very brief length of tube and short bevel. The design of the tubes in present use was made by Machray. They are placed in position under direct vision with an intubating bronchoscope of the Magill (Fig. 11) or modified Magill type. The latter is adapted to take the standard light fitting of a Negus bronchoscope (Mansfield, 1957).

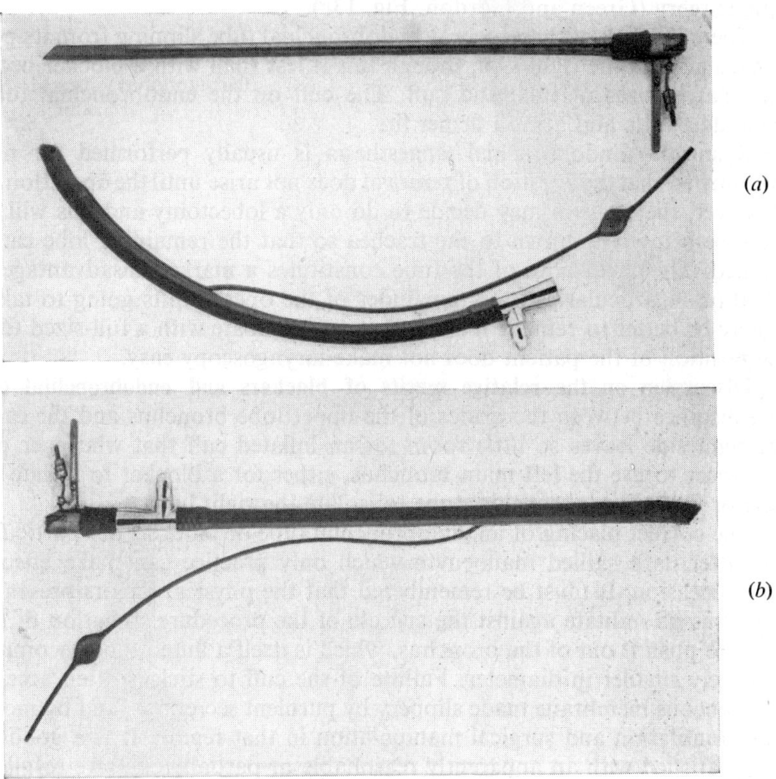

13/Fig. 11.—(*a*) Magill's intubating bronchoscope with Machray's endobronchial tube. (*b*) Bronchoscope and endobronchial tube ready for bronchial intubation.

Technique for endobronchial intubation.—The bronchoscope is greased with a little sterile lubricant paste and then placed within the endobronchial tube. This must be stretched to its full length, so that the bevel of the bronchoscope and of the tube correspond in position. There is no advantage in attempting to cut the tube to the exact distance between the major bronchi and the front teeth, and it is better to have the tube a little too long than too short. Bronchoscopy is performed and any secretions in the tracheobronchial tree are removed. For left endobronchial intubation the beak of the bronchoscope is placed well within the main bronchus, the cuff is inflated, and the bronchoscope slid from within the tube while this is firmly held in position at the mouth. On the right side the opening of the upper lobe bronchus must first be visualised and then the cuff of the endobronchial tube placed between this and the carina with the bevel

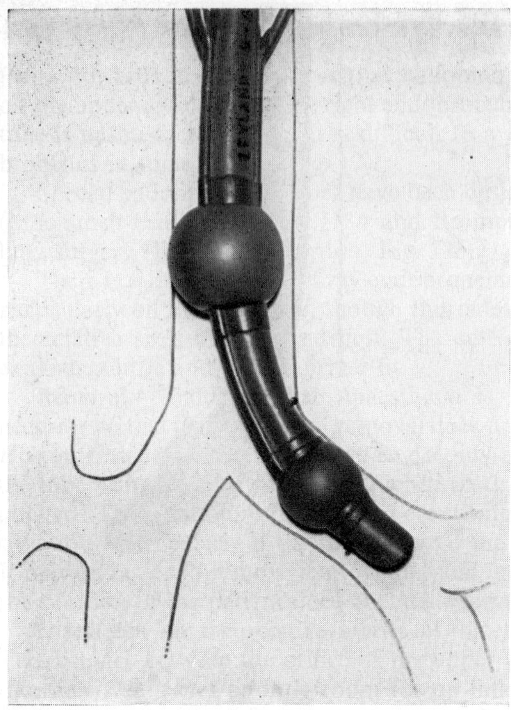

13/FIG. 13(*b*).—Brompton triple-cuffed endobronchial tube. This tube was designed for wedge resection of part of the right lung. The cuff in the left main bronchus is duplicated so that accidental puncture during operation of the outer cuff is not a disaster.

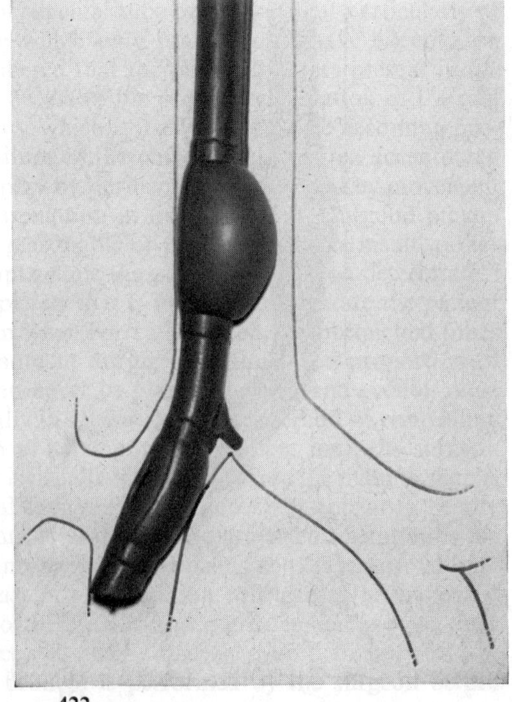

13/FIG. 13(*c*).—Green and Gordon's right endobronchial tube. The lower cuff lies in the right main bronchus. A small opening at the level of the right upper lobe bronchus prevents this lobe of the lung being obstructed. This tube is suitable for left lung surgery.

reinflation, since collapse of the whole lung with loss of air movement greatly diminishes the chance of spread from one lobe to another. The benefits in terms of a trouble-free anaesthesia performed through the sound lung are very great and the relatively short time the cuff remains in the bronchus in these circumstances decreases the chance of mucosal sloughs from pressure anaemia.

The overall advantages of endobronchial anaesthesia or bronchial blocking are not in doubt provided they are used with care and not looked upon as being fool-proof. They can be used with great advantage not only in the handling of excessive secretions, but to control or limit bleeding in the lower respiratory tract; to localise slight but infected sputum as in tuberculosis; to facilitate surgical access by collapsing the lung prior to removal for a neoplasm or other disease; and to control a broncho-pleural fistula. They may also be useful during the removal of an air cyst from the lung (see p. 429).

Anaesthesia for Endobronchial Intubation or Bronchial Blocking

When selective lung collapse is to be performed to control either excessive secretions, bleeding, or small amounts of sputum infected with tubercle bacilli, the mode of anaesthesia must allow for adequate removal of visible secretions by suction and the placing of the blocker or endobronchial tube before positive-pressure respiration in any form is carried out. Moreover, until this is accomplished it is axiomatic that the posture of the patient must be such as to retain the secretions in the affected areas once the protective cough reflexes of the patient are removed. Under local analgesia there is no need to bother about positive-pressure respiration and the patient oxygenates himself throughout the procedure. But placing either a blocker or endobronchial tube is uncomfortable for a conscious patient, puts some strain on his already diminished circulatory and respiratory reserves when the lung collapses, and is not easy to perform correctly unless the patient breathes very quietly. It does, however, encourage gentleness and avoids the need to hurry. The conditions produced by general anaesthesia with a relaxant make the procedure easier and considerably quicker, but in inexperienced hands and for those patients in whom there is little margin for error, local analgesia is less likely to lead to a dangerous situation if the procedure fails at the first attempt.

The essentials for general anaesthesia are inhalation of oxygen for about 3–4 minutes followed by induction of anaesthesia with a small dose of thiopentone and then the production of total paralysis with suxamethonium. A dose of approximately 100 mg. for an adult should be used to ensure paralysis for about 3–4 minutes, which is usually enough to complete the procedure. Pre-operative oxygen inhalation can be dispensed with in dry cases, but inflation with oxygen must then be carried out after the onset of paralysis and before bronchoscopy so that the period of apnoea does not lead to anoxia. The tracheo-bronchial tree should also be well sprayed with topical analgesic to prevent coughing with possible dislodgement of the tube on recovery from the paralysis. An alternative method of general anaesthesia is to use oxygen and halothane and to maintain spontaneous respiration until the blocker or tube is in position. Patients with broncho-pleural fistula or air cysts present special problems and must usually be treated the same way as wet cases (see p. 428 *et seq.*).

"Sleeve" Resection

The treatment of a neoplastic growth in the upper lobe of a lung cannot be effected by simple lobectomy when there is invasion of the main bronchus. A "sleeve" resection involves removing a length of the main bronchus together with the affected lobe. Following this, on the right side the end of the right bronchus is anastomosed to the trachea, while on the left side the bronchus is restored in continuity. The anaesthetist may encounter difficulty as the cut bronchus must remain open for a considerable period, but this can be overcome by the use of a blocker or double lumen tube. However, it is important to remember that a blocker or tube may be displaced due to manipulation of the bronchus and that the cuff of either may be accidentally deflated by the surgeon's knife. A reserve cuff is therefore an advantage (Pallister, 1959).

Double Lumen Tubes

There are three principal tubes available for selective control of either lung to be carried out during anaesthesia. These are the Carlens, Bryce-Smith and Robertshaw double lumen tubes, and they are illustrated in Figs. 14 *a–d.* The Carlens tube was not designed for use during operations and in many centres has been superseded by the Bryce-Smith and Robertshaw tubes which are both made in right and left forms. They are easier to manipulate than the Carlens and have a proportionately larger lumen which makes suction easier. The use of a double lumen tube enables the anaesthetist to provide at will a collapsed lung for the surgeon and to reinflate the same lung as required.

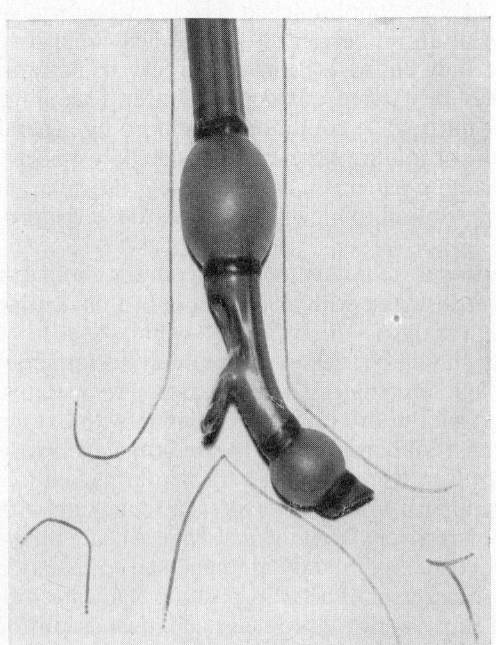

13/Fig. 14(*a*).—Carlens double-lumen endobronchial tube.

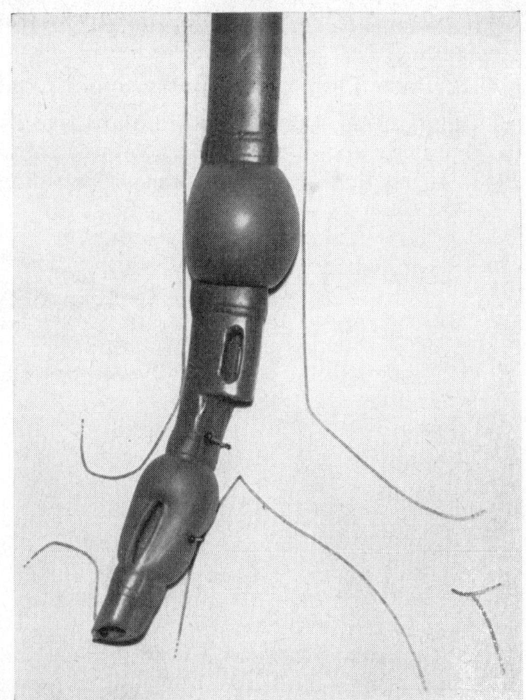

13/FIG. 14(*b*).—Bryce-Smith right endobronchial double lumen tube. The lower cuff has an opening opposite the origin of the right upper lobe bronchus.

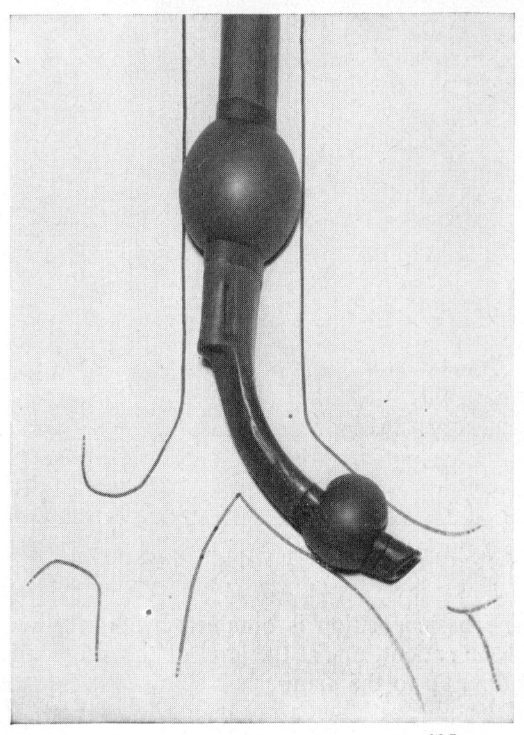

13/FIG. 14(*c*).—Bryce-Smith left endobronchial double lumen tube.

The Prone Position with Drainage of Secretions

This position was designed to allow free drainage from the diseased areas to the trachea and into the mouth without soiling the sound lung (Parry Brown, 1948). It has the further advantage of avoiding mediastinal displacement when

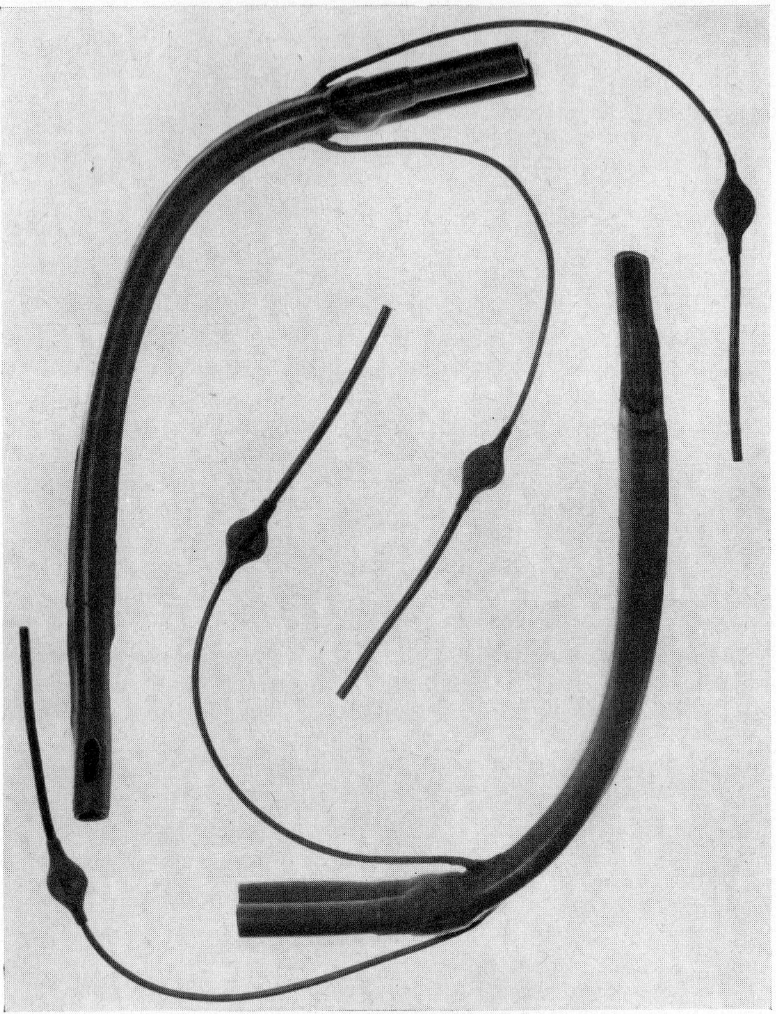

13/Fig. 14(*d*).—Robertshaw tubes—right and left.

the pleural cavity is opened. The basic position is obtained by putting two padded supports beneath the prone patient, one at the level of the pelvis and one under the lower chest extending up to the manubrium sterni. The side for operation is placed at the edge of the table with that arm hanging down (Fig. 15), and keeping the scapula away from the operation field. The upper dorsal and cervical vertebrae are flexed over the chest support and should be tilted downwards, while the lower dorsal and lumbar vertebrae are made horizontal. The head is extended at the atlanto-occipital joint and with the neck rotated to face the side of the lesion so that the trachea and bronchus of the affected lung are in a straight line. There is a danger that the bronchus on the sound side may become kinked during hilar traction at operation when the head is slanted in the opposite direction.

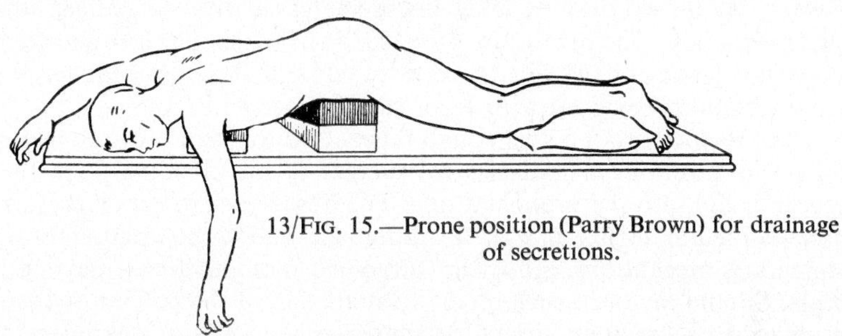

13/FIG. 15.—Prone position (Parry Brown) for drainage of secretions.

The principal objection to this position is the more limited surgical exposure which it allows. There is adequate freedom for diaphragmatic movement and the hanging arm does not suffer. The position has marked advantages in allowing free drainage of secretions. This is particularly important in children where other methods of control, such as blocking or suction, may be impracticable or inadequate, though posture alone cannot be relied upon when the secretions are copious and intermittent suction must be carried out. There is, however, a slight risk of spread either to the dependent middle or lingula lobe bronchus. Induced hypotension is dangerous in the prone position as an abnormally low systemic pressure may follow its use.

Prone Position with Retention of Secretions

In this position the patient is supported at the head, shoulders and hips so that there is no restriction of respiratory movement. The diseased side, although the patient is tilted head-downwards, is dependent to keep secretions from spreading (Overholt *et al.*, 1946).

With this method, if the secretions are copious, manipulation of the lung may cause periodic overflow. It is better, therefore, to have them flowing freely during the whole operation, as is the case in Parry Brown's position, and to aid their removal by intermittent suction.

Upright Retention Position

The flow of large quantities of secretions in young children may seriously affect the airway despite repeated suction, and even in the prone position there is a possibility of spread to the dependent middle or lingula lobe. In patients with bilateral disease this risk is greatly increased and may constitute an indication for the use of an upright retention method. Anaesthesia must be induced with the child upright, and suction used to clear as much sputum as possible from the respiratory tract.

The advantage of the method is that the secretions remain in the affected areas, thus limiting the need for suction: there is also less risk of respiratory obstruction.

Empyema

Empyemata offer many dangers to the unwary anaesthetist and for reasons of safety should be drained under local analgesia with the patient sitting in an upright position. The line of the proposed incision should be infiltrated, and the intercostal nerves of the ribs to be resected, and those immediately above and below, should be blocked with 1 per cent lignocaine.

The presence of an active cough reflex, and avoidance of the lateral, supine and prone positions, diminishes the danger of pus flooding from the infected pleural cavity into the bronchial tree. The absence—proved or presumed—of a broncho-pleural fistula makes no difference and is no excuse for neglecting elementary precautions, since the surgeon's manipulations may well make a fistula. Should factors—such as the mental state of the patient or the surgeon's desire to do more than simple drainage—make local analgesia insufficient, a method of general anaesthesia must be selected and administered as described in the next section.

Broncho-Pleural Fistula

A broncho-pleural fistula may follow a pulmonary resection, rupture of a lung abscess or may result from the spread of an untreated empyema. Whatever the origin an operation may be necessary and the presence of the fistula complicates anaesthesia and increases its dangers.

Diagnosis.—Post-operatively fistulae usually develop within the first two weeks, though they may occur after several months of convalescence when they are perhaps symptomatic of an unsuspected empyema. In their mode of onset the majority are undramatic; the usual suggestive signs are a cough which—especially after changes of position—is productive, the sputum being often blood-stained. If there is much fluid in the pleural cavity the sputum may be copious. Occasionally the onset is dramatic, as when after a bout of coughing the patient suddenly brings up large quantities of fluid. Sometimes when the fistula is small it has a valvular action—each cough forcing air into the pleural space. In this event the rising pleural pressure leads to collapse of the lung and mediastinal shift, with consequent dyspnoea, tachycardia, cyanosis and engorged neck veins—all signs of a tension pneumothorax.

In all cases the danger of a broncho-pleural fistula is overflow of infected pleural fluid into normal lung, and this risk is greatly increased by anaesthesia unless special precautions are taken. Surgical treatment usually takes one of three forms—a simple rib resection and drainage of the pleural space, thoracoplasty for chronic or grossly infected cases, or thoracotomy with closure of the fistula in early post-operative cases. A fistula occurring soon after lung resection is not necessarily associated with an infected pleural space, but this complication will soon follow unless the fistula is quickly closed.

Anaesthesia.—It is important when considering anaesthesia for simple drainage of an empyema, to have in mind the possibility that a fistula may be already present or be caused during the operation. This operation should, therefore, be performed with the patient sitting up. In the presence of a fistula the risk of spread under local analgesia is minimal, and in view of the comparatively minor nature of the operation, this technique is preferable to general anaesthesia which necessitates, in this instance, a complicated procedure.

When general anaesthesia is essential—as for instance when sepsis of the chest wall contra-indicates local injections—three points must be considered. First, that placing the patient supine, or worse still in the lateral position with the diseased side uppermost, will lead to flooding of the normal lung. These positions must never be used for the induction of general anaesthesia for this type of case. Secondly, that even with positive-pressure respiration it may be impossible to oxygenate the patient adequately in the presence of a large fistula —particularly when the surgeon enters the thorax; and thirdly, that if the hole is very small, continued positive-pressure may lead to a tension pneumothorax. The choice of technique therefore depends to some extent on a clinical evaluation of the type and size of the fistula; but unless the surgeon is prepared to guard against contralateral spread by operating in the prone position, one lung anaesthesia or the use of a double lumen tube is to be preferred. Indeed, one or other of these may be essential to ensure efficient ventilation even in the prone position when the fistula is large. A particular advantage of a double lumen tube is that when an attempt is being made to close a broncho-pleural fistula, the efficacy of the repair can be tested easily, whereas in similar circumstances an endobronchial tube would need to be withdrawn into the trachea.

Since both tubes and blockers may slip, their use should be combined with as much anti-Trendelenburg position on the operating table as possible in a further attempt to localise all fluid to the lower part of the diseased pleura. The surgeon must be prepared to clamp the bronchus as soon as he enters the thorax, or to occlude the fistula temporarily if it is a large one.

The choice between local and general anaesthesia for placing the blocker or tube must be made for reasons similar to those already described under wet lung cases. The margin of safety is so narrow with a broncho-pleural fistula and an infected pleural space that if there is any doubt about the practical problem, bronchoscopy and placing of the blocker or tube should be done under local analgesia and general anaesthesia induced afterwards. When general anaesthesia with a muscle relaxant is proposed, it must be preceded by the inhalation of oxygen as described for wet lung cases, so that positive-pressure respiration can be avoided until the affected lung has been isolated. An alternative method is to use oxygen and halothane, maintaining spontaneous respiration until the tube or blocker is in position (Francis and Smith, 1962). The induction of anaesthesia, bronchoscopy and the passage of the tube or blocker must be performed with the patient sitting up.

Lung Cysts

Gray and Edwards (1948) note that cysts of the lung occasionally have a one-way valvular mechanism (Fig. 16). Such cysts are usually congenital, but some may be acquired in emphysematous patients. As previously mentioned (pp. 416 and 428) a similar valvular mechanism sometimes occurs at the site of a small broncho-pleural fistula, or when an endobronchial blocker is incorrectly placed; if intermittent positive-pressure respiration is used in such circumstances the tension of the gases in the cyst (the pleural space or the isolated lobe as the

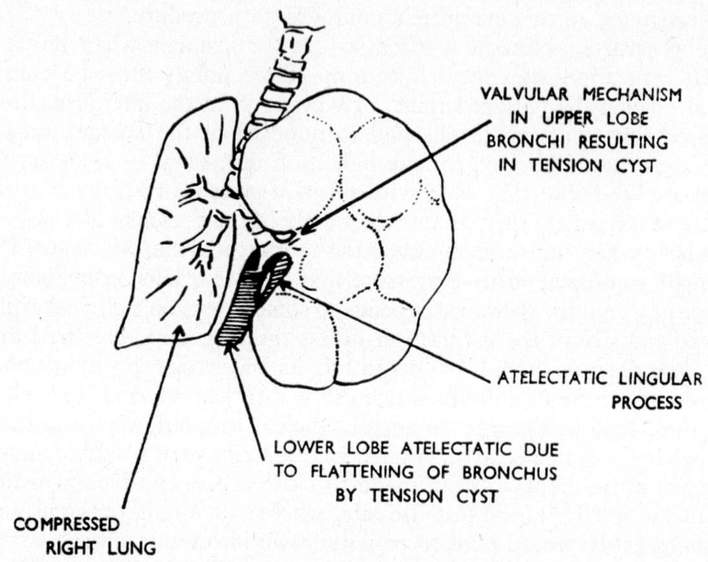

13/Fig. 16.—Tension cyst of lung.

case may be) will rise, and may eventually cause enough distension to collapse the surrounding lung tissue and displace the mediastinum and its contents with serious impairment of the patient's gaseous exchange and circulation.

When such a condition is suspected pre-operatively, spontaneous respiration must be maintained until the valve can be isolated either by a blocker or endobronchial tube, or by the surgical operation. If it is only discovered after respiration has been controlled as a result of deterioration in the patient's condition, increased pressure needed for inflation, and loss of gases in the anaesthetic breathing bag, then speedy treatment may be necessary. Either the surgeon must quickly open the pleural cavity or, if he is not prepared, a large-bore needle must be passed into it to let off the pressure.

Tuberculosis

Although several points need amplification, the principles of anaesthesia for the surgery of pulmonary tuberculosis are no different from those for other pulmonary diseases.* There is a tendency to differentiate intrapleural operations from those such as thoracoplasty, which are designed to collapse part of the

* The sterilisation of apparatus used for tuberculous patients is discussed in Appendix 3.

lung and as a result to postulate the use of general anaesthesia for the one and local analgesia for the other. Both can be, and are, performed under general anaesthesia, and there is no evidence to suggest that the general tendency to move away from local analgesia has led to an increase in operative complications, or indeed in spread of disease.

This is fortunate because major thoracic operations, thoracoplasty in particular, are at best unpleasant procedures under local analgesia.

The arguments put forward in favour of local analgesia are usually maintenance of the cough reflex, diminished bleeding, and no post-operative unconsciousness, so that breathing exercises can be started at once. The adequacy of the cough reflex under local analgesia is open to some doubt; certainly when the pleural cavity is open or when ribs have been removed at thoracoplasty, the act of coughing is useless since the lung tends to be blown into the wound and the sputum is not expelled up the trachea. It is rarely possible for the surgeon to prevent this by trying to hold back the lung temporarily with his hands, and it seems probable that under such conditions coughing may actually spread infection. It also exhausts the patient. Furthermore, very few local techniques are satisfactory unless combined with adequate general sedation and analgesia. The effect of this is to diminish the cough reflex and also depress ciliary activity. Thus, unless quite a considerable quantity of sputum is in the bronchial tree—and in normal parts of it at that—expectoration is unlikely to be attempted. Under general anaesthesia efficient suction is more likely to control the spread of secretions than inefficient coughing, and when indicated, the diseased part of the lung can be localised by one of the specific techniques already described.

There is no doubt that bleeding is slight with a local analgesic technique, but general anaesthesia can be combined with an infiltration of adrenaline and saline, or hypotension can be induced should the occasion warrant it.

A rapid return of consciousness is not difficult to accomplish after general anaesthesia; but spontaneous respiration with a conscious patient during a thoracoplasty may enable the surgeon to assess more accurately the effects of rib-resection and apical lung collapse step by step in those patients who have a very much diminished ventilatory capacity. Under general anaesthesia inadequate gaseous exchange despite high oxygen mixtures—with the patient at rest on assisted or controlled respiration—is obviously an indication that the extent of the operation must be limited. Converse findings, on the other hand, are of no significance, and then, unfortunately, the ultimate function can only be gauged after the patient has returned to spontaneous respiration and consciousness. When it is difficult to decide beforehand in borderline cases how extensive the operation should be for optimal results, there may be some advantage in using a local analgesic technique. If proper pre-operative investigations are performed, such patients are remarkably limited in number, and few physicians would care to submit a patient to an operation with reserves that are so slender. Although intubation is essential to maintain adequate control of the airway under general anaesthesia, and facilitates suction, there is no evidence to suggest that tuberculous ulceration of the larynx or trachea follows the procedure. An interesting fact following the use of general anaesthesia is that post-operative vomiting, a frequent complication after local techniques, is very much reduced in incidence and severity.

Thoracoplasty

The operation is usually carried out in two or three stages. At the first stage the first, second, and half or all the third rib are removed. An extrapleural strip of the lung is performed and the apex collapsed. At the second stage the remainder of the third and the fourth and fifth ribs are removed with further stripping of the lung. In some cases a third stage may be necessary to achieve further collapse and in this case two more ribs are removed, but in most cases a total of five suffices. Besides being a vascular one, the operation entails considerable stimulation while the lung is being stripped, and the expression of any secretions from the diseased area into the main bronchus.

REFERENCES

FRANCIS, J. G., and SMITH, K. G. (1962). An anaesthetic technique for the repair of bronchopleural fistula. *Brit. J. Anaesth.*, **34,** 817.

GRAY, T. C., and EDWARDS, F. R. (1948). The anaesthetic problems associated with giant tension cysts of the lung. *Thorax*, **3,** 237.

LUNDING, M., and FERNANDES, A. (1967). Arterial oxygen tension and acid-base status during thoracic anaesthesia. *Acta anaesth. scand.*, **11,** 43.

MALONE, D. M., GOULD, J. C., and GRANT, I. W. B. (1968). A comparative study of ampicillin, tetracycline hydrochloride and methacycline hydrochloride in acute exacerbations of chronic bronchitis. *Lancet*, **2,** 594.

MANSFIELD, R. (1957). Modified bronchoscope for endobronchial intubation. *Anaesthesia*, **12,** 477.

NILSSON, E., SLATER, E. M., and GREENBERG, J. (1965). The cost of the quiet lung: fluctuations in Pa_{O_2} when the Carlens tube is used in pulmonary surgery. *Acta anaesth. scand.*, **9,** 49.

OVERHOLT, R. H., LANGER, L., SZYPULSKI, J. T., and WILSON, N. J. (1946). Pulmonary resection in the treatment of tuberculosis. *J. thorac. Surg.*, **15,** 384.

PALLISTER, W. K. (1959). A new endobronchial tube for left lung anaesthesia. *Thorax*, **14,** 55.

PARRY BROWN, A. I. (1948). Posture in thoracic surgery. *Thorax*, **3,** 161.

STEPHEN, E. D. S. (1952). Problem of "blocking" in upper lobectomies. *Curr. Res. Anesth.*, **31,** 175.

Chapter 14

POST-OPERATIVE PULMONARY COMPLICATIONS

by

G. T. SPENCER

THERE are a large number of complications (see Table 1) which may occur in the lungs after an operation and anaesthetic, though most are rare and many representative of individual stages in the progress of a single disease. During the immediate post-operative period the lungs usually contain more secretions than normally, due in part to the absence or depression of normal reflex activity, while the vital capacity is usually subnormal. Here at the very least are the essential ingredients of what every anaesthetist knows as "cough and sputum" —a challenge to the physiotherapist and himself. Such a state is, however, in certain cases a stage on the way to bronchiole or bronchial obstruction which may, in favourable soil, lead to collapse of lung tissue and infection, with the potential, but admittedly rare, prospect of incomplete resolution and bronchiectasis as the ultimate result.

Despite the great improvement in anaesthetic techniques and increased understanding of the causes and mechanisms of post-operative pulmonary

14/TABLE 1

POST-OPERATIVE PULMONARY COMPLICATIONS (EXCLUDING THOSE DUE TO CARDIAC AND CIRCULATORY DISEASE)

Bronchitis . . .	"Cough and sputum". Simple bronchitis. Acute purulent bronchitis.
Collapse of Lung .	Obstructive: Multiple scattered lobular collapse. Collapse of segment, lobe or lung. Reflex: Acute massive collapse. Passive: Pneumothorax. Haemothorax.
Pneumonia . .	Broncho-pneumonia: Infected collapsed lung tissue. Hypostatic or terminal infection. Lobar pneumonia.
Abscess . . .	Aspiration. Secondary pyaemia.
Oedema . . .	Exudative, secondary to aspiration.
Tuberculosis . .	

complications, most studies have shown that there has been little decrease in their incidence over the past thirty years. Wightman (1968) in an extensive survey of 785 patients suggests that the reason why the advances in chemotherapy, antibiotics and surgical anaesthetic techniques appear to have had so little effect on the overall incidence of pulmonary complications is that patients are now operated on who would formerly have been rejected on grounds of age, chronic respiratory or other disease. It would seem almost certain that this explanation is correct. So much is now known about the varying and numerous aetiological factors that not only is avoidance of many of them simple, but active preventive therapy can be almost routinely carried out. In fact the key to the problem is drainage, and although infection can and does occur as a primary and acute event, it is more commonly secondary to inadequate drainage.

Normally secretions are removed from the lower to the upper bronchial tree by ciliary activity, while at the higher level an active cough reflex leads to effective expulsive efforts. Free drainage is also dependent upon aeration of all parts of the lung and hence upon an adequate minute volume of respiration. Disease, personal habits, climatic changes, surgery and anaesthesia, and indeed many other factors, can totally upset or alter these normal relationships in the lungs. It is unfortunate that in spite of all that is known about the causes of post-operative chest complications, so little is done to minimise the likelihood of their occurrence. Few patients are admitted long enough before an operation to allow pre-existing respiratory disease to be detected and treated. Improvement will probably only come from the more widespread adoption of already well-known therapeutic measures.

Factors Concerned in the Aetiology of Pulmonary Complications

The patient.—Post-operative pulmonary complications occur more frequently in men than in women, but no satisfactory explanation of this discrepancy has yet been found. They are particularly likely to occur in the winter months. This fact has a connection with the seasonal incidence of respiratory tract infection, since there is no doubt that pre-existing pulmonary disease increases the incidence. Smoking is a contributing factor, probably on account of the sputum that it causes, and it has been suggested that the occurrence of chest complications is six times more frequent in smokers than in non-smokers (Morton, 1944). Although it is widely assumed that pulmonary complications are commoner in the older age groups, recent studies (Wightman, 1968) have failed to confirm this and suggest that it is little more than a reflection of the higher incidence of pre-existing respiratory disease in the elderly. The same probably applies to obesity.

The operation.—Site of operation is the most important factor affecting the incidence of pulmonary complications. Most series show an overall incidence of 5 per cent. This rises to 21 per cent for operations on the gastro-intestinal and biliary tract, but only to 6 per cent for other abdominal operations. Non-abdominal operations are followed by a much lower incidence of pulmonary complications, usually below 1 per cent. The pain that high abdominal incisions cause in the post-operative period is a principal factor in reducing vital capacity and effective coughing, but the proximity of the operative site to the diaphragm and the way in which the operation is performed are factors of great importance. Thus retraction and handling of the bowel will lead to some post-operative swelling, while a slight leak at an anastomosis will markedly aggravate the situation. In either event there is some diaphragmatic splinting, and Mimpriss and Etheridge (1944) showed a connection between the complications of gastric surgery and post-operative pulmonary complication. Anscombe (1957) reports that pulmonary mechanical function may be decreased by 50–70 per cent after upper abdominal operations and by 25–35 per cent after lower abdominal ones.

Prolonged surgery, and the effects of posture, particularly the steep Trendelenburg and lithotomy positions, which limit total lung capacity because of the pulmonary venous engorgement they cause, are potentiating factors (Hamilton and Morgan, 1932).

The anaesthetic.—Pre- and post-operative medication must be considered here. Morphine, atropine, and their analogues can be effective instruments in the prevention of pulmonary complications if used in judicious dosage, but overdosage or underdosage can equally mitigate against the patient. All drugs of these types depress ciliary activity and therefore the normal clearing mechanism of the lower bronchial tract, but the beneficial effects of atropine in preventing excessive secretions, and morphine in relieving pain, are paramount. Excessive medication may produce viscous mucus which is difficult to expectorate and a too-sleepy patient with depressed respiration and a depressed cough reflex. It will also depress the normal "sigh" which is important in maintaining normal ventilation-perfusion ratios in the lungs.

Individual anaesthetic agents and sequences, including local analgesia, are of little importance, provided there is no pre-existing chest disease. Lucas (1944) has shown in a comparable series of cases that the incidence of post-operative pulmonary complications is the same, whatever the anaesthetic. On the other hand, the way in which the anaesthetic is administered can, like the performance of the surgical operation, be decisive. Depth of anaesthesia, inadequate ventilation and a prolonged post-operative recovery during which reflex activity is markedly depressed or absent, must be avoided. Infected foreign material, such as blood, vomit or pus, should not be allowed to reach the lower respiratory tract either fortuitously or because of bad technique, while excessive secretions, such as are often present in the lungs or the pharynx at the end of operation, and particularly after the use of neostigmine, must be removed.

A subsidiary factor is the rate of absorption of gases from the alveoli. The elimination of nitrogen during a long anaesthetic and the substitution of rapidly absorbed anaesthetic gases will increase the risk of pulmonary collapse distal to complete—or, in certain circumstances, incomplete—bronchial obstruction. If ventilation is depressed or inadequate—as in partial curarisation without assisted respiration—gases may be absorbed from peripheral lung segments more quickly than they can be replaced from above a partially blocked bronchus. Many inhalational anaesthetics, in depressing ciliary activity, may contribute to bronchial obstruction.

Hypoxaemia after anaesthesia.—Nunn and Payne (1962) have shown that a fall in arterial oxygen tension usually follows even minor general anaesthetics. It persists up to 24 hours even when the carbon dioxide tension remains normal.

The cause is not fully understood though it is almost certainly due to a combination of the factors outlined in the preceding two paragraphs. It underlines, however, the importance of oxygen therapy in the post-operative period and may be a significant cause of pulmonary complications in susceptible patients.

Pulmonary complications in neonatal life and infancy.—Rees (1958) has described the factors peculiar to neonatal life and infancy that increase the risk of a pulmonary complication occurring after an operation at this age. The baby is immobile, and has an immature respiratory apparatus. Thus coughing is relatively ineffective and the danger of aspiration is considerable, while respiration is paradoxical with the diaphragm sucking in the thoracic cage during inspiration—the mobile and soft ribs being unable to play much part in ventilation. The surgical disease may also hamper respiration, particularly when it is a hiatus hernia with a large amount of bowel in the thoracic cavity or an abdominal lesion associated with distension. Finally, dehydration may accentuate these difficulties, as some restriction of fluid intake may be part of a deliberate surgical policy following neonatal operations.

BRONCHITIS

A brief note is needed of the several post-operative pulmonary complications which are not infrequently lumped together under the general term of "bronchitis". In fact the pathology may vary from the minimal but normal accumulation of secretions that follows most operations and anaesthetics, albeit for a brief period of time, to the presence of an acute infective process with the production of purulent and excessive quantities of sputum. Moreover it may be difficult, if not impossible, to differentiate on purely physical examination between bilateral bronchial infection with associated bronchial spasm and congestion, and the presence of multiple and scattered areas of peripheral lobular lung collapse (see below). Indeed the bronchitis may be a potent cause of the latter. More often than not bronchitis is a trivial complication of anaesthesia, being little more than a slight exacerbation of a pre-existing condition. Phillips (1966) has shown that the use of contaminated endotracheal tubes and unsterile analgesic lubricant may precipitate bronchial infections.

COLLAPSE OF LUNG

In this disease there is an area of collapse which may vary in size from a small lobule to that of a segment, lobe, or whole lung.

Lobular collapse is of particular interest, not only because it may occur more often than clinical diagnosis can confirm, but because untreated it could be a precursor of more extensive lung collapse by diminishing the compliance, increasing airway resistance and therefore the work of breathing. Since there is an inter-alveolar gaseous interchange via the pores of Kohn, many people have argued that lobular collapse cannot occur; but although this may be so in normal people, under abnormal conditions, particularly when respiration is depressed, such a gaseous exchange is absent (Van Allen *et al.*, 1931).

Sooner or later in the collapsed area infection supervenes, and indeed it is probable that in the smaller lesion until this occurs there is neither constitutional upset nor even pyrexia to suggest a complication. Infection also accounts for the fact that many cases of post-operative pulmonary collapse are mistakenly diagnosed as pneumonia.

It is difficult to say when the process of collapse begins, for although most cases present clinically between 24 and 48 hours after operation there is some evidence that the disease starts much earlier—perhaps even on the operating table during the anaesthetic. Stronger (1947) found that five out of thirteen patients who developed radiological evidence of collapse had abnormal pictures as early as four hours after operation.

The processes of infection in a collapsed area of lung may lead to a sequence of events which ultimately terminate in a bronchiectatic area. But even without treatment there is a tendency for the disease to cure itself, since with infection there is liquefaction of the mucus which blocks the bronchus and a better opportunity, therefore, for the patient to clear the obstruction and aerate the distal alveoli. In less fortunate cases the process may be severe enough to lead to a mistaken diagnosis of primary pneumonia, while gross destruction of lung tissue is a rare cause of lung abscess.

Bronchiectasis is the long-term result of incomplete and delayed re-expansion of lung tissue. The walls of the bronchi or bronchioles are weakened by infection since healing is by fibrosis, while during the period of collapse the negative pressure in the pleural space is greatly increased and thus exerts traction on the lung and air passages. Peribronchial fibrosis also exerts a pull which can lead to bronchial dilatation.

Diagnosis.—The diagnosis of a sizeable area of collapse is usually readily made from an examination of the patient. The onset is often acute and associated with pain in one or other side of the chest, a dry cough and dyspnoea. It usually occurs within the first forty-eight hours after operation.

On examination temperature, pulse and respiration rate are all increased, and indeed a clinical chart which shows the sudden onset of this classical triad of signs in the immediate post-operative period is itself almost pathognomic of the condition. Although the increase in pulse and respiratory rate can easily be accounted for by the sudden change in respiratory mechanics, no satisfactory explanation has yet been given for the high rise in temperature at this early stage. Cyanosis may be present if the area of collapse is large.

Classical physical signs of collapse will be found on physical examination of the patient, while substantiation of the diagnosis may be aided by radiography (see Figs. 1*A* and *B*).

Prevention and Treatment of Bronchitis and Pulmonary Collapse

Prevention

The most essential component of the treatment of post-operative pulmonary complications is undoubtedly the wise use of preventive measures. In the first place a thorough understanding of the aetiological factors and the systematic avoidance of all possible ones should be a routine part of anaesthetic practice.

No patient should be submitted to non-emergency surgery unless an effort has been made to clear pre-existing respiratory tract disease. If cure is impossible then the patient should be presented for anaesthesia in the best possible conditions. It is sometimes preferable to wait until spring or summer rather than oper-

ate on a "chesty" patient in the winter. Ellis (1955) suggests that many operations can be carried out with little increase in the risk by the presence of a common cold, although he excludes abdominal operations and those on the chest and respiratory tract itself. Upper respiratory tract infection, irrespective of operation and anaesthesia, is a not uncommon cause of aspiration pneumonia—a condition of collapse and pneumonia of a broncho-pulmonary segment from aspiration of infected secretions—which in turn can lead to bronchiectasis in as high a proportion as 5 per cent of all such cases (Morle and Robertson, 1953). There can be little excuse for increasing such a risk by the administration of an anaesthetic if the operation can safely be delayed. This dictum applies equally to the use of general anaesthesia or local analgesia.

Loder (1955) has advocated that a chest X-ray should be taken routinely before non-emergency surgery. In a series of 1,000 pre-operative chest radiographs, 29 patients were found to have chest disease sufficient to necessitate postponement of their operation. Advanced pulmonary tuberculosis was discovered for the first time in six of these patients.

In the prevention of pulmonary complications the pre- and post-operative use of breathing exercises and postural drainage is of considerable importance, particularly for thoracic and upper abdominal operations. In the two subsequent sections these forms of therapy are described in some detail, although it will be apparent to the reader that in their entirety neither is necessary for every case submitted to operation and anaesthetic.

Breathing exercises.—Most post-operative patients, particularly those accustomed to a sedentary occupation, rely upon upper thoracic movement for aeration of their lungs and the diaphragmatic element is small. In the post-operative period ventilation is reduced as a result of fear, pain and analgesic drugs, while other factors which have already been discussed, such as an alteration in the secretion of mucus and a reduction in ciliary action, are at work.

The object of breathing exercises is to increase the vital capacity and aid drainage of the respiratory tract. This implies an increase in the capacity of all areas of the lung, including those affected by disease. Vital capacity does not in itself give an indication of respiratory efficiency, but an increase in it, with improved chest measurements, indicates that greater ventilation can take place.

More specifically, breathing exercises should be carried out with three purposes in mind:

(*a*) To encourage diaphragmatic movement so that the lung bases are well ventilated.
(*b*) To teach the patient how to produce good and controlled movement in all parts of the chest.
(*c*) To teach the patient how to cough effectively, particularly in the presence of a surgical wound.

Method.—The patient should be lying in a comfortable position in bed with the head and chest supported by pillows. Each breath should be taken quietly and slowly and expiration in particular should not be hurried. Excessively deep inspiration is not necessary. Throughout the exercises care must be taken to avoid movement of the shoulder girdle and postural changes such as rotation or arching of the thoracic spine, all of which mitigate against effective respiration, especially when localised breathing is being practised. The maintenance of a good posture should be taught coincidentally with breathing exercises, so that any tendency to deformity which may arise as a result of disease or operation is prevented.

Since the patient must know how to use the whole thorax the first important objective is to achieve mobility of it and of the dorsal spine. This can be done by repeatedly raising the arms above the head to stretch the ribs, rotating and bending the whole of the upper body from the trunk and rolling the shoulders. Secondly, control of the abdominal muscles must be taught so that relaxation and contraction can be carried out at will. Thirdly, the actual breathing exercises should consist of controlled expiratory movements which will assist the movement of secretions from the insensitive periphery of the lungs to the area of cough reflex, so that expectoration may be achieved. Good and equal movements on both sides rather than unilateral movements should be aimed at.

Progression to more spectacular exercises for localised expansion should never overshadow the importance of these bilateral movements, but localised breathing must be practised so that all parts of the thorax can be used individually or collectively. This is important after thoracic operations.

Localised breathing.—Adequate diaphragmatic breathing needs relaxation of the abdominal muscles during inspiration and contraction during expiration. Descent of the diaphragm can be roughly marked if the attendant's hand is placed just below the sternum. Lateral costal breathing should be practised against the pressure of the hand placed in the mid-axillary line, either over the lower or upper ribs, while for apical breathing the hand must be just beneath the clavicle. Both lateral costal and apical breathing should be carried out individually and unilaterally, and, when abdominal surgery is contemplated, postero-lateral expansion against the pressure of the hand behind the mid-axillary line may be included. This latter movement is less painful than lateral costal in the presence of an upper abdominal incision, though its efficiency is open to some doubt.

Postural drainage.—The object of postural drainage is not only to drain a diseased area, but also all segments of the lungs, since clinical and radiographic investigations are not invariably correct in limiting the site of the disease, and to allow sputum to accumulate in the main bronchi, where the cough reflex is

14/Table 2

Lobe	*Segment*	*Position of patient*	
Upper	Anterior	Horizontal	Supine
	Apical	Vertical	Sitting
	Posterior	Inclined forward	Sitting
Middle or Lingula		35° head-down tilt	Inclined to normal side
Lower	Apical	Horizontal	Pillow at hips. Supine
	Posterior	45° head-down tilt	Inclined to normal side
	Lateral	45° head-down tilt	Lying on normal side
	Anterior	45° head-down tilt	Supine

active and will lead to expulsion. There are eight positions necessary to drain the eight principal segments of the lung. These segments are illustrated diagrammatically in Fig. 2 and the positions needed for each are described in Table 2 (Storey, 1955).

Each position should be maintained for a few minutes while the secretions flow, and then coughing should be encouraged and percussion over the affected area started. Breathing exercises designed to increase the expansion of each segment can be usefully combined with this, but the general rule should be against working the patient over-hard, and to repeat rather than prolong the drainage. Three or four minutes are adequate for each position, though a little longer may be useful if the particular lobe is known to be diseased. The whole procedure repeated three times a day is generally sufficient, and the course should be continued until an optimum reduction in sputum is obtained or the collapsed area is completely cleared.

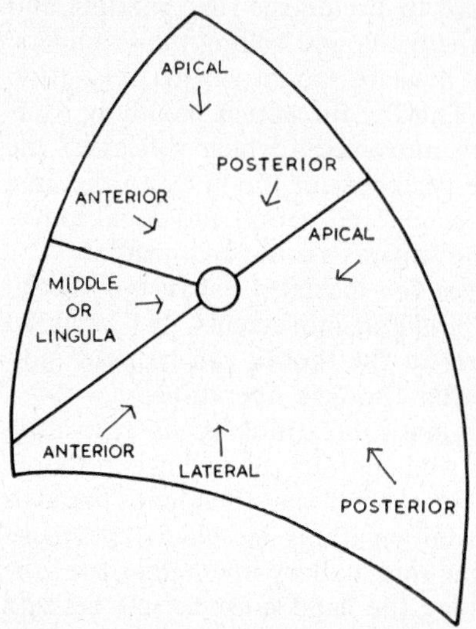

14/Fig. 2.—Composite picture to show the eight areas of the lung requiring separate postural drainage.

The treatment of pain.—The influence of post-operative pain in reducing vital capacity and preventing coughing is well-known. The use of respiratory depressants such as morphine may, paradoxically, improve the situation when used in moderate dosage by allaying pain, and, with the possible exception of morphine and morphine-antidote combinations, no other agents have yet proved so satisfactory when all factors are taken into consideration.

Nevertheless, mention must be made of local infiltration of the operation wound with a local analgesic, the continuous intravenous use of these agents, and of epidural analgesia.

The former method has fallen into disrepute because a safe long-acting local analgesic has not yet been discovered, while irrigation of the wound through a plastic catheter with a short-acting drug is cumbersome and unsatisfactory. Several people have claimed success for the use of an intravenous procaine drip after upper abdominal operations for the control of pain without further decreasing pulmonary ventilation. But contrary to expectations this method does not lead to an increase in vital capacity over the normal post-operative figures (Pooler, 1949).

Epidural analgesia need not interfere with the muscles of respiration if the concentration of local analgesic solution is carefully chosen, and it is accompanied by bronchial relaxation (Bromage, 1954). A painless operation site, unimpeded respiratory activity and bronchial relaxation are marked advantages, particularly for bronchitic and emphysematous patients, in the immediate post-operative period, but to be really valuable, they must be maintained for several hours by continuous epidural analgesia (Simpson *et al.*, 1961).

Other drugs.—Palmer and Sellick (1953), in a survey of 180 patients undergoing abdominal operations, were able to show a remarkable decrease in the incidence of pulmonary complications by the adoption of isoprenaline inhalation combined with postural drainage and with vibratory and clapping percussion to the chest wall before and after operation. In 90 patients treated in this way the incidence of lung collapse was 9 per cent compared with 43 per cent in 90 similar patients treated with breathing exercises alone before and after operation. All these patients had procaine penicillin before and after operation.

Isoprenaline has a powerful bronchodilator and vasoconstrictor action on bronchial mucosa. These workers delivered 1 ml. of a 1 per cent solution of the drug by oral inhalation by means of a hand nebuliser three times a day, and followed each treatment by fifteen to twenty minutes of postural drainage, combined with percussion during expiration. Immediately on recovery of consciousness after operation they gave another inhalation of isoprenaline, repeating the dose six-hourly, and started postural drainage when the patient's condition permitted—usually 6–12 hours after the operation. This treatment was continued for as long as sputum was produced on tipping.

The use of specific antibiotics should be reserved for cases with pre-existing respiratory tract diseases when they help to avoid the risk of exacerbation, or for part of the treatment of post-operative purulent bronchitis or infected areas of collapsed lung. Although Collins *et al.* (1968) showed a reduction of over 50 per cent in the incidence of pulmonary complications following the use of prophylactic antibiotics, this method is not generally accepted in view of the well-recognised disadvantages which accompany the administration of antibiotics on a prophylactic basis. Such drugs can never be a substitute for active treatment of the type described to deal with the mechanical factors concerned in these post-operative pulmonary complications. Expectorants are more likely to increase secretions than to aid in their efficient elimination at this stage, and the inhalation of carbon dioxide and oxygen mixtures is of little value.

In contrast to the results of Palmer and Sellick (1953), Collins *et al.* (1968) were unable to show any benefit from routine use of post-operative isoprenaline inhalations. Discrepancies of this sort are characteristic of many studies of post-operative pulmonary complications and their prophylaxis. The success of most methods depends on the enthusiasm with which they are pursued, and their value lies in their being part of a general stir-up regime. rather than in the details of methods employed. Diament and Palmer (1967) and Leiner *et al.* (1965) maintain that in order to detect pre-operatively the bronchitic patient who is particularly liable to post-operative pulmonary complications, it is necessary to perform pulmonary function tests. Even if true, this concept may be unrealistic in busy clinical practice, and Bethune *et al.* (1968) suggest that, using the classification of chronic bronchitis recommended by the Medical Research Council (1965), the initial diagnosis can be made clinically with sufficient accuracy to be of considerable value.

The Medical Research Council defined chronic bronchitis and suggested three groups which could be useful in the epidemiology of the disease. They developed a standard questionnaire for use in obtaining the patient's history, and found that it enabled the individual to be placed in one of the following groups:

Group 1. Simple chronic bronchitis—i.e. patients who have a chronic or recurrent mucoid secretion sufficient to cause expectoration.

Group 2. Chronic recurrent mucupurulent bronchitis. Patients who have chronic or recurrent mucopurulent sputum, not due to localised disease.

Group 3. Chronic obstructive bronchitis: similar patients to Group 2, but with the addition of airway obstruction.

Treatment

Once pulmonary collapse has been diagnosed, postural drainage, percussion over the affected area, and encouragement to cough must all be started or continued with redoubled effort. Morphine should be given to remove fear and pain and allow unrestrained coughing. The vast majority of cases of collapsed lung will respond to this sort of "stir-up" regime and begin to re-aerate within six to twelve hours, while occasionally dramatic results are produced in a matter of minutes. The extent of the affected area and the general state of the patient may, however, warrant more active measures at once. There is seldom difficulty in deciding when to interfere, even after serious surgical operations; bronchial suction must obviously be carried out on an acutely ill patient with a large area of collapsed lung, if no improvement follows other methods in an hour or so. Suction may also be of great value when the air passages fill up with secretions and the patient is unable to clear them properly. After thoracic operations suction may have to be speedily applied if permanent loss of a lobe or even of life is to be avoided.

Nosworthy (1944) has described how simple bronchial suction can be carried out in the ward with the patient sitting up in bed. Ideally the patient is given a lozenge of local analgesic to suck, or a lignocaine gargle, and an injection of morphine a short while before the procedure is to be performed. When ready, 2 ml. of 4 per cent lignocaine are squirted over the back of the tongue to anaesthetise the glottis, and the procedure repeated at once. The patient is best intubated sitting up with neck flexed forward and head extended at the atlanto-occipital joint, and an endotracheal tube may be passed orally under direct vision with a laryngoscope. For cases *in extremis* no analgesia is necessary. A suction catheter should be passed down the endotracheal tube and, by posturing the patient, it is possible to enter either main bronchus. A more efficient toilet may be performed by using a bronchoscope under the same form of analgesia, but if he has a full set of teeth it is more unpleasant for the patient. In either event, although plugs of mucus may in fact be removed, it seems probable that the amount of coughing that is caused is a factor of predominant importance in relatively dry cases.

In neonatal life, movement, postural drainage and gentle percussion over the affected side are often sufficient to encourage re-expansion of an area of collapsed lung, but if these fail or the baby's general condition deteriorates rapidly an endotracheal tube or suckling's bronchoscope should be speedily passed and the mucus sucked away. It may even be necessary to assist respiration for some period of time and this is best done manually by intermittent positive-pressure through a suitable anaesthetic system (Rees, 1958).

Tracheostomy and artificial ventilation.—If the above methods fail and the patient continues to deteriorate, more active interference must be considered.

Prolonged endotracheal intubation is unsuitable if repeated aspiration is required. It is unpleasant for the patient, who will usually need additional sedation in order to tolerate the tube. This further impairs coughing, depresses respiration and a vicious circle is thus created. Thus, if coughing continues to be inadequate despite vigorous physiotherapy and several episodes of endotracheal suction, a tracheostomy may have to be considered. If the patient is co-operative but too weak or in too much pain to cough effectively, a period of assisted ventilation via a mouth-piece using a triggered ventilator (see Chapter 15, p. 465) may be sufficient to tide him over a difficult period. The value of this technique lies mainly in relieving the patient of the work and discomfort of breathing. Short rest periods achieved in this way enable the patient to summon up enough energy to cough effectively and thus get out of difficulty. This method requires patience and understanding by the operator, who must train the patient to use the apparatus. In selected patients facing an elective operation, pre-operative training can be of value, particularly prior to thoracic or cardiac surgery. If the staff and facilities needed for this technique are not available or if the patient fails to respond to it, a tracheostomy becomes necessary. It should be performed under general anaesthesia with an endotracheal tube in place. Tracheostomy enables secretions to be aspirated repeatedly and effectively and facilitates the use of mechanical ventilation.

Artificial ventilation.—Sykes *et al.* (1969) have summarised well the indications for ventilatory assistance in this situation.

Ventilatory assistance is usually required if the arterial P_{CO_2} rises above 55–60 mm. Hg. In elderly patients and those who are severely ill, it may be required before this level is reached, while in those who are known to have chronic bronchitis and emphysema with a raised P_{CO_2} before operation, higher levels of P_{CO_2} may be allowed before tracheostomy is performed. When reaching a decision, it is important to take into account all the circumstance of the case and to observe the patient's morale, level of consciousness and general appearance.

Much of the improvement resulting from mechanical ventilation is due to the abolition of the work of breathing and the reduction in oxygen consumption which results (Thung *et al.*, 1963).

Drugs.—In the presence of recent pulmonary collapse the use of drugs to produce an involuntary bout of coughing may be of some value, although they must be combined with the procedures already outlined. Thus the intravenous injection of 3 ml. of nikethamide will cause a sudden deep breath and often strong coughing.

Antibiotics can be used with value to control the secondary infection which always takes place in the collapsed area and to treat all types of acute bronchitis. Antibiotics should only be used if the sputum is obviously purulent. A suitable specimen must first be obtained and dispatched to the laboratory for microscopy, culture and determination of antibiotic sensitivity of the predominant organism. The indiscriminate use of antibiotics should be deplored. It is likely to do more harm than good, by allowing overgrowth of antibiotic-resistant organisms. Antibiotics should therefore be restricted to cases where there is good evidence that the complication is or has become primarily one of infection.

A variety of mucolytic substances has recently been developed. They are

In such cases only small quantities of fluid may be concerned; in fact there may be no obvious history of vomiting or regurgitation and still less evidence of actual aspiration, while in several reported instances the patients have recovered full consciousness after the causative episode and before the onset of symptoms. Thus the connection between vomiting and this pulmonary complication may conceivably be disregarded or lost. As a syndrome it seems most commonly to occur in obstetrics, although cases have been met in other branches of surgery. This is surprising because equal opportunities for aspiration occur in general surgical emergencies, and it may be that the susceptibility of the obstetric patient to the effects of gastric inhalation is greater than others. Indeed Hausmann and Lunt (1955) have suggested that acute adrenal failure accounts for the difference. They consider that after delivery the loss of the placenta, an organ which is partly responsible for the increase in ACTH and gluco-corticoids normally found in pregnancy, the patient is in no state to stand a sudden and severe stress, such as that produced by the effects of gastric inhalation.

Treatment.—Treatment should first be aimed at prevention (see Chapters 47 and 53). Taylor and Pryse-Davies (1966) have drawn attention to the importance of the acidity of the aspirated fluid. Animal experiments have shown that when the pH of this fluid is more acid than 2·5 pulmonary oedema and bronchoconstriction result, whereas solutions which are more alkaline merely lead to acute bronchitis and broncho-pneumonia. In an investigation of 60 patients in labour, Taylor and Pryse-Davies found that the pH of the gastric contents was more acid than 2·5 in 43 per cent of the cases. Furthermore, if such patients were given as little as 15 ml. of an antacid (magnesium tricilicate) to swallow, then within fifteen minutes the pH was no longer within the danger range. The prophylactic administration of an antacid has therefore been advocated to reduce the incidence of Mendelson's syndrome in the obstetrical patient. Should aspiration be known to occur, removal by suction must be attempted, though this is disappointing when only small quantities of fluid are concerned. If the immediate general condition of the patient warrants it, bronchoscopic aspiration and flushing of the major bronchi with large quantities of saline has been recommended. As much as two or three hundred millilitres may be used, and most of this will be rapidly absorbed from the lower respiratory tract. When severe symptoms develop treatment must be more symptomatic than specific, and the use of antispasmodics and oxygen, supplemented by antibiotics to control secondary infection, are the principal stand-bys. Hausmann and Lunt (1955) have reported successful results from the immediate use of intravenous hydrocortisone to combat the potential adrenal failure. They recommend that 100 mg. should be given within four hours. In any event hydrocortisone is likely to be useful should bronchiolar spasm and oedema occur.

Unfortunately the adoption of these methods of treatment has not noticeably decreased either the incidence or the severity of the syndrome. Its occurrence is unpredictable and occasional. It by no means always follows aspiration of acid gastric contents. Bronchoscopy following known aspiration is not without risk: it may cause further episodes of inhalation and increase hypoxia. There is little evidence to support the use of bronchial lavage and it does not appear to be an effective prophylactic method (Adams *et al.*, 1969). The prophylactic administration of an antacid has also proved ineffective (Adams *et al.*, 1969) and may increase the likelihood of vomiting during induction by filling the stomach and promoting gastric secretion. If pulmonary oedema is severe, mechanical ventilation may be required for days or even weeks (McCormick *et al.*, 1966; Adams *et al.*, 1969). Extremely high inflation pressures may be required both to overcome the airway resistance and to maintain high enough minute volumes to compensate for the effects of the severe ventilation/ perfusion inequalities which occur.

TUBERCULOSIS

Cross-infection from anaesthetic apparatus contaminated through previous use on a case of pulmonary tuberculosis has not been shown to occur in practice, although, as might be expected, clinical records which could be correlated back to such an incident would be difficult, if not impossible, to obtain. Careful bacteriological examination of apparatus used on infected cases has demonstrated, however, how remarkably difficult it is to show any evidence of tubercle bacilli at all. Nevertheless, precautions must be taken to prevent any chance of cross-infection and all apparatus must be properly sterilised after use (see Appendix 3).

Pulmonary tuberculosis occurring in the post-operative period is almost always due to a latent lesion becoming active. The points concerned are not so much the use of local or general anaesthesia, nor of actual individual agents, as the impact of a large number of individual factors, such as are at work in the picture of post-operative pulmonary collapse, on a patient with latent tuberculosis. Care must be exercised in the use of intermittent positive-pressure respiration for cases with recently healed foci, since it is presumably possible to break down adhesions by excessive movement and pressure. The natural resistance of the patient is diminished in the immediate post-operative period, while any area of collapsed lung is a potential source of spread from infected sputum. Cases with known active pulmonary tuberculosis are potential candidates for spread of the disease, but it must not be supposed that the risk is greater should general anaesthesia be used in preference to local analgesia. The latter may be a more expedient method in certain circumstances, but the incidence of tuberculosis-spread, like that of all pulmonary complications, does not differ after either form of anaesthesia, provided each is competently administered.

REFERENCES

Adams, A. P., Morgan, M., Jones, B. C., and McCormick, P. W. (1969). A case of massive aspiration of gastric contents during obstetric anaesthesia. *Brit. J. Anaesth.*, **41,** 176.

Alexander, I. G. S. (1968). The ultrastructure of the pulmonary alveolar vessels in Mendelson's (acid pulmonary aspiration) syndrome. *Brit. J. Anaesth.*, **40,** 408.

Anscombe, A. R. (1957). In: *Pulmonary Complications of Abdominal Surgery*, p. 56. London: Lloyd-Luke (Medical Books).

Bethune, D. W., Edmonds-Seal, J., and Gabriel, R. W. (1968). Medical Research Council questionnaire for preoperative assessment of the chronic bronchitis patient. A comparison with spirometry. *Lancet*, **1,** 277.

Brock, R. C. (1946). Studies in lung abscess. *Guy's Hosp. Rep.*, **95,** 40.

Bromage, P. R. (1954). *Spinal Epidural Analgesia.* Edinburgh: E. & S. Livingstone.

COLLINS, C. D., DARKE, C. S., and KNOWELDEN, J. (1968). Chest complications after upper abdominal surgery: their anticipation and prevention. *Brit. med. J.*, **1**, 401.

DIAMENT, M. L., and PALMER, K. N. V. (1967). Spirometry for preoperative assessment of airways resistance. *Lancet*, **1**, 1251.

ELLIS, G. (1955). Anaesthesia and the common cold. *Anaesthesia*, **10**, 78.

FRY, I. K., and EARL, C. J. (1950). Report on preliminary investigation into incidence of inhalation of blood and other debris during dental extraction under general anaesthesia in upright position. *Guy's Hosp. Rep.*, **99**, 41.

GARDNER, A. M. N. (1958). Aspiration of food and vomit. *Quart. J. Med.*, **27**, 227.

HALMAGYI, D. F. J. (1961). Lung changes and incidence of respiratory arrest in rats after aspiration of sea and fresh water. *J. appl. Physiol.*, **16**, 41.

HALMAGYI, D. F. J., and COLEBATCH, J. H. (1961). Ventilation and circulation after fluid aspiration. *J. appl. Physiol.*, **16**, 35.

HAMILTON, W. F., and MORGAN, A. B. (1932). Mechanism of postural reduction in vital capacity in relation to orthopnea and storage of blood in lungs. *Amer. J. Physiol.*, **99**, 526.

HAUSMANN, W., and LUNT, R. L. (1955). The problem of the treatment of peptic aspiration pneumonia following obstetric anaesthesia (Mendelson's syndrome). *J. Obstet. Gynaec. Brit. Emp.*, **62**, 509.

LEINER, G. C., ABRAMOWITZ, S., LEWIS, W. A., and SMALL, M. J. (1965). Dyspnea and pulmonary function tests. *Amer. Rev. resp. Dis.*, **92**, 822.

LODER, R. E. (1955). Routine pre-operative chest radiography: analysis of 1,000 cases. *Lancet*, **1**, 1150.

LUCAS, B. G. B. (1944). Pulmonary complications following simple herniorrhaphy. *Proc. roy. Soc. Med.*, **37**, 145.

MCCORMICK, P. W., HAY, R. G., and GRIFFIN, R. W. (1966). Pulmonary aspiration of gastric contents in obstetric patients. *Lancet*, **1**, 1127.

MEDICAL RESEARCH COUNCIL REPORT (1965). Definition and classification of chronic bronchitis for clinical and epidemiological purposes. *Lancet*, **1**, 775.

MENDELSON, C. L. (1946). Aspiration of stomach contents into lungs during obstetric anesthesia. *Amer. J. Obstet. Gynec.*, **52**, 181.

MIMPRISS, T. W., and ETHERIDGE, F. G. (1944). Post-operative chest complications in gastric surgery. *Brit. med. J.*, **1**, 466.

MORLE, K. D. F., and ROBERTSON, P. W. (1953). Segmental aspiration pneumonia and bronchiectasis. *Brit. med. J.*, **1**, 130.

MORTON, H. J. V. (1944). Tobacco smoking and pulmonary complications after operation. *Lancet*, **1**, 368.

NOSWORTHY, M. D. (1944). Bronchoscopy in the prevention and treatment of traumatic and post-operative pulmonary lesions. *Proc. roy. Soc. Med.*, **37**, 303.

NUNN, J. F., and PAYNE, J. P. (1962). Hypoxaemia after general anaesthesia. *Lancet*, **2**, 631.

PALMER, K. N. V., and SELLICK, B. A. (1953). The prevention of post-operative pulmonary atelectasis. *Lancet*, **1**, 164.

PHILLIPS, I. (1966). Postoperative respiratory-tract infections with *Pseudomonas aeruginosa* due to contaminated lignocaine jelly. *Lancet*, **1**, 903.

POOLER, H. E. (1949). The relief of post-operative pain and its influence on the vital capacity. *Brit. med. J.*, **2**, 1200.

REES, G. J. (1958). Communication read at the Annual Meeting of the Association of Anaesthetists of Great Britain and Ireland.

SIMPSON, B. R., PARKHOUSE, J., MARSHALL, R., and LAMBRECHTS, W. (1961). Extradural analgesia and the prevention of postoperative respiratory complications. *Brit. J. Anaesth.*, **33**, 628.

STOREY, G. M. (1955). *Thoracic Surgery for Physiotherapists*. London: Faber & Faber.

STRINGER, P. (1947). Atelectasis after partial gastrectomy. *Lancet*, **1,** 289.

SYKES, M. K., MCNICOL, M. W., and CAMPBELL, E. J. M. (1969). In: *Respiratory Failure*, p. 227. Oxford: Blackwell Scientific Publications.

TAYLOR, G., and PRYSE-DAVIES, J. (1966). The prophylactic use of antacids in the prevention of the acid-pulmonary-aspiration syndrome (Mendelson's syndrome). *Lancet*, **1,** 288.

THUNG, N., HERZOG, P., CHRISTLIEB, I. I., and THOMPSON, W. M. (1963). The cost of respiratory effort in postoperative cardiac patients. *Circulation*, **28,** 552.

VAN ALLEN, C. M., LINDSKOG, G. E., and RICHTER, H. G. (1931). Collateral respiration, transfer of air collaterally between pulmonary lobules. *J. clin. Invest.*, **10,** 559.

WHIGHTMAN, J. A. K. (1968). A prospective study of the incidence of postoperative pulmonary complications. *Brit. J. Surg.*, **55,** 85.

FURTHER READING

ANSCOMBE, A. R. (1957). *Pulmonary Complications of Abdominal Surgery*. London: Lloyd-Luke (Medical Books).

Chapter 15

ARTIFICIAL RESPIRATION

by

G. T. Spencer

During normal spontaneous respiration air is drawn into the lungs by expansion of the thoracic cavity and expelled during passive relaxation of the respiratory muscles, aided by the elasticity of the lungs themselves. Adequate gaseous exchange is thereby maintained. Failure of any of the structures involved in this process may lead to inadequate gaseous exchange which must then be maintained artificially until the failure has been corrected. Many methods of maintaining ventilation artificially have been described and Whittenberger (1955) has classified them under five headings:

1. Manual manipulation of the thoracic cage.
2. Gas pressure applied to the upper respiratory tract.
3. Pressure changes applied to the trunk but not the head.
4. Displacement of sub-diaphragmatic structures.
5. Electrical stimulation of the respiratory muscles.

History

Chapter Four of the Second Book of Kings in the Old Testament contains a remarkable account of the resuscitation of an apparently dead Shunammite child by the Prophet Elisha. Verses 34 and 35 read:

> "And he went up, and lay upon the child, and put his mouth upon his mouth, and his eyes upon his eyes, and his hands upon his hands: and he stretched himself upon the child; and the flesh of the child waxed warm . . . and the child sneezed seven times, and the child opened his eyes".

We are not told where Elisha learnt the technique, but this possibly represents the first recorded account of resuscitation which may have been by artificial respiration.

The idea that drowned or collapsed people might be restored to life by artificial respiration recurs sporadically throughout recorded history, and has been entertainingly reviewed by Shackleton (1962). The first attempt to consider the problem constructively was made in Amsterdam in 1769, when the "Society for the Recovery of Drowned Persons" was formed. Interest in the subject rapidly increased and in 1796 Herholdt and Rafn published a monograph which has been translated into English by Poulsen (1960). The use of bellows for resuscitation was advocated by John Hunter, who invented a two-way bellows for the purpose (Hunter, 1776). The Royal Humane Society continued to recommend this method until 1837, when it was abandoned in favour of artificial ventilation by manual compression of the thoracic cage. This method persisted until Safar *et al.* (1958) showed that intermittent positive-pressure inflation of the lungs produced more efficient ventilation than manual compression.

The possibility that artificial inflation of the lungs by positive pressure might be applicable to respiratory failure during anaesthesia was missed by Hewitt (1901) who advocated the use of Sylvester's method and it was not until Gale and Waters (1932) suggested that pulmonary collapse during thoracic operations might be prevented by positive-pressure ventilation achieved by intermittent inflation of the reservoir bag, that the method was used in anaesthesia. Since the introduction of muscle relaxants it has become a standard technique. This method was first used to treat patients with long-term respiratory failure during the great epidemic of poliomyelitis in Copenhagen in 1952. Lassen (1953) working with Ibsen, used a Waters' canister and reservoir bag to give intermittent positive-pressure ventilation. This was continued for periods of up to three months by relays of medical students who were paid 30/- per 8-hour shift to squeeze the bag. He described the method as "bag ventilation" and it was applied via an endotracheal tube, or cuffed tracheostomy tube. During the subsequent years the method was extensively developed and medical students replaced by mechanical ventilators.

Artificial ventilation by intermittent positive pressure (I.P.P.R.) applied mechanically via a cuffed tracheostomy tube or endotracheal tube has now become the standard method of acute treatment for respiratory failure from many causes, some of which are outlined below. Manual manipulation of the thoracic cage was used mainly for emergency resuscitation by the methods of Holger Nielsen, Silvester and Schafer. These techniques are now obsolete. Pressure changes applied to the trunk but not the head, and displacement of subdiaphragmatic structures are still useful methods of assisting the ventilation of certain patients with permanent weakness of the muscles of respiration (see below); electrical stimulation of the respiratory muscles has rarely been found to be a useful practical procedure and has been abandoned.

FIRST AID METHODS

Resuscitation of partly drowned or asphyxiated subjects is often necessary when apparatus and equipment are not to hand. External cardiac massage by chest compression combined with simple methods of artificial ventilation has very greatly increased the chances of success in emergency resuscitation. Safar *et al.* (1958) and Poulsen *et al.* (1959) have shown convincingly that expired air or mouth-to-mouth respiration is more effective in maintaining normal, or even increased, volumes of ventilation than manual compression of the chest. Subsequent work has confirmed these findings and the following methods are now widely accepted, taught and practised. The World Federation of Societies of Anaesthesiologists (Poulsen, 1968) has recently produced an excellent manual on which teaching should be based.

Mouth-to-Mouth Resuscitation

The rescuer approaches the subject's head from the side and supports the upper airway by inserting his thumb between the teeth, grasping the mandible and pulling it forcefully upwards. The rescuer's mouth is placed on the subject's mouth and the subject's lungs are inflated by forcible expiration which the rescuer repeats 10–15 times per minute. An alternative technique in which the rescuer inflates via the subject's nose has been described. A possible advantage of this route is that there is less likelihood of inflating the stomach and therefore of regurgitation.

In addition to the observation that ventilation is more efficient by these methods, other advantages over manual compression methods are claimed:

1. If the airway becomes obstructed, the rescuer senses resistance.
2. If secretions or vomit accumulate, he feels and hears gurgling.
3. Expansion of the chest during inflation can be watched.
4. The return of spontaneous respiration can be felt.
5. Both the rescuer's hands are available for airway toilet and jaw support.
6. Positive pressure during inflation may make ventilation possible in patients with a high airway resistance caused by foreign material in the lungs.
7. It is suitable for neonates and children.

The disadvantages of mouth-to-mouth resuscitation are:

1. If the airway is not perfectly clear, or if the airway resistance is high, air may pass into the subject's stomach, thus increasing the likelihood of regurgitation or vomiting.
2. With the patient in the supine position, fluid or vomitus may enter the lungs before its presence is appreciated.
3. It is usually aesthetically unpleasant and in some circumstances may be sufficiently unacceptable to cause serious delay in starting resuscitation.
4. It cannot usually be maintained for more than 15 minutes without producing fairly severe dizziness in the rescuer.
5. It cannot be used on subjects who have inhaled noxious vapours.

It is now generally recognised that mouth-to-mouth or mouth-to-nose resuscitation is the most satisfactory method available for emergency use. Anaesthetists, therefore, have an important role to play in educating the lay public in these techniques, which should always be taught for preference.

ARTIFICIAL RESPIRATION USING SIMPLE APPARATUS

While it may be essential to perform artificial respiration at the scene of an accident with no apparatus at all, the use of simple apparatus can greatly increase the convenience and efficiency of the procedure and therefore the chances of a successful outcome. Apparatus of the type described below should be available in all hospital wards and departments, and as far as possible in ambulances, first aid posts, and general practitioners' bags.

The Brook Airway (Fig. 1*a*)

A wide variety of airways and connections have been developed in attempts to make mouth-to-mouth respiration less unpleasant to perform, and to make it

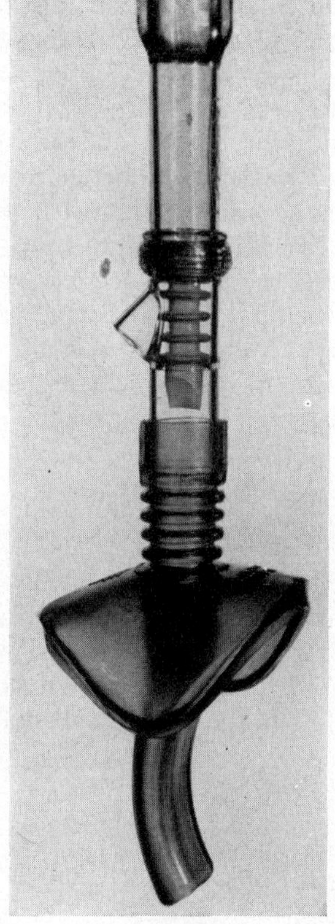

15/FIG. 1(*a*).—The Brook Airway.

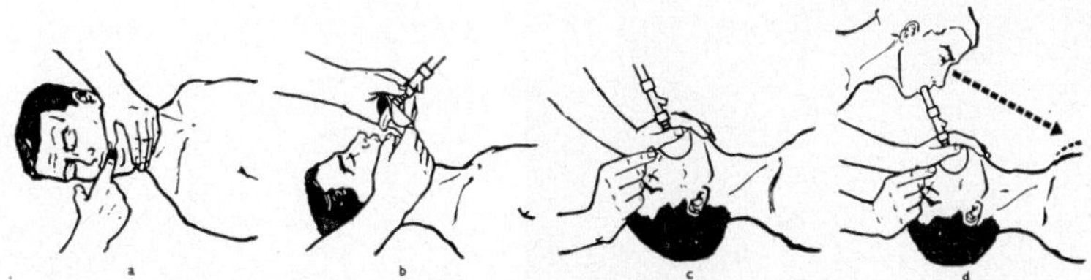

15/FIG. 1(*b*).—Mouth-to-mouth resuscitation using the Brook airway. (*a*) Place victim on back. Quickly clear mouth and throat of foreign matter with fingers. Tilt head fully back. (*b*) Insert airway over tongue until mouth-guard covers lips. (*c*) Raise the chin, and maintain this position with the same hand that holds the airway in place. Pinch nostrils closed to prevent air leakage. (*d*) Take a deep breath and blow into airway. Watch for chest rise. Between breaths listen for sound of air returning from the victim. Repeat every 3–4 seconds.

easier for untrained operators to maintain a clear airway. Of these devices, the Brook airway has particular advantages and has maintained its place since it was first described by Brook *et al.*, 1962. It consists of an intra-oral section shaped like a pharyngeal airway. This is connected to a flange designed to maintain an airtight fit on the patient's lips. A tube projects from the airway section and flange. It contains a simple one-way valve, allowing expired air from the patient to pass out through a short side-arm rather than through the operator's mouthpiece. The apparatus is constructed of transparent plastic so that the presence of vomit can be easily seen. In use the operator stands above the patient's head and inserts the airway section into the patient's mouth until the flange fits closely over the lips (Fig. 1*b*). One hand is used to support the patient's jaw and the other to close the nostrils. The operator is then conveniently placed to watch the movements of the chest as he inflates the lungs by blowing down the tube section of the device rhythmically 10–15 times a minute.

The Ambu Resuscitator (Fig. 2).

Ruben and Ruben (1957) have described a self-expanding bag attached to a Ruben non-rebreathing valve which enables intermittent positive-pressure respiration to be carried out with atmospheric air, which can be enriched with oxygen as required. The apparatus can be connected to an endotracheal or tracheostomy tube, or applied to the patient via an anaesthetic face-mask. When

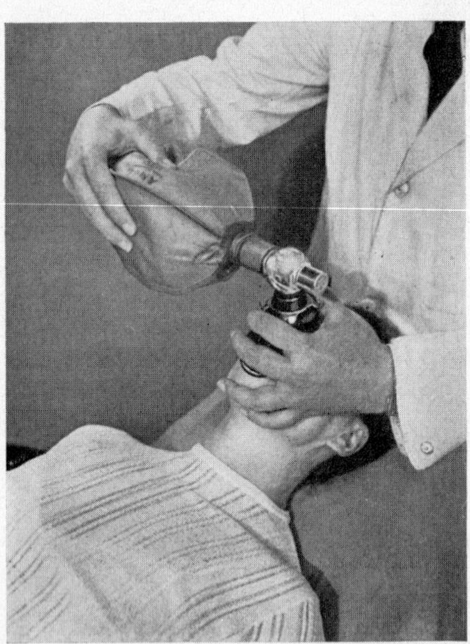

15/Fig. 2.—The Ambu resuscitator, as described by Ruben and Ruben.

the bag is squeezed, a one-way valve at the distal end closes and air is forced into the patient via the Ruben non-rebreathing valve. During expiration, expired air passes out through the expiratory part of the non-rebreathing valve, and fresh atmospheric air is drawn into the self-expanding bag through the one-way valve at the distal end. Self-expansion of the bag is achieved by lining it with sponge rubber. The apparatus has two disadvantages:

1. It is sometimes difficult for untrained people to obtain an airtight fit of the mask on the patient's face, and the mask may conceal the presence of vomit.
2. If the resistance to inflation is high (50 cm. H_2O), air in the bag is compressed into the sponge rubber rather than forced into the lungs. This effect can be partly overcome by compressing the bag against the side of the patient's face.

Modifications of this apparatus are now available in which self-inflation of the bag is achieved without the need for sponge rubber.

The Ruben non-rebreathing valve. (Fig. 3). (Ruben, 1955).—This valve has a dead space of 9 cm. and a resistance of 0·8 cm. H_2O during inspiration and of 1 cm. H_2O during expiration at flow rates of 25 litres per minute. The expiratory resistance can be reduced to very low levels by removing the disc in the outlet channel when the valve is used for positive-pressure respiration. In this form the valve is not suitable for spontaneous respiration during anaesthesia because the patient will inspire air through the expiratory part.

The Ambu Hesse Valve (Fig. 3).—This valve has advantages over the Ruben valve. It has a lower deadspace and flow resistance. At 25 litres per minute the resistance during inspiration is 0·4 cm. H_2O and during expiration 0·6 cm. H_2O. Excessive positive pressure will overcome the expiratory valve and allow excess gases to escape. In contrast to the Ruben valve it is quiet in operation and can be sterilised by autoclaving.

The Resusci Folding Bag (Mark I). (Figs. 4*a-d*)

This is a simplified version of the Ambu resuscitator which eliminates some of its disadvantages. The transparent, self-inflating, folding bag has a simple one-way valve at each end. These valves allow the recovering patient to make spontaneous inspiratory efforts as resuscitation proceeds. A supplementary oxygen point is incorporated into the distal valve, and the proximal valve has exhaust ports around its outer edge which prevent expired air from re-entering the bag (see Fig. 4*a*). The face-mask is transparent, allowing vomit to be seen at once, and mask and bag can be folded into a small box for storage and portability. A more sophisticated version of the Resusci Folding Bag, namely the Mark II, is also available. It is more suitable for hospital and anaesthetic use.

The Oxford Inflating Bellows (Fig. 5).

Macintosh (1953) has designed a small hand-unit consisting of bellows with a pair of unidirectional valves for inflating the lungs. The concertina reservoir bag contains a spiral spring so that it automatically refills after each forced inspiration, while the valves prevent rebreathing. The unit can be used in anaesthesia in conjunction with an air draw-over inhaler such as the E.M.O. (see Chapter 9), with the patient breathing spontaneously. When used for positive-pressure ventilation for more than short periods it is necessary to include a non-rebreathing valve adjacent to the patient. These bellows formed the basis of the early version of the Radcliffe ventilator (Russell and Schuster, 1953). A

weight was dropped on the bellows during inspiration, and lifted by an electric motor operating through a bicycle three-speed gear during expiration.

Mechanical Devices

In recent years a number of mechanical devices have been developed to assist ambulance and other paramedical personnel in maintaining artificial ventilation while patients are transported to hospital. They are usually pneumatically driven from an oxygen cylinder and are applied to the patient via a face-mask. This development is undesirable and should be condemned. Performing effective artificial respiration in an emergency requires the continuous attention of the rescuer. To apply and adjust a machine can only distract this attention and may delay the recognition of airway obstruction or the presence of vomit. If the airway is not perfectly clear these machines are liable to inflate the stomach and thus provoke vomiting.

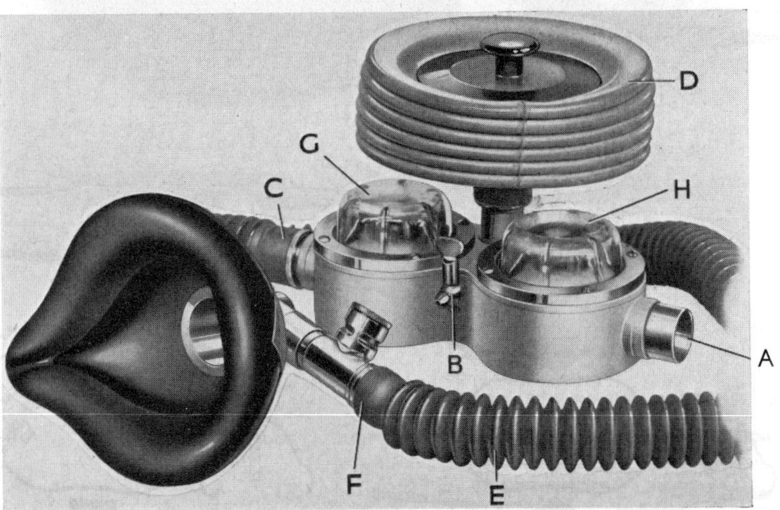

15/Fig. 5.—The Oxford inflating bellows.

A. Air inlet; B. Inlet tube and tap for oxygen; C. Air outlet to patient; D. Concertina reservoir bag; E. Corrugated tubing; F. Spring valve; G. and H. Gravity-operated unidirectional flow valves.

ARTIFICIAL RESPIRATION WITH MECHANICAL VENTILATORS

There is no doubt that a mechanical apparatus properly used is the most efficient means of ventilating the lungs for long periods. Artificial respiration, by any known method, involves a disturbance to normal respiratory physiology. By altering intrathoracic pressure relations it also causes changes in circulatory physiology. Over short periods these changes may be insignificant, but their significance increases as their duration increases. Mechanical ventilators should be designed to cause the minimum possible upset to normal physiology, and the aim of medical and nursing care must be to correct or compensate for whatever disturbance is unavoidable.

Pressure to the Outside of the Body

Tank ventilators (Cabinet respirators, "Iron Lungs").—The first power-driven tank ventilator was invented by Professor P. Drinker, an engineer of Harvard, U.S.A., and although modern tank ventilators have been modified in attempts to make them more convenient to use, and a positive phase added to the negative phase, the principles of operation remain the same. The patient is placed in a rigid tank from which only his head protrudes. Access to his body is obtained either by placing him on a couch which can be slid out of the tank, or by using a tank whose upper half will hinge open like an alligator's jaws. An airtight fit is obtained round the patient's neck using a flexible collar split into two sections. It must be carefully padded to prevent pressure sores developing and a tracheostomy is best avoided if a tank ventilator is to be used. Minor nursing attention can be carried out through ports in the side of the tank. The tank is connected to large mechanically operated bellows.

During inspiration the bellows expand, creating a subatmospheric pressure of 15–30 cm. H_2O within the tank. Air is drawn into the patient's lungs until the elastic resistance of the lungs and chest wall equals the pressure difference between the inside and outside of the tank. Inspiration must be maintained for long enough to allow equilibration to occur. This usually takes 1–2 seconds, but if the airway resistance is high due to bronchial narrowing, accumulation of secretions, or partial obstruction of the upper airway as may occur during sleep, equilibration takes longer and may not be obtained. Ventilation may therefore be seriously reduced. During expiration the bellows contract, pressure in the tank rises to atmospheric, and air flows out of the lungs passively due to their elastic recoil. Expiration may be assisted by applying a positive pressure to the inside of the tank.

With the advent of intermittent positive pressure to the upper airway, the use of tank ventilators has declined. Their disadvantages are that they are cumbersome and difficult to use. Pulmonary atelectasis and accumulation of secretions can be difficult to prevent, although this problem can be largely

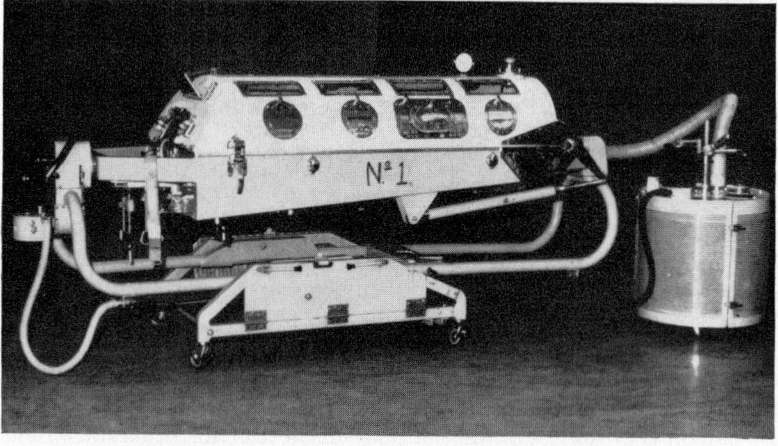

15/Fig. 6.—The Kelleher rotating tank ventilator (Kelleher, 1961).

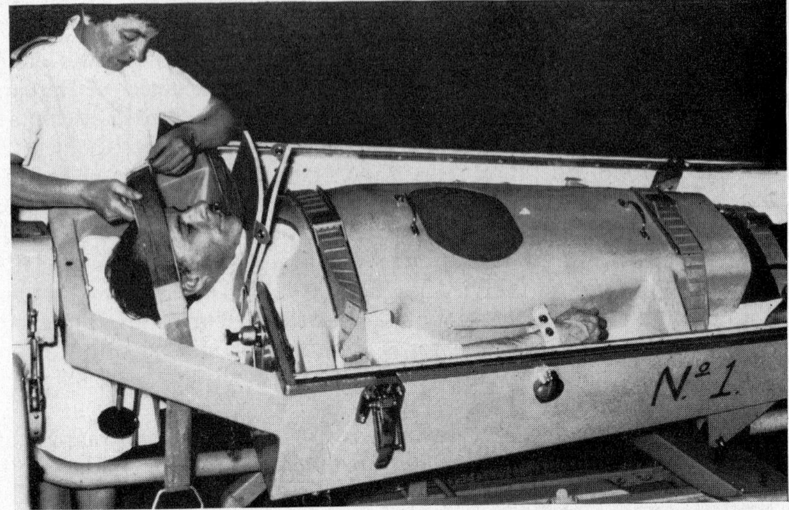

(*a*)

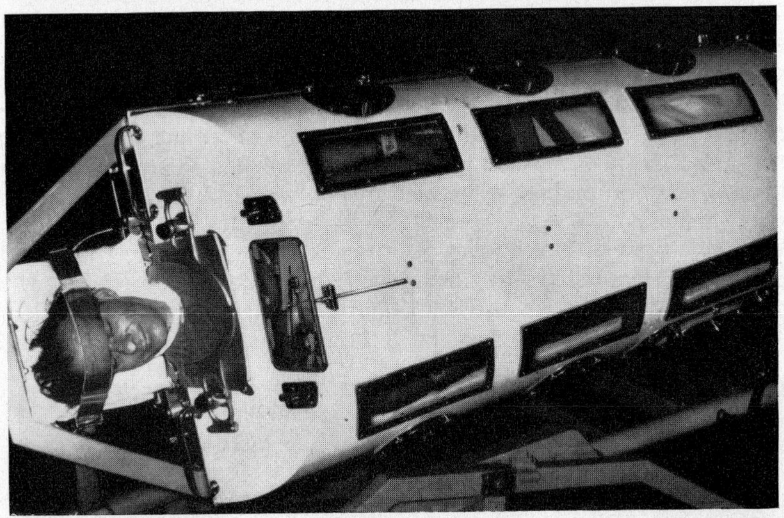

(*b*)

15/Fig. 7 (*see opposite*).

overcome by using the Kelleher rotating ventilator (Kelleher, 1961) (Fig. 6). The tank section of this machine can be rotated through a complete circle on its long axis. A section of matress can then be removed and the posterior aspect of the thorax is accessible for auscultation and physiotherapy (Figs. 7*a*–*c*).

The collar of a tank ventilator makes a tracheostomy difficult to manage. Thus, if the muscles of the pharynx and larnyx are paralysed, or if the patient is unconscious, vomiting and regurgitation become a desperate hazard. The supine patient is powerless to prevent pharyngeal contents being drawn into the lungs by the inspiratory stroke of the bellows. Even for the conscious patient

(c)

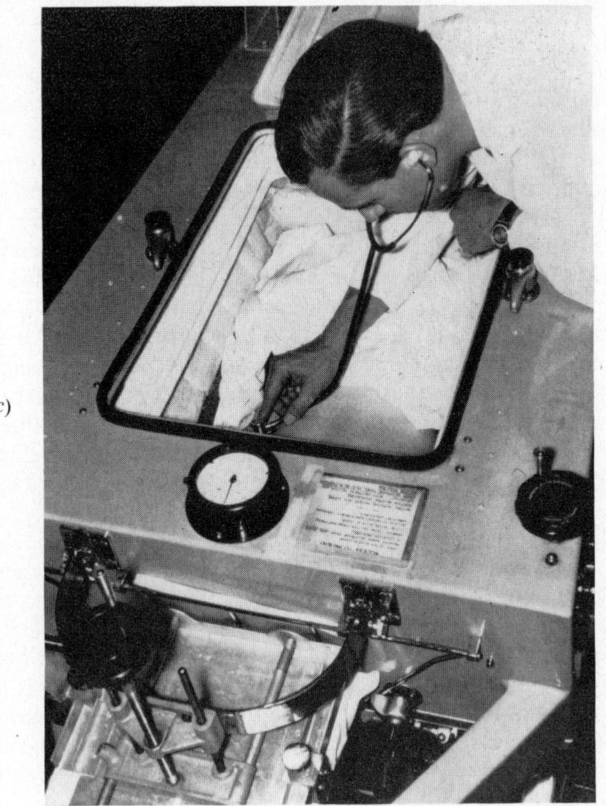

15/Fig. 7.—The Kelleher Rotating Tank Ventilator in Use.

(*a*) To rotate the patient into the prone position a shell, shaped to the body, is strapped into position inside the tank.

(*b*) The tank is rotated around its long axis with a forehead strap holding the patient's head.

(*c*) A section of mattress is removable allowing ausculation and physiotherapy to the posterior thorax.

with a normal pharynx, vomiting in a tank ventilator is hazardous. Should it occur, an access port should be opened immediately to equalise pressures and prevent aspiration.

Despite these disadvantages, there is no doubt that tank ventilators still retain a place in clinical practice (Kelleher, 1969; Spencer, 1969; Beaver, 1969). They are primarily used in the long-term management of patients with severe weakness of the respiratory muscles, but whose laryngeal and pharyngeal muscles are intact (see below under Poliomyelitis). Many such patients can breathe adequately while conscious, using techniques such as glossopharyngeal breathing (Ardran *et al.*, 1959), but require assistance during sleep. Tank ventilators may also be of value to these patients in tiding them over an acute respiratory infection. Their great advantage is that tracheostomy is avoided, normal use of the voice and the ability to perform glossopharyngeal breathing are retained, and subsequent machinery dependence is not increased.

Tank ventilators are also occasionally necessary for patients in whom tracheostomy and tracheal catheter suction are impossible, for example in haemophiliacs.

Cuirass ventilators.—The cuirass ventilator consists of a rigid shell held over the thorax and abdomen. It makes contact with the skin only at its edges with a padded rubber rim, which must fit sufficiently well to form an airtight seal. A bellows is connected to the shell and produces a subatmospheric pressure during inspiration. Unfortunately, the presence of the shell along the lateral side of the thoracic cage tends to splint the lower ribs. Inspiration is therefore mainly diaphragmatic. A modification of the cuirass which overcomes this difficulty to some extent is the Tunnicliffe breathing jacket. It incorporates a similar rigid shell, which is somewhat smaller in size than that of the cuirass. An airtight fit is achieved by enclosing the whole of the upper half of the body, except the head, in a soft jacket, with elastic tapes round the elbows, neck and waist. The Tunnicliffe jacket will produce greater ventilation for a given subatmospheric pressure than the cuirass (Spalding and Opie, 1958), but neither is as efficient as the tank and they can only be used as respiratory assistors in partly paralysed patients.

Belt ventilators.—The Bragg Paul Pneumobelt is the most widely used type and consists of an inflatable belt applied to the patient's abdomen. Inflation causes the diaphragm to rise, thus assisting expiration. Inspiration occurs by gravity, if the patient is sitting, or by what muscle power is available if the patient is lying. A belt ventilator is unobtrusive and portable, but somewhat limited in the amount of respiratory assistance which it can produce. This is because the expiratory reserve volume is only about one-third that of the inspiratory reserve volume (see Chapter 4). Bronchial calibre decreases during expiration and a belt ventilator may tend to promote atelectasis of the lower parts of the lung.

Displacement of Subdiaphragmatic Structures

Schuster and Fischer-Williams (1953) have described a motor-driven rocking bed which will produce an arc of swing of a little more than 40;. Bryce-Smith and Davis (1954) using a similar bed on a paralysed apnoeic patient in the supine position, were unable to obtain a tidal volume above 282 ml. Despite its inefficiency, some patients prefer this method of respiratory assistance to any other, because it leaves them unencumbered.

Pressure Applied to the Upper Respiratory Tract—Intermittent Positive-Pressure Respiration (I.P.P.R.)

This is now much the most widely used form of artificial ventilation. Its short term use by manual squeezing of the reservoir bag has been practised in anaesthesia for at least thirty years, and many ventilators have been designed for use during anaesthesia. Although this relieves the anaesthetist of his duties in bag squeezing, the value of mechanical ventilators during anaesthesia remains debatable. Intermittent positive-pressure respiration has become a vast subject in its own right, and as always in such instances has generated its own jargon, not all of which is either intelligible to the outsider or a credit to the English language. The peripatetic correspondent of *The Lancet* recently quoted from a published paper: "The patient was trached and respiratored machinewise".

The principle of I.P.P.R. is that the patient's upper airway is connected by tubing to a machine containing bellows. During inspiration the bellows contract—either mechanically or by gas pressure from without—and air is forced into the patient's lungs. Expiration is either passive, due to the elastic recoil of the patient's lungs and chest wall, or is assisted by applying a subatmospheric phase to the upper airway. Although the latter may be of benefit to the circulation of certain patients by reducing the intrathoracic pressure and aiding venous return, it carries a respiratory cost in that physiological dead space is increased and a larger inspiratory volume must be used.

The advantages of I.P.P.R. are that the patient is free of apparatus—apart from the connecting tubes—and can be easily nursed and cared for. Fully adequate ventilation can be produced for patients with all but the most severe forms of lung disease. Even here the limiting factor is usually circulatory embarrassment from high intrathoracic pressure, rather than an inability to achieve full ventilation (Bradley *et al.*, 1964). Although the presence of an endotracheal or tracheostomy tube is a disadvantage in some respects, it allows adequate removal of secretions by catheter suction to be carried out more efficiently than is possible with any other form of artificial respiration. There is no reason why, if treatment is properly carried out, the lungs should not remain clear and fully expanded throughout.

The disadvantages of I.P.P.R. all lie in the means by which the patient is connected to the ventilator. For long-term I.P.P.R. a tracheostomy is essential and a cuffed tracheostomy tube must be used. The patient is thus exposed to all the potential dangers and complications of tracheostomy, and in most cases is unable to use his voice. For shorter periods of I.P.P.R., such as during and after anaesthesia, an endotracheal tube may suffice, but this cannot be left in place for longer than a few days, or damage to the larynx may result. An endotracheal tube is poorly tolerated by many conscious patients and secretions may only be removed through it with difficulty. In certain circumstances it may be possible to administer I.P.P.R. through a mouthpiece or anaesthetic face-mask, but this technique is only suitable for short-term or intermittent use. The presence of a face-mask is often as distressing for the patient as that of a tracheostomy or endotracheal tube, while gastric inflation may occur if a high inspiratory pressure is needed, and inhalation of pharyngeal contents is likely if the laryngeal and pharyngeal reflexes are absent. Where the reflexes are present, the efficiency of ventilation may be impaired by the patient's inability to co-operate.

Triggered Ventilators

Many ventilators now available incorporate a device which allows the patient's respiration to be assisted rather than fully controlled. The inspiratory effort of the patient produces a slight subatmospheric pressure in the connecting tubing which—provided that the tubing is of small volume and non-expansile—can be made to trigger off the inspiratory phase of the ventilator and thereby augment the patient's respiratory efforts. To be effective, the pressure and flow rate from the ventilator must rise rapidly following the start of inspiration. In the absence of this pressure pattern the ventilator may follow the patient too slowly and resist the patient rather than assist him. Furthermore, there is evidence showing that a rapid pressure and flow rise at the start of inspiration is not the most efficient pressure pattern, particularly for a patient with chronic lung disease, yet it is for acute exacerbations of chronic lung disease that assisted respiration is most advocated. Many studies have been made of its use in this condition, and those which include arterial gas tension estimations indicate that the ventilatory benefit may be marginal.

Despite this lack of ventilatory gain there is no doubt that patient-triggered respiratory assistors often appear to be of great benefit to many patients. The benefit is greatest in conditions such as status asthmaticus, where the work of breathing is greatly increased. The early use of a triggered ventilator may stave off exhaustion and further deterioration, thus avoiding more radical therapeutic methods. Further, patients with heart or lung disease usually have a strictly limited total oxygen uptake. A reduction in respiratory work by the use of an assistor may thus have a double benefit in allowing oxygen, which would otherwise be consumed in breathing, to be available to other tissues.

Patient-triggering of the ventilator is also used in anaesthesia, where it may provide a useful guide to the degree of curarisation. However, when a patient continues to make respiratory efforts during an anaesthetic which may well have included the use of respiratory depressant drugs, as well as muscle relaxants, it suggests that carbon dioxide retention is present. Assisted positive-pressure respiration is valuable during the phase of weaning a patient suffering from respiratory paralysis from artificial ventilation. It often enables the patient to regain the use of his respiratory muscles more quickly than is possible by the alternative method of intermittent short bouts of spontaneous respiration.

An important requirement of a triggered—or patient-cycled—ventilator is that, should the patient cease to make respiratory efforts, the machine will continue to ventilate him, though usually at a slower rate than his spontaneous one. Some of the early patient-cycled ventilators did not include this feature and stopped altogether if the patient ceased to make spontaneous efforts.

Physiology of Artificial Respiration

Numerous studies of particular aspects of the physiological disturbances caused by artificial respiration have been made, notably that of Price *et al.* (1954). A comprehensive study of the subject was made by W. E. Watson, working at the respiration unit of the Churchill Hospital, Oxford (Watson, 1961), much of whose work is likely to become classical.

Intrathoracic Pressure

During normal inspiration air is drawn into the lungs by expansion of the thoracic cage, which creates a subatmospheric pressure within the thorax. The subatmospheric pressure is made greater by the elastic properties of the lungs, and is transmitted to the right atrium, which is a lax-walled structure. This has the effect of assisting venous return. All forms of artificial respiration impede venous return to some extent by raising intrathoracic pressure relative to the atmosphere; the only exception being electrophrenic respiration.

It is sometimes stated that tank ventilators are more physiological than positive-pressure ventilators because the patient's lungs are expanded by producing a subatmospheric pressure within the tank. This argument is fallacious, because the subatmospheric pressure is applied everywhere, except the head. The intrathoracic pressure is higher than the pressure in the tank, due to the elastic recoil of the lungs and chest wall. The pressure gradient between the right atrium and peripheral veins therefore remains reversed, despite the subatmospheric pressure within the tank. It is clear that the same argument applies, though rather less forcibly, to the cuirass ventilator and breathing jacket, where subatmospheric pressure is applied to the chest and abdomen during inspiration.

During I.P.P.R., the intrathoracic pressure is raised considerably, while the surface of the patient's body remains at atmospheric pressure. A marked pressure gradient therefore exists which tends to impede venous return. Attempts have been made to overcome this disadvantage by designing ventilators which apply a subatmospheric pressure to the lungs during expiration. This is known as negative phase. Opie *et al.* (1961) have shown that if a negative phase is applied throughout expiration it is possible to maintain mean intrathoracic pressure almost within normal limits. The use of a negative phase unfortunately reduces the efficiency of ventilation (see below, Physiological dead space). Opie also showed that the greatest rise in mean intrathoracic pressure occurs with ventilators which have a long inspiratory phase and slow rate of flow rise during inspiration.

Elastic Resistance during I.P.P.R.

In a paralysed unanaesthetised patient receiving I.P.P.R. the elastic resistance of the lungs is about three times normal (Smith and Spalding, 1959). In an anaesthetised patient Howell and Peckett (1957) found that the elastic resistance of the lungs was greater during paralysis than during spontaneous respiration, a finding which is in general agreement with those of Foster *et al.* (1957). Changes in elastic resistance occur within a few minutes of the start of I.P.P.R. (Watson, 1962*c*), suggesting that they are due to alterations in the distribution of air in the lungs, rather than to bronchial blockage by secretions. This is supported by the fact that during I.P.P.R. the fall in compliance is greatest when the duration of inspiration is less than one second (Watson, 1962*a*), the rapid introduction of air increasing its abnormal distribution within the lung.

During I.P.P.R. the chest wall, instead of producing inspiration, acts as an elastic resistance to it. In a totally paralysed subject this resistance is equal to about half that provided by the lungs themselves (Smith and Spalding, 1959). A patient with some respiratory power, however, often learns to assist the ventilator by expanding his chest wall during inspiration, and is more likely to do so when artificial respiration is less than adequate. Clinically such assistance is often impossible to detect.

Airway Resistance During I.P.P.R.

The greater part of the non-elastic resistance to inflation during I.P.P.R. is due to frictional resistance to the flow of air along the air passages which must include the resistance of the tracheostomy or endotracheal tube. The resistance to flow of air through a tube varies inversely with the fourth power of its diameter so that halving the diameter of a tracheostomy or endotracheal tube increases its resistance about sixteen times. This fact is of great importance during positive-pressure respiration in neonates and small babies. The fall in pressure between the ventilator and the alveoli is very large and accounts for the high pressures which must be applied if a significant ventilatory volume is to be achieved. Studies of oesophageal pressure during I.P.P.R. in babies are not at present available, but are likely to show a considerably greater pressure gradient between the trachea and oesophagus than occurs in adults. A similar situation exists in patients with chronic obstructive airways disease. The walls of the small air passages are weakened by disease and can close completely during expiration, a phenomenon known as air trapping (Campbell, 1958). The airway resistance is further increased by the presence of copious secretions in the bronchial tree. Raised airway resistance may account for the clinical observation that high tracheal pressures used to ventilate bronchitics and babies do not often produce damage to the lung parenchyma. In paralysed patients with normal lungs it has been found by Opie *et al.* (1961) that during I.P.P.R. the non-elastic resistance of the lungs is about half that of normal subjects. This may be because the airways are dilated by the positive pressure from the ventilator.

Physiological Dead-Space During I.P.P.R.

In normal subjects breathing spontaneously, physiological dead-space (V_D) is less than a quarter of the tidal volume (V_T), i.e. the V_D/V_T ratio is less than 25 per cent. Watson (1962*b*) has shown that during I.P.P.R. the V_D/V_T ratio can be kept within normal limits if the inspiratory phase lasts more than 1·5 seconds. Using shorter durations of inspiration the V_D/V_T ratio rises. When inspiration lasts half a second it may be as high as 50 per cent. This observation is in line with Watson's findings for compliance during rapid inflation, and suggests that ventilation perfusion ratios are altered under these conditions (see also Chapter 4). A negative (subatmospheric) phase during I.P.P.R. also produces a rise of 10–15 per cent in the V_D/V_T ratio. It must be emphasised that the above observations apply only to patients with relatively normal lungs and do not necessarily hold for patients with chronic lung disease.

Circulatory Effects of I.P.P.R.

Each inspiration during I.P.P.R. constitutes a mild Valsalva's manoeuvre. The effect of this upon the circulation depends upon the integrity of the patient's venous reflexes and whether there is a normal response to the raised intra-thoracic pressure (see Chapter 20). Patients with normal venous reflexes (Sharpey-Schafer, 1961) are able to compensate for increases in intrathoracic pressure of the magnitude and duration used in I.P.P.R. by increasing their venous tone. Thus in most patients venous return is not seriously impeded by I.P.P.R. and a negative phase is unnecessary and a disadvantage since it serves only to increase the V_D/V_T ratio, necessitating a larger ventilatory volume to overcome this effect.

It is sometimes suggested that a negative phase is useful when I.P.P.R. has to be used on a patient in cardiac failure. The argument is that further obstruction to venous return is undesirable and may cause circulatory collapse. But this is an er oneous theory since a patient in cardiac failure shows a square wave response to Valsalva's manoeuvre (Sharpey-Schafer, 1955) and I.P.P.R. will therefore increase the stroke output of the heart and raise the blood pressure. Clinical experience confirms that I.P.P.R. is often beneficial to patients in heart failure. The benefit is obvious although Grenvik (1966) has shown that in these patients the start of I.P.P.R. is often accompanied by a small reduction in cardiac output. This effect appears to be secondary to reduced oxygen consumption resulting from the reduction in the work of breathing, in that the mixed venous oxygen saturation is unchanged and the oxygen available to the tissues is therefore greater.

Certain patients requiring artificial ventilation show a blocked response to Valsalva's manoeuvre since they are without reflex control of venous tone. As a result the capacity vessels of the circulation behave mechanically, and a rise in intrathoracic pressure produces a proportional fall in venous return, stroke output and blood pressure. A negative phase during expiration may therefore maintain cardiac output and prevent severe hypotension. These patients include those with severe polyneuritis, cervical cord lesions, drug overdosage, oligaemia and other severe disorders (Barraclough and Sharpey-Schafer, 1963).

Unfortunately conflicting results have been obtained in studying the effect of a negative phase on cardiac output (Andersen and Kudriba, 1967; Prys-Roberts *et al.*, 1967). Most of the information comes from animal studies or fit patients undergoing anaesthesia and although impressive improvements in cardiac output in man have been claimed using a negative phase, this has not been confirmed by the comprehensive study of Auchinloss and Gilbert (1967). Comparisons are difficult as many reports do not contain enough detail of the physical characteristics of the negative phase (Norlander, 1968).

Clinical experience suggests that the beneficial effects of a negative phase are marginal. This probably accounts for both the undoubted decline in its use and the difficulty in interpreting studies on negative phase.

The effects of I.P.P.R. on the pulmonary circulation are complex because it is a low pressure system and great variations exist in different parts of the lungs. During inspiration right ventricular stroke output falls and left ventricular stroke output rises (Morgan *et al.*, 1966). This effect is reversed during expiration and accounts for the cyclical variation in systemic arterial pressure, and the axis changes on the ECG seen during I.P.P.R.

The circulatory effects of I.P.P.R. on patients with acute exacerbations of chronic lung disease and cor pulmonale are interesting and require further elucidation. During the first hours of treatment hypotension is usual (Bradley *et al.*, 1964). Unfortunately it is not possible to use Valsalva's manoeuvre in such patients as a means of obtaining information about circulatory reflexes. This is because air trapping prevents the sudden release of intrathoracic pressure which is necessary to demonstrate an overshoot. It seems unlikely, however, that hypotension in such patients is due to blocked reflexes. A more probable explanation may be the effect on the peripheral circulation of the rapid fall of carbon dioxide tension which accompanies the start of I.P.P.R.

Inspired Gases during I.P.P.R.

Physiological dead space and venous admixture are always increased during I.P.P.R. and for this reason it is usually necessary to enrich the oxygen content of the inspired air if hypoxia is to be avoided (Nunn *et al.*, 1965). These changes, however, appear to lessen as I.P.P.R. is continued and patients with muscular paralysis and apparently normal lungs, who have been maintained on I.P.P.R. with air for months or years, often have an unusually high arterial oxygen tension. One patient who has received I.P.P.R. via a tracheostomy for eleven years persistently maintains a Pa_{O_2} of between 100 and 110 mm. Hg. The mechanism of this long term adjustment is unknown but it is clear that an increased alveolar-arterial oxygen gradient normally accompanies the start of I.P.P.R. (Pontoppidan *et al.*, 1965) and it is probably for this reason that artificial ventilation is rarely of value in pure pneumonia.

An excessive inspired oxygen concentration during I.P.P.R. is also harmful. Nash *et al.* (1967) studied the lungs of 70 patients who died after prolonged artificial ventilation. Lungs ventilated with high oxygen concentrations showed severe histological changes characterised by alveolar oedema, intra-alveolar haemorrhage and fibrin exudate. The mechanism if these changes is not known but they are now widely recognised and have led to the use of the term "respirator lung" (Fig. 8).

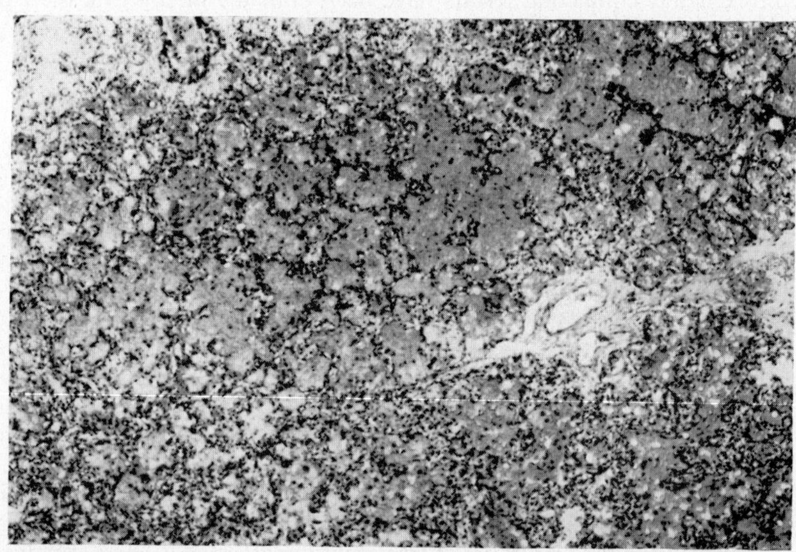

15/FIG. 8.—The "respirator lung" syndrome. Microscopic section of a lung following 5 days of I.P.P.R. with high oxygen concentration. Intra-alveolar haemorrhage is clearly seen.

The oxygen concentrations necessary to produce these changes are uncertain but experience suggests that they are almost inevitable if concentrations above 80 per cent are used for more than a few hours. Clinically they are manifested by a progressively falling arterial oxygen tension and an increasing "white out" on radiological examination of the lung fields. Once established, this condition is almost universally fatal and it is therefore of the utmost importance never to use an inspired oxygen concentration higher than is necessary to produce an arterial tension between 100 and 150 mm. Hg.

The use of nitrous oxide during prolonged I.P.P.R. is also undesirable.

Despite its safety for short-term use during anaesthesia, if administration is prolonged for more than three to four days, serious bone marrow suppression and leucopenia results (Parbrook, 1967).

MANAGEMENT OF PATIENTS RECEIVING ARTIFICIAL RESPIRATION

Tracheostomy (see also pp. 19 and 144)

The indications for tracheostomy may be summarised as follows:

1. **Upper airway obstruction.**—This applies to acute and chronic obstruction above the level of the trachea. The obstruction is bypassed and the indication is usually clear-cut.

2. **Suction.**—Tracheostomy is indicated for patients who are unable, through muscular weakness or other debility, to cough up their bronchial secretions adequately. The situation can be temporarily relieved by bronchoscopy, but unless the cause of secretion retention is fairly rapidly self-limiting, or can be kept pace with by suction down an endotracheal tube, tracheostomy is necessary.

3. **Isolation of the lower respiratory tract.**—When, for any reason, the pharyngeal or laryngeal reflexes are lost, the lungs must be isolated from the pharynx and larynx by tracheostomy. This does not, of course, apply to short-term causes such as occur during anaesthesia, but to conditions in which reflexes are absent for a significant period. Isolation can be maintained for several days using an endotracheal tube. As a result of improvements in the management of patients receiving I.P.P.R. via an endotracheal tube and improvements in the tubes themselves, it is now possible to leave them in position for up to one week (see below).

It is important to remember that this indication for tracheostomy may be present in neoplastic conditions of the pharynx, larynx and oesophagus, where mechanical interference with swallowing may be severe enough to necessitate isolation of the trachea and lungs.

4. **To maintain artificial ventilation.**—If artificial ventilation by intermittent positive pressure is necessary for more than a few days, tracheostomy is essential.

Tracheostomy is sometimes said to be of value in that it reduces respiratory dead space. This argument is fallacious, and has probably arisen from confusion between anatomical and physiological dead space. Tracheostomy has been shown in several studies to reduce anatomical dead space by 10–50 per cent. Immediately after it has been performed, the proportion of tidal volume which is effective in producing gaseous exchange, i.e. the alveolar ventilation, rises, the arterial P_{CO_2} falls, the central stimulus to ventilation is decreased, and the volume of ventilation falls until the arterial P_{CO_2} has become re-established at its previous level. The converse applies if anatomical dead space is increased by breathing through a face-mask. Ventilation rises and P_{CO_2} remains at almost its original level. These theoretical arguments have been confirmed by Froeb and Kim (1964) who showed that both in normal subjects and in patients with emphysema there is little alteration in arterial gas tensions and a reduction in respiratory minute volume following tracheostomy. The same authors found a small increase in arterial oxygen saturation following tracheostomy in subjects with a level below normal. This increase was not significant and was within the limits both of experimental error and normal variations in oxygen saturation due to alterations of the alveolar/arterial oxygen gradient within the lung. These results were confirmed in the studies of Grant *et al.* (1964).

It has also been suggested that, by reducing dead space, tracheostomy may postpone the need for artificial ventilation, but this is not so. In practice it is always found that due to hypoxia, clinical distress and possibly carbon dioxide retention, artificial ventilation is needed when vital capacity is still two or three times greater than mean tidal volume (see p. 482). If dead space reduction were to have any effect in avoiding artificial ventilation, vital capacity and tidal volume would have to be both equal and reduced. This situation represents a patient *in extremis* who should have been receiving respiratory assistance considerably earlier.

To summarise, tracheostomy produces a 10–50 per cent reduction in anatomical dead space, alveolar ventilation is unchanged, and dead space reduction *per se* is of little value to the patient.

Tracheostomy Tubes

A wide variety of tracheostomy tubes is available but none is completely satisfactory for all purposes.

Cuffed tracheostomy tubes.—A cuffed tube exposes the patient to a number of additional hazards (see below—Complications). It should not be used unless indications 3 or 4 (above) are present. The requirements of a cuffed tube are as follows:— It must have as wide a bore as possible to provide an airway with low resistance to airflow. The lumen must be smooth-walled to prevent crusting of secretions and to allow easy introduction of suction catheters. The curve of the tube must be gentle to facilitate suction. The cuff must be smooth-surfaced and inflate evenly to maintain an airtight fit in the trachea and minimise the risk of herniation. The inflatable section of the cuff should be not less than $1\frac{1}{4}$ inches (3 cm.) long to ensure a wide area of gentle contact with the tracheal mucosa, and reduce the risk of tracheal damage. It must possess a suitable flange or neck to allow it to be securely tied in position. The connection to the ventilator tubing must be light in weight and not liable to become detached in use. At the same time it must be easily disconnected to facilitate suction.

Few, if any, tubes meet all these requirements completely. Two are illustrated which come near to it.

The Portsmouth tracheostomy tube (Hodges *et al.*, 1956) (Fig. 9) is built up from a Magill cuffed endotracheal tube. A silver lining piece is inserted to maintain a suitable curve and a plastic Cobb suction union (Portland Plastics Ltd.) used as a connection. It has been found (Bradley *et al.*, 1964) to be particularly suitable for use when high inflation pressures are needed.

The Portex tracheostomy tube (Whittard and Thomas, 1964) (Fig. 10) is disposable, plastic throughout and supplied sterile in a two-layered plastic container bag. It is convenient to use and non-irritant but, as at present made, the cuff is somewhat short and the connection tends to become insecure in use. A modified version overcoming these disadvantages is shortly to be introduced.

Non-cuffed tracheostomy tubes.—The requirements of a non-cuffed tracheostomy tube are not exacting and designs are well-established. The Negus and Durham silver tubes are the most commonly used in England. Of the two, the Negus is probably the most satisfactory.

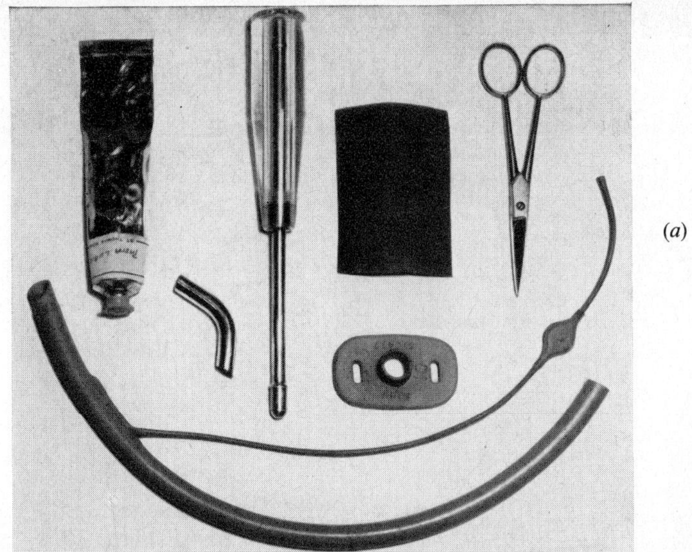
(*a*)

Component parts.

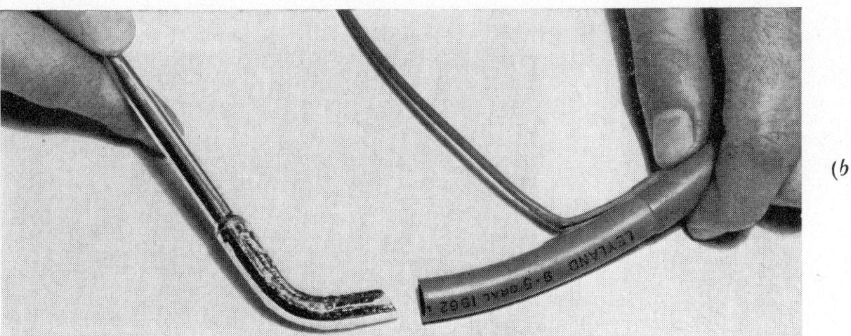
(*b*

Introducing the silver lining tube.

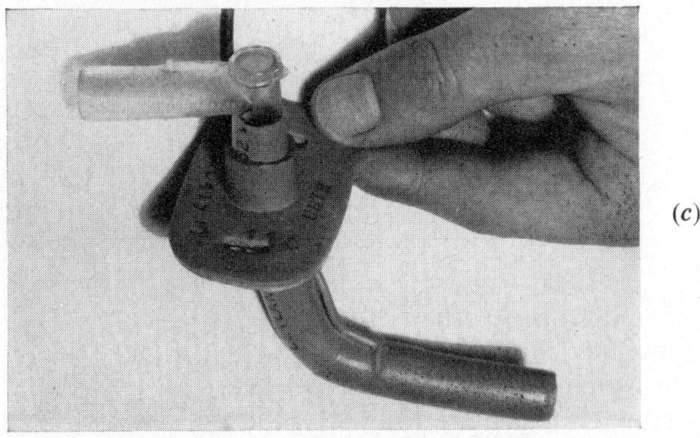
(*c*)

15/Fig. 9.—Portsmouth tracheostomy tube.

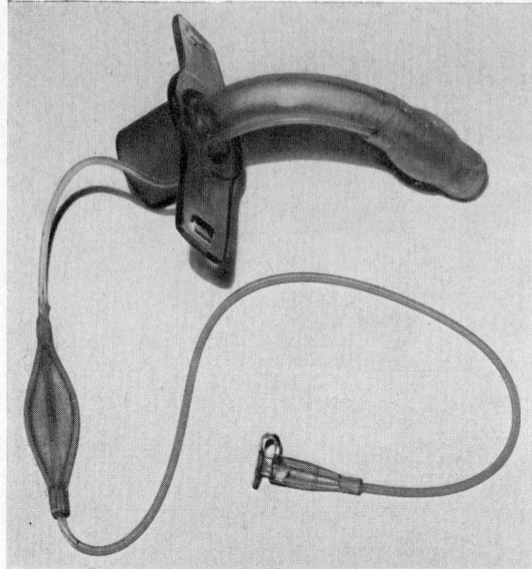

15/FIG. 10.—Portex tracheostomy tube. A pre-sterilised, all plastic, disposable tube.

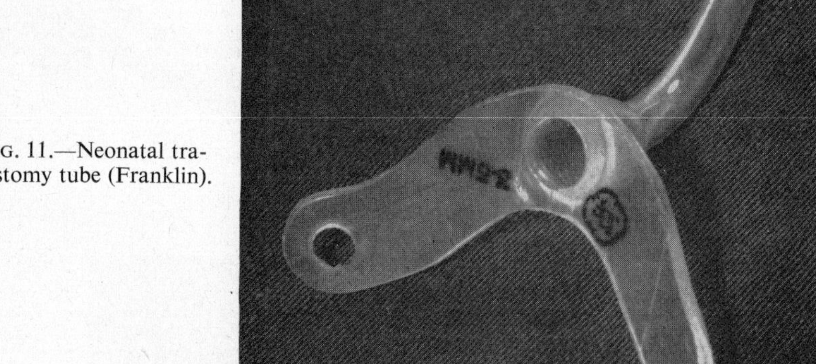

15/FIG. 11.—Neonatal tracheostomy tube (Franklin).

Neonatal tracheostomy tube (Glover, 1965). (Fig. 11).—This tube is specially shaped for infants. To maintain as large a lumen as possible it is cuffless and an airtight fit is obtained by selecting a size large enough to fit snugly into the trachea. The funnel shaped enlargement below the flange serves both to maintain an airtight fit at the site of the tracheostome and to hold in position the catheter mount connection. The flange is angled upwards to accommodate the anatomical differences of the neonate. The management of neonatal tracheostomy requires special precautions all of which are related to the small size of the bronchial tree. Serious blockage occurs more quickly than in adults and is more difficult to treat. Tracheal narrowing following decannulation is commoner and more likely to be clinically significant.

It is also clear from clinical experience and experimental studies (Okmian, 1966) that it is wrong to try to reproduce the same pattern of respiration frequency during artificial ventilation that the infant maintains spontaneously. More efficient ventilation is achieved using frequencies of between 20 and 25 breaths per minute.

Anaesthesia for Tracheostomy

Tracheostomy is best performed under general anaesthesia with an endotracheal tube in place, and it should be an elective, planned procedure so far as is possible. Local analgesia is only justifiable when it is impossible to introduce an endotracheal tube beforehand, or when an experienced anaesthetist is not available.

Complications of Tracheostomy

Most of the complications of tracheostomy can be avoided provided great care is taken to see that management is always perfect. Nevertheless, complications are surprisingly common. McClelland (1965) found evidence of complications in over 50 per cent of tracheostomies performed in a general hospital.

Obstruction of the tube.—This is usually due to inadequate humidification of the inspired gases and the accumulation of inspissated secretions.

Displacement of the tube.—This can occur if the tubes from the ventilator are allowed to pull on the tracheostomy tube during nursing attentions. In the first few days following tracheostomy it may be a serious matter since replacement may be difficult until a track has become established. Certain patterns of tube, such as the Durham metal tube, are more liable to dislodge, owing to a short intratracheal section. If it is necessary to change a tracheostomy tube during the first 48 hours, a laryngoscope and endotracheal tube must always be immediately available. If it is difficult to insert the new tube an oral endotracheal tube should be passed and the new tube inserted under good vision, possibly in the operating theatre. If this procedure is not followed, a false passage may be created (Fig. 12).

Damage to surrounding structures.—Erosion into the oesophagus or innominate artery can occur. The former is most common when metal tracheostomy tubes are used, and the latter is usually associated with a cuffed tracheostomy tube and I.P.P.R.

Infection.—Infection, either at the tracheostome or in the tracheobronchial tree, is difficult to prevent. A meticulous aseptic technique should be used at all times. The tracheostome should be kept exposed and secretions removed from around it as soon as they appear.

Granulomata.—Granulomata of the trachea (Pearce and Walsh, 1961) can occur and they may cause respiratory difficulty when the tube is removed. Infection at the tracheostome is possibly a predisposing factor.

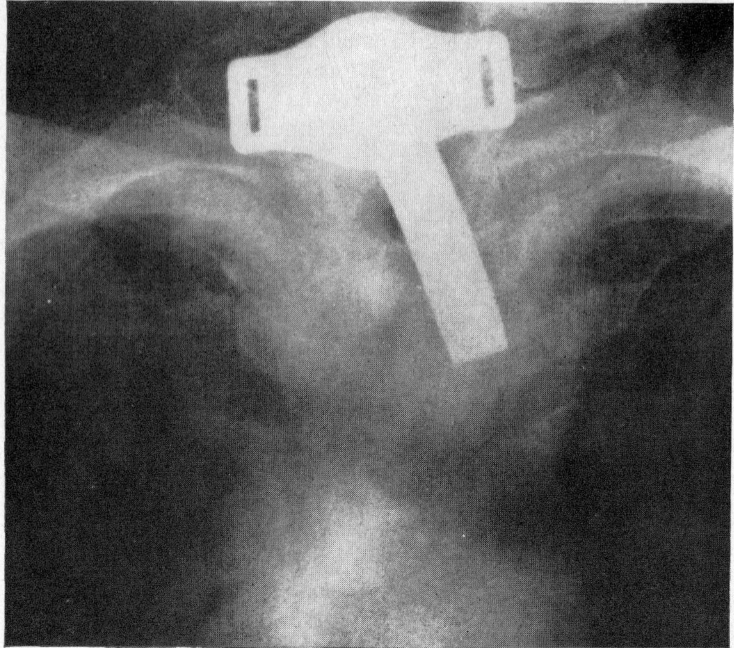

15/FIG. 12.—X-ray showing a tracheostomy tube in a false passage. This was caused by forceful tube replacement following a recent tracheostomy.

Dilatation of the trachea.—Some enlargement of the trachea at the site of the cuff is probably inevitable. If the cuff is too short, or over-inflated, the dilatation may be considerable (Lloyd and McClelland, 1964). Mucosal damage, due to pressure, is usual, but if the pressure is excessive or uneven, erosion of the cartilaginous rings may result (Fig. 13). Various routines of intermittent cuff deflation have been advocated to overcome this problem, but it is doubtful whether in themselves, they are entirely effective and they are certainly potentially dangerous (Fig. 14). The best protection against tracheal damage is meticulous management and inflation with the minimum quantity of air.

Tracheal stricture.—This is a late complication of tracheostomy which may occur at the tracheostome or lower down the trachea at the site of the cuff.

Humidification (see also Chapter I, p. 9).

In normal respiration inspired air is warmed and moistened during its passage through the nose and upper air passages. By the time it reaches the trachea the air is at 32–36° C even when breathing cold air through the nose and has a relative humidity of over 90 per cent (34-35 mg./litre at 32° C). Dry air passing straight into the trachea produces marked changes in the tracheal mucosa which becomes hyperaemic; and excessive mucus is formed which becomes dry and crusted. Cilial action is depressed or abolished (Burton, 1962). These effects can be avoided if the air or gas drawn in or blown through a tracheostomy is warmed to body temperature and adequately humidified. Most ventilators include a water bath humidifier in the inspiratory limb of the patient circuit.

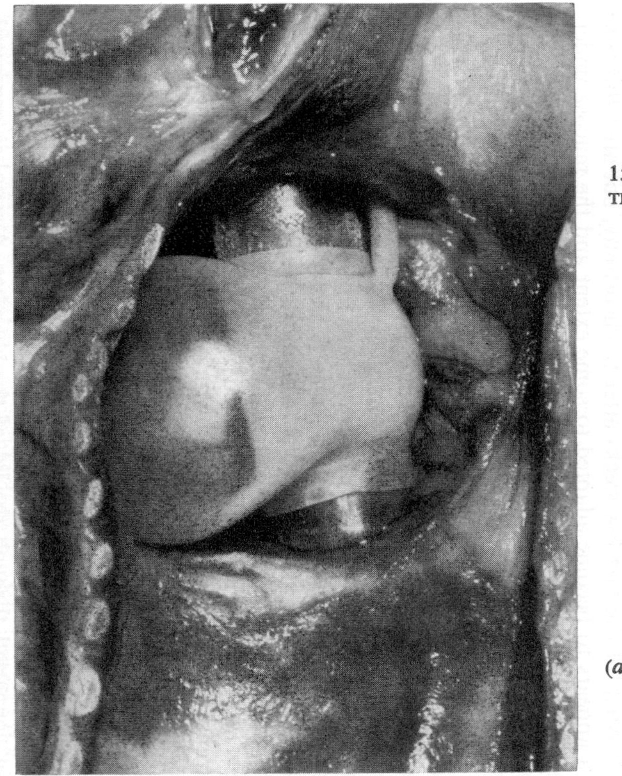

(*a*)

15/Fig. 13.—Dilatation of the Trachea.

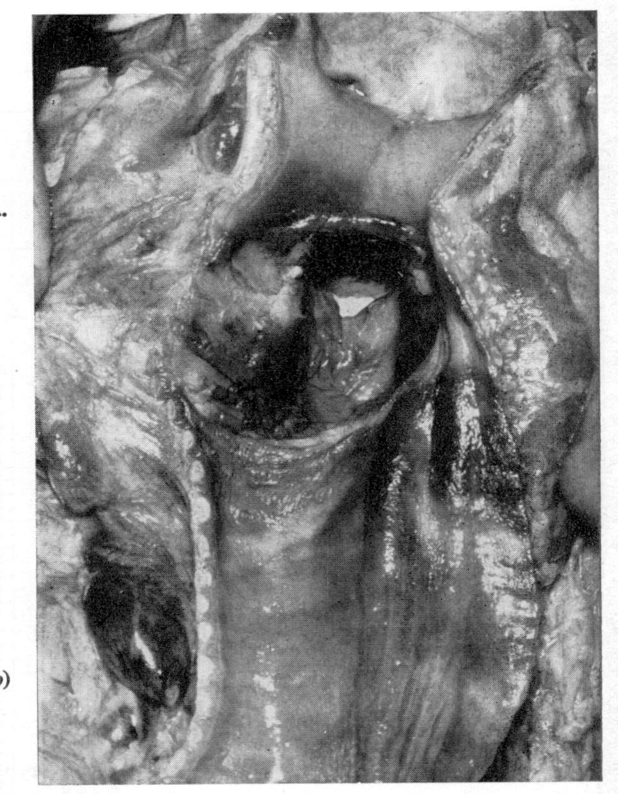

(*b*)

A trachea at autopsy, opened from behind. (*a*). Tracheostomy tube ***in situ***. Excessive and uneven pressure from the cuff has caused a sacular dilatation of the trachea. The open end of the tracheostomy tube is completely obstructed by the wall of the sac. (*b*). Trachea with tracheostomy tube removed. The cartilaginous rings of the trachea can be seen in the walls of the dilatation. They are eroded and broken.

of nursing care they receive, and this fact, coupled with the introduction of plastic tubes which appear to lessen the risks of vocal cord damage have reawakened interest in prolonged endotracheal intubation. Given a high standard of nursing care the advantages and disadvantages of the two techniques can be compared as below. It cannot be too often repeated, however, that if nursing standards are not perfect, tracheostomy is safer.

The advantages of prolonged endotracheal intubation compared with tracheostomy are:

1. Endotracheal intubation is simple, repeatable and quick.

2. Immediate operative complications of tracheostomy are avoided. These risks include: haemorrhage, surgical emphysema, pneumothorax, air embolism and cricoid cartilage damage.

3. Stricture of the trachea at the stomal site is avoided.

4. Cross infection of a surgical wound adjacent to a tracheostomy, e.g. a median sternotomy, does not occur.

5. Even using a horizontal incision a tracheostomy scar does not heal well. This uncosmetic scar may be a serious disadvantage to some patients e.g. young women who require short term I.P.P.R. following suicidal drug overdosage. A tracheostomy scar is an unwelcome reminder of an unhappy incident in their lives. An endotracheal tube avoids this problem.

6. The incidence of complications is lower than those of tracheostomy (Lindholm, 1969).

The disadvantages of prolonged endotracheal intubation compared with tracheostomy are:

1. Laryngeal damage can occur although usually the effects of this are limited to transient hoarseness of the voice.

2. An endotracheal tube is less well tolerated by the patient than a tracheostomy. This may increase the need for sedation and make weaning more difficult.

3. Fixation of an oral endotracheal tube is difficult. A Nosworthy (long shaft) connection extending between the teeth is essential to prevent the patient biting the tube.

4. The tube may become kinked in the pharynx. This difficulty is better avoided by the use of small plastic rather than nylon reinforced latex tubes, down which suction catheters can be difficult to pass.

5. Owing to the difficulties of fixation the tube may be easily displaced into the right main bronchus.

6. Though the incidence of complications is lower, when they do occur they are more severe, and approximately 1 per cent of patients need permanent tracheostomy (Tonkin and Harrison, 1966; Harrison and Tonkin, 1967, 1968; Peachey and Pease, 1971).

Some of these disadvantages can be overcome by the use of a nasotracheal tube. This technique is particularly suitable for neonates and young children because the internal diameter of the nose is greater than that of the larynx. A suitable tube has been developed by Rees and Owen-Thomas (1966). Unfortunately nasotracheal intubation is less suitable for adults and can cause damage to the external nares. Effective aspiration of tracheal secretions is even more difficult owing to the greater length and narrower bore of the tube.

In summary, prolonged endotracheal intubation has real advantages for selected patients, provided that the standard of nursing care is high. The naso-tracheal route is the most suitable for babies and the orotracheal route for adults. The subject has been comprehensively reviewed by Lindholm (1969).

Care of the Lungs

Adequate care of the lungs during artificial ventilation is the key to success. Bronchial secretions must be aspirated whenever they can be felt or heard and certainly never less than two hourly. As far as possible an aseptic technique should be employed and a fresh sterile catheter must be used for each insertion. Ideally catheters should be individually packed and sterilised by autoclaving. Despite improvements in plastic suction catheters, soft rubber whistle-tipped catheters still remain the most satisfactory for use in prolonged I.P.P.R. The whistle-tip pattern appears to be the least traumatic. In the words of one Doctor/patient, after four years of artificial ventilation in several hospitals: "It's the only type which doesn't feel like a red hot wire thrust down my trachea!—single hole catheters do a series of mucosal biopsies as they're hauled out!".

Plastic suction catheters frequently cause tracheal bleeding if they are used repeatedly. They are difficult to manipulate down plastic tracheostomy and endotracheal tubes because the two plastic surfaces tend to adhere. In a busy unit up to 500 suction catheters may be used per day. In the interests of cost, resterilisation is usually necessary and plastic catheters withstand this less well than rubber ones at present. Angulated suction catheters which can be made to enter the left main bronchus are not routinely necessary and their use has declined following improvements in physiotherapy techniques during I.P.P.R.

Physiotherapy.—Transference of secretions from the periphery of the lungs to the trachea or main bronchi usually has to be assisted during the first months of artificial ventilation by postural drainage and physiotherapy. The most effective form of physiotherapy is the technique of artificial coughing described by Sykes *et al.* (1969). The lung is hyper-inflated with oxygen by means of a reservoir bag and the squeeze on the bag is suddenly released. The moment of pressure release is made to coincide with an external squeeze and vibration produced by the physiotherapist. This procedure is repeated several times for each area of the chest until it is clear to auscultation.

If skilfully performed this technique is well tolerated even by severely ill patients and may need to be repeated several times a day. It is remarkably effective. Figure 16 *a* and *b* shows radiographs of the chest of a 3-year-old child taken half an hour apart, before and after physiotherapy.

Periodic deep breaths.—During normal spontaneous breathing Bendixen *et al.* (1964) have shown that tidal volume varies greatly, and sighs (breaths larger than three times the average tidal volume) occur regularly about ten times per hour. These writers consider that periodic deep breaths are of physiological importance, because atelectatic air spaces are reinflated and pulmonary compliance, the work of breathing and venous admixture kept within the normal range. In relating these findings to artificial ventilation a similar group of workers (Bendixen *et al.*, 1963) showed a mean fall of Pa_{O_2} during controlled ventilation of 22 per cent and suggested that the cause might be small areas of pulmonary collapse not necessarily visible on X-rays. They postulated that these changes

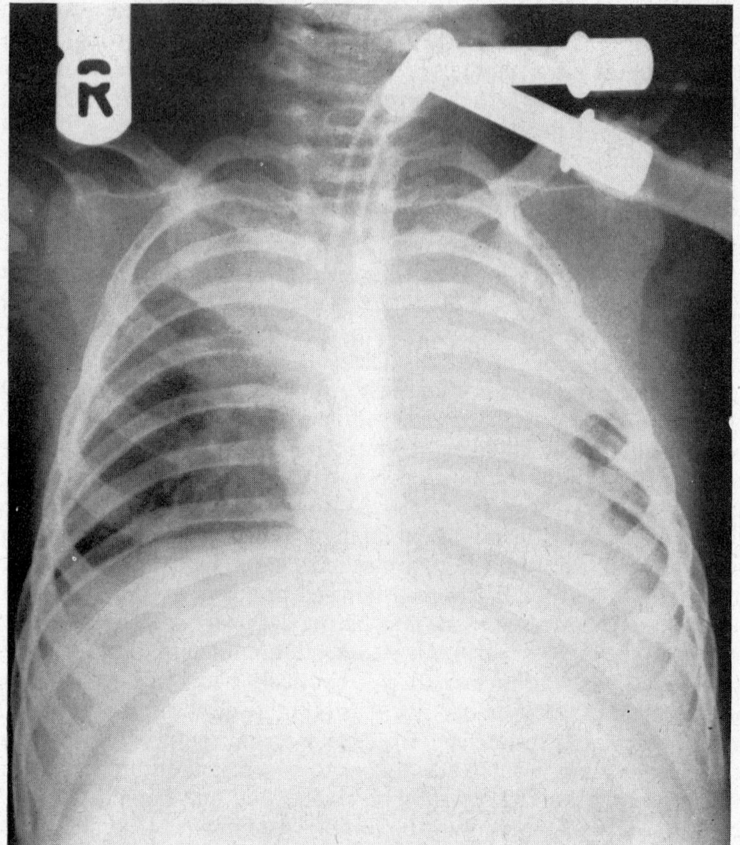

15/Fig. 16(*a*)

could be avoided during I.P.P.R. by the use of automatic periodic sighs built into the ventilator. A variety of devices have been developed to produce this effect (Feychting and Settergren, 1966). The changes described by Bendixen *et al.* have not been confirmed by subsequent work (Morgan *et al.*, 1970) and are ascribed by Norlander *et al.* (1968) to inefficient ventilators. Certainly artificial sighs have not been shown to be beneficial. Improved techniques of ventilation and physiotherapy are preferable.

Assessment of Respiration in Muscular Weakness

When are muscular paralysis and respiratory weakness severe enough to justify mechanical assistance? Generalisations on this question are no more accurate than most other clinical generalisations but individual clinical assessment of each patient remains the most valuable method for arriving at the correct answer. As respiratory paralysis progresses, a patient becomes anxious and restless, the accessory muscles of respiration are used, and frequent feeble attempts

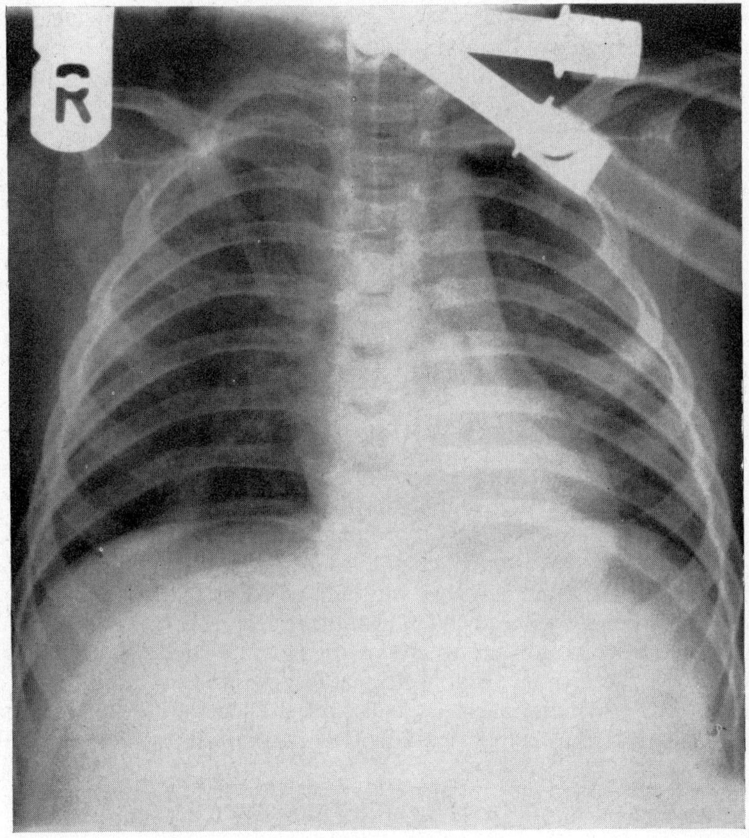

15/FIG. 16(*b*)

15/FIG. 16(*a*) and (*b*).—Chest radiographs of a child taken half an hour apart, before and after physiotherapy by "artificial coughing".

at coughing may be made. Carbon dioxide accumulation is a late sign of respiratory inadequacy due to muscular weakness. Hypoxaemia and cyanosis occur much earlier and minute volume may actually be increased from this cause, possibly due to increased venous admixture from maldistribution of ventilation and perfusion in the lung. The fact that respiratory assistance is often needed when vital capacity is still at least twice the average tidal volume may be due to the loss of this sigh mechanism. Measurements of peak expiratory flow rate may also be valuable in assessing the need for respiratory assistance, for when this flow is less than 100 litres/minute, coughing is inefficient and pulmonary complications are likely.

Volume of Ventilation

The only completely satisfactory way to ensure that a patient is receiving the correct volume of ventilation is to measure his arterial P_{CO_2} and preferably his arterial P_{O_2} as well. Unfortunately the apparatus needed for these measurements is expensive and requires care and skill in use if reliable results are to be obtained. It is not at present universally available and, in the initial period of artificial ventilation at least, approximations may have to be made without the benefit of these measurements. For patients who start off with normal lungs, respiration nomograms such as those of Radford *et al.* (1954) (see Chapter 4) or Engström and Herzog (1959) may be helpful. It is preferable to err on the side of over-ventilation rather than underventilation.

Patients receiving artificial ventilation for pulmonary disease present a special problem, since nomograms are of no value and measurement of arterial gas tensions is essential. In the early stages, however, it may be necessary to accept a less-than-ideal ventilatory volume. Ventilation may have to be set to the largest volume which does not lead to serious hypotension (Bradley *et al.* 1964).

Some Conditions in which Artificial Respiration may be Required

Artificial respiration has become an established form of therapy in an increasing range of conditions. It remains, nevertheless, a complicated and potentially dangerous treatment unless it is properly carried out in specially adapted units by staff experienced in the techniques involved. Like all forms of therapy, it cannot be considered in isolation without due consideration of the conditions for which it is being used and the indications for its use.

These conditions can be conveniently divided into four types, depending on which of the structures involved in normal respiration have failed.

Some of these conditions are now discussed, but only in respect of the need for artificial respiration in their treatment. Clinical details are not intended to be

Failure of Muscles or Neuro Muscular Junction	*Failure of The Lungs*	*Failure of The Nervous System*		*Failure of Bony Structures*
		Central Nervous System	*Peripheral Nerves*	
General anaesthesia using muscle relaxants	Chronic bronchitis and emphysema	Drug overdosage	Poliomyelitis	Crush injury to thorax
Tetanus	Neonatal respiratory distress syndrome	Status epilepticus	Polyneuritis	Respiratory infection in kyphoscoliosis
Myasthenia gravis				
Dystrophia myotonica	Status asthmaticus	Head injury		
	(Pneumonia)	Cervical cord injury		
	Post-operative pulmonary complications	After neurosurgery		After thoracotomy
	Drowning			

comprehensive since, in fact, many of the diseases are described more fully elsewhere in this book.

It should be appreciated that in addition to the above table, artificial ventilation commonly has to be used for what are primarily cardiovascular reasons. These may also apply to some of the above conditions, for example in respiratory distress syndrome and status asthmaticus where the work of breathing is enormously increased and up to 30 per cent of the cardiac output may be used in this work. In addition, if the cardiac output is severely reduced as occurs after cardiac surgery or myocardial infarction, the oxygen demands of spontaneous respiration may be too great for the patient to perform satisfactorily and artificial ventilation is of great benefit (Norlander, 1968).

Artificial Respiration in General Anaesthesia

Two separate questions must be answered when the decision to use artificial respiration during general anaesthesia is being made. Firstly, will the patient's best interests be served by allowing him to breathe spontaneously, or by controlling his respiration? Secondly, if artificial respiration is used, is it best performed manually, or by a mechanical ventilator? The first question is much the more difficult one to answer satisfactorily. For thoracic surgery and operations requiring full muscular relaxation the answer is easy. For short operations, requiring little more than the abolition of painful stimuli, the answer is equally easy. Most operations lie between these two extremes, and it is in this large intermediate group that the answer is difficult. It is doubtful whether in most cases there would be any difference in the ultimate results after either method. Many schools of anaesthesia exist which hold strongly opposed opinions concerning the benefits of one technique over the other. It is obviously impossible for widely divergent views to be held if a highly significant advantage were offered by either method in a particular situation. Nevertheless, today, when satisfactory anaesthesia can be assured by so many methods, it is important to elucidate the marginal advantages offered by a particular technique. Due to the many variables involved, these advantages may be exceedingly difficult to establish. It seems reasonable to assume that the best anaesthesia is that which involves the least disturbance to normal physiology. It is therefore necessary to compare the physiological changes which accompany artificial respiration properly performed in paralysed patients, with those accompanying equivalent anaesthesia by narcotic and inhalational agents, but with spontaneous respiration. It may be that in the long run the most significant difference will be found to be in the postoperative effects on ventilation caused by a respiratory acidosis or alkalosis existing during anaesthesia (Semple, 1965) (see Chapter 4). When artificial respiration is used, it can be performed manually or mechanically. A ventilator frees the anaesthetist's hands, so that he is able when single-handed to attend to other duties, while at the same time ensuring efficient ventilation. However the feel of the anaesthetic reservoir bag is still a valuable adjunct in clinical practice. Its loss divorces the anaesthetist from his patient and makes it harder to observe and anticipate minor variations in the patient's condition. Clutton Brock (1962) has described a device for introducing a negative phase during manual artificial respiration, but even with this device it is probably true that manual ventilation, no matter how conscientiously carried out, cannot hope to provide at all times throughout an operation the constant and physiological respiratory cycling of a good machine which has been correctly adjusted.

Tetanus

Knott and Cole (1952) describe six types of tetanus.

Type I: Purely local, usually mild, which often occurs in people who have been immunised.

Type II: Generalised tonic rigidity which intensifies and then passes off without spasm.

Type III: Tonic rigidity, intensifying and leading to reflex spasms. These too increase and finally relax if the patient has not succumbed during the crescendo.

Type IV: Involvement of the muscles of deglutition and respiration with less emphasis on generalised spasms.

Type V: Cephalic tetanus, involving principally the cranial nerves.

Type VI: Infantile tetanus from infection of the umbilical cord.

In groups I and II management by sedation and hypotonic drugs such as mephenesin and chlorpromazine (Kelly and Laurence, 1956) is usually sufficient. The use of these drugs has not been accompanied by any reduction in mortality during tetanus (Adams, 1958), whereas the value of curarisation and intermittent positive-pressure respiration—at least in groups III to VI—is clearly established (Shackleton, 1954; Ablett, 1956; Wright *et al.*, 1961; Pearce, 1961). In these groups death is most commonly due to respiratory failure, either from asphyxia during a spasm, or from chest complications following hypertonicity of the respiratory muscles or loss of the ability to swallow. Death may occur during the first major tetanic spasm, and such a spasm is a certain indication for tracheostomy, curarisation, and I.P.P.R. When chest complications occur in tetanus it is usually necessary to perform a tracheostomy because hypertonicity prevents the patient from coughing. The irritation caused by the tube however may precipitate generalised spasms, and then curarisation and I.P.P.R. become essential.

Mortality in neonatal tetanus is very high. A substantial reduction has been achieved by using curarisation and I.P.P.R. (Wright *et al.*, 1961; Smythe, 1963). That the reduction in mortality was not greater was because the treatment is technically difficult and requires a higher standard of care than usually exists in areas where the disease is common. Tetanus is a self-limiting condition although curarisation may have to be maintained for 4–5 weeks. For this reason *d*-tubocurarine has usually been found to be the most satisfactory relaxant. It can be given intramuscularly in doses of 15 mg. as often as is necessary to maintain flaccidity. Pancuronium has been advocated as an alternative to *d*-tubocurarine for the treatment of tetanus. Although it appears to have pharmacological advantages, in practice these advantages are theoretical rather than real and are outweighed by the shorter duration of action of pancuronium.

In 1967 a symposium on tetanus in Great Britain was held in Leeds (Ellis, 1967) and the results of treatment in several centres were reviewed. The best series showed an overall mortality of 4 per cent in all cases. In most published series the mortality is well above this figure.

In recent years interest in the treatment of tetanus has centered on the unexpectedly high mortality of severe cases, when compared with other similarly paralysed patients for whom artificial ventilation is used. The striking feature of these cases is the cardiovascular changes which develop shortly after the start of I.P.P.R. They include hypertension, tachycardia, cardiac arrhymias, sweating and intense peripheral vasoconstriction, sometimes of glove and stocking distribution. Various causes for this condition have been postulated, but it was not until Kerr (1967) noted its striking resemblence to the 'fight or flight' reaction of sympathetic overactivity and to the changes of phaeochromocytoma that the underlying cause became apparent. Subsequent studies by Kerr *et al.* (1968) and Keilty *et al.* (1968) have shown increased urinary and serum catecholamine levels in such patients. In an attempt to suppress these manifestations Prys-Roberts *et al.* (1969) used continuous halothane anaesthesia and blockade of adrenergic receptors with a combination of bethanidine and propranolol. At present there is insufficient experience of these methods of treatment to make it possible to decide whether any reduction in mortality due to sympathetic overactivity will outweigh increased mortality from side-effects and secondary complications from the drugs themselves. To administer β-adrenergic blocking drugs to a paralysed patient receiving I.P.P.R. is a serious step. Should inadvertent disconnection from the ventilator occur, cardiac arrest follows more rapidly and is much more difficult to reverse.

It is encouraging that sympathetic overactivity is not universally noted in all reported series. Cole and others in an extensive clinical experience over many years have never seen sympathetic overactivity (Cole and Youngman, 1969). In a previous paper they point out that most patients find tetanus and its treatment a frightening and painful ordeal (Cole and Youngman, 1968). For this reason they have used paraldehyde freely as the drug of choice for central sedation throughout their experience.

These results raise the interesting possibility that sympathetic overactivity may be due to awareness and stress. Large doses of *d*-tubocurarine, used to maintain flaccidity in severe cases, may make it more difficult to detect wakefulness.

Myasthenia Gravis

This disease is described in Chapter 33. The indications for artificial ventilation are similar to those in any disease affecting muscle power, and are discussed on page 482 *et seq*.

Dystrophia Myotonica

Myotonia of the respiratory muscles commonly occurs in dystrophia myotonica. This may lead to a large reduction in the patient's vital capacity and maximum breathing capacity (Kaufman, 1960). It has been stated by Dundee (1952) that patients with dystrophia myotonica are particularly susceptible to thiopentone, possibly due to a specific peripheral action of the drug, but further studies have not substantiated this cause. While it is true that patients suffering from dystrophia myotonica are sensitive to thiopentone—100 mg. may cause apnoea for twenty minutes—the effect is probably a central one and common to all respiratory depressant drugs. Weakness of the muscles of respiration may lead to respiratory inadequacy when depressant drugs are given, or when the work of breathing is increased.

Patients with dystrophia myotonica are sometimes presented for anaesthesia, particularly because premature cataract is one of the features of the disease. A period of artificial respiration may be necessary post-operatively, but myotonia of the respiratory muscles may make ventilation extremely difficult, if not impossible. The reaction to muscle relaxants is variable because the abnormality is in the muscle fibre itself. Quinine hydrochloride in doses of 300–600 mg. may be useful, as it is said to prolong the refractory period of the muscle fibre after contraction (Harvey, 1939).

Chronic Bronchitis and Emphysema

Pulmonary changes in chronic bronchitis and emphysema are irreversible and progressive. The progression is not uniform, however. Successive bouts of superadded acute infection occur with increasing frequency. Patients usually die during these acute exacerbations from carbon dioxide retention leading to narcosis with further secretion retention. Severe ventilation-perfusion inequalities exist in the lung and give rise to marked hypoxaemia. Possibly due to the accumulation of bicarbonate in the cerebrospinal fluid, the respiratory centre, via its chemoreceptors, becomes less sensitive to increases in carbon dioxide tension and hypoxia forms the main drive to respiration. If hypoxia is relieved, respiration is further depressed, carbon dioxide accumulates and unconsciousness supervenes. In an attempt to prevent this sequence of events, Campbell (1960) has described a method by which oxygen can be given to these patients in a controlled concentration which can be varied between 23 and 35 per cent. A special mask, working on the venturi principle, is used. This has two advantages. The high flow rate produced prevents any rebreathing from the mask and minimises a further rise in arterial carbon dioxide tension. The oxygen lack is only partly corrected and the hypoxic drive to ventilation is thereby maintained. Owing to the shape of the oxygen dissociation curve for blood this relatively small increase in inspired oxygen tension produces a much larger rise in arterial oxygen content, and with careful supervision a course can be steered between dangerous hypoxia and narcosis from carbon dioxide. In severely ill patients this method is not always successful (Satinder Lal, 1965; Warrell *et al.*, 1970). Furthermore, it seems reasonable to assume that it is best, if possible, to correct the hypoxia completely in patients so seriously ill. When this leads to severe carbon dioxide retention and narcosis, the alternatives are either to use a lower inspired oxygen concentration or to perform tracheostomy and artificial respiration. Their comparative merits cannot be finally decided until there is more data on the survival rate of patients treated by each of these two methods (Bradley *et al.*, 1964). The aim of tracheostomy and fully controlled respiration under these conditions is to produce a normal arterial P_{CO_2} during treatment. Over physiological ranges the carbon dioxide dissociation curve for blood is virtually a straight line. It is therefore possible to compensate for underventilated or non-ventilated alveoli by hyperventilating the remainder, and a normal arterial P_{CO_2} can usually be achieved by using large ventilatory volumes and high inflation pressures. This may necessitate the use of a volume-cycled machine. Unfortunately, it is not possible to relieve the hypoxia by hyperventilation, as a glance at the oxygen dissociation curve for blood will show. In fact, arterial oxygen tensions may even be reduced by artificial ventilation, due to increased maldistribution of ventilation and perfusion. It is, therefore, essential in these patients to measure the arterial oxygen tension frequently to ensure that adequate arterial tensions are maintained with the lowest possible concentration of oxygen in the inspired air.

There is an alternative way in which artificial ventilation can be used in acute exacerbations of chronic bronchitis (Sheldon, 1963). Assisted respiration using a patient-triggered ventilator is applied via an anaesthetic face-mask, mouthpiece or endotracheal tube. This technique can only be used for relatively short periods and rarely achieves a normal arterial P_{CO_2}, but it may be sufficient to enable the patient to survive his acute exacerbation. Assisted respiration may prevent respiratory failure by reducing the work of breathing, which is much increased in obstructive lung disease.

A two to three week period of fully controlled artificial ventilation via a tracheostomy, may, if the volume of ventilation is sufficient to produce a normal arterial P_{CO_2}, actually improve the patient's respiratory function after treatment is discontinued (Bradley *et al.*, 1964). Two mechanisms may be involved here. Rigidity of the thoracic cage, which is a common sequel to chronic bronchitis and emphysema, may be reduced by a period of forcible ventilation. After chronic carbon dioxide retention it may require several weeks of fully adequate ventilation for normal ionic concentrations in the cerebrospinal fluid to be restored (Semple, 1965). If this can be achieved, the patient may be able to maintain near-normal carbon dioxide tensions when artificial ventilation is stopped. This is possibly because the respiratory centre has been resensitised to carbon dioxide.

Weaning from artificial ventilation may be particularly difficult in these patients, so that it is well to decide in advance which patients are liable to become ventilator-dependant cripples. Munck *et al.* (1961) suggested that a useful guide might be obtained by assessing the patient's exercise tolerance and respiratory history prior to the acute exacerbation. Bradley *et al.* (1964) found a well-marked correlation between difficulty in weaning and the degree of emphysema detectable on the chest X-ray. This can be assessed by signs of attenuation of the peripheral pulmonary arteries and increased transradiancy of the lung fields (Fletcher *et al.*, 1963).

Jessen *et al.* (1967) in a ten-year follow-up of 111 patients with chronic lung disease treated with I.P.P.R. divided their patients into three groups based on their physical states before treatment. These important results are summarised in the table below:

Patients		*Survival rates on discharge*	*Survival rates three years after discharge*
		%	%
Patients able to work to some extent	A	85	58
Patients unable to work but able to leave home for personal needs	B	70	31
Patients confined to their homes	C	50	0

They concluded that if artificial ventilation is undertaken for patients in group C they can be expected to require lifelong intermittent or constant artificial ventilation.

Status Asthmaticus

Recent reports have suggested that mortality from asthma may be increasing (Speizer *et al.*, 1968) and that this may be associated with increased use of corticosteroids and pressurised aerosols. Lung pathology in asthma has also been studied and it is now recognised that in severe asthma bronchial plugs are formed. These plugs are tenacious and persistent and completely obstruct many of the smaller bronchi. Mechanical ventilation combined with efficient humidification, possibly by bronchial lavage, have been used to overcome this problem. The results of Marchand and Van Hasselt (1966) and Ambiavagar and Sherwood Jones (1967) testify to the effectiveness of these methods in skilled hands.

The indications for mechanical interference are still under discussion. Once collapse, coma or circulatory arrest have occurred, interference is obligatory, but more difficult and less likely to be successful. It is therefore important to recognise clinical signs which may herald a severe life-threatening deterioration. Death in asthma can occur suddenly and unexpectedly (Earle, 1953). A rising Pa_{CO_2} is a late sign of deterioration but it is possible that taken in conjunction with the respiratory effort the patient is capable of generating, it may be helpful. A useful clinical measure of this effort is the magnitude of paradoxical arterial pressure swings with breathing. In severe asthma the systolic arterial pressure can vary by as much as 40 mm. Hg with respiration. The work involved in generating such pressure swings is great and few patients can sustain it for long. Decreasing arterial paradox and a rising Pa_{CO_2} would therefore seem, at present, to be the most useful criteria for judging when mechanical assistance is necessary.

Mechanical ventilation in asthma presents many problems and requires great care. The chest is already hyperinflated due to air trapping and efforts by the patient to increase bronchial calibre. Over-enthusiastic I.P.P.R. can easily worsen this state and cause severe embarrassment to the right ventricle. Ventilation must be set to the maximum which will not cause unacceptable hypotension and increasing chest distension. It is seldom possible to achieve anything approaching a normal Pa_{CO_2} during the early stages and for this reason heavy sedation or curarization are needed to prevent the patient from fighting the machine.

Bronchial lavage by repeated instillation of 10 ml. of sterile isotonic saline has been used successfully and certainly produces a good harvest of bronchial casts from the smaller bronchi with consequent easing of the difficulties of ventilation (Ambiavagar and Sherwood Jones, 1967). There are theoretical and practical objections to this technique. In normal lungs, saline lavage has been shown to cause a sustained decrease in lung compliance and a fall in Pa_{O_2} due to increased venous admixture (Colebatch and Halmagyi, 1961; Simenstad *et al.*, 1963). Further hypoxaemia in already hypoxic patients, even though temporary, may be dangerous and the technique must therefore be used with speed, skill and caution. Provided an efficient ventilator is available it may be that other methods of humidification, using ultrasonic vibrators to generate a finely divided aerosol, are better though slower (Herzog *et al.*, 1964; Stevens and Albregt, 1966).

Neonatal Respiratory Distress Syndrome (Hyaline Membrane Disease)

Advances in the understanding of the nature of this condition and improvement in apparatus and techniques of artificial ventilation in neonates have recently enabled an improvement in mortality to be achieved.

Artificial ventilation is still the mainstay of supportive treatment though the indications for its use vary in different reports. The most important indications are:

1. Recurrent apnoeic attacks in the small premature baby.
2. Continued deterioration despite adequate conservative therapy including complete correction of fluid and acid base disturbances (Reid *et al.*, 1967).

The techniques of artificial ventilation required are similar to those used in other neonatal conditions. Opinion varies as to whether it is best performed via an endotracheal tube or tracheostomy (Reid and Tunstall, 1966; Glover, 1965). (See also p. 479, Prolonged endotracheal intubation.)

Pneumonia

Artificial respiration has occasionally been advocated as a treatment for severe lobar and bronchopneumonia. It is rarely effective and the additional hazards to which the patient is subjected are not justified by the results obtained. The consolidated area of lung acts as an A-V shunt, producing severe arterial desaturation. The drive to ventilation is increased by this hypoxia and respiratory minute volumes of 10–20 litres are usual. Arterial P_{O_2} and P_{CO_2} are both low. Under these conditions the patient is usually able to do better for himself than a machine can do for him.

I.P.P.R. in the Post-operative Period

The effects of pre-existing pulmonary disease are usually increased by surgery and anaesthesia since coughing is impaired by pain, and a tracheostomy may be needed to remove secretions. The ability of severely ill and debilitated patients to prevent pharyngeal contents from entering their lungs is greatly impaired (Gardner, 1958) and a cuffed tracheostomy tube is of value in isolating the lungs from the pharynx. Nunn and Payne (1962) showed that hypoxaemia in the post-operative period is common, even in patients with normal lungs. This effect is probably due to an increase in ventilation-perfusion inequalities. It is likely to be greater in patients with pre-existing pulmonary disease and may precipitate respiratory failure.

After cardiac surgery artificial respiration may be particularly valuable. Signs of respiratory distress, an increasing tachycardia, circulatory failure or neurological damage are the most important indications for its use. The work of breathing is removed, oxygen demands reduced and despite the potentially adverse circulatory effects of I.P.P.R. most patients are improved by its use (Zeitlin, 1965). Some authorities use artificial respiration routinely after open cardiac surgery (Dammann *et al.*, 1963). The place of artificial respiration in the post-operative period has been reviewed by Norlander (1968) and for further reading reference should be made to *Respiratory Failure* by Sykes *et al.* (1969).

Drowning

Experimental study of human drowning and semi-drowning is virtually impossible, but various mechanisms have been postulated following animal experiments. Their relevance to human drowning is open to some doubt. The remarkable recovery of a Norwegian child after twenty minutes immersion in icy fresh water (Kvittengen and Naess, 1963) exemplifies this doubt. Apparently, in this patient, ventricular fibrillation did not occur, although experimental evidence from animals suggests that it should have been present for a considerable period before resuscitation was started.

From animal experiments, different consequences have been suggested following salt and fresh water drowning.

Salt water.—Being hypertonic, inhalation of sea water causes plasma water to be drawn into the alveoli, thus the lungs increase in weight and widespread peripheral haemorrhages occur. There may follow contraction of the endothelial cells, due to osmotic gradients between intracellular fluid and the sea water in the alveoli (Halmagyi, 1961). Pulmonary compliance decreases and arterial oxygen saturation falls, due to increased venous admixture (Halmagyi and Colebatch, 1961). Haemoconcentration has been said to occur, but the experimental evidence is doubtful. It is possible that blood volume may rise as water is drawn from the tissues. Serum sodium and potassium rise, and death is probably due to ventricular fibrillation following hypoxia and electrolyte disturbance.

Fresh water.—The sequence of events in fresh water drowning is somewhat clearer. Inhaled water is rapidly lost from the alveoli and a 50 per cent rise in blood volume may occur in 2–3 minutes, which accounts for the phenomenon known as "dry drowning". Lungs free of fluid have often been noticed at post-mortem and this finding has previously been attributed to protection of the lungs by laryngeal spasm. Haemodilution causes rupture of red cells and liberation of potassium, so that death is due to ventricular fibrillation from hyperkalaemia and anoxia.

Modell (1968) has recently cast doubt on the validity of these dogmatic distinctions between salt and fresh water drowning. In a review of data from several published series Rivers *et al.* (1970) conclude that there are no significant differences in the clinical pathology that can be attributed to the salinity of the drowning fluid.

The clinical picture presented by partly drowned subjects is due primarily to secondary effects such as hypoxaemia, aspiration, pneumonitis and pulmonary oedema, rather than to the type of water aspirated.

In the clinical management of the victims of drowning, emphasis must be placed on correcting these disturbances and the severe electrolyte disorders which are invariably present. Artificial ventilation is an essential part of regimes of treatment and should probably be used more frequently and for longer periods than has been the case in the past.

Hyperventilation and drowning.—Hyperventilation and breath-holding prior to underwater swimming are dangerous. Hyperventilation causes only a small increase in arterial oxygen tension, but a considerable reduction in carbon dioxide tension. Cerebral blood flow is thereby reduced. Valsalva's manoeuvre may be maintained unintentionally during breath-holding, causing a fall in cardiac output, and a further fall in cerebral blood flow. During swimming a muscle oxygen debt is built up and glucose metabolism only proceeds to the lactic acid stage, so little carbon dioxide is formed. Cerebral hypoxia sufficiently severe to cause unconsciousness may then occur before sufficient carbon dioxide has accumulated to produce in the swimmer the desire to breathe (Dumitru and Hamilton, 1963).

Drug Overdosage

Massive overdosage with any sedative or hypnotic drug can cause respiratory or circulatory failure. Barbiturates are still the commonest group of drugs used for suicide attempts, though poisoning with newer drugs such as tranquillisers and mono-amine oxidase inhibitors is increasing. Experience has shown conclusively that the best treatment is to support respiration and circulation rather than to rely on antidotes, but it is also possible to hasten normal excretion of the drug (see also Chapter 35, p. 989). With many drugs gross oral overdosage causes gastric irritation which predisposes to vomiting and inhalation. Partial obstruction of the airway may have existed for some hours, and this makes regurgitation even more likely (O'Mullane, 1954). The first step is to pass an endotracheal tube and perform bronchial toilet. Only when this has been done is it safe to wash out the stomach. This is always worthwhile, even when it is considered that the bulk of the drug has already been absorbed. In some cases, the gastric washings may provide the only clue to the nature of the drug which has been taken. If the patient is sufficiently deeply unconscious to permit passage of an endotracheal tube without difficulty, it is best to assume that pharyngeal contents have already entered the lungs. This is often confirmed by bronchial toilet. If it is suspected, bronchoscopy should follow gastric lavage. Under these conditions bronchoscopy itself is not without hazard, since it may provoke further regurgitation during introduction or removal of the bronchoscope. The initial stages of the treatment of drug overdosage are most important and may greatly affect the chances of a successful outcome. It is easy to underestimate the severity of the condition, and unless vigorous treatment is started at the earliest possible moment, the patient may die from bronchopneumonia or other pulmonary complications a few days later.

Drug overdosage is one of the conditions in which a subatmospheric phase during I.P.P.R. may be of real value, since poisoning with many drugs appears to depress, probably centrally, the reflex mechanisms responsible for maintaining venous tone, with resultant hypotension. This can be treated with intravenous plasma expanders or it may be necessary to use a venoconstrictor agent, such as noradrenaline. This drug will increase venous tone, central filling pressure will be raised, and an acceptable stroke output and blood pressure can be maintained (Sharpey-Schafer and Ginsburg, 1962).

Head Injury with or without Cervical Cord Injury

In the majority of moderately severe head injuries, the passage of a cuffed endotracheal tube may be all the respiratory treatment necessary. A clear airway is maintained and the trachea is isolated from pharyngeal contents. In some severe head injuries respiratory assistance may be needed. This usually indicates a grave prognosis, unless respiratory failure is precipitated by a rapid rise in intracranial pressure which it is possible to relieve surgically.

Head injury is sometimes accompanied by fracture dislocation of the cervical spine. Damage to the spinal cord resulting from this may cause respiratory failure and quadraplegia. In the presence of a head injury, this condition may be missed for some time, respiratory failure being attributed to the head injury. This is particularly likely if the cord is damaged below the origin of the phrenic nerve. The diaphragmatic component of respiration continues to function, but ventilation may become inadequate and require augmentation.

Tracheostomy in head injury.—Unless there is some evidence of inhalation of pharyngeal contents, the decision to perform tracheostomy is probably best left for at least 48 hours. An endotracheal tube can be used in the interim period, provided that the inspired air is efficiently humidified and it is possible to keep the lungs clear. At the end of this time many patients have recovered sufficiently to make further measures unnecessary. The presence of a tracheostomy tube irritates the trachea and increases coughing, intracranial pressure is raised and cortical damage may be increased.

Status Epilepticus

Most patients with status epilepticus can be satisfactorily controlled by sedation and general measures, but artificial ventilation may occasionally be needed in severe cases. It must be considered if sedation fails to control the patient's fits. Under these conditions, the combination of heavy sedation, persistent unconsciousness between fits and respiratory arrest during each fit, may produce dangerous underventilation and pulmonary complications. Violent muscular activity increases the body's oxygen requirements and predisposes to respiratory insufficiency.

Poliomyelitis

Until a few years ago, poliomyelitis was the commonest single condition in which artificial respiration was needed for long periods. Many of the details of technique and management were worked out on patients with poliomyelitis. With the widespread use of effective vaccines, new cases of paralytic poliomyelitis are rare, at least in countries where the facilities for effective treatment are available.

Many patients, who contracted the disease some years ago, are still alive and remain extensively paralysed. In the acute phase of spinobulbar poliomyelitis the ability to swallow is usually lost and a tracheostomy must be performed. Swallowing commonly returns when the acute phase of the disease is over. If so, the cuff of the tracheostomy tube can be deflated, and the patient is able to talk during the inspiratory period.

The indications for artificial respiration are the same in all the paralysing diseases, and have been conveniently considered together under the section on general management of artificial ventilation. Today, the most commonly seen patients with poliomyelitis are those who have reached the chronic stage of the disease and who suffer a temporary set back due to such things as an upper respiratory infection. Respiratory assistance, physiotherapy and antibiotics are usually sufficient to help the patient over the acute episode. A tracheostomy is rarely indicated, and to perform one may seriously handicap the subsequent management of the condition. Many patients, who are afflicted with long term respiratory weakness, become expert in the management of their state, and the best advice on the therapeutic needs can often be obtained from the patient himself. Heroic efforts have been made in rehabilitating these severely handicapped patients and astonishing results achieved in the face of an almost overwhelming disability.

For rational clinical management it is convenient to divide patients with respiratory impairment after poliomyelitis into the following four categories:

Grade 1

Those patients who need respiratory assistance during minor ailments, particularly upper respiratory tract infections, but who breathe spontaneously without assistance at all other times.

Grade 2

Those patients who regularly need respiratory assistance during sleep, but are normally able to maintain adequate spontaneous respiration during the day.

Grade 3

Those patients who need full artificial respiration during sleep and who require some degree of mechanical respiratory assistance during waking hours.

Grade 4

Those patients who need totally artificial respiration at all times and who therefore rapidly succumb if this fails and immediate support is not available.

Patients in Grade 1 usually have vital capacities over 800 ml. and are able to cough adequately when well by inflating their lungs using glossopharyngeal breathing (see p. 463). During upper respiratory tract infections, secretions are increased and they are best treated in a rotating tank ventilator (see Figs. 6 and 7).

Patients in Grade 2 usually use a cuirass ventilator or rocking bed for sleeping and adopt the same techniques as those in Grade 1 during waking hours. They have vital capacities in the 400–800 ml. range.

Grade 3 patients commonly need a tank ventilator for sleeping and use pneumobelts during the day. These can be battery driven and incorporated into a wheel chair. It has recently been shown by Hamilton *et al.* (1970) that periodic deep inflations using a simple positive pressure source such as a reversed portable domestic vacuum cleaner may be helpful in maintaining normal arterial gas tensions in these patients. Their vital capacities are in the 150–400 ml. range.

Grade 4 patients have a spontaneous vital capacity below 150 ml. Permanent tracheostomy and I.P.P.R. is usually essential, though it is best avoided in the less severe grades as it is liable to increase their degree of machinery dependence.

A number of patients in this severe category have succeeded in rehabilitating themselves from hospital and leading an independent life at home. They have developed combined wheel-chair respirators (Fig. 17*a* and *b*) and talk intermittently during the inspiratory stroke of the ventilator.

Polyneuritis

This term includes what are probably a group of similar diseases. Names such as acute toxic polyneuritis, infective neuronitis and Guillian Barré syndrome have been used. When the disease is severe enough to involve the muscles of respiration, the management is similar to that of poliomyelitis, but a number of important distinctions exist. The onset of paralysis is sometimes slower and more insidious. Daily measurements of vital capacity are particularly important in assessing the need for artificial ventilation. Owing to the gradual onset and slow

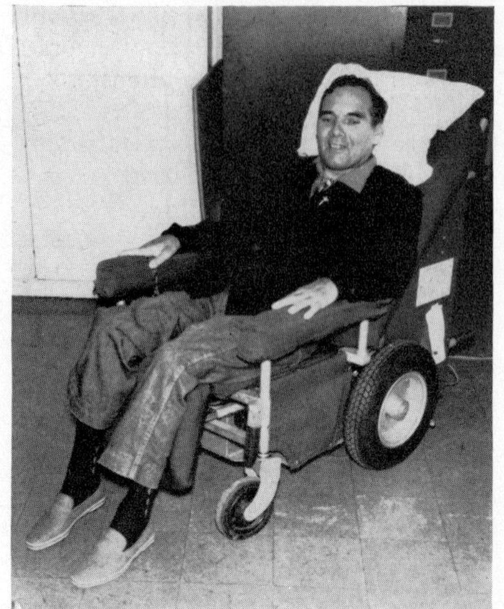

(*a*)

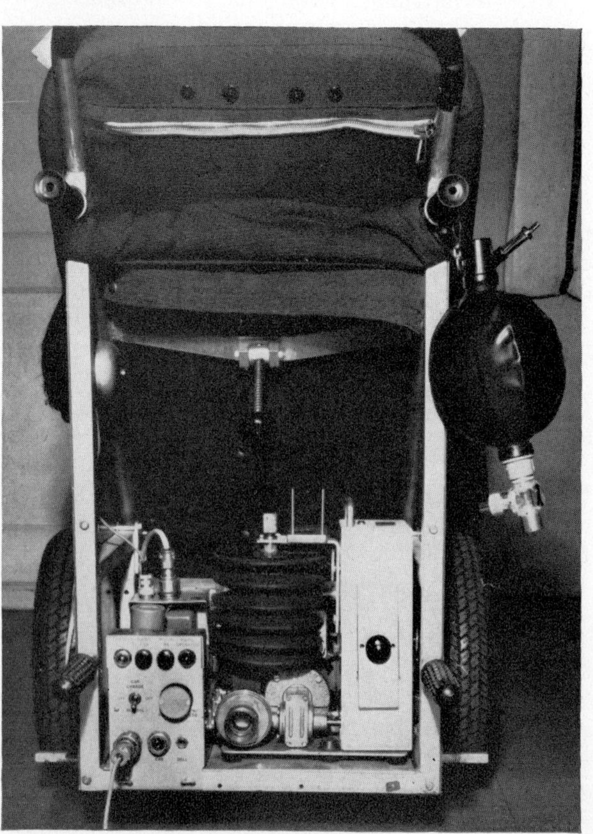

(*b*)

15/Fig. 17(*a*) and (*b*).—The "Cavendish" wheelchair/ventilator.

increase in paralysis, the patient is often less disturbed by his weakness and marked respiratory insufficiency can exist without the patient appearing distressed. In polyneuritis it is less usual for the muscles of respiration to be affected without involvement of the muscles of deglutition. A tracheostomy is therefore essential, and treatment in a tank ventilator rarely indicated. Polyneuritis sometimes affects the autonomic nervous system (Watson, 1962*d*). This may produce circulatory disturbances wholly or partly due to interruption of the autonomic reflex arcs which control the circulation, and a subatmospheric phase during the respiratory cycle is often necessary if an adequate circulation is to be maintained. Facial involvement in these patients may prevent them from closing their eyes, and protection may be needed to avoid corneal ulceration.

The prognosis in polyneuritis is usually excellent. Virtually complete recovery is usual. These patients are some of the most rewarding to treat, and to lose one must be regarded as a tragedy.

Recently evidence has been presented suggesting that patients severely affected by this condition show signs of sympathetic overactivity similar to that seen in severe tetanus (see p. 487) (Dingle, 1969).

Chest Injuries

Chest injuries, involving sufficient disruption of the thoracic cage to cause serious interference with breathing, are difficult to treat. This is partly because the injury is rarely an isolated one, but is associated with a head or neck injury. Concurrent abdominal injuries, such as a ruptured spleen or liver, frequently present additional complications. Despite the theoretical disadvantage of I.P.P.R., that of converting a pneumothorax or haemopneumothorax into a tension pneumothorax, it has proved of great value and is often life saving. The indications for artificial respiration include pain and clinical distress on breathing, retention or inhalation of secretions and signs of paradoxical movement of the chest. Hypoxaemia may be present, due to increased venous admixture in areas of damaged, non-ventilated lung. This must be corrected at once. Endotracheal intubation, curarisation and positive-pressure ventilation using a high inspired oxygen concentration is the most effective method. Paradoxical movements of the chest are stopped, and the work of breathing which may be abnormally great if the airways are partly obstructed by foreign material, is eliminated.

Accumulation of carbon dioxide is usually a late sign of respiratory insufficiency in chest injuries. Its presence indicates that artificial ventilation is long overdue (Hunter, 1964).

It is probable that in assessing these complicated problems too much emphasis has been placed on the anatomical damage to the thoracic cage and not enough on damage to the underlying lung and the physiological disturbances resulting from this damage. Ambiavagar *et al.* (1966) showed that minor rib trauma in patients with pre-existing lung disease often constitutes a severe injury whereas, if pulmonary function is previously good and little new lung trauma results from the injury, respiratory function may be surprisingly little impaired, even after extensive rib injury.

Continuous thoracic epidural analgesia has been tried as a method of pain relief in these patients. Apart from localized chest injuries, in which pain and cough impairment may be slight, it is surprisingly ineffective. The source of pain extends over too many spinal cord segments for effective relief to be possible without using doses of local anaesthetic which produce unacceptable circulatory side-effects.

Kyphoscoliosis

Severe kyphoscoliosis is accompanied by deformity of the thoracic cage. Vital capacity is greatly reduced and coughing impaired by the structural deformity. Caro and Dubois (1961) have shown that chest wall compliance is progressively reduced as age advances. Lung compliance is also reduced. The patient is prone to recurrent pulmonary infections and eventually succumbs during an acute attack.

Artificial ventilation by intermittent positive pressure is clearly valuable in this situation. The patient can be helped over acute episodes and the thoracic cage rendered more supple by a period of forcible ventilation. The possibility that the life of these patients might be usefully prolonged by a period of artificial ventilation deserves further consideration. Structural deformities may make tracheostomy technically difficult, but the potential benefits of treatment appear to justify further investigation.

REFERENCES

Ablett, J. J. L. (1956). Tetanus and the anaesthetist. A review of the symptomatology and the recent advances in treatment. *Brit. J. Anaesth.*, **28**, 258.

Adams, E. B. (1958). Clinical trials in tetanus. *Proc. roy. Soc. Med.*, **51**, 1002.

Ambiavagar, M., Robinson, J. S., Morrison, I. M., and Jones, E. S. (1966). Intermittent positive pressure ventilation in the treatment of severe injuries of the chest. *Thorax*, **21**, 359.

Ambiavagar, M., and Sherwood Jones, E. (1967). Resuscitation of the moribund asthmatic. *Anaesthesia*, **22**, 375.

Andersen, M. N., and Kudriba, K. (1967). Depression of cardiac output with mechanical ventilation. Comparative studies of intermittent positive, positive negative and assisted ventilation. *J. thorac. cardiovasc. Surg.*, **54**, 182.

Ardran, G. M., Kelleher, W. H., and Kemp, F. H. (1959). Cineradiographic studies of glossopharyngeal breathing. *Brit. J. Radiol.*, **32**, 322.

Auchinloss, J. H., and Gilbert, R. (1967). An evaluation of the negative phase of a volume limited respirator. *Amer. Rev. resp. Dis.*, **95**, 66.

Barraclough, M. A., and Sharpey-Schafer, E. P. (1963). Hypotension from absent circulatory reflexes. *Lancet*, **1**, 1121.

Beaver, R. A. (1969). Respirators in respiratory failure. *Brit. med. J.*, **4**, 494.

Bendixen, H. H., Hedley-Whyte, J., and Laver, M. B. (1963). Impaired oxygenation in surgical patients during general anaesthesia with controlled ventilation. *New Engl. J. Med.*, **269**, 991.

Bendixen, H. H., Smith, G. M., and Mead, J. (1964). Pattern of ventilation in young adults. *J. appl. Physiol.*, **19**, 195.

Bradley, R. D., Spencer, G. T., and Semple, S. J. G. (1964). Tracheostomy and artificial ventilation in the treatment of acute exacerbations of chronic lung disease. *Lancet*, **1**, 845.

Brook, M. H., Brook, J., and Wyant, G. M. (1962). Emergency resuscitation. *Brit. med. J.*, **2**, 1564.

Bryce-Smith, R., and Davis, H. S. (1954). Tidal exchange in respirators. *Curr. Res. Anesth.*, **33**, 73.

BURTON, J. D. K. (1962). Effects of dry anaesthetic gases on the respiratory mucous membrane. *Lancet*, **1,** 235.

BYRN, F. M., DAVIES, C. K., and KENT HARRISON, G. (1967). Tracheal stenosis following tracheostomy. *Brit. J. Anaesth.*, **39,** 171.

CAMPBELL, E. J. M. (1958). Mechanisms of airway obstruction in emphysema and asthma. *Proc. roy. Soc. Med.*, **51,** 108.

CAMPBELL, E. J. M. (1960). A method of controlled oxygen administration which reduces the risk of carbon dioxide retention. *Lancet*, **2,** 12.

CARO, G. C., and DUBOIS, A. B. (1961). Pulmonary function in kyphoscoliosis. *Thorax*, **16,** 282.

CHAMNEY, A. R. (1969). Humidification requirements and techniques, including a review of the performance of equipment in current use. *Anaesthesia*, **24,** 602.

CLUTTON-BROCK, J. (1962). A device for introducing a phase of subatmospheric pressure into manually performed I.P.P.R. *Brit. J. Anaesth.*, **34,** 746.

COLE, L., and YOUNGMAN, H. (1968). An attack of tetanus. *Lancet*, **2,** 567.

COLE, L., and YOUNGMAN, H. (1969). Treatment of tetanus. *Lancet*, **1,** 1017.

COLEBATCH, H. J. H., and HALMAGYI, D. F. J. (1961). Lung mechanics and resuscitation after fluid aspiration. *J. appl. Physiol.*, **16,** 684.

COOPER, E. A., SMITH, H., and PASK, E. A. (1960). On the efficiency of intragastric oxygen. *Anaesthesia*, **15,** 211.

DAMMANN, J. F., THUNG, N., CHRISTLIEB, I. I., LITTLEFIELD, J. B., and MULLER, W. H. (1963). The management of the severely ill patient after open heart surgery. *J. thorac. cardiovasc. Surg.*, **45,** 80.

DINGLE, H. R. (1969). Sympathetic overactivity in tetanus (in discussion). *Proc. roy. Soc. Med.*, **62,** 664.

DUMITRU, A. P., and HAMILTON, F. G. (1963). A mechanism of drowning. *Curr. Res. Anesth.*, **42,** 170.

DUNDEE, J. W. (1952). Thiopentone in dystrophia myotonica. *Curr. Res. Anesth.*, **31,** 257.

EARLE, B. V. (1953). Fatal bronchial asthma. A series of fifteen cases with a review of the literature. *Thorax*, **8,** 195.

ELLIS, M. (1967). Editor: *Proceedings of a Symposium on Tetanus in Great Britain*, Leeds.

ENGSTRÖM, C.-G., and HERZOG, P. (1959). Ventilation nomogram for practical use with the Engström respirator. *Acta chir. scand.*, Suppl. **245,** 37.

FELDMAN, S. A., and MONRO, J. A. (1963). A new blower humidifier. *Brit. med. J.*, **2,** 612.

FEYCHTING, H., and SETTERGREN, G. (1966). Automatic sighing device. *Lancet*, **1,** 26.

FLETCHER, C. M., HUGH-JONES, P., MCNICOL, M. W., and PRIDE, N. B. (1963). The diagnosis of pulmonary emphysema in the presence of chronic bronchitis. *Quart. J. Med.*, **32,** 33.

FOSTER, C. A., HEAF, P. J. D., and SEMPLE, S. J. G. (1957). Compliance of the lung in anaesthetised and paralysed subjects. *J. appl. Physiol.*, **11,** 383.

FROEB, H. F., and KIM, B. M. (1964). Tracheostomy and respiratory dead space in emphysema. *J. appl. Physiol.*, **19,** 92.

GALE, J. W., and WATERS, R. M. (1932). Closed endobronchial anaesthesia in thoracic surgery: A preliminary report. *J. thoracic Surg.*, **1,** 432.

GARDNER, A. M. N. (1958). Aspiration of food and vomit. *Quart. J. Med.*, **27,** 227.

GLOVER, W. J. (1965). Mechanical ventilation in respiratory insufficiency in infants. *Proc. roy. Soc. Med.*, **58,** 902.

GRANT, J. L., COOK, J., and MOULTON, P. P. (1964). Effects of tracheostomy in chronic pulmonary disease. *Amer. Rev. resp. Dis.*, **90,** 424.

GRENVIK, A. (1966). Respiratory, circulatory and metabolic effects of respirator treatment. *Acta anaesth. scand.*, Suppl. **19.**

HALMAGYI, D. F. J. (1961). Lung changes and incidence of respiratory arrest in rats after aspiration of sea and fresh water. *J. appl. Physiol.*, **16,** 41.

HALMAGYI, D. F. J., and COLEBATCH, J. H. (1961). Ventilation and circulation after fluid aspiration. *J. appl. Physiol.*, **16,** 35.

HAMILTON, E. A., NICHOLS, P. J. R., and TAIT, G. B. W. (1970). Late onset of respiratory insufficiency after poliomyelitis. *Ann. phys. Med.*, **10,** 223.

HARRISON, G. A., and TONKIN, J. P. (1967). Some serious laryngeal complications of prolonged endotracheal intubation. *Med. J. Aust.*, **1,** 605.

HARRISON, G. A., and TONKIN, J. P. (1968). Prolonged (therapeutic) endotracheal intubation. *Brit. J. Anaesth.*, **40,** 241.

HERHOLDT, J. D., and RAFN, C. G. (1796). *Life Saving Measures for Drowned Persons.* Copenhagen: Acta Anaesth. Scandinav. English translation by Henning Poulsen (1960).

HERZOG, P., NORLANDER, O. P., and ENGSTRÖM, C.-G. (1964). Ultrasonic generation of aerosol for the humidification of inspired gas during volume controlled ventilation. *Acta anaesth. scand.*, **8,** 79.

HEWITT, F. W. (1901). *Anaesthetics and their Administration*, p. 468, 2nd edit. London: Macmillan & Co.

HODGES, R. J. H., MORLEY, R., O'DRISCOLL, W. B., and MCDONALD, I. (1956). A tracheostomy tube for use in acute poliomyelitis. *Lancet*, **1,** 26.

HOWELL, J. B. L., and PECKETT, B. W. (1957). Studies of the elastic properties of the thorax of supine anaesthetised paralysed human subjects. *J. Physiol.* (*Lond.*), **136,** 1.

HUNTER, A. R. (1964). Artificial ventilation of the lungs in combined head and chest injuries. *Lancet*, **2,** 279.

HUNTER, J. (1776). Proposals for the recovery of people apparently drowned. *Phil. Trans. roy. Soc. Lond.*, **66,** 412.

JESSEN, O., SUND KRISTENSEN, H., and RASMUSSEN, K. (1967). Tracheostomy and artificial ventilation in chronic lung disease. *Lancet*, **2,** 9.

KAUFMAN, L. (1960). Anaesthesia in dystrophia myotonica. *Proc. roy. Soc. Med.*, **53,** 183.

KEILTY, S. R., GREY, R. C., DUNDEE, J. E., and MCCULLOUGH, H. (1968). Catecholamine levels in severe tetanus. *Lancet*, **2,** 195.

KELLEHER, W. H. (1961). A new pattern of iron lung for the prevention and treatment of airway complications in paralytic disease. *Lancet*, **2,** 1113.

KELLEHER, W. H. (1969). Respirators in respiratory failure. *Brit. med. J.*, **3,** 528.

KELLY, R. F., and LAURENCE, D. R. (1956). Effect of chlorpromazine on convulsions of experimental and clinical tetanus. *Lancet*, **1,** 118.

KERR, J. H. (1967). In: *Symposium on Tetanus in Great Britain*, p. 49. Edit. Ellis, M.

KERR, J. H., CORBETT, J. L., PRYS-ROBERTS, C., CRAMPTON-SMITH, A., and SPALDING, J. M. K. (1968). Involvement of the sympathetic nervous system in tetanus. *Lancet*, **2,** 236.

KNOTT, F. A., and COLE, L. (1952). "Tetanus". In: *British Encyclopaedia of Medical Practice*, Vol. 12, p. 40. London: Butterworth & Co.

KVITTENGEN, T. D., and NAESS, A. (1963). Recovery from drowning in fresh water. *Brit. med. J.*, **1,** 1315.

LASSEN, H. C. A. (1953). A preliminary report on the 1952 epidemic of poliomyelitis in Copenhagen with special reference to the treatment of acute respiratory insufficiency. *Lancet*, **1,** 37.

LINDHOLM, C. E. (1969). Prolonged endotracheal intubation. *Acta anaesth. scand.*, Suppl., **33.**

LLOYD, J. W., and MCCLELLAND, R. M. A. (1964). Tracheal dilatation. *Lancet*, **2,** 83.

MCCLELLAND, R. M. A. (1965). Complications of tracheostomy. *Brit. med. J.*, **2,** 567.

MACINTOSH, R. R. (1953). Oxford inflating bellows. *Brit. med. J.*, **2,** 202.

MAPLESON, W. W., MORGAN, J. G., and HILLARD, E. K. (1963). Assessment of condenser-humidifiers with special reference to a multiple-gauge model. *Brit. med. J.*, **1,** 300.

MARCHAND, P., and VAN HASSELT, H. (1966). Last-resort treatment of status asthmaticus. *Lancet*, **1,** 227.

MODELL, J. H. (1968). The pathophysiology and treatment of drowning. *Acta anaesth. scand.*, Suppl., **29,** 263.

MONRO, J. A., and SCURR, C. F. (1961). The Starling Pump as a ventilator for infants and children. *Anaesthesia*, **16,** 151.

MORGAN, B. C., MARTIN, W. E., HORNBEIN, T. F., CRAWFORD, E. W., and GUNTHEROTH, W. G. (1966). Haemodynamic effects of intermittent positive pressure respiration. *Anesthesiology*, **27,** 584.

MORGAN, M., LUMLEY, J., and SYKES, M. K. (1970). Arterial oxygenation and physiological deadspace during anaesthesia: effects of ventilation with a pressure preset ventilator. *Brit. J. Anaesth.*, **42,** 379.

MUNCK, O., KRISTENSEN, H. S., and LASSEN, H. C. A. (1961). Mechanical ventilation for acute respiratory failure in diffuse chronic lung disease. *Lancet*, **1,** 66.

NASH, G., BLENNERHASSETT, J. B., and PONTOPPIDAN, H. (1967). Pulmonary lesions associated with oxygen therapy and artificial ventilation. *New Engl. J. Med.*, **276,** 368.

NORLANDER, O. P. (1968). The use of respirators in anaesthesia and surgery. *Acta anaesth. scand.*, Suppl. **30.**

NORLANDER, O. P., HERZOG, P., NORDEN, I., HOSSLI, G., SCHAER, H., and GATTIKER, R. (1968). Compliance and airway resistance during anaesthesia with controlled ventilation. *Acta anaesth. scand.*, **12,** 135.

NUNN, J. F., BERGMAN, N. A., and COLEMAN, A. J. (1965). Factors influencing the arterial oxygen tension during anaesthesia with artificial ventilation. *Brit. J. Anaesth.*, **37,** 898.

NUNN, J. F., and PAYNE, J. P. (1962). Hypoxaemia after general anaesthesia. *Lancet*, **2,** 631.

OKMIAN, L. G. (1966). Artificial ventilation by respirator for newborn and small infants during anaesthesia. *Acta anaesth. scand.*, Suppl. **20.**

O'MULLANE, E. J. (1954). Vomiting and regurgitation during anaesthesia. *Lancet*, **1,** 1209.

OPIE, L. H., SPALDING, J. M. K., and SMITH, A. C. (1961). Intrathoracic pressure during intermittent positive-pressure respiration. *Lancet*, **1,** 911.

PARBROOK, G. D. (1967). Leucopenic effects of prolonged nitrous oxide treatment. *Brit. J. Anaesth.*, **39,** 119.

PEACHEY, R., and PEASE, W. S. (1971). Long term sequelae of prolonged endotracheal intubation (awaiting publication).

PEARCE, D. J., and WALSH, R. S. (1961). Respiratory obstruction due to tracheal granuloma after tracheostomy. *Lancet*, **2,** 135.

PONTOPPIDAN, H., HEDLEY-WHITE, J., BENDIXEN, H. H., LAVER, M. B., and RADFORD, E. P. (1965). Ventilation and oxygen requirements during prolonged artificial ventilation in patients with respiratory failure. *New Engl. J. Med.*, **273,** 401.

POULSEN, H., (1968). *Cardiopulmonary Resuscitation.* World Fed. Soc. Anaesth., Aarhus, Denmark.

POULSEN, H., SKALL-JENSEN, J., STAFFELDT, I., and LANGE, M. (1959). Pulmonary ventilation and respiratory gas exchange during manual artificial respiration and expired air resuscitation on apnoeic normal adults. *Acta anaesth. scand.*, **3,** 129.

PRICE, H. L., CONNOR, E. H., and DRIPPS, R. D. (1954). Some respiratory and circulatory effects of mechanical respirators. *J. appl. Physiol.*, **6,** 517.

PRYS-ROBERTS, C., CORBETT, J. L., KERR, J. H., CRAMPTON-SMITH, A., and SPALDING, J. M. K. (1969). Treatment of sympathetic overactivity in tetanus. *Lancet*, **1,** 542.

PRYS-ROBERTS, C., KELMAN, G. R., GREENBAUM, R., and ROBINSON, R. H. (1967). Circulatory influences during artificial ventilation during nitrous oxide anaesthesia in man. *Brit. J. Anaesth.*, **39,** 534.

RADFORD, E. P., FERRIS, B. G., and KRIETE, B. C. (1954). Clinical use of a nomogram to estimate proper ventilation during artificial respiration. *New Engl. J. Med.*, **251,** 877.

REES, G. J., and OWEN-THOMAS, J. B. (1966). A technique of pulmonary ventilation with a nasotracheal tube. *Brit. J. Anaesth.*, **38,** 901.

REID, D. H. S., and TUNSTALL, M. E. (1966). The respiratory distress syndrome of the newborn. *Anaesthesia*, **21,** 72.

REID, D. H. S., TUNSTALL, M. E., and MITCHELL, R. G. (1967). A controlled trial of artificial respiration in the respiratory distress syndrome of the newborn. *Lancet*, **1,** 532.

RIVERS, J. F., ORR, G., and LEE, H. A. (1970). Drowning. Its clinical sequelae and management. *Brit. med. J.*, **2,** 157.

RUBEN, H. (1955). A new non-rebreathing valve. *Anesthesiology*, **16,** 643.

RUBEN, H., and RUBEN, A. (1957). Apparatus for resuscitation and suction. *Lancet*, **2,** 373.

RUSSELL, W. R., and SCHUSTER, E. (1953). Respiration pump for poliomyelitis. *Lancet*, **2,** 707.

SAFAR, P., ESCARRAGA, L. A., and ELAM, J. O. (1958). A comparison of the mouth to mouth and mouth to airway methods of artificial respiration with the chest-pressure arm-lift methods. *New Engl. J. Med.*, **258,** 671.

SATINDER LAL (1965). Blood gases in respiratory failure. *Lancet*, **1,** 339.

SCHUSTER, E., and FISCHER-WILLIAMS, M. (1953). A rocking bed for poliomyelitis. *Lancet*, **2,** 1074.

SEMPLE, S. J. G. (1965). Respiration and the cerebro-spinal fluid. *Brit. J. Anaesth.*, **37,** 262.

SHACKLETON, R. P. W. (1954). The treatment of tetanus. Role of the anaesthetist. *Lancet*, **2,** 155.

SHACKLETON, R. P. W. (1962). In my end is my beginning. *Ann. roy. Coll. Surg. Engl.*, **30,** 229.

SHARPEY-SCHAFER, E. P. (1955). Effects of Valsalva's manoeuvre on the normal and failing circulation. *Brit. med. J.*, **1,** 693.

SHARPEY-SCHAFER, E. P. (1961). Venous tone. *Brit. med. J.*, **2,** 1589.

SHARPEY-SCHAFER, E. P., and GINSBURG, J. (1962). Humoral agents and venous tone. *Lancet*, **2,** 1337.

SHELDON, G. P. (1963). Pressure breathing in chronic obstructive lung disease. *Medicine* (*Baltimore*), **42,** 197.

SIMENSTAD, J. O., GALWAY, C. T., and MACLEAN, L. D. (1963). The treatment of aspiration and atelectasis by tracheobronchial lavage. *Curr. Res. Anaesth.*, **42,** 616.

SMITH, A. C., and SPALDING, J. M. K. (1959). Intermittent positive pressure respiration. Some physiological observations. *Proc. roy. Soc. Med.*, **52,** 661.

SMYTHE, P. M. (1963). Studies in neonatal tetanus and on pulmonary compliance of the totally relaxed infant. *Brit. med. J.*, **1,** 565.

SPALDING, J. M. K., and OPIE, L. (1958). Artificial respiration with the Tunnicliffe breathing jacket. *Lancet*, **1,** 613.

SPEIZER, F. E., DOLL, R., and HEAF. P. (1968). Observations on recent increase in mortality from asthma. *Brit. med. J.*, **1,** 335.

SPENCER, G. T. (1969). (Indications for tank ventilators.) Respirators in respiratory failure. *Brit. med. J.*, **3,** 780.

STEVENS, H. R., and ALBREGT, H. B. (1966). Assessment of ultrasonic nebulization. *Anesthesiology*, **27,** 648.

SYKES, M. K., MCNICOL, M. W., and CAMPBELL, E. J. M. (1969). In *Respiratory Failure*, p. 153. Oxford: Blackwell Scientific Publications.

TONKIN, J. P., and HARRISON. G. A. (1966). The effect on the larynx of prolonged endotracheal intubation. *Med. J. Aust.*, **2,** 581.

WARRELL, D. A., EDWARDS, R. H. T., GODFREY, S., and JONES, N. L. (1970). Effect of controlled oxygen therapy on arterial blood gases in acute respiratory failure. *Brit. med. J.*, **2,** 452.

WATSON, W. E. (1961). Physiology of artificial respiration. (D. Phil. Thesis submitted to Oxford University.)

WATSON, W. E. (1962*a*). Some observations on dynamic lung compliance during intermittent positive pressure respiration. *Brit. J. Anaesth.*, **34,** 153.

WATSON, W. E. (1962*b*). Observations on physiological dead space during intermittent positive pressure respiration. *Brit. J. Anaesth.*, **34,** 502.

WATSON, W. E. (1962*c*). Observations on the dynamic lung compliance of patients with respiratory weakness receiving intermittent positive pressure respiration. *Brit. J. Anaesth.*, **34,** 690.

WATSON, W. E. (1962*d*). Some circulatory responses to Valsalva's manoeuvre in patients with polyneuritis and spinal cord disease. *J. Neurol. Neurosurg. Psychiat.*, **24,** 19.

WHITTARD, B. R., and THOMAS, K. E. (1964). A new polyvinyl chloride cuffed tracheostomy tube. *Lancet*, **1,** 797.

WHITTENBERGER, J. L. (1955). Artificial respiration. *Physiol. Rev.*, **35,** 611.

WRIGHT, R., SYKES, M. K., JACKSON, B. G., MANN, N. M., and ADAMS, E. B. (1961). Intermittent positive pressure respiration in tetanus neonatorum. *Lancet*, **2,** 678.

ZEITLIN, G. L. (1965). Artificial respiration after cardiac surgery. *Anaesthesia*, **20,** 145.

FURTHER READING

POULSEN, H. (1968). *Cardiopulmonary Resuscitation.* Aarhus, Denmark: World. Fed. Soc. Anaesth.

SPALDING, J. M. K., and SMITH, A. C. (1963). *Clinical Practice and Physiology of Artificial Respiration.* Oxford: Blackwell Scientific Publications.

SYKES, M. K., MCNICOL, M. W., and CAMPBELL, E. J. M. (1969). *Respiratory Failure.* Oxford: Blackwell Scientific Publications.

Chapter 16

AUTOMATIC VENTILATORS

by

G. T. Spencer

Only a brief review of the principles of automatic ventilators is given here, and a few ventilators in common use are illustrated and described. For a fully comprehensive review of the subject the reader is referred to *Automatic Ventilation of the Lungs*, by Mushin *et al.* (1969).

Principles of Ventilators

Ventilators can be conveniently classified by the patterns of flow, volume and pressure which they produce in the patient's lungs. Unfortunately, this classification does not define function fully and the method by which the machine is cycled has to be considered. Thus the respiratory cycle of a ventilator can be divided into four parts:

1. The inspiratory phase.
2. The change-over from the inspiratory to the expiratory phase.
3. The expiratory phase.
4. The change-over from the expiratory to the inspiratory phase.

(Mapleson, 1969).

1. The Inspiratory Phase

Flow generators.—These are ventilators which deliver a predetermined flow during the inspiratory phase. The flow may be generated by a compressor which pumps out a fixed volume at each stroke or revolution, as in the Blease ventilator (p. 514). The flow is not necessarily constant as many ventilators deliver a near sinusoidal flow. This can be generated by a bag or bellows which is compressed directly by a cam or crank, as in the Cape (p. 507) or indirectly by pneumatic compression of a bag in a bottle as in the Engström ventilators (p. 511).

The volume delivered by a flow generator is independent of the resistance caused by the ventilator tubing, the patient's airway or the pulmonary compliance. An increase in any of these variables will produce a rise in inflation pressure rather than a fall in ventilatory volume. Flow generators are therefore particularly suitable for ventilating patients with pulmonary disease in whom they will maintain a constant minute volume despite variations in airway resistance or compliance. They are susceptible, however, to leaks in the circuit, because air so lost causes a corresponding loss to the inflation volume.

Compression volume.—Not all of the flow generated by the ventilator enters the patient's lungs and some is absorbed by air compression in the ventilator circuit. If the inflation pressure is high, or the volume of the humidifier or ventilator circuit large in relation to the tidal volume, losses from compression may be significant. Both these factors combine when small babies are being ventilated. Under these conditions the compression volume may be several times greater than the tidal volume.

Pressure generators.—These are ventilators which generate a constant pressure during the inspiratory phase. The pressure may be generated by the release of gas or air from a pressure source, as in the Barnet ventilator (p. 512) and the Bennett ventilator (p. 515) or by a weight acting on a concertina bag, as in the East Radcliffe ventilator (p. 507).

The volume delivered by a pressure generator is dependent on the resistance of the ventilator circuit, the patient's airways and the pulmonary compliance. Regular measurements of minute volume will therefore provide an indication of changes in these variables, such as occur when secretions accumulate.

Pressure generators will to some extent compensate for leaks in the ventilator circuit. A leak acts as a loss of resistance, and a correspondingly greater volume will be delivered by the predetermined pressure. Equally, volume loss due to compression in the tubing will be constant and therefore less significant than when a flow generator is used.

Owing to the limits of pressure available it may be impossible, when airway resistance is high, to achieve the desired volume of ventilation. Maximum difficulty is encountered when ventilating small babies with pulmonary abnormalities.

2. The Change-over from the Inspiratory to the Expiratory Phase

Cycling at the end of inspiration may occur in three ways.

(*A*). *Time cycling.*—In time cycled ventilators the change-over from inspiration to expiration occurs after a fixed time and is uninfluenced by the state of the patient's lungs. The timing mechanism may be operated pneumatically, as in the Bennett ventilator (p. 515), electrically, as in the Barnet ventilator (p. 512), or mechanically, as in the Engström (p. 511) and East Radcliffe (p. 507) ventilators.

(*B*). *Pressure cycling.*—Here, the change-over occurs when a predetermined pressure is reached. The mechanism can be operated magnetically, as in the Bird ventilator (p. 515), or mechanically, as in the Blease ventilator (p. 514) when this machine is set to function on a pressure cycled basis. The time taken to reach the critical pressure is influenced by the resistance offered by the patient's lungs, and will be reached more quickly when the resistance is high. An alteration in airway resistance is detectable by the alteration in respiratory rate which accompanies it.

(*C*). *Volume cycling.*—In volume-cycled ventilators, the change-over occurs when a fixed volume has been delivered from the machine. It occurs mechanically when the cam operating the bellows reaches the end of its stroke in the Cape ventilator (p. 507) and the Beaver ventilator (p. 513). It can also be made to occur by limiting the stroke of the bellows by a mechanical trip. This is the method used in the Blease ventilator (p. 514) to convert it to volume cycling.

3. The Expiratory Phase

It is possible to apply the same terminology to the expiratory phase as has been used above to describe the inspiratory phase. This is cumbersome, however, as ventilators vary a lot in their expiratory phase characteristics and several different patterns may exist in the same ventilator at different stages of the expiratory phase. The simplest method of expiration is to connect the patient's lungs to the atmosphere. This is used in the Beaver ventilator (p. 513). Most ventilators are now capable of exerting a subatmospheric pressure during the expiratory phase, which may last throughout it or only for part of it. The greatest negative pressure may occur at the start of expiration, and thereafter decline, as in the Blease ventilator, or the pressure may become increasingly negative as the expiratory phase continues, as in the Barnet and Cape ventilators. At present no data is available to suggest which is the best pattern, and a functional analysis is therefore valueless. It can be argued that it is best to apply the greatest negative pressure at the start of expiration when bronchial calibre is larger and air trapping less likely to occur. It can be argued with equal force that a sudden change from maximum positive to maximum negative pressure may predispose to air trapping, and subatmospheric pressure is therefore best applied in a gradually increasing pattern. At present the answer to these questions is unknown.

4. **The Change-over from the Expiratory to the Inspiratory Phase**

In practice only two methods are used for this change-over:

Time cycling.—Here, the changeover from the expiratory phase to the inspiratory phase occurs at a pre-set time. In some ventilators, such as the Barnet, the timing of the expiratory cycle can be varied independently of the inspiratory cycle. In others, such as the Engström, the two cycles cannot be varied independently, and the proportions of the respiratory cycle occupied by inspiration and expiration are fixed.

Patient cycling.—Ventilators which include this feature are commonly known as triggered ventilators, or assistors. A slight inspiratory effort by the patient produces a subatmospheric pressure in the ventilator tubing, which triggers off the change-over from the expiratory phase to the inspiratory phase, and the patient's spontaneous inspiration is augmented. The mechanism is operated either pneumatically, as in the Bennett and Bird (p. 515), and Blease (p. 514) ventilators, or electrically, as in the Barnet MK III ventilator. It is possible that a patient with sufficient respiratory power to operate a patient cycled ventilator may not gain significant improvement in ventilation from doing so. Spontaneous inspiratory efforts in patients with respiratory insufficiency are often short in duration and somewhat jerky. By the time air pressure changes have passed through the ventilator tubing and triggered off the inspiratory phase of the ventilator, expiration by the patient has almost certainly begun. The force of the patient's expiration, inertia of the thoracic cage, and the elastic recoil of the lungs has to be overcome by the ventilator before significant ventilation is achieved. Physiological dead space may be considerably increased in this situation, which may account for marginal improvements in ventilation, despite obviously greater movement of the patient's chest.

Efficient patient cycling may be difficult to achieve in practice and requires careful adjustment of the ventilator. It is probably most suitable for short term use, under close expert supervision.

In addition to assessing its function, a number of other factors have to be taken into account in choosing the most suitable ventilator for a particular purpose or hospital.

Motive Power

This may be provided by an electric motor or by a pressure input of gas or air. The Barnet ventilator is peculiar in that it requires a combination of the two. The bellows are filled by gas input from a pressure source, but the cycling is operated electrically. A source of gas or air at the appropriate pressure may not always be readily available, and for long-term use it is often more reliable and convenient to use a machine which will entrain its own air from the atmosphere, and which does not require a pressure source to operate it.

Most ventilators available today are functionally sound and mechanically efficient. It is usually best to choose a ventilator which has been manufactured in the country in which it is to be used, since servicing is likely to be better and the machine may be better adapted to match existing ancillary equipment and fittings.

Examples of Commonly Used Ventilators

1. Electrically Operated Ventilators

The East Radcliffe positive-negative respiration pump (Russell *et al.*, 1956). (Fig. 1). This is probably the best tried and most widely used ventilator in the United Kingdom. It is particularly suitable for patients who are permanently dependent on artificial ventilation. A number of such patients have used simple models of the Radcliffe ventilator in their own homes for up to ten years (see 15/Fig. 17*a* and *b*). The machine is robust, portable and cheap. Using non-cuffed tracheostomy tubes such patients are able to talk during the inspiratory phase by leaking air up the trachea around the tube to the vocal cords which are voluntarily held adducted at other times. Being a pressure generator the machine can compensate for this leak and maintain the previous minute volume. These simplified Radcliffe ventilators can be set to produce a longer inspiratory than expiratory phase, thus giving a usefully greater talking time.

In the model shown in Fig. 1, a constant speed electric motor lifts a variable weight which is then allowed to fall on to a bellows producing inspiration. A second bellows exerts a negative pressure during expiration. A variable leak provides control of the negative pressure applied. Mechanical valves produce cycling and a thermostatically controlled heater humidifier is included in the inspiratory limb of the circuit.

In the event of power failure, the machine can be driven either by an alternative 12-volt motor powered by an accumulator, or by a hand crank. Both motors operate via a Sturmey-Archer four-speed bicycle hub. This allows four different respiratory rates to be used. An oxygen reservoir is provided in the air intake to allow enrichment of the inspired air.

Sykes (1962) has described a modification of the East Radcliffe pump which adapts it for anaesthesia (Fig. 2).

Summary.—An air-entrainment, positive/negative, time-cycled, pressure generator. Mechanical valves preclude patient cycling.

The Cape ventilator (Fig. 3).—The Cape ventilator is a development of the

Smith-Clarke ventilator (Smith-Clarke and Galpine, 1955), and its operating principles are much the same. Motive power is provided by a constant speed electric motor driving a single cam shaft via a gear box which allows the respiratory rate to be freely adjusted between 10 and 50 cycles per minute. The cam shaft

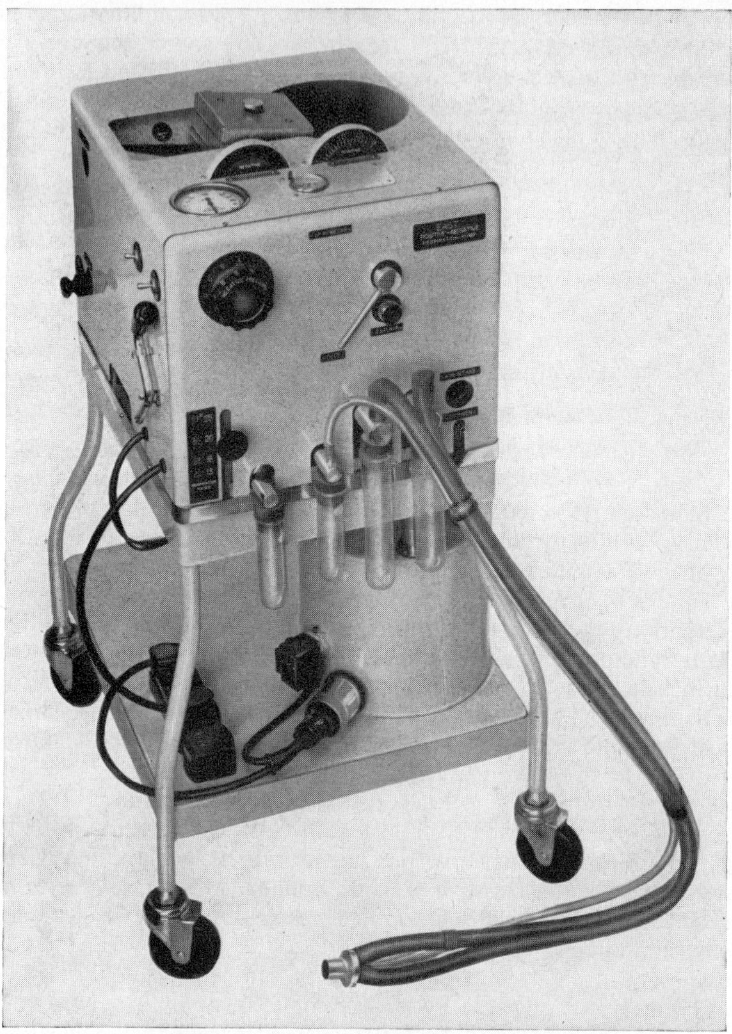

16/Fig. 1.—East Radcliffe positive-negative respiration pump.

drives inspiratory and expiratory poppet valves, and both bellows. The inspiratory bellows are compressed by a rocking beam with a movable fulcrum which allows the volume delivered by the bellows to be varied from 0·2 litres to 1·6 litres. The second bellows, which can be excluded from the circuit, provide subatmospheric pressure during expiration and this can be adjusted by a variable air leak. An

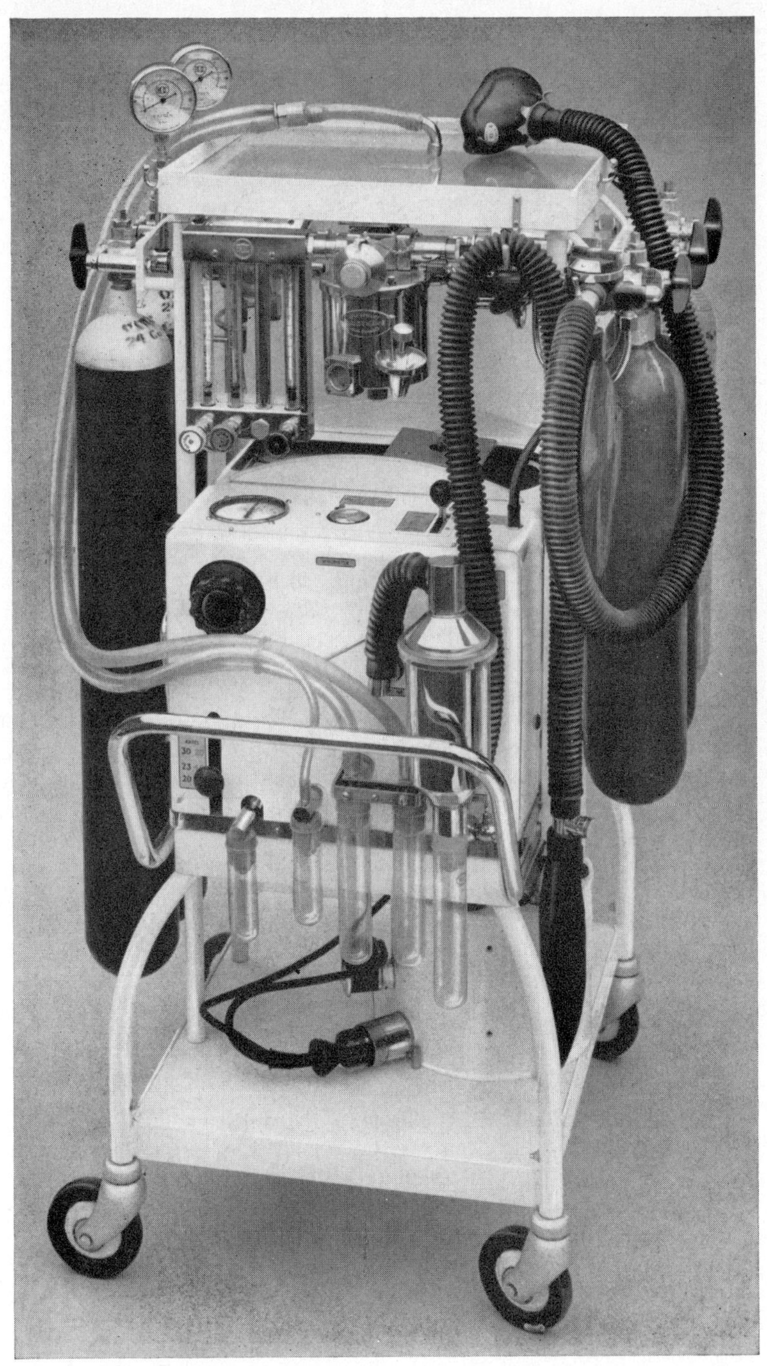

16/FIG. 2.—East Radcliffe positive-negative respiration pump adapted for anaesthesia.

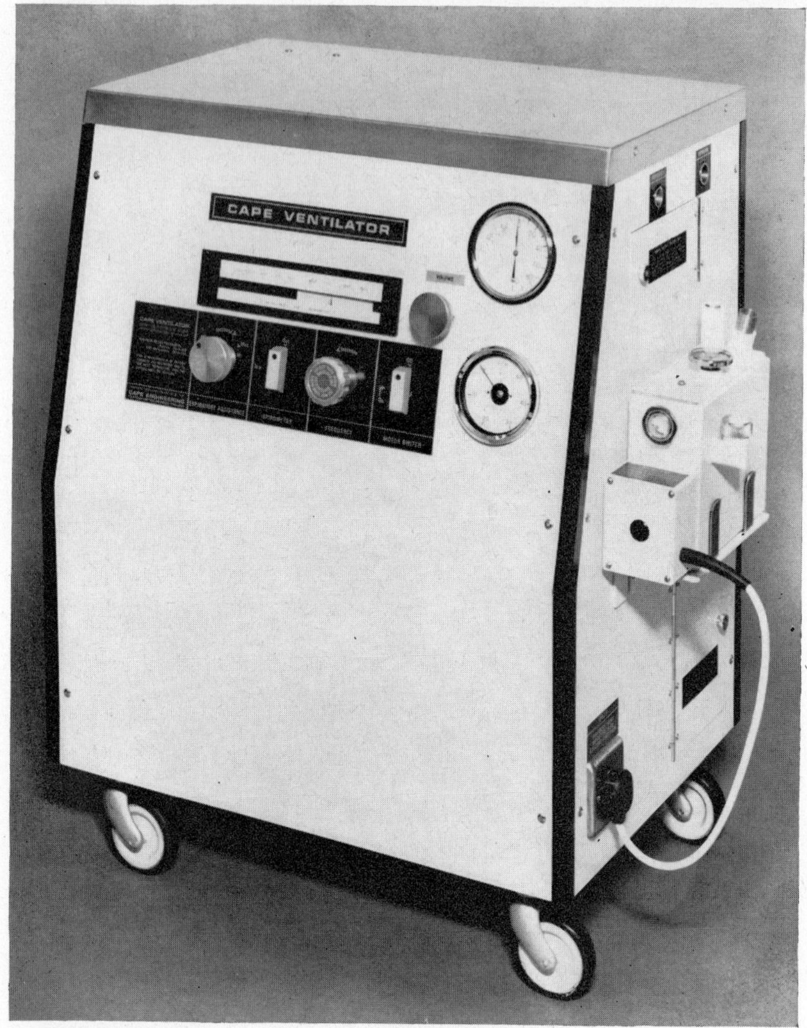

16/FIG.3.—The Cape ventilator.

oxygen reservoir can be attached to the air intake and a thermostatically controlled heater humidifier is included in the inspiratory limb of the circuit. As this is between the patient and the inspiratory valve it constitutes a compression volume.

In the event of power failure, manual operation is provided by a crank handle connected to one end of the cam shaft. Thus, one turn of the handle is equal to one respiratory cycle. The Cape-Wayne ventilator is an alternative machine which has been developed for anaesthesia (Waine and Fox, 1962).

Summary.—An air entrainment, positive/negative, time-cycled, flow generator. Mechanical valves preclude patient cycling.

The Engström ventilator (Engström, 1954).—The Engström ventilator is undoubtedly the most sophisticated and comprehensive machine available. Only its cost and size preclude it from more widespread use. Motive power is provided by a constant speed electric motor driving a piston in a two-way cylinder. During inspiration the piston compresses a reservoir bag contained in a chamber. Gas or air is forced from the bag through a pneumatically operated one-way valve via a thermostatically controlled water-bath heater humidifier into

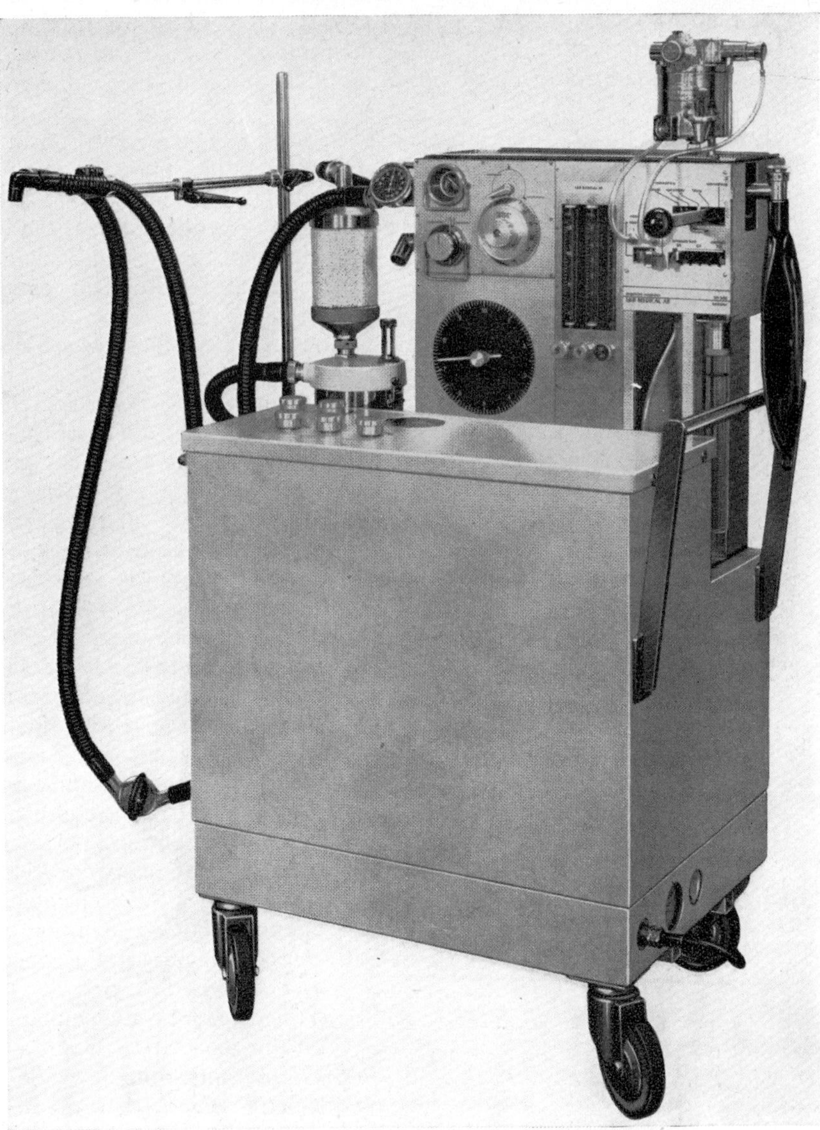

16/Fig. 4.—The Engström Model 300 ventilator.

the patient's lungs. The humidifier represents compression volume. A side-arm from the inspiratory limb of the circuit closes the expiratory valve by air pressure. At the end of inspiration the expiratory valve opens and the patient's lungs are connected to the atmosphere. A subatmospheric pressure is introduced by a venturi jet in the exhaust port driven from the double piston during its back stroke. The back stroke also serves to draw air into the reservoir bag. In the event of power failure, it is possible to include in the patient circuit a reservoir bag which can be switched in and operated manually. If the pressure gas source fails, the machine can entrain a regulated amount of room air. In normal use both air entrainment and the input of selected gases can be regulated independently, and precise control of the composition of the inspired gases is therefore possible.

Summary.—A mixed, gas input/air entrainment, time-cycled, positive/negative flow generator. Towards the end of the inspiratory phase the machine becomes a pressure generator. It is significant that despite his extensive experience (Engström, 1963) and the presence of pneumatically operated valves, the designer of this machine has not included facilities for patient cycling.

An interesting new model of the Engström ventilator has recently been introduced (Norlander *et al.*, 1968) (Fig. 4). While retaining similar principles of operation, the patient circuit can be removed and sterilised by autoclaving.

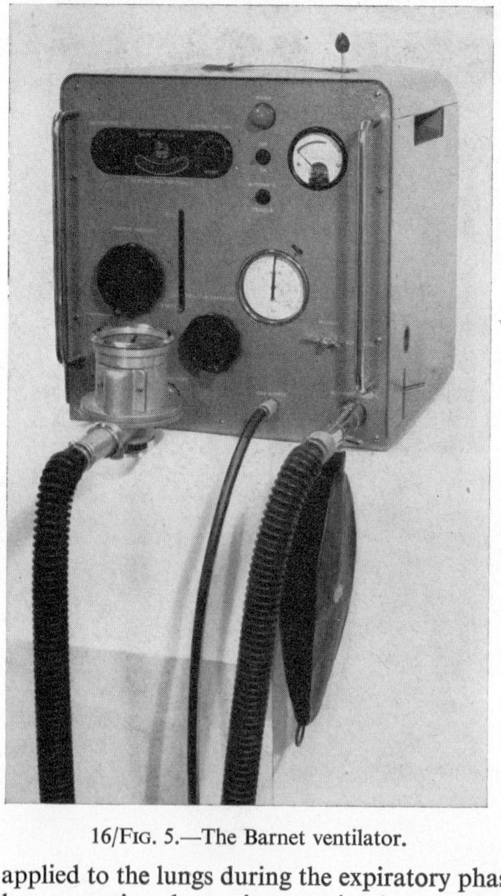

16/Fig. 5.—The Barnet ventilator.

The Barnet ventilator (Rochford *et al.*, 1958) (Fig. 5).—This machine was developed primarily for use during anaesthesia and it could be fitted between the shelves of a Boyle's anaesthetic machine. Gases from a low-pressure source flow continuously into a concertina bag. The inspiratory and expiratory valves are operated electronically at independently variable timings. During inspiration the gas in the concertina bag is delivered to the patient at a pressure maintained on the concertina bag by a variable coil spring. A variable subatmospheric pressure can be applied to the lungs during the expiratory phase. Patient cycling can be provided by connecting the expiratory circuit to a diaphragm operating a microswitch.

A thermostatically controlled water-bath heater humidifier is available as an optional extra.

If the power supply fails, the machine continues to function automatically, drawing power from an accumulator. If the source of gas pressure fails the ventilator becomes inoperative.

Summary.—A gas input, time-cycled, positive/negative pressure generator, with alternative positive pressure patient cycling.

A Mark III model of this ventilator has recently been introduced. It is exceedingly complicated and includes alternative volume cycling. It is too big to be incorporated into a Boyle's anaesthetic machine.

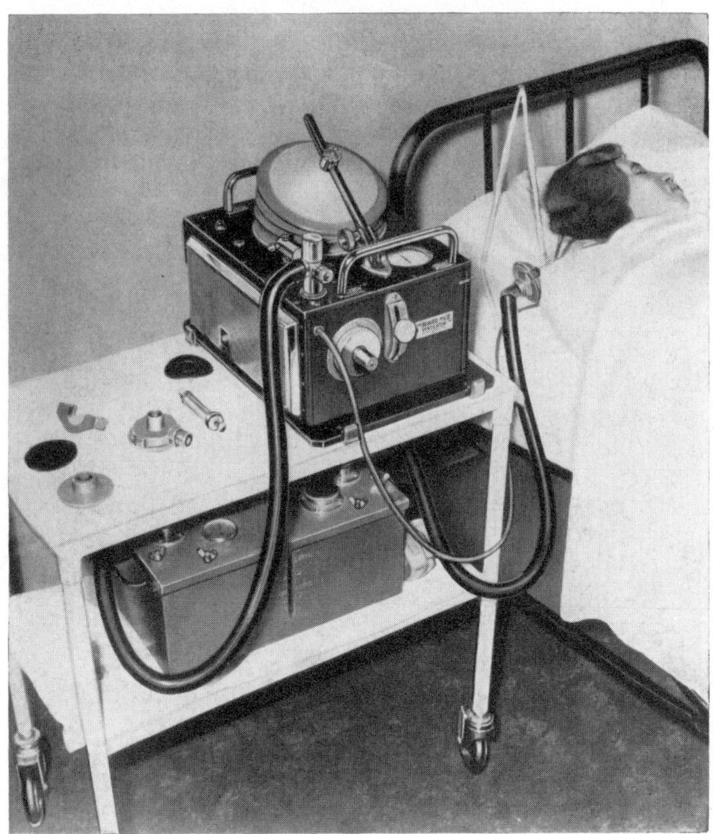

16/FIG. 6.—The Beaver ventilator and Smith-Clarke humidifier.

The Beaver ventilator (Beaver, 1956). (Fig. 6).—Air is drawn through a one-way valve into a concertina bag which is expanded and compressed by an arm driven from a variable speed motor. During inspiration the air in the concertina bag is transferred to the patient through a solenoid operated valve at the patient end of the tubing. During expiration the patient's lungs are connected to atmosphere via the solenoid operated valve.

In the event of a power failure, a link pin can be removed and the bellows arm operated by hand.

A humidifier is not normally included with this ventilator. A Smith-Clarke or similar pattern heater humidifier unit can be connected into the patient tubing, where it constitutes compression volume.

Summary.—An air entrainment, volume cycled, positive pressure flow generator.

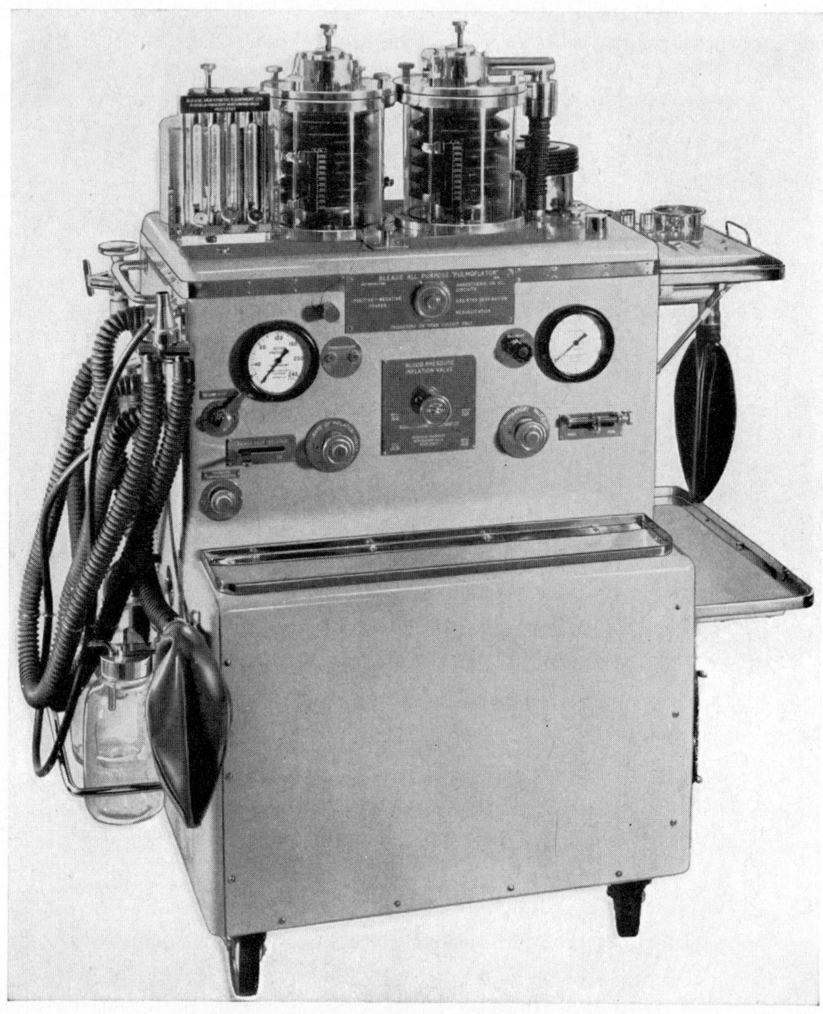

16/FIG. 7.—Blease pulmoflator.

The Blease ventilator (Fig. 7).—Various models of this machine are available, offering different facilities. The principles of operation are the same in all models. An air pump, housed in the base of the machine, supplies air to a chamber. The rise of pressure in this chamber compresses a concertina bag, from which gas or air is forced into the patient's lungs. In the models for use during anaesthesia, the concertina bag is filled from gas cylinders. As the pressure rises in the chamber a spring connected to a flexible diaphragm is compressed until, at a pre-set pressure, a valve is opened and the chamber connected to the atmosphere.

A subatmospheric phase can be introduced during expiration by using air from the pump to drive a venturi jet which creates a negative pressure in the main chamber. A device for patient cycling is also included. Some models can be converted to volume cycling by allowing the concertina bag to operate a trip mechanism. A heater humidifier is not normally included.

In the event of power failure, the anaesthetic circuit can be switched to manual operation. In the event of failure of the gas supply the ventilator becomes inoperative.

Summary.—A gas input, pressure cycled, positive/negative, flow or pressure generator, with alternative positive pressure patient cycling.

Recent developments of this machine include a patient circuit which is partly removable and can be autoclaved.

2. Pneumatically Operated Ventilators

The Bird ventilator (Fig. 8).—This machine is operated by a source of oxygen pressure at 50 lb./sq.in. If the pressure source fails the machine becomes inoperative. The entry of oxygen to the machine is varied by a needle valve which controls the flow and speed during inspiration. Air can be entrained during inspiration by passing the oxygen through a variable venturi injector.

Cycling is controlled pneumatically by alterations in pressure on opposite sides of adjustable diaphragms. The inspiratory diaphragm is placed within the main chamber of the machine and the expiratory diaphragm is contained in a valve at the patient end of the tubing. This arrangement allows efficient and sensitive patient cycling. Some degree of humidification is provided by a "nebuliser" operating on the venturi principle, at the patient end of the tubing. Many versions of the Bird ventilator are available, offering different facilities.

Summary.—With air entrainment, the machine is a pressure cycled, positive/negative, pressure generator, with alternative positive pressure patient cycling. When no air is entrained the machine becomes a flow generator.

The Bennett ventilator (Fig. 9).—This machine is operated by a high pressure source of air or gas. It contains its own reducing valve. If the pressure source fails, the machine becomes inoperative. The valves are pneumatically operated and are either time or patient-cycled. During inspiration the machine acts as a pressure generator, inflating the lungs at approximately constant pressure.

GENERAL COMMENT

The use of ventilators has increased so much in recent years that the variety and sizes available are now almost bewildering. An excellent summary of many more widely available types, including small ones for use during anaesthesia, has been compiled by Adams (1968). Of particular interest to the clinical anaesthetist are miniature ventilators driven by the gas pressure produced by the distension of an anaesthetic reservoir bag (Collis *et al.*, 1969).

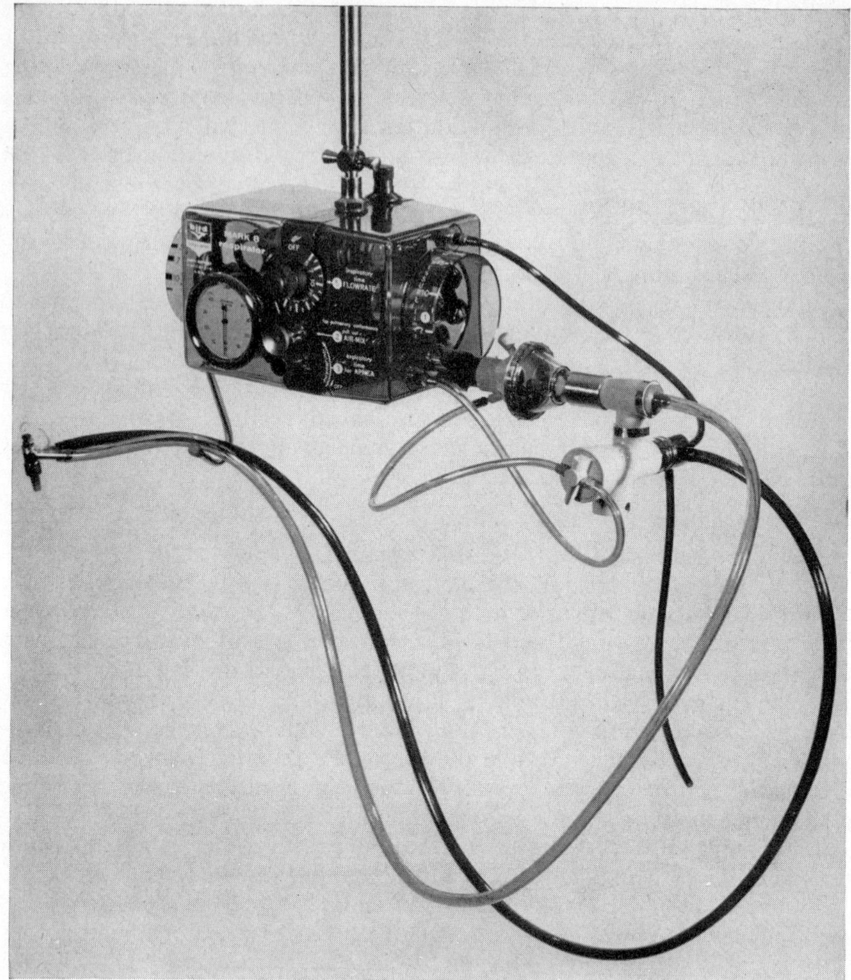

16/FIG. 8.—The Bird ventilator.

BACTERIAL CONTAMINATION AND STERILISATION OF VENTILATORS

The bacterial contamination of automatic lung ventilators is a common occurrence during prolonged artificial respiration, and the possibility of transferring bacteria from one patient to another via the ventilator has been recognised for some time (Phillips and Spencer, 1965). Nevertheless the number of adequately documented instances are few (Phillips, 1967; Wright *et al.*, 1961; Bishop *et al.*, 1962). The organism concerned is usually the *Pseudomonas aeruginosa*, which rapidly colonizes the upper respiratory tract of many patients following prophylactic antibiotic therapy and endotracheal intubation (Redman and Lockey, 1967). Although Hellewell *et al.* (1967) showed experimentally that bacteria

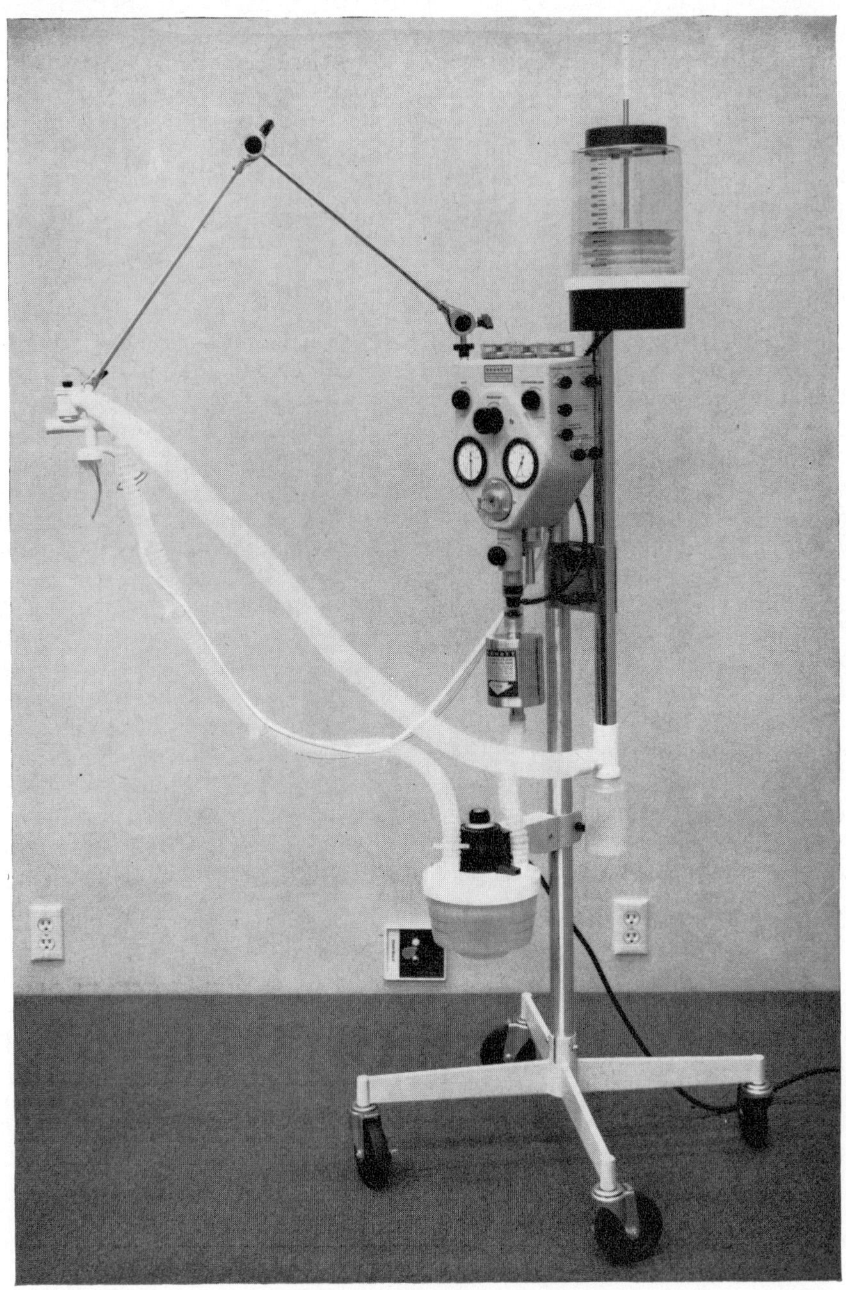

16/FIG. 9.—The Bennett ventilator.

introduced into the inspiratory limb of a ventilator did not spread in a retrograde direction, their results are in conflict with the experience of Phillips and Spencer (1965) and Reinarz *et al.* (1965). Multiplication of vegetative micro-organisms in the water bath humidifier of a ventilator can occur rapidly. This can be prevented either by filling the humidifier with a solution of 0·1 per cent chlorhexidine in distilled water, or by maintaining the water in the humidifier at a pasteurizing temperature of 60°C. (Glover, 1966).

Filters

An absolute bacterial filter has been described by Bishop *et al.* (1963) for attachment to the air intake of ventilators. This is useful in cleaning incoming air, but it does not prevent contamination of the ventilator by the patient. Ideally, filters should be placed in the inspiratory and expiratory tubing to the patient, isolating him from the ventilator. The filter described by Bishop *et al.* cannot be used in this position as it becomes blocked by water droplets condensed from the humidifier and the expired air. Blockage can be overcome by a suitable filter design (Pyle *et al.*, 1969), but unfortunately, when a volume cycled ventilator is used, filters in this position add substantially to the compression volume of the circuit.

Although filters are useful in delaying ventilator contamination by the patient, there is general agreement that they do not obviate the need to sterilise the ventilator between use in patients if it has been in action for more than a few days. (Spencer *et al.*, 1968).

Disinfection of Ventilators

A variety of methods of disinfecting ventilators between use have been described. These methods have been compared by Fisher and Kyi Kyi (1969). None is completely satisfactory and all have disadvantages. The only ideal solution is to design autoclavable ventilators (Norlander *et al.*, 1968).

Ethylene Oxide

This is a highly toxic and explosive gas which is heavier than air, freely soluble in water and rubber, and has only a faint smell. It can be used to sterilise apparatus which would be damaged by heat. Sterilisation is efficient provided the conditions are carefully controlled. It has been advocated as an agent for sterilising ventilators by Bishop *et al.* (1962), who enclosed the ventilator in a polyvinyl chloride bag containing a mixture of 10 per cent ethylene oxide in carbon dioxide—a mixture which is non-explosive. Ethylene oxide passes freely through polyvinyl chloride (Thomas, 1960) and a "Polythene" bag is preferable. It is doubtful whether the use of ethylene oxide in a plastic bag is either efficient or safe, and it is probably best restricted to specialised plant designed for the purpose.

Formaldehyde

Formaldehyde vapour can be used to sterilise ventilator circuits by introducing 100 ml. formaldehyde B.P. into the water bath humidifier and running the machine for a period. Although this method is effective, formalin can remain in the ventilator and contaminate the patient's lungs when next the machine is in use (Sykes, 1964). Residual formalin can be neutralised with ammonia vapour blown through the ventilator in a similar manner.

Alcohol Aerosol

This method was described by Peterson and Rosdahl (1966) and has proved satisfactory throughout considerable clinical experience (Spencer *et al.*, 1968; Gullers *et al.*, 1969). It has been suggested by Judd *et al.* (1968) that the alcohol method carries an explosion risk, but Herzog *et al.* (1970) have shown convincingly that this is not so.

The method depends on the generation of a finely divided mist of 70 per cent ethyl alcohol or 70 per cent isopropyl alcohol by an ultrasonic nebulizer (Herzog *et al.*, 1964). It can only be used for ventilators which are capable of conversion to a closed circuit system. It is desirable, though not essential, to fill the circuit with nitrogen before starting. The process is completed in two hours, and residual alcohol is not harmful to the next patient.

Hydrogen Peroxide

This method was described by Judd *et al.* (1968). A finely divided mist of 20 vol. per cent H_2O_2 B.P. is generated by an immersed plate ultrasonic DeVilbis nebulizer (British Oxygen Company) or Monaghan ultrasonic nebulizer (Electronic and X-ray Applications Ltd.). It is effective and probably less limited in its application than the alcohol method, although only the expiratory limb of some ventilators is disinfected. It is potentially harmful to the skin of the operator and unless the ventilator is allowed to stand for long enough to allow residual hydrogen peroxide to break down, can desquamate the trachea of the subsequent patient.

Picloxydine

This method was described by Meadows *et al.* (1968) and simplified by Nancekievill and Gaya (1969). Clinical experience is limited at present and its use has so far been confined to the Radcliffe ventilator. It appears to be effective, cheap and fairly rapid, but the disinfectant may cause damage to mechanical parts of the ventilator. It is somewhat messy in use, but residual disinfectant is probably harmless to the patient.

REFERENCES

Adams, A. P. (1968). Ventilators for use in anaesthesia. *Brit. J. hosp. Med.*, Suppl. 23.

Beaver, R. A. (1956). The Beaver Mark II Respirator. *Lancet*, **1**, 449.

Bishop, C., Potts, M. W., and Molloy, P. J. (1962). A method of sterilization for the Barnet respirator. *Brit. J. Anaesth.*, **34**, 121.

Bishop, C., Roper, W. A. G., and Williams, S. R. (1963). The use of an absolute filter to sterilize the inspiratory air during intermittent positive pressure respiration. *Brit. J. Anaesth.*, **35**, 32.

Collis, J. M., Bethune, D. W., and Tobias, M. A. (1969). Miniature ventilators: an assessment. *Anaesthesia*, **24**, 81.

ENGSTRÖM, C-G. (1954). Treatment of severe cases of respiratory paralysis by the Engström Universal Respirator. *Brit. med. J.*, **2,** 666.

ENGSTRÖM, C-G. (1963). The clinical application of prolonged controlled ventilation. *Acta anaesth. scand.*, **7,** Suppl. 13.

FISHER, M. F., and KYI KYI, K. (1969). Contamination and disinfection of lung ventilators. *Brit. Hosp. soc. Serv. J.*, 1404.

GLOVER, W. J. (1966). *Pseudomonas aeruginosa* cross infection (letter). *Lancet*. **1,** 203.

GULLERS, K., MALMBORG, A-S., NYSTRÖM, B., NORLANDER, O. P., and PETERSON, N. (1969). Clinical experience of disinfection of the Engström respirator by ultrasonic nebulized ethyl alcohol. *Acta anaesth. scand.*, **13,** 247.

HELLIWELL, J., JEANES, A. L., WATKIN, R. R., and GIBBS, F. J. (1967). The Williams bacterial filter. *Anaesthesia*, **22,** 497.

HERZOG, P., NORLANDER, O. P., and ENGSTRÖM, C-G. (1964). Ultrasonic generation of aerosol for the humidification of inspired gas during volume controlled ventilation. *Acta anaesth. scand.*, **8,** 79.

HERZOG, P., NORLANDER, O. P., and NYSTROM, B. (1970). Physical principles of ultrasonic aerosol generation for disinfection. *Proc. roy. Soc. Med.*, **63,** 911.

JUDD, P. A., TOMLIN, P. J., WHITBLY, J. L., INGLIS, T. C. M., and ROBINSON, J. S. (1968). Disinfection of ventilators by ultrasonic nebulisation. *Lancet*, **2,** 1019.

MAPLESON, W. W. (1969). In: *Automatic Ventilation of the Lungs*. Edit. Mushin, W. W. *et al.* Oxford: Blackwell Scientific Publications.

MEADOWS, G. A., RICHARDSON, J. C., FISH, E., and WILLIAMS, A. (1968). A method of sterilization for the East-Radcliffe ventilator. *Brit. J. Anaesth.*, **40,** 71.

NANCEKIEVILL, D. G., and GAYA, H. (1969). Disinfection of the East-Radcliffe ventilator. *Anaesthesia*, **24,** 42.

NORLANDER, O. P., NORDEN, I., OLOFSSON, S., and HERZOG, P. (1968). The new Engström Respirator 300. *Acta anaesth. scand.*, **12,** 213.

PETERSON, N. O. A., and ROSDAHL, K. G. (1966). Ultrasonic nebulized ethanol for the disinfection of respiratory equipment. *Opusc. med.* (*Stockh.*), **11,** 278.

PHILLIPS, I. (1967). *Pseudomonas aeruginosa* cross infection in patients receiving mechanical ventilation. *J. Hyg.* (*Lond.*), **65,** 228.

PHILLIPS, I., and SPENCER, G. (1965). *Pseudomonas aeruginosa* cross infection due to contaminated respiratory apparatus. *Lancet*, **2,** 1325.

PYLE, P., DARLOW, M., and FIRMAN, J. E. (1969). A heated ultra-high efficiency filter for mechanical ventilators. *Lancet*, **1,** 136.

REDMAN, L. R., and LOCKEY, E. (1967). Colonisation of the upper respiratory tract with gram-negative bacilli after operation, endotracheal intubation and prophylactic antibiotic therapy. *Anaesthesia*, **22,** 220.

REINARZ, J. A., PIERCE, A. K., MAYS, B. B., and SANFORD, J. P. (1965). The potential role of inhalation therapy equipment in nosocomial pulmonary infection. *J. clin. Invest.*, **44,** 831.

ROCHFORD, J., WELCH, R. F., and WINKS, D. P. (1958). An electronic time-cycled respirator. *Brit. J. Anaesth.*, **30,** 23.

RUSSELL, W. R., SCHUSTER, E., SMITH, A. C., and SPALDING, J. M. K. (1956). Radcliffe respiration pumps. *Lancet*, **1,** 539.

SMITH-CLARKE, G. T., and GALPINE, J. F. (1955). A positive-negative pressure respirator. *Lancet*, **1,** 1299.

SPENCER, G., RIDLEY, M., EYKYN, S., and ACHONG, J. (1968). Disinfection of lung ventilators by alcohol aerosol. *Lancet*, **2,** 667.

SYKES, M. K. (1962). The East Radcliffe ventilator adapted for anaesthesia. *Brit. J. Anaesth.*, **34,** 203.

SYKES, M. K. (1964). Sterilizing mechanical ventilators (letter). *Brit. med. J.*, **1,** 561.
THOMAS, C. G. A. (1960). Sterilization by ethylene oxide. *Guy's Hosp. Rep.*, **109,** 57.
WAINE, T. E., and FOX, D. E. R. (1962). A new and versatile closed circuit anaesthetic machine with automatic and manual ventilation. *Brit. J. Anaesth.*, **34,** 410.
WRIGHT, R., SYKES, M. K., JACKSON, B. G., MANN, W. M., and ADAMS, E. F. (1961). Intermittent positive pressure respiration in tetanus neonatorum. *Lancet*, **2,** 678.

FURTHER READING

MUSHIN, W. W., RENDELL-BAKER, L., THOMPSON, P. W., and MAPLESON, W. W. (1969). *Automatic Ventilation of the Lungs*, Oxford: Blackwell Scientific Publications.

Chapter 17

SPECIAL CARE UNITS

by

G. T. SPENCER

THE general hospital ward has proved a durable and flexible unit in which to care for patients and on which to base the medical and nursing staff. From an early stage in hospital development general wards have tended to become less general and more specialised in the type of patient they cater for. This has largely resulted from specialisation within the medical profession. Traditionally, therefore, wards have become restricted by the specialised work of the doctor in charge and patients have been sited in hospital by virtue of their disease rather than by the amount of attention and treatment they need. The development of complex methods of treatment which are necessary and effective in only a minority of patients has resulted in a small number of very ill patients requiring more attention, facilities and space than can conveniently be provided in a normal ward if they are to have the best chance of recovery. On the other hand, many patients require less attention and facilities than a normal ward provides.

Recognition of these developments has led to the concept of Progressive Patient Care. Under this system patients are grouped in hospital according to the severity of their illness rather than its nature. The stimulus to this development has its origin in staff shortage. By adopting progressive patient care it is hoped to make more efficient use of staff, concentrating expertise where it is really needed and thus avoiding wasteful staff deployment. In practice, progressive patient care has been found to have many disadvantages and the claimed advantages have rarely been fully realised. The provision of special areas in hospital where severely ill patients can be treated intensively has been more successful. This is the one aspect of progressive patient care which is becoming widely adopted. Such units are called, for want of a better term, Intensive Therapy Units (Planning Unit Report No. 1, 1967).

Parallel with these developments has come the recognition that many patients cannot safely be returned to a general ward immediately upon completion of any but the most trivial operation or anaesthetic. Special recovery units have been developed in an attempt to overcome this problem. They can be staffed by experienced nurses and thus effectively bridge the gap between the continuous individual medical attention inevitable during surgery and anaesthesia, and the more sporadic nursing care in a general ward (Jolly and Lee, 1957).

Within these two frameworks many variations exist, and even terminology is confused. It may be helpful to outline the principal types of unit with brief indications of advantages and disadvantages.

Recovery Units

Recovery Units can be divided into two types with different advantages and disadvantages.

Recovery Rooms

These are usually small rooms which form an integral part of an operating suite. They are conveniently sited alongside the anaesthetic room so that the patient enters the operating room via the anaesthetic room and leaves it via the recovery room. Normally one such room serves one, or at most two, operating theatres. Their particular advantage is that being close to the theatre, they allow easy supervision of the patient by the surgeon and anaesthetist who have performed the operation, and thus achieve the best possible continuity of medical responsibility. They are only suitable for short stay patients because the facilities which can be provided in a single room are space limited. If a patient is not ready to leave the recovery room by the time the subsequent operation is completed, serious congestion and disruption of the work of the theatre can result. Nurse staffing is difficult because the work load is irregular and dispersed. It is usually necessary to release a theatre nurse with limited experience to supervise the patient. This may seriously deplete staffing of the operating theatre.

Recovery rooms are most suitable for small hospitals with single theatre units, or for departments such as X-Ray or out-patients where occasional anaesthetic services only are required.

Recovery Areas (Post-anaesthetic recovery units: Post-operative Departments)

In an attempt to overcome these disadvantages, larger recovery areas have been developed which are common to a number of operating theatres. They can be more extensively equipped than a recovery room and patients can remain in them for longer periods. A separate nursing and medical staff is needed, and if the area serves four or more theatres the work load may be sufficiently sustained to justify a night staff and twenty-four hour service. While this is always desirable, it is inefficient unless regularly used.

The disadvantage of a recovery area often lies in its siting. Unless it has been included from the outset in the centre of a multiple theatre suite it may have to be sited at a considerable distance from some of the operating theatres feeding it. Transport of patients from theatre to recovery area may then be hazardous or disruptive to the work of the theatre if an anaesthetist has to accompany them.

A centrally sited recovery area in a multiple theatre suite is ideal for patient admission and supervision during the working day, but suffers from the disadvantage of being in the clean area of modern theatre design. Access to the recovery area is inconvenient once medical staff have left the theatre suite and continuity of medical and nursing care may therefore suffer. Probably the best compromise is to site the area in the junction zone near the entrance to a multiple theatre suite. Even in this situation the area may, in large theatre complexes, be at an inconvenient distance from some of the theatre suites it serves.

Patient monitoring in the recovery room.—Patient monitoring is a phrase which is both fashionable and imprecisely used. Nevertheless it is in the field of post-operative care that true patient monitoring probably offers the greatest benefit. It is important to distinguish between continuous physiological measurement and true physiological monitoring.

A continuous physiological measuring system simply displays the output of appropriate transducers on pen recorders or oscilloscopes. In its simplest form this may consist of nothing more than the oscilloscope display of an ECG. Usually, however, it is taken to include the output from pressure transducers. A typical bedside system has been described by Cowell (1967). The aim of a physiological measuring system of this type is to obtain more information about a patient's state, and particularly how that state is changing, and thus enable his treatment to be more precisely controlled. It does not in any way reduce the amount of nursing or medical surveillance that the patient needs. Indeed, it increases it, and places on the user the considerable burden of ensuring that the apparatus is properly maintained and is making accurate measurements. No measurement at all is better than an inaccurate one. It does not actively mislead. A physiological measuring system probably has greater application in the intensive therapy unit than in the recovery room.

A true monitoring system does more than this. It must be able to recognise when the measurement moves outside present limits, and then draw the attention of the user to this abnormal situation. In other words, it must have the ability to sound an alarm. It is thus aimed at reducing the need for nursing supervision and making good safe care available for the many, rather than performing miracles for the few (Wolff, 1968*a*).

The following criteria for a true monitor have been proposed by Wolff (1968*b*). It must:

Communicate: Tell someone not actually looking at it that something is going awry.

Record: Measurements are recorded on paper at suitable intervals.

Display: Current values can be seen on some sort of a dial.

These are stiff criteria and may be unobtainable for some years yet. No apparatus at present has completely fulfilled them and, more important, proved itself reliable in practice. There are many dangers in such a system (Brock, 1970). It must be completely reliable and yet not raise too many false alarms. It must be simple, cheap and unobtrusive for the patient. The nearest approach so far to this ideal is probably the Medical Research Council's "Monitron" system (Rawles and Crockett, 1969). The patient-sensor interface is the most unreliable part of the system and Crockett (1970) has shown that nearly half the technical faults which occur in use are in this area.

In an attempt to improve alarm reliability, Stewart (1969) has proposed a system of integrating signals from more than one sensor. A simple device for monitoring the circulation and integrating three signals has been developed by Sadera *et al.* (1970) and Levy *et al.* (1970) report favourably on its experimental application. Insufficient clinical experience is yet available to assess the real value of this method.

A particularly interesting development is a "Cerebral Function Monitor". There is no doubt that cerebral function is the most reliable single indication of a patient's well-being. Unfortunately it is a function of unparalleled complexity. In an attempt to monitor cerebral function Maynard *et al.* (1969) have developed a simple single channel EEG which records on slow moving paper. The trace thus appears as a solid band. Oxygen deprivation to the cerebral cortex causes a rapid reduction in amplitude (voltage) of the EEG and the band narrows, and thereby sounds an alarm. To date clinical experience with this device is encouraging (Prior *et al.*, 1971).

Respiratory monitoring has obvious application in the recovery room. Unfortunately reliable simple methods are not yet available, though interesting attempts have been made using complicated on-line computers (Beaumont *et al.*, 1968; Raison, 1970).

Despite the undoubted deficiency of equipment and techniques of monitoring at the present time (Maloney, 1968), there is no doubt that its development is of vital importance. While everybody agrees that the human computer, in the form of a nurse, is the best patient monitor, she is in increasingly limited supply. Extended use of machinery is therefore inevitable (Planning Unit Report No. 3, 1969), and its further development justifies a high priority (Taylor, 1970). Monitoring at present is at the stage of the 1910 motor car—it works some of the time! (Wolff, 1970).

Special Function Units

These units are designed to meet the needs of patients suffering from a particular disease, or type of disease.

Respiratory Units

Respiratory Units were the prototype for all special care units and many have been adapted to cater for a wider variety of conditions. Lassen (1953) was among the first to recognise the need to set aside special areas for the treatment of respiratory poliomyelitis, and the requirements of such units have now become clearly established. Their design can be specialised and their needs are well exemplified by the unit which has been described by Hercus *et al.* (1962, 1964).

Coronary Care Units

In recent years there has been considerable interest in reducing the mortality following myocardial infarction by prevention and treatment of arrhythmias and ventricular fibrillation, which are liable to occur in the first few days. Brown *et al.* (1963) and Julian *et al.* (1964) showed that deaths following myocardial infarction are mainly due to electrical disturbances of cardiac rhythm which are potentially reversible if appropriate resuscitative measures can be promptly undertaken. If treatment is to be successful, it is clear that patients who have suffered an infarct must be admitted to a unit staffed and equipped to provide continuous electrocardiographic monitoring as soon as possible after the acute episode. The design and organisation of typical units have been described by Shillingford and Thomas (1964) and Lawrie *et al.* (1967).

In theory, therefore, the problem is simple and the benefits obvious. In practice, coronary care has raised as many problems as it has solved and the benefits are less than had been hoped.

Medical resources.—Myocardial infarction in Western countries is a distressingly common condition, and full intensive care for all cases is economically unrealistic. Statistical surveys have suggested that up to 30 per cent of the occupants of acute medical beds in general hospitals are there either directly or indirectly as a result of ischaemic heart disease. It is costly to equip so many beds with ECG monitors, and virtually impossible to provide enough staff to interpret the information displayed.

The most recent estimates (Lown *et al.*, 1969) suggest that the actual total mortality reduction in myocardial infarction achieved by coronary care is 2–3 per cent, and the theoretical maximum if coronary care units were universally available no more than 10 per cent. This is because only 34 per cent of those dying suddenly from coronary artery disease survive long enough to reach hospital and 60 per cent of deaths in hospital are caused by "pump failure" due to massive infarction.

It can be argued that the research benefit from intensive coronary care is considerable. This is true but it is not an argument for its universal adoption as a routine theıapeutic measure. Moreover it is important not to concentrate too much research effort on end-stage disease (Miller, 1969) thereby deflecting it from studying the underlying causes of atherosclerosis.

Case selection.—Approximately 90 per cent of patients with myocardial infarction who reach hospital alive exhibit rhythm disorders during the first 72 hours, and the incidence declines steadily with the passage of time (Lown *et al.*, 1967). Thus it is common practice to limit the period of continuous monitoring to about 72 hours unless there is evidence that serious arrhythmias are still present or a pacemaker is *in situ*. Although it is reasonable to place a time limit on continuous monitoring in this way, it has the disadvantage that a small proportion of patients with minor infarcts do not develop serious arrhythmias for a week or more after infarction. It has been suggested that graded coronary care with telemetric monitoring continued for a longer period may help to overcome this problem. Attempts to select cases at particular risk have rarely been successful.

Staffing.—Although the staff requirements of a coronary care unit are less than those of an intensive therapy unit, they still present a major problem. Coronary care units tend to be particularly unpopular with nurses because the work is unvarying and the mortality is high. Continuous observation of one or more oscilloscopes is impossible to perform efficiently for long periods and machinery capable of pattern recognition is complex and not yet generally available. In practice, the establishment of coronary care units is limited by the availability of suitable staff.

Psychological effects of coronary care.—A doctor who believes that monitoring will help a patient can usually quite readily persuade the patient to accept the minor discomforts involved (Crook, 1970). Most patients are reassured by monitoring equipment once their initial fears have been overcome. Nevertheless, there is evidence suggesting that a proportion of the rhythm disturbances observed during coronary care are caused by the patient's fear of the circumstances in which he finds himself. It has even been suggested that the indications for hospital admission in myocardial infarction are social rather than medical; provided he can be cared for at home, he is just as well off in his own familiar environment. Telemetric ECG monitoring is of value because it is less obtrusive to the patient, and reassurance at all times is of vital importance. One death in a coronary care unit can have a devastating effect on the other patients who know they are suffering from the same disease.

Pre-hospital coronary care.—The majority of deaths from myocardial infarction occur soon after the onset of symptoms, 40 to 60 per cent being in the first hour. McNeilly and Pemberton (1968) showed that the mean time interval between onset of symptoms and hospital admission was more than eight hours. In an attempt to reduce this massive death rate, Pantridge and Adgey (1969) have established a mobile coronary care unit based on an extensively equipped ambulance. The benefits of pre-coronary care were discussed at a symposium in 1969, and the proceedings published (Goldstein and Moss, 1969). Although encouraging results were described, it is too early to assess the overall benefits to be expected from pre-hospital coronary care.

Conclusions.—Intensive coronary care is undoubtedly a therapeutic advance. Properly applied it can usefully save lives, though the economic outlay and staff requirements are heavy. The danger of needlessly and officiously prolonging the act of dying is ever present and it is vitally important to preserve a sense of proportion. It is no substitute for efficient care and adequate resuscitation services for the hospital as a whole (see Chapter 28).

Intensive Therapy Units

The essential difference between an intensive therapy unit (I.T.U.) and the various special function units from which the concept emerged is that it is a multi-discipline, and preferably central, service area.

An intensive therapy unit has been defined as a special unit providing the following:

(1) A *Facility* available to all medical staff giving more space, staff and equipment for the care of a patient than can be provided in the ordinary wards.

(2) A *Service* which provides continuous observation of the vital functions and can support these functions more promptly and efficiently than could be done elsewhere in the hospital.

Both the faculty and the service can be developed within a specialist division or ward, but the essence of the I.T.U. is that, like most operating theatres, it is communal (Planning Unit Report No. 1, 1967).

Size of Unit

The optimum size for an intensive therapy unit is 6–8 beds. Units of less than four beds are rarely viable because the work load is so variable that at many times the unit is empty, the staff become dispersed to other duties and are unavailable when a need suddenly arises (Jørgensen, 1966). Units of over ten beds are unwieldy and incoherent; it is impossible for one person to be aware of what is happening to all the patients at all times.

One per cent of acute beds in a general hospital has usually been found adequate to meet the need for intensive therapy (Lees, 1965). Thus it is hard to justify a unit in a hospital of less than 400 beds. Where a district service is shared between several smaller hospitals it is preferable to transfer patients to a single central unit. A hospital of over a thousand beds will tend to need more than one unit. In such hospitals there is usually at least one speciality or division which has sufficient need for intensive therapy to justify having its own special function unit of four or more beds (Spencer, 1970).

Cross Infection

Cross infection in an intensive therapy unit is a serious problem. The more diverse the work of the unit, the more critical it becomes. There are three main reasons for this: firstly, the patients are critically ill and any infection may tip the balance between survival and death. Secondly, patients are often unduly susceptible to bacterial infection, either as a result of their disease or the treatment they are receiving. Thirdly, the unit is bound to admit some patients whose basic problem is bacterial infection, often wildly out of control. These patients are a potent source of bacterial infection (Ridley, 1970).

Airborne cross infection can be largely eliminated by adequate air conditioning, allowing parts of the unit to be isolated. Sterilisation of equipment between use is essential. Within limits dictated by staff numbers and the needs of observation, movement of staff between patients should be discouraged, if necessary by physical barriers. Cross infection is most likely to occur when the unit is overworked or understaffed, or both.

Layout of Unit

Many layouts have been described for intensive therapy units (Rosen and Secher, 1963; Hamilton, 1964; Spencer, 1970). None has been shown to have particular advantages provided certain basic requirements are met.

Adequate space is essential (Fig. 1). 25–30 sq. meters per bed is necessary in single bed areas, and 20 sq. metres in multiple bed areas. The service area should be at least equal to the bed area. 30–50 per cent of the beds should be in single areas. Units accepting a wide variety of patients may need to be separated into clean and dirty areas. An open plan unit is easy to staff but bacteriologically unsatisfactory, except for short stay patients. A unit of single cubicles is bacteriologically ideal but extravagant to staff and sometimes undesirable for conscious patients, who may feel unduly isolated.

Staffing

This really is the heart of the matter. An intensive therapy unit succeeds if its staff have the confidence and goodwill of the hospital—whatever formal arrangements are made. Without these intangibles, the advantage of a communal site in providing a common ground for staff of all disciplines is replaced by the disadvantage of incomplete consultation, with failure to define or accept responsibility leading to illwill and indecision which endangers the life of the patient (Planning Unit Report No. 1, 1967).

Senior medical staff commitment to the unit is essential, though it should probably take the form of an administrative rather than a clinical responsibility. The development of intensive therapy as a medical speciality is not desirable (Hunter, 1967). No single doctor can be competent in all aspects of treatment of the severely ill. If the medical staff running the unit become too involved with clinical responsibility the unit tends to develop into an elite organisation separate from the rest of the hospital, and thereby loses goodwill and service function. It is also helpful if administrative responsibility rests in the hands of a doctor who does not have a vested interest in bed allocation.

Junior medical staff commitment to the unit is equally important. One

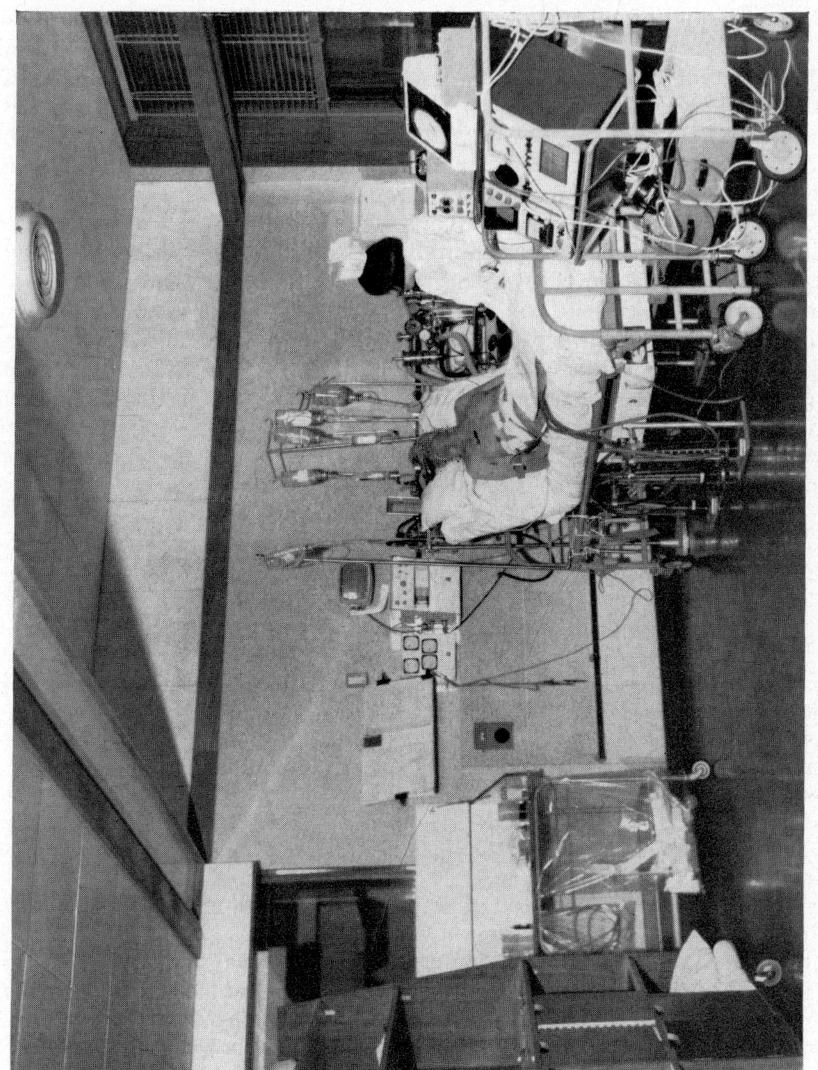

17/Fig. 1.—The Intensive Therapy Unit: space is the essential requirement.

doctor must be available at all times to act as the final common path for medical orders. This is essential in order to prevent conflicting instructions being issued to nursing staff. The chain of medical command must be clearly understood by all concerned if misunderstandings are to be avoided.

Nurse staffing is the greatest problem, and the work of most units is limited by the availability of adequate experienced staff. Overall nurse shortage, however, is only part of the problem. The work load of a unit can vary several hundred per cent over the space of a few hours; if the unit is kept fully staffed at all times there will inevitably be periods of inefficient under-employment, and if it is not fully staffed it may be unable to meet a sudden demand. Holmdahl (1962) has described a method of "on call" duties for specially trained nursing auxillaries which goes some way towards resolving this dilemma.

Conclusions.—Intensive therapy units undoubtedly save lives and make possible techniques of therapy which would otherwise be impossible. The overall mortality reduction achieved by intensive therapy, though difficult to estimate, is probably no more than 10 per cent. Due mainly to its staffing needs, the cost of running a unit is high, and medical priorities have to be considered. Over-energetic treatment may be encouraged; the fact that it is possible to maintain and prolong life does not inevitably mean that to do so is justifiable or even desirable. Patients should only be admitted to an intensive therapy unit after individual consideration, and not simply because they belong to a particular diagnostic category.

REFERENCES

Beaumont, J. O. B., Osborn, J. J., Raison, J. C. A., and Russell, J. A. G. (1968). Respiratory measurement and monitoring based on an on-line computer. *Proc. Assn. Advancement of Med. Instrument.* Houston.

Brock, Lord (1970). In "A Symposium on Patient Monitoring". *Postgrad. med. J.*, **46**, 404.

Brown, K. W. G., MacMillan, R. L., Forbath, N., Mel'grano, E., and Scott, J. W. (1963). Coronary Unit. An Intensive Care Centre for acute myocardial infarction. *Lancet*, **2**, 349.

Cowell, T. K. (1967). St. Thomas' Hospital Intensive Care Monitoring System. *Brit. Hosp. soc. Serv. J.*, p. 1630.

Crockett, G. S. (1970). The Patient Sensor Interface. *Postgrad. med. J.*, **46**, 378.

Crook, J. (1970). User needs of patients and nurses in clinical monitoring. *Postgrad. Med. J.*, **46**, 374.

Goldstein, S., and Moss, A. J. (1969). Eds. Symposium on the pre-hospital phase of acute myocardial infarction. *Amer. J. Cardiol.*, **24**, 609.

Hamilton, M. K. (1964). Workshop on Intensive Care Units. *Anesthesiology*, **25**, 192.

Hercus, V. (1962). Planning a Respiratory Unit. *Brit. med. J.*, **2**, 1604.

Hercus, V., Johnston, J. B., Rollison, R. A. A., and Hackett, R. E. (1964). The place of a respiratory unit in a general hospital. *Lancet*, **1**, 1265.

Holmdahl, M. H. (1962). The Respiratory Care Unit. *Anesthesiology*, **23**, 559.

Hunter, A. R. (1967). Intensive Care as a Specialty. *Lancet*, **1**, 1151.

JOLLY, C., and LEE, J. A. (1957). Post-operative observation ward. *Anaesthesia*, **12,** 49.

JØRGENSEN, C. C. (1966). Establishment of, and experience gained in, an intensive care unit in a Danish Regional Hospital. *Acta anaesth. scand.*, Suppl. **23,** 108.

JULIAN, D. G., VALENTINE, P. A., and MILLER, C. G. (1964). Disturbances of rate, rhythm and conduction in acute myocardial infarction. A prospective study of 100 consecutive unselected patients with the aid of electrocardiographic monitoring. *Amer. J. Med.*, **27,** 915.

LASSEN, H. C. A. (1953). A preliminary report on the 1952 epidemic of poliomyelitis in Copenhagen, with special reference to the treatment of acute respiratory insufficiency. *Lancet*, **1,** 37.

LAWRIE, D. M., GREENWOOD, T. W., GODDARD, M., HARVEY, A. C., DONALD, K. W., JULIAN, D. G., and OLIVER, M. F. (1967). A Coronary Care Unit in the routine management of myocardial infarction. *Lancet*, **2,** 109.

LEES, W. (1965). In: *Hospital Management, Planning & Equipment*, p. 690. London: H.M.S.O.

LEVY, L. S., LEE, W. R., GURASWAMY, B. A., and STEWART, J. S. S. (1970). Experimental studies with a clinical monitor and diagnostic computer. *Postgrad. med. J.*, **46,** 366.

LOWN, B., KOSOWSKY. B. D., and KLEIN, M. D. (1969). Pathogenesis, prevention and treatment of arrhythmias in myocardial infarction. *Circulation*, **40,** Suppl. 4, p. 261.

LOWN, B., VASSAUX, C., HOOD, W. B., FAKHRO, A. M., KAPLINSKY, E., and ROBERGE, G. (1967). Unresolved problems in coronary care. *Amer. J. Cardiol.*, **20,** 494.

MCNEILLY, R. H., and PEMBERTON, J. (1968). Duration of last attack in 998 fatal cases of coronary artery disease and its relation to possible cardiac resuscitation. *Brit. med. J.*, **3,** 139.

MALONEY, J. V. (1968). The trouble with patient monitoring. *Ann. Surg.*, **168,** 605.

MAYNARD, D., PRYOR, P. F., and SCOTT, D. F. (1969). Device for continuous monitoring of cerebral activity in resuscitated patients. *Brit. med. J.*, **4,** 545.

MILLER, H. (1969). Real goals for medicine. *Sci. J.*, **5a,** 90.

PANTRIDGE, J. F., and ADGEY, A. A. J. (1969). Pre-hospital coronary care; The Mobile Coronary Care Unit. *Amer. J. Cardiol.*, **24,** 666.

Planning Unit Report No. 1 (1967). *Intensive Care.* London: British Medical Association.

Planning Unit Report No. 3 (1969). *Computers in Medicine.* London: British Medical Association.

PRIOR, P. F., MAYNARD, D. E., SHEAFF, P. C., SIMPSON, B. R., STRUNIN, L., WEAVER, E. J. M., and SCOTT, D. F. (1971). Monitoring cerebral function: clinical experience with new device for continuous recording of electrical activity. *Brit. med. J.*, **2,** 736.

RAISON, J. C. A. (1970). Patient monitoring: on line computing. *Postgrad. med. J.*, **46,** 360.

RAWLES, J. M., and CROCKETT, G. S. (1969). Automation on a general medical ward: Monitron system of patient monitoring. *Brit. med. J.*, **3,** 707.

RIDLEY, M. (1970). Cross Infection in Intensive Therapy Units. In: *Progress in Anaesthesiology* (Proc. 4th World Congr. of Anaesthesiologists), p. 479. Amsterdam: Excerpta Medica Foundation.

ROSEN, J., and SECHER, O. (1963). Intensive Care Unit at University Hospital, Copenhagen. *Anesthesiology*, **24,** 855.

SADERA, T. D., PENNY, R. K., GURASWAMY, B. A., and STEWART, J. S. S. (1971). Design of a Circulatory Failure Analyser. *Proc. Soc. Eng. Sci.* (In press).

SHILLINGFORD, J. P., and THOMAS, M. (1964). Organisation of unit for intensive care and investigation of patients with myocardial infarction. *Lancet*, **2,** 1113.

SPENCER, G. T. (1970). Planning and construction of Intensive Therapy Units. In: *Progress in Anaesthesiology* (Proc. 4th World Congr. of Anaesthesiologists), p. 479. Amsterdam: Excerpta Medica Foundation.

STEWART, J. S. S. (1969). Meaningful monitoring. *Lancet*, **1**, 1305.

TAYLOR, D. J. W. (1970). Developing viable medical equipment in general and for patient monitoring. *Postgrad. med. J.*, **46**, 350.

WOLFF, H. S. (1968*a*). Bioengineering—the next few years. *Bio-med. Engng.*, **3**, 15.

WOLFF, H. S. (1968*b*). Patient monitoring in intensive care. *Brit. J. hosp. Med.*, **2**, 554.

WOLFF, H. S. (1970). Patient Monitoring—A Boon or a Burden. In: *Progress in Anaesthesiology* (Proc. 4th World Congr. of Anaesthesiologists), p. 337. Amsterdam: Excerpta Medica Foundation.

FURTHER READING

SPALDING, J. M. K., and SMITH, A. C. (1963). *Clinical Practice and Physiology of Artificial Respiration.* Oxford: Blackwell Scientific Publications.

Planning Unit Report No. 1 (1967). *Intensive Care.* London: British Medical Association.

Intensive Therapy Units. A Symposium (1970). *Progress in Anaesthesiology* (Proc. 4th World Congr. of Anaesthesiologists), p. 477 *et seq.* Amsterdam: Excerpta Medica Foundation.

Chapter 18

FIRES AND EXPLOSIONS

by

T. H. S. BURNS

IF a gauze swab is soaked in anaesthetic ether and put on the floor of a clean operating theatre, a lighted match will make it burn, but the fire may easily be smothered before any serious damage is done. In the closed system of an anaesthetic machine, seven per cent of ether vapour in oxygen will cause a dramatic explosion if brought into contact with a relatively weak "static" spark, and considerable damage may be done to apparatus and personnel. This comparison illustrates some of the problems in assessing the risk of fire or explosion in association with anaesthetic drugs. The supporting gas mixture is important; so is the energy of the ignition source; and ignition in a confined space will have a more dramatic effect than one in a large space.

There is no essential difference between a fire and an explosion. A *fire* becomes an *explosion* if the combustion is sufficiently rapid to cause pressure changes which result in the production of sound waves. For example, paraffin poured on to a red coal fire will increase the rate of combustion sufficiently to make it "roar". Ether vapour and oxygen, in certain proportions, will, if ignited in a confined space, cause an explosion. In certain circumstances, the speed of combustion may be so high that a pressure wave is produced which ignites adjacent gas mixtures by compression rather than by the speed of a flame. Such combustion is extremely violent and is known as "detonation". Ether will detonate in certain circumstances in oxygen, but not in air.

Since the Report of the Working Party on Anaesthetic Explosions by the Ministry of Health in 1956 and the introduction of halothane into anaesthetic practice in the same year, the number of fires and explosions associated with anaesthesia has fallen to almost insignificant proportions in England and Wales. In 1966 and 1967 no explosions were reported. In 1968 there was one. The last time a death occurred following an anaesthetic explosion was in 1964.

The risk of an anaesthetic explosion has never been high. Even before the introduction of full anti-static precautions, the risk of death from the explosion of a flammable anaesthetic was less than one in three million. In spite of this relatively slight risk, it is still necessary to include a chapter on fires and explosions in a textbook of anaesthesia, because ether and cyclopropane still have their uses and more detailed investigations into the flammability of newer compounds such as halothane and methoxyflurane have shown that these and older drugs are not "non-flammable" in an absolute sense. Indeed, some workers (Schön and Steen, 1968) have recently been able to make even nitrous oxide burn, given an ignition source of enormous energy (200 watts/second for 0·5–1·0 second). But such freak conditions would never be encountered in clinical anaesthetic practice.

The essential conditions for an explosion are the presence, close enough

18/TABLE 1

Drug	*Limits in air per cent v/v*		*Limits in oxygen per cent v/v*		*Limits in pure nitrous oxide per cent v/v*	
	lower	higher	lower	higher	lower	higher
Diethyl ether	1·9	48·0	2·0	82·0	1·5	24·0
Divinyl ether	1·7	27·0	1·8	85·0	1·4	25.0
Cyclopropane	2·4	10·4	2·5	60·0	—	—
Ethyl chloride	3·8	15·4	4·0	67·0	2·0	33·0
Trifluoro-ethyl-vinyl-ether, fluroxene ("Fluoromar")	3·0	—	—	—	—	—
Ethylene	3·1	32·0	3·0	80·0	1·9	40·0
Trichloroethylene ("Trilene")	non-flammable		10·0	65·0	2·0/2·5*	

18/Table 1 (*continued*)

Halothane ("Fluothane") F H F–C–C–Cl F Br	non-flammable		non-flammable		4·0/5·0*	
Methoxyflurane ("Penthrane") Cl F H H–C–C–O–C–H Cl F H	9·0*	28·0*	5·2*	28·0*	4·0*	—
Teflurane F H F–C–C–F F Br	"non-flammable" (Artusio, 1963)					
Ethrane (Comp. 347) F F F Cl–C–C–O–C–H H F F	"non-explosive in anaesthetic concentrations" (Krantz, 1964)					
Halopropane H F F Br–C–C–C–H H F F	non-flammable (Fabian *et al.*, 1960)			non-flammable		

These values are taken from the U.S. Bureau of Mines Bulletin 503, Washington 1952, except for those for fluroxene, which are given by Krantz *et al.* (1953), those marked (*) which are manufacturers' figures and those for the last three compounds, where other references are given. Although figures are given for lower limits of flammability in oxygen for trichloroethylene and in air and oxygen for methoxyflurane, it should be remembered that these concentrations cannot be obtained in unheated vaporisers at normal operating theatre temperatures (18–22° C).

Anaesthesia at hyperbaric pressures.—The manufacturers of halothane ("Fluothane") give the following recommendation for this drug when it is used with oxygen in hyperbaric conditions up to 4 atmospheres pressure and at ordinary temperatures:—"In small volumes, such as closed circuit anaesthetic equipment, the concentration of 'Fluothane' should not exceed 2 per cent v/v; in large volumes, any concentration up to that given by its saturated vapour pressure may be used." They do not recommend the use of oxygen/nitrous oxide mixtures with halothane at hyperbaric pressures.

together, of an *explosive mixture* and a spark of sufficient energy, or a surface hot enough, to cause *ignition.* Whenever ether, cyclopropane, ethyl chloride or ethylene is used in anaesthetic concentrations, an *explosive mixture* is present, and even the low energy spark provided by static electricity is sufficient to cause *ignition.* Flammability limits of other drugs shown in Table 1 are either outside the anaesthetic concentrations or cannot be obtained in unheated vaporisers at room temperature (18–22° C). This table shows the flammability limits of inhalational anaesthetic drugs in air, oxygen and nitrous oxide. It is of interest that nitrous oxide lowers the lower limit of flammability for each drug. As oxygen is added to a mixture of an inhalational anaesthetic in nitrous oxide, a wider range of the concentrations used in anasthesia becomes non-flammable. Figure 1 which is based on information supplied by the manufacturers of "Fluothane" shows the flammability limits of halothane in oxygen/nitrous oxide mixtures at 20° C. Two observations may be made by way of example. To a 70 per cent nitrous oxide/30 per cent oxygen mixture more than 8 per cent halothane would have to be added before ignition could occur and at 100 per cent oxygen, no ignition is possible at any concentration of halothane up to that corresponding with its saturated vapour pressure at room temperature. The figures were obtained using a cerium-magnesium fusehead ignition source. This is more powerful than any ignition source likely to be found in an operating theatre.

The *energy* required to ignite anaesthetic gases varies according to the nature of the gases and how nearly their concentration approaches the stoichiometric, at which ignition is most easy. The stoichiometric mixture of any fuel is that at which, theoretically, combustion can be complete and all the fuel and oxygen molecules in the mixture react to form the products of combustion. The two main sources of ignition in the operating theatre are static electricity and diathermy.

PREVENTION

Fires in operating theatres may be prevented in three main ways—the use of non-flammable gas mixtures, the elimination of every sort of spark or flame, or the separation, at a safe distance, of flammable gases from ignition sources.

The Use of Non-flammable Drugs

There is no doubt that from a physical point of view, the soundest method of preventing explosions is to use drugs which cannot be made to burn in any circumstances in the operating theatre; but the prevention of explosions is by no means the only problem for the anaesthetist. Many regard ether or cyclopropane, or both, as indispensable to the production of good anaesthesia in certain cases and there are occasions when the physiological risk to the patient of a non-explosive anaesthetic is greater than the risk of an explosion. In such circumstances, if the diathermy can be dispensed with, or its spark kept at a safe distance from the gas mixtures without increasing the risk to the patient, a flammable agent should be used. In such a case, both the surgeon and anaesthetist must be prepared to understand the other's problems.

A "non-flammable theatre".—It has been suggested that if a group of anaesthetists agreed to use only non-flammable drugs, their operating theatres

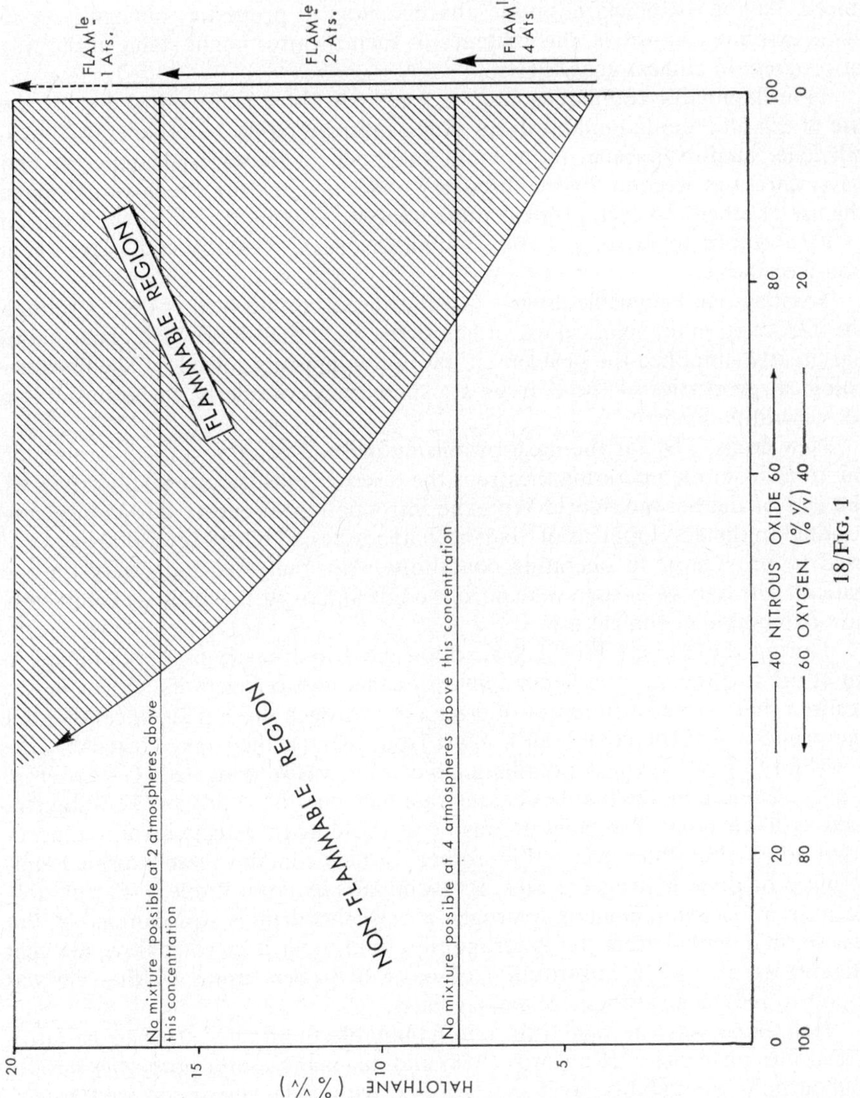
FLAM.le 1 Ats.
FLAM.le 2 Ats.
FLAM.le 4 Ats.
FLAMMABLE REGION
NON-FLAMMABLE REGION
No mixture possible at 2 atmospheres above this concentration
No mixture possible at 4 atmospheres above this concentration
HALOTHANE (% v/v)
20
15
10
5
0 20 40 NITROUS OXIDE 60 80 100
100 80 60 OXYGEN (% v/v) 40 20 0

18/Fig. 1

need not be designed to eliminate static electricity and other sources of ignition. But such a suggestion is not without risk. A visiting anaesthetist, in the habit of using ether or cyclopropane might well come to work in such theatres and not be in agreement with the view that flammable gases are unnecessary, or he might forget the limitations of the theatres. Furthermore, if a new drug were introduced, having extremely desirable pharmacological properties but ignitable in some extreme conditions, the existence of such theatres might stand in the way of progress in clinical anaesthesia.

Non-flammable techniques may be sought in three main ways, first by the use of existing non-flammable drugs such as nitrous oxide, halothane, trichloroethylene, methoxyflurane, intravenous drugs, local or regional analgesia and basal narcotics; second, by the discovery of some new drug which would make the use of ether and cyclopropane quite unnecessary; and third, by the addition of a substance to existing useful flammable drugs, which would make them non-flammable.

Existing non-flammable drugs.—All that need be said here is that, although the introduction into clinical use of halothane and other fluorinated anaesthetics has greatly simplified the problem, it has not completely solved it. The pharmacological properties of these drugs are sometimes considered to be unsuitable for certain patients.

New drugs.—By far the most promising method of removing all flammable mixtures from the operating theatre is the discovery of new drugs. Shortly after the end of the Second World War, the introduction of curare into clinical use resulted in the development of "balanced anaesthesia" where several drugs were used to provide good operating conditions with analgesia and safety for the patient. The only gases used were nitrous oxide and oxygen, which are completely non-flammable in clinical use.

During the Second World War, fluorinated hydrocarbons were studied in an effort to produce non-flammable lubricants and refrigerants. When it was realised that the substitution of fluorine for hydrogen did not significantly alter the properties of the compounds, apart from making them less "reactive", the possibility of producing a non-flammable ether was investigated. Go Lu *et al.* (1953) were among the first to demonstrate the anaesthetic properties of fluorinated hydrocarbons. The most promising of those he investigated was trifluoroethyl vinyl ether (fluroxene—"Fluoromar") which contains three fluorine atoms in place of three hydrogen atoms. Its formula is given in Table 1. Presumably because of its five remaining hydrogen atoms, this drug is still flammable, but less so than diethyl ether. Its lower ignition limit in air is given as three per cent (Krantz *et al.*, 1953). Substitution of more hydrogen atoms by fluorine was found to reduce anaesthetic potency greatly.

Halothane was the first truly non-flammable fluorinated drug to be introduced into anaesthesia (Raventós 1956) and has many useful properties besides that of non-flammability, as it may be used with soda lime in a closed system, is a potent anaesthetic and shares with ether the ability to minimise expiratory spasm in asthmatic patients. Unfortunately it cannot be claimed to be the complete answer, because there are still occasions when anaesthetists feel that ether or cyclopropane is the drug of choice.

Many more fluorinated compounds will probably be made and investigated, and possibly one or more of these will enable anaesthetists to dispense with the use of flammable drugs entirely, without prejudicing the safety of the patient or the convenience of the surgeon. In the meantime, care must be taken that new, non-flammable drugs are used on patients only if they offer a real clinical advantage and after most thorough pharmacological study. There are too many instances in medicine where drugs or techniques which appear attractive at first, prove to have totally unexpected side-effects either when used alone or in combination with some other drug. To justify its use on human patients, any new drug must claim to offer a *major* advantage over existing drugs. It is then for the anaesthetist to decide whether this advantage is sufficiently great in the case of a particular patient to outweigh the known risks of using any new compound.

Other fluorine compounds which have reached clinical practice since the introduction of halothane and fluroxene are "Teflurane" (Artusio *et al.*, 1967), which may be regarded as halothane with the chlorine replaced by fluorine, and "Ethrane" (Virtue *et al.*, 1966) which is an ethyl methyl ether of similar structure to methoxyflurane. But no new compound has so far been discovered which has fewer side-effects than halothane and yet is equally non-flammable. Hexafluorobenzene (Burns *et al.*, 1961) gave promise of avoiding the cardio-vascular and respiratory effects of halothane, while being non-flammable in air. Unfortunately, six per cent can be made to burn in oxygen and four per cent appears to be needed for induction of anaesthesia. It is interesting that a time may come when a drug like hexafluorobenzene will be used in some clinical circumstances, where its pharmacological advantages outweigh the very slight risk of an explosion.

Inert diluents added to otherwise flammable drugs.—In theory, volatile drugs such as ether and cyclopropane could be made effectively non-flammable by the addition of an inert diluent. This could work either by (a) absorbing the thermal energy of an incipient explosion or (b) absorbing free radicals. These free radicals result from the absorption of thermal energy by a molecule of an explosive gas, and, if they are not deactivated, will combine with oxygen and initiate a chain reaction, which results in an explosion (Ubbelohde, 1935; Hinshelwood, 1940).

Any added substance obviously has to satisfy certain requirements:

1. It must not be toxic to the patient.
2. It must have physical properties which enable the necessary vapour concentration to be obtained at room temperature.
3. It must not react with soda lime.
4. The concentration of the substance required to prevent an explosion must be relatively low, so that it does not interfere with the amounts of anaesthetic and oxygen which have to reach the patient.

(a) Energy absorbing diluents.—Carbon tetrafluoride is an example of this type of diluent. Jones *et al.* (1950) have shown that a concentration of 68 per cent of this substance will completely inhibit the combustion of cyclopropane/oxygen mixtures.

A more practical member of this group is nitrogen. Figure 2 is a "triple graph", showing the flammability limits for trichloroethylene/oxygen/nitrogen mixtures (Jones and Scott, 1942). As the concentration of nitrogen is increased, the upper limit of flammability is lowered. Unfortunately, there is little effect

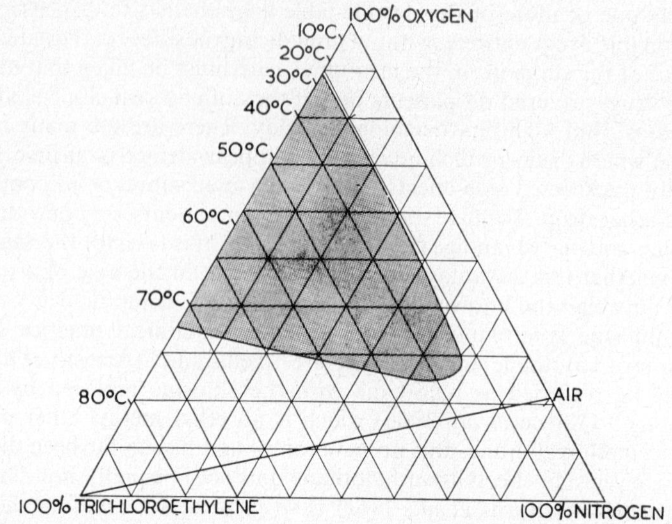

18/FIG. 2.—The flammability limits for trichloroethylene/oxygen/nitrogen mixtures.

on the lower limit, which remains at between ten and twelve per cent until the nitrogen reaches over 70 per cent. As it is the lower limit which is of most interest to anaesthetists, the use of nitrogen, or, for that matter, helium, as an inert diluent is not of much practical value.

Figure 2 also shows that no concentration of trichloroethylene will burn in a mixture of oxygen and nitrogen when the oxygen concentration is less than 21 per cent. In other words, trichloroethylene/air mixtures are non-flammable.

It should be noted from the temperature scale on the graph that ten per cent trichloroethylene vapour cannot exist in room conditions where the temperature is below 25·5° C. The temperature in the average operating theatre may be taken as being 18° and 22° C, while the anaesthetic range of trichloroethylene rarely exceeds two per cent. Hence, unless nitrous oxide is added to the mixture (see Table 1) trichloroethylene may be regarded as a non-flammable anaesthetic.

The lack of effect of increasing concentrations of nitrogen on the *lower limit* of flammability of a gas is a fairly constant phenomenon (Coward and Jones, 1952). The upper limit is affected to a much greater extent. Hence the *range* of flammability is always greater in oxygen than in air, although the *lower limit* is not significantly different. It may be useful to note here that the addition of water vapour which may occur when a patient inhales a gas does not alter the combustion limits to any useful extent. In the conditions found in operating theatres, "wet" gases are as likely to burn as "dry" ones.

(b) "Free-radical" absorbers.—The value of a free radical absorbing diluent has been investigated by adding ethylene to mixtures of cyclopropane and oxygen (Jones *et al.*, 1943). This is depicted in Fig. 3 which shows that an explosion cannot occur so long as the oxygen concentration remains below 20 per cent. A non-explosive mixture containing 30 per cent oxygen can be provided. Any reduction in the cylopropane concentration or further increase in the amount of oxygen results in an explosive mixture. Such a mixture has been tested clinic-

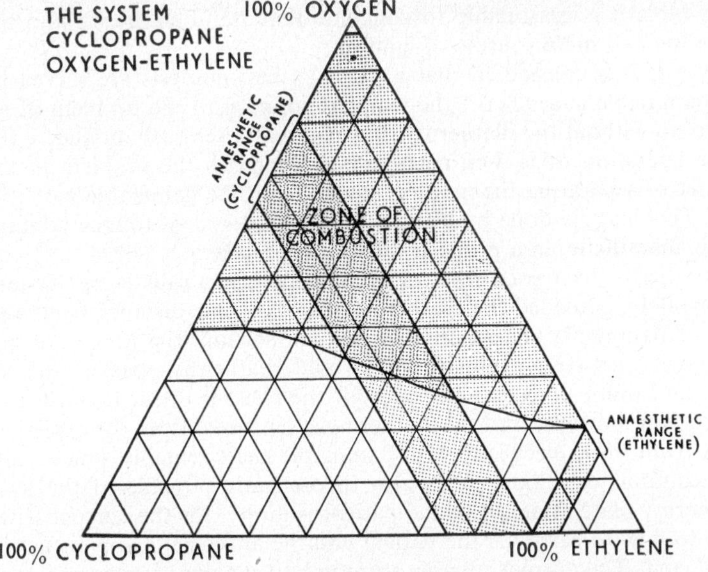

18/FIG. 3.—The system cyclopropane-oxygen-ethylene.

ally, but extremely careful control was necessary to keep it within the non-explosive limits (Horton, 1940). Coleman (1952) has shown that only about four per cent of some bromine containing fluorocarbons is necessary to inhibit the combustion of n-hexane in air. It is thus possible that a chemical could be found which would render a flammable gas non-flammable and yet leave it clinically useful. It has been shown that 7 per cent halothane will prevent the ignition of cyclopropane/oxygen mixtures (Bracken, personal communication) but as this is more than enough halothane to produce deep anaesthesia itself, the discovery is not of practical use.

The Elimination of Ignition Sources

The Report of the Working Party on Anaesthetic Explosions (H.M.S.O., 1956) lists the following probable sources of ignition in thirty-six explosions reported to the Ministry of Health from 1947 to 1954:

	Number	*Percentage*	
Static spark	22	61·1	69·4
Static spark or open gas burner . .	1		
,, ,, or electric heater . .	1	8·3	
,, ,, or smouldering towel .	1		
Diathermy	5	14·0	
Spark in switch or cut-out . . .	3	8·3	
Faulty valve in gas cylinder . .	1		
Foreign matter in valve . . .	1	8·3	
Smoking (?)	1		

From this table it is reasonable to conclude that static electricity and the diathermy are the two main sources of ignition.

Diathermy.—If it is considered that a patient's best interests are served by the use of a flammable anaesthetic, the simplest solution to the problem of an explosion is to do without the diathermy. But this might seriously prejudice the success of the operation. It is then necessary to approach the problem in the third way—that of separating the ignition source from the flammable gas by a safe distance. This may be done by using a fully closed system for the administration of the anaesthetic, in a properly ventilated theatre.

Many anaesthetists have used ether or cyclopropane in a fully closed system with complete safety, provided the diathermy spark is some distance from any possible leak of flammable anaesthetic. In this connection, the lungs are not an effective barrier between explosive gases and diathermy sparks, and so such a technique cannot be used with safety if the chest is open. It must also be remembered that, however well the diathermy is separated from the explosive gases, the risk from static electricity with flammable gases remains, unless full-anti-static precautions are taken. It is also theoretically possible, if the lead from the diathermy plate attached to the patient is faulty, for the current from the diathermy to flow to earth via the patient and the anaesthetic apparatus, or via the anaesthetist. The current, unable to return to the diathermy apparatus along the plate lead, takes the shortest path to earth. This path may well be through the anaesthetist, should he be touching the patient, and can lead to the formation of a spark between the anaesthetist's fingers and the patient, if this contact is broken while the current is flowing. It is essential that the earth lead should be known to be functioning whenever the diathermy is used.

In connection with the leak of flammable gases from anaesthetic systems, Bulgin (1953) describes three zones in operating theatres. These are:

1. The highly dangerous zone, comprising the anaesthetic machine, breathing bag, tubing, face mask, patient's head, and the immediate vicinity of the patient.
2. A zone extending from about one foot from the above items for about three feet in all directions. In this area, the gases are much more difficult to ignite.
3. A zone beyond that in (2), in which the gases will normally be below the ignition limit.

In this connection, recent work by Vickers (1970) has shown that as close as 10 cm. from an expiratory valve delivering 15 per cent ether in eight litres of air/minute, the highest concentration of ether detectable was only 0·85 per cent of the lower limit of flammability. He concluded "that, as far as the mixtures escaping in clinical anaesthesia are concerned, there seems no likelihood of explosive concentrations occurring at a distance greater than 25 cm. from the expiratory valve".

Good *ventilation* is important in operating theatres because it will clear the air of flammable gases as well as pathogenic organisms. Ideally, fresh air should be admitted from points more than six feet above floor level, and extraction should take place from openings close to the floor. In this way, explosive anaesthetics, which are all heavier than air, are kept close to the floor and away from possible sparks. Air should be extracted from the theatre at a point near the anaesthetic machine, and not drawn from the machine across the theatre.

Sparks from other electrical apparatus.—Just as it would be unreasonable to ban the use of the diathermy in order to minimise the risk of an explosion, so it would not be reasonable to ban the use of electrical apparatus, such as suckers or blood warmers, simply because they are capable of producing an electric spark. Explosions from such sparks can be prevented by the installation and regular inspection of recommended types of equipment. Some types of electrical apparatus, such as the brush gear in a motor, produce sparks, even when functioning normally. When an electric motor is used to work a suction apparatus, it must be designed to prevent any explosive gases which may be sucked from the mouth, e.g. during tonsillectomy, from coming into contact with a spark. Some electric heaters, sterilisers and cautery apparatus can become sufficiently hot to ignite a flammable mixture.

When this type of apparatus, which is capable of producing a dangerous spark, has to be used in an operating theatre, steps must be taken to ensure that the spark never comes into contact with a flammable gas mixture. In addition to the separation in space described above, three methods are used for minimising the risk.

1. *A gas-tight container* can be used to surround a particular piece of equipment and keep out the explosive mixture. An example is the moulded rubber cover used for a foot operated diathermy switch.

2. *A pressurised container* can be used when the apparatus is too bulky to be made gas tight. This involves supplying air under slight pressure to the container and so minimising the risk of an explosive mixture being drawn into it.

3. *An intrinsically safe circuit* is one in which the current is so limited that any sparking which might occur under normal or faulty conditions would be not of sufficient energy to ignite an explosive anaesthetic mixture. It is particularly suitable for instruments used for endoscopy. Their source of light should be obtained from a dry battery, or other circuit in which there is a resistor which limits the amount of current passed. Such a system is the only practical application of the theory of preventing explosions by limiting the energy of a potential spark. The danger of spark ignition is greater with alternating than with direct current. For example 6 volts D.C. require a minimum resistance of 3·25 ohms, while 6 volts A.C. require a minimum of 14 ohms (H.M.S.O., 1956). Guest *et al.* (1952) have shown that anaesthetic gases in air require a spark to ignite them of 200 times greater energy than that required when they are mixed with oxygen. However, the energy of the spark required, even in air, is of the order of only 200 μj *, and, except for apparatus which can be operated from a six-volt dry battery, this principle has no practical clinical application.

Static electricity.—It is almost impossible to ensure that a dangerous accumulation of static electricity will never occur in an operating theatre. Nevertheless most explosions due to static can be traced to a failure to observe fairly simple precautions. Anaesthetic explosions are fortunately very rare and this may sometimes be a reason for lack of thoroughness in taking proper steps to prevent their occurrence. Unfortunately, when such an explosion does take place, the patient may receive severe or fatal injuries, and others in the theatre may be injured by flying glass or be burned.

* μj = a millionth part of a joule, which is a measure of energy.

Careful design and maintenance of apparatus which could give rise to a spark and the avoidance of explosive anaesthetics when an obvious ignition risk is present, can practically eliminate the risk of explosions from *electrical apparatus*. If the surface of *every* person and piece of apparatus in the theatre could be joined together electrically, and with a very low resistance, the risk from *static electricity* could also be eliminated.

Bonding.—Even if it were possible to bond everything in the theatre at a very low resistance, theatre personnel would be exposed to the risk of electrocution should a fault develop in any piece of electrical apparatus, such as a lamp or power saw. The insulation provided by ordinary leather footwear, and most floors, is a useful protection against such a mishap.

Path to earth via resistance.—Anti-static precautions in operating theatres are, therefore, aimed at removing all articles which readily acquire static charges, and providing a path to earth through all personnel and equipment, so that any static charges that develop are dissipated as quickly as possible, without significantly increasing the risk of electrocution. In general terms it involves ensuring that there is a resistance of not more than 100 megohms* and not less than 50,000 ohms between each person or article in the theatre and earth.

Static charges may be produced by *movement*, *friction* and *induction*. Trolleys, when *moved* about the theatre, can acquire dangerous static charges. This risk used to be minimised by fitting all mobile equipment with chains which trailed across the floor and could conduct away static charges, provided they were kept clean and did not break. Nowadays a more satisfactory method is to use wheels fitted with conducting rubber tyres.

High static charges may be produced by *friction* in woollen blankets when these are quickly shaken or drawn across a trolley. Static charges may be *induced* on equipment by the presence of certain types of electrical apparatus in the theatre, and in such cases there is no contact between the source of the current and the article on which the charge is induced.

Materials.—Certain materials, such as "Perspex" and nylon, are inherently dangerous, since they readily acquire static charges. It is usually possible to find suitable alternative materials which are not so troublesome, but where this is not possible the offending materials can be treated with an anti-static wax.

Personnel.—Theatre staff should not wear clothing which readily acquires a static charge. Plastic aprons and woollen garments should therefore not be worn. Aprons of conductive rubber are available.

Conducting footwear should be worn by everyone in the theatre. Anti-static shoes or boots are most satisfactory, but light canvas shoes with anti-static rubber soles can also be worn with safety. People who enter the theatre for only a short time may put on conductive "over-shoes".

As far as personal clothing is concerned, the most important thing is to wear a close-fitting cotton or other anti-static outer garment. It should fit closely to reduce movement between the clothes and the wearer.

Woollen blankets should not be brought into the theatre. They should be replaced by cotton blankets, a towel, or some other anti-static fabric. Closely fitting woollen stockings worn by patients are not a serious static risk since they

* 1 megohm = 1 million ohms.

become moist, and provided they are not removed or roughly handled in the theatre, are not likely to acquire a charge of static electricity.

It is sometimes suggested that nurses and others should not wear nylon stockings in the theatre, as this material might insulate the wearers. Quinton (1953) has shown that this does not occur. No significant difference in resistance between the thigh and the outside of the sole of the shoe was found in a volunteer nurse who wore different types of stockings. Apparently the skin of the foot makes contact with the inside of the shoe through the mesh of the stocking.

Floors.—It is obviously essential that the floor in an operating theatre should have a conductivity of the same order as the items resting on it. The most satisfactory types of flooring in use at present are terrazzo or concrete with a resistance of from 0·1 to 10 megohms. To replace all unsatisfactory floors would be a most expensive undertaking, but it is now possible to lay conductive rubber or plastic on top of an existing floor and so render it satisfactory. Where an anaesthetic is only occasionally given, and the floor is unsuitable, it is sufficient to stand the anaesthetic trolley on a moistened sheet large enough to prevent anyone from touching the trolley without himself also making contact with the sheet.

Relative humidity.—The generation of static electricity is more difficult in a damp atmosphere, while moisture on the surface of an article renders it more conductive. It is good practice, therefore, to wet rubber breathing tubes before use if their anti-static properties are in doubt. A 1 per cent solution of "Teepol" or other wetting agent is more effective than plain water.

A high relative humidity reduces the risk of a static explosion, but cannot entirely remove the hazard. It must also be remembered that articles have to be exposed to a humid atmosphere for about ten minutes before any significant amount of moisture collects on their surfaces.

No exact figure can be given for an optimum relative humidity, and different authorities in this country recommend from 50–65 per cent. It is, however, very difficult to raise the humidity in a theatre; washing down the floor with hot water barely raises it by 8 per cent—and even if it were possible, there are few theatres in which the temperature could be kept low enough to make it comfortable to work in a high humidity. Where full air conditioning exists, a relative humidity of over 70 per cent is quite comfortable provided the temperature is not allowed to rise above 20–21° C (68–70° F).

Ideally, all operating theatres should be equipped with hygrometers of the paper or human hair type. When the humidity falls below 50 per cent the anaesthetist should be told, and he should take whatever steps he thinks necessary for the safety of the particular patient he is anaesthetising. These might involve the wetting of floor and walls, or the use of non-explosive anaesthetics.

Rubber equipment.—There is little doubt that non-conducting rubber is the main source of dangerous static electricity (H.M.S.O., 1956). Sometimes the charge is generated on the rubber, sometimes the rubber prevents the rapid discharge of static produced elsewhere. Only anti-static rubber should be used in association with anaesthetic equipment. This rubber is made by the addition of carbon to the rubber "mix". It owes its conductivity to the proximity of the carbon particles and it is thus possible for ordinary wear and tear to reduce its conducting properties. For complete safety, therefore, all anti-static rubber should be tested about once every three months.

From the practical point of view, when there is any doubt about the anti-static properties of rubber equipment, it should be kept moist. If an anti-static article does not retain all the desirable properties of its non-conductive equivalent, then an ordinary rubber one may be used, provided it is kept moist. The only anti-static item which is really markedly unsatisfactory in practice is the endotracheal tube. It is reasonable to use endotracheal tubes made of ordinary rubber, since they are kept moist when in position in the patient.

The instrument most commonly used for testing the conductivity of a material is a 500-volt D.C. insulation tester. The two leads of the apparatus are applied to different areas of the object to be tested, and the handle of the instrument is turned. A direct reading of the conductivity between the two test points is then given on a scale.

Ionisation.—Quinton (1953) has designed an apparatus which conducts away static charges by ionising the air in the neighbourhood of the anaesthetic trolley and the operating table. The ionised air is electrically conductive and serves to dissipate static charges. The apparatus is spark-proof, and the radio-active source is so arranged that theatre personnel cannot be exposed to radiation.

Quinton uses a small induction motor which blows a stream of air down a brass cylinder 10 cm. long and 5 cm. in diameter and with walls 2 mm. thick. The cylinder is lined on its inside curved surface with a metal foil incorporating radiothallium 204 at a strength of ¼ mc*/cm², making 50 mc altogether. The radiations from the thallium ionise the air, but very little radiation can escape

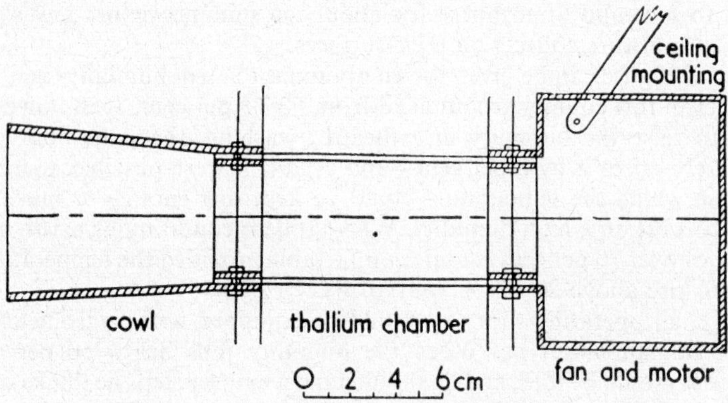

18/FIG. 4.—Diagram of radio-active thallium ion blower.

into the theatre. The apparatus is mounted about six feet from the floor and arranged so that the stream of ionised air is directed at potentially dangerous areas such as the anaesthetic trolley. It is shown diagrammatically in Fig. 4.

Anaesthetic gases are not the only sources of flammable mixtures in operating

* mc = 1/1000th of a Curie. A Curie is the quantity of any radio-active substance that is undergoing $3{\cdot}7 \times 10^{10}$ disintegrations per second.

theatres. The too speedy use of the diathermy or cautery following a liberal use of a spirit based skin cleanser may produce a fire which will burn the patient, particularly if he is lying on impervious sheeting, so that the liquid collects in a pool under him. Ether and other flammable liquids may be spilled on the floor or other part of the theatre. Their vapour may be ignited and the spread of the flame in such circumstances can be alarmingly rapid and far-reaching.

In summary, it may be said that, where a flammable gas is in the patient's best interests, full antistatic precautions should be taken, and no sparks or other ignition sources permitted within 25 cm. of any possible leak of anaesthetic gas.

REFERENCES

ARTUSIO, J. F., Jr. (1963). *Halogenated Anesthetics.* Philadelphia: F. A. Davis Co.

ARTUSIO, J. F., VAN POZNAK, A., WEINGRAM, J., and SOHN, Y. J. (1967). Teflurane. A nonexplosive gas for clinical anesthesia. *Curr. Res. Anesth.*, **46**, 657.

BULGIN, D. (1953). Factors in the design of an operating theatre free from static risks. *Brit. J. appl. Phys.*, Suppl. No. 2, S 87.

BURNS, T. H. S., HALL, J. M., BRACKEN, A., and GOULDSTONE, G. (1961). An investigation of new fluorine compounds in anaesthesia. (3) The anaesthetic properties of hexafluorobenzene. *Anaesthesia*, **16**, 333.

COLEMAN, E. H. (1952). Effect of fluorinated hydrocarbons on the inflammability limits of combustible vapours. *Fuel*, **31**, 445.

COWARD, H. F., and JONES, G. W. (1952). Limits of flammability of gases and vapors. U.S. Bureau of Mines, Bulletin 503. Washington.

FABIAN, L. W., DEWITT, H., and CARNES, M. A. (1960). Laboratory and clinical investigation of some newly synthesized fluorocarbon anesthetics. *Curr. Res. Anesth.*, **39**, 456.

"Fluothane": A report to the Medical Research Council by the Committee on Non-explosive Anaesthetic Agents. *Brit. med. J.*, 1957, **2**, 479.

GUEST, P. G., SIKORA, V. W., and LEWIS, B. (1952). Static electricity in hospital operating suites. Bureau of Mines Report of Investigation 4833 (U.S. Dept. of Interior).

HINSHELWOOD, C. N. (1940). *The Kinetics of Chemical Change.* London: Oxford Univ. Press.

H.M.S.O. (1956). *Report of a Working Party on Anaesthetic Explosions, including safety code for equipment and installations.* London: H.M. Staty. Office.

HORTON, J. S. (1940). *Bull. Amer. Assn. Nurse Anesthetists*, **8**, 285.

JONES, C. S., FAULCONER, A., Jr., and BALDES, E. J. (1950). Preliminary investigations of carbon tetrafluoride as an inert diluent gas to prevent explosions of mixtures of cyclopropane and oxygen. *Anesthesiology*, **11**, 562.

JONES, G. W., KENNEDY, R. E., and THOMAS, G. J. (1943). U.S. Bureau of Mines, Technical Paper 653. Washington.

JONES, G. W., and SCOTT, G. S. (1942). U.S. Bureau of Mines, Report of Investigation 3666. Washington.

KRANTZ, J. C., Jr. (1964). Unpublished reports.

KRANTZ, J. C., Jr., CARR, C. J. C., LU, G., and BELL, F. K. (1953). Anesthesia XL. The anesthetic action of trifluoroethyl-vinyl ether. *J. Pharmacol. exp. Ther.*, **108**, 488.

LU, G., LING, J. S. L., and KRANTZ, J. C., Jr. (1953). Anesthesia XLI. The anesthetic properties of certain fluorinated hydrocarbons and ethers. *Anesthesiology*, **14**, 466.

QUINTON, A. (1953). Safety measures in operating theatres and the use of a radioactive thallium source to dissipate static electricity. *Brit. J. appl. Phys.*, Suppl. No. 2, S 92.

RAVENTÓS, J. (1956). The action of fluothane—a new volatile anaesthetic. *Brit. J. Pharmacol.*, **11,** 394.

SCHÖN, G., and STEEN, H. (1968). Explosion limits and ignition temperatures of some inhalation anaesthetics in mixtures with various oxygen carriers. *Anaesthesist*, **17,** 6.

UBBELOHDE, A. R. (1935). Investigations on the combustion of hydrocarbons. I. The influence of molecular structure on hydrocarbon combustion. II. Absorption spectra and chemical properties of intermediates. *Proc. roy. Soc. A* , **152,** 354 and 378.

VICKERS M. D. (1970). Explosion hazards in anaesthesia. *Anaesthesia*, **25,** 488.

VIRTUE, R. W., LUND, L. O., PHELPS, M., Jr., VOGEL, J. H. K., BECKWITT, H., and HERON, M. (1966). Difluoromethyl 1,1,2-trifluoro-2-chloroethyl ether as an anaesthetic agent: results with dogs, and a preliminary note on observations with man. *Canad. Anaesth. Soc. J.*, **13,** 233.

Section Two

THE CARDIOVASCULAR SYSTEM

Chapter 19

THE HEART

THE CORONARY ARTERIES

Anatomy

THE **left coronary artery** (Fig. 1) arises from the left posterior aortic sinus below the level of the free edge of the aortic cusp. The main trunk runs forwards and to the left between the base of the pulmonary artery and the left auricle to enter the atrioventricular groove. At this point it gives off a large and important branch—the interventricular—which passes downwards in the anterior interventricular groove, then curls round the apex of the heart, and finally anastomoses with the corresponding branch of the right coronary artery. It supplies branches to both ventricles.

Meanwhile, the main trunk—called in the past the left circumflex branch of the left coronary artery—passes along the left atrioventricular groove. It continues round the left border of the heart and accompanies the coronary sinus as far as the interventricular groove where it anastomoses with similar branches from the right coronary artery.

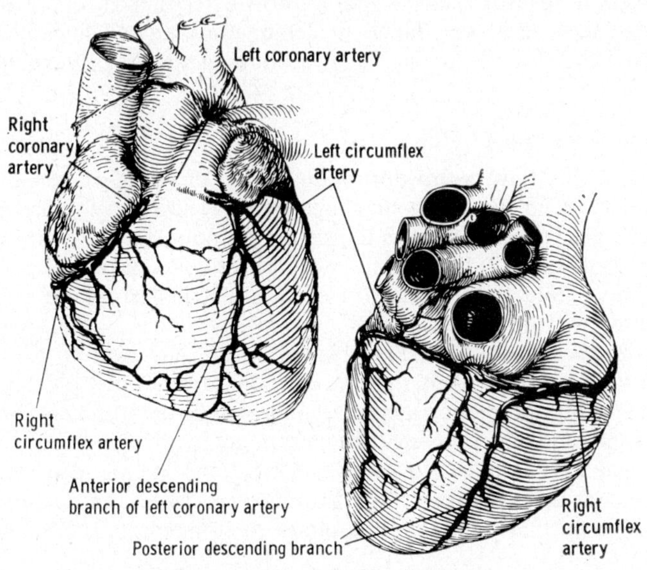

19/FIG. 1.—The coronary circulation.

The **right coronary artery** (Fig. 1) arises from the anterior aortic sinus just below the level of the free edge of the anterior cusp of the aortic valve. It passes forwards and to the right between the root of the pulmonary trunk and the right auricle and then runs in the right atrioventricular groove to the right side of the heart near its inferior margin. Here, it curls round the right border on to the posterior aspect of the heart and then runs towards the left side until it reaches the interventricular groove, where it anastomoses with the left coronary artery. It gives off two important branches; the *marginal*, which arises near the point where it curls round the right border of the heart and passes along the inferior border, supplying branches to both surfaces of the right ventricle; and the *interventricular*, which arises just before the termination of the main trunk on the posterior aspect of the heart. This branch runs downwards and forwards in the interventricular groove, giving off branches as it goes until finally it ends by anastomosing with the corresponding branch of the left coronary artery.

The blood supply to the neuromuscular tissue of the heart is of some importance. The sino-atrial (S-A) node receives a branch directly from either the right or the left coronary artery. The atrio-ventricular (A-V) node is supplied by twigs from the left coronary artery; the atrio-ventricular (A-V) bundle has an abundant blood supply, receiving branches from the left coronary artery which accompany the bundle in the moderator band and supply the right division of the bundle. The left limb of the bundle has no specific branch and is supplied by small arterioles in its neighbourhood.

It is generally believed that the vagus nerve carries constrictor fibres to the coronary arteries whereas the sympathetic nerves are responsible for vasodilatation. In the past, this led to the routine use of atropine in the treatment of coronary thrombosis, on the assumption that it prevented reflex coronary constriction. Recent investigations using improved techniques of coronary flow measurement, have, however, failed to demonstrate any significant or consistent change in the flow following vagal section in the dog (Eckenhoff *et al.*, 1947).

Coronary Artery Blood Flow

Coronary artery flow begins during the period of isometric relaxation of the cardiac muscle, when the ventricular muscle is relaxed and the pressure in the aorta is high. The inflow continues to rise up to about the mid-point of diastole and then falls off again in the second half of diastole as the aortic pressure subsides. During systole the contraction of the ventricular muscle prevents the coronary arteries from filling.

Since the circulation of blood through these channels is of such great importance it would seem likely that the coronary arteries possess some intrinsic mechanism for their protection against changes in the environment. Some of the factors that influence the coronary circulation are:

(a) *Oxygen saturation of the blood.*—Alterations in this may influence the lumen of the coronary vessels. A fall in saturation to 50 per cent results in a fourfold increase in coronary flow in an attempt to compensate for the myocardial hypoxia.

(b) *Cardiac output.*—Changes in the cardiac output have a marked effect, since the coronary flow varies inversely with it. That is to say, when the cardiac output falls the coronary flow increases and *vice versa*. In the dog the heart receives about 4–5 per cent of the total cardiac output under normal conditions, but if the cardiac output is seriously curtailed the total percentage of the blood passing through the aortic valves which goes back into the coronary circulation may be as high as 10 per cent. Such information in man is not available.

(c) *pH of the blood.*—Changes in the pH of blood in the coronary circulation also affect the flow. A fall in pH leads to an increase in the flow, but an increase in the carbon dioxide content of the perfused blood in dogs is apparently without effect.

(d) *Body temperature.*—During the early stages of hypothermia in dogs the coronary blood flow decreases relatively more than the blood pressure or cardiac output. This is probably due to a simultaneous but greater reduction in the work required of the myocardium. Such a view is supported by the finding that the hypothermic heart can respond to an increased work load by raising the coronary flow (McMillan *et al.*, 1957). It is possible, therefore, that changes in the vessel calibre may be induced directly by alterations in body temperature (Berne, 1954).

(e) *Blood pressure.*—The mean aortic blood pressure influences the coronary artery blood flow. Usually a rise in pressure leads to an increased flow and a fall to a decreased flow. Such generalisations take no account of the cause of the change in blood pressure and the associated changes in cardiac output, coronary artery diameter, and the peripheral resistance, all of which affect the flow.

Coronary artery dilators.—The coronary vessels supply the myocardium with oxygen and other substances necessary for contractile activity. The efficiency of this mechanism depends on an adequate supply of raw materials. If the heart is called upon to do more work without a corresponding increase in the coronary flow then the myocardial efficiency must suffer.

Amyl nitrite and glycerine trinitrate ("Trinitrini") are generally regarded as the most efficient coronary vasodilators in the presence of angina pectoris. Although they are claimed to produce vasodilatation of the coronary vessels, their main action is probably to reduce the general peripheral resistance and thereby to make the work of the heart easier. It is important to remember, therefore, that a reduction in the myocardial work is as important as an increase in coronary flow.

On the other hand, adrenaline and noradrenaline are believed to produce an increase in coronary flow. Berne (1958) has shown that the primary action of these amines on the coronary circulation is one of vasoconstriction but this is overruled by their secondary activity in stimulating myocardial metabolism so that the final result is an increase in coronary flow.

Digitalis, in therapeutic dosage, has no action on the coronary flow but increases the efficiency of the myocardial contraction.

Xanthine, thyroxine and theophylline are all believed to increase the coronary flow directly.

Coronary Circulation and Artificial Perfusion (see Chapter 25)

Oxygenated blood is necessary for the proper functioning of a beating or fibrillating heart and this is provided by pumping oxygenated blood through the coronary arteries through the special catheters. However, the oxygen requirements of a quiescent heart is such that long periods of ischaemic arrest can be tolerated without subsequent damage.

THE HEART RATE

Control

In the region of the floor of the 4th ventricle lie two groups of neurones, the cardio-inhibitory and the cardio-accelerator centres. The former is part of the dorsal nucleus of the vagus and the latter is intimately connected with the dorsal sympathetic outflow.

The heart rate is controlled by a balance of the inhibitory influence of the vagus and the excitatory influence of the sympathetic. At rest the heart rate is dominated by the effect of the vagus. The sympathetic system only contributes but slightly to the rate of the heart at rest. The exact extent to which the cardiac sympathetic influences the resting heart rate has been investigated by producing beta-receptor blockade in normal subjects, but this does not fully explain the nature of the control as the vagus and cardiac sympathetic are only the effector pathways of a complex servo system involving many feedback afferents from peripheral receptor sites.

The various influences affecting the heart rate may be summarised:—

1. *Peripheral stimulation.*—Hypoxia and carbon dioxide stimulate chemoreceptors and increase the heart rate.

2. *Direct stimulation.*—A rise in body temperature may increase the heart rate by increasing the rate of discharge in the sino-atrial node. Circulating catecholamines may also directly stimulate the heart.

3. *Impulses from other cranial centres.*—These may reflexly affect the pulse rate. For example, a sudden fright in a conscious subject may lead to intense vagal stimulation, vasodilatation and hypotension with slowing of the heart: i.e. a vasovagal attack.

Sinus arrhythmia is thought to occur as a result of the spread of respiratory neurone activity to adjacent cardiac centre neurones.

A rise in intracranial tension, as produced by a cerebral tumour, slows the pulse rate.

4. *Vascular reflexes.*—These are the most important. The pressor receptors are situated in the media of the roots of the great vessels; the common carotid and the subclavian arteries and the arch of the aorta. The area of the bifurcation of the common carotid arteries is dilated and is known as the carotid sinus. Other pressor receptors are situated in the atria and the great veins. Afferents from the pressor receptors pass to the medulla. An increase in blood pressure is followed by a fall in heart rate (Marey's law) and vice versa. The carotid and aortic bodies also strongly influence the cardiac centre by responding to changes in the carbon dioxide and oxygen tensions of the blood.

Abnormal Rhythm

Normal myocardial muscle exhibits characteristic physiological properties which are called automaticity, conductivity, excitability, and refractoriness. It is the effect of various agents on one or other of these properties that causes an abnormal rhythm.

Automaticity is the ability of myocardial muscle to undergo spontaneous depolarisation. Not all cardiac muscle exhibits this property, but it is seen in the sino-atrial node and in:

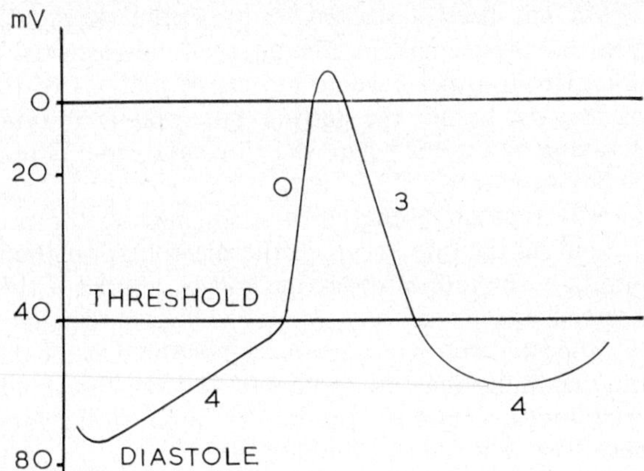

19/FIG. 2.—The action current of a pacemaker fibre recorded by an intracellular electrode.

1. adjacent venous tissue;
2. certain tracts of atrial tissue;
3. the His-Purkinje system.

These tissues are all potential pacemaker sites, though normally the sino-atrial node, having the highest rate of spontaneous depolarisation, is the pacemaker.

The stages of myocardial electrical activity are best examined by following the changes in the intracellular electrical potential. These changes are divided into four phases following depolarisation (Figs. 2 and 3).

(0) Depolarisation.
(1) Rapid repolarisation.
(2) Slow repolarisation ('Plateau').
(3) Second rapid repolarisation.
(4) Restoration of resting potential
 (or diastolic depolarisation in pacemaker tissue).

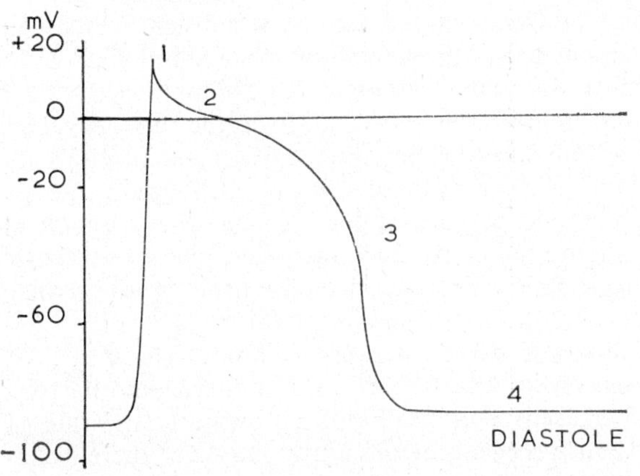

19/FIG. 3.—The action current of a ventricular muscle fibre recorded by an intracellular electrode.

As has been described, only certain parts of the myocardial muscle can perform as pacemakers. The intracellular electrical charges of pacemaker tissue differ from other cardiac muscle in phase 4 of the cycle. During diastole, in pacemaker tissue, the resting potential is not maintained but is constantly decaying to a point where the threshold level is reached, when a depolarisation 'spike' occurs.

The rate of discharge of a site having the property of automaticity will depend on the rate at which the diastolic potential is raised to threshold level. Similarly the rate of discharge will be altered if the threshold level is raised or lowered.

The *excitability* of a site is proportional to the difference in potential between the maximum diastolic potential and the threshold potential. For instance the excitability is raised if the maximum diastolic potential is raised (i.e. made less negative) or if the threshold is lowered (i.e. set at a greater negative potential).

An alteration in the state of certain areas of the myocardium has been described following ischaemic injury or in the presence of some halogenated anaesthetic agents. The altered areas show impairment of conduction of impulses, and these localised areas of impaired conduction allow *re-entry* to take place. Re-entry is said to occur when an impulse has by-passed an altered area of muscle, but re-enters this area when the normal muscle is refractive. The impulse reinitiated in the damaged area is then able to be conducted into the normal muscle when that has ceased to be refractory. This is a theory of the genesis of ectopic rhythm.

From this description, it may be seen, that an increase in the automaticity of a site other than the sino-atrial node may give rise to an abnormal pacemaker site, as in nodal rhythm when the pacemaker is situated either at the atrio-ventricular node or in the adjacent bundle of His.

Catecholamines and Cardiac Rhythm

The main action of catecholamines on the heart is to raise the rate of spontaneous diastolic depolarisation (phase 4) in pacemaker tissue. However not all pacemaker tissue is affected to the same extent and this may give rise to aberrant pacemaker sites.

Contrary to widespread belief, catecholamines do not significantly increase excitability. A dual action may be seen, characterised by a transient increase in excitability, which may be associated with potassium release, followed by a longer diminution in excitability. It should be noted that excitability is a term that should be used only in the confined sense of changes in the relative values of threshold potential and maximum diastolic potential. An increased excitability implies an approximation of one or both of these levels to each other.

The response of the sympathetic nervous system to anaesthetic agents is variable. Cyclopropane and diethyl ether produce increased plasma catecholamine levels whilst thiopentone and halothane produce little or no change (Price *et al.*, 1959).

It has been shown that halothane affects the myocardial muscle in at least two ways. Firstly it has been shown that the rate of spontaneous diastolic depolarisation (phase 4) is increased. This results in a slowing in the rate of discharge of the pacemaker, and a slowing of the pulse. However the effect is not uniform on all automatic tissue and a new pacemaker may arise. The occurrence of a "wandering" pacemaker is frequently observed during halothane anaesthesia. Secondly, the potential difference between the maximum diastolic potential and the threshold potential is decreased, or the excitability is raised. This example of halothane exhibits the futility of attempting to describe the effects in terms of sympathetic or parasympathetic overactivity.

Price has described the effects of chloroform as those of suppression rather than increased excitability. Suppression of the sinus and atrioventricular nodes in their ability to respond to a generalised increase in rate and automaticity.

THE CARDIAC OUTPUT

The term "cardiac output" denotes the volume of blood that *each* ventricle pumps out per minute. It is abbreviated in flow equations by the symbol $\dot{Q}$ in order to achieve comparative values in different individuals; it is sometimes related to the surface area and then known as the "cardiac index".

With the advent of reliable methods of estimating cardiac output at rest and during exercise, it became clear that changes in cardiac output were not solely dependent upon changes in heart rate, as a fivefold increase in cardiac output was observed to be associated with only a $2\frac{1}{2}$ times rise in heart rate. The response of the heart to an increased body metabolism is to raise its rate, to eject more blood with each beat, and to eject that volume of blood in a shorter time.

Venous Return

When the cardiac output is considered for anything but brief periods of time clearly the venous return must equal the cardiac output. However, instantaneous changes in cardiac output may take place without a corresponding increase in venous return (or vice versa). To achieve such short-term inequalities, the heart must draw on reserve volumes of blood contained in the heart itself (change in diastolic volume) or from the pulmonary circulation. Further volumes of blood may be acquired from a reduction in the capacity of larger central veins, though the mechanisms involved in venomotor reflexes are not clearly understood.

There are numerous factors commonly accepted by physiologists as playing some part in the venous return and being responsible for controlling the flow of blood to the right atrium every minute. For example:

1. The *vis a tergo* deprived from the pressure in the arterioles driving the blood through the capillary plexus on into the venous system.
2. The uni-directional valves present in the veins below the superior vena cava. There are none proximal to this level.
3. The squeezing action of the skeletal muscles during exercise.
4. The assistance of gravity in draining blood from the areas above the level of the heart.
5. The negative pressure in the thoracic cavity, varying with each phase of respiration and thus acting as an auxiliary pump.

The fact that the cardiac output is well-maintained despite intermittent positive pressure respiration, diffusion respiration, bilateral open thorax, and induced hypotension, strongly suggests that there must be some additional mechanism present. There is no doubt that a persistent high positive pressure in the closed thorax not only compresses the pulmonary capillaries but also the great veins, and thus reduces the cardiac output. This can be simply demonstrated in the dog where inflation of the lungs under pressure can be shown to reduce the blood pressure in direct proportion to the rise in intrathoracic tension. Release of this tension results in an immediate rise in the blood pressure. In the anaesthetised subject this test is sometimes used to demonstrate the presence or absence of autonomic activity, because the sudden fall in blood pressure stimulates the baroreceptors in the aortic arch. Their response brings about a rapid rise in the systemic pressure on release of the intrathoracic tension. Nevertheless, the baroreceptor activity is so sensitive that there is a temporary "overswing" and the pressure rises slightly above the control value for a few seconds before returning to the initial level. In the absence of autonomic (baroreceptor) activity the "overswing" is not observed.

During controlled respiration the systemic pressure is often slightly lower than in the presence of spontaneous respiration. Raising the intrathoracic tension during a spontaneous inspiration, e.g. "assisted respiration", tends to diminish venous return, but if adequate time is allowed for an expiration *at atmospheric pressure*, the blood pressure usually rapidly readjusts itself to the normal level. Any resistance to expiration, however, will make the raised intrathoracic tension persist during both phases of respiration, which will reduce both venous return and systemic pressure.

The lack of importance of movement of the abdominal contents and diaphragm or variations in the negative intrathoracic pressure can be demonstrated by using a continuous insufflation technique. The patient's lungs are kept mildly distended by a large flow of oxygen but, although this is sufficient to produce adequate oxygenation, it is rarely enough to wash out the carbon dioxide. The chest remains motionless for many minutes without any sign of interference in the venous return.

Probably the most important factor in controlling venous return is the tension of oxygen in the tissues themselves. Muscular activity is known to increase venous return, and this is thought to be due to vasodilatation in the tissues. It is now thought that this increase in tissue perfusion is caused directly or indirectly by a reduction in the oxygen content of the blood within the active tissue (Guyton, 1963). It thus appears that it is the oxygen requirements of the tissues themselves which regulate the level of the venous return and thus the cardiac output. The role of the autonomic nervous system in the control of the cardiac output has been described by Sarnoff (1960). The effect of sympathetic stimulation is three-fold. Firstly there is a more forceful contraction of the ventricles for any given end-diastolic pressure. Secondly there is an increased stroke volume which leads to more complete ventricular emptying and thus increases the ventricular compliance. And thirdly there is augmented atrial contraction.

The effects of the parasympathetic appear to be confined to the atria which beat with diminished vigour in the presence of vagal stimulation.

This explanation is an expansion of the *Starling-Frank* relationship of end-diastolic pressure or fibre length to the strength of ventricular contraction.

Effect of Anaesthetic Agents upon the Cardiac Output

There has been widespread confusion in the world literature on the subject of the action of the various anaesthetic drugs on the cardiac output. This is because the drugs used for premedication or induction of anaesthesia can seriously influence the action of the inhalational agents. For example, cyclopropane leads to a bradycardia in the patient premedicated with morphine, yet this action is absent when cyclopropane is used alone (Price, 1960).

Fundamentally, it can be said that all anaesthetic agents in equipotent doses depress myocardial activity in the isolated heart preparation. This direct depressant action is seldom seen in intact man because it is overshadowed by the compensatory mechanisms. The precise effect of the various anaesthetic agents appears to be closely related to their respective ability to liberate the catecholamines in the sympatho-adrenal system (Etsten and Li, 1962).

The effect of the principal anaesthetic agents on the cardiac output in man can briefly be summarised as follows:

Ether.—The cardiac output is increased due principally to the increased liberation of noradrenaline which improves myocardial activity.

Cyclopropane.—The cardiac output is reduced when morphine premedication is used (Li and Etsten, 1957), yet it is increased in the absence of premedicant drugs (Jones *et al.*, 1960). This action is due to an increase in noradrenaline liberation.

Thiopentone.—There is a reduction in cardiac output in most cases.

Halothane.—The cardiac output is reduced due principally to a block of the action of noradrenaline, thus preventing it stimulating the myocardium. Unlike most other inhalational anaesthetic agents there is no increase in noradrenaline liberation during halothane anaesthesia (Price *et al.*, 1959).

Discussion.—There would seem to be general agreement that the cardiac output falls after anaesthesia has been in progress for some time. Thus, as the skin and muscle vasodilatation of early anaesthesia gives way to vasoconstriction with the progress of the operation, so the output falls. Apart from gallamine, which has a chronotropic action, the muscle relaxant drugs do not influence the cardiac output.

Measurement of the Cardiac Output

In the *experimental animal*, the cardiac output may be measured at the aortic root by various implantable flow meters, using electromagnetic or Doppler-ultrasound principles.

In *man*, there are two main methods—the Fick and the Dye Dilution. Both utilise the dilution principle, the former of oxygen and the latter of dye. Cardiac output can also be measured by a pulse contour method.

The Fick principle.—This can be used to measure the flow of blood through any organ, whether it be heart, brain or kidney. If the concentration of the oxygen in the arterial blood to an organ is known, and also that in the venous blood leaving it, then provided one can measure the total oxygen that has been removed from or added to the blood per minute, the quantity of blood flowing through the organ in unit time can readily be calculated. When this principle is used in calculating the (total) cardiac output, the oxygen consumption is that of the whole body and is measured as oxygen uptake by the lungs. The relationship of flow to oxygen uptake is given by the equation:

$$\dot{Q} = \frac{O_2 \text{ consumption}}{\text{A-V}o_2 \text{ content difference}}$$

where $\dot{Q}$ is flow in unit time.

The fall in oxygen content is determined by measuring the oxygen content of arterial blood and that in mixed venous blood, preferably in the pulmonary artery. The oxygen consumption is measured by collecting the expired gases and estimating the uptake by comparison with the O_2 content of the inspired mixture. The concentration of oxygen may be measured in the inspired gas (F_1O_2) or assumed in the case of air. The volume and oxygen content of the expired gases (F_eO_2) are measured and the oxygen uptake obtained from the following equation:

$$\dot{V}o_2 = (\dot{V}_1.F_1o_2) - (\dot{V}e.F_e\text{-}o_2)$$

all volumes being corrected to S.T.P.D. (standard temperature, pressure and dry). With the subject breathing air, the inspired minute volume is the expired minute

$$\text{vol.} \times \frac{\text{expired nitrogen concentration}}{\text{inspired nitrogen concentration}}$$

If the body nitrogen stores are in a steady state, the inspired minute volume will equal the expired minute volume.

When the subject is breathing a gas mixture other than air, this assumption is not valid and various techniques have been devised to overcome this difficulty. One technique described by Nunn and Pouliot (1962) utilises a box-bag spirometer.

Dye dilution.—This is the method described by Hamilton and his co-workers. It consists of the injection of a known amount of dye, or detectable substance, into the bloodstream and measuring the concentration in an arterial sample during the first circulation of the dye.

The dye commonly used is indocyanine green which has superceded other dyes as its absorption spectrum is not close to either reduced or oxyhaemoglobin. It has a half life of approximately 10 minutes and repeat estimations may be performed frequently.

Other substances may be used as indicators such as cold saline or dextrose injections (Branthwaite & Bradley, 1968), and a solution of radioactive Krypton.[85]

Early methods involved the collection of a number of discrete, timed samples in order to plot the rise in concentration. Dynamic methods have been evolved (Hamer *et al.*, 1966), using cuvette densitometers through which arterial blood is drawn at a constant rate. The output of the densitometer is fed to a pen writer which records the rise and fall in concentration as a continuous curve (Fig. 4).

The cardiac output is determined from the following equation:

$$\dot{Q} = \frac{I}{ct} \text{ where } \begin{array}{l} I = \text{amount of indicator injected.} \\ c = \text{concentration of indicator.} \\ t = \text{time for one circulation.} \end{array}$$

The area beneath the curve is the function *ct* and may now be measured by laborious counting of squares or by using an instrument known as a planimeter.

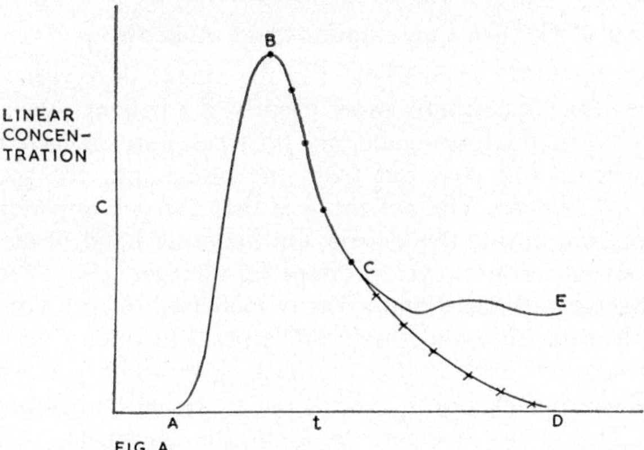

19/FIG. 4(*a*)—Curve A B C E is that produced by the output of a cuvette densitometer.

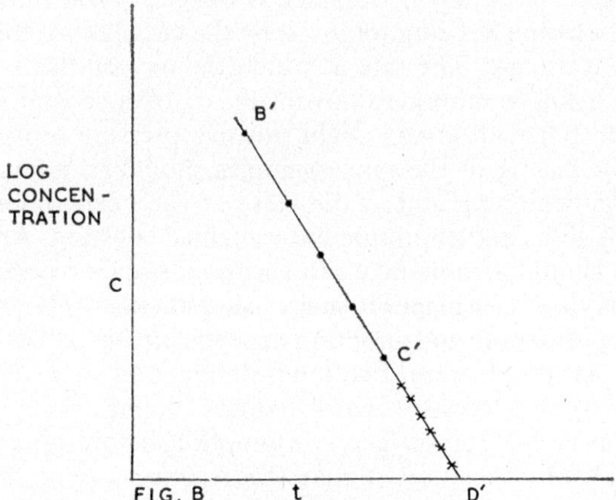

19/FIG. 4(*b*).—This is the downslope portion of the curve in Fig. 4(*a*) redrawn on semi-logarithmic paper.

The concentration of dye (C) in Fig. 4(*a*) does not fall to zero after one passage through the body due to the effect of recirculation of the dye. The effect of recirculation is ignored by re-plotting the downslope portion of the curve (BC) on a semi-logarithmic scale (B′C′). Since the downslope is an exponential decay, B′C′ will be linear and may be extrapolated to D′. Points along the line CD on the original curve may thus be obtained by reference to the semi-logarithmic plot. Thus the area beneath the curve A B C D may be obtained, free of the effects of recirculated dye.

More recently, the output of the densitometer may be fed to a computer which is able to "sense" the downslope of the curve, integrate the signal and in a properly calibrated system, produce direct values of the cardiac output.

Pulse contour method.—Continuous estimations of the cardiac output may be obtained from examination of the contour of a centrally recorded intra-arterial pressure tracing. The method has been developed to produce an on-line system of recording cardiac output, in conjunction with a digital computer (Warner, 1968).

Measurement of Oxygen Consumption under Anaesthesia

Under anaesthesia, the measurement of the uptake of oxygen is complicated by the presence of the anaesthetic gases. Clearly, if a patient—anaesthetised with cyclopropane/oxygen mixture—suddenly breathes pure oxygen from a spirometer, cyclopropane will pass out from the blood into the spirometer until equilibrium is established. The net result is that there is apparently almost no oxygen consumption during this period. On the other hand, if the spirometer is filled with a concentration of cyclopropane far in excess of that in the patient's blood, the converse will occur and a vastly increased oxygen consumption will be apparent. In order to avoid these difficulties and obtain accurate readings under anaesthesia, it is necessary to establish equilibrium between the concentrations in the spirometer and in the patient's circulation before any measurement is made. This is best achieved by filling the spirometer with an identical mixture to that respired by the patient. At the requisite moment the patient's respirations are directed in and out of the spirometer whilst the carbon dioxide is absorbed. Greater accuracy is obtained if oxygen is run into the tank at the identical rate at which it is being removed by the circulation, thus giving a horizontal line on the tracing. The rate at which the oxygen flows in may be measured, either by a finely calibrated flowmeter, or by a second spirometer filled with pure oxygen but with a very slight positive pressure replacing the normal perfect counterbalancing of the tank. Samples should be taken from the main spirometer at the beginning and at the close of each experiment to check that the percentage of gases in the mixture has remained constant. Arterial blood saturation samples should also be taken to ensure adequate oxygenation.

Values of oxygen consumption under anaesthesia.—The effect of anaesthesia on the rate of oxygen consumption depends largely on the criteria adopted for comparison. Although premedication is designed to alleviate fear and apprehension, it is rarely so successful that it reduces the metabolic rate to a normal resting level. The higher the oxygen consumption before operation, therefore, the greater the fall with the onset of anaesthesia. In a series of 23 patients Shackman and his associates (1951) noted an average fall of 15 per cent compared with the basal oxygen consumption. The values for male patients varied from 128 ml. per minute to 212 ml. per minute, with an average of 179. The comparable figures for the female patients were 120–202, with an average of 159 ml. per minute.

The rate of oxygen consumption under anaesthesia does not vary significantly with changes in the tidal volume. Even when apnoea occurs the oxygen consumption continues if there is a high enough tension of oxygen in the alveoli to maintain a diffusion gradient into the blood circulating through the pulmonary capillaries. The difference between body temperature and that in the spirometer does not appear to have any appreciable effect on the measurement of the rate of oxygen consumption under anaesthesia, but this point should be taken into account in any calculation.

Intracardiac and Main Vessel Measurements (See also Chapter 24)

A knowledge of the normal values for the various chambers of the heart is useful to the anaesthetist engaged in anaesthesia for cardiac operations. The

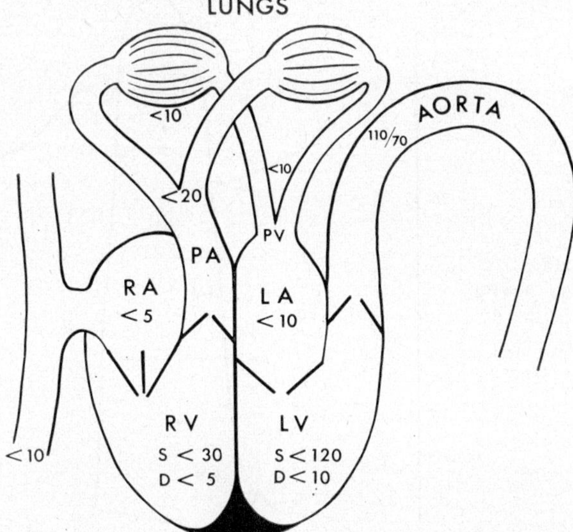

19/FIG. 5.—Normal mean intracardiac and major vessel pressures in mm. Hg.

pressure in the chambers on either side of a diseased valve will reflect the variation from normal—in other words, the degree of stenosis or incompetence of the valve. The mean normal values for the chambers of the heart and great vessels are illustrated in Fig. 5.

During pre-operative cardiac catheterisation the values of the oxygen saturation (or tension) of the blood in the various areas of the heart can be recorded. Some normal values are shown in Fig. 6. Such values do not take the haemoglobin level of the blood into account; for this reason oxygen content/100 ml. of the blood is often reported, as this enables the cardiologist to assess the amount of blood which is passing through a "shunt" e.g. atrioseptal defect.

It is often necessary to make pressure measurements within the heart and great vessels. The pressure waves as seen on the oscilloscope for a normal patient

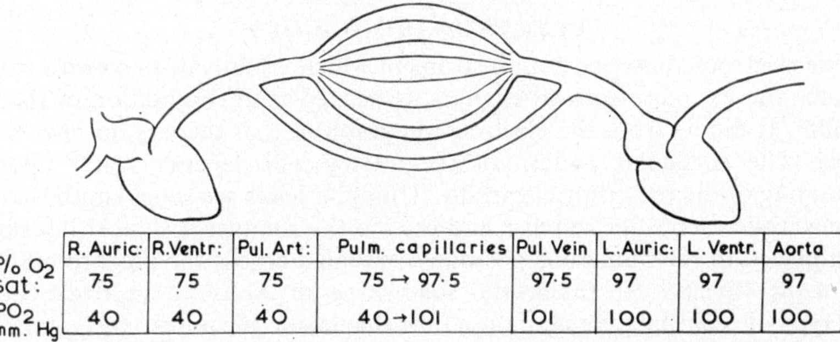

	R. Auric:	R.Ventr:	Pul. Art:	Pulm. capillaries	Pul. Vein	L. Auric:	L. Ventr.	Aorta
% O_2 sat:	75	75	75	75 → 97·5	97·5	97	97	97
PO_2 mm. Hg	40	40	40	40→101	101	100	100	100

19/FIG. 6.—Oxygen saturation and tension figures in a normal person breathing air. The fall in saturation and tension between pulmonary vein and left auricle is due to pulmonary shunting. (Adapted from Comroe *et al.*, 1962).

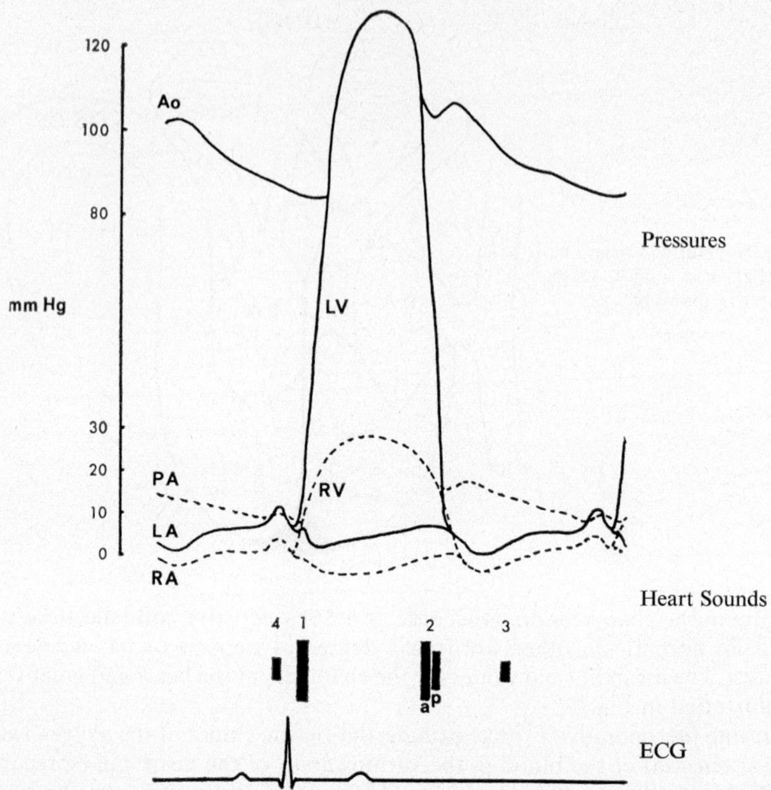

19/Fig. 7.—Typical normal pressure tracings for the various chambers of the heart superimposed on a common scale. From the relative pressures, the time of aortic and pulmonary valve opening, and the opening of the atrio-ventricular valves can be predicted. The diagram also enables the timing of murmurs in the heart to be understood.

are very characteristic and prompt recognition will permit confirmation of the site of the needle. Typical normal pressure waves are shown in Fig. 7.

ELECTROCARDIOSCOPY

The electrocardioscope is an instrument which visually displays on a cathode ray tube the various electrical changes associated with contraction of the myocardium. It differs from the electrocardiograph in that there is no final written record. The particular pattern of the tracing will depend largely upon the positioning of the recording electrodes. Unipolar leads are so arranged that only one electrode carries the impulse and used in this manner it is most informative when placed in the numerous positions—situated across the precordium in the line of the 4th and 5th intercostal spaces—as an exploring electrode (Fig. 8). This type of recording is mainly used for diagnostic purposes.

Bipolar leads, however, record from two parts of the body simultaneously and the tracing results from both. It is evident, therefore, that although greater accuracy is obtained with unipolar leads, the classical bipolar leads are more

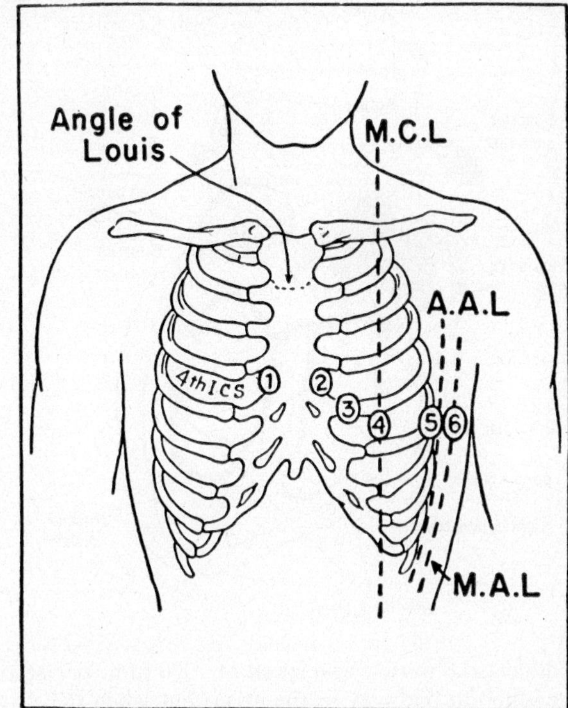

19/FIG. 8.—THE LOCATION OF THE SIX PRAECORDIAL LEADS

M.C.L., midclavicular line;
A.A.L., anterior axillary line;
M.A.L., midaxillary line.

suitable for the conditions prevailing during pulmonary or cardiac operations because the leads can be placed far away from the operation site. As far as the anaesthetist is concerned the main purpose of electrocardioscopy is continuous monitoring of the myocardial activity during intrathoracic work.

Different wave-forms are found depending upon which limbs the electrodes are placed. During anaesthesia Lead II (right arm, left leg) has been found to be the most satisfactory (see Table 1).

19/TABLE 1

SHOWING POSITIONS OF BIPOLAR LEADS ON THE PATIENT'S EXTREMITIES

Lead I	Right arm—Left arm.
Lead II	Right arm—Left leg.
Lead III	Left arm—Left leg.
Lead IV	Chest Lead—Indifferent electrode on limb or back.

The Normal Electrocardiogram

The impulse that initiates the normal heart beat arises at the sino-atrial node, situated at the junction of the superior vena cava and right atrium (Fig. 9). This specialised tissue is rich in nerve fibres and ganglia cells. The wave spreads out from this area—commonly referred to as the pacemaker— and envelops the

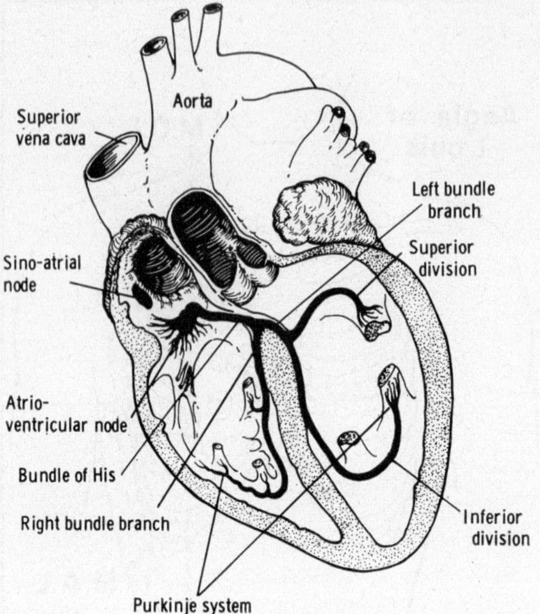

19/Fig. 9.—Conduction through the heart.

whole atrial muscle at a speed of 1000 mm. per second. There is no specialised conduction pathway in the atria, but when the wave of excitation reaches the junction between the atrium and the ventricle it excites another area of specialised nervous tissue—the atrioventricular node. From here the impulse passes down the bundle of His which is a nerve channel running into the

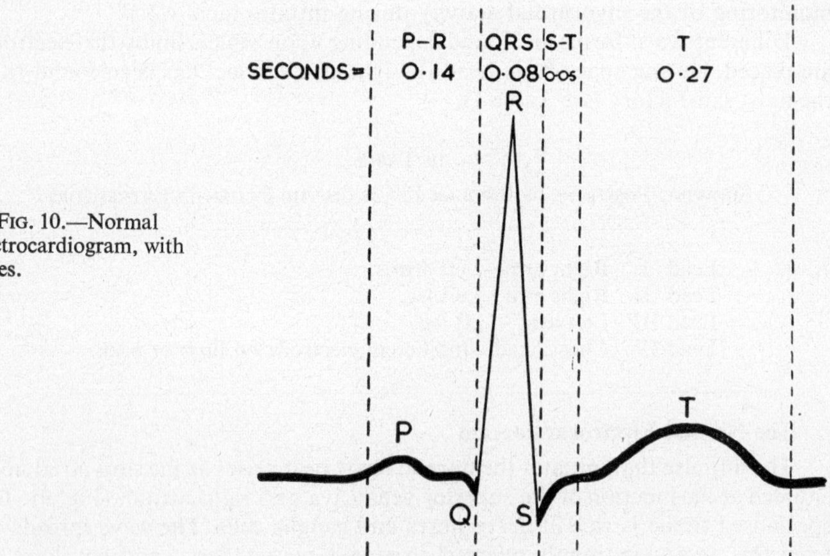

19/Fig. 10.—Normal electrocardiogram, with times.

interventricular septum where it divides into two branches—a right and a left—extending down each side of the septum. This specialised pathway continues on downwards and then spreads out into finer branches to encompass the whole mass of the ventricular muscle. These finer divisions are called Purkinje fibres and are found in great numbers near the surface of the heart.

In the electrocardiographic record (Figs. 10 and 11) the P wave represents the contraction of the atria. The width of the P wave roughly indicates the time it

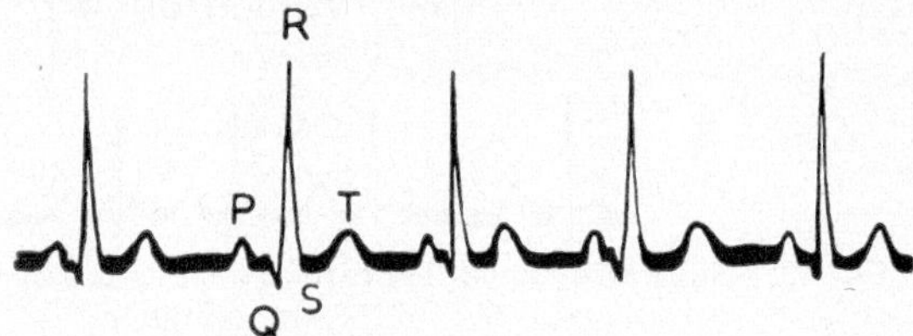

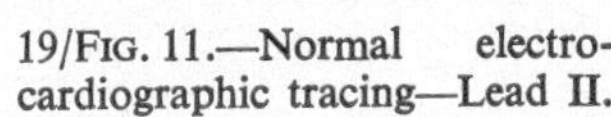
19/FIG. 11.—Normal electrocardiographic tracing—Lead II.

takes for the impulse to travel from the S-A node to the A-V node—normally this does not exceed 0·11 second.

The P-R interval indicates the time it takes the stimulus to spread from the sinus node to the ventricles. It varies slightly with the heart rate and is normally shorter in children. In adults, the P-R interval varies from 0·12 to 0·2 second, whereas in children the range is from 0·1 to 0·18 second.

The QRS complex represents the contraction of the ventricles. The height of this complex is a sign of the voltage and can be varied by repositioning the recording electrodes. Enlargement of the left ventricle—as in hypertensive heart disease—leads to left ventricular preponderance with left axis deviation. All this means is that the electrical axis has shifted because the left ventricular muscle is larger than the right. Thus in a 3-lead electrocardiogram when the highest upward initial deflection (R wave) occurs in Lead I and the lowest downward deflection (S wave) in Lead III, left ventricular preponderance is present. Note that in left axis deviation the main deflections are away from one another. In right ventricular preponderance the changes are reversed and the lowest downward wave is in Lead I and the highest upward deflection is in Lead III, i.e. the main deflections are towards one another.

The width of the QRS complex indicates the time taken for the stimulus to spread through the ventricles and normally varies from 0·06 second to 0·11 second. Widening of this complex occurs in ventricular hypertrophy, bundle branch block, and in some cases of complete heart block. The period of the QRS complex represents the stage of invasion and contraction since the upstroke of the R coincides with the onset of ventricular systole; the T wave coincides approximately with the end of ventricular systole. The average duration of this wave is 0·27 seconds.

Sinus rhythm denotes a normal regular beat originating from the sinoatrial node. Since this node is under the influence of vagal impulses, sinus bradycardia or tachycardia may occur. Slowing of the normal heart rate follows athletic training, carotid sinus pressure, intracranial lesions, jaundice, cyclopropane, chloroform or halothane anaesthesia, and drugs such as digitalis and quinidine. Sinus tachycardia is usually taken as a normal rhythm faster than 100 beats per minute, though some authorities regard 120 beats per minute as the lowest level. This occurs in children and in adults on exercise, excitement, haemorrhage, or as a result of hypoxia, atropine, and many other drugs. The rate often becomes so fast that the P waves become merged with the T waves of the preceding complex.

Sinus arrhythmia is a normal sinus rhythm in which periodic variations in the heart rate occur in relation to respiration (Fig. 12). It is due to alterations

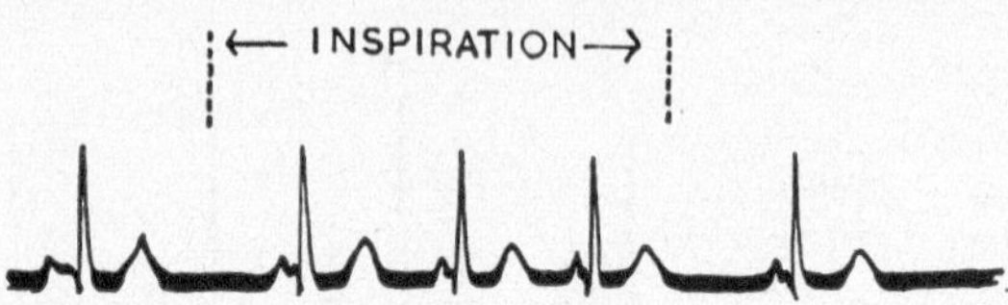

19/FIG. 12.—Sinus arrhythmia. The cardiac cycle speeds up during inspiration and slows again on expiration.

in vagal tone during the respiratory cycle, so that the heart rate quickens during inspiration and slows again on expiration. It is a normal healthy finding which can be abolished by an injection of atropine.

Abnormal Contractions of the Myocardium

In the anaesthetised subject almost every known type of arrhythmia has been recorded. Nevertheless, in this book it is not intended to delve deeply into the complex problems of interpreting electrocardiographic records, but rather to outline the more common changes that may be seen during anaesthesia.

Supraventricular tachycardia is an omnibus term used to denote that the ventricles are receiving a regular stimulus from the A-V node in the usual manner regardless of the rhythm of the auricles. It includes atrial tachycardia, nodal tachycardia, atrial flutter and fibrillation. This comprehensive diagnosis is only applied in the absence of more precise evidence, such as failing to recognise the "F" waves or "saw-toothed" appearance of auricular flutter, or the "F" waves of auricular fibrillation. Atrial tachycardia is differentiated by the presence of P waves and a fast regular rhythm, whereas in nodal tachycardia the P waves appear before, within, or after the normal QRS complex. In each case the heart rate is usually greater than 140 beats per minute. Supraventricular tachycardia should be distinguished from ventricular tachycardia by the complete absence of any sign of an atrial contraction in the latter condition.

Atrial ectopic beats (extrasystoles) may arise in any part of the auricular muscle. In normal circumstances only the sino-atrial node exercises this function. On the electrocardioscope these premature beats are difficult to detect but their presence is often suspected when the intervals between the QRS complexes become irregular (Fig. 13). The abnormal P wave is often swallowed up in the preceding QRS complex or it may occur on top of the T wave giving rise to a biphasic potential. When a beat originates in some part of the atrial muscle other than the S-A node, the impulse travels throughout the muscle; on reaching the S-A node it blocks the impulse that is in the process of being formed, and on arriving at the A-V node it brings about a full ventricular response provided this node is not in a refractory state from the previous beat. The significance of atrial

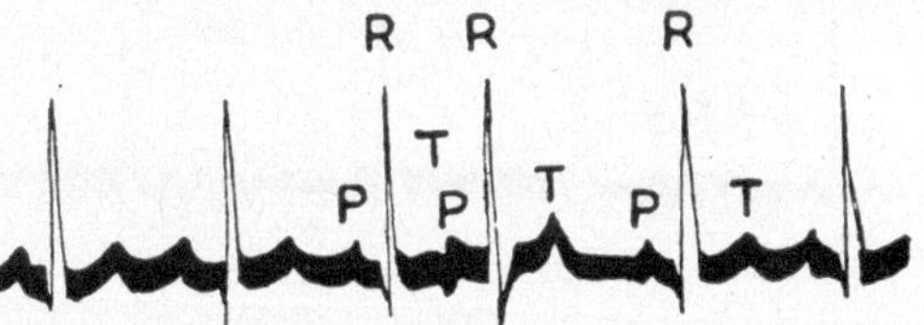

19/FIG. 13.—Atrial ectopic beats. Note the irregular interval between the QRS complexes and the presence of a P wave superimposed on a T wave.

premature contractions is not sufficiently understood, because they may occur in both conscious and unconscious patients, normal and abnormal hearts, and under all types of anaesthesia.

Atrial flutter was for many years believed to be due to an ectopic stimulus spreading round the atria in a circular manner, i.e. "circus movement". Prinzmetal and his colleagues (1951), however, have shown in recent studies with the aid of high speed photography that the flutter wave passes in every direction from its point of origin and does not, in fact, pursue a circular course. The atrial rate in this condition is generally between 200 and 350 beats per minute, but it is nearly always associated with some degree of atrioventricular block so that the ventricle only beats at half or quarter the rate of the auricle, i.e. 2:1 or 4:1 block. The electrocardioscopic pattern is notable for the "saw-toothed" appearance due to the presence of numerous "F" waves (Fig. 14). In reality these are multiple P waves of relatively high voltage. They are best seen when oesophageal leads are used, since in some of the classical leads they become distorted by the QRS complex and T waves. In atrial flutter the P-R interval is absent and the ventricular rate may be regular or irregular. When there is no A-V block the presence of "F" waves or the "saw-toothed" appearance may be difficult to recognise, and just a diagnosis of supraventricular tachycardia must then be made. To summarise, the principal features of atrial flutter are:

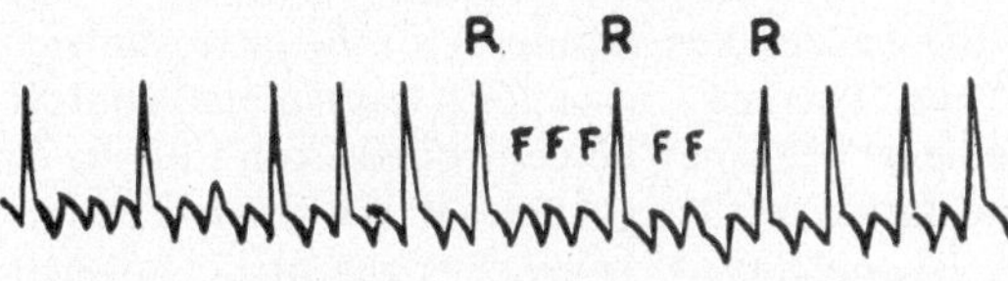

19/FIG. 14.—Atrial flutter. Presence of "F" waves.

1. The presence of "F" waves giving a "saw-toothed" appearance to the tracing.
2. Absence of the P-R interval.
3. Regular or irregular ventricular rate usually associated with some degree of heart block.

Atrial fibrillation has also been investigated with high-speed photographic methods. It has been possible to demonstrate that two main types of fibrillary twitches occur in the atrial muscle. First, the coarse and moderately irregular contraction which replaces the P wave and is called an "F" wave (Fig. 15). They have an extremely low potential and are therefore small and difficult to recognise. This response occurs at rates varying from 350–600 per minute. Secondly, minute and very irregular twitches that occur at much faster rates of 800–40,000 per minute. There is no evidence, however, to support the concept

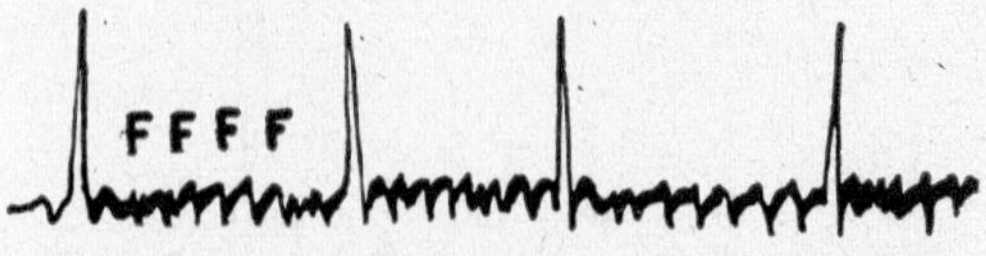

19/FIG.15.—Atrial fibrillation. Presence of "F" waves.

that a circus movement of the atrial muscle takes place. The essential difference between atrial fibrillation and flutter is that in the latter condition the atrial twitches occur at the slower rate of 200–350 per minute. In both conditions, the impulse often reaches the atrioventricular node when it is in a refractory state, so that some degree of heart block is always present. The ventricular response is grossly irregular, short and long cycles occurring without rhyme or reason. To summarise, there are three features that make it possible to recognise atrial fibrillation on the electrocardioscope:

1. Absence of P waves.
2. Presence of "F" waves.
3. Gross irregularities in the occurrence of the ventricular complex.

Nodal rhythm occurs when the pacemaker wanders to the atrioventricular node or even to the bundle of His. This may occur for a few isolated contractions or the whole rhythm of the heart beat may be controlled from this site for long periods of time. The impulse passes to the ventricles in the normal manner so that the ventricular complex is unchanged. It reaches the atria, however, in the reverse manner so the atrial contraction occurs either immediately before or just after the ventricular complex. If the focus of origin is near the atria in the A-V node it will reach the atrium rapidly and a short P-R interval will be seen on the electrocardioscope. On the other hand, if the focus of origin is low down in the bundle of His, either the impulse may not reach the atrium until after the ventricle has contracted (giving a P wave near the T wave) or it may be swallowed up in the QRS complex (no visible P wave) (Fig. 16). Despite the nodal rhythm, the S-A node sometimes continues to function so that the

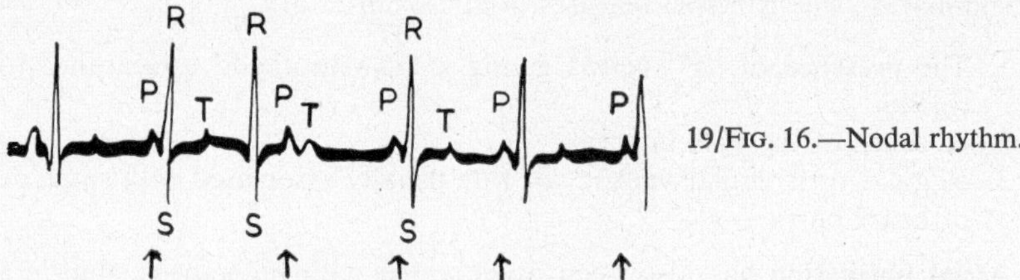

19/FIG. 16.—Nodal rhythm.

origin of the P waves is supplied by either the S-A or the A-V node, but nevertheless both types of rhythm occur at regular intervals regardless of the ventricular contraction. To summarise, nodal rhythm is exemplified by:

1. Short P–R interval.
2. Occasional absence of P waves.
3. P wave superimposed on the RS–T segment.

Nodal rhythm commonly arises under all forms of anaesthesia and leads to a reduction in cardiac output.

Heart block is a term used to designate some form of delay to the passage of impulses through the main conducting pathway of the atrio-ventricular node and the bundle of His. In a mild case the length of time (P–R interval) taken for an impulse to traverse this junctional tissue is lengthened. As the defect increases so the impulses from the auricles find it increasingly difficult to reach the ventricles, until finally one is blocked. In this manner there may be two or three atrial beats to every ventricular contraction, i.e. 2:1 or 3:1 heart block. In very severe cases the defect may be such as to block all conduction—namely, complete heart block (Fig. 17). Here the atria, dictated by the S-A node, con-

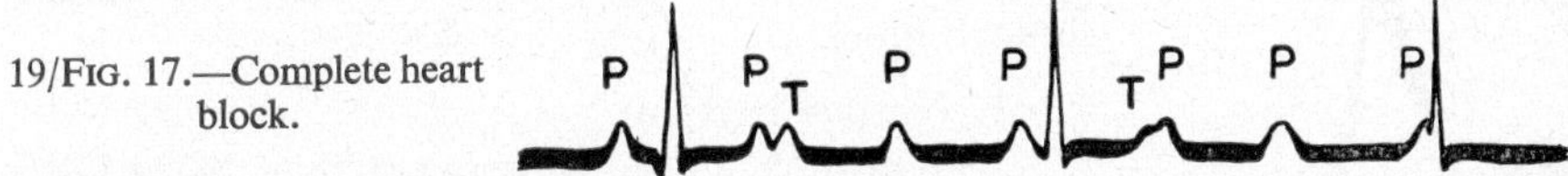

19/Fig. 17.—Complete heart block.

tinue to contract at their own rate, whilst the ventricular rhythm is controlled by a pacemaker that arises immediately below the block, somewhere in the A–V node or the bundle of His. Since the inherent rhythmicity of the ventricles is slow, the rate is only 30 beats or so a minute, but absolutely regular. Thus the atria and ventricles contract independently of each other. The differential diagnosis between complete and partial heart block is made by following the P waves. In complete block the P waves and QRS complexes occur regularly but the P wave gradually changes its relation to the R wave until it actually overtakes it.

In a partial block two or more P waves may occur to each ventricular cycle but the last one is regularly followed by a ventricular contraction.

To summarise, the three degrees of heart block are:

1. Prolonged P-R interval with normal A-V conduction.
2. Increasing P-R interval with dropped beats (Wenkebach phenomenon).
3. A-V dissociation or complete heart block with a slow ventricular rate (usually about 30 beats/minute).

Bundle branch block is caused by disease in one or other of the conducting bundles below the bundle of His (Fig. 18*a*). An impulse may start at the S–A

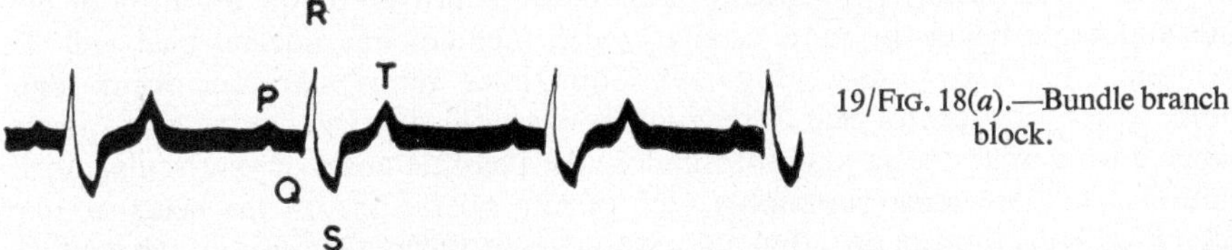

19/Fig. 18(*a*).—Bundle branch block.

node, pass to the A–V node and then down the bundle of His in a normal manner, but on reaching either the left or right bundle it may be delayed by a defect. If this obstruction arises on the left side, the impulse will travel rapidly down the right bundle but be delayed in its passage through the left. This leads to a widened QRS complex on the electrocardioscope and/or sometimes to actual notching, representing the separate contractions of the two ventricles.

The T wave usually follows immediately after the ventricular complex and is in the opposite direction to the main deflection.

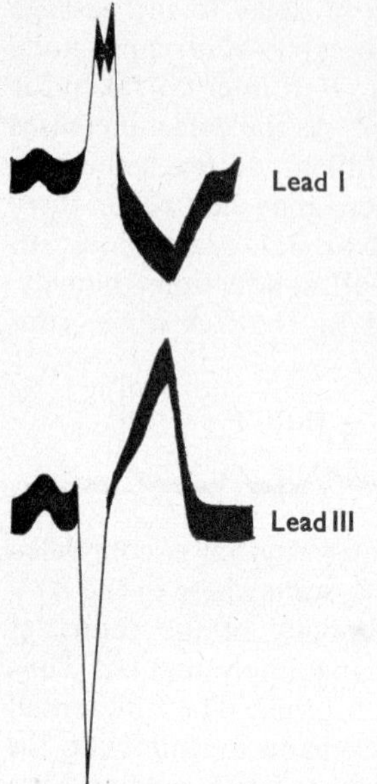

19/Fig. 18(*b*).—Left bundle branch block.

The way of telling whether the block is in the left or the right bundle is similar to that for determining the axis of deviation of the heart and, in each case, requires a knowledge of all three classical leads. If the main deflection is upward in Lead I and downward in Lead III, left bundle branch block is present. (Fig. 18*b*). Conversely, if the main deflection is downward in Lead I and upward in Lead III, right bundle branch block is indicated.

To summarise, the principle features of bundle branch block are:

1. Normal rhythm.
2. Widening, and sometimes notching, of the QRS complex.
3. T wave moves in opposite direction to the main deflection.
4. The direction of the main deflection in Leads I and III signifies whether the right or left bundle is defective.

Bundle branch block occurs most frequently in association with hypertensive heart disease, aortic stenosis, coronary ischaemia, and during hypothermia.

Ventricular ectopic beats arise from foci in any part of the ventricular muscle. The spread of this impulse is abnormal so that the resultant potential is different from normal. Its shape and size depends upon whether the impulse arises in the left or the right ventricle, and whether in the basal or apical region. Usually the complexes are large and broad, and occasionally coarsely notched with a T wave pointing in the opposite direction to the main deflection (Fig. 19). After this contraction the ventricle is in a refractory state when the atrial impulse arrives, so that this fails to bring about a ventricular contraction; the heart has therefore to wait until the next impulse arrives before it responds again. This period of inactivity is termed a "compensatory pause"; that the rhythm of the pacemaker remains undisturbed is proven by the duration of two normal beats being the same as that which includes one normal beat and the ectopic (viz. A-B = B-C; Fig. 19). Sometimes ventricular foci occur regularly with every second beat (bigeminy) or every third (trigeminy). Their appearance during anaesthesia may foreshadow the possible onset of ventricular fibrillation. They are most commonly seen during operations on the heart or may occur with cyclopropane, ethyl chloride or chloroform anaesthesia, particularly in the presence of hypoxia or a raised carbon dioxide tension.

To summarise, the essential features of ventricular ectopic beats are:

1. Large, broad, coarse and sometimes notched potential.
2. Absence of preceding P wave.
3. T wave extends in opposite direction to main deflection.
4. The rhythm of the pacemaker remains unchanged.

Effect of Drugs upon the Electrocardiogram

Digitalis principally produces alterations in the S-T segment and the T wave. With early digitilisation there is a depression of the S-T segment in all leads in the opposite direction to the main deflection of the QRS complex. As digitalis therapy proceeds, first the T wave becomes reduced in amplitude and then the S-T segment swings above or below the base line in the opposite direction to the T wave. The result is an ECG with a typical "cupping" effect (Fig. 27).

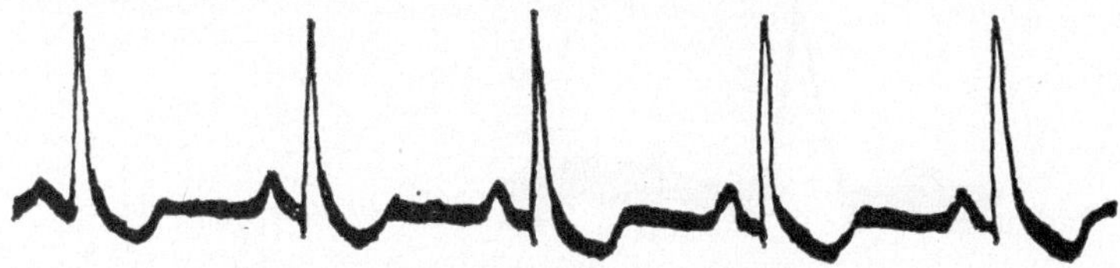

19/FIG. 27.—Effect of digitalis. Note that S–T segment is depressed and "cupping" is present. There is a low voltage T wave.

These changes can be observed within a few minutes of an intravenous dose of digoxin during anaesthesia. Overdigitilisation affects not only the rate and the rhythm of the heart by means of vagal stimulation and a direct depressant action on the conductive system, but it is capable of reproducing every known type of arrhythmia and heart block. The effects of digitalis therapy can still be observed in many cases some 2–3 weeks after cessation of therapy and they are exaggerated in the presence of a low serum potassium.

Quinidine tends to depress the electrical activity of the heart. The P wave and the QRS are increased in duration. The S wave widens and the T wave is lowered and widened (Fig. 28). In excessive dosage all types of cardiac irregularities may be observed.

Adrenergic drugs, adrenaline, ephedrine, etc. lower the amplitude of T waves and may reverse their direction. Cholinergic drugs may have the same effect.

Amyl nitrite produces marked tachycardia and reversal of the direction of the T wave.

Effects of Anaesthesia and Operation upon the Electrocardiogram

Excluding the direct stimulation of the heart by the surgeon, the main causes of a disordered rhythm during anaesthesia are the inherent toxicity of the agents used, changes in electrolyte balance, and faulty anaesthetic technique. The effects of individual anaesthetic drugs are described elsewhere in this book. The role of carbon dioxide retention and hypoxia in increasing the incidence of cardiac arrhythmia—presumably by a direct action upon the myocardium—is now so well known as to need little comment. Their importance, and the dangers of dogmatising on the part played by reflex stimulation in arrhythmia production, are illustrated by the electrocardiographic study of endotracheal intubation. This has shown, in man, that during intubation numerous ectopic beats can be recorded. Some authorities believe that this arrhythmia is due to the stimulation of vagal afferents in the trachea, whereas others consider that

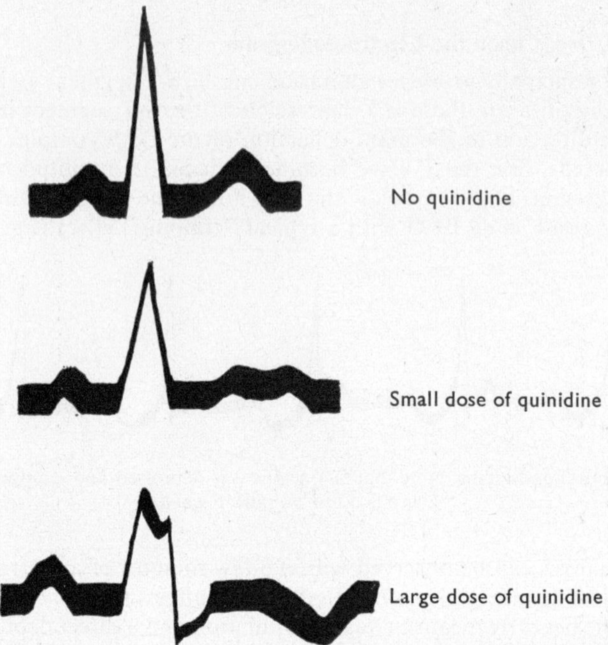

19/FIG. 28.—Effect of quinidine. Changes produced in the ECG with varying doses.

it is due to hypoxia and carbon dioxide retention and can always be abolished by adequate ventilation (Johnstone, 1955). In fact, intubation under light anaesthesia with inadequate muscular relaxation is a common cause of cardiac arrhythmia, whereas with a barbiturate induction, complete paralysis with suxamethonium and adequate ventilation it does not affect the rhythm.

A reduction in tidal volume, such as may occur during thiopentone, nitrous oxide and oxygen anaesthesia, can lead to a decrease in the voltage of the T wave and S-T segment depression, but both disturbances disappear when ventilation is improved.

Abnormal Pulse Rhythms during Anaesthesia

Sinus arrhythmia is a common and apparently normal phenomenon of the conscious state which generally disappears during anaesthesia. It is due to variations in vagal tone in relation to respiration so that the pulse slows on expiration and quickens again on inspiration.

Pulsus paradoxus is concerned with differences in the volume of the beat rather than the rate. It is nearly the converse of sinus arrhythmia in that the radial pulse becomes very weak or absent during inspiration and recovers its volume again on expiration. It may be produced by over-enthusiastic intermittent positive pressure respiration!

Pulsus alternans consists of a strong beat followed by a weak beat, the interval between the beats being equal in contrast to pulsus bigeminus. It can be induced by speeding up the rate of the heart and is commonly felt during paroxysmal tachycardia and atrial flutter. It is better detected by auscultation than by palpation of the pulse; during measurement of the systolic blood pressure, as the pressure of the occluding cuff drops, so, at first, only the strong beats are heard; later, when the pressure reaches a lower level, the pulse rate suddenly appears to double as the weak beats are heard for the first time. Slowing the heart rate abolishes pulsus alternans.

Pulsus bigeminus, or "coupling" of two beats, is usually due to the presence of a ventricular ectopic beat immediately after each normal beat. The ectopic beat blocks the next normal one so that there is a pause after each couple of beats. This can, however, be imitated by a weak ectopic heart beat following two normal beats: in this case the extrasystole is not strong enough to produce a propagated impulse at the wrist but—because of the refractory period—prevents the next normal heart beat arising.

Pulsus trigeminus is similar to coupling but three beats, rather than two, are followed by a pause.

Prevention of Arrhythmias under Anaesthesia (see also p. 665 *et seq.*)

The onset of arrhythmias during anaesthesia should always first raise the suspicion of an increased carbon dioxide level of the blood or of the effect of the anaesthetic agent. When both these factors can be excluded, specific treatment may occasionally be required for an intractable arrhythmia. Lignocaine may be given intravenously as a 1 per cent solution (1 mg./kg. body weight). If the arrhythmia is thought to be due to circulating catecholamines a receptor blocking agent can be tried, but its action is partically dependent on a local analgesic action similar to that of lignocaine; moreover there is a real danger of acute hypotension when such agents are used during anaesthesia. Recently an agent has been introduced which is said to have a specific receptor blocking action and to be free of any quinidine-like activity. This agent —"Practalol" (ICI 50, 172)—is claimed to be safe (Macdonald and McNeill, 1968; Shinebourne *et al.*, 1968).

Anaesthesia and Heart Block

Though a patient with Stokes-Adams attacks or incomplete heart block rarely requires general anaesthesia, the various effects of these agents in such circumstances have been reviewed (Ross, 1962). Chandler and Clapper (1959) have emphasised the value of the use of isoprenaline sulphate. This drug can be used intravenously in a dose of 0·01–0·025 mg. (made up in a 1:20,000 solution) to raise the pulse rate (Zoll *et al.*, 1958). However, it may cause hypotension. (See also Chapter 24).

THE CARDIAC GLYCOSIDES

Digitalis

In 1775 Withering found that extracts of the foxglove flower (digitalis purpurea) had a powerful diuretic and cardiac action. The active principle in this extract consisted of three glycosides—digitoxin, gitalin and gitoxin. Other active glycosides are digoxin, derived from *digitalis lanata*, and G-strophanthin (ouabain) from the seeds of *strophanthus gratus*.

The overall effect of digitalis on the *normal* human heart is controversial, but the majority believe that the output is either unchanged or diminished. The fall in output is explained on the basis that the heart is decreased below its optimal size by the direct myocardial action of the drug. This led some workers to suggest that digitalis was contra-indicated in heart failure with normal rhythm, but in actual fact the output in these cases is increased by digitalis.

The improvement in cardiac output in the presence of failure is achieved by increasing the force of contraction of the myocardium, whereas the other effects—namely, diminution in size of the heart and a reduction in the venous pressure, are a direct result of this improved contractility. Thus, when digitalis increases the contractile strength of a failing myocardium, the ventricle is able to empty more completely and consequently the diastolic filling is also improved. This, in turn, allows the atrium to cope efficiently with more blood so that the venous return improves and the venous pressure falls. As compensation is restored, so the heart rate slows. Animal experiments have shown that the oxygen consumption of the failing heart is greater than that of the same heart under the influence of digitalis (Peters and Visscher, 1936), suggesting that digitalis not only increases the force of contraction but also the mechanical efficiency of the myocardium.

Digitalis acts on the vagus, the pacemaker, the conducting tissue and the muscle of the ventricular wall. There has been a great deal of controversy over the exact mechanism of its action, but it is now generally believed that, except when large doses are used, the cardiac slowing of digitalis is due to a reflex vagal effect consequent upon the improved circulation. In large doses, however, it stimulates vagal activity directly. It depresses the conductivity of the A-V node and the bundle of His so that the electrocardioscope shows a prolongation of the P-R interval, and, in large doses, it leads to the signs of an atrioventricular block. Finally, it has a direct action on the ventricular muscle fibres, rendering them less sensitive to any impulses which manage to pass through the bundle of His.

Digitalis and atrial fibrillation.—The depression of conductivity of the A-V node and the bundle of His is particularly beneficial in this condition. The atria are contracting about 400 times per minute and as the A-V bundle cannot conduct more than 280 impulses a minute some degree of heart block must be present. Digitalis increases this block by slowing the conduction time in the A-V node and the bundle of His; this permits the ventricular rate to slow, the circulation improves, and then reflex vagal effects caused by this improvement slow the conduction of impulses through the bundle still further. Nevertheless, it is important to remember that the increase in the refractory period of the A-V muscle is not the primary cause of improvement if any degree of heart failure is present. In this case, the increase in the contractile force and mechanical efficiency of the myocardium, together with a reduction in ventricular excitability, is the chief cause of improvement. Early cases of atrial fibrillation can be treated by R-wave, triggered D.C. countershock under general anaesthesia.

Digitalis and atrial flutter.—A large dose of digitalis will increase the rate of the contracting atria during flutter, thus reducing the refractory period and converting the rhythm to fibrillation. It also depresses A-V conduction so that the partial block will permit the ventricle to beat more slowly. On withdrawal of the digitalis the heart sometimes returns to normal rhythm.

Summary of actions on the myocardium:

1. Improves contractile force of the myocardium.
2. Increases vagal stimulation—reflexly in small doses and directly in high doses.
3. Diminishes the conductivity of the A-V node and bundle of His.

Other actions of digitalis.—The glycoside has an action on the peripheral circulation as well as on the heart itself. It is believed to produce contraction of arteriolar smooth muscle and thus increase the peripheral vascular resistance (Ross *et al.*, 1960*a* and *b*). Furthermore, Braunwald and his colleagues (1961) administered digitalis preparations to patients on cardiopulmonary bypass and found that digitalis augmented the contractile force of the non-failing human heart and also constricted the systemic vascular bed. Other workers have failed to find any adverse effect of digitalis on the cardiac output or peripheral circulation in normal subjects (Selzer *et al.*, 1959).

The response of the human heart in failure is diminished in the presence of hypothermia (Szekely and Wynne, 1960).

Electrocardioscope changes during digitalis therapy.—See p. 577.

Anaesthesia and digitalis therapy.—See Chapter 24.

Administration.—The tinctures of digitalis are now rarely prescribed because the tablets are more stable and more convenient. Digoxin has the advantage over digitalis in that it is easier to assay; it is prepared from *digitalis lanata* and has uniform potency and absolute purity. It also is more rapidly absorbed from the gastro-intestinal tract.

The method used to bring about digitalisation depends largely upon the urgency of the treatment; thus it can be divided into rapid and slow methods.

(a) *Rapid method*

Digoxin—1 mg. intravenously for the average 70 kg. (11 stone) adult. The effect should be noticed as a slowing of the cardiac rate within ten minutes. Intravenous digoxin should not be used if the patient has been treated with digitalis in any form during the previous ten days because of its cumulative qualities.

(b) *Slow method*

1. Digoxin tablets—1·5 mg. by mouth followed by 0·5 mg. 6-hourly. The effect should be noticeable after the first six hours.

2. Digitalis tablets—200 mg. t.d.s. 1st day
150 mg. t.d.s. 2nd day
then 60 mg. t.d.s. until the heart rate is controlled.

Contra-indications

Digitalis therapy is valueless and, due to the increased irritability of the myocardium that it causes, may actually prove harmful in the following conditions—uncomplicated sinus tachycardia, peripheral circulatory failure in the presence of a normal myocardium, heart block without failure, ventricular tachycardia or fibrillation, and constrictive pericarditis.

Signs of toxicity.—One of the earliest signs of digitalis poisoning is loss of appetite, followed by headache, nausea and vomiting. Occasionally diarrhoea and blurring of vision may occur. Amongst the principal signs of the effectiveness of the treatment is a slowing of the pulse, but if this reaches a rate of 60 or less then the dose of digitalis should be reduced. The onset of ventricular extra-systoles and coupled beats is a danger sign that calls for stopping therapy for at least twenty-four hours. If treatment is continued there is a risk that the patient may suddenly develop ventricular tachycardia which may go on to fibrillation.

Ouabain

Ouabain has a similar action to digitalis on the myocardium, but since its absorption from the bowel is erratic it must be used intravenously. Since it has a rapid action Horton and Davison (1955) recommend it for the supplementary treatment of shock, when the response to intravenous fluid therapy is poor. The intravenous dose is 0·25–0·5 mg.

Quinidine

Quinidine acts upon the myocardium in a complicated manner and the final result is due to a composite effect, namely:

(a) It acts directly on the atrial and ventricular muscle, lengthening the refractory period and slowing transmission. This prolongation of the refractory period may be as much as 100 per cent.

(b) It depresses conduction in the A-V node and the bundle of His.

These actions tend to slow the rate of the heart and quinidine may be used as a preventive measure after D.C. conversion of atrial fibrillation.

The effect of quinidine upon the rate of the heart is interesting, because often it causes a quickening instead of a slowing. This again is due to its multiple actions, for not only does it depress A-V conduction, tending to slow the heart rate, but its action of diminishing vagal tone tends automatically to increase the rate. Furthermore, the action of slowing atrial transmission also tends to speed A-V conduction so that on some occasions the other actions of quinidine may overrule its direct junctional tissue depression and bring about increased conductivity with a rise in the pulse rate.

ECG Changes with Quinidine.—See p. 577.

Administration.—Occasionally a patient has an idiosyncrasy to quinidine which shows itself by nausea, vomiting, and sometimes circulatory collapse. Thus a test dose of 0·2 g. repeated once again after two hours is advisable. The maintenance dosage is from 0·2–0·4 g. daily.

The signs of toxicity are headache, tinnitus, blurring of vision, nausea, vomiting and diarrhoea.

REFERENCES

BERNE, R. M. (1954). The effect of immersion hypothermia on coronary blood flow. *Circulat. Res.*, **2,** 236.

BERNE, R. M. (1958). Effect of epinephrine and norepinephrine on coronary circulation. *Circulat. Res.*, **6,** 664.

BRANTHWAITE, M. A., and BRADLEY, R. D. (1968). Measurement of cardiac output by thermal dilution in man. *J. appl. Physiol.*, **24,** 434.

BRAUNWALD, E., BLOODWELL, R. D., GOLDBERG, L. I., and MORROW, A. G. (1961). Studies on digitalis. IV. Observations in man on the effects of digitalis preparations on the contractility of the non-failing heart and on total vascular resistance. *J. clin. Invest.*, **40,** 52.

CHANDLER, D., and CLAPPER, M. I. (1959). Complete atrioventricular block treated with isoproterenol hydrochloride. *Amer. J. Cardiol.*, **3,** 336.

ECKENHOFF, J. E., HAFKENSCHIEL, J. H., and LANDMESSER, C. M. (1947). The oxygen metabolism of the dog's heart. *Amer. J. med. Sci.*, **213,** 123.

ETSTEN, B., and LI, T. H. (1962). Current concepts of myocardial function during anaesthesia. *Brit. J. Anaesth.*, **34,** 884.

GOLDBERGER, E. (1953). *Unipolar Lead Electrocardiography and Vector Cardiography*, 3rd edit. Philadelphia: Lea & Febiger.

GUYTON, A. C. (1963). *Handbook of Physiology*, ii, **2,** 1125. Washington: Amer. Physiol. Soc.

HAMER, J., EMANUEL, R., NORMAN, J., and BURGESS, M. (1966). Use of a computer in the calibration of dye dilutation curves by a dynamic method. *Brit. Heart J.*, **28,** 147.

HAMILTON, W. F., MOORE, J. W., KINSMAN, J. M., and SPURLING, R. G. (1932). Studies on circulation; further analysis of the injection method, and of changes in hemodynamics under physiological and pathological conditions. *Amer. J. Physiol.*, **99,** 534.

HORTON, J. A. G., and DAVISON, M. H. A. (1955). Ouabain in the treatment of shock. *Brit. J. Anaesth.*, **27,** 139.

JOHNSTONE, M. (1955). Relaxants and the human cardiovascular system. *Anaesthesia*, **10,** 122.

JONES, R. E., GULDMANN, N., LINDE, H. W., DRIPPS, R. D., and PRICE, H. L. (1960). Cyclopropane anaesthesia. III. Effects of cyclopropane on respiration and circulation in normal man. *Anesthesiology*, **21,** 380.

LI, T. H., and ETSTEN, B. (1957). Effect of cyclopropane anesthesia on cardiac output and related hemodynamics in man. *Anesthesiology*, **18,** 15.

MACDONALD, A. G., and MCNEILL, R. S. (1968). A comparison of the effect upon airway resistance of ICI 50, 172 and propranalol. *Brit. J. Anaesth.*, **40,** 508.

MCMILLAN, I. K. R., CASE, R. B., STAINSBY, W. N., and WELCH, G. H. (1957). The hypothermic heart. *Thorax*, **12,** 208.

NUNN, J. F., and POULIOT, J. C. (1962). The measurement of gaseous exchange during nitrous oxide anaesthesia. *Brit. J. Anaesth.*, **34,** 752.

OSBORN, J. J. (1953). Experimental hypothermia: respiratory and blood pH changes in relation to cardiac function. *Amer. J. Physiol.*, **175,** 389.

PETERS, H. C., and VISSCHER, M. B. (1936). Energy metabolism of heart failure and the influence of drugs upon it. *Amer. Heart J.*, **11,** 273.

PRICE, H. L. (1960). General anesthesia and circulatory hemostasis. *Physiol. Rev.*, **40,** 187.

PRICE, H. L., LINDE, H. W., JONES, R. E., BLACK, G. W., and PRICE, M. L. (1959). Sympatho-adrenal responses to general anesthesia in man and their relation to hemodynamics. *Anesthesiology*, **20,** 563.

Primrose, W. B. (1954). The venous return. Physiological considerations related to heart failure during anaesthesia. *Brit. J. Anaesth.*, **26,** 100.

Prinzmetal, M., Oblath, R., Corday, E., Brill, I. C., Kruger, H. E., Smith, L. A., Fields, J., Kennamer, R., and Osborne, J. A. (1951). Auricular fibrillation. *J. Amer. med. Ass.*, **146,** 1275.

Ross, E. D. T. (1962). General anaesthesia in complete heart block. *Brit. J. Anaesth.*, **34,** 102.

Ross, J., Waldhausen, J. A., and Braunwald, E. (1960*a*). Studies on digitalis. I. Direct effects on peripheral vascular resistance. *J. clin. Invest.*, **39,** 930.

Ross, J., Waldhausen, J. A., and Braunwald, E. (1960*b*). Studies on digitalis. II. Extracardiac effects on venous return and capacity of the peripheral vascular tree. *J. clin. Invest.*, **39,** 937.

Sarnoff, S. J. (1960). Certain aspects of the role of catecholamines in circulatory regulation. *Amer. J. Cardiol.*, **5,** 579.

Selzer, A., Hultgren, H. N., Ebnother, C. L., Bradley, H. W., and Olstone, A. (1959). Effect of digoxin on the circulation in normal man. *Brit. Heart J.*, **21,** 335.

Shackman, R., Graber, G. I., and Redwood, C. (1951). Oxygen consumption and anaesthesia. *Clin. Sci.*, **10,** 219.

Shinebourne, E., Fleming, J., and Hamer, J. (1968). Haemodynamic responses to exercise in hypertension: place of sympathetic system evaluated by I.C.I. 50, 172. *Cardiovasc. Res.*, **4,** 379.

Szekely, P., and Wynne, N. A. (1960). The effects of digitalis on the hypothermic heart. *Brit. Heart J.*, **22,** 647.

Warner, H. R. (1968). Experiences with computer-based monitoring. *Curr. Res. Anesth.*, **47,** 453.

Zoll, P. M., Linenthal, A. J., Gibson, W., Paul, M. H., and Norman, L. R. (1958). Intravenous therapy of Stokes-Adams disease. *Circulation*, **17,** 325.

Chapter 20

THE PERIPHERAL CIRCULATION AND THE AUTONOMIC NERVOUS SYSTEM

CIRCULATORY efficiency depends as much on the integrity of the peripheral vasculature as it does upon the performance of the heart.

Arterial System

This is the resistive element in the circulation, most of the peripheral resistance resulting from tone in muscular arteries and arterioles. The other important factor is blood viscosity which is largely a reflection of the haematocrit.

Selective constriction and dilatation of appropriate arteries is responsible for distributing the cardiac output according to tissue requirements. Under resting conditions, approximately 50 per cent of the cardiac output flows to the kidneys and viscera whereas on exercise, the enormous increase in muscle blood flow is supplied not only by an increase in cardiac output but also by redistribution of blood flow away from the viscera. Minor degrees of readjustment can be achieved by varying local vascular tone so that overall resistance and flow do not change.

Arteriolar constriction is also one of the mechanisms available for the support of arterial blood pressure in the face of a falling cardiac output, but as will be shown later venoconstriction is a more important homeostatic mechanism, at least in the early stages of circulatory impairment. In this context, it is highly relevant that the arterial side of the circulation only contains about 15 per cent of the total blood volume.

The Capillaries

It is at the level of these smallest vessels that metabolic exchange occurs between blood and tisues, but the overall capacity of the capillary bed is so large that were all capillaries to be open simultaneously, blood would accumulate in the tissues and the circulation would soon fail. Flow into the capillaries is controlled by pre- and post-capillary sphincters. When these are constricted, blood flow by-passes the capillary bed and flows instead through short wide arterio-venous channels. It is possible that circulatory failure becomes "irreversible" when the tone of the pre-capillary sphincter is lost while the post-capillary sphincter remains constricted so that stagnant blood accumulates in the anoxic, leaking capillary bed (Lillehei *et al.*, 1964).

Unlike arteries and veins where tone is primarily controlled by the autonomic nervous system, local physical and chemical agents are predominantly responsible for the regulation of tone in the micro-vasculature. Metabolic activity and local heating cause dilatation whereas cold initially causes constriction, with extreme or maintained cold producing vascular paralysis. The effects of anaesthetics have been investigated by microscopic examination of accessible vascular beds e.g. mesentery (Baez, 1964). Light anaesthesia with ether, cyclopropane or halothane causes an increase in spontaneous periodic contraction (vasomotion) and increased reactivity to topically applied adrenaline whereas deep anaesthesia with these agents, and methoxyflurane at any concentration, depress both vasomotion and reactivity to adrenaline. Although a variety of physiological and biochemical changes are produced by anaesthesia which could themselves affect the microvasculature, at least some of the observed response is due to the direct action of the agents studied.

The Venous System

Under normal conditions 65–70 per cent of the blood volume is contained within the veins which therefore act as a capacitance or reservoir system. The compliance of this system is determined by venomotor tone, which, like arterial tone, is controlled by autonomic impulses from the vasomotor centre in the floor of the fourth ventricle.

The effects of sympathetic stimulation on the peripheral vascular bed were studied experimentally by Mellander (1960). He showed that sympathetic stimulation causes a rapid decrease in limb blood flow due to arteriolar constriction together with an equally rapid fall in limb volume due to contraction of the capacitance vessels (veins). Subsequently a further diminution in limb volume occurred more slowly; this was attributed to the slow return of tissue fluid into capillaries in which the lowered hydrostatic pressure consequent upon arteriolar constriction was exceeded by intravascular osmotic pressure. Mellander also showed that throughout the range of frequency of sympathetic discharge known to occur naturally, the effect on the veins was always greater than the effect on resistance vessels when expressed in terms of their maximum capacity to constrict.

The relevance of an increase in venous tone can best be appreciated by considering the effects of haemorrhage on the circulation. In the absence of reflex compensatory mechanisms, a fall in blood volume will cause a reduction in cardiac filling and consequently a fall in cardiac output. However if as blood volume falls venous tone increases due to sypathetic stimulation, there will be a shift of blood into the right heart so that filling pressure and therefore cardiac output can be maintained, within the limits of venoconstrictor ability. In other words, a normal blood *flow* can be provided in spite of a diminution in blood *volume*. Only at maximal rates of sympathetic stimulation does arteriolar constriction help to maintain that easily measured, but often misleading parameter, the arterial blood pressure. Teleologically, arteriolar constriction is of value in maintaining a head of pressure for the perfusion of vital organs (head and heart) and there is undoubtedly evidence that a critical closing pressure exists below which blood flow ceases (Burton, 1951; Burton and Yamada, 1951). However there is also ample evidence that prolonged arteriolar constriction from any cause ultimately results in tissue damage, and may be responsible for the irreversible nature of extreme circulatory failure (Lillehei *et al.*, 1964; Nickerson, 1964).

In summary, it is the function of the circulation to provide an adequate flow of nutrients to the tissues and the heart is the motive force for this supply. The ability of the normal heart to discharge its function is determined by the adequacy of cardiac filling and the degree of sympathetic stimulation applied to the ventricles. Cardiac filling is determined by the volume of blood available in the venous reservoir, the degree of venous tone and the compliance of ventricular muscle.

Vasomotor reflexes

A number of factors can influence autonomic discharge from the vasomotor centre, either directly or by reflex action.

1. **Chemical stimuli.**—An increase in carbon dioxide tension produces peripheral vasoconstriction by stimulating the vasomotor centre, but vasodilatation by its direct action on the vessel walls. Anoxia can transiently stimulate the centre but soon leads to direct depression. Vasomotor stimulation is produced indirectly but much more powerfully by anoxic drive from the chemoreceptors.

2. **Cortical stimuli.**—Extreme emotion is commonly responsible for considerable changes in vasomotor activity; both stimulation and depression can be provoked in this way.

3. **Baroceptor reflexes.**—Pressure sensitive receptors are situated in the arterial system (aorta, carotid bifurcation and root of the right subclavian artery), in the atria and in the ventricles (Keele *et al.*, 1965).

The systemic arterial receptors are sensitive to pulse pressure and their maximum sensitivity to small changes exists when the mean arterial pressure is normal (Keele *et al.*, 1965). An increase in pulse pressure causes reflex vasodilatation and bradycardia, and the reverse occurs when the pulse pressure decreases.

Atrial and ventricular receptors discharge in response to an increase in pressure within that chamber and may be regarded as cardiac proprioceptors (Keele *et al.*, 1965). An increased discharge from any of these receptors produces qualitatively similar effects which are bradycardia, dilatation of both arteries and veins and an overall decrease in cardiac output; however in left ventricular failure Sharpey-Schafer (1961) found that venous tone is high and he attributed this to reflex venoconstriction secondary to a high atrial pressure. In addition the atrial receptors are thought to act as volume sensors, stimulation by atrial distension causing a diuresis by inhibiting the secretion of antidiuretic hormone (Gauer and Henry, 1963).

Vasomotor reflexes can be tested in man by performing the Valsalva manoeuvre—forced expiration against a resistance (Sharpey-Schafer, 1955). The effect of this is to decrease the effective filling pressure of the heart by reversing the gradient between intra- and extrathoracic pressures. In the normal subject a diminution in stroke output is produced which after about six seconds provokes reflex vasoconstriction and a tachycardia. This compensatory change is reflected in the arterial blood pressure tracing (Fig. 1). The drop in pulse pressure is arrested and the diastolic pressure may even rise if vasoconstriction is considerable. When the expiratory resistance is removed at the end of twelve seconds there is a sudden rise in effective filling pressure and consequently in stroke output. In the presence of persisting sympathetic stimulation provoked by the manoeuvre, this produces a large pulse pressure and an "overshoot" of blood pressure which in turn causes reflex bradycardia and vasodilatation, thus returning the circulation to its original state. If facilities for intra-arterial pressure recording are absent, a normal response may be recognised by the occurrence of a bradycardia almost immediately after the manoeuvre is completed. Professor Sharpey-Schafer taught that in heart failure a "square wave" response to the

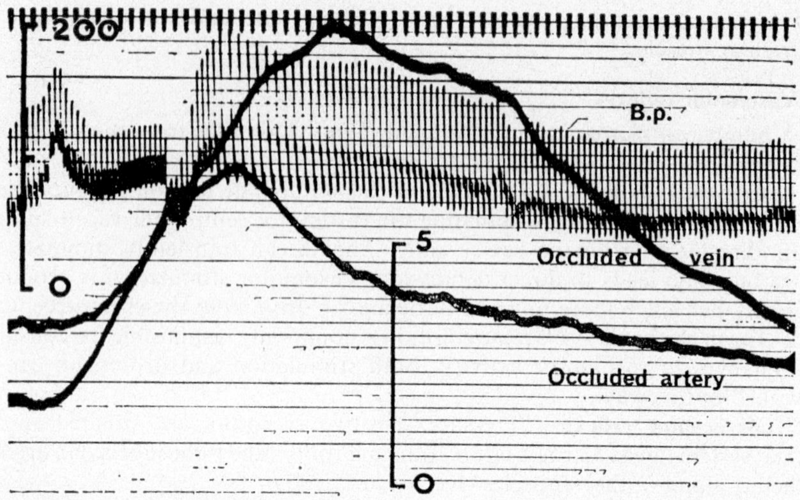

20/Fig. 1.—Effect of Valsalva Manoeuvre on Arterial and Venous Pressure.

Upper margin: time-scale (sec.)

Upper record (B.p.) is that of the arterial pressure in the left brachial artery and shows the usual changes with the Valsalva manoeuvre in a subject with a normal circulation.

The two curves are the right brachial artery pressure (occluded artery) and the right antecubital venous pressure (occluded vein). The limb has been cut off from the rest of the circulation by a high-pressure cuff on the upper arm, so that only nervous impulses can influence the vessels. The blood is stationary in the limb. After seven seconds of the Valsalva manoeuvre, reflex arterial and venous constriction is shown by the rise of pressure in both sets of vessels Reflex dilatation occurs after the overshoot.

Calibrations in mm. Hg.

Valsalva manoeuvre (Fig. 2) indicating no decrease in stroke output and therefore no compensatory changes, reflected the inability of the failing heart to respond to a change in effective filling pressure. However, it may be that the square wave response merely reflects an excessive central blood volume as it can be produced in normal subjects by rapid transfusion.

In the presence of vasomotor paralysis, reflex response to a fall in stroke output cannot occur (Barraclough and Sharpey-Schafer, 1963). In such patients, the Valsalva manoeuvre produces a progressive fall in pulse pressure and blood pressure, with a slow recovery and no overshoot when the expiratory resistance is withdrawn (Fig. 3). This abnormal response underlines the importance of providing the lowest possible intrathoracic pressure when using intermittent positive pressure ventilation in patients with vasomotor paralysis (Watson *et al.*, 1962). Some degree of impairment of vasomotor reflexes is probably produced at least temporarily by most anaesthetic agents although information on this subject is scanty.

THE AUTONOMIC NERVOUS SYSTEM

This is a predominantly motor system consisting of parasympathetic (craniosacral) and sympathetic (thoraco-lumbar) components which together control visceral function (Fig. 4). Both components contribute to the innervation of

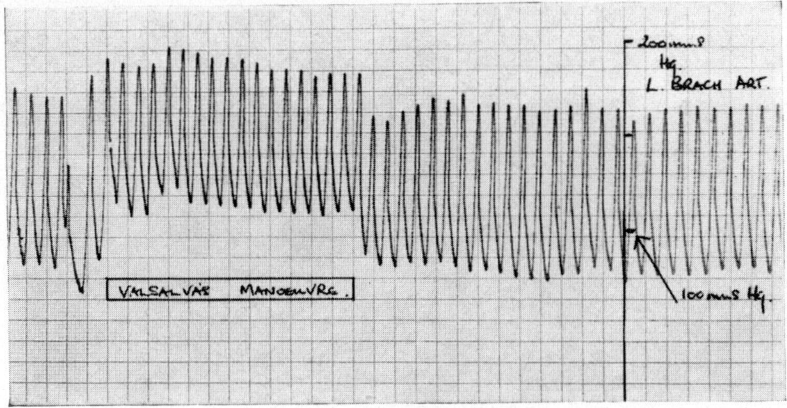

20/FIG. 2.—Square wave response to the Valsalva manoeuvre in a patient with left ventricular failure.

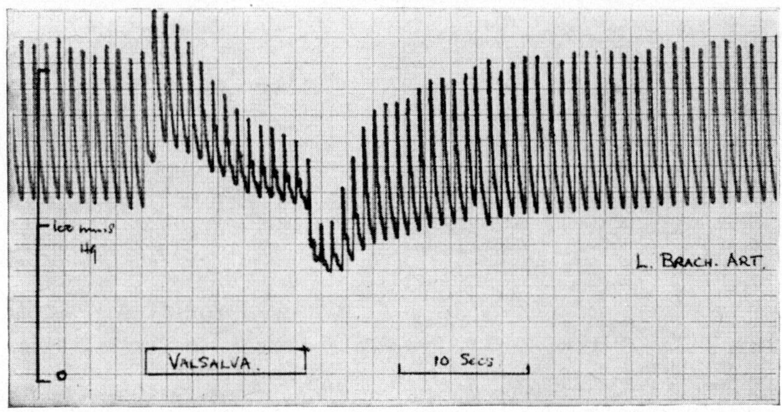

20/FIG. 3.—Effect of Valsalva manoeuvre in a patient with blocked circulatory reflexes.

each visceral system and the effects of parasympathetic and sympathetic stimulation on any one organ are generally opposite. Although the parasympathetic system is commonly regarded as cholinergic and the sympathetic system as adrenergic, there is now evidence of sympathetic cholinergic fibres (Roddie and Shepherd, 1963) and it may be that acetylcholine is responsible for the release of noradrenaline from the stores in the sympathetic nerve terminals (Burn, 1961).

During anaesthesia, the activity of the sympathetic system is of the greatest importance, particularly the effects of sympathetic stimulation or sympathomimetic drugs on the cardiovascular system. Other aspects of autonomic activity which require consideration are the control of secretions and the regulation of body temperature.

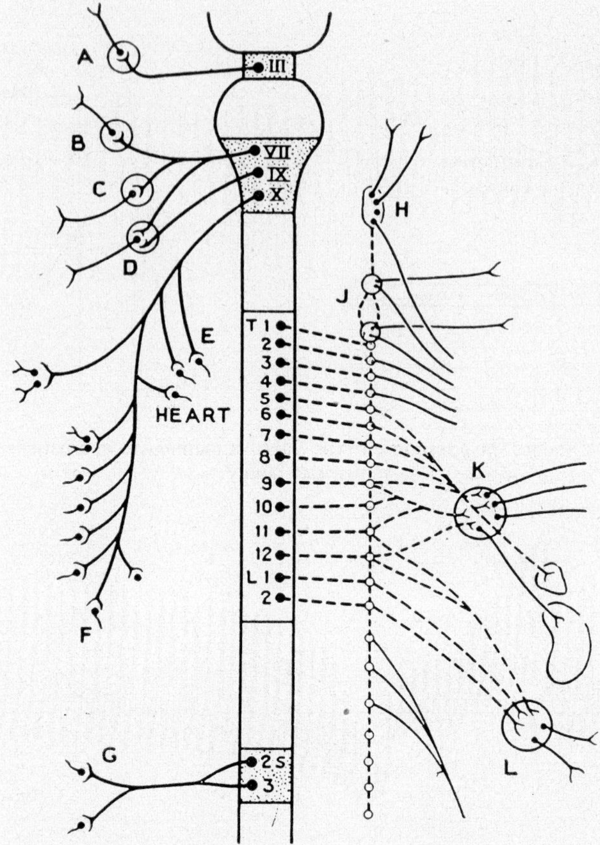

20/FIG. 4.—THE AUTONOMIC NERVOUS SYSTEM

On left: Cranial and sacral autonomic (parasympathetic) system. Thick lines from III, VII, IX, X, and S2, 3 are pre-ganglionic (connector fibres).

A—ciliary ganglion.
B—sphenopalatine ganglion.
C—submaxillary and sublingual ganglia.
D—otic ganglion.
E—Vagus excitor cells in nodes of heart.
F—Vagus excitor cells in wall of bowel.
G—sacral autonomic ganglion cells in pelvis. Thin lines beyond—post-ganglionic (excitor) fibres to organs.

On right: Sympathetic nervous system. Dotted lines from T 1–12, L 1, 2 are pre-ganglionic fibres.

H—superior cervical ganglion.
J—inferior cervical and 1st thoracic ganglia (stellate ganglion).
K—coeliac and other abdominal ganglia (note pre-ganglionic fibres directly supplying the adrenal medulla).
L—lower abdominal and pelvic sympathetic ganglia. Continuous lines beyond—post-ganglionic fibres.

Actions of Sympathomimetic Agents

The effects of sympathomimetic drugs are conveniently classified using Ahlquist's theory of alpha and beta adrenergic receptors (1948). Stimulation of alpha receptors causes vasoconstriction and mydriasis, whereas beta effects are vasodilatation, bronchial relaxation and myocardial stimulation (increased rate, contractility and excitability, and facilitation of atrioventricular conduction).

Venoconstriction is a feature of both alpha and beta stimulation (Shepherd, 1966).

The mechanism by which these effects are mediated may be either direct action on the receptor or indirectly by the liberation of noradrenaline from stores within the adrenergic nerve terminals; some drugs produce their effect both directly and indirectly (Schmidt and Fleming, 1963).

An appropriate choice of sympathomimetic drug can only be made by careful consideration of circumstance. It is inappropriate to choose an indirectly-acting drug to correct hypotension in a patient treated with reserpine which depletes tissue stores of noradrenaline. Similarly, hypotension following sympathetic blockade requires (if treatment is needed at all) an increase in blood volume or a peripheral vasoconstrictor, whereas hypotension and bradycardia following myocardial injury are more logically treated with a drug which improves cardiac output.

Table 1 lists the structure, mode of action and effects of the commonly used sympathomimetic agents.

20/Table 1

Structure, Action and Effects of Sympathomimetic Agents

	5 6 4 1—C—C--N 3 2				*Direct or Indirect Stimulation*	*Alpha Action*	*Beta Action*
Adrenaline	3—OH 4—OH	CHOH	CH_2	$NHCH_3$	Direct	+++	+++
Noradrenaline	3—OH 4—OH	CHOH	CH_2	NH_2	Direct	+++	+
Metaraminol	3—OH	CHOH	$CHCH_3$	NH_2	Both	+++	+
Isoprenaline	3—OH 4—OH	CHOH	CH_2	$NHCH(CH_3)_2$	Direct	−	+++
Ephedrine		CHOH	$CHCH_3$	$NHCH_3$	Both	+	++
Amphetamine		CH_2	$CHCH_3$	NH_2	Indirect	+	++
Methylamphetamine		CH_2	$CHCH_3$	$NHCN_3$	Indirect	+	++
Mephentermine		CH_2	$C(CH_3)_2$	$NHCH_3$	Indirect	++	+
Phenylephrine	3—OH	CHOH	CH_2	$NHCH_3$	Direct	+++	−
Methoxamine	2,5—OCH_3	CHOH	$CHCH_3$	NH_2	Mainly Direct	+++	−

Adrenaline is released endogenously from the adrenal medulla by a variety of stimuli including fear, anger, anoxia, hypercarbia and hypotension. Therapeutically it is used as a myocardial stimulant (particularly in the treatment of cardiac arrest), as a bronchodilator and to relieve anaphylactic reactions. It is an effective vasoconstrictor when infiltrated into skin and subcutaneous tissues although there is a dangerous incidence of arrhythmias if the infiltration is carried out in the presence of certain anaesthetic agents, e.g. cyclopropane or halothane.

Noradrenaline is released in small quantities from the adrenal medulla and is also the physiological transmitter at sympathetic nerve endings. It is a powerful vasoconstrictor with some inotropic action on the heart but reflex bradycardia prevents any increase in cardiac output. Prolonged infusion can cause such intense peripheral vasoconstriction that gangrene or organ damage may result.

Metaraminol ("Aramine") is similar in action to noradrenaline although less potent, longer-lasting and less liable to cause tissue damage due to excessive vasoconstriction.

Isoprenaline is a powerful beta-receptor stimulant. It raises cardiac output by increasing both stroke output and heart rate, lowers systemic vascular resistance and is an effective bronchodilator.

Methylamphetamine ("Methedrine") is a popular vasopressor producing both vasoconstriction and an increase in cardiac output. In spite of the increase in systemic vascular resistance, renal blood flow is increased. Methylamphetamine is a powerful cerebral stimulant.

Mephentermine ("Mephine") is pharmacologically similar to methylamphetamine although it is not a cerebral stimulant.

Phenylephrine ("Neosynephrine") is an effective vasopressor with no inotropic action on the myocardium. Myocardial irritability is not increased and there is no cerebral stimulation.

Methoxamine ("Vasoxyl") is similar in action to phenylephrine.

Pre-existing pathology or previous therapy can alter individual responses to these drugs and the net effect on the circulation of those which have both alpha and beta actions may vary with the dose (Laurence, 1966) or may be modified by reflexes invoked by changes in blood pressure (Aviado, 1959).

Two additional vasoconstrictor drugs deserve mention.

Angiotensin is a naturally occuring substance which causes constriction of peripheral arteries and arterioles, including cerebral and coronary vessels, but has little effect on venous tone (Gross *et al.*, 1965). There is no myocardial stimulation, in fact cardiac output and heart rate fall reflexly secondary to the rise in blood pressure. The drug is effective even when the vessels are refractory to noradrenaline.

Vasopressin only has cardiovascular effects in pharmacological as distinct from physiological doses. Systemic vascular resistance increases due to vasoconstriction (which includes the coronary vessels) and cardiac output and heart rate fall.

Adrenergic Antagonists

It is customary to restrict this term to drugs which block the adrenergic transmitter at the nerve endings, and the group is further subdivided into alpha and beta adrenergic blocking agents. The chief alpha adrenergic blocking drugs are tolazoline, phentolamine and phenoxybenzamine, the first two being short-acting and the latter of long duration.

Tolazoline ("Priscol") is used as a peripheral vasodilator although it produces greater increase in skin than in muscle blood flow. In addition to its alpha-blocking action, it is a direct vasodilator and also increases heart rate, gastro-intestinal motility and gastric acid secretion.

Phentolamine ("Rogitine") is chemically and pharmacologically very similar to tolazoline but is unreliable when used orally.

Phenoxybenzamine ("Dibenzyline") requires conversion in the body before it is effective and is therefore slow in onset. The effect may last up to two days or more and can be difficult to reverse with noradrenaline although angiotensin will produce vasoconstriction if required.

Although these are the drugs used specifically to achieve alpha-blockade, it is important to appreciate that the same lack of vasomotor control characterises patients whose circulatory reflexes are impaired by disease or therapy interfering with the sympathetic nervous system at other levels. The hazards of anaesthesia in patients on hypotensive therapy were described by Crandell (1962), but equally important are the risks of suddenly witholding this therapy. In all patients whose circulatory reflexes are impaired, particular attention must be paid to posture and the maintenance of blood volume. If controlled ventilation is required, a low mean intrathoracic pressure is essential and a negative expiratory pressure may therefore be of value. It is also probably wise to avoid anaesthetic agents which commonly produce hypotension as this effect may be enhanced.

Propranolol ("Inderal") is the principal beta-blocking agent available at present.

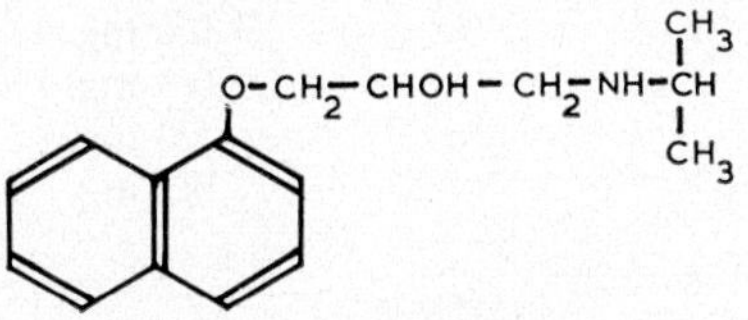

$$O{-}CH_2{-}CHOH{-}CH_2{-}NH{-}CH(CH_3)_2$$

It can be used to control cardiac arrhythmias including those occurring during anaesthesia (Payne and Sinfield, 1964), but its use may occasionally precipitate circulatory failure in patients who are relying on sympathetic stimulation to achieve adequate myocardial performance. Selective beta-blocking agents which decrease irritability without impairing contractility are currently under investigation (see Chapter 24, p. 666).

Adrenergic drugs and their antagonists are fully reviewed in a Symposium (1966) published in the *British Journal of Anaesthesia.*

ANTI-SIALOGOGUE DRUGS

The value of arresting or diminishing salivary secretions during anaesthesia is frequently questioned (Holt, 1962) and there is no doubt that an anaesthetic sequence involving no irritant inhalational agent and no intra-oral instrumentation rarely causes excessive salivation. The use of atropine-like drugs may merely submit the patient to the discomfort of a dry mouth, unpleasant tachycardia and tacky bronchial secretions which are difficult to expectorate. In conventional premedicant doses, atropine does not fully block vagal activity so that it is difficult to justify the claim that it protects the heart against reflexly-induced arrhythmias. However, instrumentation is commonly needed, albeit only an oral airway, and anti-sialogogues are therefore generally given. Scopolamine has the additional advantages of sedation and a powerful antiemetic effect, although it may cause confusion and restlessness in the aged or very young in whom it is better avoided.

Assessment of Anti-Sialogogue Drugs

In 1953 Mushin *et al.* investigated the effects of atropine sulphate and atropine mucate using lemon juice to provoke salivary secretion. They found that 0·65 mg. atropine sulphate produces 50 per cent depression of salivary activity with the maximum effect reached one hour after subcutaneous injection but only persisting for a further 30 minutes; atropine mucate was found to last slightly longer.

Wyant and Dobkin (1958) used the response to an intravenous injection of a carbachol-adrenaline solution to assess the anti-sialogogue activity of a number of drugs. Some of their results are reproduced in Table 2.

20/TABLE 2

ACTIVITY OF ANTI-SIALOGOGUE DRUGS

	Dose	*Percentage drying effect*
Atropine sulphate	0·6 mg.	96·0 per cent
l-Hyoscyamine	0·3 mg.	99·5 per cent
Methantheline bromide	5·0 mg.	95·0 per cent
l-Hyoscine (scopolamine)	0·2 mg.	97·0 per cent

Despite the multiplicity of anti-sialogogue drugs available, atropine sulphate and scopolamine remain the most popular. The choice is largely determined by the age and condition of the patient; for intravenous use immediately prior to induction of anaesthesia atropine sulphate is most commonly used.

TEMPERATURE REGULATION AND SWEATING

Normal body temperature is controlled by the balance between heat production and heat loss and there is now evidence for man as well as animals that there are two regulating systems (Cranston, 1966).

The first is a reflex system activated from skin receptors. If the circulation to an arm is occluded and the limb then immersed in cold water, reflex vasoconstriction occurs immediately in the opposite limb and may diminish heat loss sufficiently to cause a recordable increase in oral temperature.

There is also a hypothalamic centre which responds to local changes in blood temperature. A rise of 0·4° C will produce skin vasodilatation, sweating and increased respiration, whereas cooling causes vasoconstriction and shivering. It is possible that noradrenaline or 5-hydroxytryptamine play some part in the hypothalamic control system, although this is equivocal. During fever, body temperature is regulated as precisely as in health but at a higher level.

In the conscious subject sweating occurs when an increase in heat loss is required to maintain a normal body temperature, but it can also be provoked by emotional stimuli, asphyxia and anoxia. The sweat glands are innervated by cholinergic fibres of the sympathetic system, and sweating in these circumstances may merely reflect increased sympathetic activity.

The anaesthetised patient tends to become poikilothermic because of central depression and loss of vascular control. The body temperature therefore is less accurately controlled and tends to drift according to environmental conditions. Most commonly cooling occurs, particularly in small children and when a visceral cavity is opened. However a hot environment, theatre lighting, rubber sheeting and heavy drapes may combine to cause an increase in body temperature, and unless central depression is profound this will provoke sweating. Visceral stimulation also appears to cause sweating in some subjects, particularly if lightly anaesthetised. This is commonly accepted as an indication for increased analgesia or a greater depth of anaesthesia. Sweating during anaesthesia may also indicate anoxia or hypercarbia; during induction, it may be due to emotional stimuli or to increased muscular activity.

Recently a number of cases of extreme hyperpyrexia during general anaesthesia have been described (*Brit. med. J.*, 1968; Harrison *et al.*, 1968). A rapid rise in temperature is associated with tachycardia, cyanosis or flushing, hyperventilation and often abnormal muscular rigidity. Gross metabolic and respiratory acidosis is commonly present and in spite of attempts to control the temperature, cerebral oedema and irreversible circulatory failure develop. This condition is discussed in some detail in Chapter 33.

REFERENCES

AHLQUIST, R. P. (1948). A study of the adrenotropic receptors. *Amer. J. Physiol.*, **153,** 586.

AVIADO, D. M. (1959). Cardiovascular effects of some commonly used pressor amines. *Anesthesiology*, **20,** 71.

BAEZ, S. (1964). Anaesthetics on the Microcirculation. In: *Effects of Anaesthetics on the Circulation.* Eds. Price, H. L. and Cohen, P. J. Springfield, Ill.: Charles C. Thomas.

BARRACLOUGH, M. A., and SHARPEY-SCHAFER, E. P. (1963). Hypotension from absent circulatory reflexes. Effects of alcohol, barbiturates, psychotherapeutic drugs and other mechanisms. *Lancet*, **1,** 1121.

British Medical Journal (1968). Leading Article. Malignant hyperpyrexia. **3,** 69.

BURTON, A. C. (1951). On the physical equilibrium of small blood vessels. *Amer. J. Physiol.*, **164,** 319.

BURTON, A. C. and YAMADA, S. (1951). The relationship between blood pressure and flow in the human forearm. *J. appl. Physiol.*, **4,** 329.

BURN, J. H. (1961). A new view of adrenergic fibres explaining the action of reserpine, bretylium and guanethidine. *Brit. med. J.*, **1,** 1623.

CRANDELL, D. L. (1962). The anaesthetic hazards in patients on anti-hypertensive therapy. *J. Amer. med. Ass.*, **179,** 495.

CRANSTON, W. I. (1966). Temperature regulation. *Brit. med. J.*, **2,** 69.

GAUER, O. H., and HENRY, J. P. (1963). Circulatory basis of fluid volume control. *Physiol. Rev.*, **43,** 423.

GROSS, M., MONTAGUE, D., ROSAS, R., and BOHR, D. F. (1965). I. Cardiac action of vasoactive polypeptides in the rat. II. Angiotensin. *Circulat. Res.*, **16,** 155.

HARRISON, G. G., BIEBUYCK, J. F., TERBLANCHE, J., DENT, D. M., HICKMAN, R., and SAUNDERS, S. L. (1968). Hyperpyrexia during anaesthesia. *Brit. med. J.*, **3,** 594.

HOLT, A. T. (1962). Premedication with atropine should not be routine. *Lancet*, **2,** 984.

KEELE, C. A., NEIL, E., and JEPSON, J. B. (1965). *Samson Wright's Applied Physiology.* London: Oxford University Press.

LAURENCE, D. R. (1966). *Clinical Pharmacology.* London: J. & A. Churchill.

LILLEHEI, R. C., LONGERBEAM, J. K., BLOCH, J. H., and MANAX, W. G. (1964). The nature of irreversible shock. Experimental and clinical observations. *Ann. Surg.*, **160,** 682.

MELLANDER, S. (1960). Comparative studies on the adrenergic neurohumoral control of resistance and capacitance blood vessels in the cat. *Acta physiol. scand.*, Suppl. **176,** 1.

MUSHIN, W. W., GALLOON, S., and FANING, E. L. (1963). Anti-sialogogue and other effects of atropine mucate. *Brit. med. J.*, **2,** 652.

NICKERSON, M. (1964). Vasoconstriction and Vasodilatation in Shock. In: *Shock*. Ed. Hershey, S. G. Boston: Little Brown and Co.

PAYNE, J. P., and SINFIELD, R. M. (1964). Pronethalol in the treatment of ventricular arrhythmias during anaesthesia. *Brit. med. J.*, **1,** 603.

RODDIE, I. C., and SHEPHERD, J. T. (1963). Nervous control of the circulation in skeletal muscle. *Brit. med. Bull.*, **19,** 115.

SCHMIDT, J., and FLEMING, W. W. (1963). The structure of sympathomimetics as related to reserpine-induced sensitivity changes in the rabbit ileum. *J. Pharmacol. exp. Ther.*, **139,** 230.

SHARPEY-SCHAFER, E. P. (1955). Effects of Valsalva's manoeuvre on the normal and failing circulation. *Brit. med. J.*, **1,** 693.

SHARPEY-SCHAFER, E. P. (1961). Venous tone. *Brit. med. J.*, **2,** 1589.

SHEPHERD, J. T. (1966). Role of the veins in the circulation. *Circulation*, **32,** 484.

SYMPOSIUM (1966). Symposium on adrenergic drugs and their antagonists. *Brit. J. Anaesth.*, **38,** 665.

WATSON, W. E., SMITH, A. C., and SPALDING, J. M. K. (1962). Transmural central venous pressure during intermittent positive pressure respiration. *Brit. J. Anaesth.*, **34,** 278.

WYANT, G. M., and DOBKIN, A. B. (1958). Further studies of anti-sialogogue drugs in man. *Anaesthesia*, **13,** 173.

Chapter 21

SHOCK

THE term "shock" is commonly used but ill-defined. Conditions to which it is applied vary in aetiology, pathology and presentation, so that the value of the term even as a clinical description is frequently challenged (Bloch *et al.*, 1966; Thal and Kinney, 1967). However, the most widely accepted definition is a state of generalised impairment of the function of vital organs due to acute circulatory inadequacy (MacLean, 1966; Dietzman and Lillehei, 1968). It is important to recognise that "circulatory inadequacy" includes abnormalities of pressure, flow or distribution of blood supply, and that there are circumstances in which excessive metabolic demand may render inadequate an otherwise normal circulation (Roe and Kinney, 1965).

The factors which initiate and perpetuate this imbalance between supply and demand have been the source of speculation and study for many years. Both experimental work and clinical observation have contributed to the available knowledge, but a fuller understanding of the pathogenesis of the shock syndrome will depend on further detailed and accurate recording of deranged function in acute and often rapidly-changing situations.

Before the First World War, emphasis was laid on the behaviour of the peripheral circulation and its response to nervous stimuli. Crile's theory (1899) of vasomotor paralysis was widely accepted.

The high mortality of traumatic shock in the First World War led to further investigation both clinical and experimental, and intense vasoconstriction rather than vasodilatation was demonstrated in animals and man (Erlanger *et al.*, 1919*a*; Ducastaing, 1919). The possible dangers of excessive amounts of circulating adrenaline were emphasised by Bainbridge and Trevan (1917) and Erlanger *et al.* (1919*b*).

It was also shown that circulating blood volume is decreased in traumatic shock even in the absence of external blood loss (Keith, 1919). This finding, together with the observation that restoration of circulation to a crushed limb was followed by the rapid development of shock led Cannon and Bayliss (1919) to postulate that wound shock could be defined as a discrepancy between blood volume and vascular capacity, and that toxic substances liberated from damaged tissues caused a generalised increase in capillary permeability with loss of fluid from the circulation and stagnation of blood in venous reservoirs. Subsequent work by Blalock (1930) emphasised the extent of fluid loss around the site of injury and challenged the concept of generalised vascular damage. That hypovolaemia is not the sole mechanism leading to circulatory dysfunction following haemorrhage or trauma is demonstrated by the failure of transfusion to prevent progressive deterioration and death in some cases.

Renewed interest in the behaviour of the peripheral vessels followed experimental work on the effects of haemorrhage and endotoxin administration in the dog. In this animal, haemorrhagic hypotension of four to five hours duration does not respond to the return of the shed blood but the blood pressure continues to fall until death occurs. At post-mortem examination, there is striking haemorrhage and engorgement in the bowel mucosa (Lillehei, 1957) and a similar state can be produced by the administration of bacterial endotoxin (Longerbeam *et al.*, 1962) or by the prolonged infusion of adrenaline (Freeman *et al.*, 1951). Microscopy of the damaged gut shows capillary engorgement with arteriolar dilatation and venular contraction (Zweifach, 1958, 1961), possibly due to the differing ability of the pre-and post-capillary sphincters to maintain their tone during prolonged adrenergic stimulation (Lewis and Mellander, 1962). At first, both pre- and post-capillary sphincters are tightly constricted allowing little blood to enter the capillary bed. The pre-capillary sphincters then lose tone due to local anoxia and the accumulation of acid metabolites, while the post-capillary sphincters remain constricted. This leads to capillary engorgement and stagnation, with extravasation of fluid causing further depletion of the blood volume. Ultimately there is capillary destruction and loss of frank blood. According to Lillehei *et al.* (1964) the onset of this state during prolonged haemorrhagic hypotension or shock from any cause marks the change of the condition from "reversible" to "irreversible", in other words the point at which restoration of blood volume alone is insufficient to prevent progressive deterioration and death. The same authors point out that the organs showing most damage vary from one species to another but that this haemodynamic disturbance in the peripheral vascular bed is a common feature and is the result of prolonged and harmful vasoconstriction. Thus although stimulation of the sympathetic nervous system and the liberation of adrenaline can accommodate quite considerable physiological demands on the circulation by increasing venous tone, increasing the rate and force of myocardial contraction and maintaining blood pressure by arteriolar constriction, it would seem that when prolonged and intense, sympathomimetic activity either endogenous or exogenous may be harmful (Nickerson, 1963; Lillehei *et al.*, 1962).

Besides the loss of circulating volume which takes place when fluid extravasates around the site of injury or through the walls of damaged capillaries, there is some evidence of further loss of extracellular fluid by translocation into the intracellular compartment due to derangement of the sodium pump (Shires *et al.*, 1961). However the occurrence of this "sequestration" of extracellular fluid is not universally accepted (MacLean, 1968; Hardaway, 1968).

An additional factor contributing to the "irreversibility" of experimental shock has been suggested by the work of Fine (1954). In the dog, prolonged visceral ischaemia may enable gut bacteria to enter the blood stream thus adding sepsis to the original injury with consequent further detriment to circulatory performance. To what extent this mechanism is important in species where gut vasoconstriction is less prominent remains uncertain. However, cell damage in experimental shock results in the release of lysosomal enzymes (Janoff, 1964) and these can cause further cellular injury and therefore propagate tissue destruction.

In addition to the views of Lillehei and his associates on the effects of sympathetic stimulation on the microcirculation, there is evidence that flow patterns within these vessels are altered. Both Knisely (1965) and Gelin (1956) have demonstrated aggregation and sludging of red cells in human conjunctival vessels following injury. Brill and Shoemaker (1960) have shown experimentally that a similar process occurs in the liver of dogs following the use of large doses of adrenaline.

The development of platelet thrombi with consequent plugging of small vessels has been demonstrated by Robb (1963) and the importance of widespread intravascular coagulation with subsequent coagulation defects in the circulating blood has been emphasised by Hardaway *et al.* (1967) as part of the later stages of acute circulatory failure. The slowly-flowing and therefore abnormally acid capillary blood is hypercoagulable, and disseminated intravascular clotting is readily initiated by thrombogenic agents such as the products of haemolysis, bacterial toxins or the proximity of damaged tissue. Lysis of these clots *in situ* will ultimately follow but by this time there may be irretrievable cell death in the tissue beyond the obstructed vessels. The occurrence of widespread intravascular thrombosis depletes the circulating blood of a number of coagulation factors and haemorrhagic manifestations may sometimes be seen. Even in the absence of clinical evidence of this process it is often possible to document it by serial estimation of clotting factors and this information is used by Hardaway as an index of prognosis.

There is thus evidence from many sources that a variety of defects in the peripheral vascular system can contribute to acute circulatory insufficiency but equally, or possibly of greater importance, is the behaviour of the heart. Sarnoff *et al.* (1954) and more recently Guyton (1963) and Gomez and Hamilton (1964) have demonstrated deterioration in myocardial function during prolonged experimental haemorrhagic hypotension, and the contribution of some degree of cardiac failure to circulatory inadequacy in a variety of clinical disorders, often in young and previously healthy subjects, has been documented by MacLean (1966). The recognition and treatment of this aspect of circulatory failure is frequently life-saving.

The evidence presented so far has all emphasised deficiencies of blood flow (low cardiac output due to myocardial impairment or deficient blood volume; poor tissue perfusion due to excessive vasoconstriction and abnormalities within the microcirculation). This is reflected in the conventional clinical description of the "shocked patient"—hypotensive with small pulse pressure, cold, pale or cyanosed sweating extremities, oliguria or anuria, rapid respiration, anxiety, restlessness or clouding of consciousness.

However there are situations (some cases of septicaemia, some following myocardial infarction) where overall blood flow is normal or high and systemic vascular resistance low (MacLean *et al.*, 1967; Thomas *et al.*, 1966). Tissue perfusion may still be inadequate if blood flow is diverted through arteriovenous shunts, if blood pressure is lower than the critical closing pressure of small vessels (Burton, 1951) or if hypermetabolic states such as severe trauma, burns or sepsis impose an increased demand for oxygen supply.

These features underline the difficulty of applying the single term "shock" to such a variety of conditions. It is perhaps fair to accept shock or acute circulatory inadequacy as a generic term similar to respiratory or renal failure, realising that it covers a variety of conditions. Impairment of function of vital organs is a feature common to all; the circulatory defect which is responsible may differ according to the aetiology of the condition.

Classification

Attempts to classify shock (Tables 1 and 2) are generally based either on the initial precipitating event (Thal and Kinney, 1967; Dietzman and Lillehei, 1968) or on the haemodynamic diagnosis (MacLean, 1966).

The latter system is not fully comprehensive—for example, the septic patient with high cardiac output, low systemic vascular resistance and normal or low arteriovenous oxygen difference is not apparently suffering from cardiac defect, hypovolaemia or peripheral pooling. The limitation of discussing conditions in terms of the precipitating event is that several factors may coexist or there may be a transition from one variety of shock to another—for example, the coexistence of sepsis and fluid loss with the subsequent development of impaired cardiac function. However this aetiological system is the one most widely used. On this basis, it is necessary to consider hypovolaemia and the effective hypovolaemia of vasodilatation, together with the conditions of cardiac and septic shock.

21/Table 1

Classification of Shock Based on Aetiology. (From Thal and Kinney, 1967)

1. Hypovolaemic shock
   (*a*) pure
   (*b*) combined with sepsis or cardiac failure
2. Cardiogenic shock
   (*a*) failure of left ventricular ejection
   (*b*) failure of left ventricular filling
3. Septic shock
   (*a*) pure
   (*b*) combined with cardiac failure or hypovolaemia
4. Neurogenic shock (loss of vasomotor control).

21/Table 2

Classification of Shock Based on Haemodynamic Diagnosis. (From Maclean, 1966)

1. Cardiac deficit.
2. Hypovolaemia.
3. Peripheral pooling.

Hypovolaemia is still one of the commonest causes of circulatory inadequacy, especially in surgical practice. Fluid loss may be overt or concealed, and consist of blood, plasma or extracellular fluid. Sympathomimetic activity is prominent, initially maintaining cardiac output, venous and arterial pressure within the normal range, but with progressive fluid loss these indices fall. Oliguria is present, due initially to hormonally mediated retention of sodium and water and subsequently to the damaging effects of hypotension and a lowered blood flow on renal function.

It is clinical custom to include in the consideration of shock conditions in which vasodilatation is accompanied by low venous and arterial pressures although the cardiac output is relatively normal until vasodilatation is extreme. This can be described as "effective hypovolaemia"—a blood volume within the normal range but still inadequate to achieve normal filling of a dilated vascular bed. Such disorders include barbiturate overdosage, certain neurological injuries, anaphylaxis, acute adrenal steroid depletion and some cases of septicaemia. However, not all patients with these conditions can justifiably be classified as "shocked" defining the term as "impaired function of vital organs due to acute circulatory inadequacy."

Cardiogenic shock as a primary event is most commonly due to myocardial infarction. Other causes are arrhythmias or extremes of rate, sudden obstruction (pulmonary embolism) or regurgitation (ruptured cusp or papillary muscle), compression (tamponade) or trauma.

The haemodynamic findings are variable. Hypotension, tachycardia and elevation of venous pressure are common, but although some cases have a lowered cardiac output and a high systemic vascular resistance, in others, particularly those with infarcts, there is hypotension with a normal cardiac output and low systemic vascular resistance, possibly due to vasodilating reflexes arising from afferents in the coronary bed (Dawes and Comroe, 1954) or left ventricle (Braunwald, 1968; Thomas *et al.*, 1965, 1966).

Septic shock is the group in which clinical and haemodynamic findings are most variable. Both Gram-positive and negative infections may be responsible (*Lancet*, 1963; Austen and Buckley, 1967) and the effects may be attributable to circulating endo- or exotoxins rather than true bacteraemia.

The haemodynamic changes may be those of vasoconstriction with low cardiac output and high systemic vascular resistance, but the exact opposite situation, namely high cardiac output, low systemic vascular resistance and vasodilatation is also common. This hyperkinetic state may be an early response to bacterial toxins (Spink, 1962) and some suggest that the low output, vasoconstricted state only develops in the presence of hypovolaemia either preexisting (such as often occurs in sepsis complicating intra-abdominal pathology) or secondary to fluid loss due to diarrhoea, sweating and excessive capillary permeability (Austen and Buckley, 1967; MacLean *et al.*, 1967).

Dietzman and Lillehei (1968) emphasise the early contribution of peripheral pooling due to "microcirculatory stagnation" to hypovolaemia in endotoxic shock. This is said to be secondary to intense sympathomimetic stimulation and indeed sympathomimetic activity due to endotoxins can be demonstrated experimentally in kidney, lung and bowel (Hinshaw *et al.*, 1961; Kuida *et al.*, 1958; Lillehei, 1958). This effect appears two-fold—partly due to the liberation of catecholamines but possibly also due to the formation of a vasoconstrictor substance by the joint action of endotoxin and some factor present in whole blood. However, the evidence that this vasoconstrictor activity occurs and is an important contributory factor in the development of septic shock is better for dogs than for man.

In spite of vasodilatation with a high flow and low vascular resistance, metabolic demands may not be supplied as demonstrated by progressive metabolic acidosis due to the accumulation of lactic acid. The arteriovenous oxygen difference is often normal or low and the acidosis does not respond to treatment with hyperbaric oxygen, suggesting either that blood is flowing through arteriovenous shunts or that cellular utilisation of oxygen is impaired (Siegel *et al.*, 1967; Sardesai and Thal, 1966; Thal and Wilson, 1965).

Disseminated intravascular coagulation and secondary haemorrhagic phenomena are prominant features of septic shock in man and may be the result of a generalised Schwartzmann reaction (Rapaport *et al.*, 1964). This inevitably causes further impairment of tissue perfusion. Intravascular haemolysis may also develop and so diminish oxygen-carrying capacity.

Although the group of vasodilated, hyperkinetic patients may initially remain alert and with a good urinary output in spite of hypotension, evidence of widespread organ failure (heart, lungs, kidney, liver, brain and gut) will ultimately appear and may occur early in the more severe forms of septic shock, possibly reflecting the increased metabolic demands. These features, together with a progressive metabolic acidosis in spite of a normal or high cardiac output, are generally associated with a fatal outcome. Death commonly occurs from pulmonary oedema although haemodynamic evidence suggests that this is due to the excessive permeability of damaged capillaries leaking protein-rich fluid, rather than cardiac failure leading to an increase in pulmonary capillary pressure (MacLean, 1966; Riordan and Walters, 1968).

Diagnosis and Assessment

Although it is customary to subdivide "shock" into these three categories, it cannot be too strongly emphasised that these divisions are not absolute and that patients suffering from a single disease may manifest together or sequentially all three disorders; even more important is that both hypovolaemia and myocardial impairment are common features of the septic shock syndrome.

A further difficulty is the accurate recognition of "shock" bearing in mind the problems of definition. Most commonly the term is used clinically to describe hypotension although the arterial blood pressure is a notoriously poor guide to the adequacy of circulatory function. Alternatively patients are described as shocked when their skin is vasoconstricted, cold and sweating even though the arterial pressure is still within the normal range.

The two essential requirements for the management of such patients are to attempt some assessment of blood flow rather than pressure and to determine, by observing the height of the venous pressure, whether hypovolaemia is contributing to circulatory inadequacy. Some idea of blood flow may be gained by noting the level of consciousness, the rate of urine secretion and the colour, temperature and degree of superficial venous filling of the peripheral tissues.

When flow is well maintained the limbs are warm and often dry, peripheral pulses are palpable, urine flow is not interrupted and consciousness is fully maintained in spite of arterial hypotension.

Poor flow is suggested if the skin is cold, sweating and cyanosed, urine secretion reduced or absent and consciousness impaired. Peripheral pulses are weak because the pulse pressure is low and the blood pressure difficult to record using a sphygmomanometer. If recovery occurs, urine flow improves (provided the kidneys have not been too severely damaged) and warmth gradually spreads down the limbs until the skin is uniformly pink, warm and dry and the superficial veins well-filled.

In addition to the clinical assessment of tissue perfusion, there must be a careful examination of the heart, lungs and abdomen together with a brief neurological survey (for evidence of raised intra-cranial pressure, meningism or localising signs). Few patients are so desperately in need of therapeutic intervention that this initial examination cannot be made thoroughly and an accurate diagnosis of the primary event is most likely to be reached only if this examination is carried out before therapy has modified the clinical features. It is important to realise however that some physical signs may be masked by the presence of shock. In particular, severe peritonitis may be present with few if any signs in the abdomen until the circulation has been restored towards normal.

In many patients, the history and initial clinical examination are sufficient to establish the diagnosis, but if this is not so the following assessment should be made.

Measurement of Venous Pressure

Unless the central venous pressure can be accurately determined by observation of the neck veins, it must be measured in a vessel in free communication with the intrathoracic veins. This is the most important single observation which can be readily made in general clinical practice as it reflects the adequacy of both cardiac filling and cardiac performance.

Interpretation of the Venous Pressure

In the shocked patient, a value of less than zero (using the sternal angle as the reference point) indicates inadequate filling of the circulation. This may be due to fluid loss or to excessive vasodilatation of the capacitance vessels and means that in these acute situations there is no absolute value for "normal blood volume" (MacLean *et al.*, 1965; Friedman *et al.*, 1966; Daintree-Johnson, 1966; Sampson and Hutchinson, 1967). Optimal blood volume is that which provides adequate cardiac filling at any particular level of venous tone. When venous tone is high (prolonged sympathetic stimulation, heart failure) a "normal" blood volume may result in a venous pressure so high that pulmonary oedema is produced (Fig. 1). Conversely, when venous tone is low (sympathetic paralysis, barbiturate overdosage) a "normal" blood volume may still result in such a low venous pressure that cardiac filling is inadequate and cardiac output low (Starling's law). This means that the measurement of venous pressure must be interpreted in conjunction with either a measurement of blood volume or an assessment of vascular tone. There are many sources of potential error which can invalidate measurements of blood volume in the shocked patient (Heath and Vickers, 1968), quite apart fom the temptation to use the value obtained as the sole criterion of adequate circulatory filling. It is both safe and simple to interpret venous pressure in conjunction with the physical signs of vasoconstriction or vasodilatation.

Low venous pressure.—Vasoconstriction and a low venous pressure can only be produced by fluid loss. This loss may be whole blood (overt or concealed haemorrhage), plasma or protein-rich exudate (burns or inflammatory exudates) or protein-free fluid (intestinal obstruction, diabetic coma). Measurements of haematocrit, electrolytes and urea, plasma proteins and blood sugar as appropriate will help to differentiate these causes.

Vasodilatation with a low venous pressure is due to an increased vascular capacity such as may be seen in certain forms of neurological damage, barbiturate

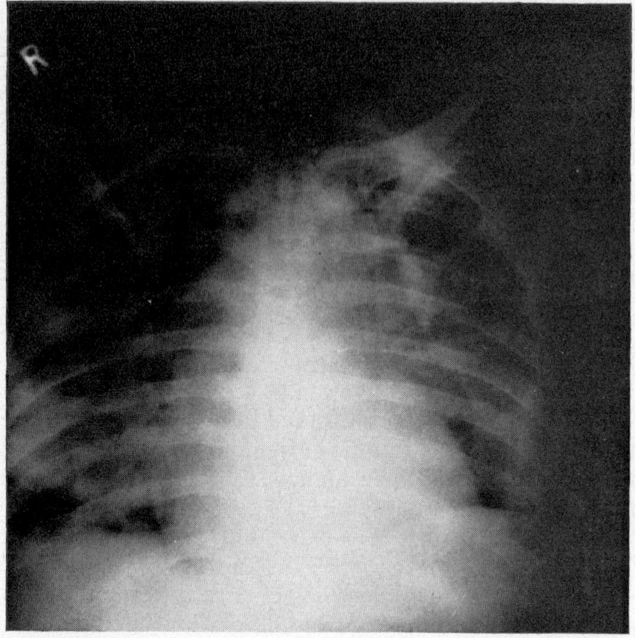

21/Fig. 1.—Chest X-ray of a 52-year-old patient with ischaemic heart disease in whom pulmonary oedema developed when the measured blood volume (3·1 litres) was increased to the predicted normal for age, height and weight (4·2 litres).

and other drug overdosage, fever and some patients with sepsis. These conditions are commonly associated with an abnormally low tone in resistance vessels so that arterial as well as venous pressure is low, but unless vasodilatation is extreme or the myocardium damaged, overall blood flow may be normal or even elevated (Fig. 2).

High venous pressure.—Elevation of the venous pressure is most commonly due to cardiac embarrassment but it can also be produced by over-transfusion. An initial difficulty is to define what constitutes dangerous elevation of the venous pressure. The normal range is given by Paul Wood (1968) as minus 5 to plus 3 cm. relative to the sternal angle. However, the fact that the venous pressure lies outside this range does not necessarily mean that circulatory function is impaired. If a normal heart is over-filled so that the venous pressure is above plus 3 cm. the cardiac output will rise (Starling's law; Fig. 3). This situation shows none of the features of shock or circulatory failure. Ultimately a point is reached where the venous pressure (both pulmonary and systemic) is so high that oedema develops, and the combination of systemic and pulmonary oedema with elevation of the venous pressure is clinically labelled "heart failure". However, it is difficult to accept this in a physiological sense as the heart is still behaving normally in response to increased filling. Finally however, true cardiac failure is produced when the hypoxia of pulmonary oedema together with functional tricuspid and mitral regurgitation due to cardiac over-distension

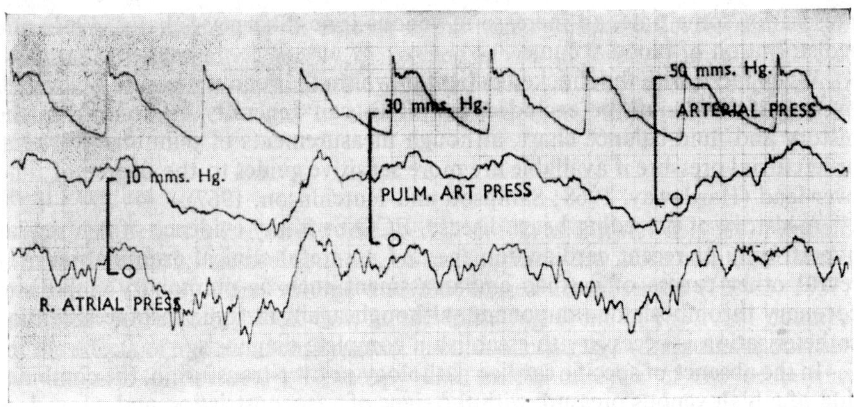

21/FIG. 2.—Haemodynamic and biochemical findings in a boy of 16 with Gram-negative septicaemia.

Cardiac output = 11·4 l./min.	Pa_{O_2} 62 mm. Hg (breathing oxygen)
Pulse rate = 130/min.	Pa_{CO_2} 41·5 mm. Hg
Stroke output = 88 ml./beat	pH_a 7·29

combine to lower the cardiac output so that blood pressure falls and reflex vasoconstriction develops.

More commonly shock associated with a high venous pressure reflects impaired cardiac performance due to myocardial damage, valvular defects, obstruction or compression. The high venous pressure is produced by a combination of factors including fluid retention in situations where heart failure has been

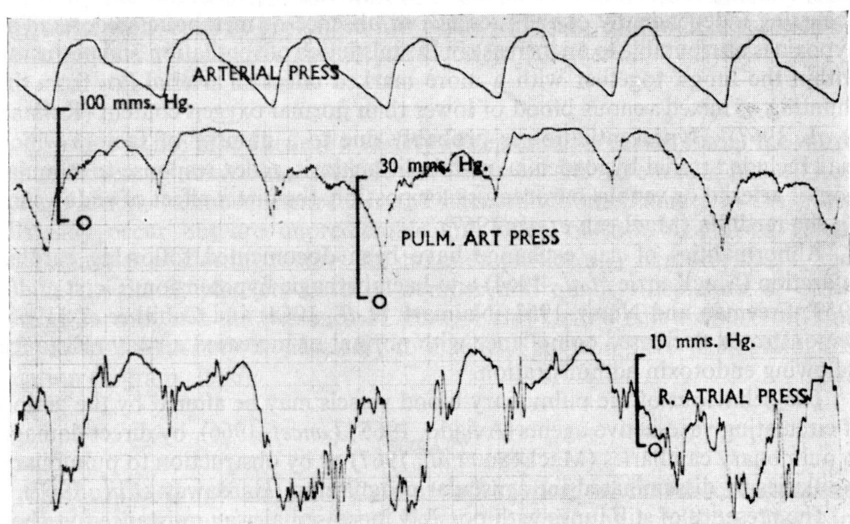

21/FIG. 3.—Haemodynamic findings in a young adult (19 years) with acute glomerulo-nephritis.

Cardiac output = 12·0 l./min.
Pulse rate = 120/min.
Stroke output = 100 ml./beat

oxygen supply at cellular level; the factors contributing to tissue oxygenation are blood flow, oxygen-carrying capacity and arterial oxygenation (Nunn and Freeman, 1964).

Hypovolaemia, effective or absolute, must be corrected using the central venous pressure in conjunction with signs of vasoconstriction or vasodilatation to assess the volume required. If hypovolaemia is the sole mechanism of circulatory inadequacy, the infusion of fluid will restore evidence of adequate tissue flow—vasodilatation will occur and the venous pressure will rise to normal. If in a patient suspected of hypovolaemia, central venous pressure is already normal but there is evidence of persistent vasoconstriction, it is safe to infuse small volumes of fluid (100–200 ml.) in a short period of time (5–15 minutes) and observe the circulatory changes this produces. If hypovolaemia is still present, a small infusion will cause the central venous pressure to rise only transitorily and signs of vasodilatation will begin to appear. If there is some other cause of circulatory impairment, central venous pressure will rise sharply and remain elevated and there will be no evidence of improved flow (Sykes, 1963).

The choice of fluid depends on the nature of the fluid lost together with serial measurements of haematocrit, plasma protein and electrolyte concentrations. Hardaway (1968) recommends the determination of red cell mass to assess the requirement for whole blood, using other fluids to continue volume repletion once the normal red cell mass has been reached even though the haematocrit may fall as a result. However measurements of red cell mass are not widely available, and it may in any case be wiser to maintain a normal haematocrit so that oxygen-carrying capacity is not reduced.

Plasma rather than blood will be required to correct protein loss due to inflammatory exudates; fresh frozen plasma supplies a high concentration of clotting factors and has the additional advantage of carrying a lower risk of hepatitis. The various dextran preparations also avoid the risk of hepatitis but when used in large volumes may interfere with cross-matching and with *in vivo* coagulation. Low molecular weight dextran not only expands the blood volume by the amount infused but also has a powerful osmotic effect so that it causes considerable expansion of blood volume at the expense of the extracellular fluid. It may also have some specific action on the red cells, minimising the tendency to sludging.

Colloid-free electrolyte solutions are needed to replace deficits in extracellular fluid but only a percentage of their volume is retained in the vascular compartment. If the plasma protein concentration of blood is decreased or the capillary walls damaged, electrolyte solutions will contribute to the formation of oedema rather than restore the blood volume to normal.

When a rapid rate of transfusion is required, all solutions should be raised to body temperature and the use of calcium salts to cover massive transfusion of citrated blood is generally recommended (Royal Society of Medicine Symposium, 1968). Once a normal central venous pressure has been reached, the rate of fluid infusion should be decreased so that the venous pressure remains constant while vasodilatation occurs. If vasodilatation and evidence of improved tissue flow does not appear, some authors (Hardaway, 1968; MacLean, 1966) recommend continued transfusion to raise the central venous pressure above normal in the hope that cardiac output will rise in response to greater diastolic filling (Starling's law). However in patients with disease affecting the left side of the heart, in those with reduced levels of plasma proteins and those suffering from septicaemia, this may lead to the development of pulmonary oedema (Guyton and Lindsey, 1959; Guyton, 1963; MacLean *et al.*, 1967). If, therefore, evidence of adequate tissue perfusion cannot be achieved when the central venous pressure is within the normal range, it may be wiser to consider other methods of increasing cardiac output or improving the distribution of blood flow. The only exception to this rule lies in the management of patients with known disease of the right side of the heart in whom elevation of the venous pressure above the normal range is justifiable and may well be desirable.

An inotropic agent will virtually always increase cardiac output whether this is inadequate because of a primary disorder of the heart or because myocardial impairment has developed during severe or prolonged shock. Isoprenaline, a powerful beta-sympathomimetic agent combining myocardial stimulation with peripheral vasodilatation, is widely used for this purpose in the treatment of all varieties of shock (MacLean *et al.*, 1965; Kardos, 1966; Elliott and Gorlin, 1966; Du Toit *et al.*, 1966; Kirklin and Rastelli, 1967). Therapy is easy to control when the drug is given intravenously although its use is occasionally limited by tachycardia or arrhythmias. In some patients, digitalis or drugs to control rate or rhythm may also be needed. Correction of acidosis may improve myocardial performance by permitting maximum effect of stimulating catecholamines even though evidence for direct myocardial depression by acidosis is conflicting (Weil *et al.*, 1957; Thrower *et al.*, 1961; Goodyer *et al.*, 1961; Anderson and Mouritzen, 1966).

The use of vasopressor agents to maintain arterial pressure and redistribute flow to vital organs (Kurland and Malach, 1952; Braunwald, 1968) has largely given way to enthusiasm for vasodilating drugs. The use of phenoxybenzamine has been widely advocated, particularly by Lillehei *et al.* (1964) who stress the value of decreasing systemic vascular resistance and increasing vascular capacity so that improved microcirculatory perfusion is combined with a lessened work load on the left ventricle. However all authorities recommending this therapy stress the importance of monitoring central venous pressure so that there is immediate recognition of the need for further volume infusion as the vascular bed dilates. Phenoxybenzamine may have additional value by interfering with the action of vaso-active and toxic substances liberated in shock (Bloch *et al.*, 1966).

Large doses of corticosteroids (50 mg./kg./day of hydrocortisone) are often recommended, particularly for septicaemic shock. Their value is uncertain and any circulatory improvement may be attributable, at least in part, to alpha adrenergic blockade (Lillehei *et al.*, 1962).

Efforts to improve overall flow and distribution of blood will be of little value if the microcirculation is obstructed by disseminated intravascular coagulation. Anticoagulants or fibrinolysins may be of some value in resolving these changes (Hardaway and Drake, 1963).

In addition to therapy directed at restoring blood flow, a high arterial oxygen content must be provided by maintaining a normal haemoglobin and full saturation. Oxygen administration is generally necessary and usually sufficient to achieve full saturation except in a few cases in whom controlled ventilation will be required. In these cases, the benefits of improved oxygenation and decreased respiratory work are generally more apparent than any deterioration due to the effects of intermittent positive pressure ventilation on cardiac output. The possible value of hyperbaric oxygen remains to be fully assessed (Whalen and McIntosh, 1965) but when oxygen requirements are high, for example due to fever or restlessness, cooling, sedation or muscular paralysis may be worthwhile.

If tissue blood flow is not rapidly restored, severe and sometimes irreversible renal failure may follow, but the prophylactic use of mannitol, an osmotic diuretic with additional actions on renal vasculature and blood flow, decreases the incidence of acute renal failure (Luke and Kennedy, 1967; Dawson, 1968).

This short review of therapy underlines some of the uncertainties surrounding the shock syndrome. Precise information on the clinical effects of a number of these agents is lacking, and few of them can be expected to benefit the hypotensive, septic patient with high cardiac output, low systemic vascular resistance and rapidly progressive acidosis. It may well be that with increasing knowledge some separation of the variants of the shock syndrome will become possible so that in each condition appropriate therapy can be chosen and the effects accurately assessed.

REFERENCES

ANDERSON, M. N., and MOURITZEN, C. (1966). Effect of acute respiratory and metabolic acidosis on cardiac output and peripheral resistance. *Ann. Surg.*, **163,** 161.

AUSTEN, W. G., and BUCKLEY, M. J. (1967). Treatment of various forms of surgical shock. *Progr. cardiovasc. Dis.*, **10,** 97.

AVIADO, D. M. (1965). The pulmonary circulation. In: *Shock and Hypotension.* Eds. Mills, L. C. and Moyer, J. H. New York: Grune and Stratton.

BAINBRIDGE, F. A., and TREVAN, J. W. (1917). Some actions of adrenalin upon the liver. *J. Physiol.* (*Lond.*), **51,** 460.

BLALOCK, A. (1930). Experimental shock: cause of low blood pressure produced by muscle injury. *Arch. Surg.*, **20,** 959.

BLOCH, J. H., DIETZMAN, R. H., PIERCE, C. H., and LILLEHEI, R. C. (1966). Theories of the production of shock. *Brit. J. Anaesth.*, **38,** 234.

BORDEN, G. W., and HALL, W. H. (1951). Fatal transfusion reactions from massive bacterial contamination of blood. *New Engl. J. Med.*, **245,** 760.

BRAUNWALD, E. (1968). The pathogenesis and treatment of shock in myocardial infarction. *Bull. Johns Hopk. Hosp.*, **121,** 421.

BRILL, N. R., and SHOEMAKER, W. C. (1960). Studies on the hepatic and visceral microcirculation during shock and after epinephrine administration: a preliminary report. *Surg. Forum*, **11,** 119.

BURTON, A. C. (1951). On the physical equilibrium of small blood vessels. *Amer. J. Physiol.*, **164,** 319.

CAHILL, J. M., JOUASSETT-STRIDER, D., and BYRNE, J. J. (1965). Lung function in shock. *Amer. J. Surg.*, **110,** 324.

CANNON, W. B., and BAYLISS, W. M. (1919). Notes on muscle injury in relation to shock. *Med. Res. Comm.*, **81,** 19.

CRILE, G. W. (1899). *An Experimental Research into Surgical Shock.* Philadelphia: J. B. Lippincott.

DAINTREE-JOHNSON, H. (1966). Central venous pressure and blood volume. *Lancet*, **2,** 701.

DAWES, G. S., and COMROE, J. H., Jr. (1954). Chemoreflexes from the heart and lungs. *Physiol. Rev.*, **34,** 167.

DAWSON, J. L. (1968). The etiology and prevention of acute renal failure in surgical patients. *Proc. roy. Soc. Med.*, **61,** 1163.

DIETZMAN, R. H., and LILLEHEI, R. C. (1968). The nature and treatment of shock. *Brit. J. hosp. Med.*, **1,** 300.

DUCASTAING, R. (1919). La vaso-constriction peripherique chez les shockés. Action du nitrite d'angle. *Presse méd.*, **27,** 782.

DU TOIT, H. J., DOMMISSE J., THERON, M. S., DU PLESSIS, J. M. E., RORKE, M. J., and DE VILLIERS, V. P. (1966). Treatment of endotoxic shock with isoprenaline. *Lancet*, **2,** 143.

ELEY, A., HARGREAVES, T., and LAMBERT, H. P. (1965). Jaundice in severe infections. *Brit. med. J.*, **2,** 75.

ELLIOTT, W. C., and GORLIN, R. (1966). Isoproterenol in treatment of heart disease. *J. Amer. med. Ass.*, **197,** 315.

ERLANGER, J., GESELL, R., and GASSER, H. S. (1919*a*). Studies in secondary traumatic shock. I: The circulation in shock after abdominal injuries. *Amer. J. Physiol.*, **49,** 151.

ERLANGER, J., GESELL, R., and GASSER, H. S. (1919*b*). Studies in secondary traumatic shock. III: Circulatory failure due to adrenaline. *Amer. J. Physiol.*, **49,** 345.

FINE, J. (1954). *The Bacterial Factor in Traumatic Shock*. Springfield, Ill.: Charles C. Thomas.

FREEMAN, J., and NUNN, J. F. (1963). Ventilation-perfusion relationships after haemorrhage. *Clin. Sci.*, **24,** 135.

FREEMAN, N. E., FREEDMAN, H., and MILLER, C. C. (1951). The production of shock by the prolonged continuous injection of adrenalin in unanesthetized dogs. *Amer. J. Physiol.*, **131,** 545.

FRIEDMAN, E., GRABLE, E., and FINE, J. (1966). Central venous pressure and direct serial measurements as guides in blood volume replacement. *Lancet*, **2,** 609.

GELIN, L. E. (1956). Studies in the anaemia of injury. *Acta chir. scand.*, Suppl. **210,** 1.

GERST, P. H., RATTENBORG, C., and HOLADAY, D. A. (1959). The effect of haemorrhage on pulmonary circulation and respiratory gas exchange. *J. clin. Invest.*, **38,** 524.

GOMEZ, O. A., and HAMILTON, W. F. (1964). Functional cardiac deterioration during development of haemorrhagic circulatory deficiency. *Circulat. Res.*, **14,** 327.

GOODYER, A. V. N., ECKHARDT, W. F., OSTBERG, R. H., and GOODKIND, M. J. (1961). Effects of metabolic acidosis and alkalosis on coronary blood flow and myocardial metabolism in the intact dog. *Amer. J. Physiol.*, **200,** 628.

GUYTON, A. C. (1963). *Circulatory Physiology; Cardiac Output and its Regulation.* Philadelphia: W. B. Saunders.

GUYTON, A. C., and LINDSEY, A. W. (1959). Effect of elevated left atrial pressure and decreased plasma protein concentration on the development of pulmonary oedema. *Circulat. Res.*, **7,** 649.

HARDAWAY, R. M. (1968). *Clinical Management of Shock*. Springfield, Ill.: Charles C. Thomas.

HARDAWAY, R. M., and DRAKE, D. C. (1963). Prevention of irreversible haemorrhagic shock with fibrinolysin. *Ann. Surg.*, **157,** 39.

HARDAWAY, R. M., JAMES, P. M., Jr., ANDERSON, R. W., BREDENBERG, C. E., and WEST, R. L. (1967). Intensive study and treatment of shock in man. *J. Amer. med. Ass.*, **199,** 779.

HAYES, M. A. (1957). The influence of shock without clinical renal failure on renal function. *Ann. Surg.*, **146,** 523.

HEATH, M. L., and VICKERS, M. D. (1968). An examination of single-tracer, semi-automated blood volume methodology. *Anaesthesia*, **23**, 659.

HINSHAW, L. B., SPINK, W. W., VICK, J. A., MALLET, E., and FINSTAD, J. (1961). Effect of endotoxin on kidney function and renal haemodynamics in the dog. *Amer. J. Physiol.*, **201**, 144.

INGRAM, G. I. C. (1966). The clinical investigation of a bleeding tendency. *Hosp. Med.*, **1**, 57.

JANOFF, A. (1964). Alterations in lysosomes (intracellular enzymes) during shock; effects of preconditioning (tolerance) and protective drugs. In *Shock*. Ed. Hershey, S. G. Boston: Little Brown.

KARDOS, G. G. (1966). Isoproterenol in the treatment of shock due to bacteraemia with gram-negative pathogens. *New Engl. J. Med.*, **27**, 868.

KEITH, M. N. (1919). Report of shock committee. English Medical Research Committee, No. 27.

KELMAN, G. R., NUNN, J. F., PRYS-ROBERTS, C., and GREENBAUM, R. (1967). The influence of cardiac output on arterial oxygenation: a theoretical study. *Brit. J. Anaesth.*, **39**, 450.

KIRKLIN, J. W. and RASTELLI, G. C (1967). Low cardiac output after open intracardiac operations. *Progr. cardiovasc. Dis.*, **10**, 117.

KNISELY, M. H. (1965). Intravascular erythrocyte aggregation (blood sludge). In: *Handbook of Physiology*, Section 2, Circulation, Vol. 3, 2249. Washington: Amer. Physiol. Soc.

KUIDA, H., HINSHAW, L. B., GILBERT, R. P., and VISSCHER, M. B. (1958). Effect of gram-negative endotoxin on pulmonary circulation. *Amer. J. Physiol.* **192**, 335.

KURLAND, G. S., and MALACH, M. (1952). The clinical use of norepinephrine in the treatment of shock accompanying myocardial infarction and other conditions. *New Engl. J. Med.*, **247**, 383.

Lancet (1963). Annotation. Septic shock. **2**, 1265.

Lancet (1966). Leading Article. Cor pulmonale in endotoxin shock. **1**, 863.

LEWIS, D. H. and MELLANDER, S. (1962). Competitive effects of sympathetic control and tissue metabolites on resistance and capacitance vessels and capillary filtration in skeletal muscle. *Acta physiol. scand.*, **56**, 162.

LILLEHEI, R. C. (1957). The intestinal factor in irreversible haemorrhagic shock. *Surgery*, **42**, 1043.

LILLEHEI, R. C. (1958). The intestinal factor in irreversible endotoxic shock. *Ann. Surg.*, **148**, 513.

LILLEHEI, R. C., LONGERBEAM, J. K., BLOCH, J. H., and MANAX, W. G. (1964). The nature of irreversible shock: experimental and clinical observations. *Ann. Surg.*, **160**, 682.

LILLEHEI, R. C., LONGERBEAM, J. K., and ROSENBERG, J. C. (1962). The nature of irreversible shock: its relationship to intestinal change. In: *Shock; Pathogenesis and Therapy* (Ciba Internat. Symp.) Ed. Bock, K. D. Berlin: Springer-Verlag.

LONGERBEAM, J. K., LILLEHEI, R. C., SCOTT, W. R., and ROSENBERG, J. C. (1962). Visceral factors in shock. *J. Amer. med. Ass.*, **181**, 878.

LUKE, R. G., and KENNEDY, A. C. (1967). Prevention and early management of acute renal failure. *Postgrad. med. J.*, **43**, 280.

MACKENZIE, G. J., TAYLOR, S. H., FLENLEY, D. C., MCDONALD, A. H., STAUNTON, H. P., and DONALD, K. W. (1964). Circulatory and respiratory studies in myocardial infarction and cardiogenic shock. *Lancet*, **2**, 825.

MACLEAN, L. D. (1966). The clinical management of shock. *Brit. J. Anaesth.*, **38**, 255.

MACLEAN, L. D. (1968). Shock and metabolism. *Surg. Gynec. Obstet.*, **126**, 299.

MacLean, L. D., Duff, J. H., Scott, H. M., and Peretz, D. I. (1965). Treatment of shock in man based on haemodynamic diagnosis. *Surg. Gynec. Obstet.*, **120,** 1.

MacLean, L. D., Mulligan, W. G., McLean, A. P. H., and Duff, J. H. (1967). Patterns of septic shock in man: a detailed study of 56 patients. *Ann. Surg.*, **166,** 543.

Naimark, A., Dugard, A., and Rangnor, E. (1968). Regional pulmonary blood flow and gas exchange in haemorrhagic shock. *J. appl. Physiol.*, **25,** 301.

Nickerson, M. (1963). Sympathetic blockade in the therapy of shock. *Amer. J. Cardiol.*, **21,** 619.

Nunn, J. F., and Freeman, J. (1964). Problems of oxygenation and oxygen transport in anaesthesia. *Anaesthesia*, **19,** 120.

Perlmuter, M., Grossman, S. L., Rothenberg, S., and Dobkin, G. (1959). Urine-serum urea nitrogen ratio: simple test of renal function in acute azotaemia and oliguria. *J. Amer. med. Ass.*, **170,** 1533.

Rapaport, S. I., Tatter, D., Coeur-Barron, N., and Hjort, P. F. (1964). Pseudomonas septicaemia with intravascular clotting leading to the generalized Schwartzmann reaction. *New Engl. J. Med.*, **271,** 80.

Riordan, J. F., and Walters, G. (1968). Pulmonary oedema in bacterial shock. *Lancet*, **1,** 719.

Robb, H. J. (1963). The role of microembolism in the production of irreversible shock. *Ann. Surg.*, **158,** 685.

Roe, C. F., and Kinney, J. M. (1965). The caloric equivalent of fever. II. Influence of major trauma. *Ann. Surg.*, **161,** 140.

Royal Society of Medicine Symposium (1968). Massive blood transfusion. *Proc. roy. Soc. Med.*, **61,** 681.

Sampson, J. H., and Hutchinson, J. C. (1967). Heart failure in myocardial infarction *Progr. cardiovasc. Dis.*, **10,** 1.

Sardesai, V. M., and Thal, A. P. (1966). Myocardial glucose metabolism in endotoxin shock. *Fed. Proc.*, **25,** 634.

Sarnoff, S. J., Case, R. B., Waithe, P. E., and Isaacs, J. P. (1954). Insufficient coronary blood flow and myocardial failure as a complicating factor in late haemorrhagic shock. *Amer. J. Physiol.*, **176,** 439.

Sharpey-Schafer, E. P. (1961). Venous tone. *Brit. med. J.*, **2,** 1589.

Shires, T., Williams, J., and Brown, F. (1961). Acute changes in extracellular fluid associated with major surgical procedures. *Ann. Surg.*, **154,** 803.

Siegel, J. H., Greenspan, M., and del Guercio, L. R. M. (1967). Abnormal vascular tone, defective oxygen transport and myocardial failure in human septic shock. *Ann. Surg.*, **165,** 504.

Spink, W. W. (1962). Pathogenesis and therapy of shock due to infection: experimental and clinical studies. In: *Shock; Pathogenesis and Therapy* (Ciba Internat. Symp.) Ed. Bock, K. D. Berlin: Springer-Verlag.

Sykes, M. K. (1963). Venous pressure as a clinical indication of adequacy of transfusion. *Ann. roy. Coll. Surg. Engl.*, **33,** 185.

Thal, A. P., and Kinney, J. M. (1967). On the definition and classification of shock. *Progr. cardiovasc. Dis.*, **9,** 527.

Thal, A. P., and Wilson, R. (1965). Shock. In: *Current Problems in Surgery*, Vol. 9. Chicago: Yearbook Publishers.

Thomas, M., Malmcrona, R., and Shillingford, J. P. (1965). Haemodynamic changes in patients with acute myocardial infarction. *Circulation*, **31,** 811.

Thomas, M., Malmcrona, R., and Shillingford, J. P. (1966). Circulatory changes associated with systemic hypotension in patients with acute myocardial infarction. *Brit. Heart J.*, **28,** 108.

THROWER, W. B., DARBY, T. D., and ALDINGER, E. E. (1961). Acid-base derangements and myocardial contractility. *Arch. Surg.*, **82,** 56.

WEIL, M. H., HOULE, D. B., BROWN, E. B., Jr., CAMPBELL, G. S., and HEATH, C. (1957). Influence of acidosis on the effectiveness of vasopressor agents. *Circulation*, **16**, 949.

WHALEN, R. E., and MCINTOSH, H. D. (1965). Hyperbaric oxygenation. Potentials and problems. *Amer. Heart. J.*, **69,** 725.

WOOD, P. (1968). *Diseases of the Heart and Circulation*, 3rd edit. London: Eyre and Spottiswoode.

ZWEIFACH, B. W. (1958). Microcirculatory derangements as basis for lethal manifestations of experimental shock. *Brit. J. Anaesth.*, **30,** 466.

ZWEIFACH, B. W. (1961). *Functional Behaviour of the Microcirculation.* Springfield, Ill.: Charles C. Thomas.

FURTHER READING

HARDAWAY, R. M. (1966). *Syndromes of Disseminated Intravascular Coagulation with special reference to Shock and Hemorrhage.* Springfield, Ill.: Charles C. Thomas.

WEIL, M. H., and SHUBIN, H. (1967). *Diagnosis and Treatment of Shock.* Baltimore: Williams & Wilkins.

MOYER, C. A., and BUTCHER, H. R. (1967). *Burns, Shock and Plasma Volume Regulation.* St. Louis: C. V. Mosby.

SHOEMAKER, W. C. (1967). *Shock: Chemistry, Physiology and Therapy.* Springfield, Ill.: Charles C. Thomas.

Review articles:

HAMIT, H. F. (1965). Current trends of therapy and research in shock. *Surg. Gynec. Obstet.*, **120,** 835.

Cardiogenic and other forms of Shock. *Progr. cardiovasc. Dis.*, **9,** No. 6, and **10,** Nos. 1 and 2.

Chapter 22

CEREBRAL CIRCULATION AND BRAIN METABOLISM

THE importance of the blood supply to the brain is well known and is emphasised by the frequency with which neurological damage is the factor limiting full recovery after an episode of circulatory arrest.

ANATOMY

The arterial supply to the brain is derived from the internal carotid and vertebral arteries on each side. The left common carotid artery arises directly from the aorta, whereas the right is a branch of the innominate artery. The vertebral vessels arise from the subclavian artery on their respective sides and join together at the lower border of the pons to form the basilar artery. The circle of Willis (Fig. 1) is formed by an anastomoses between the terminal branches of the basilar and two internal carotid arteries.

Kramer (1912) using a methylene blue technique, first suggested that the streams of blood passing to the circle of Willis do not normally mix but are

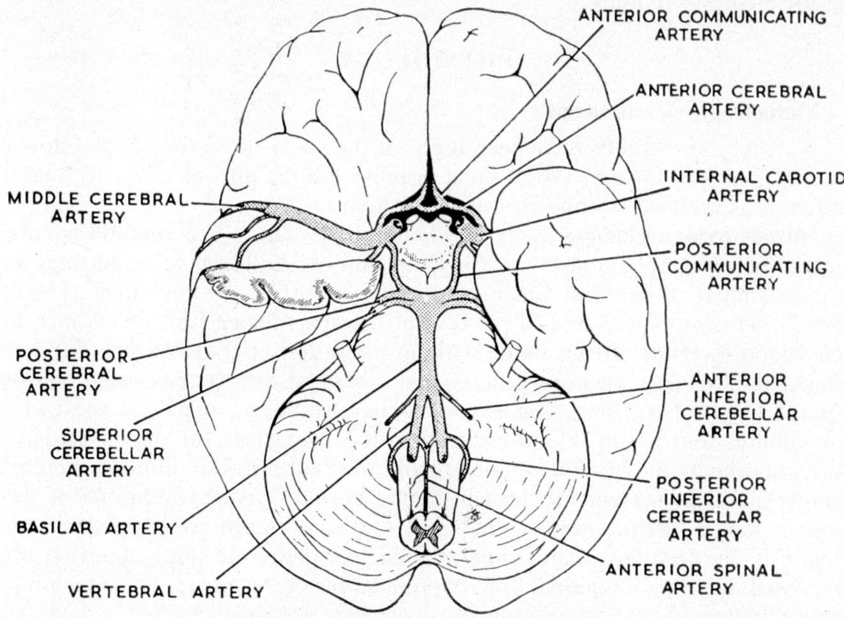

22/FIG. 1.—The circle of Willis.

distributed to sharply demarcated areas of brain on the same side, and work with cerebral angiography (McDonald and Potter, 1951) has confirmed this. Flow across the anastomotic communications does occur though, and the importance of the circle of Willis was underlined by Brain (1957) who stated "the purpose served by the circle of Willis is to guarantee that whatever the position of the head in relation to gravity and to the trunk, and however from one moment to another the relative flow through either carotid or vertebral artery may vary as a result, these variations are always compensated for distal to those vessels, and within the cranial cavity, by the freest possible anastomosis before the brain is reached." However the adequacy of the anastomotic channels in pathological states is limited as is shown by the fact that after ligation of one internal carotid artery, the pressure distal to the ligature is about half its previous value (Sweet and Bennett, 1948). Although in young people one internal carotid artery may be ligated with no diminution in total cerebral blood flow, a reduction may occur with symptoms of cerebral ischaemia in older subjects (Shenkin *et al.*, 1951).

Cerebral venous drainage, even in health, does not follow the unilateral pattern of the arterial supply (Batson, 1944). About two-thirds of the blood in the superior jugular bulb comes from the ipsilateral side and there is also a small (approximately 3 per cent) extra-cerebral contribution at this level (Shenkin *et al.*, 1948). This may be important when a sample from one jugular bulb is taken as representative of the entire cerebral venous drainage. Kety and Schmidt (1948*a*) concluded that for most purposes, unilateral sampling is adequately representative, although Munck and Lassen (1957) recommend bilateral sampling for greatest accuracy.

PHYSIOLOGY

Methods of Measurement

A variety of methods have been used for the study of cerebral blood flow in man (Ingvar and Lassen, 1965); most popular are the nitrous oxide technique, and various cerebral isotope clearance methods.

Nitrous oxide technique (Kety and Schmidt, 1948*a*).—This method is based on the Fick principle, and the assumption that cerebral uptake of an inert gas is independent of cerebral function. A mixture of 15 per cent nitrous oxide with 21 per cent oxygen and 64 per cent nitrogen is inhaled (this giving measurable blood levels of nitrous oxide without alteration of consciousness) and the integral of the arteriovenous difference is obtained over a ten-minute period. Uptake by the brain has been shown to be virtually complete at the end of ten minutes and as the blood-brain partition coefficient for nitrous oxide is unity, uptake by the brain is obtained from the concentration in mixed cerebral venous blood at the end of the ten-minute period. Under conditions of slow flow, a longer period may be required for equilibrium to be reached and obviously the technique cannot be applied to rapidly changing states. It also gives no indication of regional flow. Modifications of the nitrous oxide technique using Krypton 85 as the inert indicator have been described (Lassen and Munck, 1955) and with this substance continuous estimation of cerebral blood flow is possible (Lewis *et al.*, 1955*a* and *b*).

Cerebral isotope clearance methods.—These techniques allow regional cerebral blood flow to be measured. The isotope, most commonly Krypton 85 or Xenon 133, is injected intra-arterially and detected by external gamma-counting (Lassen and Ingvar, 1963; Hoedt-Rasmussen *et al.*, 1966). External counting following the inhalation of Xenon 133 has also been used (Veall and Mallett, 1963) but non-cerebral structures contribute to the observed count making interpretation difficult.

Heat clearance methods.—Several techniques have been described for the measurement of cerebral blood flow using heat as an indicator. Meyer and Gotoh (1964) described a thermovelocity method for the measurement of flow within the internal jugular vein, while others (Gibbs, 1933; Carlyle and Grayson, 1956) have applied heat directly to the cortical surface and deduce blood flow from heat clearance. Calibration of the instruments to provide quantitative information is difficult, and with the tissue probes, proximity to large vessels can produce non-linearity between heat clearance and tissue blood flow.

Other methods which have been used include dye-dilution techniques with Evans Blue (Gibbs *et al.*, 1947*b*; Shenkin *et al.*, 1948), isotopically labelled red cells instead of dye (Nylin and Blömer, 1955; Nylin *et al.*, 1960), impedance plethysmography (Jenkner, 1962) and direct measurements on exposed vessels during surgery (Kristiansen and Krog, 1962).

Normal Values and Physiological Variation in Cerebral Blood Flow

Cerebral blood flow measured by the nitrous oxide technique is 50–55 ml./100 g./minute in normal adults, indicating a total cerebral flow of approximately 750 ml./minute (Kety and Schmidt, 1948*a*). The flow rate is greater in the first decade of life, falling at puberty towards the adult values (Kennedy and Sokoloff, 1957). Although most evidence suggests that cerebral blood flow tends to fall from middle age onwards (Shenkin *et al.*, 1953), this does not necessarily occur (Sokoloff, 1959*a*). Sleep, exercise, mental arithmetic and a raised body temperature cause no change in total cerebral blood flow which cannot be attributed to simultaneous changes in arterial carbon dioxide tension (Lambertsen *et al.*, 1959; Hedlund *et al.*, 1962; Mangold *et al.*, 1955; Sokoloff *et al.*, 1955; Heyman, *et al.* 1950). There is however evidence of regional variation in flow with alterations of cerebral activity (Sokoloff and Kety, 1960).

Factors Controlling Cerebral Blood Flow

The Munro-Kellie doctrine of 1783 postulated that because the nearly incompressible brain is housed within a rigid cranium, the quantity of blood in the cerebral circulation will remain constant and flow through it will respond passively to changes in arterial pressure. In 1890, Roy and Sherrington suggested that in addition to the effects of the systemic arterial pressure, the calibre of the cerebral vessels could vary in response to chemical changes in their environment, and it is now accepted that intrinsic regulation of the cerebrovascular resistance is the most important determinant of cerebral blood flow under normal conditions (Sokoloff and Kety, 1960). The many factors which can influence cerebral blood flow do so either by altering the pressure gradient across the vessels, or by changing the resistance within them.

1. Factors Affecting the Pressure Gradient Across the Cerebral Vessels

(a) Arterial blood pressure.—In the absence of hypotension, the systemic blood pressure is believed to play little part in the regulation of the cerebral blood flow, and until the blood pressure is less than 60–70 mm. Hg the cerebral blood flow is maintained (Finnerty *et al.*, 1954). This autoregulation of cerebral flow in response to changes in arterial pressure has been demonstrated by a variety of techniques and over a wide range of both high and low abnormal pressures, spontaneous and induced (Lassen, 1959). However, the autoregulatory response is abolished by elevation of the arterial carbon dioxide tension (Harper and Glass, 1965) and by deep anaesthesia, extensive surgery, arterial hypoxaemia and circulatory arrest (*Lancet*, 1968). A transitory failure of autoregulation can also follow sudden changes in pressure (Schneider, 1963).

The mechanism of autoregulatory control of the cerebral vessels is obscure—Bayliss (1902) postulated a direct effect of pressure on the musculature of the blood vessels whereas Lassen (1959) suggests that the tissue carbon dioxide tension is the regulating factor. The existence of conditions under which the mechanism fails may explain the discrepancy between some reports of the effect of arterial pressure on cerebral blood flow, and also provides a warning that only moderate hypotension occurring during some of the circumstances met in clinical anaesthesia may endanger cerebral perfusion. In addition, it is important to recall that the critical pressure at which autoregulation begins to fail even in the conscious subject may well be higher in the elderly and arteriosclerotic, and Bromage (1953) has produced electroencephalographic evidence in support of this.

(b) Venous pressure.—The effect of the pressure in the great veins is normally insignificant even in heart failure (Novak *et al.*, 1953) but when coughing or straining or during occlusion of the great veins, much higher pressures may be reached. Moyer *et al* (1954) demonstrated no change in cerebral blood flow when the internal jugular venous pressure of man was elevated to 23 cm. of water, and Jacobson *et al.* (1963*a*) have produced evidence to suggest that autoregulation of cerebral blood flow can occur in response to changes in venous pressure.

2. Factors Affecting the Cerebrovascular Resistance

(a) Chemical control.—Arterial carbon dioxide tension is the most important single factor controlling cerebral blood flow. The inhalation of 7 per cent CO_2 increases cerebral blood flow by 100 per cent while overventilation to an arterial CO_2 tension of 26 mm. Hg reduces cerebral blood flow by 35 per cent (Kety and Schmidt, 1948*b*). However these changes in flow are not accompanied by any alteration in cerebral oxygen consumption, arteriovenous oxygen difference changing reciprocally with alterations in cerebral blood flow. Although Patterson *et al.* (1955) reported a threshold for the increase in cerebral blood flow on the administration of carbon dioxide, this was not observed by Harper and Glass (1965). The latter authors also reported that in anaesthetised, normotensive dogs, maximum change in cerebral blood flow is produced by varying the arterial carbon dioxide tension between 20 and 90 mm. Hg. Beyond these limits, changes in carbon dioxide tension produce no further change in cerebral blood flow. Harper and Glass also demonstrated that the response to carbon dioxide is diminished in the presence of hypotension and abolished when the systemic blood pressure reaches 50 mm. Hg. Similarly, Lennox and Gibbs (1932) showed that the response of the cerebral blood flow to carbon dioxide is diminished in the presence of arterial hypoxaemia.

The effect of carbon dioxide on cerebral flow is not mediated by changes in arterial pressure or pH and is unaltered by spinal transection, decerebration or cervical sympathectomy (Schieve and Wilson, 1953; Lambertsen *et al.*, 1961; Wolff, 1936). A direct action on the smooth muscle of the vessel wall seems the most probable mechanism, possibly mediated by pH changes in the surrounding tissue fluids (Lassen, 1966).

Although alterations in arterial pH have been claimed to alter cerebral blood flow, alkalosis producing constriction and acidosis dilatation of cerebral vessels, Harper and Bell (1963) showed no change in regional cerebral blood flow in dogs when the arterial carbon dioxide tension was held constant during infusions of sodium bicarbonate and lactic acid. There is undoubtedly an increase in cerebral blood flow in severe diabetic ketosis (Kety *et al.*, 1948*d*) but in experimental acidosis (Schieve and Wilson, 1953) and in diabetic ketosis short of coma, cerebral vasoconstriction due to secondary hyperventilation predominates so that cerebral blood flow is low.

The effects of changes in arterial oxygen tension on cerebral blood flow are opposite to those produced by carbon dioxide. The inhalation of 10 per cent oxygen causes a 35 per cent increase in cerebral blood flow (Kety and Schmidt, 1948*b*) and this occurs even if the carbon dioxide tension is held constant (Turner *et al.*, 1957). Although the overall oxygen consumption of the brain is unaltered, symptoms of hypoxia occur suggesting regional inadequacy. However Harper, McDowall and Jacobson could demonstrate no diminution in cortical flow in dogs until the arterial Po_2 had reached 40 mm. Hg (Harper, 1965).

Higher than normal arterial oxygen tensions, including oxygen under increased pressure, cause a diminution in cerebral blood flow which is partly mediated by a concomitant fall in arterial CO_2 tension (Lambertsen *et al.*, 1953; Turner *et al.*, 1957; Jacobson, Harper and McDowall, 1963*b*). In 1965, Harper, McDowall and Ledingham showed that in hypotensive dogs, there was no change in cortical blood flow with the administration of oxygen under pressure but oxygen uptake was restored to normal.

(b) Neurogenic control.—In spite of evidence to the contrary in certain animals (Forbes *et al.*, 1939; Schmidt, 1944), there is no evidence in man of direct action of the autonomic nervous system on the cerebral blood vessels (Harmel *et al.*, 1949; Sokoloff and Kety, 1960). This statement is difficult to reconcile with the arteriographic appearance of "spasm" of cerebral vessels after emboli (Ecker and Riemenschneider, 1951) and although this has been attributed to multiple thromboses (Fisher and Cameron, 1953) or hypotension in critically narrowed vessels (Eastcott *et al.*, 1954), it could also represent local changes in vessel calibre which are so compensated that overall flow is unaltered. Such a mechanism could be mediated by the local release from brain cells of vaso-active materials which are known to be stored in some parts of the brain (Schmidt, 1960).

(c) Intracranial pressure.—At pressures up to about 500 mm. water, increases of intracranial pressure produce no change in cerebral blood flow because of the associated increase in arterial pressure. Above this level there is a considerable fall in the cerebral circulation (Kety *et al.*, 1948*c*).

(d) Viscosity.—Cerebral blood flow was found by Kety (1950) to be less than half normal in polycythaemia and it can be significantly increased in severe anaemia (Robin and Gardner, 1953).

Effects of Drugs on the Cerebral Circulation

Many of the conflicting reports on the effects of drugs on cerebrovascular resistance and some of the variations in response are attributable to choice of species or the dose and route of administration. Thus aminophylline in man causes cerebral vasoconstriction, the effect of the falling carbon dioxide tension predominating over the direct vasodilator effect seen in other species (Wechsler *et al.*, 1950; Shenkin, 1951). Adrenaline given intravenously in doses which raise the mean arterial pressure by 20 per cent causes an increase in cerebral blood flow, whereas with noradrenaline the vasoconstrictor effect predominates and the cerebral blood flow falls in spite of the rise in blood pressure (King *et al.*, 1952). A review of the effects of drugs on the cerebral circulation is given by Sokoloff (1959*b*) and of the effects of anaesthetic drugs by McDowall (1965)—see Table 1. McDowall points out the many ways in which changes induced by anaesthetic drugs may affect the cerebral circulation, and emphasises the difficulty of attributing observed changes in cerebral blood flow to the direct action of the anaesthetic drugs. However the effects of barbiturates can be

22/Table 1

Effects of General Anaesthetic Drugs on Cerebral Blood Flow

Agent	*Cerebral blood flow*	*Cerebral metabolic rate*	*Cerebrovascular response to* CO_2
Barbiturates	↓	↓ ++ proportional to depth of GA	unchanged
Ether	↑	↓ +	unchanged
Chloroform	↑	↓ +	unchanged
Trilene	no change	↓ +	unchanged
Halothane	probably ↑	↓ +	unchanged

(Derived from McDowall, 1965)

shown to differ from those of the volatile anaesthetic agents. The barbiturates cause a reduction in cerebral metabolic rate and blood flow proportional to the depth of anaesthesia so that the tensions of oxygen and carbon dioxide in cerebral venous blood are unaltered. It has also been shown (Landau *et al.*, 1955) that the inequalities of regional cortical blood flow in conscious cats are greatly decreased during light thiopentone anaesthesia, this levelling out being due mainly to selective decrease in those areas with the greatest flow in the conscious state. The volatile agents produce little decrease in oxygen uptake, and cerebral blood flow is either unaltered or increased. With both volatile and non-volatile agents the cerebrovascular responses to changes in arterial P_{CO_2} are unaltered.

EFFECTS OF HYPOTHERMIA

Both cerebral blood flow and cerebral metabolic rate fall in dogs with decrease in body temperature (Rosomoff and Holaday, 1954; Kleinerman and Hopkins, 1955). Rosomoff (1956) showed a diminution in cerebral blood flow in dogs of 6–7 per cent for each degree centigrade fall in temperature. At a temperature of 28° C, a fall in cerebral blood flow of 50 per cent was recorded and Kleinerman and Hopkins reported that at temperatures between 22 and 27° C the reduction in cerebral blood flow exceeded the diminution of cerebral oxygen consumption. Albert and Fazekas (1956) reported five cases of induced hypothermia in man; in two of these the diminution in cerebral blood flow exceeded the decrease in cerebral metabolic rate. However, Rosomoff and Holaday reported a parallel reduction in both metabolic rate and blood flow in dogs cooled to 26° C and in clinical practice the technique is widely and successfully used to prevent cerebral damage during procedures which may jeopardise cerebral blood flow.

HYPERVENTILATION AND ANAESTHESIA

Hyperventilation raises the pain threshold in conscious volunteers and appears to reduce requirements for central depressant drugs during anaesthesia. It has been shown that hypocapnia does not alter anaesthetic requirements in man (Bridges and Eger, 1966) and greater depth of anaesthesia during hyperventilation may be due to the higher alveolar tension of anaesthetic agent which develops when increased ventilation occurs at constant inspired concentration (Eger *et al.*, 1965). There is conflicting evidence on the possible occurrence of cerebral hypoxia secondary to cerebral vasoconstriction and shift of the oxygen dissociation curve due to a low arterial carbon dioxide tension (Clutton-Brock, 1957; Sugioka and Davis, 1960; Robinson and Gray, 1961; Allen and Morris, 1962; Pierce *et al.*, 1962; Bollen, 1962; Wollman *et al.*, 1965). Many of these authors support the view that mild degrees of cerebral hypoxia can be produced by hyperventilation, but despite this theoretical disadvantage there is no clinical evidence that moderate hyperventilation of the anaesthetised patient produces cerebral damage and the benefits of controlled respiration, circulatory stability and minimal central depression have made the technique widely popular. Full arterial saturation throughout is obviously essential to minimise any possible hypoxic hazard.

Value of Hyperventilation in Neurosurgery

Although it is sometimes claimed that hyperventilation can "shrink" the normal brain, Rosomoff (1963) showed in dogs that hyperventilation does not reduce the volume of the brain tissue and that intracranial pressure is unaffected provided the carbon dioxide tension is normal before the onset of increased ventilation. The spontaneously breathing, anaesthetised patient is almost always underventilating to some extent so that controlled ventilation is likely to provide better and safer operating conditions. Likewise in head injuries or patients with cerebral oedema, controlled ventilation with a guaranteed airway may be more satisfactory than possibly inadequate spontaneous respiration and an airway jeopardised by coma. Recently (Lassen, 1966; *Lancet*, 1968) it has been suggested that definite benefit may be gained from hyperventilation in cases of cerebral injury. Lassen uses the term "luxury perfusion syndrome" to describe the increase in cerebral blood flow which occurs after a local cerebral anoxic episode. Unlike reactive hyperaemia seen elsewhere after ischaemia, luxury perfusion lasts longer and oxygen uptake of the affected tissue is diminished. The vasomotor paralysis appears complete in that there is no vascular response to changes in P_{CO_2}, blood pressure or aminophylline in the area involved, and Lassen suggests this may be due to acute metabolic acidosis localised within the damaged brain tissue. Under these circumstances, a raised arterial carbon dioxide tension may give an intra-cerebral "steal" effect by causing vasodilatation in the normal cerebral vessels and thereby lowering the perfusion pressure in the pressure-passive area of the lesion; conversely, a low arterial P_{CO_2} induced by hyperventilation will produce cerebral vasoconstriction in areas capable of responding to this stimulus, and this will tend to promote blood flow into the area of the lesion.

If the cerebral vessels in the damaged area react in this passive manner, the possible hypoxic risks occasioned by hypocapnia discussed above cannot operate in the already damaged area, so that the evidence at present suggests that moderate hyperventilation is of benefit to those with an anoxic cerebral insult (Alexander and Lassen, 1970).

CEREBRAL METABOLISM

Measurements of overall cerebral metabolism depend on the determination of cerebral arteriovenous differences and total blood flow. The venous sample is drawn from the superior jugular bulb in man (Myerson *et al.*, 1927) and this provides blood which is almost exclusively representative of cerebral activity.

The brain is unique in that it relies entirely on carbohydrate utilisation and under normal circumstances the oxidation of glucose to carbon dioxide and water is the only energy-producing mechanism which can be demonstrated *in vivo*. Small quantities of lactate and pyruvate may also be formed (Himwich and Himwich, 1946) and during hypoxia, lactate production is considerably increased (McGinty, 1929). The oxygen consumption of the brain is normally high (3·5 ml./100 g./minute) and is independent of cerebral blood flow, there being no diminution in oxygen consumption until cerebral flow has been reduced to 60 per cent by hypotension (Finnerty *et al.*, 1954).

Available stores of glucose and oxygen in the brain are so small that an uninterrupted circulatory supply is essential—oxygen deprivation by total circulatory arrest causes loss of consciousness in ten seconds (Rossen *et al.*, 1943) and hypoglycaemia produces all degrees of functional disturbance progressing to coma, the degree of hypoglycaemia correlating well with the level of impairment (Kety *et al.*, 1948*e*).

Relationship to Functional Activity

Physiological variations of cerebral activity produce no change in the overall metabolic rate or cerebral blood flow (Mangold *et al.*, 1955; Sokoloff *et al.*, 1955), but regional variations in flow induced by changes in cerebral activity may well account for this (Landau *et al.*, 1955; Sokoloff, 1957). It is also possible to correlate depression of mental activity in a variety of pathological conditions affecting consciousness with cerebral metabolic rate (Fazekas and Bessman, 1953; Kety, 1950; Freyhan *et al.*, 1951).

Changes in Pathological Conditions

Circulatory deficiency rapidly causes irreversible metabolic changes as witnessed by prolonged unconsciousness and a lowered cerebral oxygen consumption even after cerebral blood flow has been restored (Fazekas and Bessman, 1953). Lesser degrees of anoxia cause an increase in glycolysis and depletion of energy-rich phosphate compounds together with an increased production of lactic acid (Gurdjian *et al.*, 1944). Young animals have a greater capacity for withstanding cerebral anoxia without harm because of prolonged retention of the foetal ability to metabolise anaerobically (Himwich, 1951).

During hypoglycaemic coma, a persistent low level of oxygen consumption together with a respiratory quotient which is still unity suggests that other carbohydrate stores can be utilised slowly (Kety *et al.*, 1948*e*). When these are exhausted, hypoglycaemic coma becomes irreversible and as with prolonged anoxic damage, coma and a low oxygen consumption persist even when higher than normal blood sugar levels have been restored (Fazekas *et al.*, 1951).

THEORIES OF ANAESTHESIA

Anaesthesia may be defined as a progressive reversible depression of nervous tissue, or more simply as the controlled production of unconsciousness.

There is no simple theory explaining the mechanism of the anaesthetic state, nor any means of predicting which substances will produce anaesthesia. In addition to the well known chemical agents, apparently unrelated factors such as cold, hypoxia, hypercarbia, bromine and magnesium, the rare gases and the passage of an electric current through the brain can all produce reversible unconsciousness.

Anaesthetic agents have no chemical specificity and many of them are not metabolised in the body and can be recovered practically *in toto*. For many substances, anaesthetic potency is related to vapour pressure, oil/water partition coefficient, surface activity (i.e. the ability to lower surface tension) and water solubility, and all these depend on the thermodynamic activity of the molecule. The following theories have been based on physical or chemical properties of the anaesthetic agents.

Colloid Theory

In 1875 Claude Bernard suggested that anaesthetic agents produced a modification of the cell protoplasm and this he called coagulation. Bancroft and Richter (1931) elaborated the theory and noted that the Brownian movement which could be seen in yeast cells with the ultra-microscope diminished during narcosis with chloroform, ether and chloral hydrate and returned during recovery, along with the ability of cells to ferment carbohydrate and to multiply.

In 1950 Seifriz revived this theory and called the protein change gelatinization which is reversible, as opposed to coagulation which is regarded as irreversible. His observations were made on the streaming of protoplasm in slime mould and were conducted using various agents to produce this change.

Lipid Theory

In 1899 and 1901 Meyer and, independently, Overton advanced a theory which has become known as the Meyer-Overton law. This states that there is a direct relationship between the affinity of the anaesthetic for lipid and its depressant action, in other words the higher the oil/water partition coefficient, the more powerful the anaesthetic.

The theory arose from the observation that when a series of chemical substances are arranged in the order of the oil/water coefficient it is found that with a few exceptions they are in the order of anaesthetic potency. Despite the apparent attractions of this theory, there are six possible objections. First, the measurements on which it rests were made using vegetable lipids and water, not animal lipids and body fluids; secondly a number of anaesthetics do not fit into the pattern; thirdly, it does not apply to the alkaloids or the inorganic ions; fourthly, many organic compounds having similar oil/water coefficients to those of powerful anaesthetic agents have no anaesthetic potency; fifthly different stereo-isomers with the same oil/water coefficient have different actions on the brain and sixthly, one cannot predict whether any given substance has anaesthetic properties from the ratio. Although possibly accounting for the affinity of the substances for the cells and their membranes, this theory does not explain the mechanism of their action.

Wulf and Featherstone (1957) suggest that van der Waal's constants agree better with anaesthetic potency than other physical properties of the substances It must be remembered however that merely arranging a series of related compounds in a particular order due to one property, probably automatically ensures a similar relationship to some other and different property (Butler, 1950).

Surface Tension or Adsorption Theory

This theory equates the potency of anaesthetics with their ability to lower surface tension. It is assumed that the presence of the substances in the cell membrane alters its function in some way and disturbs the metabolic processes of the cell, but as with the previous theories it does not fully explain anaesthetic action. Many substances lower surface tension and are not anaesthetics and many anaesthetics do not lower surface tension.

Cell Permeability Theory

This is an elaboration of the surface tension theory and postulates that once the anaesthetic agent is adsorbed, it causes a decrease in the permeability of the cells of the central nervous system. It has been shown that stimulation of nerve cells has the opposite effect, and these changes may be mediated by an alteration in the state of the lipids of the cell membrane.

Inhibition of Oxidation

As a result of *in vitro* studies using cortical brain slices, Quastel (1952) has suggested that depression of oxidation is the mechanism by which the anaesthetic state is produced, but many drugs which produce stimulation of the brain also decrease oxygen uptake by nerve cells. The criteria necessary before inhibition of oxidation can be said to cause the effect of the drug have been described by

Butler (1950). McIlwain (1959) has demonstrated that anaesthetics depress the uptake of oxygen by active cells but have no effect on the basal oxygen consumption.

Electrical Theory

The observed decrease in negative potential of the cerebral cortex and the lessened conductivity of impulses through the cerebrospinal axis when the nervous system is depressed by drugs have been postulated as the cause of the anaesthetic state (French *et al.*, 1953). However this is merely descriptive of the changes in electrical activity which occur and provides no explanation of their cause.

Pauling (1964) postulated that narcosis caused by non-hydrogen bonding substances was due to an increase in the impedence of the neuronal network rather than a decrease in the activity of the exciting mechanism. The increase in impedance is said to occur mainly in the synaptic regions because of the formation of hydrate microcrystals in the fluid of the brain. The microcrystals become attached to some of the electrically charged side-chain groups of proteins and also trap some of the ions, thus interfering with their mobility and with their contribution to the electrical oscillations.

More recently, attention has been focused on the properties of the central nervous system and the mechanisms of sleep and arousal (Eccles, 1953; Feldberg, 1959; Buxton Hopkins, 1961; Dunkin, 1965). It seems likely that until this aspect of neuro-physiology can be more clearly elucidated the processes by which the anaesthetic state is produced will remain largely obscure.

ELECTRO-ENCEPHALOGRAPHY

The electroencephalogram (EEG) is conveniently recorded from multiple symmetrically paired electrodes placed on the skull, although monitoring during anaesthesia is commonly performed with only two electrodes (frontal and occipital). A number of extraneous signals may interfere with the recording of these very small potentials (tens of microvolts only); excessive sweating, eye movements and contraction of scalp or limb muscles can all produce artefacts, and arterial or venous pulses, respiratory changes and the electrocardiogram can be superimposed on the EEG, particularly if the electrodes or earth lead are poorly applied or incorrectly sited. Proximity to other apparatus frequently causes interference and it may be necessary to perform the recording in a screened room.

Normal Activity

A wide variety of patterns may be recorded from normal individuals and the following wave forms have been recognised.

Delta waves, 0·5–3·5 c./sec., occur in infants and sleeping adults with an amplitude of about 100 microvolts. They are largest in the frontal lobes, symmetrical but asynchronous.

Theta waves, 4–7 c./sec., occur in children with an amplitude of 50 microvolts and in adults with an amplitude of 10 microvolts. They are diffuse in children but become localised to the parietal and temporal regions in adults.

Alpha waves, 8–13 c./sec., occur in infants with an amplitude of 20 microvolts, in children with an amplitude of 75 microvolts and in adults with an amplitude of 50 microvolts. These, like the theta rhythms, are diffuse in children but become localised to the parietal and occipital areas in adults. They are symmetrical and synchronous. The alpha waves are augmented by closing the eyes and during mental repose, and are reduced by visual and mental activity, sometimes to the extent of total removal or "blocking".

Beta waves, 14–15 c./sec., of about 20 microvolts, usually occur in the fronto-central areas in children and are symmetrical and asychronous.

Gamma waves, 26 or more c./sec., usually have an amplitude of 10 microvolts and are rare in normal subjects.

Some Abnormal Patterns

It is very rare to obtain a record of a major convulsive seizure free from artefact but minor seizures are frequently well recorded, especially when a stimulus such as over-breathing is used (Fig. 2–*4*). Seizures produced in this way are often less severe than those usually suffered by the patient and are called "larval". About 50 per cent of people subject to "fits" have an "abnormal" EEG record between attacks—that is they show patterns which are never seen in normal subjects (Fig. 2–*5*). Hysterical fits do not affect the EEG.

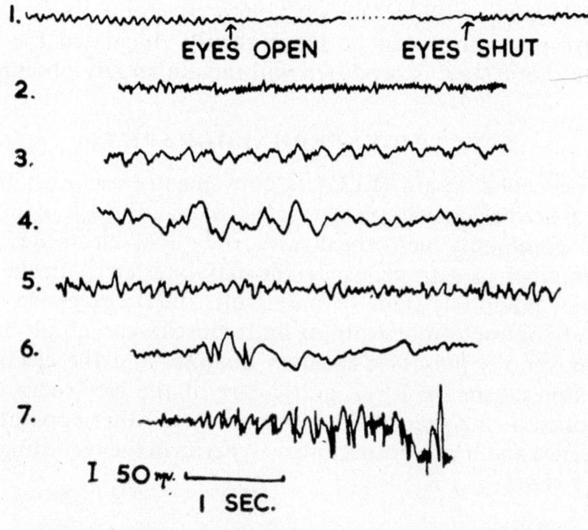

22/Fig. 2.—Some Electro-encephalographic Patterns

1. Normal *alpha* rhythm showing effect of opening the eyes; 2. Normal fast activity; 3. Normal slow activity; 4. Slow activity in a child of 10 produced by hyperventilation; 5. Typical inter-seizure record; 6. Wave and spike activity; 7. Pre-convulsion trace.

As the disturbances arise in differing parts of the brain, the pattern of the electro-encephalogram will vary from lead to lead. A minor seizure pattern is characterised by "wave and spike" activity containing a very large component up to 1 millivolt at a frequency from 1·5 to 3·5 c./sec. (Fig. 2–*6*). The spike component lasts from 0·02 second up to 0·1 second. In organic diseases the relationship between the spike and wave varies from moment to moment.

The pattern of a major convulsion appears to be an all-or-none phenomenon and it is not much altered by drugs. The pattern depends on the site of onset and route of spread of the electrical disturbance but is symmetrical and synchronous when it is fully developed. It starts to alter thirty seconds or so before the onset of the convulsion is manifest, as shown by rhythms of 2–7 c./sec. which increase in amplitude and are most prominent in the pre-motor regions (Fig. 2–7). The tonic stage of the convulsion is characterised by the abrupt onset of spikes of moderate amplitude. The spikes then become "grouped" and there is a slow component at 1·5–3 c./sec. which bears a constant time relationship to the groups of spikes. Towards the end of the convulsion, the spikes occur only in synchronised groups on the crest of a rhythmic slow wave. The frequency of this wave slows to 1 c./sec. with no decline in amplitude, and then it suddenly ceases. After the convulsion there is random slow activity with an occasional spike which is followed by the gradual reappearance of the normal pattern.

The Effect of Anaesthetic Drugs on the Electro-encephalogram

It is difficult to correlate the classical Guedel signs of anaesthesia with changes in the EEG and there is some variation in the changes which are produced by different anaesthetic agents. Sadove and his colleagues (1967) state as a broad outline that the following changes occur. When there is only slight mental impairment with mild analgesia and amnesia, low voltage fast activity is increased and the record resembles the normal "attention" trace. With the onset of light anaesthesia, fast activity of high voltage predominates. Slowing of the electrical activity occurs with deepening of the anaesthetic, followed by brief periods of inactivity and finally, total electrical silence. The stage of brief periods of inactivity may be reached transitorily after a rapid intravenous induction.

Common sedatives (barbiturates, chloral hydrate and paraldehyde) can produce variable changes in the EEG but there is no correlation with the clinical effect of the drug. All sedatives producing sleep, even those used clinically as anticonvulsants, tend to activate seizure discharges in epileptic or predisposed persons (Gibbs *et al.*, 1947*a*). Atropine, pethidine and morphine used in conventional doses produce no change in the EEG and curare likewise has no effect provided respiration is controlled (Kiersey *et al.*, 1951). Spinal anaesthesia produces no change in the EEG although coincidental sleep or sedation may have some effect on the record.

Effects of Hypoxia

Slowing of the wave frequency of the EEG is the most characteristic change associated with hypoxia, but cerebral venous oxygen tensions of 18 mm. Hg may be reached before there is any alteration of the record. An initial increase of frequency and amplitude lasting 1 to 2 seconds occurs sometimes with the onset of sudden and complete anoxia. By ten seconds there is slow cortical activity of 1 to 3 cycles per second which becomes slower and of greater amplitude. When it reaches 1 cycle per second the amplitude decreases so that by 18 to 20 seconds after complete anoxia, the EEG becomes a straight line. If hypoxia is rapidly relieved the EEG returns to normal in the reverse order, but changes may persist long after the oxygen tension has been restored to normal if the period of hypoxia was prolonged. Following a long period of hypoxia, a flat trace with superimposed low voltage (5 microvolts), fast (50 c./sec.), spiky activity may occur (Gronquist *et al.* 1952). This is known as "file pattern" and carries a poor prognosis.

It has been suggested that the EEG may be used to identify "cerebral death" in patients requiring support of cardiorespiratory function, and Hockaday *et al.* (1965) were able to predict with considerable accuracy from the EEG whether anoxic damage following cardiac or respiratory arrest would prove fatal or non-fatal. However Haider *et al.* (1968) have reported survival with complete normality in patients with a persistently flat EEG for many hours after barbiturate intoxication and it must therefore be realised that the EEG alone is insufficient evidence on which to decide whether supportive therapy should be continued or withdrawn from a patient with severe cerebral damage. Serial recordings, considered in conjunction with clinical assessment of the function of the central nervous and other systems and the aetiology of the condition, may be of some value in making these individual and difficult decisions.

Effects of Hypercapnia

Moderate increases in carbon dioxide tension (5 per cent inspired CO_2) cause an increase in frequency of cortical activity. Greater increases (more than 10 per cent CO_2) reverse this acceleration and slow waves appear (Sadove *et al.*, 1967). High carbon dioxide tensions also potentiate the effects of barbiturates and other anaesthetic drugs (Clowes *et al.*, 1953).

Effects of Hypocapnia

Voluntary hyperventilation in man produces high voltage slow waves in the EEG which Brazier (1943) concluded are due to the direct effect of a low P_{CO_2} and are not secondary to hypoxia due to cerebral vasoconstriction. Holmberg (1953) however found that voluntary hyperventilation with oxygen produced less alteration in brain potentials than voluntary hyperventilation with air, and Bollen (1962) considered that the slow wave activity and accompanying analgesia of hyperventilation were indicative of mild cerebral hypoxia. The relevance of this clinical practice is discussed in the section on hyperventilation and anaesthesia.

Effects of Hypotension

The electro-encephalographic pattern during hypotension depends not only on the level of blood pressure but also on the rate of fall to that level. At a rate of under 10 mm./Hg minute, a fall of 100 mm. Hg in a hypertensive patient produced no electro-encephalographic change (Bromage, 1953), whereas a rapid but smaller decrease in blood pressure can produce slow, high amplitude waves or even temporary cessation of cortical activity (Fig. 3). These effects may be due to delay in the response of the cerebral blood vessels to sudden changes in blood pressure.

Effects of Hypothermia

Little change occurs in the EEG until the temperature has fallen to 35–31° C when some decrease in amplitude and frequency takes place. At 25° C the ampli-

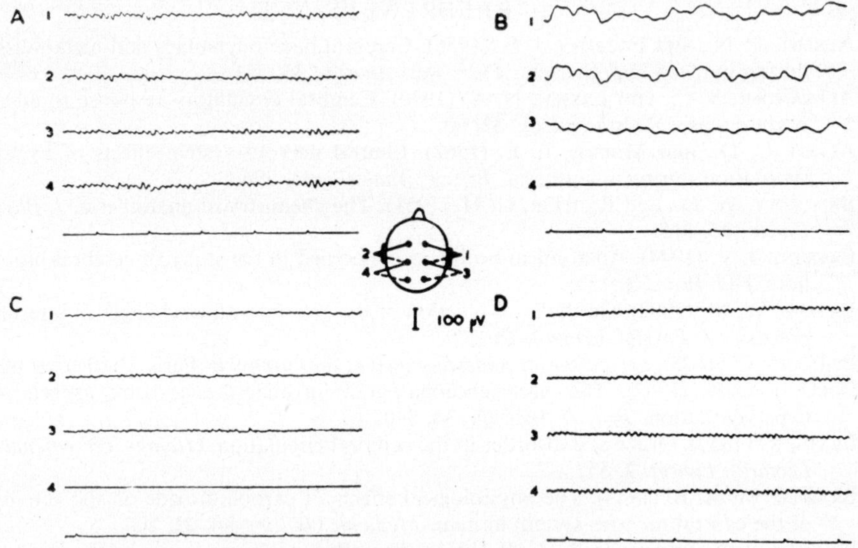

22/FIG. 3.—THE EFFECTS OF HYPOTENSION ON THE ELECTRO-ENCEPHALOGRAM

EEG records of normal man, aged 38.
Time marker: 1 second intervals.
A—Normal resting rhythm of 9 c/s. B.P. 130/80.
B—During acute fall of B.P. to unrecordable levels, after 100 mg. C5 and 45 degrees foot-down tilt. Subject unconscious.
C—One minute after B, 10 degrees head-down. B.P. 40/? Consciousness returning.
D—Four minutes after C. B.P. 105/70. Conscious. Normal α-rhythm.

tude is further decreased and at 20° C there is no appreciable activity in either parietal or occipital regions, and only a very low amplitude wave remains at 2 cycles per second in the frontal regions. Prolonged maintenance at low temperatures produces no further alterations. With rewarming the changes occur in the reverse order but at one or two degrees higher than on cooling and there are no permanent changes (Wilson, 1957).

The effect of circulatory arrest in the hypothermic patient is to produce a flat record but this appears more slowly than would be the case at normal temperatures. "File pattern" low voltage fast activity may be seen in these circumstances, but it is not of grave significance (Pearcy and Virtue, 1959).

Effects of Surgery and Cardiopulmonary By-pass

Studies before and after major surgery show that in a high percentage of cases, changes are produced which generally last for two or three days but which can persist for up to two weeks (Sadove *et al.*, 1967). During cardiopulmonary by-pass, transitory slowing of the EEG may occur with the onset of perfusion, possibly due to differences in temperature, chemistry or drug content of the blood in the apparatus, but subsequently the EEG may be used to monitor the adequacy of cerebral perfusion.

REFERENCES

ALBERT, F. N., and FAZEKAS, J. F. (1956). Cerebral haemodynamics and metabolism during induced hypothermia. *Curr. Res. Anesth.*, **35,** 381.

ALEXANDER, S. C., and LASSEN, N. A. (1970). Cerebral circulatory response to acute brain disease. *Anesthesiology* **32,** 60.

ALLEN, C. D., and MORRIS, L. E. (1962). Central nervous system effects of hyperventilation during anaesthesia. *Brit. J. Anaesth.*, **34,** 296.

BANCROFT, W. D., and RICHTER, G. H. (1931). The chemistry of anaesthesia. *J. Phys. Chem.*, **35,** 215.

BATSON, O. V. (1944). Anatomical problems concerned in the study of cerebral blood flow. *Fed. Proc.*, **3,** 139.

BAYLISS, W. M. (1902). On the local reaction of the arterial wall to changes of internal pressure. *J. Physiol.* (*Lond.*), **28,** 220.

BERNARD, C. (1875). *Leçons sur les Anaesthesiques et sur l'asphyxie*. Paris: Baillière et fils.

BOLLEN, A. R. (1962). The electroencephalogram in anaesthesia; some aspects of hyperventilation. *Brit. J. Anaesth.*, **34,** 890.

BRAIN, R. (1957). Order and disorder in the cerebral circulation. (*Harvey Tercentenary Lecture*). *Lancet*, **2,** 857.

BRAZIER, M. A. B. (1943). The physiological effects of carbon dioxide on the activity of the central nervous system in man. *Medicine* (*Baltimore*), **22,** 205.

BRIDGES, B. E., and EGER, E. I., II (1966). The effect of hypocapnia on the level of halothane anaesthesia in man. *Anaesthesiology*, **27,** 634.

BROMAGE, P. R. (1953). Some electro-encephalographic changes associated with induced vascular hypotension. *Proc. roy. Soc. Med.*, **46,** 919.

BUTLER, T. C. (1950). Theories of general anaesthesia. *Pharmacol Rev.*, **2,** 121.

BUXTON HOPKINS, D. A. (1961). Some suggestions for the neural basis of the anaesthetic state. *Brit. J. Anaesth.*, **33,** 114.

CARLYLE, A., and GRAYSON, J. (1956). Factors involved in the control of cerebral blood flow. *J. Physiol.* (*Lond.*), **133,** 10.

CLOWES, G. H. A., KRETCHMER, H. E., MCBURNEY, R. W., and SIMEONE, F. A. (1953). Electroencephalogram in evaluation of effects of anaesthetic agents and carbon dioxide accumulation during surgery. *Ann. Surg.*, **138,** 558.

CLUTTON-BROCK, J. (1957). The cerebral effects of over-ventilation. *Brit. J. Anaesth.*, **29,** 111.

DUNKIN, L. J. (1965). Mechanisms of anaesthetic sleep. *Anaesthesia*, **20,** 157.

EASTCOTT, H. H. G., PICKERING, G. W., and ROB, C. G. (1954). Reconstruction of the internal carotid artery. *Lancet*, **2,** 994.

ECCLES, J. C. (1953). *The Neurophysiological Basis of Mind.* Oxford: Clarendon Press.

ECKER, A., and RIEMENSCHNEIDER, P. A. (1951). Arteriographic demonstration of spasm of intracranial arteries with special reference to saccular arterial aneurysms. *J. Neurosurg.*, **8,** 660.

EGER, E. I., II, SAIDMAN, L. J., and BRANDSTATER, B. (1965). Minimum alveolar anaesthetic concentration: a standard of anaesthetic potency. *Anesthesiology*, **26,** 756.

FAZEKAS, J. F., ALMAN, R. W., and PARRISH, A. E. (1951). Irreversible post-hypoglycaemic coma. *Amer. J. med. Sci.*, **222,** 640.

FAZEKAS, J. F., and BESSMAN, A. N. (1953). Coma mechanisms. *Amer. J. Med.*, **15,** 804.

FELDBERG, W. (1959). A physiological approach to the problems of general anaesthesia and unconsciousness. *Brit. med. J.*, **2,** 771.

FINNERTY, F. A., WITKIN, L., and FAZEKAS, J. F. (1954). Cerebral haemodynamics during cerebral ischaemia induced by acute hypotension. *J. clin. Invest.*, **33,** 1227.

FISHER, M., and CAMERON, D. G. (1953). Concerning cerebral vasospasm. *Neurology (Minneap.)*, **3,** 468.

FORBES, H. W., SCHMIDT, C. F., and MASON, G. I. (1939). Evidence of vasodilator innervation in the parietal cortex of the cat. *Amer. J. Physiol.*, **125,** 216.

FRENCH, J. D., VERZEANO, M., and MAGOUN, H. W. (1953). A neural basis of the anaesthetic state. *Arch. Neurol. Psychiat. (Chic.)*, **69,** 519.

FREYHAN, F. A., WOODFORD, R. B., and KETY, S. S. (1951). Cerebral blood flow and metabolism in psychoses of senility. *J. nerv. ment. Dis.*, **113,** 449.

GIBBS, F. A. (1933). A thermo-electric blood flow recorder in the form of a needle. *Proc. Soc. exp. Biol. (N.Y.)*, **31,** 141.

GIBBS, F. A., GIBBS, E. L., and FUSTER, B. (1947*a*). Anterior temporal localisation of sleep induced seizure discharges of the psychomotor type. *Trans. Amer. neurol. Ass.*, **72,** 180.

GIBBS, F. A., MAXWELL, H., and GIBBS, E. L. (1947*b*). Volume flow of blood through the human brain. *Arch. Neurol. Psychiat. (Chic.)*, **57,** 137.

GRONQUIST, Y. K. J., SELDON, T. H., and FAULCONER, J., Jr. (1952). Cerebral anoxia during anaesthesia. Prognostic significance of electroencephalographic changes. *Ann. Chir. Gynaec. Fenn.*, **41,** 149.

GURDJIAN, E. S., STONE, W. E., and WEBSTER, J. E. (1944). Cerebral metabolism in hypoxia. *Arch. Neurol. Psychiat. (Chic.)*, **51,** 472.

HAIDER, I., OSWALD, I., and MATTHEW, H. (1968). EEG signs of death. *Brit. med. J.*, **3,** 314.

HARMEL, M. H., HAFKENSCHIEL, J. H., AUSTIN, G. M., CRUMPTON, C. W., and KETY S. S. (1949). The effect of bilateral stellate ganglion block on the cerebral circulation in normotensive and hypertensive patients. *J. clin. Invest.*, **28,** 415.

HARPER, A. M. (1965). Physiology of the cerebral blood flow. *Brit. J. Anaesth.*, **37,** 225.

HARPER, A. M., and BELL, R. A. (1963). The effect of metabolic acidosis and alkalosis on the blood flow through the cerebral cortex. *J. Neurol. Neurosurg. Psychiat.*, **26,** 341.

HARPER, A. M., and GLASS, H. I. (1965). The effect of alterations in the arterial carbon dioxide tension on the blood flow through the cerebral cortex at normal and low arterial blood pressure. *J. Neurol. Neurosurg. Psychiat.* **28,** 449.

HARPER, A. M., MCDOWALL, D. G., and LEDINGHAM, I. (1965). The influence of hyperbaric oxygen on the blood flow and oxygen uptake of the cerebral cortex in hypovolaemic shock. *Proc. 2nd Internat. Conf. on Hyperbaric Oxygen*, Vol. 2.

HEDLUND, S., NYLIN, G., and REGNSTRÖM, O. (1962). The behaviour of the cerebral circulation during muscular exercise. *Acta physiol. scand.*, **54,** 316.

HEYMAN, A., PATTERSON, J. L., and NICHOLS, F. T. (1950). The effects of induced fever on cerebral function in neurosyphilis. *J. clin. Invest.*, **29,** 1335.

HIMWICH, H. E. (1951). *Brain Metabolism and Cerebral Disorders.* Baltimore: Williams and Wilkins.

HIMWICH, W. A., and HIMWICH, H. E. (1946). Pyruvic acid exchange of the brain. *J. Neurophysiol.*, **9,** 133.

HOCKADAY, J. M., POTTS, F., EPSTEIN, E., BONAZZI, A., and SCHWAB, R. S. (1965). Electroencephalographic changes in acute cerebral anoxia from cardiac or respiratory arrest. *Electroenceph. clin. Neurophysiol.*, **18,** 575.

HOEDT-RASMUSSEN, K., SVEINSDOTTIR, E., and LASSEN, N. A. (1966). The inert gas intra-arterial injection method for determining regional cerebral blood flow in man through the intact skull. *Circulat. Res.*, **18,** 237.

HOLMBERG, G. (1953). The electroencephalogram during hypoxia and hyperventilation. *Electroenceph. clin. Neurophysiol.*, **5,** 371.

INGVAR, D. H., and LASSEN, N.A. (1965). Methods for cerebral blood flow measurements in man. *Brit. J. Anaesth.*, **37,** 216.

JACOBSON, I., HARPER, A. M., and MCDOWALL, D. G. (1963*a*). Relationship between venous pressure and cortical blood flow. *Nature* (*Lond.*), **200,** 173.

JACOBSON, I., HARPER, A. M., and MCDOWALL, D. G. (1963*b*). The effects of oxygen under pressure on cerebral blood flow and cerebral venous oxygen tension. *Lancet*, **2,** 549.

JENKNER, F. L. (1962). *Rheoencephalography*. Springfield, Ill.: Charles C. Thomas.

KENNEDY, C., and SOKOLOFF, L. (1957). An adaptation of the nitrous oxide method to the study of the cerebral circulation in children; normal values for cerebral blood flow and cerebral metabolic rate in childhood. *J. clin. Invest.*, **36,** 1130.

KETY, S. S. (1950). Circulation and metabolism of human brain in health and disease. *Amer. J. Med.*, **8,** 205.

KETY, S. S., POLIS, B. D., NADLER, C. S., and SCHMIDT, C. F. (1948*d*). The blood flow and oxygen consumption of the human brain in diabetic acidosis and coma. *J. clin. Invest.*, **27,** 500.

KETY, S. S., and SCHMIDT, C. F. (1948*a*). The nitrous oxide method for quantitative determination of cerebral blood flow in man: theory, procedure and normal values. *J. clin. Invest.*, **27,** 476.

KETY, S. S., and SCHMIDT, C. F. (1948*b*). The effects of altered arterial tensions of carbon dioxide and oxygen on cerebral blood flow and cerebral oxygen consumption of normal young men. *J. clin. Invest.*, **27,** 484.

KETY, S. S., SHENKIN, H. A., and SCHMIDT, C. F. (1948*c*). The effects of increased intracranial pressure on cerebral circulatory functions in man. *J. clin. Invest.*, **27,** 493.

KETY, S. S., WOODFORD, R. B., HARMEL, M. H., FREYHAN, F. A., APPEL, K. E., and SCHMIDT, C. F. (1948*e*). Cerebral blood flow and metabolism in schizophrenia; effects of barbiturates, semi-narcosis, insulin coma and electroshock. *Amer. J. Psychiat.*, **104,** 765.

KIERSEY, D. K., BICKFORD, R. G., and FAULCONER, A., Jr. (1951). Electroencephalographic patterns produced by thiopentone sodium during surgical operations. Description and classification. *Brit. J. Anaesth.*, **23,** 141.

KING, B. D., SOKOLOFF, L., and WECHSLER, R. L. (1952). The effects of l-epinephrine and l-nor-epinephrine upon cerebral circulation and metabolism in man. *J. clin. Invest.*, **31,** 273.

KLEINERMAN, G., and HOPKINS, A. L. (1955). The effects of hypothermia on cerebral blood flow and metabolism in dogs. *Fed. Proc.*, **14,** 410.

KRAMER, S. (1912). On the function of the circle of Willis. *J. exp. Med.*, **15,** 348.

KRISTIANSEN, K., and KROG, J. (1962). Electromagnetic studies on the blood flow through the carotid system in man. *Neurology* (*Minneap.*), **12,** 20.

LAMBERTSEN, C. J., KOUGH, R. H., COOPER, D. Y., EMMEL, G. L., LOESCHKE, H. H., and SCHMIDT, C. F. (1953). Oxygen toxicity: effects in man of oxygen inhalation at 1 and 3.5 atmospheres upon blood gas transport, cerebral circulation and cerebral metabolism. *J. appl. Physiol.*, **5,** 471.

LAMBERTSEN, C. J., OWEN, S. G., WENDEL, H., STROUD, M. W., LURIE, A. A., LOCHNER, W., and CLARK, G. F. (1959). Respiratory and cerebral circulatory control during exercise at 0.21 and 2.0 atmospheres inspired P_{O_2} *J. appl. Physiol.*, **14,** 966.

LAMBERTSEN, C. J., SEMPLE, S. J. G., SMYTH, M. G., and GELFAND, R. (1961). H^+ and P_{CO_2} as chemical factors in respiratory and cerebral circulatory control. *J. appl. Physiol.*, **16,** 473.

Lancet (1968). Annotation. Cerebral blood flow and cerebrospinal fluid. **2,** 206.

LANDAU, W. M., FREYGANG, W. H., ROWLAND, L. P., SOKOLOFF, L., and KETY, S.S. (1955). The local circulation of the living brain; values in unanaesthetised and anaesthetised cats. *Trans. Amer. neurol. Ass.*, **80,** 125.

LASSEN, N. A. (1959). Cerebral blood flow and oxygen consumption in man. *Physiol. Rev.*, **39,** 183.

LASSEN, N. A. (1966). The luxury perfusion syndrome and its possible relation to acute metabolic acidosis localised within the brain. *Lancet*, **2,** 1113.

LASSEN, N. A., and INGVAR, D. H. (1963). Regional cerebral blood flow measuremen in man. *Arch. Neurol.* (*Chic.*), **9,** 615.

LASSEN, N. A., and MUNCK, O. (1955). The cerebral blood flow in man determined by the use of radioactive Krypton. *Acta physiol. scand.*, **33,** 30.

LENNOX, W. G., and GIBBS, E. L. (1932). The blood flow in the brain and the leg of man and the changes induced by alteration of blood gases. *J. clin. Invest.*, **11,** 1155.

LEWIS, B. M., SOKOLOFF, L., and KETY, S. S. (1955*a*). Use of radioactive krypton to measure rapid changes in cerebral blood flow. *Amer. J. Physiol.*, **183,** 638.

LEWIS, B. M., SOKOLOFF, L., WENTS, W. B., WECHSLER, R. L., and KETY, S. S. (1955*b*). Determination of cerebral blood flow using radioactive krypton. *Fed. Proc.*, **14,** 92.

MCDONALD, D. A., and POTTER, J. M. (1951). The distribution of blood to the brain. *J. Physiol.* (*Lond.*), **114,** 356.

MCDOWALL, D. G. (1965). The effects of general anaesthetics on cerebral blood flow and cerebral metabolism. *Brit. J. Anaesth.*, **37,** 236.

MCGINTY, D. A. (1929). Variations in the lactic acid metabolism in the intact brain. *Amer. J. Physiol.*, **88,** 312.

MCILWAIN, H. (1959). *Biochemistry and the Central Nervous System.* London: J. & A. Churchill.

MANGOLD, R., SOKOLOFF, L., CONNER, E. L., KLEINERMAN, J., THERMAN, P. G., and KETY, S. S. (1955). The effects of sleep and lack of sleep on the cerebral circulation and metabolism of normal young men. *J. clin. Invest.*, **34,** 1092.

MEYER, J. S., and GOTOH, F. (1964). Continuous recording of cerebral metabolism, internal jugular flow and E.E.G. in man. *Trans. Amer. neurol Ass.*, **89,** 151.

MOYER, J. H., MILLER, S. I., and SNYDER, H. (1954). Effect of increased jugular venous pressure on cerebral haemodynamics. *J. appl. Physiol.*, **1,** 245.

MUNCK, O., and LASSEN, N. A. (1957). Bilateral cerebral blood flow and oxygen consumption in man by use of Krypton 85. *Circulat. Res.*, **5,** 163.

MUNRO, A. (1783), quoted by WEED, L. H. (1929). Some limitations of the Munro-Kellie hypothesis. *Arch. Surg.*, **18,** 1049.

MYERSON, A., HALLORAN, R. C., and HIRSCH, H. L. (1927). Technique for obtaining blood from internal jugular vein and internal carotid artery. *Arch. Neurol. Psychiat.* (*Chic.*), **17,** 807.

NOVAK, P., GOLUBOFF, B., BORTIN, L., SOFFE, A., and SHENKIN, H. A. (1953). Studies of the cerebral circulation and metabolism in congestive heart failure. *Circulation*, **7,** 724.

NYLIN, G., and BLÖMER, H. (1955). Studies on distribution of cerebral blood flow with thorium-B labelled erythrocytes. *Circulat. Res.*, **3,** 79.

NYLIN, G., SILVERSKIÖLD, B. P., LÖFSTEDT, S., REGNSTRÖM, O., and HEDLUND, S. (1960). Studies on cerebral blood flow in man, using radioactive labelled erythrocytes. *Brain*, **83,** 293.

PATTERSON, J. D., HEYMAN, A., BATTEY, L. L., and FERGUSON, R. W. (1955). Threshold of response of the cerebral vessels of man to increase in blood carbon dioxide. *J. clin. Invest.*, **34,** 1857.

PAULING, L. (1964). The hydrate microcrystal theory of general anaesthesia. *Curr. Res. Anesth.*, **43,** 1.

PEARCY, W. C., and VIRTUE, R. W. (1959). The electroencephalogram in hypothermia and circulatory occlusion. *Anesthesiology*, **20,** 34.

PIERCE, E. C., LAMBERTSEN, C. J., DEUTSCH, S., CHASE, P. E., LINDE, H. W., DRIPPS, R. D., and PRICE, H. L. (1962). Cerebral circulation and metabolism during thiopental anaesthesia and hyperventilation in man. *J. clin. Invest.*, **41,** 1664.

QUASTEL, J. H. (1952). Biochemical aspects of narcosis. *Curr. Res. Anesth.*, **31,** 151.

ROBIN, E. C., and GARDNER, F. H. (1953). Cerebral metabolism and haemodynamics in pernicious anaemia. *J. clin. Invest.*, **32,** 598.

ROBINSON, J. S., and GRAY, T. D. (1961). Observations on the cerebral effects of passive hyperventilation. *Brit. J. Anaesth.*, **33,** 62.

ROSSEN, R., KABAT, H., and ANDERSON, J. P. (1943). Acute arrest of cerebral circulation in man. *Arch. Neurol. Psychiat.* (*Chic.*), **50,** 510.

ROSOMOFF, H. L. (1956). Some effects of hypothermia on the normal and abnormal physiology of the nervous system. *Proc. roy. Soc. Med.*, **49,** 358.

ROSOMOFF, H. L. (1963). Distribution of intracranial contents with controlled hyperventilation: implications for neuro-anaesthesia. *Anesthesiology*, **24,** 640.

ROSOMOFF, H. L., and HOLADAY, D. A. (1954). Cerebral blood flow and cerebral oxygen consumption during hypothermia. *Amer. J. Physiol.*, **179,** 85.

ROY, C. S., and SHERRINGTON, C. S. (1890). On regulation of blood supply of brain. *J. Physiol.* (*Lond.*), **11,** 85.

SADOVE, M. S., BECKA, D., and GIBBS, F. A. (1967). *Electroencephalography for Anaesthesiologists and Surgeons*. Philadelphia: J. B. Lippincott Co.

SCHIEVE, J. F., and WILSON, W. P. (1953). The changes in cerebral vascular resistance of man in experimental aklalosis and acidosis. *J. clin. Invest.*, **32,** 33.

SCHMIDT, C. F. (1944). The present status of knowledge concerning the instrinsic control of the cerebral circulation and the effects of functional derangements in it. *Fed. Proc.*, **3,** 131.

SCHMIDT, C. F. (1960). Central nervous system—circulation, fluids and barriers. In: Amer. Physiol. Soc. *Handbook of Physiology*, Section I, Vol. 3, Chap. 70. Baltimore: Williams & Wilkins.

SCHNEIDER, M. (1963). Critical blood pressure in the cerebral circulation. In: *Selective Vulnerability of the Brain in Hypoxaemia*. Eds. Schade, J. P. and McMeney, W. H. Oxford: Blackwell Scientific Publications.

SEIFRIZ, W. (1950). Effects of various anaesthetic agents on protoplasm. *Anesthesiology*, **11,** 24.

SHENKIN, H. A. (1951). Effects of various drugs upon cerebral circulation and metabolism of man. *J. appl. Physiol.*, **3,** 465.

SHENKIN, H. A., CABIESES, F., VAN DEN NOORDT, G., SAYERS, P., and COPPERMAN, R. (1951). Symposium—Intracranial vascular abnormalities; haemodynamic effect of unilateral carotid ligation on cerebral circulation of man. *J. Neurosurg.*, **8,** 38.

SHENKIN, H. A., HARMEL, M. H., and KETY, S. S. (1948). Dynamic anatomy of the cerebral circulation. *Arch. Neurol. Psychiat.* (*Chic.*), **60,** 240.

SHENKIN, H. A., NOVAK, P., GOLUBOFF, B., SOFFE, A. M., and BORTIN, L. (1953). The effects of aging, arteriosclerosis and hypertension upon the cerebral circulation. *J. clin. Invest.*, **32,** 459.

SOKOLOFF, L. (1957). In: *New Research Techniques of Neuroanatomy*. Ed. Windle, W. F. Springfield, Ill.: Charles C. Thomas.

SOKOLOFF, L. (1959*a*). *Proc. Conference on the Process of Aging in the Nervous System.* Springfield, Ill.: Charles C. Thomas.

SOKOLOFF, L. (1959*b*). The action of drugs on the cerebral circulation. *Pharmacol. Rev.*, **11,** 1.

SOKOLOFF, L., and KETY, S. S. (1960). Regulation of cerebral circulation. *Physiol. Rev.*, **40,** 38.

SOKOLOFF, L., MANGOLD, R., WECHSLER, R. L., KENNEDY, C., and KETY, S. S. (1955). The effect of mental arithmetic on cerebral circulation and metabolism. *J. clin. Invest.*, **34,** 1101.

SUGIOKA, K., and DAVIS, D. A. (1960). Hyperventilation with oxygen: a possible cause of cerebral hypoxia. *Anesthesiology*, **21,** 135.

SWEET, W. H. and BENNETT, H. S. (1948). Changes in internal carotid pressure during carotid and jugular compression and their clinical significance. *J. Neurosurg.*, **3,** 178.

TURNER, J., LAMBERTSON, C. J., OWEN, S. G., WENDEL, H., and CHIODI, H. (1957). Effects of 0.08 and 0.8 atmospheres of inspired P_{O_2} on cerebral haemodynamics at a "constant" alveolar P_{CO_2} of 43 mm. Hg. *Fed. Proc.*, **16,** 130.

VEALL, N., and MALLETT, B. L. (1963). Measurement of cerebral blood flow. *Lancet*, **1,** 1081.

WECHSLER, R. L., KLEISS, L. M., and KETY, S. S. (1950). The effects of intravenously administered aminophylline on cerebral circulation and metabolism in man. *J. clin. Invest.*, **29,** 28.

WILSON, S. M. (1957). Electro-encephalography in relation to anaestheisa. *Proc. roy. Soc. Med.*, **50,** 105.

WOLFF, H. G. (1936). The cerebral circulation. *Physiol. Rev.*, **16,** 545.

WOLLMAN, H., ALEXANDER, S. C., COHEN, P. J., SMITH, T. C., CHASE, P. E., and VAN DER MOLEN, R. A. (1965). Cerebral circulation during general anaesthesia and hyperventilation in man. *Anesthesiology*, **26,** 329.

WULF, R. J., and FEATHERSTONE, R. M. (1957). A correlation of van der Waal's constant with anaesthetic potency. *Anesthesiology*, **18,** 97.

Chapter 23

HYPOTENSION IN ANAESTHESIA

THE problem of a patient with a low blood pressure may confront the anaesthetist in several ways. Hypotension may be present in the conscious state; it may be a natural phenomenon peculiar to that subject, it may have been caused by some abdominal or thoracic emergency, or due to accidental trauma, or it may be due to disease in the heart or its pericardial sac. An unwanted fall in systemic pressure may occur during the anaesthesia or operation, or the hypotension may be *deliberately* induced by the anaesthetist. Finally, the commonest—yet often the least suspected—occasion is during the early post-operative period.

PRE-OPERATIVE HYPOTENSION

The absolute value of a patient's immediate pre-operative blood pressure must be considered against the patient's general condition and knowledge, if any, of his previous blood pressure. Thus a "normal" blood pressure may represent hypotension, as may occur following a myocardial infarct in a hypertensive patient, or alternatively, a "normal" blood pressure may be being sustained only by extreme vasoconstriction when the abolition of this compensatory mechanism by anaesthesia will result in a profound fall in pressure.

The induction of anaesthesia in a patient with a naturally low systemic pressure presents no special problems beyond the normal precaution against the too rapid intravenous injection of drugs which are likely to lower it still more.

When the pre-operative hypotension is due to a low filling pressure, either the result of hypovolaemia or of peripheral vasodilatation, steps can be taken to correct this before embarking on anaesthesia. Replacement of the appropriate fluid while monitoring the central venous pressure usually restores the situation to normal. If hypotension is the result of extreme vasodilatation, which may be the sequel to infection or to drug therapy, provided the cardiac output is good and the peripheral tissues well perfused, it may be better to accept a low pressure than to administer vasopressor drugs, remembering that any further fluid losses will have to be promptly replaced. Generally, however, it is probably futile to operate when there is no response to resuscitation with a systolic pressure of 50 mm. Hg unless the operation is for uncontrolled haemorrhage (see also Chapter 21).

Where the hypotension is the result of a fixed low-output cardiac disease, which is usually associated with vasoconstriction in the peripheral vessels, the induction of anaesthesia and the consequent peripheral vasodilatation may be fatal, particularly when it is sudden. For such people it is far safer to induce anaesthesia with an inhalational agent in a high oxygen atmosphere from the start (see also Chapter 24).

Hypotension During Anaesthesia and Operation

A real problem in considering the blood pressure during anaesthesia is the absence of information on what the normal blood pressure is during deep sleep. In a small series of patients who had normal blood pressure while awake (Richardson *et al.*, 1964), it has been demonstrated that systolic pressures of 90 or even 80 are normal while deeply asleep, in which case ideas about normal blood pressure during anaesthesia need perhaps to be revised downwards. There is increasing recognition that the blood pressure is not the cardinal sign of circulatory well-being. Moderate falls in blood pressure with the body performing its own regulation of distribution of flow are preferable to a blood pressure sustained at an arbitrary level by drugs which alter the distribution of blood flow, often in a deleterious manner.

Surgical stimulation in the early stages of an operation in the lightly anaesthetised patient frequently induces a rise in the systemic pressure, but during abdominal and thoracic surgery a fall in blood pressure may follow various manipulations and this has always been believed to be due to a visceral reflex. A more common cause is obstruction to the flow of blood in the inferior vena cava due to a retractor, a gall-bladder bridge or indirect pressure in the prone position. A reduction in blood volume is, however, probably by far the commonest cause of hypotension. This may be acute and obvious enough to warrant immediate notice but more commonly the loss is either insidious or concealed. Proper estimation of blood loss, by weighing of the swabs or the colorometric estimation of haemoglobin, added to the sucker loss plus the blood observed on the towels and surgeons' gowns should help prevent this complication. Measurement of the filling pressure of the right heart with a saline manometer connected to a catheter fed from the neck or arm to the superior vena cava is technically easy and will add useful information. Prompt treatment of blood loss is advisable as up to one fifth of the total blood volume may be lost before significant changes in the systemic pressure of an anaesthetised patient are produced. Thus hypotension represents a late stage in the body's reaction to haemorrhage.

The action of drugs and the institution of intermittent positive pressure ventilation, particularly if the carbon dioxide level of the blood is markedly reduced, can both result in hypotension—this is considered below in greater detail.

Hypotension from a sensitivity reaction due to the injection of a foreign protein is believed to be rare during anaesthesia and the test dose of an anti-serum (e.g. tetanus) is often omitted when a patient is unconscious. There is insufficient information available to permit a dogmatic statement on the subject, but reports of reactions under such conditions are few. An incompatible blood transfusion may even pass unnoticed until the patient recovers consciousness.

INDUCED HYPOTENSION AND CIRCULATORY CONTROL

That an incision through skin or muscle causes a greater degree of haemorrhage in the unconscious than the conscious state has already been discussed (Chapter 20). It will be recalled that the principal factor at work is believed to be widespread dilatation of the peripheral vascular bed attending the onset of anaesthesia. Narcosis is also often associated with an increase in cardiac output without any appreciable change in the blood pressure. The increased bleeding is simply due to an increased flow of blood through the cut vessels. In the past, clinical experience taught anaesthetists that light anaesthesia caused more bleeding than deep, and also that anaesthetic agents which lowered the blood pressure—such as chloroform—were the most effective in the prevention of bleeding. Studies based on the flow of blood through skin and muscle during anaesthesia have substantiated these impressions.

One of the functions of anaesthesia and the anaesthetist is to provide optimum operating conditions for the surgeon. Blood loss, by obscuring the surgical field, or even by the sheer magnitude of the loss, may make surgery difficult or even impossible and it is a part of good anaesthesia to provide as bloodless a field as possible. In the past this has too often been considered under the heading of "induced hypotension". Eckenhoff (1966) has described the term "deliberate hypotension" as being both misleading and poorly descriptive, because in the production of a bloodless field a specific degree of hypotension is not required, nor is ganglionic blockade always necessary. It also obscures the concept that much blood loss is venous in origin and he therefore suggests the use of the term "circulatory control" to cover all those points of technique which are used to ensure a good operating field.

The factors which give rise to increased wound bleeding usually result in either venous engorgement or an increased cardiac output.

(a) **Hypercapnia.**—Principally by increasing the output of catecholamines the blood pressure and the cardiac output are increased.

(b) **Hypoxia.**—Produces vasodilatation and by chemoreceptor stimulation increases the cardiac output.

Anaesthesia tends to produce deleterious alterations in the lung ventilation-perfusion ratios, changes which are accentuated by reduction in blood pressure or cardiac output. The anaesthetist must compensate for these alterations, if necessary with controlled ventilation with an increased oxygen content of the inspired mixture.

(c) **Respiratory obstruction.**—Besides the effect on blood oxygen and carbon dioxide levels the alterations in intrathoracic pressure can result in a raised central venous pressure. With spontaneous respiration any resistance to expiration—the use of too small an endotracheal tube, or a half-closed valve—will increase venous pressure and the amount of bleeding.

(d) **Improper posture** is the most important factor in promoting venous bleeding (see below).

(e) **Inadequate analgesia** results in a raised cardiac output as a consequence of peripheral circulatory stimulation.

(f) **Ether and cyclopropane** both cause secretion of catecholamines and a raised cardiac output.

(g) **Very deep anaesthesia**, now seldom used, to the point of cardiac failure produces hypoxia and venous engorgement.

The good anaesthetist thus provides adequate unobstructed ventilatory exchange, a light but fully analgesic anaesthetic avoiding those agents which provoke catecholamine secretion in a patient who is properly postured. Larson (1964), in an excellent review, comments that induced hypotension must never be considered a panacea for indifferent anaesthesia but rather that anaesthesia must first be perfect in all respects and hypotension induced as a complementary measure only.

Further reduction of blood supply to the operative field can then be produced in a number of different ways.

(a) *Tourniquet*—Obviously restricted in its application but producing complete ischaemia for a limited period.

(b) *Use of local vasoconstrictor solutions.*—Used mainly for skin infliltration before operation (thyroidectomy) or topically, during eye or ear, nose and throat operations.

(c) *Vasoconstriction.*—This method is based on a study of the sequence of events that follows haemorrhage—namely, blood loss leading to a reduction in blood volume which in turn elicits compensatory vasoconstriction in an attempt to maintain an adequate systemic pressure. This constriction in the skin and muscle throughout the body results in a diminished blood flow at the operation site. The technique, which consists of either arteriotomy or venotomy, requires great clinical experience to estimate the exact point at which the blood loss has reached its permissible maximum. There is now no indication for this technique.

Vasodilatation

The three principles involved are the production of vascular relaxation with a decreased peripheral vascular resistance, a decrease in the cardiac output, and a lowering of the transmural pressure in the vessels.

Vascular Relaxation

This can be produced by specific ganglionic blockade, by spinal or epidural analgesia or by the effects of anaesthetic drugs such as halothane or the phenothiazines.

Paralysis occurs in the arteriolar resistance vessels leading to a drop in blood pressure but more importantly paralysis occurs in the capacitance vessels on the venous side and blood can be made to pool in different parts of the body. The decreased filling pressure of the heart then leads to a reduction in the cardiac output. In its simplest form this is practised daily by anaesthetists, using halothane anaesthesia or halothane added to a curare-induced paralysis, who do not necessarily regard this as "induced hypotension".

The basic mechanism of this technique results in a vascular tree which is unresponsive to the effects of low cardiac output or haemorrhage. With dilated inelastic capacitance vessels quite small blood losses can produce large alterations in the filling pressure of the heart, and thus the cardiac output. Much prompter action is required than in the normal patient to raise the filling pressure by alteration in posture or by blood transfusion in the event of haemorrhage.

1. Subarachnoid and epidural block.—For many years some anaesthetists and surgeons have favoured "high" spinal analgesia not only for the excellent muscular relaxation but also for the relatively bloodless field which ensues. A "high" spinal extending from the first thoracic segment downward leads to total sympathetic paralysis.

The technique and choice of drug is discussed elsewhere (Chapters 42 and 43).

The mechanism whereby spinal and epidural block produce a fall in blood pressure is similar. Bromage (1967), reviewing the pharmacology of epidural analgesia, considers that the fall is the result of four separate processes:

i. The dilatation effect on resistance and capacitance vessels with a consequent fall in cardiac output.
ii. β-receptor blockade and smooth muscle depression which results from the vascular absorption of the local analgesic drug.
iii. A reduction in the noradrenaline output in the segmental distribution of the block.
iv. In the case of block affecting the first to fourth thoracic segments, the paralysis of the cardiac sympathetic nerve producing bradycardia and a decreased cardiac output.

Although continuous epidural analgesia is technically more difficult, it greatly extends the usefulness of the technique.

Normally the patient is anaesthetised before the block is induced because the position and the fall in blood pressure produce considerable discomfort. Also, as inadequate respiration and hypoxia are so dangerous during hypotension, respiration is usually assisted or controlled.

Immediately after the injection the patient is turned on his back in a fairly steep Trendelenburg position until the systolic pressure has fallen to 80–90 mm. Hg and then the patient is suitably postured.

Two facts sometimes adduced in favour of the technique are that with suitable analgesic concentration only the sympathetic fibres can be blocked and secondly that compensatory vasoconstriction and reduction in bleeding occurs in those vessels whose sympathetic supply is not blocked. In practice it seems logical, when other methods of vascular relaxation are available, to use the techniques of spinal and epidural analgesia only when surgery is being performed on those areas which are rendered analgesic by the block.

A clinical impression exists that epidural analgesia produces a reduction in bleeding due to the qualities of the block itself and this belief often accounts for surgical requests for epidural analgesia in those patients in whom induced hypotension is contra-indicated. Donald (1969) showed that in pelvic floor surgery induced hypotension produced a highly significant reduction in blood loss, irrespective of whether respiration was spontaneous or controlled, and that this reduction was similar whether the hypotension was produced with trimetaphan or by epidural block. As epidural analgesia always produced some fall in blood pressure as compared to the standard technique, it was impossible to isolate the effect of the epidural alone. In two further papers, a series by Bond (1969) had no correlation between mean operative systolic blood pressure and blood loss, while Moir (1968) did not quote blood pressures. This emphasises the many factors which influence surgical haemorrhage and the difficulty in controlling these variables in an experimental study.

2. Drug induced.—Vasodilatation in anaesthesia is normally produced by drugs which block either the autonomic ganglia or the adrenergic nerves. Hexamethonium (C.6), pentamethonium (C.5), pentolinium ("Ansolysen"), trimetaphan ("Arfonad") and phenactropinium ("Trophenium") are good examples of the former, though the action of trimetaphan is more complex than that of pure ganglion block. Pentamethonium is less consistent in action than hexamethonium and rarely used. Guanethidine ("Ismelin") blocks adrenergic nerves. Vasodilatation is also produced by halothane, and this action, coupled with other hypotensive effects associated with deepening anaesthesia, makes this drug a useful medium for reducing bleeding. In clinical practice halothane is particularly valuable in the presence of a ganglion-blocking drug since its concentration can quickly be varied to control the exact level of the systemic blood pressure.

Hexamethonium is usually given initially in a small intravenous test dose (10 mg.) in the horizontal position before proceeding with the main injection, as occasionally a patient will be found to be hypersensitive, in which case the hypotension will be profound. Provided this is not so an intravenous dose of 25–50 mg. should be given. Thereafter these doses can be repeated after five minutes if the extent of the fall in systolic pressure is not sufficient. Enderby and Pelmore (1951) have described how in fit, young, healthy adults it may be difficult to induce or maintain hypotension with hexamethonium on account of a tachycardia which often follows the use of this drug.

Pentolinium, or pentamethylene-1:5 bis-(1-methylpyrrolidinium hydrogen tartrate), has about five times the activity of hexamethonium bromide (Wien and Mason, 1953) and a longer duration of action. The initial intravenous dose varies from 3 to 20 mg. depending upon the age and physical state of the patient. Enderby (1954*a*) notes that pentolinium causes a slow fall in blood pressure, that the hypotension it produces is more easily potentiated by posture and controlled respiration than that of hexamethonium, and that a single dose is effective for up to 45 minutes and rarely leads to tachycardia. But in fact the blood pressure may take several hours to return to normal.

Trimetaphan, one of the short-acting thiophanium group of drugs, has a marked ganglion-blocking effect (Randall *et al.*, 1949) but it also has a direct vasodilator action in dogs (McCubbin and Page, 1952), while its intravenous injection leads to the release of histamine both in man (Payne, 1956) and in dogs (Randall *et al.*, 1949). Histamine release could account for some of the hypotension that trimetaphan produces. The extremely short length of action of this drug is believed to be partly due to its destruction by the enzyme cholinesterase. It can be given either as a continuous steady infusion (1 mg./ml.) or by the intermittent injection of 2·5 to 5 mg. The latter technique has the small advantage that it obviates the use of a drip and also allows each successive dose to wear off before the next one is repeated. One of the principal disadvantages of the continuous drip technique is that a "base-line" may be reached in which the systolic pressure will fall no further unless the posture or blood volume of the patient are altered. If the drug is then continuously infused, the final recovery of blood pressure will be very much prolonged. It is important, therefore, periodically to stop the infusion and check that the blood pressure does soon start to rise again.

Phenactropinium appears to exert its hypotensive effect almost entirely by ganglion block (Robertson *et al.*, 1957) and has a short duration of action. For these reasons Robertson and his colleagues (1957) consider that it produces a readily controllable hypotension; they recommend a concentration of 2 mg./ml. for continuous intravenous infusion.

Guanethidine acts by blocking post-ganglionic sympathetic transmission. It prevents either the production or the release of noradrenaline at the nerve-ending, but has no effect on the output of noradrenaline from the adrenal gland. It acts like reserpine. However, it has the advantage that it does not cross the blood-brain barrier and affect the brain: for, whilst depression and melancholia (presumably due to reduction of noradrenaline and hydroxytryptamine in the brain) are characteristic of reserpine therapy, these symptoms are not observed when the patient is taking guanethidine (Burn, 1961). Holloway and his colleagues (1961) have described the use of guanethidine as a hypotensive agent in anaesthesia. By itself it is unsatisfactory, but it is helpful when hexamethonium produces a tachycardia and inadequate or fluctuating hypotension. In these circumstances, guanethidine produces a bradycardia and usually a further fall in blood pressure. The dose range is from 10 to 20 mg. given intravenously. Guanethidine has a prolonged action, and hypotension, once attained, may be prolonged.

Opinions differ about the technique of induced hypotension by ganglion blockade. There are those who recommend posturing the patient for the surgical operation—even though this necessitates the use of the head-up position—before giving any hypotensive drug, and there are others who induce vasodilatation in the horizontal position and only make use of posture should it be needed to aid or sustain the fall in pressure. The latter technique is safest and to be preferred, and should normally be combined with an initial small dose of the hypotensive drug to assess the reaction of the patient.

Young, normotensive people are more resistant to induced hypotension than the aged or those with hypertension. An initial fall in blood pressure may be quickly followed by a rise to the normal level in the former; further doses of ganglion-blocking agent may then have little effect even with the aid of posture. For such people halothane or controlled respiration may assist in controlling the level of blood pressure. Controlled respiration with hyperventilation and a raised mean airway pressure has a marked hypotensive effect, particularly in the period immediately after a ganglion-blocking drug has been administered (Enderby, 1958). Eckenhoff and his colleagues (1963) have investigated pulmonary gas exchange under these conditions, and find that respiratory physiological dead space is markedly increased i.e. from 35 to 80 per cent of the tidal volume, particularly when the patient is placed in the head-up position. Their results indicate that as much as three-quarters of the tidal volume may be ineffective and demonstrate the need for maintenance by controlled ventilation of a respiratory exchange well above normally adequate levels with an oxygen content of inspired gases of at least 35 to 40 per cent. The same principle also applies in cases of hypotension due to haemorrhage.

Apart from the relative resistance of many people to ganglion blockade, tachyphylaxis (or a decreasing response to the same dose) may also occur with the result that an initial fall in pressure cannot be sustained by repetitive doses. This is most likely to occur with hexamethonium, but has been described with all the hypotensive agents. It is best avoided by administering an initial large dose of the chosen drug, though such a technique undoubtedly enhances the risk of acute circulatory failure; it must therefore not be used for elderly or hypertensive patients. Under the influence of ganglion blockade the patient has lost many of his powers of compensation, so that even a mild haemorrhage or a brief period of anoxia may lead to a fatal result. The importance, therefore, of a good airway and adequate anaesthesia and ventilation cannot be stressed too strongly.

Tachycardia can be a troublesome complication of drug-induced hypotension particularly in younger fit men in whom the tachycardia may be sufficient to prevent much fall in the blood pressure. The exact mechanism of this response is not clear. It may represent an attenuation of vagal control by the ganglion blocker or be the result of carotid and aortic baroceptor stimulation. Other causative factors are atropine premedication, gallamine used as a muscle relaxant, surgical stimulus under too light anaesthesia, and carbon dioxide retention or hypoxia. In a healthy patient the tachycardia may be only troublesome in that it prevents much fall in the blood pressure. In the presence of any coronary artery or cardiac disease—when induced hypotension is probably contra-indicated anyway—tachycardia in the face of a lowered blood pressure may be dangerous and must be promptly controlled.

To combat the tachycardia, procaine amide or guanethidine have been recommended in the past but once hypotension has been produced with either of these drugs the action may be prolonged. Halothane possesses the great advantage of flexibility in its administration and is now the method of choice for controlling tachycardia. Propranalol has been advocated by a number of authors (Hellewell and Potts, 1966; Hewitt *et al.*, 1967) and is no doubt effective. The doses recommended (between 1·0 and 2·5 mg. repeated if necessary) produce a profound β-blocking action whose effects could be serious if some catastrophe, such as cardiac arrest secondary to profound hypotension or acute cardiac failure, occurred (see p. 665).

Reduction in Cardiac Output

Reduction in cardiac output occurs mainly as a consequence of a diminished filling pressure of the heart. Blood is made to pool under the influence of gravity in the relaxed capacitance vessels. Further reduction in output may be provoked by reduction in cardiac rate as with halothane or procaine amide, or by the use of intermittent positive pressure respiration. This may cause its effect either by impeding venous return or by the cardiac depressant action of hypocapnia.

It is this reduction in cardiac output which probably affects the amount of bleeding much more than the actual lowering of the blood pressure.

Lowering of Transmural Pressure

The relaxed vessels, carrying only the reduced cardiac output, are easily influenced by posture and tend to collapse easily. This results in a virtual disappearance of venous bleeding and marked reduction in arterial bleeding.

Posture

In the conscious subject alterations in position from the horizontal to the upright produce little change in the cerebral blood flow. For example, if a conscious person is suddenly tilted head upwards from the horizontal, the arterial pressure falls slightly more than the flow—although neither changes very much (Scheinberg, 1949). On the other hand, lowering the head to an angle 20° below the horizontal (i.e. head-down tilt) brings about a slight reduction in cerebral blood flow (Shenkin *et al.*, 1948). In the conscious state the head-down tilt is extremely uncomfortable, and few people—apart from acrobats and children—can maintain this position for long. The discomfort is due to a markedly increased pressure in the cranial veins, with retrograde extension into the capillaries, possibly leading to oedema and petechial haemorrhages. Great relief can be obtained by the simple expedient of a forced inspiration against a resistance (i.e. inspiring with shut lips and occluded nose). This manoeuvre lowers the arterial pressure, and subsequently reduces the venous congestion (Wilkins *et al.*, 1950).

Enderby (1954*b*) stressed the importance of taking into account the effect on the brain of any tilt away from the horizontal. For example, the blood pressure is usually measured in the arm, with the limb on a level with the heart; if the patient is tilted into the head-up position the pressure in the arm may remain the same, but the effect of the weight of the column of blood must be taken into account in both the head and the feet. Thus, in this position, the pressure in the feet may be 180 mm. Hg or more yet in the head it may be only 80 mm. Hg. Examples of the effect of changes in position on the local blood pressure are shown in Fig. 1. As a general rule the difference in pressure in a particular area may be calculated on the basis of allowing + or − 2 mm. Hg for every one inch (2·5 cm.) of tilt below or above the level of the heart. This is the reason why posture has come to play such an important part in reducing bleeding during surgery. If the operation site is raised above the level of the heart the effect of gravity reduces the pressure in the arterial system and also empties the venous channels. In some cases posture alone has not been found to produce a sufficient reduction in bleeding, and the hypotensive technique—with the deliberate removal of vasoconstrictor tone—has therefore been developed.

Changes of posture in the immediate post-operative period are particularly dangerous, as the patient's circulation may be unstable. The sitting position encourages venous pooling of blood in the dependant limbs and tends to lead to or accentuate hypotension, with consequent cerebral anaemia. The disadvantages of the sitting position must be weighed against the advantage, namely reduced pulmonary congestion. When it is essential to put the patient upright soon after an operation, a compromise can usually be obtained by also raising the legs slightly (Fig. 2).

Dangers of Induced Hypotension

The most serious complications are those involving the brain, heart and kidneys. While the circulation to these organs is usually capable of adaptation to alterations in blood pressure and cardiac output, these compensatory mechanisms may fall down in the face of abnormally low perfusion pressures or in the presence of diseased unreactive blood vessels. Cerebral thrombosis is sometimes encountered, and this may either prolong unconsciousness, appear as a hemiplegia, or even develop after consciousness has been regained. Thrombosis of the central artery of the retina, leading to unilateral blindness, may also occur. These cerebrovascular complications are almost all confined to patients with signs of arteriosclerosis, and the few in normal patients only occur when excessive degrees of hypotension (i.e. 60 mm. Hg and below) have been produced.

Coronary thrombosis has been reported but the fact that the generalised vasodilatation reduces the work of the heart will in some measure compensate for

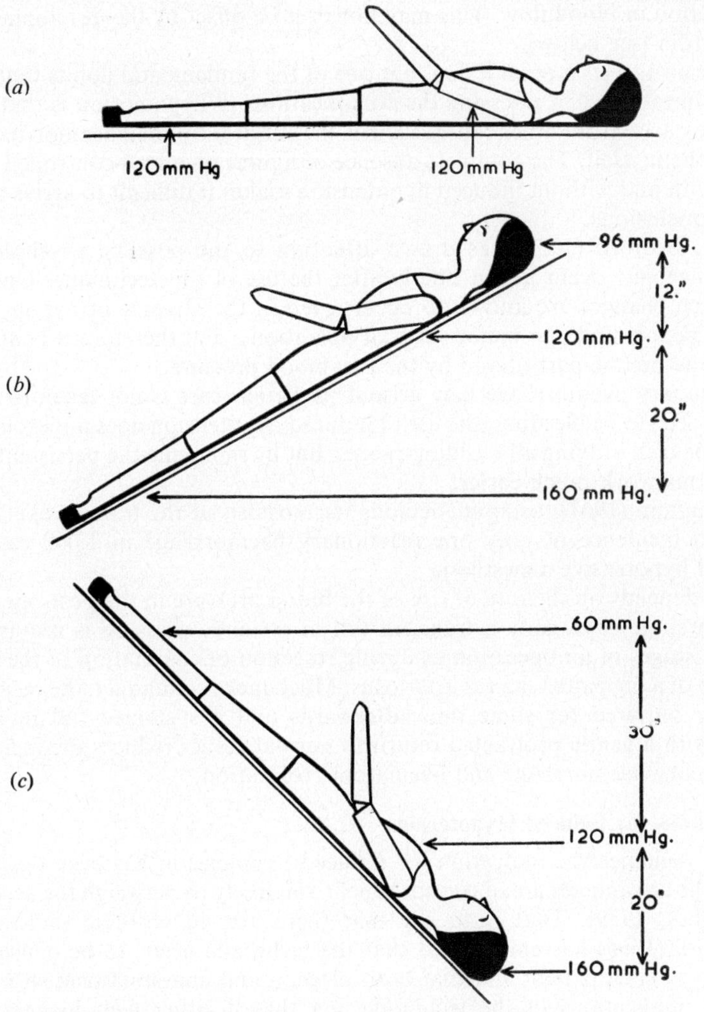

(a)

120 mm Hg 120 mm Hg

96 mm Hg.

12."

120 mm Hg.

(b)

20."

160 mm Hg.

60 mm Hg.

30"

(c)

120 mm Hg.

20"

160 mm Hg.

23/FIG. 1.—THE EFFECTS OF POSTURE ON LOCAL BLOOD PRESSURE

(*a*) Horizontal position. B.P. equal in chest and legs.
(*b*) Reverse Trendelenburg. B.P. lower in the head and higher in the feet.
(*c*) Trendelenburg. B.P. low in the feet and high in the head.

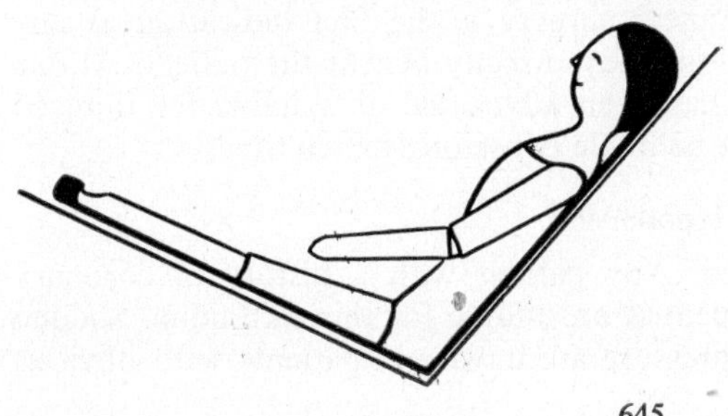

23/FIG. 2.—Post-operative posture.

any reduction in blood flow. This may however be offset by the development of a tachycardia (see below).

Oliguria suggests a renal lesion, but one of the fundamental points that must be borne in mind when assessing the complications of hypotension is that these lesions may arise from other causes such as the surgical trauma, haemorrhage, or the anaesthetic itself. The complete absence of figures on a well-controlled series of cases with and without induced hypotension makes it difficult to arrive at any definite conclusions.

Again, Bedford (1955) has drawn attention to the possible psychological changes that may occur in the elderly after the use of this technique. Unfortunately, such changes are known to occur, even in the absence of hypotension, when old people undergo major surgical operations, and therefore it is difficult to assess the precise part played by the low blood pressure.

Reactionary haemorrhage may arise if particular care is not taken to ligate any vessel seen to be bleeding; the use of induced hypotension does not excuse the surgeon the task of tying all bleeding-points, but by removing the persistent ooze it makes this work much easier.

McLaughlin (1961), using meticulous haemostasis at the time of operation, reports an incidence of only one reactionary haemorrhage in 1,000 cases of controlled hypotensive anaesthesia.

Much depends on the rate of rise of the blood pressure in the post-operative period. In some cases only a transient fall in systemic pressure is required at particular stages of an operation as during resection of coarctation of the aorta or ligation of a big patent ductus arteriosus. Much more commonly, the beneficial effects are required for some time afterwards and a sustained fall in blood pressure with a gentle protracted return to normal values reduces the incidence of reactionary haemorrhage and haematoma formation.

Indications for Induced Hypotension

In one sentence the indication for induced hypotension has been described as where the advantages are of certain benefit and likely to outweigh the accepted risks (Gillies, 1959). That is to say that there are no absolute indications. McLaughlin (1966) has emphasised that the technique needs to be considered in relation to each patient and that both surgeon and anaesthetist must understand the implications of the technique and that if either feels incapable of mastering these, hypotension should not be induced.

The claimed benefits of induced hypotension are a reduced blood loss, thus avoiding the dangers of massive blood transfusion, a more accurate surgical technique, and in cases where large raw areas are produced, as in reconstructive surgery, better wound healing. Cancer surgery is the first indication as any improvement in operating conditions may directly benefit the patient. At one time or another every operation has been advocated as suitable for induced hypotension but the decision must be made consciously each time.

Contra-indications to Induced Hypotension

These can be simply expressed. Any patient with a history of coronary ischaemia or cerebrovascular accident is unsuitable for this technique. Sudden or profound alterations in blood pressure are unwise in patients with obvious vascular disease of any vital organ. Conditions which interfere with the transport of oxygen, such as anaemia, respiratory inefficiency, hypovolaemia and cardiac failure, are all contra-indications. Obstructive airway disease is probably also a contra-indication as the high inflation pressures required may severely reduce the cardiac output. Due to the need for special post-operative care (see below) absence of good immediate post-operative supervision may well be a contra-indication.

Post-operative Care after Induced Hypotension.

To avoid the danger of reactionary haemorrhage, blood pressure is usually allowed to rise gently, although the return to consciousness normally causes some elevation. If the cardiac output and blood pressure are low, pain and restlessness may increase the body oxygen demand above the level of supply, a situation which is aggravated by respiratory obstruction or lung dysfunction in a patient breathing air.

With a vascular system still unresponsive to haemorrhage quite small blood losses will result in acute drops in blood pressure. Blood loss and replacement need to be as carefully monitored and controlled, using central venous pressure measurement if necessary, as they were in theatre.

Combining the results of 16 papers representing 13,264 cases of induced hypotension, 110 deaths (97·3 per cent of the total) were reported to have occurred in the post-operative period (Larson, 1964).

Discussion

The arguments for and against induced hypotension (Enderby, 1958; Armstrong Davison, 1958) have continued unabated since its introduction. Many feel that this technique only adds an unjustifiable risk to the patient's life and intellectual capacity. Others argue that in skilled hands it carries no great risk. Wyman (1933) reported on its use in 1,000 patients with 5 deaths. Two were believed to be due to the patient's disease and three to faulty technique. If the technique is understood he claims it should not offer any additional risks at an operation. Larson (1964) in a comprehensive review of controlled hypotension points out that though the complication risk is higher than normal, in skilled hands a very high degree of proficiency with a low morbidity can be obtained. Among the factors which he lists as militating against success are inexperience with the technique and lack of teamwork between surgeon and anaesthetist. The best results are obtained by careful selection of patients, control of ventilation, sustained gentle changes in blood pressure, the careful maintenance of blood volume and adequate post-operative care.

One of the great difficulties in assessing results is that like is not always compared with like. Ideally, we would consider operations with and without hypotension performed by the same surgeon and anaesthetist, using the same technique for blood loss measurement and replacement, but, as was discussed at the start of this chapter, the aim of the technique is to produce good operating conditions by reducing haemorrhage and with so many other factors influencing wound bleeding there is no constant relationship between blood pressure and amount of haemorrhage. As Eckenhoff has pointed out, there is very little data on the surgical benefits of hypotension so it is hard to know how much one can offset an increased morbidity.

Figures for mortality and morbidity need to be accepted with caution. If some of the early large series are examined in the light of current thought about technique, about monitoring of blood loss and blood replacement, about the relationship of flow and pressure, about proper selection of cases and post-operative care, then one may arrive at quite different conclusions from the original authors.

Eckenhoff and his colleagues (1969) have compared 18 patients undergoing hypotension with 18 patients operated on at normal pressures and have been unable to show any change in brain function as demonstrated by psychometric testing. This study was on young patients but Rollason *et al.* (1968) reached a similar conclusion in a group of elderly men undergoing prostatectomy. In another comparison involving 301 patients Eckenhoff and Rich (1966) demonstrated an appreciable saving in blood loss with no death directly attributable to deliberate hypotension.

The final assessment and decision on the use of induced hypotension must rest with a balance of the relative risks and merits to a particular patient. The size of that risk depends on the state of that patient's vascular tree, the degree of hypotension attained, and the skill of the administrator. It would be unwise however, to dismiss completely a most useful adjunct to the anaesthetist's armament, but it is imperative to proceed with circumspection.

Post-operative Hypotension

One of the most illogical situations in present day anaesthesia is the immense amount of expert skill and care that is lavished upon the patient in the operating theatre, often only to be abruptly abandoned the moment the anaesthetic is stopped. During a period when a rapid physiological transition is taking place, the patient may be submitted to gross alteration in posture and environment and transported to some far corner of the hospital where, although observed for the gross complication, he is rarely tested for the earliest premonitory signs of them (*Lancet*, 1958).

Hypotension in the post-operative period is common. It is not always important but the value of the blood pressure needs to be considered against the patient's general condition, in particular his cardiac output as evidenced by the tissue perfusion, the degree of peripheral vasoconstriction or vasodilatation and the urine output.

Probably the two commonest causes of hypotension are hypovolaemia and the residual action of anaesthetic agents—the two frequently combining. The amount of blood lost is frequently underestimated and in the event of post-operative hypotension the blood loss and replacement figures should be re-examined, consideration also being given to concealed losses, and the central venous pressure measured. Most patients respond to correct replacement therapy although the residual action of drugs such as halothane or chlorpromazine may result in a low pressure despite a normal blood volume. In this case, when oligaemia has been treated or excluded, moderate hypotension can be safely treated expectantly by keeping the patient flat or by raising the foot of the bed.

If the patient is on the edge of hypovolaemia, hypotension may be precipitated if the patient is rolled over onto his side or sat up prematurely.

Disorders of acid-base balance, although usually producing hypertension, when extreme may cause the blood pressure to fall. Circulatory depression occurs as an aftermath of a high blood carbon dioxide due to inadequate ventilation during anaesthesia.

Myocardial insufficiency due to cardiac disease will produce hypotension secondary to a low cardiac output, while quite severe hypotension may follow an operation and anaesthetic when a patient fails to compensate by the normal output of adrenocortical hormones (see Chapter 50). This is particularly liable to happen after previous treatment with cortisone or related steroids, or it may occur in patients who have been suffering from prolonged or severe disease.

Unrelieved pain will cause hypotension, but before administering potentially hypotensive drugs other causes of hypotension should be eliminated. The essentials of post-operative care therefore are the proper relief of pain, the correct replacement of fluid and the ensuring that respiration, both oxygenation and CO_2 elimination, is adequate.

REFERENCES

BEDFORD, P. D. (1955). Adverse cerebral effects of anaesthesia on old people. *Lancet*, **2,** 259.

BOND, A. C. (1969). Conduction anaesthesia, blood pressure and haemorrhage. *Brit. J. Anaesth.*, **41,** 942.

BROMAGE, P. R. (1967). Physiology and pharmacology of epidural anaesthesia. *Anesthesiology*, **28,** 592.

BURN, J. H. (1961). A new view of adrenergic nerve-fibres, explaining the action of reserpine, bretylium and guanethidine. *Brit. med. J.*, **1,** 1623.

DAVISON, M. H. A. (1958). The disadvantages of controlled hypotension in surgery. *Brit. med. Bull.*, **14,** 52.

DONALD, J. R. (1969). The effect of anaesthesia, hypotension and epidural analgesia on blood loss in surgery for pelvic floor repair. *Brit. J. Anaesth.*, **41,** 155.

ECKENHOFF, J. E. (1966). Circulatory control in the surgical patient. *Ann. roy. Coll. Surg.*, **39,** 67.

ECKENHOFF, J. E., CROMPTON, J. R., LARSON, A., and DAVIES, R. M. (1969). Assessment of the cerebral effects of deliberate hypotension by psychological measurements. *Lancet*, **2,** 711.

ECKENHOFF, J. E., ENDERBY, G. E. H., LARSON, A., EDRIDGE, A., and JUDEVINE, D. E. (1963). Pulmonary gas exchange during deliberate hypotension. *Brit. J. Anaesth.*, **35,** 750.

ECKENHOFF, J. E., and RICH, J. C. (1966). Clinical experiences with deliberate hypotension. *Curr. Res. Anesth.*, **45,** 21.

ENDERBY, G. E. H. (1954). Pentolinium tartrate in controlled hypotension. *Lancet*, **2,** 1097.

ENDERBY, G. E. H. (1954*b*). Postural ischaemia and blood pressure. *Lancet*, **1,** 185.

ENDERBY, G. E. H. (1958). The advantages of controlled hypotension in surgery. *Brit. med. Bull.*, **14,** 49.

ENDERBY, G. E. H., and PELMORE, J. F. (1951). Controlled hypotension and postural ischaemia to reduce bleeding in surgery. Review of 250 cases. *Lancet*, **1,** 663.

GILLIES, J. (1959). In: *General Anaesthesia*, p. 55. Ed. by Evans, F. T., and Gray, T. C. London: Butterworth.

HELLEWELL, J., and POTTS, M. W. (1966). Propranalol during controlled hypotension. *Brit. J. Anaesth.*, **38**, 794.

HEWITT, P. B., LORD, P. W., and THORNTON, H. L. (1967). Propranalol in hypotensive anaesthesia. *Anaesthesia*, **22**, 82.

HOLLOWAY, K. B., HOLMES, F., and HIDER, C. F. (1961). Guanethidine in hypotensive anaesthesia. *Brit. J. Anaesth.*, **33**, 648.

LANCET (1958). Post-operative hypotension (Annotation). *Lancet*, **1**, 575.

LARSON, A. G. (1964). Deliberate hypotension. *Anesthesiology*, **24**, 682.

MCCUBBIN, J. W., and PAGE, I. H. (1952). Nature of hypotensive action of thiophanium derivative (Ro 2–222) in dogs. *J. Pharmacol. exp. Ther.*, **105**, 437.

MCLAUGHLIN, C. R. (1961). Hypotensive anaesthesia in plastic surgery: a surgeon's view. *Brit. J. plast. Surg.*, **14**, 39.

MCLAUGHLIN, C. R. (1966). Hypotensive anesthesia. A surgeon's view. *Anesthesiology*, **27**, 239.

MOIR, D. D. (1968). Blood loss during major vaginal surgery. *Brit. J. Anaesth.*, **40**, 233.

PAYNE, J. P. (1956). Histamine release during controlled hypotension with Arfonad. *Proc. World Congress of Anesthesiologists*, 1955, p. 180. Minneapolis: Burgess Pub. Co.

RANDALL, L. O., PETERSEN, W. G., and LEHMANN, G. (1949). The ganglionic blocking action of thiophanium derivatives. *J. Pharmacol. exp. Ther.*, **97**, 48.

RICHARDSON, D. W., HONOUR, H. J., FENTON, G. W., STOTT, F. N., and PICKERING, G. W. (1964). Variation in arterial pressure throughout day and night. *Clin. Sci.*, **26**, 445.

ROBERTSON, J. D., GILLIES, J., and SPENCER, K. E. V. (1957). The use of a homatropinium derivative to produce controlled hypotension. *Brit. J. Anaesth.*, **29**, 342.

ROLLASON, W. N., ROBERTSON, G. S., and CORDINER, C. M. (1968). Effect of hypotensive anaesthesia on mental function in the elderly. *Brit. J. Anaesth.*, **40**, 477.

SCHEINBERG, P. (1949). The effects of postural changes, stellate ganglion block, and anaemia on the cerebral circulation. *J. clin. Invest.*, **28**, 808.

SHENKIN, H. A., HARMEL, M. H., and KETY, S. S. (1948). Dynamic anatomy of cerebral circulation. *Arch. Neurol. Psychiat.* (*Chic.*), **60**, 240.

WIEN, R., and MASON, D. F. J. (1953). The pharmacological actions of a series of phenyl alkane *p*-ω-bis-(trialkylammonium) compounds. *Brit. J. Pharmacol.*, **8**, 306.

WILKINS, R. W., BRADLEY, S. E., and FRIEDLAND, C. K. (1950). Acute circulatory effects of the head down position (negative G) in normal man, with notes on some measures designed to relieve cranial congestion in this position. *J. clin. Invest.*, **29**, 940.

WYMAN, J. B. (1953). Discussion on hypotension during anaesthesia. *Proc. roy. Soc. Med.*, **46**, 605.

Chapter 24

ANAESTHESIA AND CARDIAC DISEASE

CARDIAC disease covers a wide spectrum of both anatomical and physiological disturbance. How cardiac disease affects and is affected by anaesthesia and surgery is discussed in the following pages. However, the basic principles for successful management of cardiac patients derive, in the first place, from a proper understanding of the haemodynamic effects of the patient's lesion. The anaesthetist needs, therefore, to be able to diagnose the lesion and to assess correctly the effect that it has had on the patient's haemodynamic state.

THE ASSESSMENT OF THE PATIENT WITH CARDIAC DISEASE

Objects.—The main objects in the assessment of patients with cardiac disease are:

(a) to determine the capability of the heart and circulation to withstand the stresses which accompany anaesthesia and surgery, not only during the operative period but equally in the post-operative period;

(b) to make a logical choice of anaesthetic techniques and supportive therapy, based on an understanding of the patient's haemodynamic state.

Diagnosis.—Assessment involves firstly the diagnosis of the nature and severity of the specific lesion present. From this the haemodynamic consequences and likely complications can be predicted and therefore sought. The complications of a lesion are often more important than the actual disease itself.

An assessment, therefore, includes consideration of:

(a) the state of the myocardium—which may be shown by low cardiac output, congestive cardiac failure, or by the occurrence of arrhythmias;

(b) the state of the systemic vessels—particularly in respect of coronary artery disease or systemic hypertension;

(c) the condition of the lungs—both the ventilatory function which may be impaired by pulmonary oedema, chronic bronchitis and emphysema, and the pulmonary vascular tree in which pulmonary arterial obstructive disease can occur;

(d) the function of other organs—particularly of the liver and kidneys—which may be affected by tricuspid valve disease, venous engorgement or a low cardiac output.

Clinical assessment.—A thorough history and clinical examination of the patient will provide most of the information needed in the assessment of the fitness of patients to withstand the operation and post-operative period.

Observation of the Patient

A simple estimation of what the patient can do is valuable. The ability to carry out housework normally in the case of a woman, to climb a flight of stairs without stopping, to walk up a hill or even to dress, in some measure gives an indication of whether or not the heart can increase its output in response to demand.

Symptoms.—The symptoms of cardiac disease result from physiological disturbances. These disturbances are:

i. *Raised left atrial pressure* giving rise to dyspnoea and cough and may be due to left heart failure, mitral or aortic valve disease.
ii. *Raised systemic venous pressure* giving rise to peripheral oedema. This is due to right heart (congestive) failure, itself the consequence of lesions of the pulmonary valve, or pulmonary hypertension, or secondary to left ventricular failure. Hepatic pain occurs particularly if there is associated tricuspid incompetence. A raised systemic venous pressure, without right ventricular failure, may also be the result of pericardial disease or tricuspid stenosis.
iii. *Low cardiac output* which produces the symptoms of fatigue and syncope on exertion and which results from cardiac failure, valvular stenosis, raised pulmonary vascular resistance, tamponade or constrictive pericarditis.
iv. *Myocardial ischaemia*, of which the principal symptom is angina, and which is usually due to coronary artery disease.
v. *Arrhythmias* felt by the patients as palpitations, and which arise either from disturbances of pacemaker activity or disorders of the conducting tissue. These result principally from ischaemia or electrolyte disturbances and may be provoked by drug therapy.

Angina.—Angina is due to inadequate oxygen supply to the myocardium. This may follow narrowing of the coronary arteries, severe anaemia, thyrotoxicosis, or increased myocardial demands for oxygen which exceed the supply, as may occur in the hypertrophic ventricle of aortic stenosis or in the rapid heart rates of paroxysmal tachycardia. There are four major features of anginal pain:

i. it is situated maximally behind the sternum or across the front of the chest;
ii. the pain is described as "crushing" or as a "tight constricting sensation";
iii. it radiates characteristically to the angle of the jaw and down the inside of the left arm, but may also spread into the shoulders and neck and down the other arm to the hand;
iv. the pain comes on during exertion, anger or excitement, and when the stimulus is discontinued the pain wears off in two to three minutes.

Dyspnoea.—Dyspnoea is probably the most common symptom of cardiac disease and is usually the result of a raised pulmonary venous pressure. Rises of pressure in the left atrium and pulmonary veins are transmitted back to the pulmonary capillaries increasing the transudation of fluid from the capillaries into the interstitial tissues of the lungs. This reduces the ventilation and increases the effort needed to inflate and deflate the lungs.

Orthopnoea and paroxysmal nocturnal dyspnoea are specific types of dyspnoea. Orthopnoea means dyspnoea which occurs when lying flat and which is relieved by sitting up and is due to the increase in blood volume of the lungs that occurs in the supine position. Paroxysmal nocturnal dyspnoea wakens the patient from sleep, forcing him to sit upright or stand out of bed for relief, and is due to the blood volume increasing as interstitial fluid returns to the blood during the night. Should the pressure in the pulmonary veins rise above the osmotic pressure of the plasma, pulmonary oedema will occur; dyspnoea is then acute and is accompanied by a cough and copious pink or frothy white sputum. The upright position lowers the right atrial pressure which in turn diminishes the right ventricular output and leads to a decrease in pulmonary congestion and consequently ventilation becomes easier with less dyspnoea. Chronic congestion leads to fibrosis in the interstitial tissue of the lung between the alveoli and the capillaries, and tends to prevent transudation into the alveoli so that frank pulmonary oedema is less evident at this stage. Pulmonary oedema thus occurs essentially early in the progress of cardiac disease and is often precipitated by the stress of effort or emotion or by uncontrolled atrial fibrillation or tachycardia.

Useful information about the severity of heart disease is obtained by grading the severity of the dyspnoea:

Grade 1. Dyspnoea while undertaking unusual exertion (running, walking up hill, scrubbing).
Grade 2. Moderate walking on the level causes dyspnoea.
Grade 3. Unable to continue walking, even slowly, on the level. All but the lightest housework has to be given up.
Grade 4. The slightest effort produces breathlessness: the patient is practically confined to bed by dyspnoea.

A history of nocturnal dyspnoea or acute pulmonary oedema places the patient in grade 4 irrespective of effort tolerance. Dyspnoea may also occur in conditions which give rise to a low cardiac output when the tissue anoxia is responsible for a mild dyspnoea. Breathlessness on exertion is present in all right-to-left intracardiac shunts as the reduced oxygen content of the arterial blood stimulates the chemoreceptors at the carotid body. Dyspnoea occurring in patients with cardiac disease may also be due to an associated chronic lung lesion such as emphysema.

Cough may be precipitated by a rise in pulmonary venous pressure during exertion, causing engorgement of the bronchial mucosa. This gives rise to a troublesome dry cough. Chronic elevation of the bronchial venous pressure results in an oedematous mucosa offering less resistance to infection and prone to repeated attacks of chronic bronchitis.

Haemoptysis.—Haemoptysis is an important symptom in cardiac disease. It commonly occurs from the rupture of a small engorged vein in conditions which give rise to a raised left atrial pressure. The source of bleeding may be a pulmonary infarct and haemoptysis is common in chronic bronchitis. The patient may also describe "coughing up blood" when suffering from acute pulmonary oedema.

"Palpitations".—This is a commonly used term for any increased awareness of the heart beat. The sudden onset of fast palpitations may represent the onset of an attack of paroxysmal tachycardia or of atrial fibrillation.

Syncope.—Syncope as a symptom of cardiac disease may accompany complete heart block. Occasionally the cardiac output is acutely reduced at the onset of a fast arrhythmia and syncope results. Sudden attacks of loss of consciousness are not uncommon in children suffering from Fallot's tetralogy. They commonly occur as a result of emotional stress when they are thought to be due to spasm of the infundibulum of the right ventricle. If the attack is prolonged, death may occur. Effort syncope occurs as a characteristic symptom of aortic stenosis.

Peripheral oedema.—Congestive cardiac failure is one of the causes of peripheral oedema and is due to an abnormal retention of salt and water. The fluid tends to settle under the influence of gravity into the most dependent parts of the body.

Hepatic pain follows the enlargement and distension of the hepatic capsule which is secondary to a high systemic venous pressure in right heart failure. It causes a dull ache in the epigastrium and right hypochondrium and is often aggravated by exertion which further increases the systemic venous pressure.

Examination of the Patient

Examination of the cardiovascular system is carried out in a standard order so that no detail is missed. The patient is placed reclining against the pillows of the bed so that the thorax is at an angle of 45° to the horizontal and the head is supported so that the sterno-mastoid muscles are relaxed.

General appearance.—The general appearance of the patient is noted, especially emaciation which might accompany chronic heart failure, stunted growth which may be the result of congenital cyanotic heart disease, or obesity which may aggravate cardiac disease. Any anatomical abnormalities which are known to accompany congenital heart disease are sought for. Patients with a chronically low cardiac output have a dusty mauve flush with telangiectases on their cheeks known as a malar flush, most commonly seen in mitral valve disease complicated by pulmonary hypertension.

Cyanosis indicates an excess of reduced haemoglobin in the blood and the critical distinction must be made between peripheral and central cyanosis. Peripheral cyanosis due to increased oxygen extraction by the tissues as a compensation for low cardiac output is best seen in the lobes of the ear, the nose, and in the fingers. Central cyanosis, which is caused by reduction in oxygen content of the systemic arterial blood due to intracardiac or pulmonary right-to-left shunts, is characteristically seen in warm mucous membrane, such as the tongue, lips and conjunctivae. In cyanotic heart disease, bacterial endocarditis or left atrial myxoma there may be clubbing of the fingers, although this may be the consequence of lung disease.

The signs of anaemia and thyrotoxicosis are sought for as these two conditions both aggravate cardiac disease or may even precipitate cardiac failure.

Arterial pulse.—The arterial pulse is analysed for the four characteristics of rate, rhythm, amplitude and wave form. The brachial is a larger and more convenient artery for study than the radial. The main peripheral pulses are palpated to confirm their presence and to exclude the diagnosis of a coarctation of the aorta. A very rapid rate is likely to lead to cardiac failure, whereas a slow rate of 60 per minute or less in the absence of heart block is the most frequent precursor of ventricular extrasystoles, and this may slow even further after anaesthetic premedication. If an arrhythmia is present it will require ECG confirmation of its type. Pulsus alternans should be sought as this is good evidence of left ventricular failure. Pulsus paradoxus, in the absence of an increased inspiratory effort due to asthma or laryngeal stridor, is an indication of tamponade or constrictive pericarditis.

Blood pressure.—The blood pressure, systolic and diastolic, is measured with particular attention being paid to the width of the sphygmomanometer cuff which has to be appropriate to the circumference of the arm.

Jugular venous pressure.—The jugular venous pressure is assessed with the patient lying at 45° to the horizontal and the pulsations in the internal jugular vein in the neck are sought. The venous pulse is analysed for its height above the sternal angle and for its wave form. The normal mean pressure is 0 to 2 cm. of water above the sternal angle and the wave form reveals both "a" and "v" waves of approximately equal height. A raised jugular venous pressure with "v" waves will be apparent in right ventricular failure and in some high output states as a consequence of increased blood volume. This can be confused with the wave form (sharp "y" descent) which occurs in patients with cardiac tamponade or constrictive pericarditis. Distended veins which do not pulsate may simulate a raised jugular venous pressure and result from superior vena caval obstruction as may occur in bronchial carcinoma or enlargement of the thyroid gland.

Palpation.—The most reliable evidence of cardiac enlargement comes from the chest radiograph, but a good estimate of the heart size can be made by palpating the apex beat which should lie in the fifth intercostal space within the mid-clavicular line. Apex beats outside these boundaries indicate cardiac enlargement provided the heart is not displaced by pulmonary disease. The characteristic of the apical impulse is assessed to estimate left ventricular hypertrophy while the left sternal edge is palpated to assess right ventricular hypertrophy. Loud murmurs may be felt as palpable vibrations (thrills) which are maximal where the murmur is loudest. Loud heart sounds can also be felt—in mitral stenosis the loud first sound (the tapping impulse) and the second sound in the pulmonary area if the pulmonary arterial pressure is raised.

Auscultation.—In each area the appropriate heart sound is listened to individually and separately and additional heart sounds—ejection click, opening snap, third and fourth heart sounds—are sought. When the timing and characteristics of the heart sounds have been clearly established, murmurs are sought. A full description of any murmur includes its timing—systolic or diastolic, the site of its maximal intensity and conduction, its loudness and quality, and the influence on it of respiration. Mitral murmurs are heard loudest in the region of the apex beat with the patient turned on the left side with the breath held in expiration. Tricuspid murmurs are localised to the fourth left interspace at the sternal edge and are accentuated by inspiration which increases flow across the valve. Aortic murmurs are heard loudest in the aortic area, at the apex and over the carotid arteries in the neck. The diastolic murmur of aortic regurgitation is heard at the left sternal edge during full expiration with the patient leaning forward. Sounds from the pulmonary valve are usually localised and heard best over the pulmonary area and are accentuated during inspiration with the increased blood flow into the lungs.

Lungs.—The lungs are examined for the presence of a pleural effusion, which is not uncommon in heart failure, and for the presence of crepitations or râles at the lung bases. Left ventricular failure does not always cause sufficient excess bronchial secretions to give rise to râles and crepitations and the absence of these sounds does not exclude the diagnosis. Sounds will also frequently be suppressed by positive-pressure respiration. Widespread crepitations caused by fluid in the bronchi and alveoli are heard in the pulmonary oedema.

Liver.—The liver is palpated to determine whether it is enlarged below the costal margin and whether it is tender as well as enlarged. The oedema fluid of cardiac failure settles under the influence of gravity and is most commonly found as pitting oedema of the ankles and feet in ambulant patients, or as a pad of oedema overlying the sacrum in patients who have been confined to bed.

Signs of Cardiac Failure

(*a*) *Left ventricular failure.*—The physical signs of early left ventricular failure are sinus tachycardia, a slightly raised jugular venous pressure and a third sound at the apex. The congestion of the pulmonary capillaries leads to dyspnoea and orthopnoea and, on auscultation, moist sounds can be heard at the bases of the lungs.

(*b*) *Right ventricular failure.*—The signs of right ventricular failure may exist by themselves or be superimposed on those of left ventricular failure. The main sign of right sided failure is a raised jugular venous pressure with a large "v" wave. A right ventricular third sound may be audible. The liver is enlarged and may be tender. Oedema collects at the ankles and sacrum, and pleural effusions and ascites may be present.

Chest Radiography

Clinical examination of the patient continues with an interpretation of the straight X-ray of the heart in the standard posterior-anterior view. Penetrated posterior-anterior and penetrated left lateral chest X-rays may also be valuable for the detection of valvular or pericardial calcification but oblique films of barium swallow are used only in special circumstances as most information may be obtained by the straight posterior-anterior film.

Having checked that the patient is not rotated and that the film is straight, the heart is scrutinised in an orderly fashion. First, the right border working from above downwards. The superior vena cava is seen as a vertical line at the upper border of the heart medial to the sterno-clavicular angle. Below this lies the ascending aorta which if dilated projects to the right and distorts the normal smooth line of the S.V.C. This suggests post-stenotic dilatation, due to aortic valve disease, or an aneurysm of the ascending aorta. Below the ascending aorta the right atrium forms the right border of the heart, terminating at the diaphragm. A prominent or bulging right wall of the heart may be due to right atrial enlargement, to enlargement of the left atrium displacing the right atrium laterally or to a pericardial effusion.

Second, the left border of the heart. At the top, this is composed of the arch of the aorta, seen as a rounded knuckle at the upper left margin of the cardiac silhouette. This may be prominent in aortic incompetence or lesions causing dilatation of the aorta, or it may be inconspicuous in low cardiac output states such as severe aortic stenosis. The pulmonary trunk lies immediately below the aortic knuckle and is dilated in pulmonary valve stenosis or in conditions leading

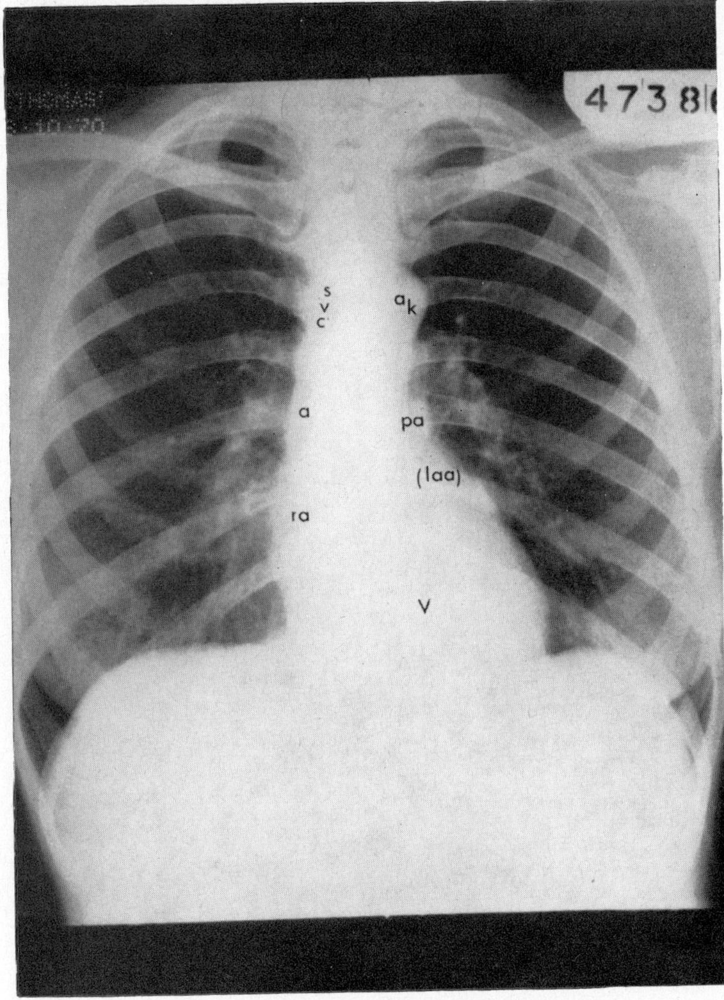

NORMAL CHEST X-RAY

V—Ventricular mass
r.a.—Right atrium
a—Ascending aorta
S.V.C.—Superior vena cava
a.k.—Aortic knuckle
p.a.—Pulmonary artery
(laa)—Position of left atrial appendage

24/FIG. 1(*a*)

to an increased flow or pressure in the pulmonary artery. Below the pulmonary artery is the atrial appendage and this is not normally visible on chest radiography unless enlarged. Enlargement of the left atrium usually accompanies enlargement of the appendage and this chamber can usually be seen as a circular shadow lying centrally behind the heart and of a slightly higher density. This is seen best on a penetrated posterior-anterior picture.

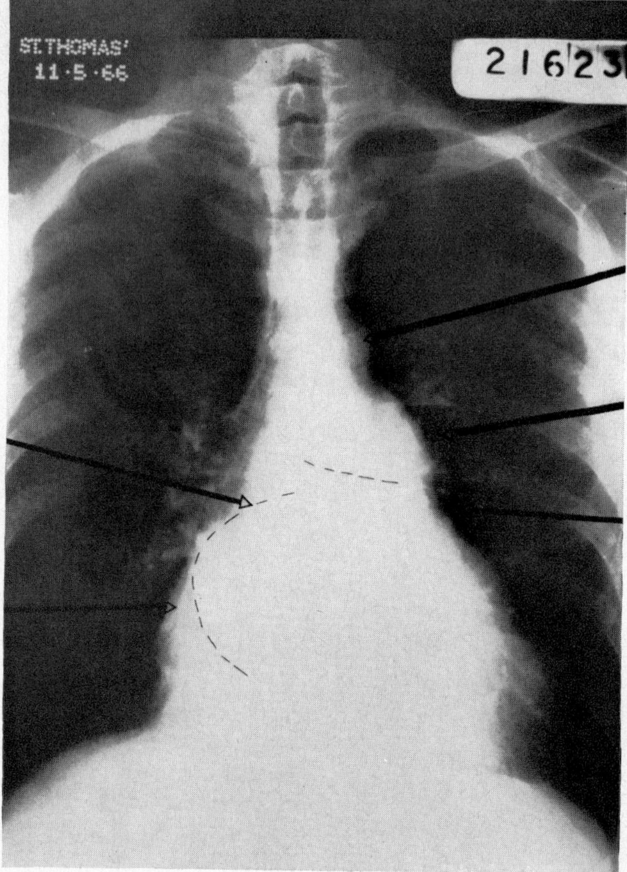

MITRAL STENOSIS
24/FIG. 1(*b*)

Differentiation of left and right ventricular hypertrophy is not easy on a chest X-ray, being better appreciated by palpation of the precordium and on the ECG.

Examination of the chest radiograph is completed by consideration of the lung fields. The larger branches of the pulmonary arteries and main pulmonary veins responsible for the normal lung markings dilate and the smaller vessels become visible when the blood flow through the lungs is increased. This is a characteristic of a left to right cardiac shunt.

If the pulmonary vascular resistance is raised (pulmonary hypertension) the proximal pulmonary arteries are large but the peripheral vessels become almost invisible leaving the lung fields abnormally clear and translucent. With decreased pulmonary blood flow (pulmonary atresia, pulmonary stenosis, Fallot's tetralogy) the vascular markings are small and sparse and the lung fields abnormally clear. In pulmonary venous congestion, secondary to a raised left atrial pressure, the

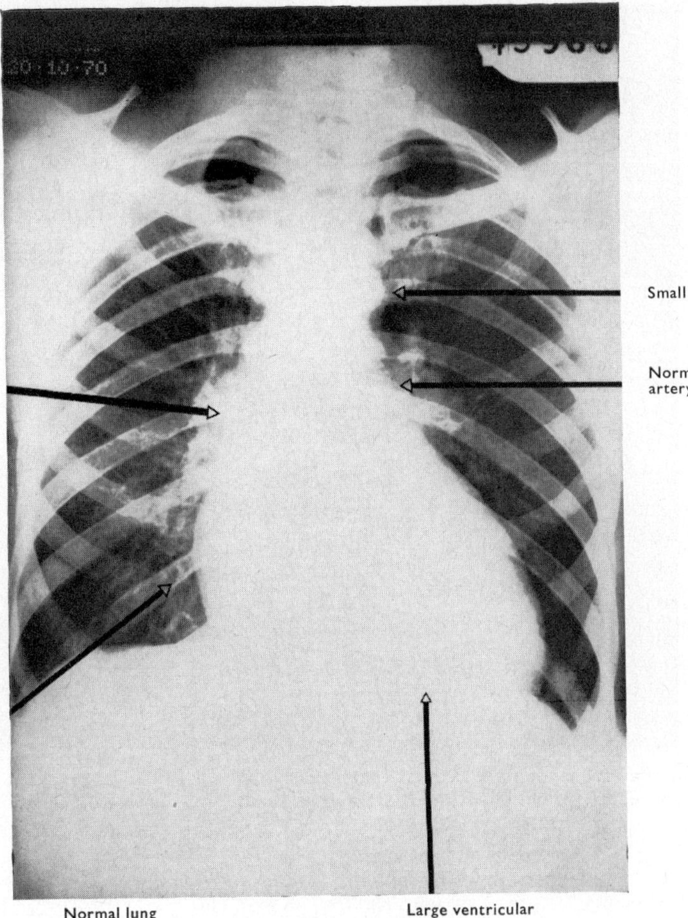

AORTIC STENOSIS
(with slight incompetence)
24/FIG. 1(*c*)

veins are dilated and more easily seen. The increased interstitial fluid produces an overall ground-glass appearance, a peri-hilar flare and fine horizontal lines in the costo-phrenic angle (Kerley lines). Pulmonary oedema represents extreme pulmonary venous congestion and patchy shadowing is seen around the hilum extending out into the surrounding lung.

Electrocardiography

After the clinical examination and examination of the chest radiograph, the examination is completed by consideration of the electrocardiogram. This is inspected principally for evidence of arrhythmias, conduction disturbances, myocardial disease and ventricular strain, and is discussed in detail in Chapter 9. A normal ECG does not, however, exclude cardiac disease.

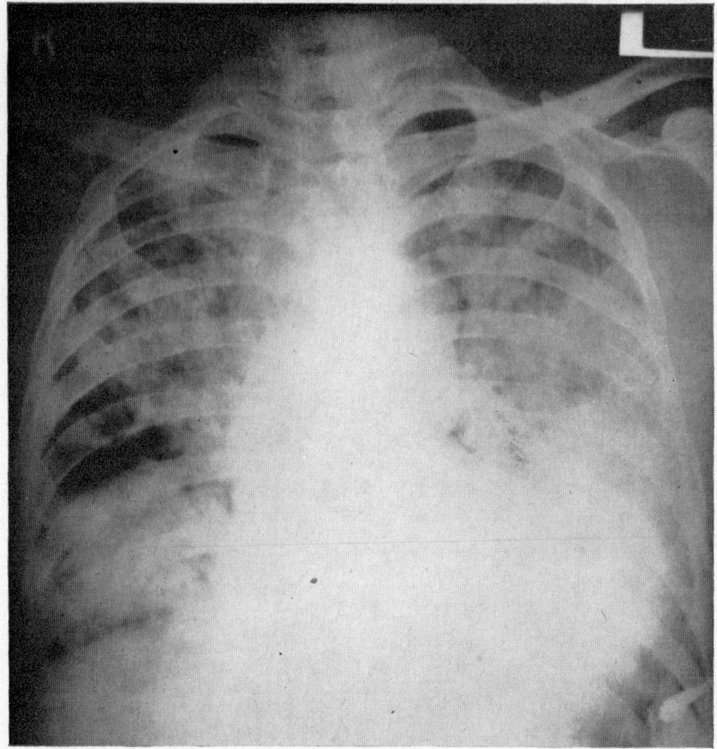

Severe bilateral pulmonary oedema, particularly marked in the lower lobes, following a myocardial infarction. Note that the heart is quite small. Physical signs at this time:

Patient dyspnoeic, sweating, confused, cyanosed, hypotensive.
Moist sounds all over chest.
Copious pink frothy sputum.
pH 7.31, Pa_{CO_2} 30 mm. Hg, Pa_{O_2} 46 mm. Hg

24/Fig. 1(*d*)

In certain circumstances, the clinical examination is supplemented by special investigations such as cardiac catheterisation and angiocardiography. This is considered in detail on page 661.

Comment

In assessing a patient with cardiac disease for anaesthesia, consideration must be given not only to the effects of anaesthesia but also to the effect of surgery and the possible complications which may arise both in the operative and post-operative period. At the time of assessment the need is to recognise firstly whether the patient is in the optimum condition for surgery. The most common complication to be found is the presence of cardiac failure and surgery ought not to be performed except of an emergency nature until the patient has been properly treated: the ability to treat cardiac failure correctly is a valuable asset for an anaesthetist. There are certain situations which ought to be easily recognised—in particular, the fixed low cardiac output, the presence of pulmonary hypertension, a propensity to dangerous arrhythmias, the likelihood of impairment of flow through the vital organs and the presence of intracardiac shunts which are dependent on normal systemic and pulmonary vascular resistances for their direction.

Against this knowledge of the patient's lesions and their complications the anaesthetist can consider the possible effects of anaesthesia and surgery. Decisions can then be made on the pre-operative treatment and how this should be modified over the operative period.

A choice can also be made of the monitoring techniques which will best facilitate continuous assessment of the circulation and what supportive therapy will be necessary to sustain the cardiovascular system.

The severity of the cardiac disease is probably of greater importance than the nature of the operation and the principles for successful management of cardiac patients in relation to the severity of their disease are needed regardless of the type of surgery.

Cardiac Catheterisation and Angiocardiography

A thorough history and clinical examination supplemented by examination of the ECG and chest radiograph will enable the precise diagnosis to be made in most cases of cardiovascular disease. In some instances, however, the diagnosis may remain in doubt and in other cases the diagnosis may be known but its quantitative effects not be clearly apparent. Cardiac catheterisation and angiocardiography are undertaken to confirm the diagnosis accurately and to provide the information on which future treatment can be based. There is an appreciable morbidity and mortality with cardiac catheterisation, higher when the left side of the heart is entered than the right (*Lancet*, 1968) and it is therefore a procedure which should not be undertaken unless there is likely to be obvious benefit to the patient.

Right heart catheterisation entails the passage of a catheter which enters the circulation through a vein, usually in the groin or elbow, and passes through the vena cava to the right atrium. It can then be passed through the tricuspid valve to the right ventricle and out through the pulmonary valve into the pulmonary arteries. If the catheter is pushed as far as possible into the lung fields the tip will wedge and it is then possible to make an indirect measurement of left atrial pressure. The coronary sinus can also be entered from the right atrium.

Left heart catheterisation can be performed in three ways. The left heart may be entered in the presence of a septal defect during right-sided cardiac catheterisation. If there is no patent foramen ovale it is possible to perforate the inter-atrial septum with a special needle during right-sided catheterisation and a catheter can then be threaded over the needle into the left atrium and thence to the left ventricle. Alternatively, aortic catheterisation can be performed by the retrograde passage of a catheter up the aorta and thence across the aortic valve and into the left ventricle.

During cardiac catheterisation, two main types of information are elicited: first is the pressure recorded in the chamber in which the tip of the catheter lies. This absolute pressure may be important: thus the pulmonary artery pressure is significant when surgery is contemplated, for some operations have a much higher mortality in the presence of pulmonary hypertension. Similarly, a high end-diastolic pressure within a ventricle may indicate myocardial failure. Valvular obstruction, as for instance mitral or aortic stenosis, can be demonstrated by measuring the pressure gradient across the valve in the presence of a reasonable cardiac output.

The second type of information relates to the oxygen tension or saturation of the blood in the various chambers, and this may be useful as a demonstration of the presence and site of an intracardiac shunt and in the measurement of cardiac output.

Information about incompetence of valves is harder to obtain from simple cardiac catheterisation and in some instances anatomical abnormalities may not be fully demonstrated by this technique. Selective angiocardiography is then required to complete the diagnosis. Radio-opaque dye is injected under pressure into the appropriate chamber of the heart and its passage recorded either on X-ray cine film or on multiple cut films. Anaesthesia for cardiac investigations is considered in detail under "Anaesthesia for Special Situations" (see p. 679)

Pre-operative Treatment

Pre-operative treatment depends both on the nature of the cardiac disease and the nature of the operation to be performed. Treatment prior to cardiac or major vascular surgery is different in emphasis from that prior to some incidental operations. All treatment should be considered under two headings: first, the treatment which is necessary to gain control of the patient and to render him in the best possible condition for surgery, and second, how this treatment should be modified in the immediate operative and post-operative period.

In general, such treatment is directed to the correction of cardiac failure, the prevention or treatment of arrhythmias, the symptomatic management of coronary artery disease, and the treatment of hypertension.

The Treatment of Cardiac Failure

Regardless of its cause, no patient should be submitted to anaesthesia or surgery while in cardiac failure. Every effort must be made to ensure that the cardiovascular system is brought to an optimal state. Sometimes a patient presents in cardiac failure with a condition requiring an emergency operation. Much can still be done to treat the failure quickly, but whenever possible operation is delayed to allow for adequate pre-operative medical treatment.

(*a*) **Bed rest** is the mainstay of treatment. As long as failure continues there should be strict bed rest and the patient only allowed up very cautiously once control has been gained.

(*b*) **Low salt diet.**—A normal diet contains 50 to 60 mEq of salt per day. Patients being treated for cardiac failure are advised not to add salt to their food and to avoid salty dishes. This reduces the intake to around 40 mEq per day. Only as a last resort, when digitalis and diuretics are unable to control the failure, is a low salt diet (less than 10 mEq per day) prescribed.

(*c*) **Digitalis.**—The primary function of digitalis is to increase the contractility, and thus the cardiac output, of the failing heart. Regardless of whether or not the heart is failing, digitalis is also used in the control of ventricular rate in atrial tachycardia and atrial fibrillation (see also p. 677). In the treatment of cardiac failure the principle is to digitalise the patient fully, raising the dose until the desired effect is obtained. If the patient shows signs of digitalis toxicity (nausea, bradycardia, ventricular arrhythmias), the drug is stopped until the symptoms cease, and then restarted at a reduced level. Normally the initial digitalising dose of 0·03 mg./kg. is given as Tabs. digoxin in divided doses over 24 hours, this being safer than the intravenous route which is reserved for use in emergencies. In the control of atrial fibrillation the dose is maintained at that level which controls the ventricular rate. Digitalis administration is contra-indicated in the presence of a low serum potassium, ventricular arrhythmias, partial heart block and in cardiac operations where any potential interference with the conducting tissue is anticipated.

The main hazard of pre-operative digitalis administration is in the possibility of the patient developing digitalis toxicity during or after surgery. Concurrent use of diuretics will increase this danger. If the patient has been receiving pre-operative digitalis and diuretics both drugs are stopped one to three days before operation, and cardiac failure is kept under control by strict bed rest alone. The opportunity is taken to push potassium supplements in an effort to replenish the body stores. In patients with tricuspid incompetence, however, it may be necessary to continue diuretics until nearer the operation, because marked fluid retention may occur. If the patient has been receiving digitalis without diuretics the digitalis can be safely administered up to the day before operation.

Prophylactic pre-operative digitalisation is sometimes advocated for patients who have a tendency to develop atrial fibrillation during or after the operation (particularly pneumonectomy or mitral valvotomy) because the onset of fibrillation is usually accompanied by ventricular rates which embarrass cardiac output. This is quite safe provided the patient has not received oral diuretics previously. If an undigitalised patient develops uncontrolled atrial fibrillation on the operating table, digoxin 0·01 mg/kg. is diluted in 10 ml. of saline and given intravenously over fifteen minutes, provided the serum potassium is normal. This is followed by intramuscular or oral administration of 0·25 mg. digoxin six-hourly until the ventricular rate is reduced and the cardiac output improved.

(*d*) **Diuretics**.—The other mainstay in the treatment of cardiac failure is the use of diuretics. The best index of fluid retention is the weight of the patient, and daily weighing is the most accurate chart of progress in the treatment of cardiac failure. The jugular venous pressure and ankle or sacral oedema are less reliable because pure left ventricular failure can exist in the presence of an almost normal right atrial pressure, although sinus tachycardia and apical gallop (3rd sound) may point to the diagnosis. Diuretics are prescribed initially to reduce the weight and thereafter to maintain it constant, while keeping the haematocrit, serum sodium and blood urea at normal levels.

Thiazides.—These are potent non-mercurial diuretics which are well tolerated and which can be given by mouth. Their mode of action is to inhibit proximal tubular reabsorption of sodium and chloride, in contrast to mercurials which act primarily by inhibiting chloride reabsorption. There are now a number of these drugs whose effectiveness is comparable and which differ only in dose and price. Bendrofluazide is cheap and effective. The dose is initially 5–10 mg. with a maintenance of 2·5–5·0 mg. daily. Diuresis starts two hours after ingestion and lasts for twelve hours.

Frusemide is a monosulphanyl diuretic which acts similarly to the thiazides but is much more potent. It is both quicker-acting and of shorter duration and possesses the advantage that it can be given intravenously. The initial oral dose is 40 mg. but up to 160 mg. can be given daily. The intravenous dose is 20 mg.

Ethacrynic acid is a desulphanyl compound which is even more potent and, like frusemide, can be given intravenously in a dose of 50 mg.

Both frusemide and ethacrynic acid have been advocated for use in the treatment of acute pulmonary oedema. Given intravenously, both produce a response within 10 minutes which may be very effective. Their potency gives rise to two dangers—the diuresis is accompanied by potassium loss and the very size of the diuresis after intravenous ethacrynic acid may produce hypovolaemic hypotension.

(*e*) **Potassium and diuretics** (see also p. 677).—All the above diuretics, besides causing inhibition of salt and water retention, lead to excessive loss of body potassium. This may be a chronic state following long-continued diuretic therapy, an acute response to a sudden diuresis, or, most dangerously, an acute loss superimposed on a chronic deficiency. All patients who have been on continued diuretic therapy will have a total body potassium content which may be reduced by 30–50 per cent despite replacement therapy and a normal serum potassium level. A low serum potassium or an otherwise unexplained metabolic alkalosis suggests a very severe deficiency. Potassium depletion potentiates arrhythmias due to digitalis and may lead to ventricular tachycardia or fibrillation.

Patients who are receiving diuretic therapy should receive potassium supplements in some form which contains chloride, such as "Slow K" (8 mEq/tablet) or "Cloref" (6·7 mEq/tablet). The dose depends slightly on diet, but because not all is absorbed and the minimum loss in urine is about 30 mEq/day, patients may require 50–100 mEq daily. If the potassium level falls below 3·5 mEq/1. as a result of an acute diuresis and the patient develops ventricular arrhythmias, intravenous potassium is given in 5 mEq increments until the arrhythmia disappears, when a slow infusion of potassium 50–100 mEq/day can be used to restore the potassium balance. Because of the loss of potassium which accompanies the use of the diuretics already described, two other diuretics—spironolactone and triamterene—which promote potassium reabsorption are sometimes prescribed in conjunction with the thiazides.

Spironolactone is an aldersterone antagonist, and by decreasing the reabsorption of sodium in the distal tubule in exchange for potassium, when used in conjunction with bendrofluazide, produces an increased diuresis with a reduction in potassium loss. The minimum effective dose is 100–150 mg. daily, but due to its blocking action further increments do not enhance its effect.

Triamterene which is an aminopteridine, increases excretion of sodium and chloride but it also acts on the distal tubule to decrease potassium loss, but not by antagonism of aldersterone (dose 50 mg. b.d.).

Effusions.—In the medical treatment of cardiac failure, pleural effusions or ascites are rarely tapped. However, large pleural effusions may embarrass cardiac and pulmonary function, particularly if the patient is to be placed in the lateral position on the operating table. These are best tapped the day before operation so that the patient has 24 hours to readjust, as on rare occasions acute pulmonary oedema may develop when the fluid is removed too quickly.

The Treatment of Arrhythmias

Patients may present for anaesthesia with some arrhythmia or may be already receiving treatment to control rhythm disturbances. The extremes of ventricular rate (bradycardia; tachycardia) both produce a reduction in cardiac output and the best output occurs when the contraction of atrium and ventricle have their normal time relationships (i.e. sinus rhythm). Certain arrhythmias are dangerous, as they are precursors of ventricular fibrillation.

Supraventricular arrhythmias.—These occur most frequently as atrial fibrillation or paroxysmal atrial tachycardia, more rarely as nodal tachycardia.

Although *atrial fibrillation* can often be converted by synchronised shock (see below) a patient who has been fibrillating either continuously or intermittently will often revert from sinus rhythm to atrial fibrillation during anaesthesia and operation. These patients are normally controlled with digitalis. Some patients may have had a D.C. cardioversion and be then maintained with oral quinidine. This drug is a myocardial depressant and in toxic doses will produce ventricular arrhythmias. Quinidine is normally continued over the operative period.

The same considerations apply to *atrial flutter.*

If the patient suddenly develops a supraventricular tachycardia, the fast rate may produce a low cardiac output and acute hypotension. These patients are cardioverted to gain immediate control and then digitalised in case the tachycardia recurs.

Attacks of paroxysmal tachycardia can often be aborted by some vagal stimulating action (carotid compression, etc.) and prior to surgery these patients are controlled with either digitalis or quinidine. Care is taken to ensure that the patient does not have paroxysmal atrial tachycardia with block which may be a sign of digitalis toxicity.

Nodal rhythm is an uncommon pre-operative discovery. It may represent digitalis toxicity but more usually is a vagal response to fear. Treatment is to stop the digitalis and reassure the patient. At operation a small dose of atropine will often restore sinus rhythm.

Ventricular ectopics are not at all uncommon. They may arise as a result of organic heart disease or in otherwise asymptomatic patients, as a result of potassium deficiency, too much smoking or black coffee. Coupled beats are often a manifestation of digitalis toxicity. If there is a specific cause (e.g. low K, digitalis) this should be remedied. Otherwise increased potassium intake is combined with suppression of ventricular excitability with quinidine or procaine amide. The latter can be used intravenously in an emergency although lignocaine is the drug of choice. Propranolol is only used very rarely in the suppression of arrhythmias, although the more recently introduced drug practolol will probably be used more often (see below).

The use of β-blocking agents before and during anaesthesia.—A possible use of propranolol is for the control of arrhythmias before anaesthesia. Its use has also been advocated for the control of arrhythmias during anaesthesia and to prevent the tachycardia which accompanies induced hypotension. The effect of β blockade on the normal healthy person is small; there is only a mild drop in blood pressure and pulse rate. Patients who are in heart failure depend on their enhanced sympathetic drive for the maintenance of their cardiac output and propranolol given to these people often results in acute reduction in cardiac output. The danger of propranolol administration to healthy patients lies in the possibility that a situation may arise subsequently in which the sympathetic effects of increased heart rate and myocardial contractility are needed. This may occur should the patient develop a cardiac arrest from any cause, suffer a myocardial infarction, or go into cardiac failure. In these instances resuscitation would prove difficult, if not impossible. It would seem that the control of arrhythmias during anaesthesia is better achieved by good oxygenation and carbon dioxide elimination, reduction in concentration of volatile arrhythmogenic agents and, if necessary, the use of lignocaine.

Propranolol may be indicated in the medical treatment of angina (see below) and outflow tract obstruction (Fallot's tetralogy with infundibular stenosis, hypertrophic obstructive cardiomyopathy). Sometimes, also, it is useful in patients with phaeochromocytoma. Normally it is discontinued at least 48 hours pre-operatively.

Propranolol is contra-indicated in patients with asthma and caution must be exercised in patients with diabetes on long-acting oral hypoglycaemic agents.

The latest β-adrenergic blocker to become available is practolol. Like propranolol it has been used in the treatment of supraventricular and ventricular dysrhythmias and in the management of hypertension and of angina. Practolol is a pure β-adrenergic receptor blocking drug which also has weak sympathomimetic properties. It lacks local analgesic and quinidine-like actions and might be expected to have little adverse effect on the myocardium, although a negative inotropic effect has been shown to result from large intravenous doses. Certainly the possibility of provoking or aggravating cardiac failure appears to be considerably less than with other drugs, such as propranolol, which have a direct myocardial depressant action. Practolol has the additional advantage that it produces no significant effect on the β-receptors of vascular and bronchial smooth muscle and can be used in asthmatic patients.

Cardioversion.—Cardioversion is used to terminate both supraventricular and ventricular tachycardias. Conversion of ventricular tachycardia and ventricular fibrillation are considered elsewhere, only supraventricular arrhythmias being considered here.

Cardioversion may be performed as an emergency procedure when some rhythm is life-threatening and other treatment will take too long to be effective. Thus the sudden onset of fast atrial fibrillation in a patient with heart disease may reduce cardiac output severely and cardioversion is performed while digitalisation takes effect.

More commonly, cardioversion is performed where an arrhythmia has persisted after the precipitating cause has been removed and it is thought likely that sinus rhythm will be stable. Thus it is performed post-operatively after cardiac surgery, or after pneumonia or thyrotoxicosis which have been treated. Quinidine is no longer used to attempt conversion of atrial fibrillation to sinus rhythm because of its myocardial depressant action, but a maintenance dose ("Kinidin durules" 750 mg. b.d.) is given for 24 hours prior to defibrillation and if successful this is continued for 18 months afterwards or until the patient reverts to atrial fibrillation. Digitalis is normally stopped 48 hours prior to cardioversion.

The contra-indications to attempted cardioversion are when the tachycardia is sinus in origin and when the patient is suffering from digitalis toxicity. Fast atrial fibrillation itself, paroxysmal atrial tachycardia with block, and nodal tachycardia may all be manifestations of digitalis toxicity and further administration of digitalis or cardioversion may be dangerous. If a shock is deemed life-saving it is preceded by intravenous lignocaine (1 mg./kg.) and is of smaller amplitude than usual. Sometimes reversion to sinus rhythm may bring out latent digitalis toxicity and rapid administration of intravenous potassium and lignocaine is then necessary.

Cardioversion is not usually performed if the patient has had a recent history of systemic embolism unless he has been anticoagulated for a month. A large heart, long-standing fibrillation and ischaemic heart disease are relative contra-indications and decrease the chance of successful reversion.

A D.C. shock of 75–300 joules is administered with two electrodes so positioned that the shock passes through the atria. The principal danger is the production of ventricular fibrillation should the shock fall on the T-wave upstroke although this should be avoided by proper synchronisation with the R-wave. Other complications are the appearance of digitalis toxicity, sudden development of cardiac failure with acute pulmonary oedema and electrical failures which can lead to the patient's attendents being shocked should they be touching him.

(Anaesthesia for cardioversion is considered on p. 679.)

The Treatment of Coronary Artery Disease

Drug therapy aimed at producing coronary vasodilatation is unsatisfactory. Hypoxia itself is the most potent vasodilator but the diseased vessels are incapable of response. Symptomatic relief of angina can be produced by reducing the work of the heart either by lowering the peripheral resistance with glyceryl trinitrate or by diminishing the ventricular contractility with propranolol.

Glyceryl trinitrate tablets are normally crushed in the mouth and absorption occurs through the oral mucosa. Because of the time taken for absorption their main value is in prophylactic use before exercise. Direct vasodilatation of the diseased coronary artery is unlikely and the effect is probably due to reduction in cardiac output and blood pressure which reduces myocardial work.

β-blockade reduces the heart rate and the velocity of contraction of the myocardial fibres. This reduces cardiac work and myocardial oxygen requirements so that the limited coronary blood flow is used to the best advantage. It also prevents the rise in work associated with exercise or emotion. There is, however, a risk of producing cardiac failure in patients with serious disease of the left ventricle, a risk which is greater with propranolol than with practolol, although the former is the more effective drug.

Surgical treatment of coronary artery disease used to consist either of sympathectomy or the creation of adhesions between the surface of the heart and some adjacent vascular structure. Two operations are now gaining favour—the Vineberg operation to implant the internal mammary artery into the myocardium, and the use of a saphenous vein graft between the aorta and a coronary artery.

In the immediate pre-operative period glyceryl trinitrate can be continued, although angina will normally be avoided by bed rest and generous sedation to prevent emotion, pain or anxiety. Propranolol will normally be discontinued. If the patient is in failure the treatment of this will be modified as suggested above.

The Treatment of Hypertension

Antihypertensive drugs have long been used in the treatment of malignant hypertension where they have clearly been shown to have a beneficial effect both on mortality and on the incidence of complications. There is more debate about the treatment of non-malignant hypertension, but as the mortality rates rise with increasing elevation of both the systolic and diastolic pressure the current tendency is to treat lesser grades of hypertension more frequently than formerly.

The usual aim of treatment is to produce a standing diastolic pressure of 100 mm.Hg or lower. This aim is not always possible either because of the troublesome side-effects of treatment or because of the danger of impaired renal function after excessive reduction in blood pressure. A higher level of blood pressure may have to be accepted to make the patient's life tolerable. Once started, antihypertensive drug treatment must in most cases be continued indefinitely.

According to the severity of the hypertension, different drug combinations are employed.

Diuretics.—The thiazide diuretics promote salt and water excretion and, by reducing plasma volume, may be sufficient therapy for some mild hypertensives. It is possible that they have some direct vasodilator action because the blood pressure remains low when the plasma volume returns to normal. In mild hypertension diuretics alone may be used but in more severe cases they may also be employed to potentiate the anti-adrenergic drugs. The usual reduction in total body potassium does not seem to give rise to trouble unless the patient develops cardiac failure or requires digitalisation for some other reason, when digitalis toxicity may be easily precipitated.

Rauwolfia.—Several active alkaloids have been extracted from rauwolfia, of which reserpine is the most popular. The hypotensive action is due to peripheral vasodilatation, probably the result of depletion of storage sites of catecholamines. Given orally, a maximal effect is reached in two to six weeks and the blood pressure returns to its previous level after up to three weeks from the time of discontinuation. Depression is the principal complication and is not uncommon, although it can be reduced in incidence by keeping the daily dose as low as possible.

Methyldopa.—More severe hypertension is treated with methyldopa which interrupts the normal synthesis of noradenaline and also depletes the adrenergic neurones of noradrenaline, thus inhibiting vasoconstrictor impulses. After oral administration an effect is achieved in three to five hours and lasts up to twenty-four hours. Renal blood flow and glomerular filtration are well maintained but tolerance, fluid retention, tiredness and depression are complications. A diuretic is usually added to combat fluid retention.

Anti-adrenergic drugs.—Bethanidine, guanethidine and debrisoquine all block post-ganglionic adrenergic neurones and deplete catecholamine stores. They have different rates of onset and duration of action but all produce a postural hypotension which may be troublesome in the morning and on exercise. Hot weather, and factors which deplete blood volume, will potentiate their effects. Side-effects are bradycardia, dry mouth, impotence, diarrhoea and fluid retention.

Other drugs.—Certain other drugs are used rarely but may cause problems in association with anaesthesia. Pargyline is a mono-amine oxidase inhibitor sometimes used as an antihypertensive. β-blockers are being used increasingly and very large doses may be employed.

For the acute treatment of hypertensive encephalopathy or eclampsia both pentolinium and trimetaphan are used. Intravenous anti-adrenergic drugs should not be used for this purpose as they produce an initial transitory rise in blood pressure.

Antihypertensive Drugs and Anaesthesia

Once antihypertensive therapy has started, even temporary discontinuation may be dangerous. Fortunately, with the wide variety of anaesthetic techniques available continued antihypertensive therapy is quite compatible with anaesthesia. At the same time, care must be taken to avoid those drugs which will potentiate the hypotensive action and the circulation must be properly monitored and supported. Blood loss is measured and promptly replaced to maintain an adequate ventricular filling pressure. If a vasopressor drug is needed it must be one which is effective in the face of anti-adrenergic drugs.

Excessive reduction in pressure in hypertensive patients may impair renal function or precipitate cerebral or coronary thrombosis, while excessive rises in pressure can result in cerebral haemorrhage.

General Considerations of Anaesthesia and Operation For Patients with Cardiac Disease

Although both anaesthesia and operation lead to specific alterations in the haemodynamics of the heart and circulation, the tolerance of the circulation in a healthy patient is considerable. It is in the presence of disease that minor upsets become accentuated and occasionally lead to cardiac or circulatory failure and death.

Effects of Anaesthesia

The effects of anaesthesia result from the administration of anaesthetic drugs and from alterations in ventilation, including positive pressure ventilation, which may accompany anaesthesia.

Anaesthetic drugs.—Some effects of drugs which may cause concern in cardiac patients are vasodilatation, depression of myocardial contractility, and alterations in rhythm and rate.

Vasodilatation is a property of many anaesthetic drugs (halothane, thiopentone, pethidine, etc.) and affects both arteries and veins. Dilatation of the arteries leads to a drop in arterial pressure which may have serious consequences if the coronary or cerebral arteries are affected by disease. The greater part of the fall in blood pressure is secondary to a reduction in cardiac output caused by blood pooling in the dilated capacitance vessels. It is the inability of the diseased heart to react to these two effects which makes the induction of anaesthesia, particularly with intravenous barbiturates, so hazardous.

Depression of myocardial contractility, which may result from halothane and the intravenous barbiturates, reduces cardiac output and decreases the response to an increased filling pressure.

In many cardiac conditions the stroke volume is relatively fixed and the cardiac output is rate sensitive. A fairly fast rate is then necessary to maintain an adequate output. Slow cardiac rates—produced by vagal stimulation, drug action or digitalis overdose—result in a decreased output and pave the way for the development of ectopic beats. At the same time, very fast pulse rates—caused by sympathetic stimulation, atropine or gallamine administration, or an arrhythmia—reduce the diastolic filling time and may result in a decreased cardiac output. In some conditions, particularly aortic stenosis, atrial contraction is needed to fill the stiff-walled ventricle and a good output is dependent on the patient being in sinus rhythm.

Ventilation.—Patients with cardiac disease frequently suffer from associated respiratory problems. The cardiac disease itself may be secondary to chronic lung disease. The lungs may have interstitial oedema from acute rise in left atrial pressure or long-standing congestion may have led to thickening and fibrosis in the lung. The effect is that the work of breathing is increased but at the same time, owing to abnormal ventilation-perfusion relationships within the lung, arterial oxygenation may be incomplete. Reductions in cardiac output will increase the arterial hypoxaemia (Kelman *et al.*, 1967).

Positive pressure ventilation is usually beneficial to these patients. The work of breathing ceases and the inspired oxygen tension can be raised (up to 50 per cent O_2) to compensate for the ventilation-perfusion abnormalities. The cardiac output may become depressed if the carbon dioxide level is lowered excessively (Prys-Roberts *et al.*, 1967) or if, because of a non-compliant chest, excessive inflation pressures are necessary. The restricted pulmonary blood flow in pulmonary stenosis and pulmonary hypertension is very vulnerable to right ventricular depression secondary to drug action and to the mechanical effects of increased airway pressure. Rarely, in patients with tabes, diabetes or drug overdosage, the circulatory reflexes may be blocked and positive pressure ventilation will reduce the cardiac output. Rises in carbon dioxide tension increase the work of the heart and add to the incidence of arrhythmias. The principal danger of these effects is that although they may be only transitory in themselves, the reduction in cardiac output which they cause leads to arterial hypoxaemia and decrease in ventricular performance. The patient then enters a vicious circle of increasing hypoxia and metabolic acidosis which is now independent of its original cause.

Effects of Operation

Haemorrhage.—Surgical haemorrhage, while in theory tending to improve congestive failure by reducing venous pressure, is in fact likely to be more dangerous because it will be additional to the pre-existing pharmacological venesection of anaesthesia and most patients, except the rare emergency, will have had their failure treated adequately before surgery. Blood loss should be prevented if possible and immediately and adequately replaced to maintain a reasonable filling pressure for the heart.

Reflex stimulation.—In the presence of inadequate anaesthesia or inadequate analgesia in the post-operative period, excessive sympathetic stimulation may produce tachycardia. Visceral reflexes may provoke vagal stimulation.

Posture and venous return.—The position on the operating table may lead to venous pooling in the periphery or, in the case of a head down tilt, excessive filling pressure of the heart. The venous return may be interfered with during retraction of the liver or by the pregnant uterus pressing on the inferior vena cava.

Chest and heart operations.—During operations on the chest and heart, two factors are added to the general effects of operation. The chest being opened leads to further alterations in lung function and possible impairment of venous return if the mediastinum becomes displaced.

Actual interference with the heart reduces the cardiac output by impairing diastolic filling or by the development of arrhythmias. Temporary interruption of the circulation, as by the introduction of a finger or dilator into the orifice of a valve, may result in severe deterioration in the patient's condition.

Conclusions

Most patients who have had adequate pre-operative preparation arrive at the operating theatre in reasonable condition and are able to perfuse themselves adequately provided the circulatory reflexes are intact and their metabolism not raised by excessive respiratory work or sympathetic stimulation secondary to pain or fright. Fortunately, these patients require very little anaesthesia. Sleep, once induced, can be maintained with minimal doses. Furthermore, operations on the heart and great vessels in the thoracic cavity, like those upon the lungs, do not appear to involve the stimulation of reflex activities akin to those in the upper abdomen. Nor is profound muscular relaxation necessary.

Deterioration in the efficiency of the cardiovascular system is best prevented by meticulous attention to avoiding depression by anaesthetic drugs or by hypoxia and hypercarbia.

Small amounts of anaesthetic result in a rapid return to consciousness with little respiratory depression at the end of operation, thus facilitating assessment of the cardiovascular system. These considerations apply whether the operation is for the relief of heart disease or for some other condition in a patient with heart disease.

Anaesthesia for Patients with Cardiac Disease

Surgery in patients with cardiac disease will include some patients with mild heart disease having major surgery, some with severe heart disease having minor surgery, and a few bad risk cases undergoing major surgery. The need is to assess the patient and the effects of anaesthesia and operation together. For the relatively mild case the principles and techniques of anaesthesia are fundamentally the same as for other patients. It is in the seriously disabled patient that there is so little margin for error. Normal patients have immense physiological reserves to cope with the stresses imposed; severe cardiac patients have lost their reserves and any trespass by anaesthesia or surgery, particularly those which result in hypoxia, may be lethal. In these patients it would seem most logical to choose those anaesthetic agents and techniques which have a minimal effect on the circulation and its reflexes.

Premedication

Mental sedation is of special importance for patients with cardiac disease, as the stresses of fear and emotional upset can be sufficient to induce an anginal attack or precipitate the acute onset of pulmonary oedema. Although drugs are of undoubted value in this respect, excessive use of them, particularly in the immediate pre-operative period, may add to the dangers of the subsequent anaesthetic, so that other less truly pharmacological but effective remedies must be used to the full. A few days rest in the atmosphere of a well-run ward with a friendly nursing staff; the presence of a nurse from this ward right up to the moment of loss of consciousness, and again on waking; movement from ward to anaesthetic room in the ward bed, to avoid those unpleasant moments of transfer to the theatre trolley and the frequent imposition of a horizontal position that goes with it; and the induction of anaesthesia while still propped up in the position of greatest comfort; all these can work wonders for most patients.

The choice of premedication is influenced not only by the condition of the patient but by the choice of anaesthetic technique to be used subsequently. Patients have a smoother induction and anaesthetic if well premedicated.

Morphine is well tolerated by cardiac patients in whom its calming effect is particularly valuable. In very anxious patients it can be preceded by an oral barbiturate if necessary. Pethidine has little sedative effect and is liable to reduce the blood pressure, as may the phenothiazines. The respiratory depressant effects of narcotics are less important with the greater use of positive pressure ventilation in the post-operative period.

It has been argued that belladonna alkaloids are contra-indicated in heart disease because modern anaesthetic techniques do not lead to profuse reactions, excessive dryness may increase the discomfort of dyspnoea, and tachycardia may be dangerous by reducing diastolic filling time. There remains the danger of vagal stimulation following suxamethonium and intubation. In practice, hyoscine used in combination with morphine rarely produces a tachycardia; indeed, once positive pressure ventilation with nitrous oxide is started, patients often develop a bradycardia. In patients who are fully digitalised it may be impossible to provoke a tachycardia and if, as a result of premedication, the patient develops a bradycardia unresponsive to atropine, it may be better to abandon the operation until more of the digitalis has been excreted.

If the effect of premedication is very unsatisfactory—either ineffective or markedly depressant—it may be advisable to postpone the operation to a subsequent day, rather than hazard the patient's life. Another indication for postponement at this stage is a marked deterioration in the patient's condition, such as the onset of incipient or acute pulmonary oedema or a profound fall in systemic blood pressure.

Induction of Anaesthesia

The induction and establishment of anaesthesia can easily mean the subsequent success of the surgical procedure. A stormy, anoxic induction can, in a few moments, undo all the good of several weeks' patient medical treatment.

The anaesthetic room should be quiet and not over-bright. All drugs, tubes, drips, are prepared before the patient enters the room so that he is not disturbed by continued activity. With the very worst patients who may arrest during induction, this should be carried out actually in the theatre, but otherwise induction is best performed in the anaesthetic room with the patient on the operating table in the knowledge that the surgeon is nearby, already changed. Before starting, the blood pressure and pulse are checked and the ECG leads attached. The disturbance this causes is far outweighed by the disadvantage of not having this information. The patient is induced in the position in which he is comfortable and is laid flat once he is unconscious.

Prior to induction the patient is preoxygenated for a full three minutes. In healthy patients with congenital abnormalities or mild heart disease induction can be performed with an intravenous barbiturate. This must be given slowly to allow for prolongation of the circulation time.

Severely ill patients with a fixed cardiac output are unable to respond to the peripheral vasodilatation and myocardial depression caused by intravenous barbiturates (Conway *et al.*, 1968; Rowlands *et al.*, 1967), indeed the cardiac output may decline further secondary to poor coronary flow, dilatation of the heart and functional valve incompetence. Patients with shunts across septal defects may have the shunt altered or even reversed if the balance of resistances between pulmonary and systemic circuits is altered. Even the smallest dose of thiopentone is best avoided in preference for an inhalational induction with cyclopropane and oxygen. Tolerance of the procedure can be increased by good premedication or by a small dose of intravenous diazepam (Baker, 1968) immediately prior to induction. Respirations are assisted or controlled as soon as unconsciousness occurs. Most patients will be intubated and ventilated, in which case a large dose of non-depolarising relaxant may make for a smoother induction than using suxamethonium. Curare may cause profound hypotension in ill patients and pancuronium is to be preferred (McDowell and Clarke, 1969).

Maintenance of Anaesthesia

Anaesthesia is normally maintained with intermittent positive pressure respiration using nitrous oxide and a muscle relaxant. The dose of muscle relaxant required is often small and with moderate hyperventilation (Pa_{CO_2} 30–35) breathing can easily be controlled, sometimes without a relaxant, by the use of small doses of respiratory depressant (phenoperidine 1 mg.) or low concentrations of halothane. Gross hyperventilation is avoided because of the reduction in cardiac output (Prys-Roberts *et al.*, 1967), the reduced cerebral blood flow (Woolman *et al.*, 1965) and the deleterious effect which it has on the pulmonary circulation, particularly in the presence of a right-to-left shunt or pulmonary hypertension.

Owing to the ventilation-perfusion abnormalities which exist in the lungs of cardiac patients and the profound effects which "shunting" and reductions in cardiac output have on alveolar-arterial gas gradients, the nitrous oxide/oxygen mixture should contain at least 30 per cent oxygen and in some cases up to 50 per cent. Fortunately, the more severely ill the patient, the less the quantity of anaesthetic agent that is required.

Supplemental Drugs

These are best avoided for cardiac operations. The indications for them are often more theoretical than real although a case for the use of a narcotic (pethidine, morphine, phenoperidine) can be made on the grounds of a long operation with a progressive decrease in the effectiveness of the premedication and hence less residual analgesia in the post-operative period. Narcotics also help in the maintenance of controlled respiration as the total dose of muscle relaxant is reduced. This is particularly so where only an inhalational induction has been used and there is no residual effect from the thiopentone. The contra-indication of post-operative respiratory depression is less important now that positive pressure ventilation is commoner in the post-operative period and if post-operative ventilation is envisaged the use of phenoperidine will enable control of ventilation without resort to the muscle relaxants, despite the prompt return of consciousness when the nitrous oxide is discontinued.

Neostigmine

If spontaneous respiration is desired at the end of the operation and curare or pancuronium has been used, the dangers of neostigmine and atropine are far outweighed by the dangers of partial paralysis and inadequate breathing. Administered together, slowly, while the ECG is watched, they seldom produce any untoward effects in the properly maintained patients. Troubles in cardiac rhythm during the administration are principally related to hypoxia, rises in carbon dioxide tension being much less important in this respect.

Heart block, extreme tachycardia, extreme cardiac irritability, or a period of arrest with successful resuscitation, are all conditions in which the use of these drugs should be cautious, but in most instances these conditions would indicate a need for post-operative ventilation to ensure oxygenation and carbon dioxide removal, in which case reversal is not desirable.

Management of the Circulation during Anaesthesia and Operation

Monitoring.—There is no substitute for accurate information about the patient's condition when decisions are to be made about therapy. Immediately after (or in some cases before) induction a large, reliable drip is set up incorporating a blood warmer in the circuit. For the simplest cases the patient can then be managed with digital recording of pulse and blood pressure, a continuous ECG and observation of the patient's peripheral tissues. The ease with which the central venous pressure can be measured via a neck vein should make this a routine. It also provides a route for intravenous therapy if the blood drip is required for rapid transfusion. It is most unwise to allow surgery to commence unless the channels for fluid therapy and monitoring are satisfactory and reliable. Arrangements are also made for the proper recording of blood loss. In more complicated surgery the recording of body temperature and urine output and the estimation of blood gases and acid-base state may be indicated.

As yet, continuous measurement of the cardiac output during anaesthesia is not a clinical possibility. The anaesthetist must make an inspired guess as to the adequacy of the cardiac output. No one measurement gives a precise indication and the anaesthetist's estimate is based collectively on the blood pressure, pulse rate, tissue perfusion, urine output, arterial and venous oxygenation and metabolic state.

Venous pressure monitoring.—The measurement of the venous pressure is a technique deriving initially from cardiac surgery but now being used for a much wider selection of patients during anaesthesia, resuscitation and post-operative care. As with many other numerical values (e.g. acid/base estimations) the absolute value at any one time is only of use if the estimation is correctly performed and if the value is considered against other confirmatory observations of the patient's condition. Taken by itself with no other knowledge of the patient's condition the value may suggest therapy which may be wrong or even dangerous.

Technique: Any of the commercially available catheters can be advanced into the superior or inferior vena cavae after percutaneous puncture of either the femoral, internal or external jugular or an arm vein (English *et al.*, 1969). Accurate readings can only be made if the tip of the catheter is within the chest. It must be possible to aspirate blood, the level must fall freely and, once settled, must fluctuate with respiration before the readings are taken as valid. Actual measurements can be made with strain gauge or U-tube manometers relative to a defined zero point (usually the sternal angle) and expressed in defined units (e.g. cm. H_2O). In most instances the value obtained will approximate to a mean right atrial pressure and results from (*a*) the blood available for cardiac filling; (*b*) the ability of the heart to deal with this blood.

The blood available for cardiac filling depends on the blood volume and on the tone of the capacitance vessels. Hence knowledge of drugs or anaesthetic agents which the patient is receiving and of the state of the peripheral veins is vital. Peripheral vasoconstriction may be sustaining the venous pressure as a compensation for haemorrhage or as a result of cold, pain, or fright.

Under normal circumstances the heart will eject the blood presented to it and maintain the right atrial pressure at its normal level. With a healthy heart attempts to raise the venous pressure tend to result in a higher cardiac output with little rise in the venous pressure. This is not so of diseased hearts nor always under anaesthesia, when the heart may be incapable either partially or completely of responding to a raised filling pressure.

Account must be taken of two other factors:

The heart consists of two ventricles which are functionally different, although in health the right sided and left sided filling pressures are very similar and tend to increase in the same proportion. This is not necessarily so in disease. In left-sided heart disease the filling pressure of the ventricle may be higher than that on the right and quite small increases in right-sided filling pressure may produce disproportionate rises on the left side. Thus pulmonary oedema can be provoked by fluid therapy at low levels of measured central venous pressure.

The filling pressure of the ventricle is affected by changes in cardiac rhythm. In the presence of sinus rhythm a good atrial contraction will fill the ventricle at a low measured central venous pressure. A higher measured pressure will be necessary for the same output in auricular fibrillation and a much higher pressure still if the patient is in nodal rhythm. Transition from sinus to noda rhythm is usually marked by a rise in measured venous pressure but a fall in arterial pressure.

Complications

1. **Hypotension.**—Mild hypotension by itself, if the cardiac output is maintained, is not serious but a falling output with systemic hypotension must not be tolerated without a diagnosis of its cause. A slight, but frequently progressive, deterioration can be expected during the manipulative part of a cardiac operation in patients with severe disease. More noticeably marked and successive falls in pressure may occur after the establishment of controlled respiration—particularly if the pulmonary vascular resistance is already high—during the thoracotomy with its attendant haemorrhage and trauma, and when the heart is handled at the time of examination and cardiotomy. The results of surgical manipulation of the heart are often especially disturbing, particularly when rotation or retraction of the organ and its great vessels from their normal position is essential. Arrhythmias are very likely to occur at this stage and, should they be persistent, increase the hypotension.

The distinction must be made between hypotension secondary to cardiac failure, in which case the filling pressure (central venous pressure) will be high, and that secondary to a low filling pressure. The latter may be due to peripheral vasodilatation with a normal blood volume or to inadequately replaced blood loss. In either case the correct treatment is to restore the filling pressure to normal with the appropriate fluid.

The treatment of low cardiac output secondary to cardiac failure is directed firstly to removing the cause of the failure if possible. It may be secondary to trauma and manipulation of the heart by the surgeon, in which case a rest period is indicated. Progressive slow deterioration is to be feared more than sudden transitory deterioration which accompanies some manipulation. Abnormal cardiac rates and arrhythmias may worsen the output (see below). Metabolic acidosis, itself a consequence of low output, will depress cardiac response to sympathetic stimulation. Sympathomimetic amines will not produce any effect—this includes isoprenaline—in the presence of a metabolic acidosis.

Initial treatment is to restore the filling pressure to normal if it is low. It can then be raised further to see if the heart is capable of increasing its output. The amount of fluid which can be infused may be limited by the development of tricuspid incompetence or pulmonary oedema. As the cardiac output is frequently rate dependent, isoprenaline (1 mg. in 500 ml. dextrose as a slow infusion) can be used to adjust the rate to its optimum level. The contractility of the heart will be increased by the inotropic action of isoprenaline, or digitalis can be given (provided the serum potassium is normal) to obtain the same effect. Metabolic acidosis is corrected by the administration of sodium bicarbonate.

The use of vasopressors is not recommended for hypotension secondary to a reduced cardiac output except in an emergency situation when, either as a result of a very low pressure or abnormal systemic arteries, coronary artery perfusion is reduced to a life-threatening level. In these circumstances a vasopressor may be necessary to support the circulation until the other measures have had time to work; choice should be made of a drug such as metaraminol which has β-stimulating activity as well as vasoconstrictor action.

2. **Cardiac rate and arrhythmias.**—Excessively fast and excessively slow rates

are equally undesirable. Attention is paid to adequate analgesia and the elimination of hypoxia and hypercarbia.

Slow cardiac rates may represent residual pre-operative digitalisation in the patient with atrial fibrillation, or may be a temporary response to direct interference with the heart. Bradycardia paves the way for the development of ectopic beats. Transitory bradycardia requires no treatment. In the digitalised patient, if the serum potassium level is low, cautious potassium administration is indicated. Otherwise, atropine to eliminate vagal effects or ultimately isoprenaline infusion is necessary. Similar treatment will be indicated if the patient changes from sinus into nodal rhythm.

Sinus tachycardia is less common and, if all the simple remedies are ineffective, may be difficult to control. If the blood pressure is sufficiently high a small amount of halothane may gain control. More commonly fast cardiac rates are the result of some arrhythmia.

Nearly every variety of arrhythmia has been reported during anaesthesia and surgery. Ventricular extrasystoles are common, nodal rhythm and atrial extrasystoles more rare. The first step is to diagnose the type of rhythm disturbance on the ECG and then to assess whether it is having a deleterious effect on the cardiac output. General measures are the correction of hypoxia and hypercarbia, the elimination of anaesthetic agents which increase myocardial irritability, the provision of adequate analgesia and the correction of the metabolic state. Naturally slow cardiac rates will allow more time for abnormal rhythms to develop and speeding the natural rate with atropine or isoprenaline will cure some nodal and ventricular rhythms.

Ventricular arrhythmias may arise, particularly in digitalised patients, due to alterations in the serum potassium level. These arrhythmias may be provoked by a diuresis, by the administration of calcium to cover the anticoagulant in bottled blood, or by alteration in the acid-base state. Positive pressure ventilation which reduces the carbon dioxide level will elevate the pH, and for each rise of 0·1 in the pH value the serum potassium will fall 0·2 mEq/litre. The serum potassium is measured and either elevated by slow administration of potassium chloride or lowered by diuresis, ion-exchange resin, or, if it is dangerously high, with intravenous glucose and insulin. If ventricular arrhythmias persist, myocardial excitability can be depressed with lignocaine (1 mg./kg. body weight). This can be continued as an infusion (1–2 mg./min.). For intractable life-threatening rhythms β-blockade, with practolol rather than propranolol, may be indicated.

Atrial flutter and atrial fibrillation may develop suddenly. If the cardiac output is well maintained despite the fast rate then the best course is to digitalise the patient. If the cardiac output is severely compromised, then cardioversion is indicated. The patient is digitalised at the same time in case he later reverts to atrial fibrillation.

3. **Pulmonary oedema*.**—The pressure in the pulmonary artery during diastole is only 8 mm. Hg rising to 20 mm. Hg during systole, and by the time the blood reaches the capillaries these pressures have dropped even further (2–8 mm. Hg).

* Pulmonary oedema may also occur in oxygen poisoning (p. 219), certain lesions of the central nervous system (p. 1146) and as a result of chemical irritation of the pulmonary epithelium (p. 447).

The capillary endothelium acts as a semi-permeable membrane but in normal circumstances the osmotic pressure exerted by the plasma proteins keeps the fluid within the vessel walls. In conditions, such as mitral stenosis, which lead to an increase in pulmonary capillary pressure, oedema may result. Once present this leads to some local anoxia which damages further the pulmonary epithelium and causes breakdown of the semi-permeable membrane so that plasma proteins and electrolytes pass into the tissue spaces and attract fluid from the vessels. Excessive transfusion of fluid can, particularly in the presence of left heart disease, produce sufficient rise in pulmonary capillary pressure to precipitate pulmonary oedema.

The treatment of acute pulmonary oedema during anaesthesia is:

1. Positive pressure ventilation preferably with a positive pressure remaining during expiration. A high oxygen content of the inspired mixture is needed. The pressure will help reabsorption of the transudate thus improving oxygenation while other measures take effect.

2. Lowering of the left atrial pressure. This can be achieved in a number of ways.

(*a*) Anti-Trendelenburg position encourages pooling in the dependent limbs.
(*b*) Vasodilation drugs—e.g. halothane, promethazine, ganglionic blockade, to enlarge the capacitance vessels.
(*c*) Diuretics—frusemide or ethacrynic acid given intravenously (see p. 663).
(*d*) Improvement of left ventricular function with digitalis or isoprenaline.
(*e*) Venesection. The surgical approach will, however, probably result in as much blood loss as is needed, bearing in mind that the peripheral vasodilation of general anaesthesia will already have accounted for a fair reduction in effective circulatory volume.

Removal of the oedema fluid by suction is quite useless. Fluid merely accumulates as fast as it is removed and the action of sucking impairs ventilation. Continuous positive pressure ventilation must not be discontinued until the measures to lower left atrial pressure have had time to work.

In general, good anaesthesia decreases the risk of acute pulmonary oedema, but in those patients whose circulatory equilibrium is finely balanced, even a change of posture—from the upright to the lateral horizontal—may induce failure. Pregnant women with cardiac disease are especially liable to this complication after delivery of the placenta at the moment when the contracting uterus displaces a large volume of blood into the general circulation. The intravenous use of ergometrine enhances the risk.

Cardiac arrest.—This is discussed in Chapter 28.

Post-operative Care of Cardiac Patients

The post-operative period is now the commonest time for patients to suffer serious complications. Careful monitoring and support of the circulation must be continued, as it was for the operation, until the situation is quite stable. Blood loss is promptly replaced to maintain the ventricular filling pressures at the optimum level for a reasonable cardiac output.

Cardiac patients are only allowed to breathe spontaneously if they are obviously capable of performing the work necessary to ventilate themselves (Zeitlin, 1965). After operation, particularly if the chest has been opened, ventilation-perfusion inequalities in the lung result in very inefficient ventilation so that much respiratory work still results in a hypoxic patient. In a group of cardiac patients the mean increase in oxygen consumption was 13 per cent (range 2–29 per cent) when respiration became spontaneous (Thung *et al.*, 1963). This rise may be too great for patients with a limited cardiac output. The decision to continue ventilation in the post-operative period nolonger depends on a tracheostomy being performed and thus if any doubt exists ventilation can be continued via the endotracheal tube for several days if necessary.

ANAESTHESIA FOR SPECIAL SITUATIONS

Cardioversion

Electrical countershock to convert atrial arrhythmias to sinus rhythm is too painful to be performed on the conscious patient. The effects of sympathetic and parasympathetic balance under various types of anaesthesia and their effect on the likelihood of success of the treatment has been reviewed (Wagner and McIntosh 1969). In practice, two anaesthetic techniques are popular. One is to give a small dose of intravenous barbiturate; the other is to give intravenous diazepam (Kahler *et al.*, 1967) until the patient is unconscious. In either event it is worth continuing with nitrous oxide and oxygen in case more than one shock is required. Neither premedication nor succinylcholine is necessary. As when any intravenous agent is used, facilities must be available to ventilate the patient if respiratory depression occurs. Post-conversion arrhythmias may require treatment with atropine, intravenous potassium chloride or lignocaine, all of which should be immediately available.

Cardiac Catheterisation and Angiocardiography

Cardiac catheterisation is not a painful procedure except for the introduction of the catheter through the skin and this can be adequately covered by local anaesthesia. The passage of the catheter through the veins should provide no sensation but the mental strain and the discomfort of lying continously in the dark X-ray room on a hard table for any length of time may make it unacceptable to the patient. Angiocardiography is more unpleasant; the injection of the dye rapidly produces a sensation of great warmth throughout the patient usually with flushing of the face and neck, a feeling of suffocation and choking together with an intense desire to cough, and some constriction and pain in the chest. All this may be followed by a feeling of faintness because there is nearly always a period of hypotension immediately after the injection and arrhythmias are not uncommon. These effects, however, pass off very rapidly.

The choice for cardiac catheterisation is either local analgesic, local analgesic combined with basal sedation, or general anaesthesia. The argument in favour of avoidance of general anaesthesia is mainly on the grounds that changes in cardiorespiratory function during anaesthesia are unpredictable and that unpremedicated, unanaesthetised patients breathing air are likely to be in a more physiological condition. The technique of cardiac catheterisation without sedation is well described (Mendel, 1968) and produces perfectly satisfactory results, if the staff work hard at reassuring the patient beforehand and avoid upsetting him during the procedure.

Anaesthesia tends to be indicated for the following groups of patients:—

1. Those patients in whom catheterisation without sedation is impossible due to the presence of a language barrier or the patient having such a low mentality that one is unable to communicate with him properly.

2. If the patient has had a previous catheterisation of which he has unpleasant memories, he may express unwillingness to have a second performance without the benefits of general anaesthesia.

3. Children (see Adams and Parkhouse, 1960).

When an investigation is being performed merely to demonstrate the anatomy of a lesion rather than its physiology—e.g. to demonstrate patent ductus arteriosus, coarctation—anaesthesia can easily be offered to the patient. Hence the exact nature of the investigation and the lesion is the most important factor in the choice of whether or not to anaesthetise the patient. Up to the age of about 12 years, good results with heavy sedation can be obtained for catheterisation and angiocardiography.

The schedule recommended by Graham (1966) is: Sodium phenobarbitone 2 mg./kg. given the previous evening and again three hours before the procedure. Half an hour before the procedure an intramuscular injection of 1 ml./10 kg. of a compound injection of pethidine, which contains in 1 ml. chlorpromazine 6·25 mg., prometh-azine 6·25 mg. and pethidine 25 mg.

It may be that diazepam will find increasing application for sedation of children during cardiac investigations (Healey, 1969).

Special Considerations.—(*a*) *Alteration in cardiac output.* During catheterisation inferences are drawn from numerical values for pressures in chambers, and for pressure changes across orifices. If the cardiac output is seriously altered by anaesthesia, extrapolation of figures from the anaesthetised patient to his normal state is not possible.

(*b*) *Alterations in systemic and pulmonary vascular resistance.* Alteration in the two main resistances may produce abnormal values for pressure measurements and in the presence of inter-chamber communications can seriously alter or even reverse the flow across the hole.

(*c*) *Gas analyses.* Gas analyses on blood samples may not be possible if the patient is receiving nitrous oxide. Fortunately, oxygen saturation using a haemoreflector or oxygen tension measured in an electrode are not affected by anaesthetic agents.

(*d*) *Ventilation.* Alterations in carbon dioxide tension will affect the circulatory state. Deviation of inspired oxygen tension from that found in air will make estimations of cardiac output or shunt across a defect difficult.

(*e*) *Apnoea* may be requested while the angiocardiograms are performed.

(*f*) The patients are usually ill with some serious cardiac lesion.

(*g*) A steady state is required as measurements at various sites are made consecutively not simultaneously.

All forms of anaesthesia have been described for use during cardiac catheterisation and according to the skill of the anaesthetist so the results. It is essential to confer first with the cardiologist so that the aims and restrictions of the investigation and the anaesthesia are known to both.

The technique preferred at St. Thomas's Hospital is to ventilate patients with nitrous oxide and 20 per cent oxygen after paralysis with pancuronium, aiming at a normal carbon dioxide tension. It is felt that the minor deviations of cardio-respiratory performance induced by positive pressure ventilation (Manners and Codman, 1969) are more than offset by the avoidance of other agents which affect myocardial contractility, peripheral resistance and the likelihood of arrhythmias.

Extracorporeal Circulation

The general principles for anaesthesia and management of patients with cardiac disease, paying particular attention to the problems of specific lesions, apply to operations performed with the aid of extracorporeal circulation. The peculiar problem posed is that of keeping the patient unconscious during the period of bypass. Ventilation of the lungs is normally discontinued and all gas exchange occurs in the oxygenator. Small quantities of halothane are sometimes vaporised in the gas flow to the oxygenator. Alternatively, combinations of narcotic and muscle relaxant can be added to the pump prime. If the patient is hypothermic this will prevent the return of consciousness. Neuroleptanalgesia has been described for this purpose. No one method appears to have a particular advantage over any other.

Some Aspects of Different Cardiac Diseases in Relation to Anaesthesia and Operation

It is not intended to describe all the individual diseases comprehensively but rather to pick out some and to discuss their special aspects which are of prime concern to the anaesthetist. The principles of anaesthesia described apply irrespective of the particular disease in the heart, but certain lesions may suggest a variation of technique or the use of an ancillary such as induced hypotension, hypothermia, or the extracorporeal circulation. Moreover, increasing experience of the behaviour of patients with certain lesions during anaesthesia and operation gives a clue to expected morbidity and mortality. Such facts as these and brief descriptions of those rarer diseases and operations, which are only likely to be seen in specialised clinics, are included to give the anaesthetist a broad background to the subject.

Three conditions which are of particular importance to the anaesthetist can occur as complications of other lesions.

Raised pulmonary vascular resistance (Pulmonary hypertension).—The pulmonary artery pressure may be raised, with no change in the pulmonary vessels, as a result of a raised left atrial pressure. A raised pulmonary vascular resistance is due to medial hypertrophy and intimal thickening in the walls of the pulmonary arterioles. This change, which may be irreversible, occurs in 30 per cent of those conditions which are characterised by a chronically raised left atrial pressure or a large left-to-right shunt. A similar effect may be produced by recurrent pulmonary emboli. The right ventricle is unable to compensate for this obstruction to its outflow and the patient enters a fixed low cardiac output state. The patient is particularly sensitive to:

i. Myocardial depressant effects of anaesthetic drugs.
ii. Vasodilatation induced by anaesthesia.
iii. Hypoxia.
iv. The mechanical effects of positive pressure ventilation.

The anoxia may be the result of poor ventilation or be the secondary effect of a reduction in cardiac output produced by haemorrhage, arrhythmias, manipulation and trauma to the heart or myocardial depression. The pulmonary vascular resistance is raised further by the effects of anoxia and metabolic acidosis, thus reducing the cardiac output further; a vicious circle is then entered with progressive deterioration in the patient's condition. As treatment for this state, apart from supportive bypass (*q.v.*), is so relatively useless, every effort must be made to maintain the circulation and to prevent entry into the circle of progressive deterioration.

Fixed low output.—This is a situation in which the heart is just capable of supporting life. Characteristically the patient is intensely vasoconstricted and the ventricular stroke volume is constant regardless of the filling pressure. The patient is particularly sensitive to the effect of myocardial depression, vasodilatation and to alteration in cardiac rhythm and rate. The common causes are cardiac failure, myocardial ischaemia, valvular lesions, particularly mitral or pulmonary stenosis, constrictive pericarditis, and pulmonary vascular disease including pulmonary embolism.

Stiff lungs.—Raised left atrial pressure leads to interstitial oedema and ultimately thickening and fibrosis in the lungs. Ventilatory function is impaired and high inflation pressures and minute volumes may be required to maintain normal gas tensions in the arterial blood.

Left-to-Right Shunt

The three common congenital conditions which lead to an increased flow through the lungs are patent ductus arteriosus, atrial septal defect and ventricular septal defect. Patent ductus leads to an overload of the left ventricle, atrial septal defect to an overload of the right ventricle, while a ventricular septal defect loads both ventricles. Anaesthesia for all three types of case presents no problem unless the patient is suffering from a complication and they can be treated as relatively healthy patients with good cardiorespiratory reserve. The two complications which may occur are:

i. Cardiac failure—which should be treated with the appropriate measures before surgery. Sometimes in neonates the size of the shunt is so large that only closure of the ductus or banding of the pulmonary artery will enable the failure to be controlled. Frequently severe cardiac failure in neonates with left-to-right shunts is complicated by the presence of multiple circulatory abnormalities.
ii. The development of pulmonary hypertension. When the pulmonary vascular resistance exceeds that of the systemic circuit the shunt will be reversed (Eisenmenger situation) and corrective surgery is no longer

possible. With lesser degrees of pulmonary hypertension anaesthesia must be conducted with care (see above).

Patent ductus arteriosus.—Narrow or long ductuses are easily ligated but a broad short one requires careful dissection to avoid a tear, and its tense pulsations can be reduced at the time of ligation with a short-acting hypotensive agent such as trimetaphan. After ligation the patient develops a rise in diastolic pressure and a bradycardia (Bramham phenomenon). The left recurrent laryngeal nerve may be damaged at the time of operation and give rise to post-operative respiratory problems.

Pulmonary Stenosis

Until severe, pulmonary stenosis produces little effect, then right ventricular failure occurs and the cardiac output falls. Normally, the stiff hypertrophied ventricle requires a good filling pressure, and preferably sinus rhythm, for an adequate output and attention must be directed towards maintaining the blood volume. When severe, anaesthetic management falls under the heading of fixed low output (*q.v.*) and operative intervention at this stage is associated with a high mortality. Patients with severe pulmonary stenosis are very vulnerable to right ventricular depression secondary to anaesthetic or drug action and to the mechanical effects of positive pressure respiration.

Fallot's Tetralogy

In this combination of pulmonary stenosis, patent ventricular septal defect, overriding aorta and enlarged right ventricle, the defect between the ventricles is usually large and the pressures in the right and left ventricles are identical. The degree of shunt, which is normally right to left, depends on the balance between the resistance due to the obstruction in the pulmonary outflow and the systemic vascular resistance. An increase in the right to left shunt may be provoked by pulmonary infundibular shutdown in association with pain, fear or emotion, or by a reduction in the systemic vascular resistance. The principles of anaesthesia thus include generous sedation and maintenance of a high peripheral resistance with vasopressor drugs (e.g. metaraminol) if necessary. Sedation needs to be ample in the post-operative period even if a corrective operation has been performed, as the muscle of the infundibulum may still go into spasm, and in the face of a closed VSD, will produce severe reduction in the cardiac output.

Operations for Fallot's tetralogy may be corrective, which entails relief of the pulmonary stenosis and closure of the VSD, or palliative. The latter, which includes subclavian-pulmonary artery and aorta-pulmonary artery anastomoses, are designed to improve the arterial oxygenation until the child or its pulmonary arteries are large enough to stand a corrective operation.

In patients who are undergoing or who have had palliative operations, certain difficulties arise. The subclavian artery may be interrupted and the blood pressure cannot be recorded in that arm. After an anastomotic operation this pulmonary artery may thrombose and at a subsequent operation, if this is not known, the other pulmonary artery may be clamped with complete reduction in the cardiac output.

All patients with Fallot's tetralogy have a low lung blood flow and induction with inhalational agents may be protracted. High concentration of induction agents (e.g. cyclopropane) are well tolerated because of the slow rise of blood level.

The problems of cyanosis are considered below.

Central Cyanosis

Among the lesions which are commonly associated with central cyanosis are Fallot's tetralogy, pulmonary stenosis with an atrial septal defect and transposition.

The cyanosis cannot be relieved by increasing the inspired oxygen tension and gaseous anaesthetic agents attain equilibrium very slowly.

Normally the packed cell volume (haematocrit) is high, leading to a marked rise in viscosity of the blood. There is a danger of spontaneous thrombosis occurring if the patient becomes dehydrated. As a consequence of the small plasma volume there is a small renal plasma flow and renal problems occur. To compensate for the danger of spontaneous thrombus formation these patients develop a very active fibrinolytic mechanism and blood loss is higher and coagulation difficulties more common at surgery.

In the management of cyanotic patients with a high haematocrit fluid balance must be well maintained to avoid dehydration. Initially, blood lost can be replaced with plasma or plasma-substitute with frequent checks made of the packed cell volume. Coagulation difficulties are best dealt with by meticulous surgical haemostasis as use of antifibrinolytic drugs may be accompanied by serious thrombus formation in the vascular tree.

Transposition

Children with transposition only survive if some mixing occurs between the two circuits. This mixing can be enhanced by the creation of an atrial septal defect either at open chest operation (Blalock-Hanlon) or during cardiac catheterisation (Rashkind operation). Total correction is performed during the Mustard operation.

Problems of anaesthesia are those of high viscosity and cyanosis (see above), very slow uptake of gaseous agents due to the poor mixing between the circuits and the very deleterious effect which arrhythmias have on the circulation.

Coarctation

Coarctation which occurs proximal to the ductus arteriosus (preductile) is always associated with an open duct and the lower limbs are perfused with unoxygenated blood from the pulmonary artery. These children usually present in failure and have other associated congenital abnormalities.

Adult (post-ductile) coarctation results in the development of a collateral circulation principally through the internal mammary, subscapular and intercostal arteries.

There is hypertension in the upper limbs but a normal or low pressure in the lower extremities; as a result of the rise in pressure, the left ventricle is enlarged. If the disease is untreated heart failure or a cerebrovascular accident will supervene. Most patients will fall into the age group 10–30 years, but surgical correction is being increasingly undertaken in younger children, when the operation is technically easier to perform, there now being evidence that the anastomosis is capable of further growth with the aorta.

The operation consists of resection of the stricture with end-to-end anastomosis or, if the resultant gap is too great, with the placing of a graft. Unless heart failure has already ensued, most patients will be otherwise physically fit and the mortality is very low. The special factors to be noted are:

1. Excessive bleeding may be encountered from the chest wall during the thoracotomy incision.
2. The enlarged intercostal arteries are easily torn during the freeing of the descending aorta in the neighbourhood of the stricture. This again may lead to excessive bleeding.
3. During the period of resection and anastomosis the aorta will be clamped above and below the stricture. The left subclavian artery may be clamped also, and will not, therefore, be available for blood pressure readings during this period.
4. When the subclavian, which through its branches normally carries a large proportion of the anastomotic flow of blood, is clamped there is usually a further increase in the level of hypertension.
5. The clamps have little effect on circulatory haemodynamics until they are removed upon completion of the anastomosis, when the sudden decrease in resistance is likely to lead to a considerable drop in blood pressure.
6. Haemorrhage is likely to occur in some degree from the anastomosis in the immediate period after the clamps are removed.

The foregoing factors strongly favour the use of induced hypotension to control rather than abolish excessive haemorrhage and to ease the surgeon's task during thoracotomy and the anastomosis. Moreover a reduction in the pressure during the period when the clamps are in position lessens the risk—albeit a very slight one—of intracranial haemorrhage from excessive hypertension. It is advisable, however, to allow the blood pressure to rise before closing the chest and to observe the patient closely for post-operative reactionary haemorrhage. Adequate blood replacement must be available at all times.

If the coarctation is very mild, good anastomotic vessels may not have developed and clamping of the aorta, besides producing marked hypertension in the upper extremity, will endanger the spinal cord and kidneys. For these patients surface hypothermia or left atriofemoral bypass may be required.

Mitral Valve Disease

Mitral stenosis has its principal harmful effects on the lungs (Arnott and Withering, 1964) causing dyspnoea as its main symptom. Ultimately, right ventricular failure occurs and the patient develops a low fixed-output state. Mitral valvotomy is performed to relieve the stenosis even when it is only mild, as this reduces the incidence of systemic embolism.

Normally the patient's digitalis will have been stopped three days prior to surgery. If he presents for anaesthesia with a bradycardia which is resistant to atropine or isoprenaline, surgery is postponed until more digitalis has been excreted. The cardiac output is so dependent on an adequate rate that bradycardia is extremely dangerous.

Venous cannulation or even intravenous injection may present problems due to the extreme peripheral vasoconstriction, but a good drip and preferably also a venous pressure line are essential before starting surgery.

Vasodilatation, particularly if produced by intravenous barbiturates which also cause myocardial depression, causes an acute drop in output and induction is best performed with cyclopropane and oxygen.

High inflation pressures may be required to produce adequate gaseous exchange due to fibrosis or thickening of the lung.

It may be difficult to maintain the blood pressure between induction and valvotomy. Adjustment of the rate with atropine or isoprenaline may help but inotropic drugs are of less use and in this circumstance metaraminol is best used in small intravenous increments. Excessive transfusion of fluid may precipitate pulmonary oedema but as a sharp loss occurs as the atrium is opened it is worth having 100 ml. of positive blood balance at the moment of the atrial incision and thereafter blood loss should be immediately replaced. At the time of cardiac manipulation clot may be thrown off and the anaesthetist is called on to temporarily compress the carotid arteries. Cardiac manipulation produces acute falls in blood pressure, particularly when the surgeon's fingers or the dilator are blocking the stenosed orifice and the pulse must be kept under continual observation and the blood pressure frequently recorded. Immediately the valvotomy has been performed the circulation usually improves but, if not, the surgeon is requested not to manipulate the heart further until the cardiac output, which is now more responsive to inotropic drugs, has improved. Digitalis can be safely given if the ventricular rate is too fast provided the serum potassium is normal. Before awakening the patient the peripheral pulses should be palpated to exclude embolism at the time of surgery.

The hazards of mitral stenosis are worsened once the pulmonary vascular resistance is raised.

Mitral incompetence is a disease of the left ventricle and although the patients develop cardiac failure they seldom present for surgery in the low output state seen with the stenotic valve. Although they require careful anaesthesia they do not seem to be the same problem, unless the mitral incompetence is associated with aortic valve disease or the development of pulmonary hypertension.

Aortic Valve Disease

Aortic stenosis occurs as a congenital abnormality or as the result of rheumatic fever or calcification of a tricuspid valve. Patients develop a thickened hypertrophied ventricle which may outgrow its own blood supply, leading to ischaemia and angina. Commonly they present for surgery with a relatively low cardiac output. Vasodilation and myocardial depression are particularly dangerous as, if the cardiac output and blood pressure drop, coronary filling becomes inadequate and the heart stops from hypoxia.

The small cavity of the thickened ventricle is only filled with difficulty to maintain an adequate cardiac output if the atrium produces a good contraction.

The production of arrhythmias or nodal rhythm results in an acute drop in cardiac output and is the common cause of sudden death in these patients.

The cardiac output under anaesthesia can sometimes be sustained with isoprenaline although this is contra-indicated in obstructive cardiomyopathy. It will also assist in preventing the development of nodal rhythm and in the maintenance of a good cardiac rate. Patients with aortic incompetence are also vulnerable to changes in rhythm and rate. In free incompetence the diastolic pressure is very low but the coronary filling is impaired if the peripheral run off is enhanced by further vasodilatation. Direct myocardial depressants again produce severe drops in cardiac output.

In both types of aortic valve disease ventricular filling pressure must be adequately sustained by avoidance of vasodilatation and by the prompt replacement of blood loss.

Pulmonary Embolism

Patients with pulmonary embolism may present for anaesthesia for pulmonary angiogram, for pulmonary embolectomy, or for ligature of the inferior vena cava or the femoral veins.

With major degrees of block to the pulmonary circuit these patients represent the extreme examples of a fixed low output state and are highly vulnerable to all forms of myocardial depressant, vasodilatation and to the mechanical effects of positive pressure ventilation.

For pulmonary embolectomy it is unwise to start the anaesthesia unless the theatre is ready and the surgeon is scrubbed ready to continue should the patient arrest on induction. Everything that can be done, positioning of drips, pressure monitoring lines, both venous and arterial, should be performed under local anaesthesia before induction. In the extreme case supportive bypass after cannulation of the femoral vein and artery under local anaesthesia may be necessary.

Pulmonary angiogram is frequently associated with acute deterioration due to the toxic effect of the contrast medium and is best performed without anaesthesia. Preferably it is carried out in the operating theatre so that the patient does not have to be moved before surgery is commenced.

Constrictive Pericarditis

The essential effect of this disease is to limit the diastolic expansion of all the chambers of the heart. Thus both ventricles have their stroke output reduced. Eventually the pressures rise in both atria and venous congestion follows.

The risk during anaesthesia is essentially similar to that of other diseases in which the cardiac output is reduced to a stage when compensation for sudden falls in peripheral resistance cannot take place. These patients must be treated in a manner similar to those with mitral stenosis and great caution exercised in the use of thiopentone.

Operative removal of the fibrous constricting layers of pericardium often leads to considerable haemorrhage, since these are ill defined. Indeed the lack of a sharp demarcation between the pericardium and the cardiac muscle in this condition usually leads to considerable trauma and manipulation of the heart. The circulatory dynamics of the heart may also be greatly upset by the rotation of the organ that is necessary during the approach to the pericardium around its base and the right atrium. Arrhythmias are frequent, hypotension common, and ventricular fibrillation a real danger. Rest periods coupled with adequate replacement of blood are the best remedies.

Coronary Artery Disease

Patients with coronary artery disease may present for incidental surgery or for operations designed to improve the blood supply to the myocardium.

Hypotension is best avoided in the presence of coronary disease. It is true that there is evidence that a satisfactory perfusion of the coronary tree can be maintained despite a lowered systemic blood pressure simply because the correlation between the oxygen consumed by the myocardium and the work necessary to maintain the blood pressure is linear. However, since coronary artery flow takes place during diastole and is dependent on mean blood pressure, this pressure must be maintained at near normal level to ensure an adequate flow in the presence of obstructive coronary artery disease.

Myocardial infarction.—Previous myocardial infarction may add materially to the risks of surgery and anaesthesia. Skinner and Pearce (1964) reported a mortality rate of 40 per cent in patients in whom an infarct had occurred less than three months prior to surgery, compared with 14 per cent in the greater than three months group.

Papper (1965) comments that if a patient has a healed myocardial infarction of more than three months' duration, if the ECG is stable and resembles his pre-infarct pattern and if there is no angina or sign of cardiac failure, he is for practical purposes an essentially normal risk for anaesthesia and surgery.

Topkins and Artusio (1964) reviewing 12,712 male patients over 50 years old, found an incidence of 6·5 per cent for post-operative infarction in patients who had had a previous myocardial infarct compared with 0·66 per cent in previously normal patients. The likelihood of recurrence was directly related to the interval between the first infarct and surgery, being over 50 per cent if this was less than six months. Both this study and Arkins *et al.* (1964) comment on the much higher mortality which occurs in post-surgical recurrent infarcts as compared with infarction occurring at some other time.

Surgery of coronary heart disease.—Anaesthesia for internal mammary implant surgery has been described by Viljoen (1968). The technique is based on the principles of generous pre-operative medication, liberal use of coronary vasodilators, suppression of ventricular excitability, prolonged post-operative sedation and positive pressure ventilation.

Atrio-ventricular block.—This is usually caused by coronary artery ischaemia or rheumatic disease affecting the conducting tissue of the myocardium. It may be congenital in origin and is then sometimes associated with other anomalies of the heart. It can, too, occur during surgical correction of heart lesions. The block may be partial or complete, the former showing several variants. Stokes-Adams attacks—bouts of syncope, vertigo or occasionally convulsions—occur most commonly in patients with a pulse rate below 40 per minute. An attack is due to cardiac standstill and recovery often takes place spontaneously and rapidly when the heart starts beating again. A feature of this type of heart disease is the ever-present risk of further changes in the rate and rhythm of the heart.

Bradycardia may get worse, cardiac arrest is not uncommon, and ventricular arrhythmias, though rarely fibrillation, often occur without apparent immediate predisposing cause.

Patients may present for anaesthesia under three situations. Patients with complete block may present for incidental surgery or for implantation of a pacemaker, or alternatively they may present for surgery with an indwelling pacemaker already in use.

Patients with complete heart block having incidental surgery are obviously very vulnerable to vasodilatation or myocardial depression. Before anaesthesia the effect of atropine or isoprenaline can be gauged, but if there is any doubt about the patient a temporary pacemaker electrode can be inserted via a peripheral vein under local analgesic.

When anaesthesia is required for the insertion of indwelling artificial pacemakers there is general agreement that despite meticulous anaesthetic care the incidence of cardiac complications is high (Ross, 1962; Howat, 1963; Wrigley, 1964). The most reliable course is to insert a pacemaker intravenously by cardiac catheter under local analgesia and to pace the heart at an adequate rate before general anaesthesia is induced. Failing this, an external pacemaker should be kept to hand during general anaesthesia until the internal pacemaker is working.

Anaesthesia for incidental surgery in patients who are already being paced has been reviewed by Scott (1970). The general principles which he cites are avoidance of reduction in cardiac output, full oxygenation, reduction in blood loss, avoidance of damage to the pacemaker and its electrodes, no diathermy, and the avoidance of sudden postural change. Sudden cessation of response to the pacemaker is an emergency. The cardiac output may be maintained at an adequate level by the idioventricular rate, stimulated by isoprenaline, if necessary (Finck *et al.*, 1969). If the output is inadequate then external cardiac compression must be carried out until temporary external pacing can be started. The myocardial threshold to stimulation is affected by the serum potassium level which must be clearly observed.

REFERENCES

ADAMS, A. K., and PARKHOUSE, J. (1960). Anaesthesia for cardiac catheterisation in children. *Brit. J. Anaesth.*, **32,** 69.

ARKINS, R., SMESSAERT, A. A., and HICKS, R. G. (1964). Mortality and morbidity in surgical patients with coronary artery disease. *J. Amer. Med. Ass.*, **190,** 485.

ARNOTT, W. M., and WITHERING, W. (1964). Physiological problems in mitral stenosis. (Editorial). *Amer. Heart J.*, **68,** 145.

BAKER, A. B. (1968). Induction of anaesthesia with diazepam. *Anaesthesia*, **24,** 388.

CONWAY, C. M., ELLIS, D. B., and KING, N. W. (1968). A comparison of the acute haemodynamic effects of thiopentone, methohexitone and propanidid in the dog. *Brit. J. Anaesth.*, **40,** 756.

ENGLISH, I. C. W., FREW, R. M., PIGOTT, J. F., and ZAKI, M. (1969). Percutaneous catheterisation of the internal jugular vein. *Anaesthesia*, **24,** 521.

FINCK, A. J., FRANK, H. A., and ZOLL, P. M. (1969). Anaesthesia in relation to permanently implanted cardiac pacemakers. *Curr. Res. Anesth.*, **48,** 1043.

Graham, G. R. (1966). In: *Intravascular Catheterization*, 2nd edit. Ed. by H. A. Zimmerman. Springfield, Ill.: Chas. C. Thomas.

Healey, T. E. J. (1969). Intravenous diazepam for cardiac catheterisation. *Anaesthesia*, **24,** 537.

Howat, D. D. C. (1963). Anaesthesia for the insertion of indwelling artificial pacemakers. *Lancet*, **1,** 855.

Kahler, R. L., Burrow, G. N., and Felig, P. (1967). Diazepam-induced amnesia for cardioversion. *J. Amer. med. Ass.*, **200,** 987.

Kelman, G. R., Nunn, J. F., Prys-Roberts, C., and Greenbaum, R. (1967). The influence of cardiac output on arterial oxygenation. *Brit. J. Anaesth.*, **39,** 450.

Lancet (1968). Editorial. Hazards of cardiac catheterisation. **2,** 547.

McDowell, S. A., and Clarke, R. S. J. (1969). A clinical comparison of pancuronium with *d*-tubocurarine. *Anaesthesia*, **24,** 581.

Manners, J. M., and Codman, V. A. (1969). General anaesthesia for cardiac catheterisation in children. *Anaesthesia*, **24,** 541.

Mendel, D. (1968). *A Practice of Cardiac Catheterisation.* Oxford: Blackwell Scientific Publications.

Papper, E. M. (1965). Selection and management of anaesthesia in those suffering from diseases and disorders of the heart. *Canad. Anaesth. Soc. J.*, **12,** 245.

Prys-Roberts, C., Kelman, G. R., Greenbaum, R., and Robinson, R. H. (1967). Circulatory influences of artificial ventilation during nitrous oxide anaesthesia in man. *Brit. J. Anaesth.*, **39,** 533.

Ross, E. D. T. (1962). General anaesthesia in complete heart block. *Brit. J. Anaesth.*, **34,** 102.

Rowlands, D. J., Howitt, G., Logan, W. F. W. E., Clarke, A. D., and Jackson, P. W. (1967). Haemodynamic changes during methohexitone anaesthesia in patients with supraventricular arrhythmias. *Brit. J. Anaesth.*, **39,** 554.

Scott, D. L. (1970). Cardiac pacemakers as an anaesthetic problem. *Anaesthesia*, **25,** 87.

Skinner, J. F., and Pearce, M. L. (1964). Surgical risk in the cardiac patient. *J. chron. Dis.*, **17,** 57.

Thung, N., Herzog, P., Christlies, I., Thompson, W. M., and Dammann, J. (1963). The cost of respiratory effort in postoperative cardiac patients. *Circulation*, **28,** 552.

Topkins, M. J., and Artusio, J. F. (1964). Myocardial infarction and surgery. *Curr. Res. Anesth.*, **43,** 716.

Viljoen, J. F. (1968). Anaesthesia for internal mammary implant surgery. *Anaesthesia*, **23,** 515.

Wagner, G. S., and McIntosh, H. D. (1969). The use of drugs in achieving successful D. C. cardioversion. *Prog. cardiovasc. Dis.*, **11,** 431.

Woolman, H., Alexander, S. C., Cohen, P. J., Smith, T. C., Chase, P. E., and Van Der Molen, R. A. (1965). Cerebral circulation during general anesthesia and hyperventilation in man. *Anesthesiology*, **26,** 329.

Wrigley, F. R. H. (1964). Anaesthesia in Stokes-Adams disease. *Canad. Anaesth. Soc. J.*, **11,** 291.

Zeitlin, G. L. (1965). Artificial respiration after cardiac surgery. *Anaesthesia*, **20,** 145.

Chapter 25

THE EXTRACORPOREAL CIRCULATION

EXTRACORPOREAL circulation has now progressed to the point where it is undertaken routinely in many centres with a very low morbidity and mortality attributable to the technique itself. Unfortunately, this good clinical result has been the consequence of greater technical dexterity by the surgeon, anaesthetists and perfusionists and stricter manufacturing tolerances in the apparatus rather than the consequence of a more profound understanding of the physiological effects of bypass. It is to be hoped that now most clinical problems can be solved on the empirical basis of experience, time can be taken to study scientifically the unexplained problems. Perhaps in the field of post-operative care this generalisation is untrue and thanks to a greater understanding of circulatory physiology and its interaction with respiratory physiology, many patients can be carried through the difficult immediate post-operative period.

HISTORICAL NOTE

In 1812 Legallois wrote "If one could substitute for the heart a kind of injection of artificial blood, either naturally or artificially made, one would succeed in maintaining alive indefinitely any part of the body whatsoever." This armchair experimentation became a near-reality nearly fifty years later, when the physiologist Brown-Séquard (1858) attempted, with moderate success, to perfuse the decapitated head of a dog. He was one of the first workers to emphasise the importance of cerebral blood flow and, in fact, showed that a period of five minutes' ischaemia of the brain was sufficient to cause death in dogs.

The development of the various methods of oxygenating blood has been a slow process and those in use today are similar to many that were tried over eighty years ago. The difference between the present-day success and the failures of yesterday seems to lie in the realisation of the enormous surface of blood that must be exposed if adequate oxygenation is to occur. Amongst the first reports of a mechanical oxygenator is that of Ludwig (1865), who tried shaking blood in a balloon filled with air. Later, other workers tried bubbling air through blood, but although they achieved adequate oxygenation they were hampered by foaming (Schroder, 1882; Jacoby, 1890; Brodie, 1903).

Frey and Gruber (1885) were amongst the first to exploit the idea of a thin film of blood exposed to oxygen. Their apparatus consisted of a cylinder and the blood was allowed to flow along the inner walls and thus take up oxygen on its way. This principle of a thin film of blood was brilliantly adapted by Gibbon (1937) and has become the basis of one of the most successful heart-lung machines in use today.

Discovery and Development of Heparin and Protamine

An inability to prevent clotting of the blood was one of the principal causes of failure in the early experiments on the extracorporeal circulation. The discovery of *heparin*—the principal anticoagulant in use today—represents one of the rare "accidental finds" in modern medicine. Before 1916 there was no known substance which could prevent coagulation of the blood. Howell, who is well-known for his contribution to the theories on the clotting mechanism, assigned the task of purifying certain phosphatides to a second-year medical student—one Jay McLean—at Johns Hopkins University, Baltimore. At that time, Howell was looking for a substance that would speed up rather than slow down the clotting process. McLean found that one phosphatide (cuorin) extracted from the heart muscle of dogs actually prevented coagulation. Howell recognised immediately the importance of this substance and in the following year, at an Harveian Oration in London, he described this substance as an anti-prothrombin. Later, it was found that this substance could be extracted in abundance from dog's liver, and thus it came to be called *heparin.*

More recent work has shown that heparin originates in the granules of mast cells of both animals and man; these cells are found not only in the liver and lungs, but also in the connective tissue surrounding capillaries and in the walls of blood vessels throughout the body.

The role of protamine in restoring the coagulating mechanism after the use of heparin was soon identified. As long ago as 1880 Schmidt-Mulheim described the effect of "peptone shock" in dogs; this condition is characterised by circulatory collapse followed by a temporary loss of clotting power in the blood. This latter effect is believed to be due to the release of heparin from the mast cells. Waters and his colleagues (1938) conclusively demonstrated the value of protamine when they showed that it prevented the failure of clotting which is the characteristic of this condition.

Indications for Extracorporeal Circulation

Certain operations can be performed on the heart or great vessels while the heart continues to maintain circulation and to perfuse the vital organs. Thus mitral valvotomy, atrial septostomy, or closure of patent ductus arteriosus, can all be performed without the use of special apparatus. Other operations, however, can only be performed on the open dry heart and some other means of supporting the circulation must be found. Of the number of solutions which have either been suggested or tried over the years, only a few have survived into extended clinical practice.

1. Inflow Occlusion with Mild Hypothermia

If the vena cavae are snared and the aorta clamped, the heart can be temporarily isolated from the circulation whilst a brief operation is performed. No perfusion of the vital organs occurs during the period of occlusion, which would, therefore, only permit three minutes' operating time at normal temperatures. By reducing the patient's temperature to 30° C using surface hypothermia (see p. 1273) inflow occlusion can be prolonged to eight minutes. Few intracardiac lesions can be repaired in this time and the better operating conditions provided by extracorporeal circulation, together with the comparable operative risk, has resulted in inflow occlusion with mild hypothermia being generally abandoned for cardiac surgery if extracorporeal circulation is available.

2. **Inflow Occlusion with Profound Hypothermia**

By reducing the body temperature to 10–15° C, the period of inflow occlusion can be prolonged to up to one hour. As the heart fails, or the ventricle fibrillates at around 30° C, profound hypothermia has to be achieved while the circulation is supported artificially. This can be done in two ways:

(*a*) The Drew technique (Drew *et al.*, 1959) (Fig. 1) involves cannulation of the right atrium and pulmonary artery to bypass the right ventricle and of the left atrium and a systemic artery to bypass the left ventricle. The patient's own lungs are used for oxygenation and carbon dioxide elimination. This method has achieved considerable success, particularly in the treatment of congenital

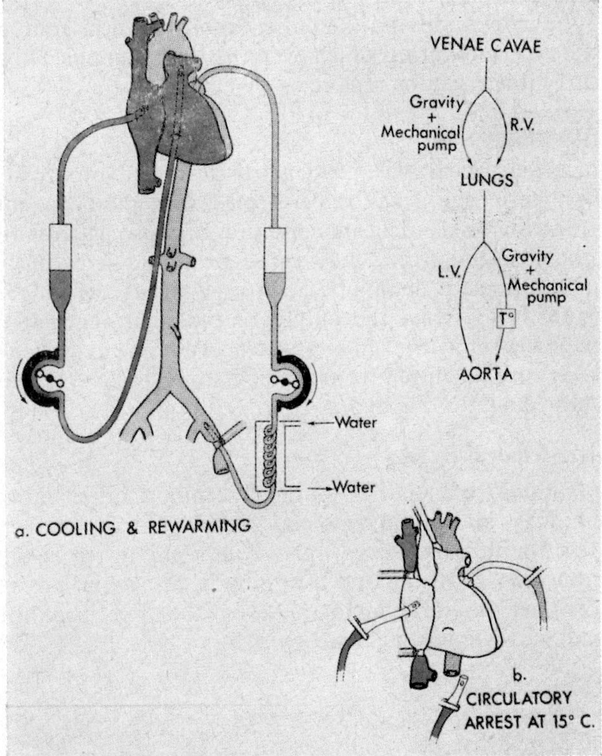

25/FIG. 1—Profound hypothermia (Drew technique).

heart disease. It has the disadvantages of requiring multiple vessel cannulations, of being time-consuming, as both cooling and rewarming are slow to avoid the development of temperature gradients within the body and yet, at the same time, placing a restriction on intracardiac operating time. It is also technically difficult in the presence of severe aortic incompetence. The merit of this method lies in the very good oxygenation of the patient's blood when compared with the performance of early oxygenators but with the development of machines capable of fully oxygenating high flows of blood, the need for this type of profound hypothermia has decreased.

(*b*) Profound hypothermia can also be produced with a normal extra-corporeal circuit, involving an oxygenator and a heat exchanger, removing blood from the right side of the heart and returning it to a systemic artery. This is sometimes indicated for operations on the great vessels where continuous perfusion would involve multiple cannulations, perhaps of the carotid and subclavian arteries. The time limit remains the same and there are similar disadvantages in the time of cooling and warming.

3. Extracorporeal Circulation using a Pump Oxygenator

This is the current method of choice for supporting the circulation during the performance of open intracardiac and great vessel surgery. The heart can be isolated from the circulation and the patient maintained in good condition for up to six hours, a period during which even the most complicated acquired and congenital heart disease can be repaired.

4. Supportive Bypass

Some intracardiac operations, particularly mitral valvotomy in the presence of pulmonary hypertension, can be performed with the heart supporting the circulation but owing to the delicate condition of these patients the manipulations which accompany surgery may cause profound hypotension. The low output and its consequent metabolic acidosis worsens the pulmonary hypertension which further reduces the output of the right ventricle. This vicious circle can only be broken with the use of extracorporeal circulation to transfer a proportion of the cardiac output from the right atrium to a systemic artery. This technique is termed supportive bypass (Fig. 2).

5. Left Atrio-femoral Bypass

During operations for aneurysms of the descending thoracic aorta the arterial supply to the kidneys and spinal cord may be temporarily interrupted, leading to renal failure or paraplegia. These organs can be supported by taking oxygenated blood from the left atrium and returning it, at arterial pressure levels, to the aorta below the clamp. The major vessels of the upper part of the body are supplied normally by the beating heart (Fig. 3).

Apparatus

Anaesthetised adult patients consume approximately 110–130 ml. O_2 per square metre of body surface area per minute, with a higher rate in infancy. To provide a full flow of completely oxygenated blood, an oxygenator needs to be capable of adding this quantity of oxygen to the venous blood for an indefinite period. Sufficient reserve capacity is also needed to cope with patients who initially are hypoxic or who develop an oxygen debt before bypass or during rewarming.

In the human lung, blood is efficiently oxygenated because of the huge surface area and the very intimate contact between the red cells and the alveolus (see Table 1). Thus oxygenation is achieved despite a low oxygen tension

25/Fig. 2.—Supportive bypass without thoracotomy.

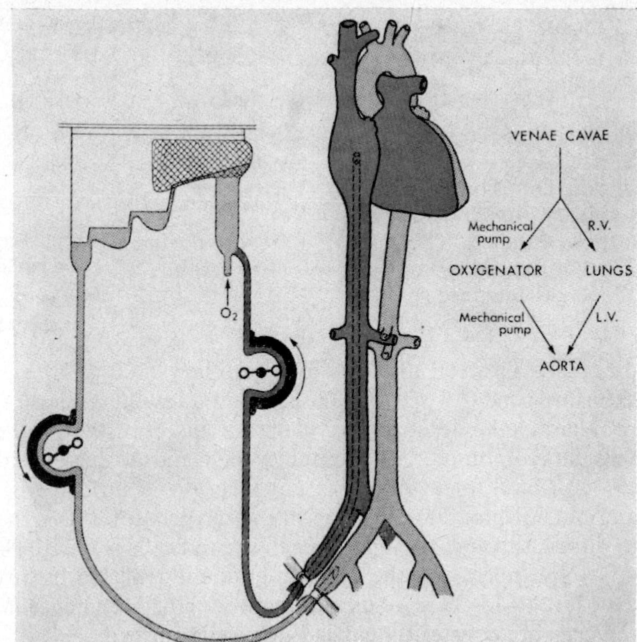

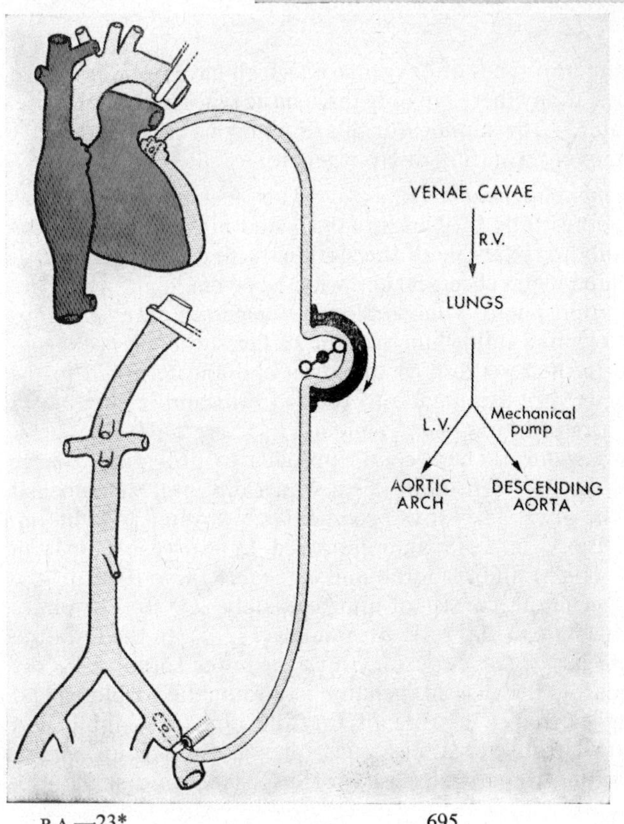

25/Fig. 3.—Left atriofemoral bypass.

25/TABLE 1

DIFFERENCE BETWEEN NORMAL LUNG AND ARTIFICIAL OXYGENATORS

Thickness of Blood Film	Monocorpuscular	20–60 r.b.c. thick (0·1–0·3 mm.)
Surface Area	50–200 sq. metres	2–10 sq. metres
Plasma Diffusion Distance	Very short	Long (N.B. Turbulence)
Capillary Membrane Diffusion	Yes	No
Oxygen Gradient	100−40=60 mm. Hg	673−40=633 mm. Hg
Time of Exposure	0·1–0·8 seconds	15–30 seconds
Blood/gas Interface	No	Yes (except membrane oxygenators)

difference between alveolus and capillary (100 − 40 = 60 mm. Hg), a short exposure time (0·1 sec. to 0·3 sec.) and a low lung blood volume. The principal problem in the design of oxygenators has been the production of a sufficiently thin film of blood. Most filming oxygenators have a film of 0·1 to 0·3 mm. (30–60 r.b.c.) thick. As a consequence, if the surface area is large, considerable amounts of blood are held up in the oxygenator. Also, the distance oxygen has to diffuse through plasma to reach the red cells is great. These disadvantages are offset by increasing the oxygen gradient tenfold, by prolonging the time of exposure to 15–30 seconds and by producing turbulence in the blood so that the red cells are constantly carried up to the surface.

Oxygenators

Despite the large number of types of oxygenators which have been described and used at different times, today there are only three basic types in common use.

The thin film oxygenator.—The support for this film may be either stationary (screen oxygenator) or moving (rotating disc oxygenator).

(*a*) *Mayo-Gibbon pump oxygenator* (Fig. 4).—This machine, which was developed and used so successfully by Kirklin (1957) and his colleagues at the Mayo Clinic, is an outstanding example of the stationary screen oxygenator. It consists of a series of coated metal sheets 30 cm. wide by 60 cm. high, which are encased in high oxygen atmosphere. Venous blood is dispersed along the tops of the sheets and flows down in a stable film over the surfaces where it is oxygenated. It is then collected in the reservoirs at the lower end and returned to the patient. This oxygenator is very atraumatic to the red cells and is capable of oxygenating large flow rates of blood.

(*b*) *Rotating disc oxygenator.*—The second approach to providing a large surface area thin film is the use of rotating discs which dip into a channel of blood as it flows under the discs. They thus become partly covered with blood. Originally designed by Björk in 1948 and improved by Melrose (1953) in England and Kay *et al.* (1958) and Osborne and his colleagues (1960) in the United States. Most oxygenators consist of approximately 100 to 120 plates 11 cm. in diameter which rotate at 100 revs. per minute (Fig. 5). In the Osborne oxygenator, the discs are larger (21 cm.) and run at a lower speed. Like the stationary screen oxygenator, the disc oxygenator is atraumatic to blood and has a large oxygenating capacity. Because of the difficulty in cleaning and sterilising disc oxygenators made of stainless steel, they are now being manufactured of plastic and supplied ready sterilised for disposal after a single use.

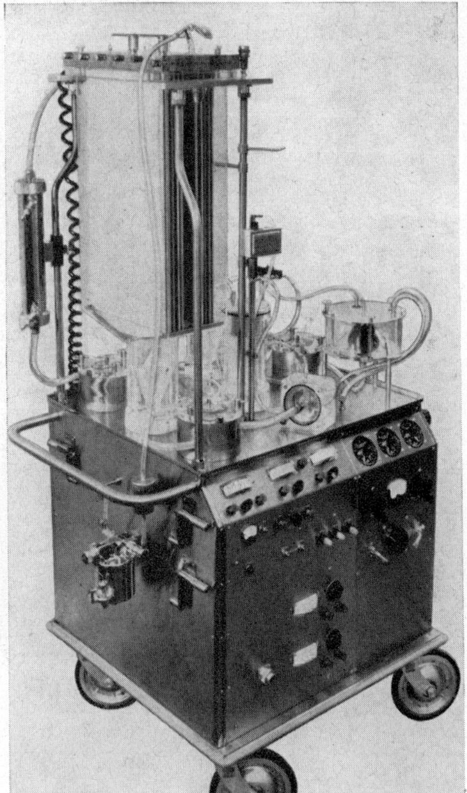

25/Fig. 4.—The Mayo-Gibbon pump-oxygenator.

The bubble oxygenator.—The bubble oxygenator was originally associated with the names of DeWall and his colleagues (1957) and is now widely available in three forms:

The "Temptrol" oxygenator (Kalke *et al.*, 1969) and
The "Travenol" oxygenator, from the United States.
The "Rygg-Kysgaard" from Denmark (Rygg *et al.*, 1964).

The basic principle is the same. Blood and gas flow together at the bottom of the column which is thus filled with ascending froth (Fig. 6). The size of the bubble is important. Small bubbles produce a large surface area and thus good oxygenation, but are difficult to eliminate before the blood is returned to the patient. A proportion of larger bubbles is necessary for the adequate elimination of carbon dioxide. At the top of the column the froth comes into contact with a large surface area coated with silicone-type anti-foam, which causes the bubbles to burst. Any residual bubbles are trapped at the surface of settling reservoirs or helices before the blood is returned to the patient. Modern bubble oxygenators are highly efficient and can cope with large flows of blood. They are slightly more traumatic to blood than the screen oxygenators. Bubble oxygenators are generally made of plastic, and are supplied pre-sterilised and designed to be used

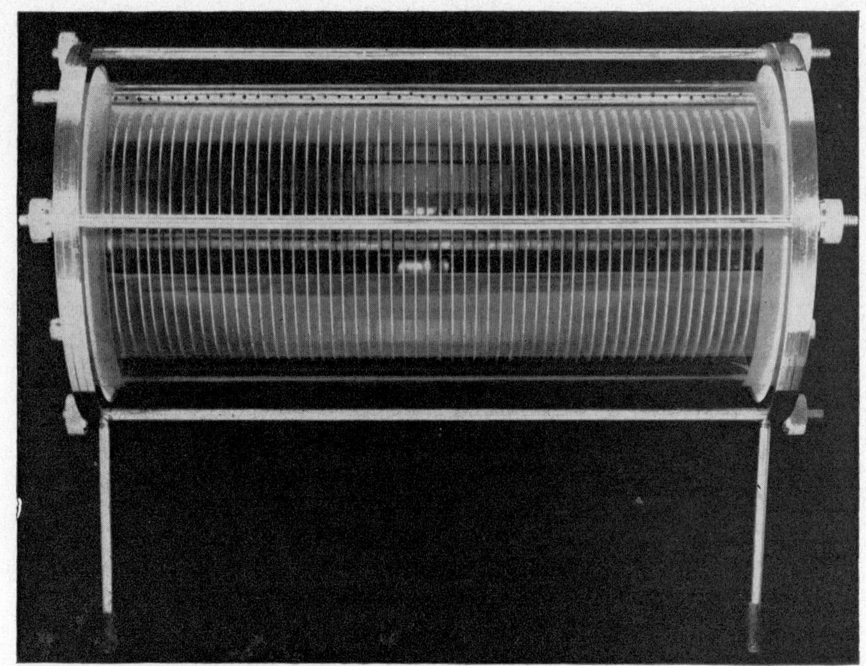

25/Fig. 5.—Oxygenator discs.

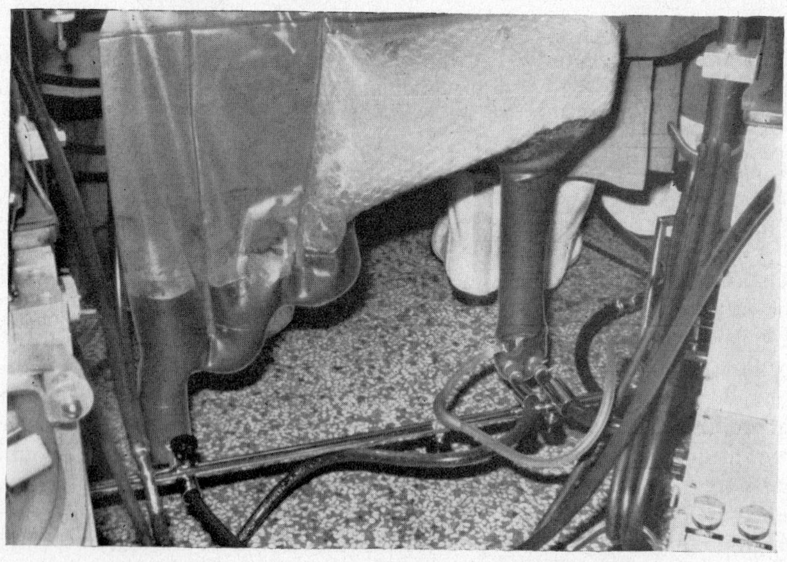

25/Fig. 6.

only once. Because of their small priming volume, the use of blood is frequently unnecessary.

The membrane oxygenator.—One of the main criticisms of the types of oxygenators described above is the presence of a blood gas interface which leads to denaturation of the plasma proteins and places a limit on the time for which bypass can be continued. The membrane oxygenator, originally described by Clowes, and now developed by Bramson and his colleagues (1965), utilises a silicone rubber membrane, permeable both to carbon dioxide and oxygen, between the gas space and the blood. It has a good capacity for oxygenation and CO_2 elimination but the technical problems of assembly and sterilisation, when set against the good performance of other types of oxygenator, mean that the membrane oxygenator is currently enjoying restricted use. Its future would appear to lie with long-term perfusion (2–6 days) to help patients with severe myocardial infarcts or acute lung disease although, if the logistic problems can be overcome, the absence of a blood gas interface and the small priming volume will make it the oxygenator of choice for cardiac surgery.

Pumps

Pumps are used in the extracorporeal circuit to return the oxygenated blood to the systemic arterial tree at high pressure levels and to provide suction to remove blood from the operative field. Pumps need to be simple, robust, easily calibrated and adjusted, and atraumatic to blood. Those parts actually in contact with the blood are usually disposable.

Of the many types of pump described, only the roller pump has survived for widespread use (DeBakey, 1934). These may have single, double (Fig. 7), or, less commonly, triple arms. Correctly adjusted for minimal occlusion with good quality tubing, they are relatively atraumatic to blood. The rate of haemolysis is directly related to the number of passages the roller makes over the tube and large bore tubing in a slow running pump is to be preferred.

Blood flow, pulsatile or continuous.—Most pumps in use today, which are robust and simple, produce a predominantly continuous flow. Pulsatile flow can be produced by a pump which is more complicated and, in some cases, more traumatic to the blood. However, the principal difficulty in producing the pulsatile flow to the patient lies in the size of the arterial cannula. This is normally the smallest point in the arterial line and commonly imposes a large resistance if high flow rates are used. To produce a pulsatile flow distal to this restriction would entail very high pressure swings proximal to it and intermittent high velocity jets through it, both of which would result in substantial damage to the blood and plasma proteins. Arguments that pulsatile flow is non-essential, based on comparisons with aortic stenosis and coarctation, are probably not valid because these are long-term conditions and the patient has become accustomed to the flow patterns over many years. In the short term, the only faintly pulsatile flow produced by most pumps does not seem to be harmful although there is some evidence that kidney function is better maintained with a pulsatile flow. If long-term perfusion for several days, as, for instance, after a myocardial infarction, becomes a practical possibility, then the desirability of a pulsatile flow may become more obvious.

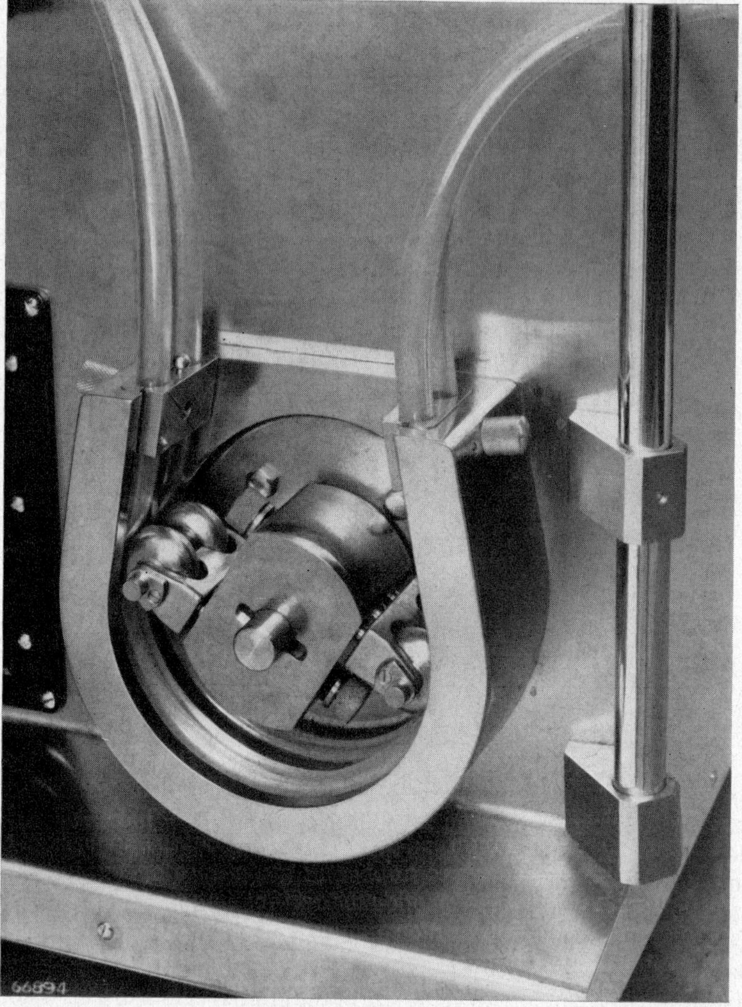

25/FIG. 7.—Roller pump.

Choice of Materials, Cleaning and Sterilisation

Though at first sight the matter of cleanliness of the machine would seem a relatively simple one, in practice it has been proved to be of the utmost importance in the development of the extracorporeal circulation. It can be shown that on almost every surface that has been in contact with blood a thin layer of protein substance remains (Bahnson, 1958). Minute scratches on the interior surface of the apparatus lead to the deposition of fibrin and platelets in this area which could be transferred from patient to patient.

One approach to the problem is to make as much of the apparatus disposable as possible. All tubing, both connecting and that used within the pumps, is normally used once only. The bubble oxygenators are usually supplied pre-sterilised by gamma radiation for single use only and other pieces of apparatus, heat exchangers, filters, even disc oxygenators, are following this pattern. This is a very expensive process because despite their short life they need to be manufactured with a high degree of precision to provide smooth atraumatic surfaces from high purity materials free from the danger of chemical toxicity (Duke and Vane, 1968).

Lately, interest has been aroused by the possibility of bonding heparin directly on to glass or on to plastic surfaces pre-treated with graphite to produce a non-thrombogenic surface.

Polycarbonate is also gaining favour as a material (Gott *et al.*, 1963; Hersh and Weetall, 1969) with a fine finish and high degree of inertness.

Those parts of the circuit which are not disposable are commonly manufactured from stainless steel which can be given a highly polished and lasting surface that is chemically inert. This can be cleaned with haemolytic compounds, acids and alkalis, or ultrasonic vibrations.

Sterilisation varies with the facilities available. Disposable parts are commonly irradiated or exposed to ethylene dioxide gas. An autoclave technique is used for glass and stainless steel parts. The total circuit of separately sterilised parts is then assembled using a full sterile technique.

Anaesthesia and Monitoring

Anaesthesia and monitoring for patients undergoing extracorporeal circulation is considered in greater detail in Chapter 24, Anaesthesia and Cardiac Disease.

Monitoring during Extracorporeal Circulation

It has been said that the more experienced the surgical team, the less the need for monitoring. Alternatively, if monitoring can be achieved with no increased morbidity the extra information is always available when needed for making decisions and for teaching or research. Melrose (1969) has expressed this viewpoint, saying "the maximum security of a perfusion system follows the meticulous monitoring of many parameters".

Percutaneous catheterisation by the anaesthetist of the radial artery, the internal or external jugular vein, and the femoral vein for cannulation of the inferior vena cava, are all technically easy. Indwelling catheters enable continuous display of arterial and venous pressures and samples are easily obtainable for blood gas, electrolyte and coagulation estimations. A display ECG is mandatory and an EEG is often included. Finally, the urine output is recorded hourly. The routine use of a wide but specific range of monitoring enables the anaesthetist continually to reassess the patient's condition on some basis other than mere clinical instinct.

Physiology of the Extracorporeal Circulation

At first sight, the withdrawal of blood from a patient with subsequent oxygenation and then retransfusion would appear to be a simple matter, but in practice it is fraught with difficulties. Each machine has its own characteristics but the most important single factor for success is the organisation of the team, which is fully conversant with all the aspects of extracorporeal circulation. Some of these problems are considered individually below.

Clotting of Blood

When blood is removed from a patient, it starts to clot within a few minutes unless some steps are taken to prevent this process. Contact of blood with any part of the machine, even if it is thoroughly siliconised, is sufficient to start the coagulation process and may ultimately lead either to the infusion of a fatal embolus or to the complete defibrination of the blood, followed by intractable bleeding. Complete reversible inhibition of the coagulation process is required and this is produced with heparin. Before cannulation of the vessels, heparin is given in a dose approximately 300 units per kilogramme body weight with the aim of producing a blood level of 4 to 5 units per ml. A similar concentration is used in the priming solution of the oxygenator. The half-life of heparin is approximately one hour at normal temperatures and, as the dangers of under-heparinisation are so great, heparin is repeated at half the original dose (150 units per kilo) at hourly intervals while bypass lasts.

After the extracorporeal circulation has been discontinued, it is important to restore normal coagulation as soon as possible to prevent persistent oozing from all cut surfaces, which is such a dominant feature of the heparinised patient. As soon as the cannulae are removed from the thoracic vessels, protamine sulphate is given. The quantity may be determined, prior to administration, by a protamine-heparin titration of the sample, or a predetermined amount (e.g. 6 mg. per kilo body weight) may be given, and the calcium thrombin time compared with the pre-bypass specimen. Protamine is always given slowly as a rapid injection can cause profound hypotension, particularly if the patient is slightly underfilled. Unfortunately, the heparin-protamine complex is sometimes broken down by sulphases in the blood before it is excreted and an hour or so after protamine administration coagulation may again become prolonged and further administration of protamine is necessary. This reappearance of free heparin should always be proved before more protamine is given as a similar effect is produced clinically by the breakdown of fibrinogen. The continued exact correction of the coagulation mechanism is required for minimal blood loss. Only very rarely is major fibrinolysis a problem and then usually in patients with severe polycythaemic heart disease (Fallot's tetralogy). The anti-fibrinolytic agents (Trasylol and Aminocaproic acid) are best reserved for administration when major fibrinolysis is demonstrated by coagulation tests. Other substances involved in coagulation (e.g. fibrinogen, vitamin K) are sometimes administered, but usually on an empirical rather than scientific basis. Patients who have been on long-term anticoagulation prior to operation normally have their prothrombin time reduced to normal over the operative period.

Cannulation of the Vessels

The heart and great vessels may be approached through either a left or right thoracotomy, or by a midline sternal split incision. The superior vena cava and inferior vena cava are normally cannulated with catheters passed though the right atrium, although when operating on the left heart, a single tube in the right atrium can be used. The size of the venous catheters is chosen to be adequate for the drainage of blood through them during bypass but, at the same time, they must not be so large as to obstruct the venous return before the onset of perfusion (Fig. 8). Once bypass has commenced, venous drainage is achieved with a gravity siphon, the rate of flow being controlled by an adjustable clamp on the main venous line. If the venae cavae of the patient are 20–30 cm. higher than the oxygenator or venous reservoir, siphonage produced by this difference in height is sufficient to maintain a good flow. In some cases, the siphonage may become excessive when it only defeats its own end by collapsing the vessel walls against the orifice of the tubes.

Blood also enters the heart from three other possible sources (Fig. 9). (1) Coronary venous return mostly re-enters the heart through the coronary sinus which drains into the right atrium. If the venous pressure is low, this blood then flows backwards into the venae cavae and down the main tubes. Alternatively, if the venous pressure is high or the venae cavae are snared up, this blood is aspirated with coronary suckers. (2) The bronchial arteries, which in Fallot's tetralogy can take up the 20 per cent of cardiac output, anastomose with the pulmonary circulation and drain to the left side of the heart where the blood is aspirated with suckers or with the left ventricular vent. (3) In the presence of aortic incompetence, blood can also pass retrogradely across the aortic valve and will have to be aspirated with suckers from the left ventricle.

The arterial return was commonly placed in the femoral or external iliac artery, but direct return to the aorta is becoming more common. The size of the cannula chosen is the largest the peripheral vessel will accept or, in the case of aortic cannulation, a large cannula which only produces a low pressure drop across it for the desired blood flow.

Left heart venting.—Under certain circumstances (aortic incompetence, hypothermia, acute heart failure), the left ventricular end diastolic pressure may rise excessively. In some patients this leads to overdistension of the ventricle and damage to the myocardium. Back pressure effects are also transmitted via the left atrium to the pulmonary capillaries where they cause pulmonary engorgement and, ultimately, pulmonary oedema. These deleterious effects can be prevented by decompressing the left ventricle, or the left atrium if the mitral valve is incompetent, with a left heart vent. This blood is returned to the pump oxygenator. The vent must be clamped or removed before attempting to discontinue bypass.

Priming Solutions

(*a*) **Volume.**—It is possible to construct an oxygenator system with a minimal priming blood volume. In such a system, however, any interference with the venous return results either in the reduction of flow or in the almost instantaneous emptying of the oxygenator into the patient with consequent risk of air embolism. For safety, therefore, most open systems have a reserve volume of about 25 per cent of the minute volume flow over and above the volume in the connecting tubes, and thus priming volumes of between two and four litres for adults are usual.

(*b*) **Composition.**—The factors which have to be taken into consideration include oxygen carrying capacity, viscosity, tonicity, electrolyte balance and clotting ability.

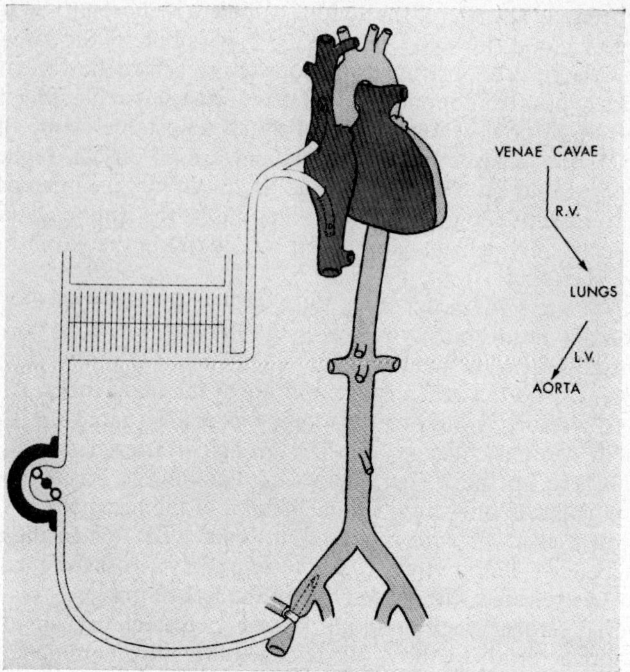

25/Fig. 8.—Before cardiopulmonary bypass.

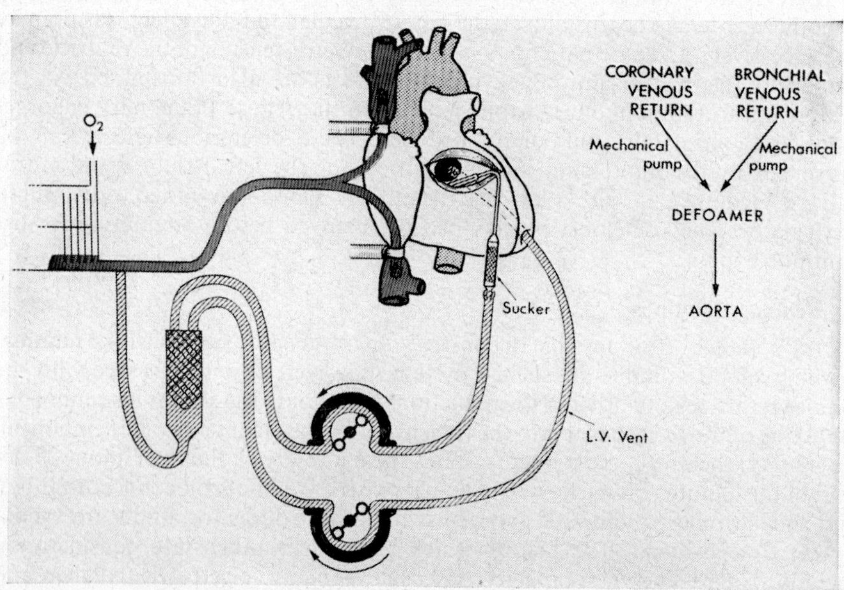

25/Fig. 9.—Return of blood from bypassed heart.

Oxygen carrying capacity.—Provided the flow rate is adequate, it is quite possible to maintain a near-normal mixed venous oxygen tension in the face of a reduced oxygen carrying capacity. The lower limit for P.C.V. once mixing between patient and prime has occurred, is usually put at 28–30 per cent. In an adult patient with, say, a blood volume of 4600 ml. and 2000 ml. r.b.c. it is possible to prime a machine with 2000 ml. of clear fluid and still have enough oxygen carrying capacity.

Blood.—Whereas blood was originally thought to be the most physiological fluid to prime a heart lung machine, today the opposite view is more common. Blood is only used to raise the oxygen carrying capacity of the priming solution to an acceptable minimum. It has fallen out of favour, partly because of the immense difficulties of finding the quantities of blood required each day for the many operations performed. The homologous blood syndrome (Gadboys *et al.*, 1962), although seen only in dogs in its most florid form, also occurs to some extent in humans. Post-operatively there is a much greater incidence of poor lung function after a blood prime than if the prime is with non-sanguinous fluid. Coagulation difficulties are also provoked by the use of large quantities of blood. These dangers are added to all the normal problems (incompatibility, wrong bottle, serum hepatitis) of blood transfusion in general.

When blood is required, and this occurs most commonly in infants in whom the ratio of priming volume to patient's blood volume is large, this is provided as normal A.C.D. blood, usually one to two days old, which is heparinised and recalcified before use.

Haemodilution technique.—The reduction in viscosity achieved by using isotonic solutions leads, under the artificial conditions of extracorporeal circulation, to a better tissue perfusion: there is also very little difficulty in obtaining the venous return sufficient to attain the ideal flow rate. Where hypothermia is used, this decrease in viscosity also offsets the rise in viscosity which normally occurs when the temperature drops.

The very multiplicity of fluids advocated and actually used indicates that no one priming solution is ideal. The large molecular dextrans are not used because of the interference with the clotting mechanisms and this is true also of low molecular dextrans in amounts in excess of 20 ml. per kilo body weight. A lactated Ringer's solution or 5 per cent dextrose plus certain electrolytes (usually calcium and potassium) are the most common. If the solution is to be fully re-infused, the water load is usually restricted to 30–40 ml./kg. body weight; this fluid is usually rapidly excreted and the haematocrit returns to normal in the early post-operative phase (Zuhdi *et al.*, 1964).

Other substances, e.g. mannitol, vitamin C, occasionally form part of a priming solution, although the precise indications are hard to find.

Control of Perfusion and Flow Rates

In the early days of heart surgery, due to the inadequacy of oxygenators, only a low flow of blood was used. With the advent of oxygenators capable of adding 250 to 300 ml. of oxygen per minute to the blood flow, low flow has become unacceptable. While the minimal acceptable venous oxygen tension is approximately 25 mm. Hg (Optiz and Schneider, 1950), ideally $P\bar{v}_{O_2}$ should not fall below the normal physiological level of 40 mm. Hg which, in the patient with normal blood, represents saturation of approximately 70 per cent and an oxygen content of 15 ml./100 ml. blood. Assuming the arterial blood to be fully oxygenated and thus to have an oxygen content of approximately 20 ml. per 100 ml. blood, the arteriovenous oxygen content difference for oxygen will be 5 ml. of oxygen per 100 ml. blood. If the oxygen consumption is 130 ml. oxygen per square metre per minute, this entails a flow of 2·4 litres per square metre per minute of blood. This flow will need to be slightly higher in children because of their higher metabolic rate relative to the surface area and can be lower in large patients whose surface area exceeds about 1·8 sq. metres. It must also be raised in the presence of haemodilution. Perfusing patients at this flow rate results in normal blood gas tensions and the absence of metabolic acidosis. Under-perfusion produces hypoxia of the tissues recognisable by low $P\bar{v}_{O_2}$ and the development of metabolic acidosis. Over-perfusion does not improve the tissue oxygenation and may lead to greater trauma to blood in the pump oxygenator.

The gas flow through the oxygenator is only roughly predictable. In theory a relatively low oxygen flow should be adequate to oxygenate the blood and by careful monitoring to remove the carbon dioxide. In practice, the control of carbon dioxide tension is much easier if the oxygenator is flushed out with a flow of gas two to three times that of the flow of blood, and which contains approximately $2\frac{1}{2}$ per cent to 3 per cent carbon dioxide. Fine adjustment of carbon dioxide tension to physiological values is made after blood gas measurements once bypass has achieved a steady state. The disadvantages of a low carbon dioxide tension in shifting the oxygen dissociation curve and in reducing tissue and cerebral blood flow (Woolman *et al.*, 1966) are so great that a slightly raised carbon dioxide level is to be preferred during bypass.

Now that oxygenators are capable of producing oxygen tensions of the order of 300 mm. Hg, the effect of high oxygen tension in raising peripheral vascular resistance and impairing tissue perfusion becomes relevant, and the oxygen tension should perhaps be limited to that which produces full oxygen saturation of the blood.

During cardiopulmonary bypass, the arterial pressure is generally said to be less important than the flow rate. Low perfusion pressures, either accidental or deliberate, are not uncommon, the result partly of anaesthetic drugs and partly from the low viscosity of the blood in the haemodilution technique. Current practice tends to confirm the observations made during induced hypotension that provided a patient has a good cardiac output and his tissues appear pink and warm, the arterial pressure is relatively unimportant.

"Partial" and "Total" bypass (Figs. 10 and 11).—A distinction used to be made between "partial" and "total" bypass according to whether or not the venous snares were tightened. "Partial" bypass means a flow rate of anywhere between 0–100 per cent of the desired flow with the cava unsnared. "Total" bypass implies that the venae cavae are snared and the flow must be at the desired level. In practice, when working on the left heart there is an advantage in remaining on "partial" at the desired flow, because if the venous pressure is low, the coronary sinus blood will drain into the cavae rather than through the lungs to the left atrium.

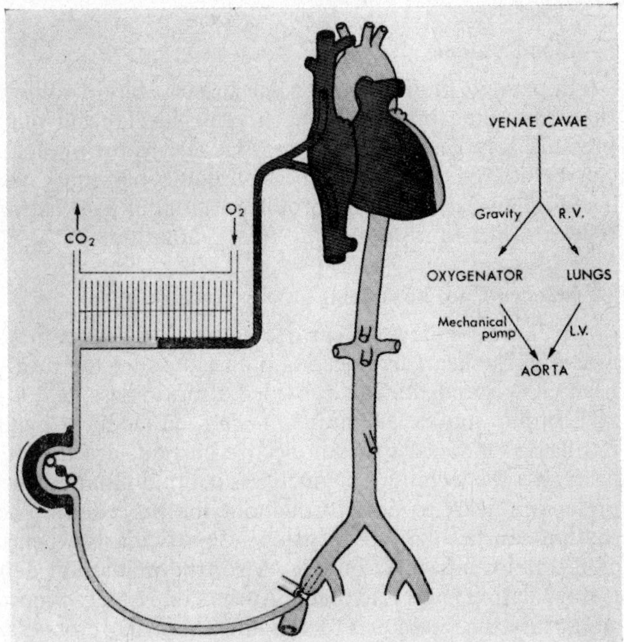

25/FIG. 10.—Partial bypass.

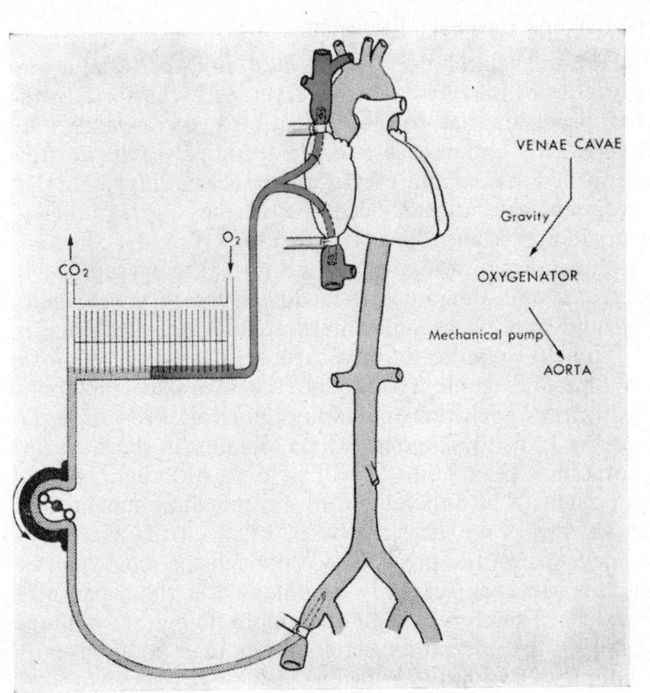

25/FIG. 11.—Total bypass.

Blood Volume

In patients undergoing cardiac surgery, blood volume is much less important than the filling pressure in each ventricle. During full flow bypass, the filling pressure is largely irrelevant and the venous pressure, and hence blood volume, can be altered to provide the optimum operating conditions for the surgery. These changes should be produced gradually so as not to invoke vasomotor reflexes which can produce a "faint" situation.

Induced Cardiac Arrest

In the early days of cardiac surgery, it was common practice to stop the action of the heart by injecting potassium into the root of the aorta after it had been cross-clamped. This provided a motionless field but had the disadvantage of being an anoxic technique. Today, either local hypothermia or ventricular fibrillation induced with an electric current, are used to provide a motionless heart, but the technique is much less common than formerly, and many surgeons prefer the heart to beat throughout the procedure. The advantage is that the rhythm can be observed constantly, particularly when operating in the region of the atrioventricular bundle. Also, the potassium depletion which occurs in the fibrillating heart is avoided. At the same time, a vigorously beating heart may embarrass the surgeon and the aorta is often cross-clamped intermittently to produce a relaxed heart with a reversibly diminished force of contraction (see below).

Myocardial Preservation and Coronary Perfusion

During simple extracorporeal circulation the myocardium is perfused normally from the coronary arteries by the blood which is returned to the aorta by the heart-lung machine. This perfusion may be interrupted for two reasons:

(*a*) **Aortic valve surgery.**—To obtain access to the aortic valve, the aorta is cross-clamped and then opened between the clamp and the heart. This means that no perfusion of the coronary arteries can occur unless they are cannulated separately (Fig. 12). It would appear most physiological to perfuse the coronary arteries continuously with a normal flow of blood at normal temperatures. In practice this is not always easy and sometimes, to facilitate surgery, the coronary perfusion is interrupted and may occur only intermittently for, say, three in every thirteen minutes. To help preserve the myocardium during these anoxic periods, hypothermia is sometimes employed to reduce the myocardial metabolic demands. Alternatively, it may be felt that the unphysiological effects of hypothermia are worse than the transitory anoxia which obtains if the aorta is clamped continuously for a short period of, say, half an hour. Although the ideal solution to this problem ought to be apparent from theoretical arguments and the experience of research, this is not necessarily so. Much of the success of intracardiac operations depends on the precision with which the repair can be effected and sometimes this precision can only be obtained at the expense of transitory myocardial hypoxia. Therefore, a somewhat unphysiological technique may, in the long term follow-up, give rather better results than an apparently more physiological technique of coronary perfusion.

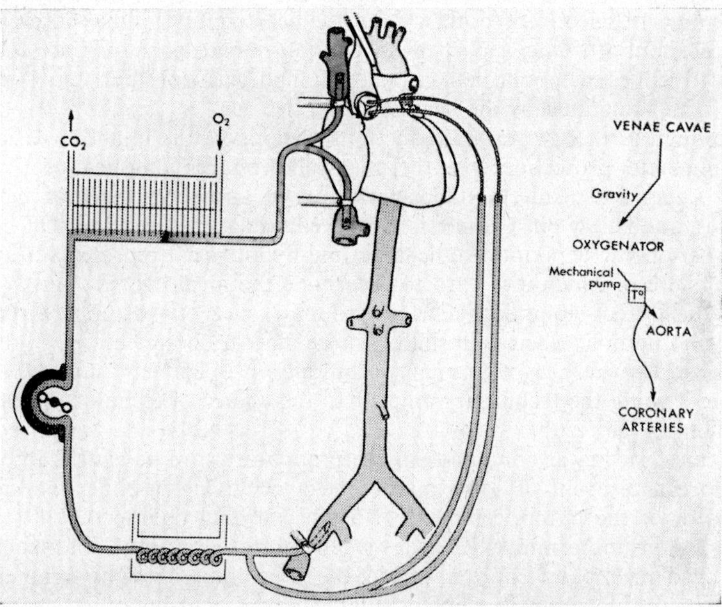

25/FIG. 12.—Circuit for aortic valve surgery.

(*b*) **Aortic cross-clamping.**—As for the aortic valve, precision of surgery is important in all branches of cardiac surgery and, to facilitate this precision, the aorta is sometimes cross-clamped. The effects of this are:

i. The cessation of coronary arterial perfusion stops blood pouring out of the coronary sinus to flood the operative field.
ii. If there is any aortic incompetence present, it prevents blood regurgitating through the aortic valve to obscure the operative field.
iii. As the heart becomes hypoxic, the muscle relaxes and the heart is more easily displaced and retracted to provide better access for surgery.
iv. If there is any danger from air embolism from a beating heart, cerebral air complications can be prevented by the presence of an aortic clamp.

Hypothermia

In cardiac surgery, hypothermia has been used in four ways:

1. Surface hypothermia to prolong the circulatory interruption time of inflow occlusion.
2. Profound hypothermia as part of the "Drew" technique.
3. Selective hypothermia of the heart.
4. Mild hypothermia as an adjunct to extracorporeal circulation.

Surface hypothermia is referred to on page 692 and covered in greater detail on page 1273.

The Drew technique has already been referred to on page 693 and is a useful method of enabling cardiac surgery to be performed in the absence of good apparatus for extracorporeal circulation.

The aims of selective hypothermia of the heart and of mild hypothermia, i.e. down to about 30° C as a part of an extracorporeal technique, are the same, namely to reduce metabolic demands so that inadequate or interrupted perfusion can be better tolerated by the heart.

Although in theory greater reductions of temperature might be desirable as providing better protection, hypothermia itself produces complications. Vascular spasm occurs and leads to under-perfusion of tissue, viscosity of the blood increases, and below 30° C there is a markedly increased incidence of bleeding in the post-operative period. At the same time, hypothermia represents an unphysiological state in which it is hard to determine the ideal pH, P_{O_2} and P_{CO_2}, and what is the correct blood flow. This has led many surgeons to adopt the principle that normothermia, albeit with slightly unsatisfactory perfusion, is a preferable alternative. However, as with many techniques in open heart surgery, it is the team performing the technique rather than the choice of technique itself which often dictates the results.

Fortunately, major complications with apparatus are nowadays rare but in the unfortunate event of some major defect occurring in either the lines, the oxygenator or the pump, cerebral perfusion can only be interrupted for three minutes at normothermia, whereas if the temperature is at 30° C the machine can be changed or repairs effected within the time limit of eight minutes. This provides a distinct improvement in safety margin, and hypothermia down to 30° C is not marked by additional complications.

Temperature control during extracorporeal circulation is normally effected by the passage of blood through heat exchangers, which are large surface areas of a high conductivity material over which the blood is filmed. The temperature in the water jacket can then be altered to affect the temperature of the blood. In some instances the heat exchanger is incorporated into some other piece of apparatus such as the oxygenator. Cooling can usually be effected more rapidly than rewarming because of the larger temperature gradient possible between blood (37° C) and the circulating fluid (0° C), whereas during rewarming the highest possible water temperature is approximately 40° C. Slow rewarming is desirable to avoid islets of cold tissue remaining in the body which cause the patient to cool again, perhaps dangerously, after bypass has been discontinued.

Renal Preservation

The preservation of renal function during extracorporeal circulation now seems to be much less of a complication than it used to be. Under conditions of high flow, particularly when associated with haemodilution, urine output is normally sustained at a high level during cardiac surgery. This is particularly so if dextrose is used in the priming solution due to its osmotic effect. If the urine output falls below 30 ml. of urine per hour, mannitol (25 g.) is commonly added to the perfusate. A high urine output also helps to excrete the products of haemolysis. The urine production commonly ceases if the patient becomes acidotic and then returns to normal on correction of the metabolic acidosis. Post-operative renal problems appear to stem not so much from the bypass procedure but from a low cardiac output produced by the patient after surgery.

COMPLICATIONS

Haemolysis

Trauma to the formed elements of the blood can be a major complication of extracorporeal circulation. The most easily measurable result is the appearance of free plasma haemoglobin, but presumably other deleterious effects occur at the same time, particularly the denaturation of the plasma proteins which results from the presence of blood-gas interface in the oxygenator. Haemolysis can be reduced to a minimum by the use of high quality tubing, by the siliconing of parts which come into contact with the blood, by the use of roller pumps which are carefully adjusted and which have large bore tubing over which the roller only passes very slowly. Haemolysis is commoner in bubble oxygenators than in stationary screen and rotating disc oxygenators, but the principal source of haemolysis in fact lies in the suckers which are used to aspirate spilt blood from the heart (Osborne *et al.*, 1962). These should be of a wide bell-mouthed type and the surgical assistant should, wherever possible, suck pools of liquid blood, rather than a mixture of blood and air. Haemolysis normally increases almost linearly with the passage of time. However, with current-day well-maintained apparatus, it is rare for plasma haemoglobins to exceed approximately 100 mg. per 100 ml. blood even at the end of long perfusions. This is a level which is not normally associated with renal damage.

Air Embolism

Air embolism is one of the major hazards of open heart surgery. The air normally gains access to the heart during an intracardiac manoeuvre and is then ejected out into the systemic circulation when the heart is reconnected to the general circulation. Every effort, therefore, is made to ensure that the heart is free of air before the heart is reconnected to the circulation.

The following manoeuvres are employed:

i. Whilst the aortic clamp is still applied, the venous pressure can be raised so that blood passes through the pulmonary capillaries, fills the left atrium and then the left ventricle, whilst the air passes outwards through a needle placed through the base of the aorta.
ii. Alternatively, air can be aspirated from the chambers of the heart, using a syringe and needle, from the left ventricle after up-ending the apex of the ventricle, or from the left atrium after the patient is positioned on his left side so that the left atrium lies above the ventricle and the mitral valve rendered incompetent.

Despite all these manoeuvres, air is commonly ejected into the aorta and the brain can be to some extent protected by positioning the patient with head downwards and also by making multiple holes or leaving needles through the arch of the aorta at its highest point. The bubbles then pass up the needles whilst the blood continues in the vessels.

During intracardiac manoeuvres, air commonly gains access to the pulmonary veins and this is often not dislodged until the pulmonary veins are perfused by raising the venous pressure and positive pressure ventilation begins. Before the aortic clamp is removed, the lungs should be inflated several times while aspirating the ventricle.

Flooding the operative site with carbon dioxide has been advocated on the grounds that if this gains access to the circulation, being highly absorbent, it will not cause significant embolism. In practice, with the motions of the heart, the patient's lungs and the surgeon's hands, it is virtually impossible to obtain local high concentrations of carbon dioxide.

Post-perfusion Lung

Post-perfusion lung is the name given to a collection of syndromes which result from different causes. The common feature is that lung function is disturbed and there is a large alveolar-arterial difference in oxygen tension. Whereas in normal lungs the venous admixture effect in the lung is approximately 3 per cent of the cardiac output, after extracorporeal circulation this figure may rise as high as 30 per cent (Fordham, 1965). In the face of a low cardiac output the (A–a) O_2 tension difference may be large enough to make the patient hypoxic despite ventilation with pure oxygen.

The causes of lung disturbance are:

i. Simple lung collapse, usually of the left or right lower lobe and much commoner than usually thought. This will always respond to physiotherapy but is better prevented than treated.

ii. Overdistension of pulmonary capillaries at operation. Before the routine use of a left heart vent to decompress the left heart at operation, damage used to occur to the lung capillaries and at post-mortem the lungs appeared liver-like with the alveoli filled with haemorrhagic exudate.

iii. High left atrial pressure. Gross damage to the pulmonary capillaries is now rare but pulmonary engorgement due to an excessively high left atrial pressure is common. This results from efforts to increase the cardiac output by raising the filling pressure of the ventricles while measuring only the right atrial pressure. Quite huge and unpredictable differences can exist between the functions of the two ventricles and quite small increases in right atrial pressure can produce increases in the left sided pressure which will result in pulmonary oedema (Sarin *et al.*, 1970).

iv. Blood prime. Sykes *et al.* (1966) have shown that lung function is much less affected after pure haemodilution prime than after a bypass with a blood-containing prime. This is perhaps due to an immune response of white cells to the foreign protein in the donated blood (Melrose *et al.*, 1965).

If all these causes are eliminated, lung function is still altered in the post-operative period but to a much smaller extent. This small degree of change might properly be termed "post-perfusion lung" and is perhaps due to some alteration in the patient's own blood plasma proteins or lung surfactant.

Cerebral Complications

Central nervous system abnormalities after open heart surgery occur with distressing frequency. Brierley (1967) reported an 80 per cent incidence of brain damage in 46 patients, while Javid and his colleagues (1969) in a prospective study found a 53 per cent incidence of neurological abnormalities. Other authors have reported an incidence between 13 per cent and 70 per cent of psychological disturbance in the post-operative period.

Clinically, there are three recognisable syndromes. Patients may develop some psychological defect. This may occur by itself or concurrently with signs of another neurological lesion. When it occurs by itself the suggested causes are low cardiac output with reduced cerebral perfusion, or because patients, while in the recovery or intensive care area, suffer from sleep and sensory deprivation.

More serious neurological defect usually presents either as a hemiplegia or coma. The possible causes are cerebral anoxia, cerebral embolism or intracranial haemorrhage. Anoxia arises either at the time of a cardiac arrest or as a consequence of reduced cerebral blood flow secondary to a low cardiac output. The situation will be aggravated by hypoxaemia secondary to lung dysfunction.

Cerebral emboli may arise from calcium off calcified valves, blood clot, fibrin, aggregated cell elements, fat or silicone antifoam, but the most common cause is air. A number of theoretical dangers exist whereby air may be carried over from a bubble oxygenator or oxygen come out of solution when blood re-enters the patient either as a result of cavitation or temperature change. Most air undoubtedly enters the heart or pulmonary veins at the time of surgery and is not removed before the circulation is re-established.

REFERENCES

BAHNSON, H. T. (1958). "Discussion on oxygenators". In: *Extracorporeal Circulation*, p. 114. Ed. J. G. Allen. Springfield, Ill.: Charles C. Thomas.

BJÖRK, V. O. (1948). Brain perfusions in dogs with artificially oxygenated blood. *Acta chir. scand.*, **96**, Supp. 137.

BRAMSON, M. L., OSBORNE, J. J., MAIN, F. B., O'BRIEN, M. F., WRIGHT, J. S., and GERBODE, F. (1965). A new disposable membrane oxygenator with integral heat exchange. *J. thorac. cardiovasc. Surg.*, **50**, 391.

BRIERLEY, J. B. (1967). Brain damage complicating open-heart surgery. *Proc. roy. Soc. Med.*, **60**, 858.

BRODIE, T. G. (1903). The perfusion of surviving organs. *J. Physiol. (Lond.)*, **29**, 266.

BROWN-SÉQUARD, E. (1858). Du sang rouge et du sang noir, et de leurs principaux éléments gazeuses, l'oxygène et l'acide carbonique. *J. Anat. (Paris)*, **1**, 95.

DE BAKEY, M. E. (1934). Simple continuous-flow blood transfusion instrument. *New Orleans med. surg. J.*, **87**, 386.

DE WALL, R. A., WARDEN, H. E., VARCO, R. L., and LILLEHEI, C. W. (1957). Helix reservoir pump oxygenator. *Surg. Gynec. Obstet.*, **104**, 699.

DREW, C. E., KEEN, G., and BENAZON, D. B. (1959). Profound hypothermia. *Lancet*, **1**, 745.

DUKE, H. N., and VANE, J. R. (1968). An adverse effect of polyvinylchloride tubing used in extracorporeal circulation. *Lancet*, **2**, 21.

FORDHAM, R. (1965). Hypoxaemia after aortic valve surgery under cardiopulmonary bypass. *Thorax*, **20**, 505.

FREY, M., and GRUBER, M. (1885). Ein Respirationsapparatus für isolirte Organe. *Arch. Anat. Physiol.*, **9**, 519.

GADBOYS, H. L., SLONIM, R., and LITWAR, R. (1962). Homologous blood syndrome. *Ann. Surg.*, **156**, 793.

GIBBON, J. H. (1937). Artificial maintenance of circulation during experimental occlusion of the pulmonary artery. *Arch. Surg.*, **34**, 1105.

GIBBON, J. H., MILLER, B. J., and FINEBERG, C. (1953). An improved mechanical heart and lung apparatus. *Med. Clin. N. Amer.*, **37,** 1603.

GOTT, V. L., WHIFFEN, J. D., and DUTTON, R. C. (1963). Heparin bonding on colloidal graphite surfaces. *Science*, **142**, 1297.

HERSH, L. S., and WEETALL, H. H. (1969). Heparin ionically linked to glass. *J. biomed. Mater. Res.*, **3,** 471.

JACOBY, C. (1890). Apparat zur Durchblutung isolirter überlebender Organe. *Naunyn-Schmiedeberg's Arch. exp. Path. Pharmak.*, **26,** 388.

JAVID, H., TUFO, H. M., NAJAFI, H., DYE, W. S., HUNTER, J. A., and JULIAN, O. C. (1969). Neurological abnormalities following open heart surgery. *J. thorac. cardiovasc. Surg.*, **58,** 502.

KALKE, B. R., CASTANEDA, A., and LILLEHEI, C. W. (1969). A clinical evaluation of a new disposable blood oxygenator. *J. thorac. cardiovasc. Surg.*, **57,** 679.

KAY, E. B., GALAJDA, J. E., LUX, A., and CROSS, F. S. (1958). The use of convoluted discs in the rotating disc oxygenator. *J. thorac. Surg.*, **36,** 268.

KIRKLIN, J. W., PATRICK, R. T., and THEYE, R. A. (1957). Theory and practice in the use of a pump oxygenator for open intracardiac surgery. *Thorax*, **12,** 93.

LEGALLOIS, J. J. C. (1812). *Expériences sur le principe de la vie, notamment sur celui des mouvements du coeur, et sur le siège de ce principe.* Paris.

LUDWIG, C. F. W. (1865). *Die physiologischen Leistungen des Blutdrucks.* Leipzig: S. Hirzel.

MELROSE, D. G. (1953). A mechanical heart-lung for use in man. *Brit. med. J.*, **2,** 57.

MELROSE, D. G. (1969) In: *Medical and Surgical Cardiology.* Edited by Cleland, Goodwin, McDonald and Ross. Oxford: Blackwell Scientific Publications.

MELROSE, D. G., NAHAS, R., ALVAREZ, D., TODD, I. A. D., and DEMPSTER, W. J. (1965). Postoperative hypoxia after extracorporeal circulation: a possible graft against host reaction (preliminary communication). *Experientia* (*Basel*), **21,** 47.

OPTIZ, E., and SCHNEIDER, M. (1950). Über die Sauerstoff-versorgung des Gehirns und der Mechanismus von Mangelwirkungen. *Ergebn. Physiol.*, **46,** 126.

OSBORNE, J. J., BRAMSON, M. L., and GERBODE, F. (1960). A rotating disc blood oxygenator and integral heat exchanger of improved inherent efficiency. *J. thorac. Surg.*, **39,** 427.

OSBORNE, J. J., CONN, K., HAIT, M., RUSSI, M., SALEL, A., HARKINS, G., and GERBODE, F. (1962). Hemolysis during perfusion. *J. thorac. cardiovasc. Surg.*, **43,** 459.

RYGG, I. H., FREDERIKSEN, T., and JORGENSEN, M. (1964). Gas exchange in the Rygg-Kyvsgaard bubble oxygenator. *Thorax*, **18,** 220.

SARIN, C. L., YALAV, E., CLEMENT, A. J., and BRAIMBRIDGE, M. V. (1970). The necessity for measurement of left atrial pressure after cardiac valve surgery. *Thorax*, **25,** 185.

SCHMIDT-MULHEIM, A. (1880). Beitrage zur Kenntniss des Peptons und seiner physiologischen Bedeutung. *Arch. Anat. Physiol., Lpz.* (Physiol. Abt.), p. 33.

SCHRODER, W. (1882). Ueber die Bildungstatte des Harnstoffs. *Naunyn-Schmiedeberg's Arch. exp. Path. Pharmak.*, **15,** 364.

SYKES, M. K., ROBINSON, B., MELROSE, D. G., and NAHAS, R. (1966). Pulmonary changes after extracorporeal circulation in dogs. *Brit. J. Anaesth.*, **38,** 432.

WATERS, E. T., MARKOWITZ, J., and JAQUES, L. B. (1938). Anaphylaxis in the liverless dog, and observations on anticoagulant effect of anaphylactic shock. *Science*, **87,** 582.

WOOLMAN, W., STEPHEN, G. W., CLEMENT, A. J., and DANIELSON, G. K. (1966). Cerebral blood flow in man during extracorporeal circulation. *J. thorac. cardiovasc. Surg.*, **52,** 558.

ZUHDI, N., CAREY, J., SHELDON, W., and GREER, A. (1964). Comparative merits and results of primes of blood and 5 per cent dextrose in water for heart lung machines: analysis of 250 patients. *J. thorac. cardiovasc. Surg.*, **47,** 66.

FURTHER READING

BRAIMBRIDGE, M. V., and GHADIALI, P. E. (1969). *Post-operative Cardiac Care.* Oxford: Blackwell Scientific Publications.

CLELAND, W., GOODWIN, J., MCDONALD, L., and ROSS, D. (1969). *Medical and Surgical Cardiology.* Oxford: Blackwell Scientific Publications.

GALLETTI, P. M., and BRECHER, G. A. (1962). *Heart-lung Bypass. Principles and Techniques of Extracorporeal Circulation.* New York: Grune & Stratton.

NORMAN, J. C., ed. (1967). *Cardiac Surgery.* New York: Appleton-Century-Crofts.

Chapter 26

PARENTERAL FLUID THERAPY

IN order to understand how present schedules of intravenous fluids for surgical patients have evolved one must go back over the last fifty years. To begin with the practice of giving such fluids largely as isotonic saline became established and a good example of this was described by Jones and Eaton (1933): their patients received about 350 mEq of sodium daily for a week after major surgery, equivalent to 2½ litres of saline a day, and most of them became oedematous on about the seventh day. Stewart and Rourke (1942) described a patient undergoing colporrhaphy who was given over 6 litres of isotonic saline a day for each of the first four post-operative days. Her convalescence was uneventful and she did not become oedematous. Gamble (1958), commenting on this case, was particularly impressed that there was no change whatever in serum sodium concentration in spite of a positive sodium balance of more than 1000 mEq. From these and other studies one can deduce that surgical patients with no cardiovascular or renal disease can tolerate large volumes of isotonic sodium infusions and that individual tolerances vary widely and are quite unpredictable. All surgical patients given such therapy go into positive sodium balance, maintain normal levels of serum sodium concentration and eventually become oedematous. It is against such a background that recent developments in parenteral fluid therapy must be judged.

As the post-operative patient's propensity to retain sodium and to become oedematous became more generally recognised, solutions of isotonic dextrose (5 per cent) were given in place of the large volumes of saline. Coller and Maddock (1933, 1940) did much to influence management at this time. They assessed insensible loss as two litres daily (though they subsequently reduced this) and recommended that a urine volume of 1 to 1½ litres a day should be aimed at from the day of surgery. It must be remembered that patients were routinely purged and given enemas before operation and received ether or chloroform with consequent likelihood of prolonged post-operative vomiting. Heat was universally regarded as beneficial for shock and there is little doubt that extrarenal losses were often appreciably higher than they are now. In this way schedules prescribing three or more litres of water a day, mostly as 5 per cent dextrose, became established. Unfortunately, the inability of the kidneys to secrete solute-free water normally was not appreciated, and it was not until ten years later that a series of papers appeared drawing attention to this (Cooper *et al.*, 1949; Ariel *et al.*, 1950; Zimmermann and Wangensteen 1952; Moore *et al.*, 1952). These workers provided conclusive evidence that in the post-operative period the kidneys retained water avidly. The mechanisms underlying this are discussed more fully on page 718, but from this time on it has been known that the administration of three litres of 5 per cent dextrose a day always puts the patient into positive water balance and occasionally can result in signs and symptoms of frank water intoxication within 48 to 72 hours of surgery.

The next phase saw the application of new and more accurate methods of metabolic balance studies by numerous workers. Accurate bed scales, the flame photometer and radio-isotopes all helped to unravel some of the many unanswered problems. Thus the role of the adrenal cortex in response to stress was elucidated and aldosterone was discovered. Clinical management was strongly influenced to curtail the amount of sodium given to surgical patients and so emerged what may be termed the present orthodox schedule of parenteral fluid therapy. The greatest single advance was the recognition of the importance of giving potassium to all patients maintained on clear fluids for more than 48 hours. The schedule prescribes two or two and a half litres a day of 5 per cent dextrose together with half a litre of isotonic saline (75 mEq sodium) and about four grams of potassium chloride (50 mEq potassium). Such a schedule has been and still is successfully used in the management of patients undergoing all types of elective surgery. The small volumes of concentrated urine passed in the first two or three days after surgery became accepted as part of the normal response to trauma and were not thought to be harmful. From that time surgeons have increased the severity and duration of operations and anaesthetists have accepted patients who twenty years ago would not have been considered as operative risks. Post-operative renal failure began to be recognised more frequently and it was inevitable that the oliguria consequent on orthodox management should be critically reappraised. It was soon realised that considerable falls in glomerular filtration rate and renal blood flow occurred during operation, and that the oxygen demands of the kidneys were closely related to renal sodium conservation.

The most recent phase began ten years ago when Shires and his colleagues in Dallas challenged the accepted doctrines by asserting that all major surgical trauma was accompanied by loss of large volumes of sodium-containing extracellular fluid and that this should be replaced (Shires *et al.*, 1961). The measurements were made during and immediately after surgery using an isotope dilution method with sulphate and allowing 20 minutes for equilibration. These workers claimed that the "functional" extracellular fluid contracted by several litres in a three or four hour operation and they gave equivalent amounts of Ringer-lactate ("Balanced Salt") solution. Very soon anaesthetists began to give patients litres of Ringer-lactate during and after surgery. The wheel had come full circle.

In the last few years attempts to confirm these large reductions in extracellular fluid have failed to do so (Anderson *et al.*, 1967; Gutelius *et al.*, 1968; Roth *et al.*, 1969). It is now agreed by many that the conclusions of Cleland *et al.* (1966) are valid and that equilibration of ^{35}S is not complete for long after the 20 minute period that Shires allowed. Cases of obvious over-transfusion began to be reported (e.g. Fieber and Jones, 1966) and these together with failure of subsequent investigators to substantiate the original work made adherents of orthodox management unwilling to abandon their well established methods. Nevertheless some who had done most to establish these methods have become convinced that in major surgery there is an accumulation of sequestered interstitial fluid in the traumatised tissues, forming the so-called "Third Space". No orthopaedic surgeon would operate on a limb and enclose it within an unpadded or unsplit plaster, or on a hand without elevating it. Similarly, prolonged and vigorous retraction of the abdominal wall and the infliction of scores of small burns by diathermy is bound to be followed by an accumulation of interstitial fluid from the freely mobilised part of the extracellular fluid which is in dynamic equilibrium with plasma. This is now acknowledged not only to occur, but to be allowed for in intra-operative fluid therapy by workers such as Hayes (1968) and Dudley (1968). Moore has given his support to the use of Ringer-lactate during major surgery in a joint editorial with Shires (1967), but they warn against uncritical use of the large volumes originally recommended. From this has developed a schedule which prescribes Ringer-lactate at rates of 5 ml. per kg. per hour of surgery, up to a maximum of 1½ to 2 litres. An excellent account of current practice is given by Crandell (1968).

If this schedule is used, it results in a positive sodium balance which is variable, but is of the order of 100 mEq of sodium. Patients with cardiovascular, renal or liver disease in whom this would be undesirable should receive smaller volumes. Protagonists point to evidence that small and concentrated urine volumes are replaced by larger volumes of less concentrated urine, and they therefore claim that renal perfusion is better and renal oxygen requirements are reduced; they further claim, and here are on less sure ground, that tissue perfusion in general is improved and that patients stand up to the trauma of major surgery better than those whose sodium intake is curtailed.

It is salutary to reflect that after 50 years we still do not really know the optimum sodium intake for the day of surgery. Shires may have been right in using the 20 minute ^{35}S space and the demonstration that hours later the isotope has a larger volume of distribution may simply mean that it has penetrated the "sequestered" pool. The result is that there is still disagreement about which is the more appropriate schedule. The present trend would seem to be towards the use of Ringer-lactate (or isotonic saline) in moderate amounts during major surgery, together with not more than 1 litre of 5 per cent dextrose in the first 24 hours and then to revert to a total fluid intake of 2 litres a day, reducing the sodium given to ½ litre of saline or Ringer-lactate.

It should be noted that the whole of the foregoing account applies to afebrile patients at rest in temperate ambient temperatures.

The Metabolic Response to Trauma

In the course of evolution mammals have developed a series of mechanisms whose purpose would appear to be designed to ensure short-term survival after injury. These involve the anterior and posterior pituitary and the adrenal cortex: they have been extensively investigated and lucidly described by Zimmermann (1965).

The anterior pituitary secretes increased amounts of ACTH in response to surgical trauma. The afferent pathways are the peripheral somatic nerves from the site of injury and also autonomic afferents arising from intravascular pressor receptors. The main effect of ACTH is to stimulate the adrenal cortex to secrete cortisol (also called Compound F or hydrocortisone), but it is now also known to produce an increase in the adrenal secretion of aldosterone. Previously the anterior pituitary had been thought not to be concerned with aldosterone release, but two types of aldosterone activity are now recognised. The first is mediated by ACTH and results in proportionally similar increases in both cortisol and aldosterone. The other is mediated by volume sensitive receptors thought to be in the renal juxtaglomerular bodies and results in increased levels of aldosterone and has no effect on cortisol levels. Zimmermann believes that in most surgical patients aldosterone release is predominantly due to the cortico-trophin mechanism.

Posterior Pituitary and Release of Antidiuretic Hormone

The first two or three days after an operation are characteristically associated with progressive dilution of the plasma and therefore with falling levels of serum sodium concentration. At the same time urine osmolarity is usually 700 to 1000 mOsmol/1.—two to three times the plasma level. This has been called the "sodium paradox" by Moore and has for long been thought to be due to secretion of anti-diuretic hormone (ADH), but only in the last few years has this been confirmed by direct hormone assays in the blood. Zimmerman (1965) has shown that ADH output is always raised during surgery and that levels fluctuate from minute to minute in response to surgical manipulations. Traction of abdominal viscera is a particularly potent stimulus and results in a 40–50 fold increase over pre-operative levels: ADH levels fall at the end of operation but remain well above control concentrations until three to five days after surgery.

Zimmermann and his colleagues at West Virginia (Moran and Zimmermann, 1967; Ukai *et al.*, 1968) have shown that the normal control of ADH activity by the osmoreceptors described by Verney (1948) can be overridden by afferent impulses originating in left atrial stretch receptors and also by pain impulses transmitted by somatic nerves. This effectively accounts for the "sodium paradox" and explains the extreme intolerance of the surgical patient to excess hypotonic fluids in the immediate post-operative period.

MAINTENANCE OF BODY OSMOLARITY

In health the body fluids, both cellular and extracellular, are maintained at a concentration of approximately one seventh molar:* this is chiefly due to the presence of potassium in the intracellular fluid (ICF) and sodium in the extracellular fluid (ECF), each milli-equivalent of which will hold 7 ml. of water in the cells or the extracellular fluid respectively. This water "binding" is shared equally between the cations and the anions which necessarily accompany them, but the cations are the vital constituents which determine the relative volume of the two major divisions of the body fluid. It is now generally accepted that no sustained osmolar gradient can exist between the ECF and the cells of non-secretory tissues. This has several important implications. Firstly, water will distribute itself in the two compartments in proportion to their relative volumes. As the intracellular fluid is approximately twice the volume of the extracellular fluid,† a positive water balance will result in twice as much water

* This is true for electrolytes which are completely dissociated. Strictly speaking the body fluids are about M/3·5. Thus isotonic solutions of electrolytes are M/7 and of non-electrolytes M/3·5. Both contain 286 mOsmol/1.

† Most estimates of the size of the extracellular fluid space are based on the volume of dilution of mannitol, sucrose or inulin. These substances probably underestimate the true volume of the space due to their very slow penetration into dense connective tissue (such as cartilage and ligaments), bone and gastro-intestinal luminal fluid (Edelman and Leibman, 1959). The part of the extracellular fluid concerned with rapid changes in volume is approximately half the volume of the cellular fluid.

entering the cells as will remain outside them. Secondly, a rise in serum Na will cause water to shift from the cells to the ECF and a fall in the serum Na, if due to sodium loss, will cause water to pass into the cells. Thirdly, a rise and fall in intracellular K will have precisely the opposite effects. The contribution of K loss to the expansion of the ECF and therefore the production of oedema has been documented clinically and experimentally (Black and Milne, 1952). Finally, the serum Na is an indication of the intracellular as well as the extra-cellular osmolarity and therefore a fall in serum Na may well be due to loss of K or to an increase in total body water with no change in the external balance of Na or K.

Water

Earlier estimates of total body water, expressed as a percentage of body weight, were higher than they are now thought to be. Edelman and Leibman (1959) give the following figures for adults of average build:

Water content expressed as a Percentage of Body Weight

	Ages 17 – 39	*Age* 60 +
Men	60·6%	51·5%
Women	50·2%	45·5%

For practical purposes, total body water can be assessed as half the body weight in kilograms.

Fluid Balance Charts

Accurately kept balance charts are essential whenever intravenous fluids are given. One must not however expect to balance the intake and output columns like a cash account. A daily reckoning will frequently show oscillations of water balance of one or occasionally two litres which eventually balance out over a period of days. The variable rates of tissue catabolism with associated production of water in the body make the net insensible loss very difficult to compute. Balances are the result of a mixture of measurement and guesswork and one must strive for the one to be accurate and the other to be informed. In a temperate climate an afebrile patient should be managed on the basis that the net un-measured loss (losses from skin and lungs minus water formed in the body) is 750 ml./day. If the patient is on a ventilator and inspired gases are saturated with water vapour at body temperature there is no pulmonary water loss and the allowance for unmeasured losses should be reduced to 500 ml./day.

Water Requirements

Water requirements of an adult are satisfied by a daily intake of about 30 ml./kg. of lean body weight: this can conveniently be rounded off to two litres a day provided there are no abnormal losses. Such an intake should not be exceeded until the third post-operative day at which time most patients will have no need for further parenteral maintenance. If fluids are given parenterally after this time, considerations of the need for more calories arise and the daily allowance can then be increased to three litres.

Figure 1 (Hayes, 1968, based on work by Kerrigan *et al.*, 1955) shows very clearly that the human kidney's tolerance for water varies with the excretory solute load and that the provision of 100 grams of dextrose a day reduces this to levels far below those associated with a normal diet. When this is added to the increased ADH activity attendant upon surgery, the ceiling for water is little above the minimum requirements.

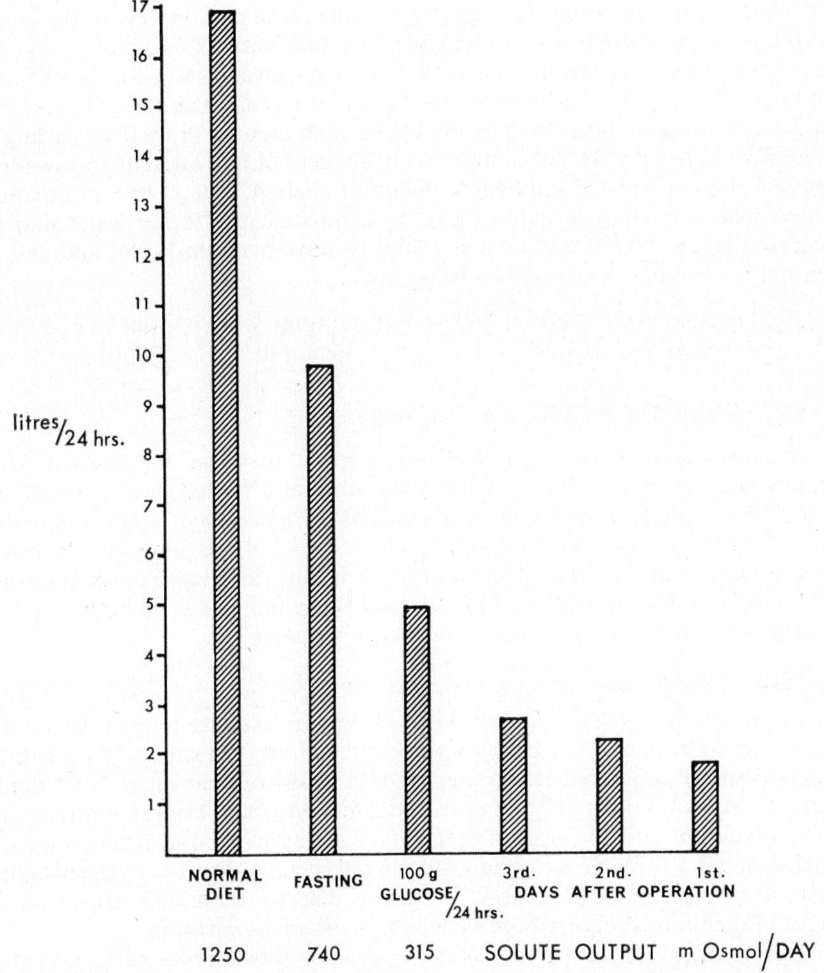

26/FIG. 1.—The ordinate shows the ceiling for water. The columns on the abscissa show how this is reduced by diminished excretion of solutes (urinary Na, K, NH_4 and urea). There is considerable individual variation. (After Hayes, 1968.)

Water Depletion

Water depletion without sodium depletion is uncommon in surgical patients. So effective is the sensation of thirst in its prevention that it is only likely to be seen in infants, in prolonged unconsciousness or those who are too feeble or too breathless to satisfy their need for water. Occasionally dysphagia due to lesions of the pharynx or the oesophagus can result in water depletion.

Patients suffering from prolonged unconsciousness due to head injuries or cerebrovascular accidents are more liable than most to become water depleted as they are often febrile and tend to hyperventilate. They may develop diabetes insipidus after head injuries or operations in the vicinity of the hypothalamus (see Chapter 39).

Water depletion is characterised by extreme thirst and dryness of the mouth with little or no change in cardiovascular function until its terminal stages. The rise in blood urea, if exogenous protein is not being given, is slow: its biochemical hallmark is a progressive rise in serum Na and Cl and it is the only common cause of such a finding. Man is unable to take care of himself physically or mentally when water deficits amount to 10 per cent of body weight and swallowing and talking become impossible (Schmidt-Nielsen, 1964). The approximate water deficit can be calculated from the estimated total body water and the observed serum Na. If a patient is found to have a serum Na of 160 and his normal body water is assessed to be 40 litres:

$$\text{Actual body water} \times 160 = \text{Normal body water} \times 140$$
$$\text{Actual body water} = \frac{40 \times 140}{160} = 35 \text{ litres}$$
$$\text{Water deficit} = 40 - 35 = 5 \text{ litres}$$

Treatment.—Five per cent dextrose is given to cover the normal water requirements plus the deficit. Unlike the dramatic response of extracellular depletion to appropriate treatment, the results of replacement seem disappointing in the first 12 hours. Very rapid restitution should not be aimed at: the calculated water deficit should be divided into thirds, one third being given in the first six hours, one third in the first 24 hours and the remainder in 48 hours. For the management of infants with hypernatraemia see page 732.

Water Excess

From the foregoing account of ADH activity in response to operation it will readily be appreciated that patients subjected to long and extensive operations are particularly liable to receive water loads in excess of their capacity to excrete them. Intakes of 3 litres of 5 per cent dextrose a day may result in a progressive accumulation of body water during the first 3–4 days after operation: when this reaches about 5 litres or the serum sodium falls below 120 mEq/1., the patient is likely to be confused and restless. Nocturnal disorientation and jerking movements of the limbs should arouse suspicion of water intoxication.

Treatment.—Fifty to 100 ml. of 5 per cent or molar (5·85 per cent) saline should be given slowly intravenously. There is no danger in this if the serum Na is below 120 mEq/1. and it will rapidly improve the mental disorientation and usually produce a brisk diuresis.

Sodium and Potassium

Certain aspects of the metabolism of sodium and potassium can conveniently be considered together. They both exist in an adequate diet greatly in excess of the body's minimum needs and they are both predominantly excreted in the urine. Fruit, vegetables and raw meat contain up to 100 times as much potassium as sodium, nearly all the sodium in the food being added as salt in the process of cooking. Thus salt-free diets are not difficult to achieve whereas potassium-free diets are not a practical proposition. The kidneys, if renal function is not impaired, can retain sodium quickly and effectively so that the urinary concentration falls to less than 20 mEq/l. within 48 hours of sodium deprivation. By contrast renal conservation of potassium develops much more slowly and potassium may be found in the urine in ten or twenty times its plasma concentration several days after complete cessation of potassium intake. The chloride concentration in the urine (Fantus test) is a very fallible guide to sodium requirements as it tends to fall when renal tubular conservation of potassium is operating (Black and Milne, 1952). It is of little value and likely to be positively misleading in the post-operative period.

Large positive balances of either sodium or potassium tend to cause large negative balances of the other ion: for this reason withholding of potassium post-operatively prolongs and intensifies the tendency for sodium to be retained. Much is written about sodium entering the cells in abnormal amounts, the evidence for which is largely inferential: however Danowski (1951) has pointed out that in many circumstances it is useful to look upon changes in cell sodium and cell potassium as occurring reciprocally in terms of direction if not of magnitude.

There is a wide variation even amongst healthy subjects in the ability to compensate for excesses or deficits of either sodium or potassium. In the absence of abnormal losses the daily requirements can be met with half a litre of isotonic saline (75 mEq) and four grams of potassium chloride (50 mEq of potassium).

Sodium and the Extracellular Fluid

The concentration of sodium in the extracellular fluid is 135 to 140 mEq/l. in health—figures which are well known thanks to the ease and accuracy of flame photometry. It is less well appreciated that knowledge of the plasma sodium concentration is no sure guide to the total body stores of sodium: if the plasma sodium concentration is raised the most likely cause is water depletion. If it is lowered it may be due to loss of sodium, but it is more commonly the result of several factors of which water retention and potassium loss are important contributory causes. Moore (1960), speaking of surgical patients, states that "most hypotonicity is dilutional" and plasma sodium must be interpreted with this in mind. This is particularly likely to apply to patients who have to be re-operated upon after several days of parenteral fluid therapy. Such a patient will often be found to have a plasma sodium concentration of 125 to 130 mEq/l. and this should only be accepted as an indication for giving sodium if there is a likelihood of unreplaced sodium loss having occurred, or if it is associated with signs of impaired cardiovascular function.

Pre-operative Losses of Extracellular Fluid

Alimentary losses due to vomiting or diarrhoea usually contain sodium in concentrations of about 80 to 100 mEq/l.: if water is drunk and absorbed the plasma sodium concentration will fall, but the more fulminating the losses the less change will there be in plasma sodium concentration. Since sodium is for practical purposes confined to the extracellular fluid of which plasma forms a part, plasma volume will fall with the contraction of the extracellular fluid space. There will be a variable loss of cell water, depending upon renal excretion of potassium and water ingestion, but the life-threatening depletion which demands urgent replacement is the loss of sodium and water from outside the cells.

Signs of Depletion of Extracellular Fluid

The term "dehydration" is too well established to be discarded. Moore (1960) has adopted the terms "dehydration desiccation" to signify pure water depletion and "desalting water loss" to signify extracellular fluid depletion. Insofar as most surgical patients with body fluid losses suffer from a mixture of the two, "dehydration" by common usage has come to be applied to such states; it is a label all too readily attached to any patient whose illness is accompanied by low blood pressure, peripheral vasoconstriction and a dry tongue.

Until losses exceed 2 litres in an adult, signs of fluid depletion are unlikely to be present. The most reliable sign is dryness of the mucous membranes not exposed to evaporative water loss: in practice this is best detected by running a finger along the bucco-labial groove. The tongue is often dry because of the prevalence of mouth breathing in ill patients, but a shrunken and wrinkled tongue is good corroborative evidence. Retraction of the eyes is always present and is a valuable sign in young patients and one of the earliest to disappear as repletion progresses. It may be difficult to assess in the elderly.

Cardiovascular system.—If large losses of water and sodium occur they will lead to a diminished plasma volume. The signs of this are a rapid pulse of poor volume, low blood pressure and peripheral vasoconstriction. All these signs may be present as a result of infection without a decrease in blood volume. The distinction of the two common causes of cardiovascular disorder is not always easy: in general, pulse rates above 130, respiratory rates above 30 and extreme hypotension all favour infection rather than fluid loss as the cause. When there is doubt it may be resolved by giving a rapid infusion of plasma or a plasma substitute, e.g. dextran 70 in saline. Obvious improvement will follow if the cause is extracellular fluid depletion provided the plasma is given quickly enough, i.e. 2 bottles in 20–30 minutes.

Biochemical findings.—The plasma electrolyte concentrations may not prove very helpful in substantiating a diagnosis of body fluid loss. By contrast, the urea concentration and haemoglobin and haemotocrit may be very informative. This point is well illustrated in Table 1 which shows the average plasma sodium and urea concentrations of fifty patients. Of these twelve were assessed as being severely dehydrated and thirty-eight as being moderately dehydrated. The third column shows the percentage of each group in whom the haemoglobin concentration was over 120 per cent.

26/Table 1

The Average Plasma Sodium and Urea Concentration of Fifty Dehydrated Patients

Assessed degree of dehydration	*Average plasma Na (mEq/1.)*	*Average plasma Urea (mg. per cent)*	*Percentage of patients with Hb of 17·5 g. per cent*
Severe (12 patients)	139	109	40
Moderate (38 patients)	135	78	10

Note particularly the higher sodium concentration in the severely depleted group and the considerable changes in urea and haemoglobin concentrations. The highest blood urea encountered was 260 mg. per cent and figures of 400 to 500 mg. per cent are described and do not necessarily indicate that intrinsic renal damage has occurred. The plasma sodium concentration is therefore a very poor guide to the size of the sodium deficit. A patient assessed to be dehydrated should be assumed to be suffering from predominant loss of extracellular fluid unless the history is of a disorder known to be associated with pure water depletion or the plasma sodium concentration is unequivocally above the normal range.

Assessment of the Magnitude of the Loss

It is unwise to make an initial assessment of the total volume of fluid required and not be prepared to alter it as treatment is given. Cardiovascular signs thought to be solely due to dehydration are not uncommonly due in part to the presence of bacterial infections such as peritonitis or to endotoxaemia arising from non-viable bowel. In such cases the response to treatment helps to establish the diagnosis—if fluid depletion is the sole cause of the signs appropriate therapy will rapidly restore circulatory efficiency. A useful rough guide to the probable size of the fluid deficit is given by Hardy (1954):

Mild	4 per cent of body weight, i.e. 2·8 litres for a 70 kg. man
Moderate	6 per cent „ „ „ „ 4·2 litres „ „ „ „ „
Severe	8 per cent „ „ „ „ 5·6 litres „ „ „ „ „

If the body weight is assessed in kilograms, these percentages are readily calculated, and in this context the weight in kilograms can be taken as half the weight in pounds. Even if the guessed weight is as much as a stone (6·5 kg.) in error, it will not affect the derived therapy significantly.

Only in rare cases should all this fluid be given as isotonic saline or Ringer-lactate. In general, saline is as effective as Ringer-lactate unless amounts in excess of 2 litres are judged to be necessary. If they are, Ringer-lactate is to be preferred as the more physiological solution. A safe practice is to give saline or Ringer-lactate until half the estimated deficit has been replaced and then to re-assess the position. Generally the remainder can be given as 5 per cent dextrose with or without further saline. The initial replacement should be given boldly and in really severe cases the fluids should be replaced from "within out" i.e. plasma, then saline and finally 5 per cent dextrose. Although European practice in a temperate climate seldom requires the administration of as much as 5 litres of sodium-containing fluids in the initial replacement, much larger volumes may be required in other parts of the world. Thus White (1961) has given up to 18 litres in six hours to Rhodesian Africans and greatly reduced the mortality of intestinal obstruction since such massive infusions were realised to be necessary. It is wise to regard 5 litres and 500 mEq of sodium as the upper limit which is likely to be required during the first twelve hours of repletion and most cases will require substantially less than this.

When replacing such losses pre-operatively the aim should be to defer operation until the initial infusion of plasma or saline no longer produces further improvement in signs of cardiovascular function. This may take two or three hours, but it is time well spent and it is never wise to administer an anaesthetic in the presence of hypotension (systolic pressure below 90–100 mm. Hg) and vasoconstriction due to water and sodium loss. Most cases can be managed without monitoring of the central venous pressure, but it may be a very helpful guide to the safety of infusing really large volumes of fluid (see Chapter 21). In its absence, very careful watch should be kept on the neck veins and the bases of the lungs.

Selective Plasma Loss in Acute Abdominal Lesions

Certain abdominal lesions, of which perforated peptic ulcers are the most common, are sometimes accompanied by large losses of plasma: this may also occur in pancreatitis, bacterial peritonitis and obstructive lesions of the mesenteric veins, e.g. volvulus. The haematocrit may rise above 60 and as Moore (1960) says "elevation of the haematocrit over 60 due to acute plasma loss alone represents a life-endangering emergency." The plasma loss is partly intra-peritoneal but mostly into the wall of the bowel and therefore not obvious. The plasma volume may become seriously reduced within a few hours without any external losses occurring at all. It is in such cases that repeated estimations of haemoglobin or haematocrit can be of most help, as there is unlikely to be any significant change in the concentration of the plasma electrolytes.

Potassium and Intracellular Fluid

Potassium depletion.—Potassium is found in the cells at a concentration of approximately 150 mEq/l. and in the extracellular fluid at a concentration of 3·5 to 5 mEq/l. The daily intake is from 60–100 mEq and a similar amount is excreted, mostly in the urine. Intestinal juices always contain potassium at an average concentration of 10 mEq/l. This is very variable and when large losses occur, the potassium concentration should be measured and accurately replaced. It is important to remember that potassium excretion continues in spite of no potassium intake and an operation causes a loss of potassium of 50–100 mEq in the first 48 hours—the loss in general varying with the severity of the operation. When protoplasm is broken down in the immediate post-operative period, each gram of nitrogen is excreted with about 2·5 mEq of potassium.

The K:N ratio is said to be 2·5. This loss occurs in starvation and is not a selective loss of potassium. If potassium is lost in excess of a K:N ratio of 2·5 the excess represents true potassium loss and this alone will affect intracellular osmolarity and accordingly be reflected by a fall in plasma sodium concentration. A patient maintained on potassium-free parenteral fluids will gradually reduce his urinary potassium loss until it stabilises at 20–30 mEq a day—in this way deficits of 200 mEq of potassium may readily be incurred within a few days of operation if no potassium is given. The presence of potassium deficiency is easy to infer but less easy to substantiate because the plasma potassium concentration may well be above its normal lower limit of 3·5 mEq/l. when there is a large overall deficit. The most reliable proof of the existence of cellular potassium depletion is provided by measuring potassium intake against urinary excretion. As long as less than 60 per cent of the intake appears in the urine, a deficit may be presumed to exist.

When potassium salts are given intravenously, they equilibrate extremely quickly with extracellular fluid if tissue circulation is normal. Equilibration is 95 per cent complete in a single transit of the circulation (Black *et al.*, 1955) and this makes venous sampling an unreliable guide to the safety of potassium infusion. Cellular penetration is rapid when a potassium deficit exists, but occurs at different rates in different tissues—liver, lungs, heart and skeletal muscles having a rapid uptake, brain and red cells a much slower one.

If the plasma potassium concentration is below 3·5 mEq/l. a potassium deficit is probable and if below 3 mEq/l., it can be assumed with certainty. Electrocardiographic changes consist of flattening of T and the occasional appearance of a small positive U wave immediately after it (see p. 575 *et seq.*).

Effects of potassium depletion.—Deprivation of potassium for 48 hours is harmless if intake has previously been adequate: deprivation beyond this time is associated with progressive apathy, muscular weakness and sodium retention with a tendency for oedema to form. There is experimental evidence that intestinal distension progressing to ileus results from potassium deficits (Darrow, 1950) and this may occur in man. Renal function is always affected and the kidneys lose their ability to concentrate the urine. Histological changes occur in the tubular cells and prolonged potassium depletion results in permanent renal damage. The heart is adversely affected and severe mental symptoms may appear.

Low levels of plasma potassium concentration are by no means always accompanied by obvious muscular weakness and the response to curare and other non-depolarising drugs is not necessarily altered. It is wise, if curare is to be used, to give a test dose of 5 mg. and observe the effect before giving larger doses. Potassium deficiency is more likely to produce muscular weakness in acidotic patients, probably because the potassium ion and the hydrogen ion have opposite effects on neuromuscular conduction (Black and Milne, 1952). The anti-curare action of potassium has been well established (Wilson and Wright, 1936), but potassium salts should be given only with the greatest circumspection to apnoeic patients in an attempt to reverse neuromuscular block produced by curare.

Loss of potassium at a K:N ratio greater than 2·5 is an invariable response to water depletion and is essential if the cells are to give up their water (Elkinton and Winkler, 1944). Whenever potassium leaves the cells, it is partially replaced by sodium and hydrogen ions: this results in a fall in extracellular hydrogen ion concentration (rise in pH) which is reflected by a rise in bicarbonate concentration. If the bicarbonate is found to be raised in a surgical patient, potassium deficiency is the most likely cause.

Daily requirements.—If parenteral fluids are required for more than 48 hours after operation, potassium should be given. Ampoules containing 1 gram of potassium chloride* (13·4 mEq potassium) can be added to each half-litre bottle. Four grams daily (approximately 50 mEq) of potassium chloride is adequate to prevent progressive potassium loss and 8 grams for the treatment of established depletion.

The correction of large sodium deficits is urgent and the total amount given is aimed to restore a large part of the presumed deficit: this does not apply to potassium deficits and quantitative replacement is achieved slowly. Fortunately relatively small amounts of potassium—far less than the overall deficit—produce improvement in muscle power and general well-being which is sometimes astonishing.

Potassium toxicity.—The dangers of rapid infusion of potassium salts are real and levels above 7 mEq/l. in the plasma are dangerous, particularly in states of acidosis. Hypoxia and an increase in hydrogen ion concentration (fall in pH) from whatever cause will result in potassium leaving the cells and in such circumstances potassium should not be given. The accepted criteria for safety are:

1. No potassium on the day of operation.
2. A urine volume of at least 500 ml. in the previous 24 hours.
3. Infusion fluids should never contain more than 1·5 grams potassium chloride per 0·5 litre bottle (i.e. 40 mEq potassium per litre).
4. Not more than 15 mEq should be given in an hour (1 gram potassium chloride contains just under this amount).

These figures are well within the limits of safety and dangerous levels of plasma potassium concentration will not occur if renal and adrenal function is normal. The electrocardiograph provides the most informative evidence of potassium toxicity, the earliest changes being high, peaked T waves, followed by disappearance of P waves and widening of the QRS complex. The changes are not solely dependent upon the plasma potassium concentration and high concentrations of sodium and ionised calcium may result in a normal ECG when the plasma potassium concentration is high (see 19/Fig. 26).

If the plasma concentration is found to be above 7 mEq/l. the immediate treatment is to give 10 ml. of 10 per cent calcium gluconate slowly intravenously, followed by 25 grams of glucose and 15 units of soluble insulin. An infusion of 50 ml. of molar (8·4 per cent) sodium bicarbonate should then be given at 1 ml. per minute.

Magnesium

Magnesium occurs in concentrations of 20 mEq per litre of cell water and the plasma range is 1·5–2·5 mEq/l. A normal diet contains 10–20 mEq a day

* Note that 1 g. of KCl. contains approximately 0·5 g. of potassium.

and renal conservation is so efficient that balance can be maintained on 1 mEq/day. The excess is excreted in the urine.

The skeleton provides a large store of magnesium and even several weeks of parenteral fluid therapy with magnesium-free fluids may not cause plasma magnesium to fall significantly. Magnesium given intravenously causes vasodilation and central nervous depression associated with some degree of myoneural block. This block is due to magnesium preventing the release of acetyl choline at the myoneural junction.

This property and the associated effect on the central nervous system led Peck and Meltzer (1916) to use intravenous magnesium sulphate to produce general anaesthesia. One of their cases received over 200 mEq of magnesium in fifty minutes and this produced respiratory arrest which was treated by pharyngeal insufflation of oxygen with recovery. It is apparent that the heart must be very tolerant to great increases in plasma magnesium concentration and the small rises known to occur in hypothermia are unlikely to have any significance.

The only likely cause of significant magnesium depletion is surgical removal of most of the small intestine. Occasional cases are recorded in which hypotonia, tetany and fibrillary muscle twitching have responded to intramuscular magnesium sulphate. The surgical implications of magnesium balance have been well reviewed by Barnes (1962).

PARENTERAL FEEDING

Standard regimes of parenteral fluids only provide about one fifth of a resting patient's total calories—the remainder being supplied by catabolism of tissue proteins and fat. The hundred grams of dextrose provided in the daily intake are however extremely important in reducing to a minimum the breakdown of tissue proteins to provide energy. This is often forgotten when blood has to be given, or when saline is given to replace extrarenal losses. If more than half a litre of saline is given it should be given as 0·9 per cent saline in 5 per cent dextrose, and Ringer-lactate similarly should be dissolved in 5 per cent dextrose. Care must be taken to impress on the nursing staff the difference between 5 per cent dextrose in water and the same solution in saline.

If parenteral fluids are to be continued for more than five days the calorie deficit must not be allowed to progress. In the presence of severe sepsis and its associated hypercatabolic state the provision of at least 2000 calories a day should be aimed at within two days of surgery. Modern management of parenteral feeding involves the use of fat emulsions and amino-acid preparations both of which are very expensive so that maintenance can cost £8 to £10 a day.

Fat Emulsions

Fat emulsions represent the most suitable source of calories as the fat is rapidly metabolised and has no osmotic activity—isotonicity is due to glycerol or sorbitol. They promote protein anabolism and do not cause thrombophlebitis (Reid and Ingram, 1967). Soya bean emulsions (Intralipid) are now preferred to emulsions of Cottonseed Oil as they can safely be given at rates of 3 g./kg./day for long periods (Lawson, 1967). Immediate reactions include nausea, headache, fever and palpitations and can be minimised by beginning the infusion very slowly. These so-called "colloid" reactions occur in about 10 per cent of patients

(Hadfield, 1965). Some authorities recommend the addition of heparin to accelerate the rate of uptake of the fat but this is unnecessary (Johnston, 1969). No drugs, vitamins or other substances should be added to the fat emulsions and the giving sets should be changed after each bottle has been run in.

Amino-acid Solutions

There are two types of amino-acid solutions, those formed by enzymatic hydrolysis of casein such as Aminosol, and solutions of crystalline amino-acids such as Trophysan. Both cause a high incidence of thrombophlebitis and have similar effects on nitrogen balance. The synthetic amino-acids in Trophysan are a mixture of D and DL forms, whereas naturally occuring amino-acids are all in the L forms. Present evidence suggests that the ideal parenteral solution of amino-acids would be one which contained synthetic amino-acids in the L forms.

The solutions available are usually given with both sugar and alcohol to increase their calorie content. Fructose has some advantages over dextrose and is the hexose sugar used in Aminosol.

Administration.—There are many schemes which do not differ in essentials and the following is based on that of Peaston (1968). Half litre bottles are given in the following sequence:

	Calories	Na	K	N
1. 20 per cent Intralipid	1000	Nil	Nil	Nil
2. Aminosol/fructose/alcohol—1½ g. KCl	435	27	20	2·1 g.
3. Aminosol/fructose/alcohol—1½ g. KCl	435	27	20	2·1 g.
4. Either 10 per cent Aminosol or	160	80	Nil	6·4 g.
5 per cent Dextrose	100	Nil	Nil	Nil
5. 20 per cent Intralipid	1000	Nil	Nil	Nil
6. Aminosol/fructose/alcohol—1½ g. KCl	435	27	20	2·1 g.

N.B. 6 g. Protein ≃ 2 g. Urea ≃ 1 g. Nitrogen.

This provides approximately 3,500 calories and either 6·5 or 13 grams of nitrogen a day, depending on the substitution of 5 per cent dextrose for 10 per cent Aminosol. Patients with raised extra-renal losses of water are best managed with 5 per cent dextrose as the 10 per cent Aminosol represents a considerable solute load. Vitamins must be added and often repeated blood transfusions are required as haemoglobin levels invariably tend to fall.

FLUID THERAPY IN INFANTS AND SMALL CHILDREN

The management of fluid and electrolyte balance in infants is very much more critical than it is in adults. Requirements vary with age and the permissible margins of error are narrow. Many of the fluid schedules prescribed for surgical causes of body fluid depletion are identical to those which are appropriate in the management of acute gastro-enteritis. This has resulted in over-generous amounts of water being given which are particularly undesirable in surgical cases. Infants with intestinal obstruction are not usually febrile and surgery corrects their lesions and induces post-operative release of antidiuretic hormone. In these circumstances too much water readily provokes water intoxication.

Infants, particularly in the first few months of life, have a greatly increased rate of turnover of water. Their body water content is greater than an adult's when related to body weight, but it is about half the adult figure if related to surface area: as surface area is more closely related to insensible loss, an infant loses water twice as fast as an adult when intake ceases.

Maintenance Requirements—Infants and Children

After the first week of life and until a child weighs 25 kg. (4 stone) maintenance requirements are adequately covered by doubling the adult intake expressed as a function of body weight. The daily adult intake of approximately 30 ml. and 1 mEq each of sodium and potassium per kg. of body weight is therefore increased to 70 ml. per kg. together with approximately 2 mEq per kg. of sodium and potassium. It will be found that if the fluid is given as "fifth normal saline in dextrose" (0·18 per cent NaCl in 4·3 per cent dextrose) and if one gram of potassium chloride is added to each 500 ml. of fluid given, the amounts of sodium and potassium will be correct (Atwell, 1971).

Example.—A baby weighing 3 kg. would receive 210 ml. water: 6·2 mEq sodium: 5·7 mEq potassium.

This schedule can be given from the day of operation onwards, except that the potassium is omitted for 48 hours after surgery. It is easy to remember and does away with the need to refer to charts most of which are designed for medical management and necessitate various corrections to be applied to infants undergoing surgery. The only exception to the general application of this regime applies during the first week of life when the intake of fluid and electrolytes is reduced by being multiplied by

$$\frac{\text{Age in days}}{7}$$

For babies 24–48 hrs. old this will result in a daily fluid intake of 50 ml. or even less and it is all too easy to give far too much if explicit instructions as to rate and volume are not written down. Whenever fluids are given to babies the giving set should always incorporate a small volume graduated burette so that large volumes of fluid cannot accidentally be infused.

If the 24-hour volume in litres is multiplied by 12, the approximate drip rate per minute is obtained. Thus 12 drops a minute will deliver approximately one litre and if it is desired to give only 250 ml., the approximate rate would be

$$\frac{12 \times 250}{1000} = 3 \text{ drops per minute}$$

Assessment of Magnitude of Body Fluid Depletion

Body fluids lost or sequestered by babies and small children all contain sodium in approximately isotonic concentration just as they do in adults. An unfortunate belief has come to be accepted that sodium should never be given to babies in a greater concentration than 30 mEq/1. (fifth normal).

In a review of the causes of death in children with appendicitis Pledger and Buchan (1969) considered that inadequate or inappropriate fluid therapy to be the commonest single cause of death. The mortality in children under 5 was eight times that of older children and this is undoubtedly related to the reluctance to treat such small children boldly. No child with peritonitis should be considered too ill for operation without an attempt being made to replenish its plasma and extracellular fluid volume.

The approximate volume of the deficit can be obtained from Table 2.

26/TABLE 2

BODY FLUIDS LOST EXPRESSED AS PERCENTAGE OF BODY WEIGHT

Age	*Mild*	*Moderate*	*Severe*
0–6 months	5	10	15
6/12–6 years	5	7·5	10
Older children (as for adults)	4	6	8

Note. Weight taken is observed weight. Assessment of degree depends on state of circulation. Mild implies good cardiovascular function, moderate early and severe gross disturbance of circulation. (Finberg, 1967.)

Replacement

The fluid first given should contain sodium in isotonic concentration and 40 ml./kg. is given in the first 40–60 minutes (Finberg, 1967). Very ill children can with advantage receive half their initial replacement (20 ml./kg.) as plasma or dextran 70 in saline and the rest as either normal saline, Ringer-lactate or sixth molar sodium lactate. Further replacement depends on cardiovascular signs: generally the rate may be reduced to replace the rest of the calculated deficit in 4–6 hrs and the sodium concentration reduced to 30–75 mEq/1. (fifth or half normal saline).

Hypernatraemic Dehydration

Raised serum sodium concentrations are comparatively common in babies: they are usually the result of loss of both water and sodium, the water loss being proportionally the greater. Cardiovascular function is not usually severely affected and it is extremely important to correct this disorder very slowly with fluids containing sodium in concentrations of 50–75 mEq/1. (one third to half normal saline). If 5 per cent dextrose is given convulsions due to water intoxication are readily provoked (Hughes-Davies, 1967).

Metabolic Acidosis

Normal nutrition in a healthy infant ensures that a large proportion of its food is incorporated into its growing tissues and Slater (1961) has shown that up to 50 per cent of the food protein may be used for growth and therefore impose no demand on the kidneys for excretion. This buffer provided by anabolism no longer operates and is invariably superseded by tissue catabolism in any infant requiring surgery: if extracellular fluid is lost as well, there will be a rapid development of metabolic acidosis. There is convincing evidence that correction of this with sodium lactate (which is converted into bicarbonate) or with bicarbonate itself drastically reduces the mortality (Illingworth, 1963). With the important exception of pyloric stenosis, any severely ill infant can be expected to be acidotic and should receive 1 to 2 mMol of sodium bicarbonate per kg. body weight added to the fluid given in the first hour. If the standard bicarbonate is known, the bicarbonate given can be calculated from the

$$\text{Base deficit in mEq/l.} \times 0{\cdot}3 \times \text{body weight in kg.}$$

CONTROL OF HYDROGEN ION REGULATION

In this account acidosis is used to describe any condition which increases, or tends to increase, the hydrogen ion concentration of the extracellular fluid. Alkalosis has the opposite effect.

Life is an acidogenic process and from birth until death the body is under a constant obligation to balance hydrogen ion output against hydrogen ion intake; the diet normally contains hydrogen ions, mostly in the form of sulphur-containing amino-acids of proteins, and the urine is the sole channel of hydrogen ion excretion. The average intake is 50–80 mEq/day—much the same as sodium and potassium: the important difference, which has tended to obscure the precisely adjusted external balance of hydrogen ions, is that intermediate metabolism can give rise to relatively enormous hydrogen ion loads. Such release of hydrogen ions is normally followed by rapid neutralisation before excretion and therefore has no net effect on hydrogen ion balance (Christensen, 1962). Certain circumstances, of which tissue hypoxia is the commonest, give rise to acidosis because the stage of hydrogen ion production outstrips the stage of hydrogen ion neutralisation and the various buffer systems in the cells and extracellular fluid are the body's only means of defence against such accumulations. The acute buffer storage capacity is capable of absorbing up to 10 mEq of hydrogen ions per kg. body weight, i.e. 500–700 in an adult, or nearly ten times the average daily intake (Talbot *et al.*, 1959). If hydrogen ion intake ceases, hydrogen ion production continues as is made evident by the gradually progressive acidosis which develops in anuric patients. It is of practical importance that hydrogen ion concentration does not reach lethal levels for 7–10 days or even longer. During this time the hydrogen ions produced by metabolism are absorbed by the various buffer systems in the cells and extracellular fluid. Renal control of hydrogen ion output is slow to develop and several days are needed for urinary excretion of hydrogen ions to increase from average to maximal amounts: the kidneys make no significant contribution to the control of sudden fluxes in hydrogen ion concentration. Tissue hypoxia, starvation and diminished ventilatory reserve are accompaniments of many surgical operations: all will tend to strain the buffer capacity of the body and it is therefore important that patients are brought to surgery with the least possible encroachment of their capacity to deal with acute rises in hydrogen ion concentration. For this among other reasons diabetes, heart failure and uraemia should all be brought under control as far as is practicable before operation. The contribution of haemoglobin to the buffer capacity of blood is considerable and tends to be overlooked on account of its more obvious importance to oxygen carriage.

Metabolic alkalosis is rarely encountered before operation and cannot arise spontaneously during surgery. In the absence of previous treatment the only possible cause of alkalosis is the loss of chlorhydric gastric juice as a result of pyloric or high intestinal obstruction. The disturbances which arise are complex (de Wardener, 1961), and a high level of plasma bicarbonate is likely to be caused by urinary loss of potassium. It seldom demands treatment with salts such as ammonium chloride, which in the course of metabolism release hydrogen ions.

The Bicarbonate-Carbonic Acid Buffer Pair

The body fluids may be regarded as aqueous solutions containing a mixture of weak acids and their highly dissociated salts of sodium and potassium. In such a solution, the ratio of the concentration of all undissociated acids to dissociated salts must satisfy the ionic relationships of reversible reactions. Study of one such buffer pair gives information about all the others and the most convenient for this purpose is the bicarbonate-carbonic acid pair. Many approximations are involved in the derived association between hydrogen ion concentration, free carbonic acid and bicarbonate concentration, but clinical management is a practical possibility when based upon its use. The various equations linking the three variables are all basically expressions derived from the Law of Mass Action and of them the one proposed by Campbell (1962) is the simplest. This makes use of nanoequivalents or micromilliequivalents and hydrogen ion concentration is expressed in them. The pH scale was designed to convert gram equivalents into a convenient scale: insofar as most disturbances of hydrogen ion concentration take place within a range of pH between 8 and 7, they could be expressed as 10^{-8} and 10^{-7} gram equivalents of hydrogen ions per litre; multiplication by 10^9 converts gram equivalents into nanoequivalents and therefore most body fluids contain between 10 and 100 nanoequivalents per litre. Strictly speaking one should refer to "hydrogen ion activity" rather than hydrogen ion concentration, but the use of concentrations is established by precedent and makes no practical difference to treatment. Campbell's formula is the simplest possible expression of the Henderson-Hasselbalch equation, achieved by the elimination of logarithms and reciprocals.

$$\text{nEq H} = \frac{24\ P_{CO_2}}{\text{mEq HCO}_3}$$

For its derivation see Campbell (1962) or Wood-Smith and Stewart (1968).

The CO_2 tension of the body fluids is determined by effective alveolar ventilation. It is more often raised than lowered so that both respiratory and metabolic changes result in increases in hydrogen ion concentration more commonly than decreases. The bicarbonate concentration is controlled chiefly by renal tubular excretion or reabsorption of bicarbonate ions, but over the range of 18–30 mEq/l. may be varied directly as a result of changes in P_{CO_2}. These are the bicarbonate concentrations which occur when the P_{CO_2} is 20 and 80 respectively—about the limits of its range when air is being breathed. Reference to Fig. 2 will show that more extreme changes in bicarbonate concentration imply that a metabolic element must be present.

Sudden acute increase in hydrogen ion liberation will be reflected by an immediate fall in bicarbonate concentration which implies, in this context, that the hydrogen ion acceptors of the buffer systems have been swamped with hydrogen ions. This will produce an increased concentration of the weakly ionised buffer acids.

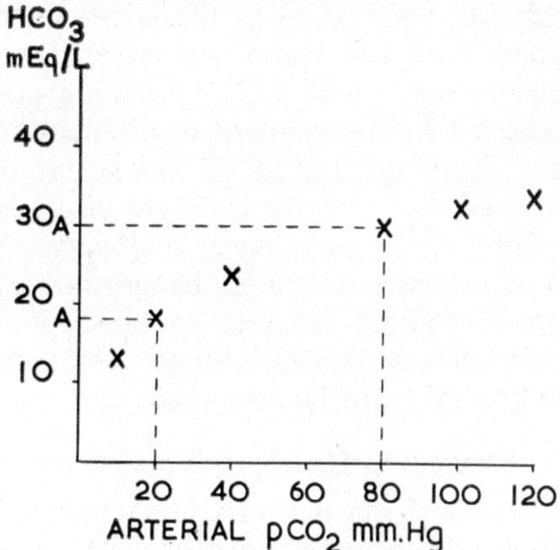

26/Fig. 2.—The bicarbonate-P_{CO_2} graph. P_{CO_2} is plotted against HCO_3 in mEq/1. Note that the higher the P_{CO_2}, the less change there is in bicarbonate concentration. A-A represents the normal range of bicarbonate values when air is breathed.

$$H^+ + HCO^-_3 \rightleftharpoons H_2CO_3$$

If the hydrogen ion load is excessive, as for example it may be following cardiac arrest at 38° C, myoneural conduction will be depressed and spontaneous breathing may cease altogether so that the compensatory elimination of CO_2, which makes the carbonic acid/bicarbonate buffer so extremely effective, will not occur.

$$H_2CO_3 \rightleftharpoons CO_2\uparrow + H_2O$$

Compensatory Changes

Whenever either P_{CO_2} or HCO_3 varies in either direction, it is followed in time by a similar change in whichever was not primarily affected. This means that whenever a compensatory change occurs, it will increase, not lessen the change that has already occurred in bicarbonate concentration. This may be illustrated by taking the example of a case of impaired alveolar ventilation resulting in a P_{CO_2} of 80.

$$\text{nEq H} = \frac{24 \times 80}{30} = 64 \text{ nEq/l.}$$

A pH of 7·4 corresponds to a hydrogen ion concentration of 40 nEq/l., so if bicarbonate is to be increased to compensate completely for the rise in P_{CO_2} from 40 to 80, the equation becomes

$$40 = \frac{24 \times 80}{HCO_3} \quad \therefore\ HCO_3 = \frac{24 \times 80}{40} = 48 \text{ mEq/l.}$$

The respiratory component produces a rise in HCO_3 of 6 mEq/l. (from 24 to 30) and the compensatory metabolic change has added a further 18 mEq/l.

Before P_{CO_2} could be easily measured, it was customary to use the bicarbonate concentration alone as the indication of the disturbance in hydrogen ion concentration. In order to nullify any change which might have occurred as a result of alteration in P_{CO_2}, the blood or plasma was equilibrated with oxygen containing carbon dioxide at a partial pressure of 40 mm. Hg. Such artificial alteration resulted in the bicarbonate value due to the metabolic component and this was referred to as the alkali reserve or standard bicarbonate, depending upon how the blood was treated before equilibration. The alkali reserve (synonymous with CO_2 combining power) may be inaccurate and should be replaced by the standard bicarbonate in which whole blood is fully oxygenated and equilibrated at 38° C with a P_{CO_2} of 40 mm. Hg (Astrup, 1959). It must be realised that even the standard bicarbonate will only indicate appropriate treatment *if the primary change is of metabolic origin*. Even more than is the case with sodium and potassium, changes in bicarbonate concentration cannot be interpreted without accurate appraisal of the clinical circumstances which altered them (Schwartz and Relman, 1963). Accuracy demands that two of the three unknowns must be measured.

Changes in Hydrogen Ion Concentration due to Alterations of P_{CO_2}

Anaesthesia is invariably associated with changes in P_{CO_2}. If the patient is allowed to breathe spontaneously, the P_{CO_2} will tend to rise and levels of 50–60 mm. Hg are common even in light anaesthesia; if relaxation for abdominal surgery is achieved, it can only be done at the expense of ventilatory depression which may result in P_{CO_2} tensions of 100 mm. Hg or more. Such physiological trespass is at best undesirable and in the elderly ill patient may well be lethal.

If relaxants are used and ventilation controlled, the anaesthetist should aim to provide a minute volume which will result in a fall in P_{CO_2}; it is now established that even several hours of overventilation associated with P_{CO_2} levels of 15–20 mm. Hg and falls of hydrogen ion concentration to 20 nEq/l. (pH of 7·7) are relatively innocuous when compared with similar changes in the opposite direction. Recent reports of workers using cardio-pulmonary by-pass have stressed the importance of maintaining hydrogen ion concentration and P_{CO_2} at as nearly normal levels as possible if deleterious effects on the heart are to be avoided. Such reports are interesting in that they represent "testing under load" and it is likely that as hydrogen ion concentration and P_{CO_2} measurements become more generally applied, there will be more emphasis on homeostasis of CO_2 tensions and their resulting changes in hydrogen ion concentration. If prolonged overventilation is employed in elderly poor-risk patients, the return of spontaneous breathing must be carefully observed, as it is occasionally associated with a period of Cheyne-Stokes breathing which can be effectively treated by a very slow injection of 0·25 g. aminophylline intravenously.

Metabolic Changes in Hydrogen Ion Concentration during Anaesthesia

No metabolic condition can reduce hydrogen ion concentration during anaesthesia. The recent developments of cardiovascular surgery have drawn attention to the invariable rise in hydrogen ion concentration which follows any episode of tissue anoxia. Brooks and Feldman (1962) first described metabolic acidosis as a possible cause of failure to re-establish adequate ventilation after operation and subsequent experience has lent support to their contention. Solutions of sodium bicarbonate are now readily available and safe amounts are more likely to be used if 8·4 per cent solutions alone are stocked. This is a molar solution and therefore contains 1 mEq of Na and 1 mEq of HCO_3 per millilitre. This can be given undiluted if it is given slowly (1 ml./minute) and up to 1 mEq per kg. can be so given with safety; in cases of known severe metabolic acidosis

2 mEq per kg. with a maximum of 150 can be given and this dosage is appropriate in cases of cardiac arrest (Stewart, 1964). The limiting factor is the amount of sodium which can be given with impunity and in the absence of sodium depletion 200 mEq should be regarded as the maximum in the first 24 hours unless accurate biochemical control is possible.

Hobsley (1963) has shown that respiratory acidosis is common in the first 8–24 hours after operation and that it is usually accompanied by a comparable degree of metabolic acidosis, both changes being unrelated to the severity of the operation. Norman and Clark (1964) report six cases of severe metabolic acidosis developing during or after surgery, all of which benefited from receiving large amounts of sodium bicarbonate.

Astrup Micro-assay of Acid/Base Balance

Brewin *et al.* (1955) first showed that if P_{CO_2} is plotted on a logarithmic scale against pH a straight line is obtained. Astrup (1959), and with his co-workers (1960), developed a micro-assay method by which the pH of blood is measured

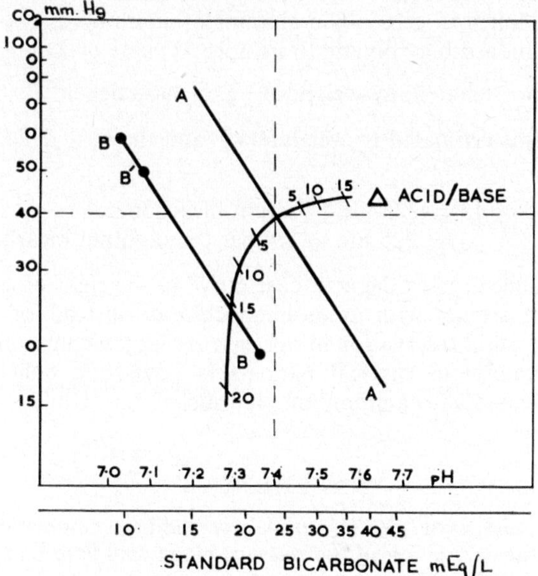

26/FIG. 3.—THE pH/P_{CO_2} GRAPH.

A-A represents the buffer line of normal blood. The pH of the patient's blood is found to be 7·1. It is then equilibrated at CO_2 tensions of 60 and 20 mm. Hg and its pH determined at each tension. The results are plotted at B-B, and the line joining them is the buffer line of the patient's blood. B^1 is then marked on the line at the point corresponding to a pH of 7·1. The following data are then read off from the graph:

P_{CO_2} = 50 mm. Hg
Standard
Bicarbonate = 12 mEq/1.

A mild degree of respiratory acidosis is therefore present, associated with a severe metabolic acidosis. The base deficit is 15 mEq/1, the point at which the buffer line crosses Δ acid/base.

(After Andersen and Engel, 1960.)

at the actual P_{CO_2} and at two known CO_2 tensions above and below the actual P_{CO_2}. These points all lie on a straight line and all data relevant to the respiratory and metabolic state of the blood can be obtained from the pH/P_{CO_2} graph. The method requires less than 0·25 ml. of capillary blood and the estimation takes about five minutes. It has become widely accepted as the most practical method of obtaining repeated information during surgery and in recovery wards.

The pH/P_{CO_2} graph has been ingeniously developed by Andersen and Engel (1960) so that the amount of base excess or base deficit can be directly read. A curve has been constructed on the graph (Fig. 3) and the point at which the patient's pH/P_{CO_2} buffer line crosses it determines the degree of metabolic acidosis or alkalosis present. Astrup refers to this as Δ acid/base. The figures on the curve to the right of the normal buffer line AA signify a metabolic alkalosis and represent base excess. Those to the left represent a metabolic acidosis and therefore base deficit.

The volume of dilution of sodium bicarbonate given intravenously is approximately equivalent to 30 per cent of body weight (this is roughly the extracellular fluid volume as would be expected from the slow penetration of the bicarbonate ion into cells). The amount of sodium bicarbonate necessary to restore the standard bicarbonate to its normal value of 24 mEq/l. is given by

$$0{\cdot}3 \times \text{body weight in kg.} \times \text{base deficit.}$$

If the patient is estimated to weigh 50 kg. and the base deficit is 15 mEq/l., this becomes

$$\begin{aligned} 0{\cdot}3 \times 50 \times 15 &= 225 \text{ mEq sodium bicarbonate} \\ &= 225 \text{ ml. of } 8{\cdot}4 \text{ per cent sodium bicarbonate.} \end{aligned}$$

If the buffer line crosses the acid/base curve to the right of the line AA, the same calculation applies with ammonium chloride instead of sodium bicarbonate. The important reservation in this case is that the commonest cause of an extracellular alkalosis in surgical patients is potassium deficiency and this should not be treated with ammonium chloride.

REFERENCES

ANDERSEN, O. S., and ENGEL, K. (1960). A new acid-base nomogram. An improved method for the calculation of the relevant blood acid-base data. *Scand. J. clin. Lab. Invest.*, **12,** 177.

ANDERSON, R. W., JAMES, P. M., BREDENBERG, C. E., COLLINS, J. A., LEVITSKY, S., and HARDAWAY, R. M. (1967). Extracellular fluid and plasma volume studies on casualties in the republic of Vietnam. *Surg. Forum*, **18,** 32.

ARIEL, I. M., KREMEN, A. J., and WANGENSTEEN, O. H. (1950). An expanded interstitial (thiocyanate) space in surgical patients. *Surgery*, **27,** 827.

ASTRUP, P. (1959). In: *pH and Blood Gas Measurement*. Ed. R. F. Woolmer. London: J. & A. Churchill.

ASTRUP, P., JØRGENSEN, K., ANDERSEN, O. S., and ENGEL, K. (1960). The acid-base metabolism. *Lancet*, **1,** 1035.

ATWELL, J. D. (1971). Personal communication.

BARNES, B. A. (1962). Current concepts relating magnesium and surgical disease. *Amer. J. Surg.*, **103,** 309.

BLACK, D. A. K., DAVIES, H. E. F., and EMERY, E. W. (1955). The disposal of radioactive potassium injected intravenously. *Lancet*, **1,** 1097.

BLACK, D. A. K., and MILNE, M. D. (1952). Experimental potassium depletion in man. *Clin. Sci.*, **11,** 397.

BREWIN, E. G., GOULD, R. P., NASHAT, F. S., and NEIL, E. (1955). An investigation of acid-base equilibrium in hypothermia. *Guy's Hosp. Rep.*, **104,** 177.

BROOKS, D. K., and FELDMAN, S. A. (1962). Metabolic acidosis. *Anaesthesia*, **17,** 161.

CAMPBELL, E. J. M. (1962). RIpH. *Lancet*, **1,** 681.

CHRISTENSEN, H. N. (1962). Current concepts of neutrality regulation. *Amer. J. Surg.*, **103,** 286.

CLELAND, J., PLUTH, J. R., TAUXE, W. N., and KIRKLIN, J. W. (1966). Blood volume and body fluid compartment changes seen after closed and open cardiovascular surgery. *J. cardiovasc. Surg.* (*Torino*), **52,** 698.

COLLER, F. A., and MADDOCK, W. G. (1933). Water requirements of surgical patients. *Ann. Surg.*, **98,** 952.

COLLER, F. A., and MADDOCK, W. G. (1940). Water and electrolyte balance. *Surg. Gynec. Obstet.*, **70,** 340.

COOPER, D. R., IOB, V., and COLLER, F. A. (1949). Response to parenteral glucose of normal kidneys and kidneys of post-operative patients. *Ann. Surg.*, **129,** 1.

CRANDELL, W. B. (1968). Parenteral fluid therapy. *Surg. Clin. N. Amer.*, **48,** 707.

DANOWSKI, T. S. (1951). Newer concepts of the role of sodium in disease. *Amer. J. Med.*, **10,** 468.

DARROW, D. C. (1950). The role of potassium in clinical disturbances of body water and electrolytes. *New Engl. J. Med.*, **242,** 978.

DE WARDENER, H. E. (1961). *The Kidney*, 2nd edit. London: J. & A. Churchill.

DUDLEY, H. A. F. (1968). Personal communication.

EDELMAN, I. S., and LEIBMAN, J. (1959). The anatomy of body water and electrolytes. *Amer. J. Med.*, **27,** 256.

ELKINTON, J. R., and WINKLER, A. W. (1944). Transfers of intracellular potassium in experimental dehydration. *J. clin. Invest.*, **23,** 93.

FIEBER, W. W., and JONES, J. R. (1966). Intraoperative fluid therapy with 5 per cent dextrose in lactated Ringer's solution. *Anesth. Analg. Curr. Res.*, **45,** 366.

FINBERG, L. (1967). Dehydration in infants and children. *New Engl. J. Med.*, **276,** 458.

GAMBLE, J. L. (1958). *Chemical Anatomy, Physiology and Pathology of Extracellular Fluid* (A Lecture Syllabus), 6th edit. Cambridge, Mass.: Harvard Univ. Press.

GUTELIUS, J. R., SHIZGAL, H. M., and LOPEZ, G. (1968). The effect of trauma on extracellular water volume. *Arch. Surg.*, **97,** 206.

HADFIELD, J. I. H. (1965). In: *Symposium on Parenteral Feeding*, p. 35. Chairman Prof. J. Anderson. London: Roy. Soc. Med.

HARDY, J. D. (1954). *Fluid Therapy*. Philadelphia: Lea & Febiger.

HAYES, M. A. (1968). Water and electrolyte therapy after operation. *New Engl. J. Med.*, **278,** 1054.

HOBSLEY, M. (1963). Respiratory disturbances caused by general surgical operations. *Ann. roy. Coll. Surg. Engl.*, **33,** 105.

HUGHES-DAVIES, T. H. (1967). Hypernatraemic dehydration. *Brit. med. J.*, **2,** 737.

ILLINGWORTH, C. (1963). Bedside biochemistry in surgical care. *Lancet*, **1,** 1275.

JOHNSTON, I. D. A. (1969). Personal communication.

JONES, C. M., and EATON, F. B. (1933). Post operative nutritional edema. *Arch. Surg.*, **27,** 159.

KERRIGAN, G. A., TALBOT, N. B., CRAWFORD, J. D. (1955). Role of the pituitary-antidiuretic hormone-renal system in everyday clinical medicine. *J. Clin. Endocrinology*, **15,** 265.

LAWSON, L. J. (1967). Parenteral nutrition in surgery. *Hosp. Med.*, **1,** 899.

MOORE, F. D. (1960). *Metabolic Care of the Surgical Patient.* Philadelphia: W. B. Saunders Co.

MOORE, F. D., HALEY, H. B., BERING, E. A., BROOKS, L., and EDELMAN, I. S. (1952). Further observations on total body water. *Surg. Gynec. Obstet.*, **95,** 181.

MOORE, F. D., and SHIRES, G. T. (1967). Editorial "Moderation". *Ann. Surg.*, **166,** 300.

MORAN, W. H., and ZIMMERMANN, B. (1967). Mechanisms of antidiuretic hormone control of importance to the surgical patient. *Surgery*, **62,** 639.

NORMAN, J. N., and CLARK, R. G. (1964). Metabolic acidosis in general surgery. *Lancet*, **1,** 348.

PEASTON, M. J. T. (1968). Parenteral nutrition in serious illness. *Hosp. Med.*, **2,** 707.

PECK, C. H., and MELTZER, S. J. (1916). Anesthesia in human beings by intravenous injection of magnesium sulphate. *J. Amer. med. Ass.*, **67,** 1131.

PLEDGER, H. G., and BUCHAN, R. (1969). Deaths in children with acute appendicitis. *Brit. med. J.*, **2,** 466.

REID, D. J., and INGRAM, G. I. C. (1967). Changes in blood coagulation after infusion of intralipid. *Clin. Sci.*, **33,** 355.

ROTH, E., LAX, L. C., and MALONEY, J. V. (1969). Ringer's lactate solution and extracellular fluid volume in the surgical patient: a critical analysis. *Ann. Surg.*, **169,** 149.

SCHMIDT-NEILSEN, K. (1964). *Desert Animals.* Oxford: Clarendon Press.

SCHWARTZ, W. B., and RELMAN, A. S. (1963). A critique of the parameters used in the evaluation of acid-base disorders. *New Engl. J. Med.*, **268,** 1382.

SHIRES, T. J., WILLIAMS, J., and BROWN, F. (1961). Acute changes in extracellular fluids associated with major surgical procedures. *Ann. Surg.*, **154,** 803.

SLATER, J. E. (1961). Retention of nitrogen and minerals by babies 1 week old. *Brit. J. Nutr.*, **15,** 183.

STEWART, J. S. S. (1964). Management of cardiac arrest. *Lancet*, **1,** 106.

STEWART, J. D., and ROURKE, G. M. (1942). The effect of large intravenous infusions on the body fluid. *J. clin. Invest.*, **21,** 197.

TALBOT, N. B., RICHIE, R. H., and CRAWFORD, J. D. (1959). *Metabolic Homeostasis.* Cambridge, Mass.: Harvard Univ. Press.

UKAI, M., MORAN, W. H., and ZIMMERMANN, B. (1968). Role of visceral afferrent pathways on vasopressin secretion and urinary secretory patterns during surgical stress. *Ann. Surg.*, **168,** 16.

VERNEY, E. B. (1948). Agents determining and influencing the functions of the pars nervosa of the pituitary. *Brit. med. J.*, **1,** 119.

WHITE, A., (1961). Intestinal obstruction in the Rhodesian African. *E. Afr. med. J.*, **38,** 525.

WILSON, A. T., and WRIGHT, S. (1936). Anti-curare action of potassium and other substances. *Quart. J. exp. Physiol.*, **26,** 127.

WOOD-SMITH, F. C., and STEWART, H. C. (1968). *Drugs in Anaesthetic Practice*, 3rd edit. London: Butterworth & Co.

ZIMMERMANN, B. (1965). Pituitary and adrenal function in relation to surgery. *Surg. Clin. N. Amer.*, **45,** 299.

ZIMMERMANN, B., and WANGENSTEEN, O. H. (1952). Observations on water intoxication in surgical patients. *Surgery*, **31,** 654.

Chapter 27

BLOOD TRANSFUSION

GENERAL CONSIDERATIONS

RECENT advances in surgery have made the transfusion of very large volumes of blood a relatively commonplace procedure. This has been made possible by a highly efficient transfusion service which, in the United Kingdom, is based on voluntary donations from over a million donors. It is likely that future developments will increase the demand for massive transfusions and that blood will become less readily available as donors become more difficult to recruit. The transfusion centres are reducing wastage by producing separate fractions of blood to meet specific needs such as antihaemophiliac factor (AHG) and platelet concentrates. This is achieved by the use of double plastic bags which make it possible to separate the red cells and plasma and re-constitute the blood after removal of the AHG or platelets. The centres will probably supply packed cells with a storage life of three weeks which is a more rational preparation for many patients who at present receive whole blood. Such economies will need to be matched by a more critical appraisal of the need for blood in operations associated with losses of up to a litre. There is an increasingly strong case to be made for the use of solutions other than blood for patients not known to be anaemic.

It is generally held that before an elective operation such as hysterectomy or prostatectomy a haemoglobin concentration of at least 10·5 g. per cent (70 per cent Haldane) is the minimum acceptable and many teams regard 11·6 g. per cent (80 per cent Haldane) as their lower limit. Nunn and Freeman (1964) have reminded anaesthetists of the importance of thinking of the factors governing the amount of oxygen available to the tissues. These are the cardiac output, the percentage saturation of arterial blood and the oxygen carrying capacity of the blood. No surgeon can guarantee that unexpected haemorrhage will not occur, and no anaesthetist can guarantee that both cardiac output and arterial oxygen saturation will never fall during anaesthesia. It is therefore good practice to ensure that the oxygen carrying capacity of the blood is not unduly low before operation. Quite apart from its predominant role in oxygen carriage, haemoglobin constitutes the most important buffer to pH changes as a result of changes in P_{CO_2}.

Figures are not available of the mortality attributable to blood transfusion. It is probably at least as great as that associated with anaesthesia for an elective operation of moderate severity and only high standards of serological control in the laboratory have made the use of stored blood as safe as it is now. Although it is in many important respects a very different tissue from circulating fresh blood, by far the commonest cause of this mortality is that a patient receives blood intended for someone else. An anaesthetist working in an unfamiliar hospital should immediately make himself aware of the methods in use for identifying patients and for checking cross-matched blood. A high "index of suspicion" should be cultivated and the patient's names alone should never be accepted as sufficient proof of identity. If a number has not been allocated, the date of birth should be used.

Good admission notes should include a record of previous transfusions and allergies, both of which may be relevant if blood is to be given. If blood is given during an operation it should be recorded in the permanent notes together with the serial numbers of the bottles actually given.

Pre-operative Anaemia

If anaemia is discovered immediately pre-operatively the operation should be postponed. It is essential to investigate the type of anaemia and not to assume it is due to iron deficiency. If time allows, iron should be given by mouth and a rise of haemoglobin concentration of 1 per cent per day can be expected. Intramuscular and intravenous preparations cannot produce a more rapid rise in haemoglobin synthesis and should only be prescribed by physicians if there are specific contra-indications to oral iron. If the operation cannot be postponed, packed cells should be given unless twenty-four hours can elapse between the end of the whole blood transfusion and surgery. The need for sleep on the night before operation should not be forgotten—few patients receiving blood, particularly if this involves splinting of the arm, will sleep well.

COLLECTION AND STORAGE OF BLOOD

Donors are accepted between the ages of 18 and 65 years. A detailed questionnaire has to be completed, and a history of viral hepatitis, malaria, venereal disease or severe allergic reactions will lead to their rejection. At each donation the blood is grouped and serological tests for syphilis and a screening test for anaemia is done. The latter is based on the Van Slyke copper sulphate method, which determines the specific gravity of a drop of blood. It ensures that on collection the donor's blood has at least 12·5 per cent of haemoglobin (85 per cent Haldane).

Blood is collected into bottles or plastic bags containing 2 grams of disodium citrate and 3 grams of dextrose in 120 ml. of water. This is the acid citrate dextrose (ACD) mixture which inactivates ionic calcium. It is very acidic (pH 5) and both this and its dextrose content result in the first part of the drawn blood being subjected to an osmotic and acidic environment far outside the normal range. In spite of this, ACD mixture has stood the test of time and blood preserved by it is based on the standard that at least 70 per cent of the red cells will remain in the recipient's blood stream for more than 24 hours when transfused on the twenty-first day (Grove-Rasmussen *et al.*, 1961).

Immediately after transfusion there is rapid extravascular destruction of non-viable red cells by the cells of the reticulo-endothelial system. This is complete within a few hours and the remaining cells then behave as they would have done in the donor's circulation and therefore disappear at just under 1 per cent per day.

Changes in Stored Blood

During storage various changes occur which only become of importance in massive transfusions (*q.v.*) and in rare instances such as liver failure and haemophilia. The changes which should be noted are shown in Table 1.

27/TABLE 1

	Blood immediately after collection	*Blood stored for 21 days*
Percentage red cell survival 24 hours after transfusion	99	75–80
Plasma potassium concentration	4 mEq/1.	25–30 mEq/1.
pH	7·1–7·2	6·7
Labile clotting factors (V and VIII)	Active	Inactive
P_{O_2}	As in mixed venous blood	20 or less
P_{CO_2}	35–40	200 or more
Ammonia	100 μg./100 ml.	900 μg./100 ml.

The change in partial pressure of oxygen and carbon dioxide is due to metabolism in the red cells at 4° C.

Other Anticoagulants

Exchange transfusion in infants and cardiopulmonary by pass are two instances when there are advantages in avoiding the use of unmodified ACD blood. Both heparin and EDTA ("Sequestrene") are used and are considered in Chapter 25.

Prolonged Storage of Blood

Red cells mixed with a glycerol-citrate-phosphate solution under certain conditions may be stored at −20° C for several months and still show good post-transfusion survival (Mollison, 1967). Techniques such as these are still in the experimental stage and are not available for routine purposes.

Plastic Bags versus Glass Bottles

There is no convincing evidence that plastic bags make any difference to red cell survival. There is a real risk that minute puncture holes may remain undetected and cause contamination of the blood. The main difference in use is that air need not displace blood in the bags and the danger of massive air embolism is eliminated.

On a practical note, plastic bags can prove troublesome in certain specific circumstances if blood has to be transfused rapidly. As mentioned previously, stored blood has a very high P_{CO_2} level (200 mm. Hg or more). If a plastic bag is warmed to body temperature then most of this carbon dioxide will come out of solution due to the difference in solubility in blood at the higher temperature. With a glass bottle this presents no problem, as the excess carbon dioxide rapidly diffuses away into the atmosphere through the air vent. But an air vent is not normally used in a plastic bag so that the first time the warmed blood comes in contact with the atmosphere is when it reaches the air in the drip chamber. When the bag is compressed, as in rapid transfusion therapy, the net result is that the level in the drip chamber is rapidly depressed and, in fact, can disappear altogether at the most vital moment. This problem can be avoided if an "in-line" rather than a "source" (see p. 747) method of warming the blood is used because the blood in the bag remains cool and the carbon dioxide remains in solution.

Giving Sets

Plastic giving sets (Fig. 1) have relatively small filters and it is essential to make use of the entire filtering surface by squeezing the filter chamber and displacing all air from it. It is usually necessary to change the giving set after three or four units of blood have been given and in any case giving sets should be changed at least daily. When blood precedes or follows a solution of 5 per cent dextrose, the giving set should first be flushed with isotonic saline in order to prevent clumping of the red cells.

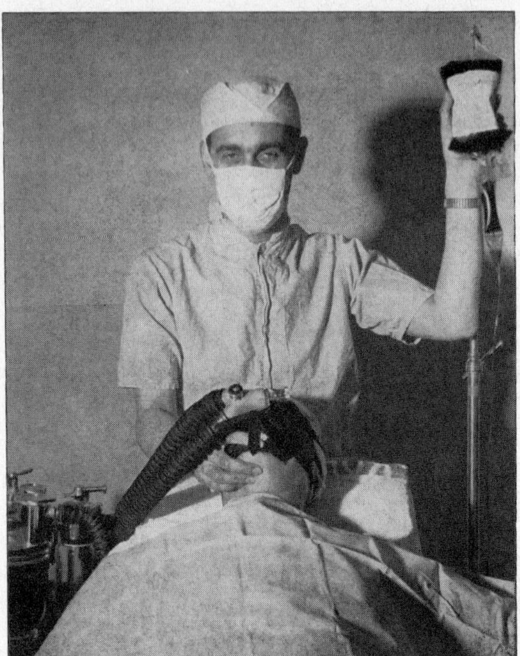

27/FIG. 1.—Plastic transfusion-giving set.

Prevention of Thrombophlebitis

Now that plastic giving sets have replaced rubber ones, by far the most important factor in the development of chemical thrombophlebitis is the length of time a particular vein is used. The site of infusion should be changed every 48 hours and if hypertonic solutions, e.g. urea or amino-acid preparations are given it should be changed daily.

BY-PRODUCTS OF BLOOD

Plasma

Plasma is made from pools of not less than eight and not more than ten donors, of whom not more than four are Group O. It is made from time-expired blood and dried and bottled in an atmosphere of nitrogen. On reconstitution it contains usually 18–20 mEq/l. of potassium and 4–4·5 g. protein together with most of the sodium citrate of the ACD originally present. Although the risk of transmitting serum hepatitis should theoretically be 8–10 times that of an equivalent volume of blood, there is no evidence that there is any material difference between the two.

Platelet Concentrates

Platelet concentrates are prepared by centrifuging fresh ACD blood at 1000 rpm. The platelet-rich plasma is aspirated from the top and then spun very rapidly so that the platelets collect at the bottom of the container from which the supernatant plasma is then aspirated.

Cryoprecipitate

If fresh plasma is frozen very rapidly some of the globulins do not re-dissolve on warming. This is the cryoprecipitate and it contains the fibrinogen and most of the antihaemophiliac factor.

Correction of some Specific Deficiencies (Table 2)

27/TABLE 2

COAGULATION FACTORS

I	Fibrinogen
II	Prothrombin
III	Thromboplastin
IV	Calcium
V	Proaccelerin (Labile)
VII	Proconvertin
VIII	Antihaemophilic globulin (Labile)
IX	Christmas factor
X	Stuart-Prower factor
XI	Plasma prothrombin antecedent
XII	Hageman factor
XIII	Fibrin stabilising factor.

Haemophilia and Christmas Disease

These are rare diseases due to inherited deficiency of Factor VIII and Factor IX. They cannot be differentiated clinically, and patients suffering from them will give a history of spontaneous bleeding or of prolonged bleeding after operations such as tooth extraction. It is the duration of bleeding, not its amount, which should arouse suspicion that a defect of coagulation may be responsible. Any such history demands an expert haematological investigation and admission to hospital for any surgery, however minor. In no circumstances can routine "bleeding and clotting time" tests be regarded as a substitute for this.

Haemophilia.—This is caused by deficiency of antihaemophiliac factor (Factor VIII, AHG or AHF). The prothrombin time is normal however severe the disease. When Factor VIII concentration falls to 25–35 per cent of normal it becomes significant clinically, and if surgery is required the aim of management is to raise it to this level and keep it so for at least a week. This can be done by daily infusions of very large volumes of fresh frozen plasma ($1\frac{1}{2}$–2 litres/day) or by injection of much smaller volumes of cryoprecipitate. Both products expose the patient to a high risk of serum hepatitis.

Christmas disease.—This accounts for about 15 per cent of cases which appear to be haemophilia and is due to Factor IX deficiency. Factor IX is comparatively stable and fresh blood or plasma can be used as sources of supply.

Platelet Deficiency

Operations such as splenectomy may be performed on patients with thrombocytopenia. Platelet concentrates made from 6 to 10 units of blood should be given at the end of operation.

HAZARDS OF BLOOD TRANSFUSION

Infections

Serum hepatitis, malaria and syphilis may all be transmitted from donor to recipient.

Serum hepatitis.—This is the most serious of the diseases which can be transmitted by stored blood. The causative virus is extremely resistant to freezing, long storage and drying. It is destroyed by moderate heat, but of the various by-products of blood only albumin can be prepared by a method which is believed to be viricidal (60° C for ten hours) without undergoing significant denaturation.

In the United Kingdom the incidence of icteric serum hepatitis is of the order of one case per 500 units of blood transfused and the mortality is high—about 10 per cent. It is now thought that many non-icteric cases occur for every jaundiced patient and that the seriousness of the disease varies with the state of health of the recipient.

Syphilis.—*T. pallidum* is killed by storage for three to four days at 4° C. As every unit of blood is serologically screened for syphilis, the risk of transmission is small.

Malaria.—All forms of malarial parasites will survive storage for three weeks at 4° C. Donors with a history of malaria are rejected.

Bacterial infection of blood after collection.—Most common organisms are killed by storage at 4° C, but certain Gram-negative bacilli can survive and multiply at this temperature. Usually, but not invariably, the red cells are haemolysed by such organisms and the plasma becomes a mauve permanganate-like colour. Examination of the colour of the blood and evidence of the presence of haemolysis should be included in the checking routine. Blood should never be returned to the refrigerator if it has been at room temperature for more than half an hour, and packed cells (if packed by hospital laboratories) should be used within six hours of preparation.

Infected blood transfused during anaesthesia is likely to manifest itself by a sudden profound fall in blood pressure and occasionally by uncontrolled bleeding.

Incompatible Transfusion

The first 100 to 200 ml. of blood given to an anaesthetised patient should be considered a "test dose" and a careful watch on cardiovascular function is essential. The signs of incompatibility are the same as those of infected blood—sudden fall of blood pressure and the development of a consumption coagulation process which sometimes progresses to the stage of uncontrolled pathological bleeding. Once it is known that incompatible blood has been given a sample of blood should immediately be taken from the recipient and put into a citrate container. Five to ten thousand units of heparin should then be given intravenously whether or not abnormal bleeding has occurred. Any blood deficit should at once be made good with compatible blood, and half to one litre of isotonic saline or Ringer-lactate given rapidly followed by a test dose of 20 g. of mannitol. For further management if anuria develops see Chapter 49.

Air Embolism

Air embolism is a rare but preventible cause of death. The use of a Higginson syringe or similar method of pressurising glass bottles is no longer justifiable. If roller pumps are used vigorously they always entrain the air of the drip chambers and in rare instances the few millilitres so injected have caused death (Bewes, 1961). One should always assume that recipients of blood may have widely patent interatrial defects and squeeze all air from the filter and drip chambers before using roller pumps.

Allergic Reactions

Any patient with a definite history of severe allergy is liable to manifest it if given blood or plasma. Piriton (chlorpheniramine maleate) 10 mg. may be given slowly intravenously, or the same dose can be injected into the first bottle of blood. Such reactions are now uncommon and should not necessitate stopping the transfusion.

Physico-chemical Dangers of Massive Transfusion

If stored blood were to perfuse the coronary tree undiluted it would stop the heart for many reasons. The danger of cardiac arrest only arises in massive transfusions—a term which implies consideration of both rate and volume, and is most simply defined as any transfusion (in an adult) at a rate of 500 ml. in five minutes or less, or replacement of half the calculated blood volume in less than an hour. The problems involved have been reviewed by Churchill-Davidson (1968) and Burton (1968). Various measures can be taken to reduce the risks.

Warming the blood.—To bring the temperature of the stored blood near to body temperature is the single most important safety measure. This is most simply done by immersion of a coil of the tubing in a water bath kept at 38–40° C. This "in-line" heating has the disadvantage that it increases the resistance of the giving set tubing and also the cold, and therefore more viscous, blood is not heated until it has been through the filter and drip chambers. These objections are overcome if the bottle or pack is heated by radio-frequency induction, by which a unit of blood can be warmed to body temperature in less than 5 minutes (Besseling *et al.*, 1965). This induction heating has proved disappointing in practice and at the present the "in-line" method is the one of choice. Whatever means are employed, the greatest care is needed to ensure that the blood is not exposed to a temperature of more than 40° C. The practice of warming bottles or packs of blood in basins of water is dangerous and should never be used.

Calcium.—Although some authorities disagree (Howland *et al.*, 1957), most now maintain that calcium should be given. Jennings *et al.* (1965) have provided convincing evidence that ACD is toxic in the dog, and it seems reasonable to replace an absent ionic element known to be essential to myocardial function. Apart from this consideration, calcium is the physiological antagonist to high serum potassium levels as well as protecting against the toxic effects of citrate (Mollison, 1967). Calcium salts are potentially dangerous and must be given slowly.

If calcium is to be given, 5 ml. of 10 per cent calcium gluconate should be injected with every 500 ml. of blood. Provided that blood is being given at rates of 100 ml./minute (and calcium should not be necessary with slower rates than this) the injection can be made into the transfusion line without causing clotting. When large masses of muscle have been injured the danger of hyperkalaemia is a very real one, and in such cases there is added reason to give calcium if massive transfusion is required.

Sodium bicarbonate.—The ultimate effect of a massive transfusion *per se* is to cause a metabolic alkalosis as a result of the metabolism of the citrate to bicarbonate. The immediate effect is a transient metabolic acidosis: if the patient is in shock and more than 4 units of blood have to be given, one gram of sodium bicarbonate (12 mMols) should be given for each unit of blood transfused.

Dilution.—There is both clinical and experimental support for giving isotonic sodium solutions in addition to whole blood in the management of massive bleeding. Ringer-lactate is more appropriate than saline and it should be warmed to body temperature. Up to one litre may be given while blood is being cross-matched and a further ½ to 1 litre is given for every 4 units of blood. The schedule was adopted by an Australian surgical team treating civilian battle casualties (Dudley *et al.*, 1968) and the benefits it is thought to confer are due to better tissue perfusion as a result of the fall in the viscosity of the blood and the protective effects of the induced sodium diuresis on the kidneys.

ECG monitoring.—Whenever the likelihood of massive transfusion can be foreseen, an ECG oscilloscope should be used. The changes to be looked for are usually those ascribed to hyperkalaemia—peaking of the T waves and widening of the QRS complex. If these are seen, calcium gluconate should be given and blood temporarily replaced by either a plasma substitute or Ringer-lactate.

DEXTRAN

Dextran 110 or dextran 70 ("Macrodex") are suitable plasma volume expanders if blood is either not available or considered to be unnecessary. Both preparations are available as 6 per cent solutions in either 0·9 per cent saline or 5 per cent dextrose and the saline preparation is the more physiological substitute for plasma. Most authorities consider 1 to 1½ litres as the maximum that should be given as larger amounts tend to interfere with blood clotting in ways which are not fully understood. Blood should be taken for cross-matching before dextran 110 is given; dextran 70 is less liable to interfere with interpretation of laboratory tests (Salsbury, 1967).

Dextran 40 ("Lomodex", "Rheomacrodex") can be used as a 10 per cent solution, and according to Hardaway (1968) it will expand the plasma volume by about double the volume given. The effect is short-lived as up to 70 per cent is excreted by the kidneys within 24 hours: it should be noted that the very viscous urine which results will have an extremely high specific gravity—figures of 1050 and above are common—but there will be a negligible increase in urine osmolarity. Dextran 40 should be given in conjunction with Ringer-lactate or saline in order to maintain a urine output of at least 50 ml./hr. If there is any doubt about renal function it should be withheld.

The Normal Blood Volume

Normal blood volumes vary over a wide range if they are expressed as a function of any readily measured characteristic. The red cell volume can be shown to be closely related to total body water and to total exchangeable potassium. The most practical association relates blood volume to body weight but there is a wide variation, as shown in Table 3 by the figures quoted from three authorities.

27/TABLE 3

BLOOD VOLUME AS A PERCENTAGE OF BODY WEIGHT

	Men	*Women*
Moore	7	6·5
Mollison	7·7	6·6
Massachusetts General Hospital	9	8

The sex difference is due to body fat content which has about one-eighth the blood content by weight of lean tissue. In practice one can assume that 90 per cent of blood volumes will fall within the range of 5 litres $\pm \frac{1}{2}$–1 litre in adults.

Blood Volumes in Babies and Children

The blood volume at term is high—about 85 ml./kg. with a haematocrit of 60 per cent and haemoglobin concentration of 18–20 g. per cent. There is a rapid loss of red cells in the first three months, so that haemoglobin concentration falls to 11–12 g. per cent (75–82 per cent Haldane). The wide range encountered during this time must be appreciated before a baby is considered to be anaemic.

The approximate blood volume of older babies and children up to 2 years can be taken as 75 ml./kg. and when anaesthetising them it is a good practice to work out their blood volume beforehand and the volume of blood which corresponds to a unit of blood in an adult.

The blood loss in infants is not easy to predict and when there is any possibility that blood may be needed intravenous access must be secured before surgery begins. The subject has been well documented by Davenport and Barr (1963).

Plasma Volume

The considerable variation in blood volume in a normal subject is due to changes in plasma volume. This is mostly postural—lying down for 2 hours after prolonged standing results in expansion of the plasma volume which is reflected in a 5 per cent fall in haemoglobin concentration. This, together with the diurnal variation and small errors in measurement can produce alterations in haemoglobin concentration of 0·5–1 g. per cent.

Plasma volume is controlled, in ways which are not fully understood, so that any alteration of total blood volume tends to be compensated for. Any overexpansion of the blood volume will therefore be followed by what Moore calls "plasma dispersal"—movement of water, sodium and albumin out of the intravascular compartment. Each gram of albumin takes with it nearly 20 ml. of water. This is the mechanism by which a chronically anaemic patient's haemoglobin concentration is raised by the administration of whole blood, even if the haemoglobin concentration of the transfused blood is little greater than that of the recipient. The recipient, as it were, packs the red cells. This takes time and a clear 24 hours should be allowed between transfusion and surgery if it is to be complete: if time does not allow this, the cells must be packed before transfusion. In this clinical setting, and in this alone, is the clinical aphorism that a unit of blood raises the haemoglobin concentration by 1 g. per cent approximately true.

If large volumes of blood are given to replace acute blood loss the resulting haemoglobin concentration in the recipient will reflect the haemoglobin concentration and haematocrit of the stored blood as it constitutes more and more of the recipient's circulating blood. After one blood volume has been given, over 60 per cent will consist of donor blood and after two blood volumes nearly 90 per cent. As a result of dilution with anticoagulant solution and rapid destruction of non-viable cells such massive transfusions will result in haemoglobin concentrations 9·5–10 g. per cent and haematocrits of 35–40 per cent. This is Moore's indeterminate hacmatocrit of the severely injured transfused patient. "Such a haematocrit is meaningless as an indication of the circulating blood volume. It may coexist with a severe volume deficit, a normal blood volume or a dangerously overtransfused blood volume" (Moore, 1960). It follows that the more blood transfused the less reliable become the haemoglobin concentration and haematocrit as indications of the need for further transfusion.

The Response to Haemorrhage

If one or two litres of blood are lost rapidly the blood volume is made good by intravascular migration of albumin, water and electrolytes from the interstitial fluid. Fit subjects with good cardiovascular function can mobilise fluid at a maximum rate of 100 ml./hour, the rate falling progressively so that final haemodilution takes usually 36 to 48 hours. During this time the haemoglobin concentration, haematocrit and red cell count all fall progressively and such a fall should not be interpreted as an indication of further haemorrhage. Post-operative estimation of the haemoglobin concentration should therefore be deferred to the second day if operative blood loss has not been replaced. In this context (and provided that no hypertonic infusions have been given) the haemoglobin concentration, haematocrit and red cell count are all different ways of expressing the same ratio and there is nothing to be gained by measuring more than one index of this ratio.

Moore *et al.* (1966) have shown that when Ringer-lactate is infused rapidly into volunteers bled approximately 10 per cent of their blood volume, more of the infused solution remains within the vascular tree than in unbled controls. It is commonly believed that saline or Ringer-lactate causes albumin to be "washed out" of the intravascular compartment, but these workers showed the opposite to be true and that there was mobilisation of protein into the plasma during the time that considerable volumes of Ringer-lactate were passing from the vascular to the interstitial compartment.

Acute Massive Haemorrhage

Once blood loss amounts to 20–30 per cent of blood volume the fine balance between alveolar perfusion and alveolar ventilation is seriously disturbed. The fall in both pressure and output of the right ventricle results in the uppermost parts of the lungs receiving little or no blood although they remain well ventilated. The corresponding fall in left ventricular output results in increased extraction of oxygen by the tissues so that the arteriovenous oxygen difference is greatly increased. The result of this is to increase the "shunt effect" of those alveoli which normally have a low ventilation/perfusion ratio and which are therefore critically influenced by the alveolar/arterial oxygen gradient. Freeman and Nunn (1963) have shown that both the increased dead-space effect and arterial desaturation occur in dogs and Nunn and Freeman (1964) have reviewed the clinical implications. Firstly, drugs such as morphine should be given with the greatest care and only if pain is a prominent symptom. Oxygen in concentrations of 30 per cent or more will be beneficial in some cases and finally infusion of any fluid such as dextran, plasma or saline should be given rapidly until blood becomes available.

Transfusion of Severely Anaemic Patients

Severe cases of chronic anaemia may become extremely sensitive to circulatory overload if transfused with whole blood. This is because they may be in a state of high output cardiac failure with raised central venous pressure. They are usually dyspnoeic on slight exertion and have haemoglobin levels of less than 5·8 grams per cent (40 per cent Haldane). Such patients should be given small volumes of packed cells very slowly (1 ml./kg./hr.) and carefully observed. The most reliable guide is provided by a quarter-hourly pulse rate chart; incipient right heart failure and pulmonary oedema is indicated by a rising heart rate. Pulmonary oedema may develop several hours later if this warning sign is disregarded.

Sickle Cell Anaemia

This is a genetically determined disease affecting Negro races. Any patient of African descent found to be anaemic should have a sickling test done before operation. The haemoglobin levels are usually 5 to 8 g. per cent and if transfusion is essential fresh blood should be given together with two grams of sodium bicarbonate per unit transfused. Sickling, with blocking of capillaries, is provoked by hypoxia and particular care must be taken to ensure that this does not occur. Metabolic alkalosis decreases the tendency to sickling, and during operation Ringer-lactate may be infused at 5 to 10 ml./kg./hr. with one gram of sodium bicarbonate added to each $\frac{1}{2}$ litre. The problems have been discussed by Gilbertson (1966).

Liver Failure and Transfusion

If anaemia is present before operation, fresh packed cells should be given (Oberman, 1967). Operative blood loss should ideally be replaced with EDTA preserved blood within five days of collection. If ACD blood is used it should not be more than one week old and calcium, 5 ml. of 10 per cent calcium gluconate, given with each unit.

Defibrination Syndrome

(*Synonyms:* Consumption Coagulopathy; Disseminated Intravascular Coagulation)

Until recently it was thought that profuse bleeding associated with very low levels of fibrinogen was a rare complication of some types of surgery and of antepartum haemorrhage in obstetrics. It is now known that disturbances of the normal enzymatic "cascade" involved ultimately in the conversion of fibrinogen to fibrin can be expected in many other clinical contexts, including some forms of shock.

The first step is activation of Factor XII (Hageman factor) by a variety of agents—tissue thromboplastins, bacterial endotoxins, intravascular haemolysis, hypoxia and endothelial damage have all been implicated (McKay, 1968). If the normal inactivation of clotting factors by the liver and the cells of the reticulo-endothelial system is impaired, thrombin will be formed with resulting conversion of fibrinogen to fibrin. Fibrin then forms widespread intravascular clots in small vessels, hence the term "Disseminated Intravascular Coagulation". Note that the process has up to this point been one of abnormal coagulation and involved increased consumption of clotting factors and platelets.

Intravascular fibrin clots are normally dissolved by the action of plasmin, a proteolytic enzyme also referred to as fibrinolysin. If plasmin (fibrinolytic) activity is excessive both fibrinogen and fibrin are broken down with the release of polypeptide split products with powerful vasodepressor effects. The process which began as enhanced coagulation is therefore followed by abnormal failure of coagulation. In rare instances, activation of fibrinolytic activity may be the primary fault in which case substances such as EACA and Trasylol which inhibit the fibrinolytic enzyme system would constitute specific therapy.

In the present state of knowledge one should assume that all acutely developing abnormal bleeding states are primarily thrombotic (Ingram, personal communication) and therefore neither EACA nor Trasylol should be given without expert advice or without evidence that primary fibrinolysis is occurring. In practice this means taking a sample of blood into a citrate container for platelet count and a fibrinogen titre test. Meanwhile the only therapy to be given unadvised is an infusion of 6 to 8 grams of fibrinogen. The rapid blood loss should be replaced with fresh frozen plasma as well as stored blood.

Surgery on Patients Taking Anticoagulant Drugs

There is now good evidence that surgery can be performed safely on patients taking coumarin or indanedione drugs provided the prothrombin time is maintained at the lower border of the therapeutic level. This will usually be 1½ to 2½ times the control time (Guralnick, 1968), but will vary with different laboratories. In order to achieve this level the drugs must usually be stopped 36 to 48 hours before operation.

Vitamin K should only be given in an emergency, as a single dose may interfere with control of these drugs for a week or more. The dose of vitamin K should be decided in consultation with a haematologist as much will depend on whether coumarin drugs are to be resumed or stopped altogether (Ingram and Richardson, 1965).

APPENDIX TO CHAPTER 27

Cross Matching Techniques

The object of these techniques is to detect any antibody in the recipient's serum which will react with blood group antigen in the donor cells. The technique must be capable of detecting both naturally occurring and immune types of antibody. The principle is to incubate the donor cells with the recipient's serum, in a small tube, under optimal conditions for antigen-antibody reaction to take place.

Three techniques are used:

1. One drop of the recipient's serum is mixed with one drop of a 2 per cent suspension of the donor's red cells in saline in two tubes and the mixtures are incubated at room temperature and at 37° C, after which they are examined for agglutination. This technique will detect naturally occurring antibodies such as anti-A and anti-B but should never be used alone.
2. One drop of the recipient's serum is mixed with one drop of a 2 per cent suspension of the donor's red cells in 30 per cent albumin and the mixture incubated at 37° C after which it is examined for agglutination. This technique will detect immune type of antibodies but is only moderately sensitive.
3. Three drops of the recipient's serum are mixed with a 50 per cent suspension of the donor's red cells in saline and the mixture incubated at 37° C. The red cells, which remain unagglutinated by immune antibodies, are then washed three times in saline and the presence of antibody on the red cells shown by agglutination after the addition of antihuman globulin serum (Indirect Coombs Test). This is the most sensitive method of cross matching and will pick up all types of antibody even in weak concentration.

The time of incubation depends on the degree of clinical urgency, but as a routine is 2 hours.

Useful Data

Drip Rate.—The time taken by the contents of a bottle (540 ml.) to run into a patient can be roughly predicted from the following figures:

40 drops a minute	4 hours
60 drops a minute	2½ hours
200 drops a minute	45 minutes

Blood Group Incidence

O Rh(D) positive	39 per cent.	O Rh(d) negative	8 per cent.
A Rh(D) positive	34 per cent.	A Rh(d) negative	7 per cent.
B Rh(D) positive	7·5 per cent.	B Rh(d) negative	1·5 per cent.
AB Rh(D) positive	2·5 per cent.	AB Rh(d) negative	0·5 per cent.

often not produce fully saturated arterial blood and despite apparent hyperventilation the carbon dioxide level rises. It is not possible to inflate the lungs at the same time as cardiac compression is carried out and ventilation normally alternates with cardiac compression in the ratio 1:5.

Closed chest cardiac massage.—The efficacy of closed chest cardiac massage in compressing the heart between the sternum and vertebral column was first reported by Kouwenhoven and his associates (1960). The technique is effective whether the heart is in asystole or ventricular fibrillation and produces a satisfactory central aortic pressure (Gurewich *et al.*, 1961; Oliver *et al.*, 1964), although this is not a good index of the amount of flow. Indeed, ventricular fibrillation may cease spontaneously and a normal beat follow as a result of closed chest massage (Wetherill and Nixon, 1962). Lateral displacement of the heart does not occur and while there is some ventilation of the lungs it is not enough to obviate the need for simultaneous artificial respiration.

Technique.—Immediately the diagnosis is made and the airway has been cleared the patient is laid flat and external cardiac compression started. Although ideally the patient should lie on a firm surface, in practice it is more important to start the massage first and then, at a convenient moment, slip a wooden board, fracture board or even a tray under the patient during a pause while the patient is ventilated.

Compression is applied through the heel of one hand which is placed over the lower half of the sternum while the operator's other hand rests on the top of the hand directly on the chest. No force is transmitted through the fingers so that compression of the lateral part of the thorax, which produces rib fractures, is avoided. In an adult the sternum is depressed for 4–5 cm. (1½″–2″) towards the spine—this requires a force of 50–70 lbs. and it is necessary for the operator to be well above the patient, kneeling on the bed if necessary, so as to use his body weight rather than the arm muscles alone, which is both fatiguing and ineffective. The cardiac output produced is only 20–40 per cent of normal and is rate-dependant. Cardiac compression is applied at between 80 and 100 beats per minute—this rate allowing adequate time for the heart to fill in diastole.

In children compression is with one hand only, producing proportionately less sternal displacement, and is at a faster rate.

The cardiac output depends on the heart refilling in between beats and pressure must be completely removed from the chest between compressions. The venous return is augmented by tipping the bed head downwards or by elevating the feet on a pillow or chair. Fracturing of the ribs which impairs the elastic recoil of the chest and the transient negative pressure which this produces, results in a decreased venous return and a lower output.

To be effective, external cardiac compression must produce a palpable pulse in the carotid or femoral artery. In cases where a direct arterial pressure recording is possible systolic pressures of 100 mm. Hg are commonly seen during massage, although of course this near normal pressure does not signify a near normal cardiac output. The pupils will diminish in size and sometimes consciousness and spontaneous respiration will return when the patient may have to be restrained so that resuscitation can continue.

External cardiac compression has to be interrupted to allow ventilation to occur, as it is impossible to inflate the chest while cardiac compression is occurring. Usually every sixth compression is missed to allow a positive pressure ventilation to be performed. When working single-handed a ratio of two inflations to fifteen compressions is easier.

The exact technique of cardiac compression which produces the optimum output is unfortunately only learnt with experience. Too quick a compression while producing a good systolic pressure results in little forward flow, too slow a compression results in a low systolic pressure and too slow a rate, thus producing a low output. Practice on a "Ressusianne" or similar manikin with an experienced teacher is invaluable.

Internal cardiac massage.—External cardiac compression has replaced internal cardiac compression because of its greater feasibility and efficiency. In most cases when external compression is ineffective it is unlikely that direct cardiac compression will be any more so. There are, however, certain indications for the internal rather than the external technique.

1. If the chest is already open during cardiac or thoracic surgery.
2. In the presence of intrathoracic pathology causing the arrest, e.g. pneumothorax, cardiac tamponade.
3. Air embolus—when air can be aspirated from the heart.
4. Excessively stiff thoracic cage, as in emphysematous patients, which prevents effective external cardiac compression.

The incision is made in the fourth left interspace lateral to the internal mammary artery and the space pulled open with the hands. In the absence of a rib spreader an anaesthetic mouth gag can be used. After the pericardium has been incised, the heart is compressed, between two hands or, failing this, with the flat of one hand behind the heart and the thumb and thenar eminence in front, taking care not to perforate any of the chambers with the fingers.

If cardiac arrest occurs during abdominal surgery, closed chest massage is preferable to massage through the diaphragm.

Restoration of Cardiac Function

In cases of transient circulatory arrest such as Stokes-Adams attacks, or arrhythmias associated with myocardial infarction, the prompt institution of external cardiac compression and artificial ventilation may result in the return of an effective spontaneous heart beat. If they do not, definitive therapy is required as an emergency, because the chances of success diminish as time passes.

First, the patient should be intubated and ventilated with pure oxygen with proper elimination of carbon dioxide.

A diagnosis of the cardiac rhythm is made by electrocardiography.

An adequate venous return is ensured by rapid fluid replacement via a drip into a large vein (femoral or internal jugular) which is started as soon as possible, thereby also providing a route for drug therapy. If the catheter can be advanced to the vena cava it can also be used to measure central venous pressure as a guide to transfusion therapy.

Blood is withdrawn for estimation of the acid-base state and for serum electrolytes, especially the serum potassium if the aetiology of the arrest is thought to be associated with any electrolyte imbalance.

Drug therapy

1. **Correction of metabolic acidosis.**—The circulatory stagnation of cardiac arrest always leads to some degree of metabolic acidosis and this may be so severe that it depresses the circulatory effects of catecholamines or even prevents restoration of a normal beat. In an intensive care unit where cardiac arrest is treated within thirty seconds and a normal circulation is quickly restored no alkalinizing agent may be required, but generally an initial dose of 1–2 mEq/kg. body weight of sodium bicarbonate is necessary. Thereafter the correction of metabolic acidosis is best controlled by serial estimations of the acid-base state of the arterial blood bearing in mind that the fluid compartment accessible for correction under the conditions of cardiac massage may be quite small. Once a normal beat is restored and the tissues become perfused a much larger acidosis is revealed which will then require correction.

2. **Inotropic drugs.**—Inotropic drugs are given both for cardiac asystole, in an attempt to provoke a return to a spontaneous heart beat, and for ventricular fibrillation, to improve the tone of the myocardium before attempting electrical defibrillation. In the case of an arrhythmia, definitive treatment of the arrhythmia should precede use of inotropic drugs.

The drug of choice is adrenaline in a dose of 1 mg. (10 ml. of 1:10,000 solution) given intravenously, preferably into a central vein. Attempted intracardiac injection may produce a pneumothorax or an injury to a coronary artery and should be avoided where possible if the heart is not directly exposed for surgery. The adrenaline can be repeated every two to five minutes. Calcium is also frequently used and is best given as an intravenous injection of $CaCl_2$ in doses of up to 1 g., unless the arrest is thought to be hypokalaemic in origin.

Cardiac standstill.—Asystole will usually respond to effective cardiac massage and ventilation together with correction of the acidosis and the administration of inotropic drugs. In cases of complete heart block or refractory bradycardia which do not respond to an infusion of isoprenaline it may be necessary to resort to electrical pacing. In the emergency this can be started using two electrodes applied over the praecordium, although this is sufficiently painful that the patient must be anaesthetised if it is continued and, as soon as possible, internal pacing is substituted using a pacemaker placed in the right ventricle via an intravenous catheter.

Ventricular fibrillation.—Fibrillation may be present as the initial form of circulatory arrest or it may arise during the emergency treatment. In a coronary care unit sudden fibrillation may be treated by instant electrical defibrillation but more commonly the first step will be cardiac compression, ventilation with oxygen, bicarbonate and drug therapy to improve the tone of the heart. Defibrillation is then attempted.

Clinical opinion now favours direct rather than alternating current in the treatment of ventricular fibrillation. For direct current defibrillation up to 2500 volts are needed (Kouwenhoven and Knickerbocker, 1961) and these are provided by charging a capacitor which can be made to provide a single output energy discharge of up to 400 joules (watt-seconds). An induction coil is usually incorporated in the discharging circuit to prevent myocardial damage (Lown *et al.*, 1962; Peleska, 1963). Most alternating current defibrillators also have an output discharge in the region of 400 joules, but the time taken for the energy to pass into the heart is about 100–200 msecs. as compared with 2–4 msecs. from a capacitor (Beard, 1964). As a result direct current is less likely than alternating current to damage the heart: it is also said to be more effective in the treatment of ventricular fibrillation. A direct current defibrillator can be charged quickly from the mains and needs only a small amount of current. It can be battery operated. Direct current defibrillators are extremely dangerous to the operator because of the high voltages built up, and this danger exists even when the apparatus is disconnected from the mains.

Direct current defibrillation through the closed chest requires an energy release in the region of 200–400 joules. For direct defibrillation of the exposed heart only 20–40 joules is sufficient.

One electrode is placed behind the right scapula and the other held over the apex.

When alternating current is to be used for defibrillation through the closed chest a shock of 400 to 500 volts should be passed for 0·2 sec. If a single shock is not successful then a run of three or four should be tried with an interval of two seconds between each. If there is a high electrical resistance between the two electrodes due to poor contact with the patient, then as much as 800 volts may be required to achieve success. Internal defibrillation of the heart requires voltages ranging from 110 to 250, each shock lasting for about 0·2 second.

In the event of defibrillation not occurring or the heart repeatedly refibrillating due to extreme irritability of the myocardium, this can be suppressed without depressing myocardial contractility by lignocaine given intravenously (dose 1 mg./kg.). If defibrillation is subsequently successful but recurrent arrhythmia is a problem, the lignocaine is continued as an infusion at 1 to 2 mg. per minute. This drug has largely replaced the use of quinidine and procaine amide. While propranolol is used to suppress ventricular arrhythmias after myocardial infarction, its use in the treatment of ventricular fibrillation is very hazardous and if the patient is restored to normal rhythm the heart may not be capable of producing a sufficient output.

In cardiac patients or patients with electrolyte imbalance, disturbances of serum potassium may cause cardiac arrest, and defibrillation may not be possible until the serum has returned to normal. Hypokalaemia is easily treated with intravenous potassium. The effects of hyperkalaemia can be partially antagonised by administration of $CaCl_2$ and the level of K^+ can be quickly lowered by the intravenous administration of glucose and insulin (100 ml. 50 per cent glucose with 12·5 units soluble insulin) while cardiac massage is continued.

After Treatment

Once a normal beat has been restored the patient is carefully monitored to ensure that the circulation is adequate. This may necessitate further periods of external cardiac compression if the pulse becomes feeble. The output is best supported by an infusion of isoprenaline (1 mg. in 200 ml. dextrose with a microdrop giving set), rather less importance being placed on vasopressor drugs and the actual value of the blood pressure. Lignocaine (1–2 mg./min.) may be needed to control arrhythmias, the rhythm being observed on an electrocardioscope. The filling pressure of the heart is measured via a central venous line as a guide to fluid replacement, the acid-base state estimated on arterial samples, the urine output charted and the pulse and blood pressure recorded.

Frequently the respiration is inadequate after cardiac resuscitation, either because of damage sustained by the rib cage or because of poor lung function. Large shunts occur in the lung which, in the face of a low cardiac output, lead to arterial hypoxaemia despite a high inspired oxygen concentration. In these circumstances positive pressure ventilation via an endotracheal tube is indicated until the circulation is restored to normal.

Cerebral dehydration and other forms of therapy following a period of cardiac arrest are discussed in Chapter 45.

Comment

All too often, cardiac arrest is the end-result of a derangement of physiology which has been either unnoticed or untreated for some time. It is much better to prevent a cardiac arrest than to treat it, however effectively.

Also, the treatment defined above covers only the essential practical details of resuscitation. Resuscitation will often be ineffective if the precipitating cause is not recognised and treated. It requires a calm logical mind with a good understanding of medicine to sort out and treat the underlying condition while at the same time performing emergency resuscitation.

However, accepting that cardiac emergencies may arise suddenly, the successful treatment must depend to some extent on the provision of proper facilities and the adequate training of personnel.

Basic resuscitation kits should be kept available in all wards and departments of the hospital. There should be a well-rehearsed plan of action so that no time is wasted on inessential manoeuvres. The ultimate result for a patient will depend on the brevity of the interval between cardiac arrest and the restoration of an effective circulation, and every anaesthetist should know what can and what should be done in that period.

Primary resuscitation must be carried out *at once* by the nurse or doctor who is immediately available, but an emergency call system is essential to ensure that suitably trained staff and specialised apparatus can get to the bedside, or site where the patient collapses, before irreparable harm has been done. Many such systems have been described, but that in use at St. Thomas's Hospital is operated as follows: When assistance is required an emergency internal telephone number is used to contact the hospital lodge. From here a spoken message is broadcast, via a multitone short-wave radio, to the anaesthetist carrying the receiver unit. This anaesthetist immediately goes to the scene of the incident. Trolleys of resuscitation apparatus (Fig. 1) are strategically sited in the hospital and one of these is fetched by the nursing staff.

EMBOLISM

Embolus translated literally means a plug. Various substances may be carried along in the bloodstream until they ultimately obstruct one or more blood vessels but those of particular interest are air, fat, tumour, blood clot, and amniotic fluid.

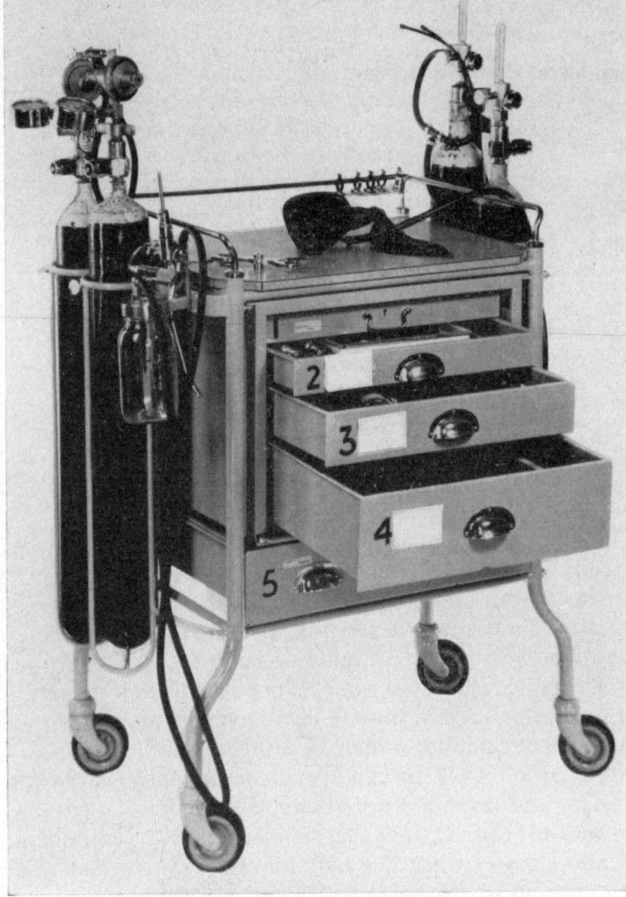

28/FIG. 1.—Emergency resuscitation trolley.

Air Embolus

This may be venous or arterial, but a combination of both can result should any quantity of air enter the venous circulation of a patient with either an atrial or ventricular septal defect. Air embolus does not occur commonly. Death may follow so quickly after the entry of air into a peripheral vein that its true cause may be missed unless a careful post-mortem is carried out under conditions which do not allow the entrapped air to leave the heart and vessels unseen. An X-ray taken immediately after death may show air in the veins or right heart. The principal sources of air embolus are summarised in Table 1.

Venous Air Embolus

Air which enters a peripheral vein rapidly reaches the right side of the heart and the pulmonary circulation. The quantity of air that is needed to cause death

28/Table 1

The Principal Sources of Air Embolus

Surgical (danger increased by low central venous pressure)	Operations involving the veins of the head, neck, thorax, abdomen or pelvis. Operations on an open, dry heart. Operations for lacerations of the liver or cavae.
Obstetrical and Gynaecological	Delivery in the presence of placenta praevia. Insufflation of the fallopian tubes. Criminal abortion.
Diagnostic	Air encephalography. Angiocardiography.
Therapeutic	Intravenous therapy. Maxillary antrum washout. Pneumothorax and pneumoperitoneum. Vaginal insufflation of powder.
Accidental	Rupture of alveolus during positive-pressure respiration.

(Adapted from Nicholson and Crehan, 1956.)

depends upon the state of the patient, but as little as 10–15 ml. may be fatal when the heart is already handicapped by such factors as disease or oligaemia (Simpson, 1942). Massive venous air embolism fills the vascular bed of the lungs, the heart and the venae cavae and leads to death from anoxia. There is, in fact, pulmonary arterial obstruction with acute cor pulmonale, consequent hypotension and cerebral anoxia. Smaller quantities of air may pass through the right side of the heart without disrupting its beat but are likely to cause some obstruction in the pulmonary arterial circulation, which is ultimately reflected in the systemic circulation. Small amounts of air can also cross the pulmonary capillaries and reach the coronary and cerebral arterial circulations.

The two prominent clinical signs that rapidly follow the entry of a reasonable volume of air into a vein are marked hypotension and irregular respiration. At this stage, auscultation of the heart will reveal a loud murmur due to the air being broken up in the blood and forming a frothy mixture. If the patient is unanaesthetised, convulsions may precede loss of consciousness. Circulatory failure and respiratory arrest rapidly follow, but the heart usually continues to beat for several minutes. It is this last fact that encourages immediate treatment.

The most important factor in treatment is undoubtedly speedy recognition of the complication, and this in some measure necessitates anticipation. In certain situations which enhance the opportunities for air to enter a vein—such as the sitting position for neurosurgical procedures in the posterior fossa—trouble can be expected when the surgeon approaches the venous sinuses. Then prevention by avoiding deep breathing, particularly when this follows coughing, and temporary pressure on the jugular veins in the neck are obviously indicated, but so also is especially careful observation of the patient for the earliest signs of air embolism. Occasionally the hiss of air entering a vein can be heard, but usually the general signs are the first indication of the complication. Then the source of entry must be closed immediately, and the patient rapidly placed in the left lateral position and tilted head downward. This position encourages the air to remain in the right atrium. Artificial respiration with 100 per cent oxygen should be carried out. This also avoids increase in the size of the bubble by preventing diffusion inwards of nitrous oxide (Munson and Merrick, 1966). When the peripheral pulse does not return within a minute, the chest must be opened and, if the heart is beating, air aspirated from the right side of the heart. Cardiac massage may help to restore an effective circulation at this stage, and should, of course, be carried out at once if the heart has already stopped (Durant *et al.*, 1947; Hamby and Terry, 1952). When a pressure chamber is immediately available the air bubbles can be made to shrink in size by increasing the ambient pressure around the patient by one atmosphere (Kylstra, 1963).

Arterial Air Embolus

Air is most likely to reach the left side of the heart during intracardiac operations or as a result of lung puncture and entry into the pulmonary veins. It may also arise paradoxically from the right side of the heart when one or other septum is patent, a risk which is greatly increased in the presence of right-to-left shunts, when all intravenous therapy and injections must be scrupulous in technique in regard to air bubbles.

Death is usually due to air emboli obstructing a coronary artery which quickly leads to ventricular fibrillation. It is very difficult to remove air from the coronary arteries although it can be forced through to the venous side if a sufficiently high pressure can be produced in the aorta (Geoghegan and Lam, 1953). The aorta is clamped, the ventricle aspirated and cardiac compression applied. The aortic pressure can be raised further by the intra-aortic infusion of blood, but this technique is probably only applicable when coronary air embolism arises during extracorporeal circulation.

Fat Embolus

This usually follows fracture of a bone—typically a long bone or rib—or rupture of the liver or kidney. It may result from an operative procedure on a bone and rarely may follow sudden decompression in a deep sea diver or high altitude flier.

Sevitt (1960; 1962*a*) has shown that pulmonary fat embolism is very common after injury and he believes it to be almost universal after fracture of a marrow bone. Clinically fat embolism can be divided into three groups; first the fulminating case, secondly the classical syndrome with cerebral, neurological and respiratory symptoms, and thirdly the incomplete or partial case. A fulminating embolus may occur within a few hours or days of a severe traumatic injury and is generally only diagnosed when the brain is sectioned after a post-mortem. Fat embolism may be suspected when the patient fails to respond to adequate resuscitation therapy, and when a period of normal consciousness subsequent to the injury is followed by coma. The classical syndrome can be expected to occur suddenly some twenty-four hours after an injury, and is typified by a mixture of mental confusion, often with localising neurological symptoms and signs, and respiratory distress with pyrexia. It seems probable that the respiratory complications are neurogenic in origin and not due to pulmonary fat embolism (Sevitt, 1960). Finally, the picture is completed by the appearance of a petechial skin eruption on the arms, chest and abdomen. An incomplete or partial case is normally mild in its course but shows some of the symptoms and signs already described.

The diagnosis of fat embolism is usually made from a clinical assessment, but examination of the retina may reveal fat globules in the vessels. Some substantiation of the diagnosis may be made from the finding of free fat in the urine or in the sputum. Sevitt suggests that a needle biopsy of the kidney to demonstrate glomerular fat embolism is useful in obscure cases of coma. The presence of petechial haemorrhages on the head, neck and thorax is said to be an important diagnostic point and histological examination of a petechia will demonstrate fat.

Recently fresh theories of the origin of fat emboli have been put forward which help to explain some of the surprising features of fat embolism, in particular the mechanism whereby systemic embolism occurs and the fact that the emboli globules have a quite different cholesterol content from bone fat (Ellis and Watson, 1968).

After injury the blood lipid level rises, reaching a peak at around three days. While clinical fat embolus can occur very shortly after injury, the time of greatest incidence coincides with the peak in the blood lipid level (O'Driscoll and Powell, 1967). The hyperlipaemia appears to be the result of reduced ability to disperse colloids in the blood. At the same time excess fat enters the blood stream as a result of trauma and in the event of hypovolaemic shock, mobilisation of tissue fluid results in quantities of fat entering the circulation via the thoracic duct.

The rise in blood lipids leads to a supersaturation of the blood with fat and a "crystallising out" of aggregations of chylomicrons which affect principally the lungs but which, when severe, occurs in the systemic arterial tree.

Treatment.—To prevent fat embolism in patients at risk, hypovolaemia and shock should be treated vigorously and clofibrate ("Atromid-S") can be used to depress the lipaemia which follows injury (dose 750 mg. initially, 500 mg. 8-hourly reducing over a week).

In the established case heparin has been suggested, based on the hypothesis that it can improve the solubility of fat in blood (Freeman, 1962). It is increasingly reported that many of the symptoms, particularly in the central nervous system, are the result of a severe unrecognised arterial hypoxia which regularly accompanies fat embolism and that relief follows the use of IPPR with oxygen and chest physiotherapy. Established cerebral coma can be treated with hypothermia, vasodilators and flow improvers, and corticosteroids (Larson, 1968; Galloon and Chakravarty, 1967).

Tumour Embolus

Tumour embolism may occur spontaneously or at operation, and, should the pieces of growth be big enough, can obstruct the pulmonary arterial or the systemic circulation, depending upon the site of the growth. Sudden death may occur from pulmonary obstruction or obstruction of the outflow tract of the left heart. Probert (1956) describes a patient who died suddenly during exploration of a carcinoma of the bronchus due to tumour embolism in the pulmonary veins.

POST-OPERATIVE VENOUS THROMBOSIS AND PULMONARY EMBOLISM

Deep Vein Thrombosis

So many factors can contribute to venous thrombosis in the post-operative period that it is probably unwise to dogmatise unduly on the importance of any one. The association of several conditions such as a severe operation in the pelvis of an old, obese patient in cardiac failure who has varicose veins, and a protracted period of immobilisation after operation, may well culminate in venous thrombosis. Although perhaps the most important predisposing factor is a previous history of deep vein thrombosis, too often a fatal pulmonary embolism occurs unexpectedly soon after a trivial operation in a fit, young patient, and is the first indication of venous thrombosis (Sevitt, 1962*b*).

Both anaesthetic and operation are conducive to venous stasis. Certain positions on the operating table and some anaesthetic techniques favour venous pooling of the blood. The removal of all skeletal muscle tone and the direct effects of surgical trauma—as in pelvic operations—are normal accompaniments of many operations, and may be accentuated should the operation be prolonged or associated with oligaemia. Most deep vein thromboses start either during surgery or in the immediate post-operative period, that is within the first 24 or 48 hours after surgery. Which factors are of prime importance is hard to prove, but in the post-operative period, the venous stasis consequent on immobilisation or restricted muscular movement has added to it the metabolic changes initiated by surgery and in this period the normal balance between thrombosing and antithrombosing factors in the blood may be upset, leading to a tendency to thrombosis. This tendency is accentuated in the presence of an infection.

Diagnosis.—The diagnosis is not always obvious, 70 per cent of deep vein thromboses having neither signs nor symptoms. The most reliable sign when it occurs is ankle oedema; less reliable but much commoner are tenderness of the calf or a slight rise in temperature, and diagnosis depends partly on a suspicious mind in the doctor.

The diagnosis is now made more frequently since the introduction of scanning techniques such as the ultra sound flow meter applied over the femoral or iliac vessels, and the use of ^{125}I-labelled fibrinogen (Kakkar *et al.*, 1970). A more exact knowledge of the extent of the thrombus within the vessels can be obtained by the use of phlebography performed on unanaesthetised patients.

Pulmonary Embolism

The common sites of origin for a pulmonary embolism are the veins of the pelvis and lower extremities—small emboli arising from the calves while large emboli come from the ilio-femoral venous segment. In cardiac disease thrombi may originate on the right side of the heart. The total incidence of pulmonary embolism is very high—in unselected post-mortem examinations as many as 70 per cent of cases can be shown to have some degree of pulmonary emboli—but the incidence of clinically detectable pulmonary embolism in post-operative patients is probably less than 1 per cent. This incidence is of course much higher in groups of patients particularly at risk, notably those with a previous history of thrombo-embolism and those undergoing orthopaedic operations or splenectomy.

The common time of occurrence is some days—3 to 21—after an operation, but this depends on the patient being fit and well previously. If the predisposing factors have existed for some time pre-operatively the time scale is shifted—the embolism may even occur at the time of operation. Fractured neck of femur followed by late reduction in an elderly patient—a situation full of predisposing factors—may well result in a pulmonary embolus at the time of reduction.

Diagnosis.—Sudden pain in the chest and dyspnoea are the classical symptoms, and if the blood clot is large enough to obstruct the pulmonary arterial circulation materially, death may rapidly follow from acute cor pulmonale. Smaller degrees of obstruction produce a less catastrophic picture but evidence of right ventricular failure—dyspnoea, tachycardia, venous engorgement, hypotension—may be present to some degree. The ECG may show right ventricular strain and the chest X-ray shows the "pruning" of the affected pulmonary vessels.

Small emboli usually cause little more than pain and dyspnoea in the first place, but these symptoms may be followed after twenty-four hours by haemoptysis, fever, and signs of pulmonary infarction. The ultimate circulatory result of a simple pulmonary embolus in a given patient is influenced partly by the size of the embolus and partly by the preceding state of the patient's heart and pulmonary vasculature—thus some patients may survive a single large pulmonary embolism, while others die from the effects of repeated small ones.

Treatment.—The best treatment is prophylactic. The prevention of venous stasis, both during the operation, whenever this is possible, and particularly in the post-operative period, is important. Recently intra-operative electrical stimulation of the calf muscles to increase venous blood flow has been tried apparently with good effect. The classical prophylactic measures are not proven in their efficacy except in major operations in the elderly (Flanc *et al.*, 1969), but elevation of the foot of the bed to promote venous return to the heart, early ambulation, and avoidance of any factor—such as a donkey pillow beneath the knees—that might impede venous drainage and movement of the lower limbs in bed, would seem reasonable precautions.

In high risk patients, particularly after trauma or during orthopaedic or gynaecological operations the prophylactic use of anticoagulants may be indicated (Sarnoff, 1969). The limited popularity of this technique, despite its proven value, is indicative of the logistic and other difficulties which ensue.

Simple Deep Vein Thrombosis

The initial treatment of simple deep vein thrombosis is to anticoagulate the patient with an intravenous dose of 12,000 units of heparin followed by 10,000 units four-hourly (i.v.). Choice of treatment then lies between the long term (6 months) use of anticoagulants either alone or preceded by thrombectomy, although this is only suitable for thrombosis in the ilio-femoral region. It is possible that in the future the use of parenteral streptokinase may become the most effective treatment for established deep vein thrombosis (Kakkar, 1969). For continued anticoagulation therapy 35 mg. warfarin sodium is given orally at the same time as the initial dose of heparin and the prothrombin time estimated after 48 hours. Subsequent doses of warfarin are chosen on the basis of the prothrombin time—the aim being to increase this twice or threefold. Routine blood prothrombin times must be estimated during the course of treatment.

Deep Vein Thrombosis with Pulmonary Embolism

As with simple deep vein thrombosis the initial treatment is with heparin. A phlebogram is performed to define the thrombi. If the thrombus appears old and well fixed long-term anticoagulation is the only treatment necessary; if however the clot appears fresh and loose and is thought likely to cause further emboli then more radical treatment is required. Thrombectomy is possible for thrombi lying in the major vessels, but where the smaller vessels, such as the calf veins, are affected, then either peripheral vein ligation or streptokinase therapy are indicated, although recent surgery may prohibit the latter. Thrombectomy or peripheral vein ligation may be performed under general anaesthesia when the anaesthetist may be called upon to perform a Valsalva manoeuvre to reverse the flow in the inferior vena cava at the moment the vein is opened. The anaesthetist should also remember that positioning on the table, perhaps even the muscle fasciculations of succinylcholine, may precipitate a further larger pulmonary embolus during anaesthesia and careful monitoring of the patient is necessary despite the apparent simplicity of the surgical procedure.

Pulmonary Embolism

The treatment of pulmonary artery embolism depends on the degree of pulmonary artery obstruction and the pre-existing state of the patient. The immediate treatment consists of the administration of heparin, the use of oxygen to prevent hypoxia, and the administration of digitalis and vasopressor drugs when indicated to support the circulation and in particular the right ventricle.

The extremes of pulmonary embolism provide no problem in treatment. The patient who is severely disabled, dyspnoeic, and in imminent danger of death, needs surgical removal of the embolus. This is preceded wherever possible by pulmonary angiography to define the affected vessels. It may be necessary to use supportive bypass, in addition to the other supportive measures, at the time of investigation, which is best carried out on an X-ray table in the theatre. It is then possible to continue the operation, with cardiopulmonary bypass if necessary, without delay. These patients are best investigated by pulmonary angiography without anaesthesia, but when anaesthesia is necessary it represents an extreme hazard for the patient and a most taxing demand on the anaesthetist (see Chapter 24).

Patients with small pulmonary emboli are treated with anticoagulants and the deep vein thrombosis considered separately for special treatment as defined above. The difficulty in choice of treatment lies in those patients who have had major pulmonary emboli but who are not so ill as to require immediate pulmonary embolectomy. These are probably best investigated with a pulmonary angiogram and then treated with streptokinase.

REFERENCES

BEARD, A. J. (1964). Cardiac arrest. *Proc. roy. Soc. Med.*, **57,** 365.

COOLEY, D. A. (1950). Cardiac resuscitation during operations for pulmonic stenosis. *Ann. Surg.*, **132,** 930.

DURANT, T. M., LONG, J., and OPPENHEIMER, M. J. (1947). Pulmonary (venous) air embolism. *Amer. Heart J.*, **33,** 269.

ELLIS, H. A., and WATSON, A. J. (1968). Studies on the genesis of traumatic fat embolism in man. *Amer. J. Path.*, **53,** 245.

FLANC, C., KAKKAR, V. V., and CLARKE, M. B. (1969). Postoperative deep vein thrombosis. *Lancet*, **1,** 477.

FREEMAN, M. A. R. (1962). Heparin in the treatment of fat embolism. *Lancet*, **1,** 1302.

GALLOON, S., and CHAKRAVARTY, K. (1967). Fat embolism treated with intermittent positive pressure ventilation. *Brit. J. Anaesth.*, **39,** 71.

GEOGHEGAN, T., and LAM, C. R. (1953). The mechanism of death from intracardiac air and its reversibility. *Ann. Surg.*, **138,** 351.

GUREWICH, V., SASAHARA, A. A., QUINN, J. S., PEFFER, C. J., and LITTMAN, O. (1961). Aortic pressures during closed-chest cardiac massage. *Circulation*, **23,** 593.

HAMBY, W. B., and TERRY, R. N. (1952). Air embolism in operations done in the sitting position; a report of five fatal cases and one of rescue by a simple maneuver. *Surgery*, **31,** 212.

KAKKAR, V. V. (1969). The problems of thrombosis in the deep veins of the leg. *Ann. roy. Coll. Surg. Engl.*, **45,** 257.

KAKKAR, V. V., NICHOLAIDES, A. N., RENNEY, J. T. G., FRIEND, J. R., and CLARKE, M. B. (1970). ^{125}I labelled fibrinogen test adapted for routine screening for deep vein thrombosis. *Lancet*, **1,** 540.

KOUWENHOVEN, W. B., and KNICKERBOCKER, G. G. (1961). The development of a portable defibrillator. *Trans. Amer. Inst. elect. Engrs.*, **81,** Part III, p. 428.

KOUWENHOVEN, W. B., JUDE, J. R., and KNICKERBOCKER, G. G. (1960). Closed chest cardiac massage. *J. Amer. med. Ass.*, **173,** 1064.

KYLSTRA, J. A. (1963). Air embolism. *Lancet*, **1,** 720.

LARSON, A. G. (1968). Treatment of cerebral fat embolism with phenoxybenzamine and surface cooling. *Lancet*, **2,** 250.

LOWN, B., NEWMAN, J., AMARASINGHAM, R., and BERKOVIT, B. V. (1962). Comparison of alternating current with direct current electroshock across the closed chest. *Amer. J. Cardiol.*, **10,** 223.

MUNSON, E. G., and MERRICK, H. C. (1966). Effect of nitrous oxide on venous air embolism. *Anaesthesiology*, **27,** 283.

NICHOLSON, M. J., and CREHAN, J. P. (1956). Emergency treatment of air embolism. *Curr. Res. Anaesth.*, **35,** 634.

O'DRISCOLL, T. M., and POWELL, F. J. (1967). Injury, serum lipids, fat embolism and clofibrate. *Brit. med. J.*, **4,** 149.

OLIVER, G. C., Jr., GAZETOPOULOS, N., and HYWEL DAVIES, D. (1964). Effect of closed-chest cardiac massage on the aortic pulse during ventricular fibrillation. *Lancet*, **1,** 1303.

PELESKA, B. (1963). Résultats des recherches faites sur le méthode de défibrillation à l'aide des décharges d'un condensateur. *Rev. Agressologie*, **4,** 483.

PROBERT, W. R. (1956). Sudden operative death due to massive tumour embolism. *Brit. med. J.*, **1,** 435.

SARNOFF, J. G. (1969). Prevention of sudden cardiopulmonary arrest in the postoperative period with prophylactic heparin. *Lancet*, **2,** 292.

SEVITT, S. (1960). The significance and classification of fat embolism. *Lancet*, **2,** 825.

SEVITT, S. (1962*a*). *Fat Embolism*. London: Butterworth & Co.
SEVITT, S. (1962*b*). Venous thrombosis and pulmonary embolism. *Amer. J. med.*, **33,** 703.
SHILLINGFORD, J. P. (1964). The differential diagnosis of conditions leading to acute cardiac arrest outside the operating theatre. *Brit. J. Anaesth.*, **36,** 550.
SIMPSON, K. (1942). Air accidents during transfusion. *Lancet*, **1,** 697.
SYKES, M. K. (1964). Organisation of a resuscitation service and results of treatment. *Proc. roy. Soc. Med.*, **57,** 372.
WEINBERGER, L. W., GIBBON, M. H., and GIBBON, J. H., Jr. (1940). Temporary arrest of circulation to central nervous system; physiologic effects. *Arch. Neurol. Psychiat.* (*Chicago*), **43,** 615.
WETHERILL, J. H., and NIXON, P. G. F. (1962). Spontaneous cessation of ventricular fibrillation during external cardiac massage. *Lancet*, **1,** 993.

Section Three

THE NERVOUS SYSTEM

Chapter 29

NORMAL NEUROMUSCULAR TRANSMISSION

Nerve Conduction

During a period of rest the surface membrane of a nerve cell is described as being in a state of polarity. That is to say, a potential difference exists between the outside and the inside of the cell. This difference is due to the relative concentrations of ions on either side of the cell membrane. Thus, potassium (K^+) and chloride (Cl^-) ions predominate on the inside, and sodium (Na^+) and chloride (Cl^-) on the outside. The cell membrane, however, is selective and impedes the flow of some ions more than others. This property is described as permeability. Normally only small quantities of ions are permitted to traverse the barrier, so that the concentration of potassium (K^+) ions inside the cell is some 20–50 times greater than that on the outside. Conversely, the amount of sodium (Na^+) ions on the outside of the cell is 3–15 times greater than on the inside (Hodgkin, 1951).

The net result of this difference in ionic concentration between the two sides of the membrane is that there is a preponderance of negatively charged ions on the inside. In other words the interior of the cell is negatively charged in relation to the outside. This potential difference is termed the resting membrane potential.

In terms of electrical charges the resting membrane potential of a nerve fibre is approximately 60–90 millivolts* (inside negative). Before activity commences this negative charge drops to a level of 45 millivolts (inside negative); thus the threshold for activity represents a change of some 15 millivolts from the resting state. Once this threshold has been reached the membrane momentarily loses its powers of permeability and it explodes into activity as ions pass freely from one side to the other. The result of this activity is to produce an electrical change much greater than the resting potential. This response is termed an *action potential* and at its peak it represents about 100 millivolts. In other words, the potential inside the cell of some 60 millivolts (negative) has now become changed to about 40 millivolts (positive)—a total alteration of at least 100 millivolts. The whole process involving the production of an action potential is called *depolarisation*, although it is, in fact, merely a reversal of polarisation.

During the resting phase both sodium and potassium ions are slowly traversing the surface membrane; radio-active isotope studies suggest that the potassium ions move slightly faster than the sodium (Keynes, 1949). The reason for this is probably that the surface membrane is relatively less permeable to sodium than it is to the potassium ions. It has been suggested that the balance between sodium and potassium ions is maintained by an active extrusion of the sodium ions from within the cell. This process is sometimes referred to as the sodium pump.

The whole process of conduction of a nerve impulse along either a nerve or a muscle fibre has been reviewed by Katz (1966). Conduction depends on two main

* 1 millivolt (mV) = 1 thousandth of a volt.

factors—the continuity of the cable-like structure of the cell and also an automatic system of amplification which is built into the cell's surface-membrane. The cell membrane itself has a low electrical conductivity and were it not for this amplification system a brief stimulus in the line would fade away within a few millimetres.

When the potential across the membrane is displaced by a certain critical amount (i.e. 15–45 millivolts) the so-called "threshold" is reached and the stability of the membrane potential is temporarily destroyed. At this point, sodium ions pour into the interior whilst after a fractional delay potassium ions pass outwards.

During the act of local depolarisation sodium ions pour into the interior of the cell in an attempt to establish equilibrium, but they are soon thwarted by the restoration of permeability to the cell membrane and are then actively extruded again. Meanwhile, the role of the potassium ions tends to become more prominent and these pass back into the cell to re-establish the resting conditions. The time relationship between these ionic changes has been excellently summarised by del Castillo and Katz (1956).

"Both Na and K permeabilities increase when the membrane is depolarised, but the sodium change precedes in time and is transient, while the K change is delayed and maintained. The important point is that the two specific permeability changes have different time-lags and are out of phase. In the normal course of events the rise of the action potential is brought about by the rapid entry of Na into the fibre, while the accelerated outflow of potassium serves to re-establish the resting condition and to ensure a quick decline of the action potential, followed by a slower recovery of the normal conductances."

The electrical energy suddenly released by this local act of depolarisation leads to a large transient amplification of the initial potential change. This amplified signal is then passed on to the neighbouring region of the fibre by cable linkage and the whole process is repeated. In this manner the response travels rapidly down the nerve fibre or along the muscle fibre without any diminution in the amplitude of the signal. The final outcome is an "all or none" response which ignites an explosive amplification of the potential that is continuously propagated to the end of the cell.

Pre-junctional or Pre-synaptic Area

The arrival of an impulse or nerve action potential at the end of the cable system (i.e. nerve) gives rise to a special situation. Despite arguments to the contrary, it is now almost universally accepted that the conduction of an impulse from nerve to muscle is not a simple electrical response but relies on the release of acetylcholine at the nerve ending to bridge the gap. This is the chemical theory of neuromuscular transmission as propounded by Dale *et al.* (1936). The work of Katz and Miledi (1965) has produced convincing evidence to support this theory because they demonstrated that there was a measurable time lag between the arrival of an impulse at the nerve ending and the release of the transmitter substance (acetylcholine).

The area of the nerve ending is obviously a very important one because at this point the formation, storage and finally liberation of acetylcholine have a very special significance. For purposes of description, therefore, these roles of acetylcholine are best considered as three separate compartments, though in reality they must be intertwined (Fig. 1).

(*a*) **Synthesis of acetylcholine.**—Acetylcholine is formed by the acetylation of choline with the help of the enzyme of cholineacetylase*. In normal circumstances there is an abundance of both choline and the enzyme available at the

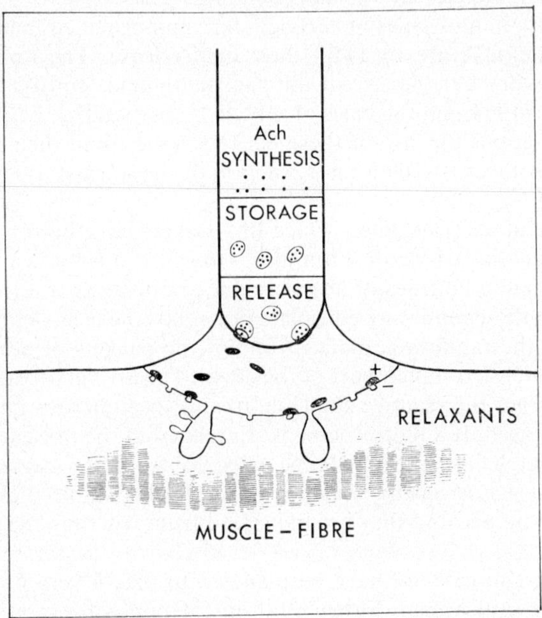

29/Fig. 1.—Diagram to show the three compartments at the nerve-ending. Note the packets or quanta of acetylcholine molecules in the storage region and their subsequent rupture on release.

nerve terminals because large quantities of choline can be absorbed from the extracellular space (Birks and Macintosh, 1957 and 1961). The discovery of a compound—hemicholinium—has thrown further light on this matter as it is capable of interfering with the transport of choline to the nerve-ending for manufacture into acetylcholine. It is, therefore, experimentally possible to reduce the amount of acetylcholine formed at the nerve-ending. The result of poisoning the nerve-ending with hemicholinium is that whilst electrophysiologically a single stimulus can be recorded, the demand of fast or tetanic rates of stimuli is too great and neuromuscular transmission fails. In normal circumstances, however, the factory for acetylcholine has immense powers of recovery and even though output is exhausted by a period of tremendous demand (i.e. very rapid stimulation), provided a few seconds rest are given, it can recuperate and respond normally. Under the influence of hemicholinium this is no longer possible, so that the phenomenon of post-tetanic exhaustion is observed. This means there is a failure to re-establish normal neuromuscular transmission (even at slow rates of stimulation) after a burst of tetanic stimulation. Such a condition is only

* The enzyme aids the transfer of an acetyl group from acetyl-CoA to choline in the presence of the enzyme (cholineacetylase).

observed in the experimental animal under the influence of hemicholinium and clinically in patients with severe myasthenia gravis (Desmedt, 1966) and in the premature infant under the influence of a depolarising drug (Churchill-Davidson and Wise, 1964).

(*b*) **Storage of acetylcholine.**—The advent of electronmicroscopy has revealed the presence of vesicles at the nerve-ending. These packets, or quanta, are believed to contain molecules of acetylcholine. In normal circumstances they are stored after manufacture to await their final release. The number of quanta available may vary but the size of the packets remains constant. Elmquist and his co-workers (1964), on the basis of muscle biopsy studies, have suggested that in myasthenia gravis the size of these packets rather than their total number is reduced so that there is only a mere fraction of the normal amount present (see p. 911).

(*c*) **Release of acetylcholine.**—Once the packets have been formed and duly stored, all awaits the arrival of a stimulus. However, it is known that even in the resting state small quantities of acetylcholine are being sporadically released. It is believed that these miniature end-plate potentials (i.e. acetylcholine molecules) are caused by the random contact of one of the packets of acetylcholine with a critical spot on the terminal part of the nerve. The arrival of an impulse (action potential) enlarges the reactive site (Fig. 6) and so numerous packets of acetylcholine are released. If a motor nerve is stimulated in the presence of *d*-tubocurarine, then acetylcholine will still be released from the nerve-ending in the normal amount (Krryević and Mitchell, 1961) but these molecules fail to produce a muscle response because they are prevented from reaching the post-junctional receptors.

Magnesium and calcium have been shown to play a very important role in the *release* of acetylcholine. Either a fall in calcium concentration or a rise of magnesium will greatly reduce the number of acetylcholine molecules that are liberated from the nerve-ending (del Castillo and Engbaek, 1954; Katz and Miledi, 1964 and 1965). Other substances which are believed to interfere with the release of acetylcholine are some of the mycin group of antibiotics (for details see p. 839), botulinus toxin and possibly procaine. The probability, however, is that the local anaesthetics affect the synthesis of acetylcholine more than the actual release of the molecules. The pathological condition called the myasthenic syndrome, which is sometimes found in patients with a bronchial carcinoma, is also believed to be associated with a difficulty in release of acetylcholine. The whole process is summarised in diagrammatic form in Fig. 2.

The Neuromuscular Junction

On leaving the pre-junctional area (i.e. the nerve-ending) the acetylcholine molecules traverse a minute gap before arriving at the post-junctional area on the muscle membrane. The term "neuromuscular junction", therefore, includes both pre- and post-synaptic areas. The post-synaptic area, however, is sometimes also referred to as the motor end-plate. Evidence for the function of this area again outstrips a knowledge of its structure but in recent years the advent of the electron microscope has thrown new light on the possible relationship between structure and function. Much of the basic information has been provided by the remarkable studies of Couteaux (1955 and 1958) and Robertson (1956).

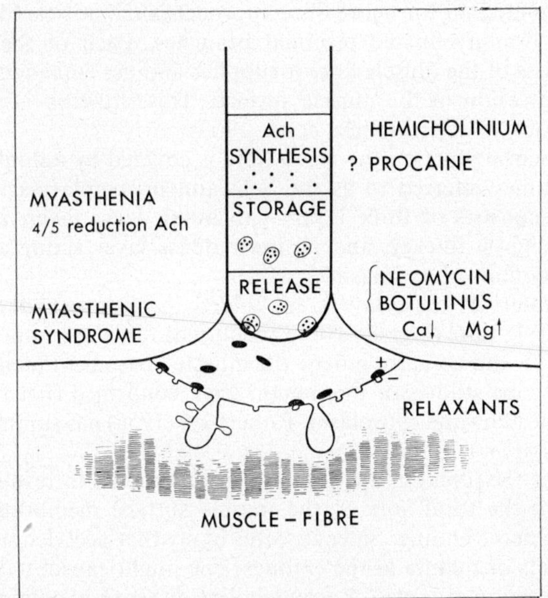

29/FIG. 2.—Diagram to summarise the possible sites of action of various drugs and diseases at the nerve-ending.

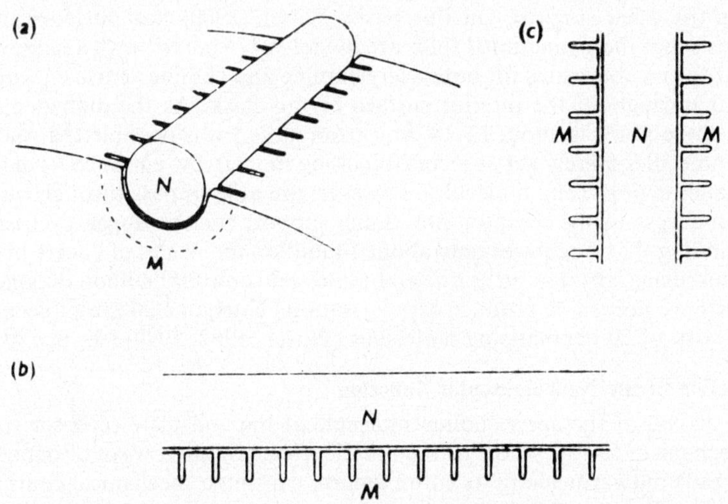

29/FIG. 3.—DIAGRAM OF NEUROMUSCULAR JUNCTION.

(*a*) Shows a small portion of the terminal axon branch N lying in a gutter formed by the surface of the muscle fibre M. The semi-circular post-junctional folds are illustrated.

(*b*) Same in longitudinal section.

(*c*) Same in tangential section.

As the myelinated motor nerve fibre approaches the muscle fibres, it divides into numerous non-myelinated terminal branches. Each of these fibres runs parallel to the axis of the muscle fibre it supplies and lies embedded in a shallow "gutter" or depression in the muscle surface. This situation is represented in diagrammatic form in Fig. 3 (Birks *et al.*, 1960).

At the myoneural junction the nerve fibre is covered by a double-membrane complex, sometimes referred to as the Schwann or axoplasmastic membrane. Essentially this consists of three layers—an outer dense layer, a middle clear zone which is slightly thicker, and an inner dense layer acting as a boundary margin for the contained axoplasm.

At regular intervals these layers are folded inwards to make indentations towards the muscle fibre (Fig. 4). These junctional folds are important because they pass close to and actually indent the muscle "basement membrane" itself. Electron microscope studies of this region have confirmed that these folds are involutions of the Schwann cytoplasm. Robertson (1956) has summarised the importance of this area as follows:

"The folds of the junction are admirably constructed to bring about a very great increase in the total area of the muscle surface membrane complex in contact with the nerve ending. Since it seems likely that acetylcholine is secreted in discrete packets or quanta at the endings, one might expect to see something analogous to secretion granules of acetylcholine either in axoplasm, sarcoplasm or within the junctional membranes. It seems reasonable to speculate that the tubular or vesicular bodies of terminal axoplasm might represent such packets of acetylcholine."

Electron microscopic studies of this region demonstrate the close proximity of the vesicles (containing acetylcholine) on the one hand with these junctional folds on the other (Fig. 5). On this basis, Waser (1960) has put forward the hypothesis that these junctional folds are in fact only "pores" with a narrow neck and that the receptor sites for both acetylcholine and cholinesterase enzymes are scattered throughout the interior surface of this flask. As the diameter of the neck of these pores is about 12–14 Ångstrom units,* it is possible that the large curare molecules merely act as a cork blocking the narrow entrance to the flask. The smaller depolarising molecules, however, are able to pass through the neck and gain access to the receptor site. Some support for this suggestion is given by the finding that it requires only about 14 million molecules of curare to block neuromuscular transmission at one end-plate, yet some 300 million depolarising molecules are needed to produce depolarisation. Thus, one curare molecule can do the work of 20 depolarising molecules (Waser, 1962, 1970) (see p. 789).

Function of the Neuromuscular Junction

The arrival of the acetylcholine molecule at the end-plate receptor triggers off a mechanism for the whole of the muscle fibre, so that a wave of depolarisation spreads outwards along its entire length, causing a mechanical contraction in its wake. The acetylcholine molecules are destroyed by a specific enzyme—cholinesterase—almost as rapidly as they are produced. Fortunately they do not have far to travel because recent electron-microscope studies have revealed that the distance between the nerve membrane and the motor end-plate is in the

* Å = Ångström Unit. This is a unit of length, 1 being equivalent to 0·1 micro μ.

(a)

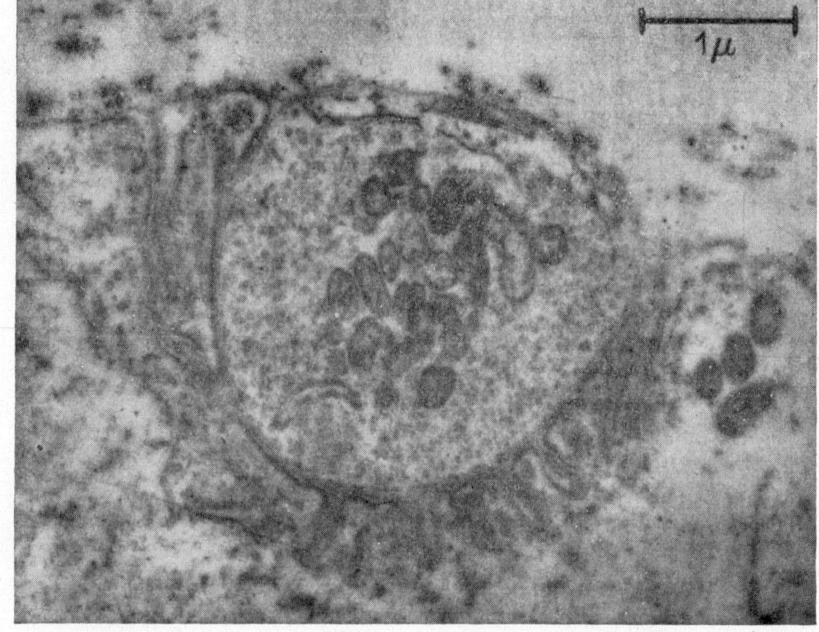

(b)

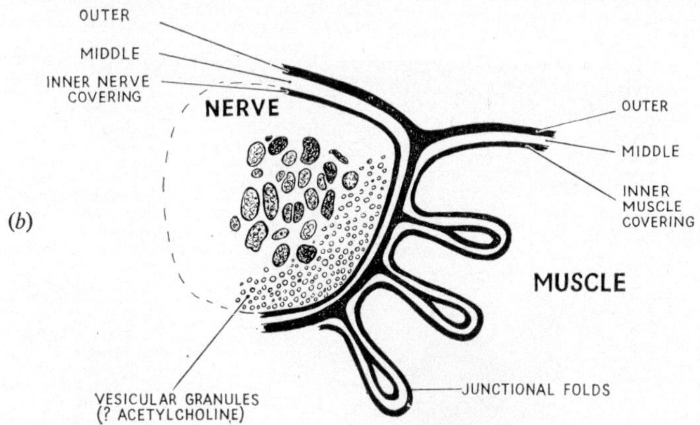

29/Fig. 4.—The Neuromuscular Junction.

(*a*) Electron microphotograph of a reptilian neuromuscular junction.
(*b*) Diagrammatic representation of the neuromuscular junction.

region of 1μ. This short range enables the acetylcholine molecules to excite the end-plate before being hydrolysed by cholinesterase. The existence and function of this enzyme can be verified by inhibiting its activity with an anticholinesterase drug (e.g. neostigmine) and thus permitting the concentration of acetylcholine ions to multiply.

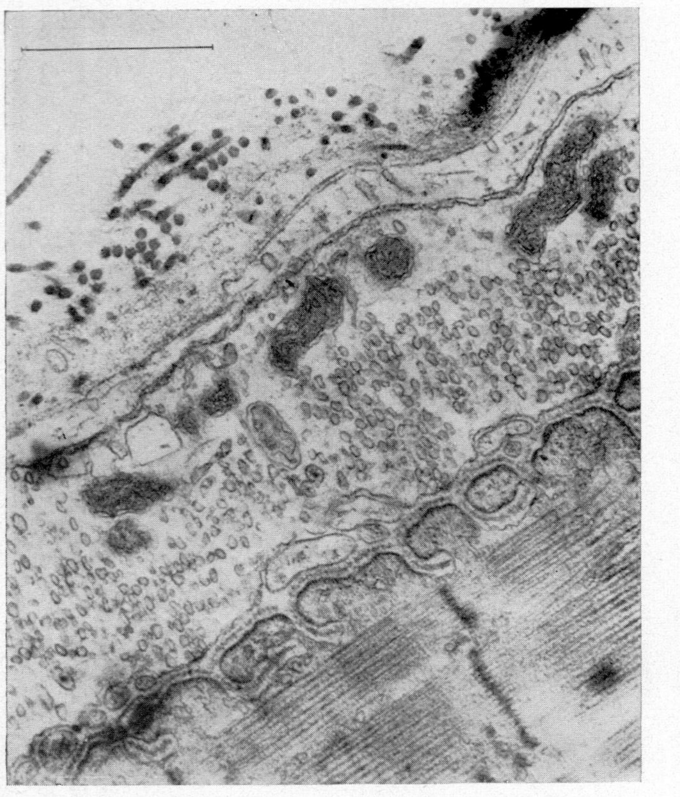

29/FIG. 5 (*a*).—Longitudinal section through the neuromuscular junction (frog).

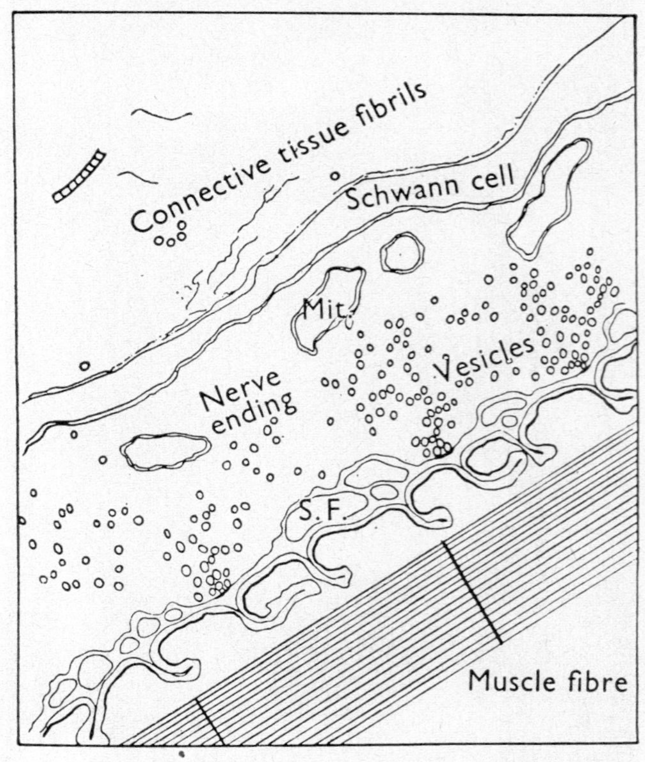

29/FIG. 5 (*b*).—Diagram of the various structures seen in (*a*).

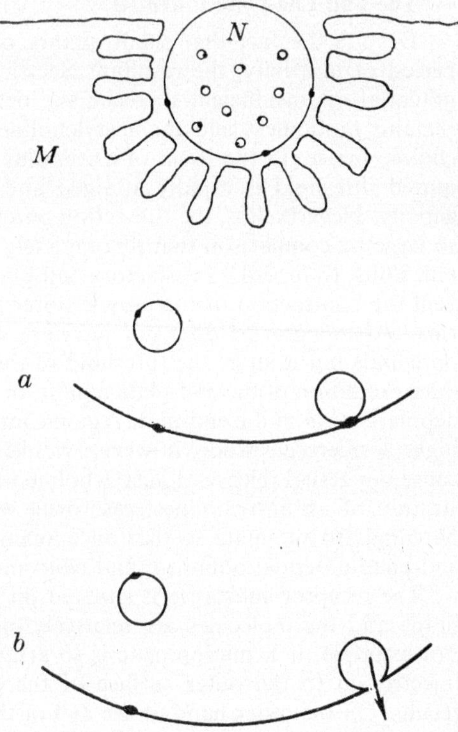

29/FIG. 6.—Diagram of vesicular hypothesis. N represents the nerve terminal with vesicles of acetylcholine contained within its lumen. M is the muscle fibre with synaptic folds. The reactive sites on both the surface of the vesicle and the terminal axon membrane are shown as black dots. When two reactive surfaces meet (as in *a*) then rupture and the release of acetylcholine molecules occurs (as in *b*).

The Resting End-plate Potential

When a micro-electrode is inserted at random into the middle of a resting muscle fibre, a steady potential of about 60–90 millivolts (inside negative) will be recorded. If the electrode is now moved gradually towards the end-plate region a point is finally reached where small potential changes of about 0·5 millivolts are recorded. These *miniature end-plate potentials* represent the release of the small packets of acetylcholine as each vesicle ruptures. Such miniature potentials occur at fairly regular intervals (about one per second) and are only observed in the resting state. The amplitude of one of these miniature potentials is insufficient to reach the threshold necessary to trigger off depolarisation of the end-plate itself.

The frequency of these miniature potentials (i.e. the rate of rupture of vesicles) depends on the conditions prevailing in the pre-synaptic region of the nerve-ending. For example, hemicholinium interferes with the synthesis of acetylcholine whilst botulinus toxin prevents the release of the transmitter substances. Both these agents reduce the frequency of the miniature potentials.

The amplitude of these miniature potentials, on the other hand, depends on the conditions at the post-synaptic membrane, i.e. on the muscle fibre. Here the principal controlling factors are the number of unblocked receptor sites available and also the degree of activity of the true cholinesterase enzyme.

The Full End-plate Potential

Despite the fact that small quanta of acetylcholine are released during a period of inactivity, the resultant electrical potential—the miniature end-plate potential—is insufficient to reach the necessary threshold so the muscle fibre remains motionless and the acetylcholine molecules are rapidly hydrolysed by cholinesterase. In the event of a stimulus passing down the nerve fibre, the required threshold is rapidly attained and the whole muscle fibre is fired into activity. Nevertheless, the full action potential of the contracting muscle fibre is so large by comparison that it completely swamps the original end-plate potential. Thus, to record a satisfactory end-plate potential it is necessary first to prevent the contraction of the muscle fibre: this is achieved by giving *d*-tubocurarine. *d*-Tubocurarine does not interfere with the liberation of these end-plate potentials but it alters the threshold of the muscle membrane necessary to produce excitation of the end-plate region. In a complete curare paralysis the act of depolarisation of the end-plate region cannot occur, because the threshold is too high. A micro-electrode, however, would record a true end-plate potential because the actual release of acetylcholine molecules is not impeded. The administration of an anti-cholinesterase drug would permit the miniature end-plate potentials to summate so that once again the threshold can be reached, a full end-plate potential obtained, and neuromuscular transmission restored.

The receptor substance is situated on the external surface of the cell membrane and the molecules are relatively insensitive to stimulation from within. For example, if a micropipette is so arranged that acetylcholine molecules are injected on to the outer surface of the end-plate region, then great activity results. On the other hand, if the end of the pipette is advanced slightly so that it now lies within the muscle cell, then the acetylcholine molecules are no longer effective (del Castillo and Katz, 1955).

The Role of the Inorganic Ions in Neuromuscular Transmission

The part played by potassium and sodium in the conduction of a nerve impulse has already been mentioned. The release of potassium from within both nerve and muscle cell is one of the most significant features of depolarisation. Apart from these two ions which behave in the muscle fibre in a similar fashion to that described in the nerve fibre, both magnesium and calcium can influence neuromuscular activity. Magnesium blocks neuromuscular transmission, probably by interfering with the pre-synaptic release of acetylcholine (del Castillo and Engbaek, 1954). If given in increasing quantities magnesium finally produces complete blockade. Similarly, withdrawal of calcium produces the same effect. The role of calcium is to oppose the neuromuscular blocking action of the magnesium and these two ions appear to be antagonistic. Del Castillo and Katz (1956) point out that this antagonism is spread over a wide range of concentrations so that a balance between the two effects is attained and the inhibition of the pre-synaptic release of acetylcholine is prevented. This antagonism between calcium and magnesium is only encountered in this connection because in nerve and muscle cells both these ions have a similar activity. These authors also emphasise that although at one time both sodium withdrawal and procaine were believed to reduce the pre-synaptic output of acetylcholine, more recent observations have shown that they lead to desensitisation of the end-plate receptor (Nastuk, 1954). Glucose is necessary for the synthesis of acetylcholine (Feldberg, 1945).

Removal of Acetylcholine

That acetylcholine molecules only have a minute distance (1μ) to travel before reaching their target has already been emphasised. Their subsequent fate, however, is a little more obscure. The majority are certainly hydrolysed by the specific enzyme—cholinesterase—to acetic acid and choline. The molecules of choline are then available for resynthesis by the nerve terminal. Nevertheless, some of the acetylcholine molecules probably diffuse into the interstitial space and are then no longer available to take part in the resynthesis process. Evidence for this diffusion process is based on the finding that acetylcholine molecules can be collected from the perfusion fluid of a nerve-muscle preparation that has been protected from hydrolysis by an inhibitor such as eserine (Brown *et al.*, 1936).

Alteration in the Sensitivity of the Motor End-plate Response

In considering the ultimate disposal of acetylcholine molecules, no account is taken of any possible alteration in the sensitivity of the motor end-plate region to the acetylcholine molecules. Originally it was believed that all drugs that acted by depolarisation produced a pure response at the motor end-plate. For example, the administration of decamethonium (a drug believed to act like acetylcholine) in the cat led first to an unco-ordinated contraction (fasciculation) followed by a prolonged paralysis due to depolarisation (Burns and Paton, 1951; Zaimis, 1951). In the same year, however, Jenden and his colleagues (1951), working on the isolated rabbit lumbrical muscle, obtained results with decamethonium that suggested this simple conception might not be correct.

Zaimis showed that the response of muscle to decamethonium varied remarkably, depending on the species selected for investigation. In fact it even varied from muscle to muscle in the same animal. Decamethonium was used in these investigations, not because it was a muscle relaxant but because it was believed to act like acetylcholine: it could therefore be used to study neuromuscular transmission. The results indicated that the muscles of man and the cat showed a persistent depolarisation in the presence of decamethonium: on the contrary, the muscles of the monkey, dog and hare produced a different type of response. At first, the block possessed the characteristics produced by acetylcholine, i.e. depolarisation, but subsequently the response changed, and though the motor end-plate appeared to have recovered its normal activity, neuromuscular transmission was still absent because the threshold of activity necessary to excite the muscle fibre had been greatly increased. In other words, decamethonium now appeared to be producing a block similar to that found after giving *d*-tubocurarine. This complex situation prompted Zaimis (1952) to state: "It is now clear that the results obtained from the muscles of any one mammalian species are valid only for this species". This statement is often forgotten by anaesthetists, yet it applies to all the actions of the muscle relaxants, even at sites other than the neuromuscular junction. Briefly, in clinical practice the only relevant studies with this group of drugs are those undertaken in man.

From the pharmacological evidence available the anaesthetist assumed that the depolarising relaxants acted by persistent depolarisation in man. This assumption proved incorrect. Gradually a number of cases were observed in which the paresis persisted longer than normally anticipated, yet an anti-cholinesterase appeared to improve rather than worsen neuromuscular transmission.

The reversal of a depolarisation block by an anti-cholinesterase drug could not be explained on the basis of a simple depolarisation of the end-plate. However, suitable techniques for measuring end-plate potentials in man were not readily available. Nevertheless, Churchill-Davidson and Richardson (1952) demonstrated electromyographically that an alteration in the response of the motor end-plate to depolarising drugs also occurred in man. Conclusive evidence for the appearance of a dual block (see p. 824) in man came when Churchill-Davidson and his co-workers (1960) demonstrated the deliberate production of this type of block, which was subsequently reversed by an anti-cholinesterase drug. In 1963, Katz and his co-workers confirmed these findings. It has also been shown that a similar type of block is produced in man by a single dose of a depolarising drug in the first few weeks of life (Churchill-Davidson and Wise, 1963).

Thesleff (1955), working with acetylcholine on an animal nerve-muscle preparation (frog) was able to throw some light on this problem. He showed that the local potential change in the end-plate region produced by the external application of acetylcholine molecules gradually declined despite the fact that there were ample supplies of acetylcholine molecules available. In other words, the end-plate region becomes less and less responsive to the depolarising action of acetylcholine, and finally a stage may be reached where a nerve impulse fails to produce a response of the muscle. A state of block without depolarisation is present.

Maclagan (1962) attempted to determine whether any difference existed in the results obtained with the muscle relaxants in the intact, perfused animal and *in vitro* specimens of the same muscle studied under artificial conditions in an ionic solution. Using the tenuissimus muscle of the cat, she found a disturbingly different response between the *in vivo* and the *in vitro* situations. *In vivo* decamethonium produced a steady depolarisation which persisted as long as the drug was administered. However, *in vitro* maximum paralysis developed quickly but recovery subsequently took place despite the continued presence of the drug in the bath. The conclusion was reached, therefore, that the artificial conditions produced by immersing the muscle in an ionic concentration must in some way be responsible for these different responses. As much of the pharmacological data on the effect of the muscle relaxants in animals is obtained in this manner, it is necessary to interpret their results with caution.

Further progress in understanding this complex process was made with the introduction of the radioactive muscle relaxants.

The Radioactive Muscle Relaxants

The object in preparing a radioactive form of a muscle relaxant is that this then permits the passage and the final destination of the drug to be studied. When injected into the mouse, this agent can be shown to occupy a specific area (the motor end-plates) on the diaphragm soon after injection. The technique involves

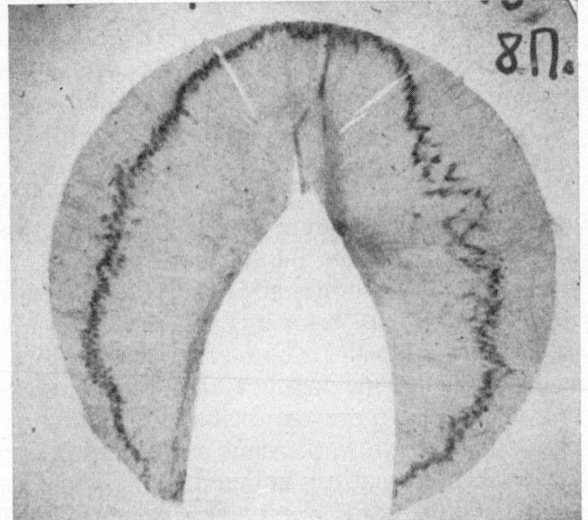

29/Fig. 7.—Effect of C^{14} toxiferine on the mouse diaphragm (Waser, 1960). Note the localised fixation of the toxiferine in the end-plate region.

killing the animal soon after apnoea has developed and then removing the diaphragm and placing it in contact with an ultra-sensitive film for a number of weeks. At the end of this time the film is developed (Fig. 7).

Using this technique combined with the electron microscope, it has been possible to distinguish individual end-plates and also to assess how molecules of toxiferine are bound to a single end-plate. These results have indicated that only a few highly differentiated receptors—widely distributed on the muscle membrane—are actually occupied by the muscle relaxant.

In contrast, the depolarising drugs have also been studied (Waser, 1960). A tagged form of decamethonium (C^{14} decamethonium) with six radioactive methyl groups has been used. The same technique demonstrated the direct action of these drugs on the motor end-plate. There were, however, some important differences. The density of the end-plate region was far greater after the de-

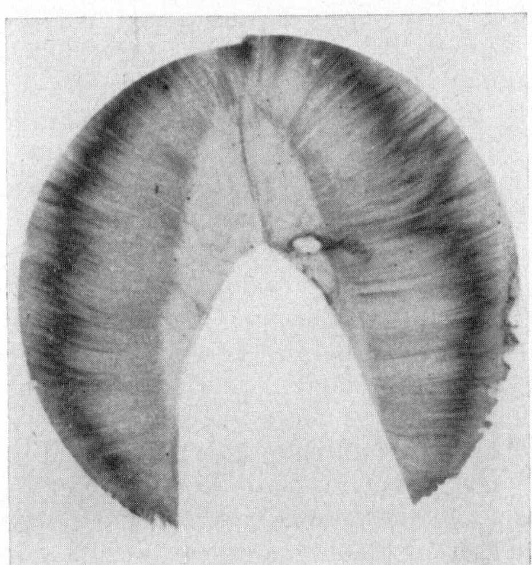

29/Fig. 8.—Effect of C^{14} decamethonium on the mouse diaphragm. Note the diffuse fixation of the drug in the end-plate region as contrasted with the localisation of toxiferine.

polarising than after the non-depolarising drug (Fig. 8). In fact, it appeared that 50 times as many depolarising molecules were taken up by the receptors compared with the non-depolarising ones. Furthermore, the clear-cut halo effect found with toxiferine gives way to a diffuse and blurred effect. It appears that decamethonium not only reaches the motor end-plate but may diffuse into the interior of the muscle cell.

Taylor (1959), using another labelled depolarising drug which is closely related to decamethonium (i.e. I^{131} iodocholinium dichloride) found a similar state of affairs. Using the rat lumbrical preparation, he found that the neuromuscular block produced by the depolarising drug always occurred in two phases with an interval for recovery between. The first phase of the block is characteristic of depolarisation and is both of rapid onset and short duration. If *d*-tubocurarine is given prior to the decamethonium it will inhibit the uptake of the depolarising molecules and so prevent the block from taking place. The second phase of the block does not show the signs of depolarisation but resembles that produced by curare itself in that it is antagonised by anti-cholinesterases, potassium ions and a fall in temperature, but it differs from a curare-block in that it takes 5–10 times as long to develop.

Taylor (1962) believes this delay in the development of the second phase is related to the penetration of the muscle fibre by the labelled depolarising drug. The point of entrance is the end-plate because a small dose of curare will close the door. *d*-Tubocurarine, however, does not appear to have any action in preventing the molecules from leaving the fibre once access has been attained, suggesting that the entrance and exit of the depolarising drug are by different means. Nevertheless, these results suggest that the depolarising drug must first enter the fibre before a Phase II block can develop.

In these experiments the muscle fibre was able to take up large quantities of the labelled depolarising drug and this uptake was closely associated with the development of a non-depolarising type of block. Furthermore, an anti-cholinesterase drug given after a large amount of depolarising drug had been stored led to an immediate improvement in neuromuscular transmission despite the fact that the muscle was unable to rid itself of the drug. The suggestion is made that neuromuscular transmission depends on the state of affairs prevailing at the end-plate irrespective of the condition of the interior of the fibre. Nevertheless the actual performance of the fibre under these conditions may be reduced.

More recently, studies have been carried out in rats using radioactive *d*-tubocurarine, gallamine and decamethonium iodide (Cohen *et al.*, 1968).

The Acetylcholine Receptor

The nature of this important structure is still in dispute. It is known that when a muscle is denervated new receptors appear, but instead of concentrating in the end-plate region as before, they spread out along the surface membrane of the muscle fibre. Waser (1960), using radioactive curare, took this matter a stage further and demonstrated that the curare molecules became attached to the new receptors. This led him to suggest that the nature of the receptor material might be a mucopolysaccharide. Other authors have contended that mucopolysaccharides do have an affinity for curare but they are an integral part of the basement membrane structure and not a physiological acetylcholine receptor (Chagas, 1962; Zacks and Blumberg, 1961).

Further suggestions have been made that it must be of a phosphate nature (Nastuk, 1967), or a polypeptide or protein (Gill, 1965).

The use of radioactive muscle relaxants has enabled investigators to estimate the amount of uptake of the various compounds in the vicinity of the motor end-plate. Labelled depolarising drugs such as decamethonium are taken up in far greater quantities than the non-depolarising drugs. Waser (1970) has drawn attention to the importance of acetylcholinesterase molecules. These are found in the end-plate region in similar numbers to those found with labelled curare molecules. He has suggested that the mouth of the pore permitting ionic flux (i.e. responsible for depolarisation) is guarded by two molecules of acetylcholinesterase with four active centres. Under normal conditions acetylcholine combines with its own cholinergic receptor surrounding the pore: this action pulls open the mouth and allows ionic movement to take place. In the presence of *d*-tubocurarine, the molecule of relaxant combines with the active centres of the acetylcholinesterase molecules and effectively blocks the opening of the pore. This theory would concede that the receptors for *d*-tubocurarine need not be the same as those for the depolarising drug, but they must be strategically placed (Fig. 9).

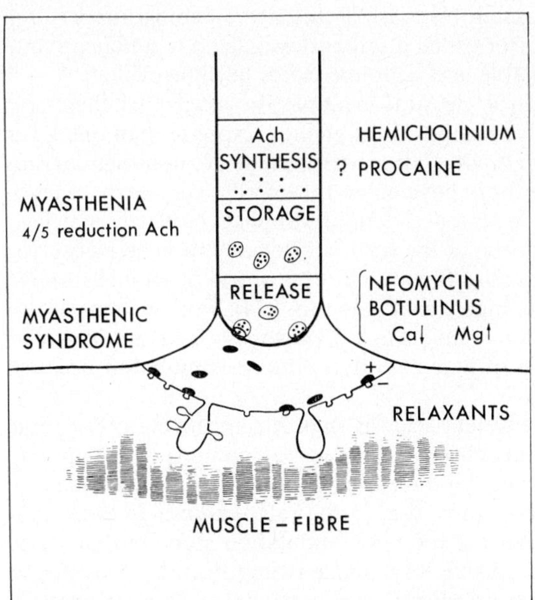

29/FIG. 9.—Diagram to summarise the possible sites of action of various drugs and diseases at the nerve-ending.

TERMINOLOGY AND NEUROMUSCULAR TRANSMISSION

Much confusion has arisen over the multiplicity of terms that are in use to describe phenomena occurring at the neuromuscular junction. This is largely due to a failure on the part of authors to agree an international nomenclature. The following may help the reader:

Term	*Alternative Names*	
Non-depolarisation block	"Curare block"	"Competitive inhibition"
Desensitisation block	"Dual block"	"Phase II block"
Post-tetanic potentiation	"Post-tetanic facilitation"	"Post-activation facilitation"
Post-tetanic exhaustion		
Wedensky inhibition	"Fade"	"Neuromuscular depression"

Some of these terms can be best understood by considering the possible behaviour of acetylcholine molecules. An exception to this is the "dual" or "desensitisation" block already mentioned. It is clear that the complex nature of this block is imperfectly understood at present. In normal neuromuscular transmission, however, it is known that the *rate* of the stimulus passing down the nerve influences the number of acetylcholine molecules that are produced. Thus, whether one is measuring the muscle response by an electrical or a mechanical method, it will be observed that the response to tetanic stimulation is greater than to a single or twitch stimulus. If this rate is excessive then the store of acetylcholine molecules available is exhausted, fresh synthesis is unable to produce enough new molecules, so fatigue takes place. The maximum speed at which impulses can pass down a nerve in normal physiological circumstances (i.e. generated by the brain) is about 50 per second. Over the first few stimuli of this train there is a gradually increasing response as the nerve-ending adapts itself to the fast rate of stimulation, after which it settles down again to a plateau until signs of exhaustion of the available acetylcholine stores become evident.

Post-tetanic potentiation.—In a classical example the single twitch *after* a period of tetanic stimulation (five seconds) is of greater response than one given just beforehand. It is always seen in association with the fade of a non-depolarising block. For this reason some authors have come to describe very early cases as "a single twitch response after a period of tetanic stimulation which is at least twice the height of the last response of the train". Clinically, it is best observed as an improvement of neuromuscular function after a period of tetanic stimulation using the movement of the fingers as a guide (p. 824). For this reason it is better to administer at least four or five single twitches both before and after the tetanus so that the abolition of fade at twitch rates of stimulation becomes obvious.

The probable reason for the potentiation is that during the period of rapid stimulation the "factory" for acetylcholine at the nerve-ending is called upon to step up production. As it happens, the increased productivity is inadequate to improve conduction during the tetanus, due to the raised threshold caused by the non-depolarisation block, but the moment stimulation stops the increased production of acetylcholine is available for a single twitch stimulus. The degree and duration of the potentiation are directly proportional to both the rate of nerve stimulation (i.e. 30, 40, or even 100/second) and the duration of tetanisation. In normal circumstances post-tetanic potentiation does not persist for more than five to ten seconds, being maximal 1–2 seconds after the termination of the tetanic stimulation, and gradually disappears over the next ten seconds.

Wedensky inhibition.—This phenomenon was described some fifty years ago and signifies a "fade" in the successive responses. It is particularly well seen in the presence of a partial *d*-tubocurarine block (see p. 822). In this instance the threshold for the number of molecules necessary to produce depolarisation of a muscle fibre has been raised to a point where the number available and the number required is critical. The result is that although a number of muscle fibres can respond if a very slow rate of stimulus (i.e. twitch rate) is used, when rapid stimuli are used there are not enough molecules available to overcome the raised threshold of the non-depolarisation block. Anti-cholinesterase drugs can remedy this deficit.

The Motor Unit

The term "motor unit" comprises the anterior horn cell in the spinal cord and its corresponding motor nerve fibre passing peripherally to divide into numerous branches, each one of which terminates at a single muscle fibre. The point of branching takes place near the skeletal muscle fibres and is an important landmark in electromyographic recordings. Stimulation below this point leads to the initial contraction of an individual muscle fibre (fibrillation potential) whereas stimulation of the motor nerve above this point leads to the simultaneous contraction of all the muscle fibres in the motor unit (a motor unit action potential) (Fig. 10).

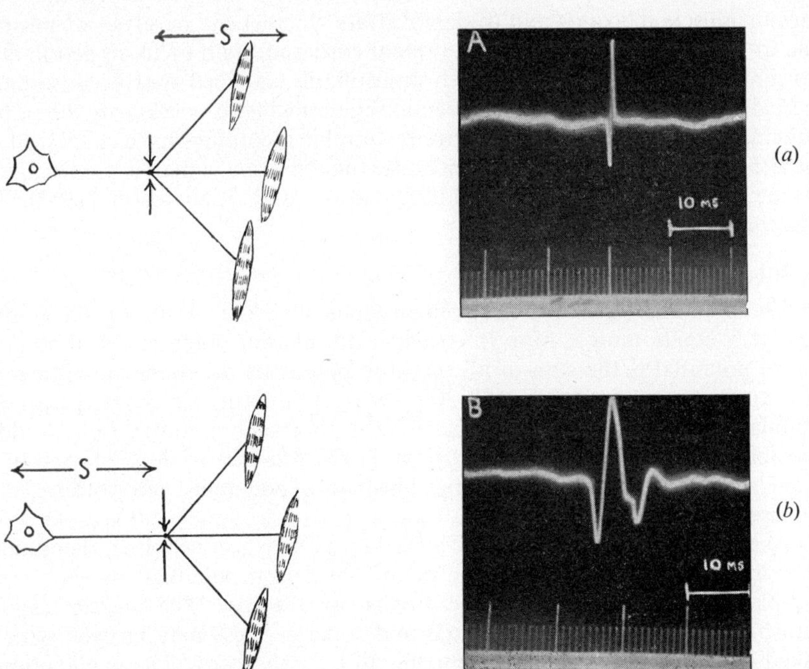

29/Fig. 10.—Electromyographic appearances from stimulation of the motor unit. (*a*) Stimulation (S) below the point of branching of the lower motor neurone produces a single fibre potential (A) or a motor unit potential. (*b*) Stimulation (S) above the point of branching of the lower motor neurone produces a motor unit potential (B).

Nevertheless, the remaining fibres of the motor unit are stimulated antidromically (Masland and Wigton, 1950) and can be recognised as the remnants of the motor unit following rapidly after the single-fibre potential.

The number of muscle fibres supplied by each anterior horn cell varies widely, depending largely on the delicacy of its function. In the highly specialised skeletal muscles such as those moving the eyeball, relatively few fibres are present in each unit (5–15), whereas in the large muscles of the back or limbs the numbers are far greater (up to 300 per unit). Similarly both the height (amplitude) and the width (duration) of the action potential (as detected by the electromyograph apparatus) differ characteristically. Thus:

	Number per unit	*Duration*	*Amplitude*
Eye muscles . .	5– 15	1 millisecond	100 microvolts or less
Large limb muscles .	150–300	5–10 millisecond	300 microvolts to 1·5 millivolts

Electromyography can also be used to demonstrate lesions affecting the motor unit and it is widely employed on this basis in the diagnosis of neurological conditions. It can be used, therefore, to determine the site of action of the various muscle relaxants and to demonstrate whether the paralysis of muscle is due to a pure central action on the spinal cord and brain or to an action at the neuromuscular junction. It is often unjustifiably assumed that because one of these drugs has a particular site of action in animals it is necessarily the same in human subjects. Fortunately, electromyographic recordings have confirmed that the site of action of decamethonium and *d*-tubocurarine in man is predominantly at the motor end-plate (Churchill-Davidson and Richardson, 1952). (See Chapter 31.)

Fibrillation Potential

The potential (recorded electromyographically) that occurs on the contraction of a single muscle fibre is termed a fibrillation potential. A motor unit action potential is the sum of all the fibre potentials occurring simultaneously in a single motor unit (i.e. 150–300 fibres). Ordinarily, it is not possible to stimulate a single muscle fibre, and besides this, such a contraction would be invisible to the naked eye. Nevertheless, in the presence of degeneration of the lower motor neurone, spontaneous fibrillation potentials can readily be recognised on the electromyograph.

As the depolarising drugs are believed to act like acetylcholine, theoretically their injection should create a shower of fibrillation potentials as each motor end-plate is depolarised. However, this is not the case. The muscle responds with numerous full action potentials and some of these may be seen with the naked eye as "fasciculations" occurring all over the body. The explanation of this phenomenon is probably that on stimulation of the first motor end-plate, an antidromic impulse sweeps backwards to the point of branching and then excites all the other fibres in that unit (Masland and Wigton, 1950).

Occasionally spontaneous fibre or fasciculation potentials are observed electromyographically following the administration of a depolarising drug. Gradually, on volition, there is a progressive disintegration of the full motor unit so that both the amplitude and the duration of its potential are diminished. Finally, when the block is established, the picture resembles a severe case of myopathy.

Fasciculations

The spontaneous contraction of a single or a group of motor units leads to a visible contraction of skeletal muscle. In all probability the contraction of a single unit produces too small a response to be recognised with the naked eye. Nevertheless, all the depolarising drugs produce this type of response in some form. Most prominent is the rapid injection of suxamethonium which leads to widespread fasciculations or twitches that can be clearly seen all over the body. Decamethonium is less spectacular but most conscious subjects comment on the peculiar twitching sensation in the back muscles, often spreading to involve the proximal muscles of the limbs.

The speed of onset of fasciculations depends on the blood flow, and the concentration and rate of injection of the drug. In a severely ill patient the poor peripheral circulation and low cardiac output may mean that it takes many minutes for the relaxant drug to reach the limb musculature.

Fasciculations, particularly after suxamethonium, are believed to be intimately concerned with the origin of post-relaxation muscle pains. The exact nature of the pains varies with the drug used. Thus, after decamethonium the pains occur almost immediately and are prominent in the jaw and calf muscles. They persist for a few hours and are partly relieved by exercise. The pains of suxamethonium are far more incapacitating; they arise particularly in association with the ambulant patient and are described as "rheumaticky" and similar to "the stiffness after the first game of tennis for the season". Unlike those following decamethonium, they do not usually appear until the morning following the injection. A typical example is a patient who receives suxamethonium during the course of a dental extraction as an out-patient. On returning home the patient notices no untoward effects and later retires to bed. On attempting to rise in the morning intense stiffness is felt in all the limb muscles and there is often a severe ache in the muscles in the xiphisternum region. In some cases the pains may persist for three to four days in gradually diminishing intensity and the substernal ache is usually the last to disappear.

The fasciculations of suxamethonium, and to a large extent the muscle pains, can be prevented by the previous injection of a small dose of a non-depolarising relaxant, e.g. 5 mg. of *d*-tubocurarine. One of the most interesting features of the fasciculations with suxamethonium is that they are rarely observed on the second injection. There are two possible explanations. First, it takes many minutes (4–10) for the limb muscles to show complete recovery of their normal activity using electromyography. Nevertheless, the exact time relationship as to when the fasciculations reappear has never been established, but it is probably a matter of fifteen minutes or more. Secondly, a possible explanation may lie in some change in response on the part of the motor end-plate (dual block), so that succeeding doses of suxamethonium no longer elicit pure depolarisation.

In disease, fasciculation may arise from two primary causes. First, when there is progressive degeneration of the anterior horn cell as is most commonly seen in cases of motor neurone disease. Secondly, when some condition affects the remainder of the motor neurone; this may, for example, be pressure on the nerve from a ruptured intervertebral disc, or some metabolic upset—such as calcium or magnesium deficiency—that directly involves the nerve fibre. Included in the last group is the rare condition of benign myokymia in which the stimulus apparently arises (for no obvious reason) in the peripheral nerve fibre. The anaesthetist can play an important part in locating the source of all such fasciculations, for they persist after paralysis of the motor fibres with spinal analgesia or blockade of the main nerve-trunk, yet they are abolished by a non-depolarising relaxant drug, thus suggesting that the site of origin is somewhere between these two points.

Fatigue

In the isolated nerve-muscle preparation of the frog, fatigue is associated with a large drop in the production of acetylcholine molecules per nerve impulse. Del Castillo and Katz (1956) concluded that during prolonged stimulation of a nerve some disorganisation of the normal acetylcholine release mechanism occurs, forestalling any exhaustion in the true sense of the intracellular acetylcholine supply. These authors suggest that in mammalian muscle the situation may be different, for the steady production of intracellular acetylcholine depends on adequate supplies of glucose being available; there is no evidence, however, of the amount of acetylcholine released in a glucose-deprived mammalian muscle.

In man fatigue is a common feature of severe muscular exercise. If a subject exerts a maximal squeeze on the hand-bulb of an ergometer this activity can be maintained at a high pitch only for a matter of a minute or so before the muscle power starts to fade. Merton (1956), in a series of tests based on the nature of fatigue, found that a subject could write for only two minutes when the circulation to the limb was stopped. If, prior to the occlusion, the subject had been busily engaged in writing, then he could only continue for 30 seconds after the circulation had ceased.

If the motor nerve is stimulated electrically at a slow twitch rate (1 per second) then this level of activity can be maintained indefinitely. But if a high tetanic rate (50 per second) is used the muscle power fades after about 30 seconds. A particularly characteristic feature of tetanic stimulation is that as the muscle power fades so an intense pain develops in the corresponding muscles. This increases in crescendo as an inverse relationship with the falling muscle activity; its origin in man would appear to be based on ischaemia of the muscle fibres. For comparison, it should be remembered that during a maximal volitional effort between 25–50 stimuli pass down the motor nerve every second. Fatigue in man, therefore, would appear to be a combination of reduced production of acetylcholine (possibly due to inadequate supplies of glucose) and ischaemia of the muscle fibres.

Contracture

Contracture is the term used to define the localised but sustained shortening of the muscle fibre that follows the intra-arterial injection of acetylcholine in birds and certain reptiles. It must be clearly differentiated from a normal *contraction* of the muscle fibre which is found in mammalian muscle. Nevertheless, if the nerve supply to mammalian muscle is cut and the nerve fibre allowed sufficient time to degenerate, then the intra-arterial injection of acetylcholine produces a typical contracture. The mechanism of this muscle power would therefore appear to be the primitive forerunner of normal neuromuscular transmission as found in mammalian muscle.

An example of the phenomenon of contracture has been observed in a patient with unilateral ptosis due to degeneration of the motor nerve supplying the eyelid muscles. On the injection of suxamethonium a "see-saw" response was observed. The normal eyelid twitched and then closed as the muscles became paralysed by the relaxant: the affected eyelid, however, gradually opened as the levator palpebrae superioris underwent a contracture of the muscle fibres. The eyelid remained wide open (something the patient could not achieve volitionally) for about one minute before finally beginning slowly to close. This process could be repeated. A similar case has been described by Marshall (1964). Axelsson and Thesleff (1959) have shown that the supersensitivity to acetylcholine which develops in chronically denervated muscle is due to the whole of the muscle fibre membrane becoming as sensitive to acetylcholine as the end-plate region.

In the young chick, the intravenous injection of either acetylcholine or decamethonium produces a state of generalised contracture in which the animal assumes a position of opisthotonos. Provided the dose has not been excessive, the bird continues to breathe but the head and neck are held forcibly retracted and the spine is curved in such a manner that the tail nearly touches the back of the neck. So typical is this response that Buttle and Zaimis (1949) have used it as the basis of their test for the presence of depolarising properties in a muscle relaxant.

The Muscle Fibre

A striated muscle fibre possesses three principal components: (1) the myofibril which contains the contractile element; (2) the mitochondria and nuclei; and (3) the cell membrane and intercommunicating systems. These latter aqueous channels have recently assumed a much greater importance as their role in relation to function can now be partly surmised (Page, 1968).

A closer study of the myofibril reveals that it contains a series of two important overlapping bands—the A and the I bands (Fig. 11). The I bands are attached to another important structure which runs transversely round the fibre and is called the Z line. The area between two Z lines is referred to as a sarcomere. The A band, on the other hand, is darker and contains the important enzyme adenosine triphosphatase (ATPase) which is essential for the breakdown of ATP in order to release energy.

A muscle contraction takes place when two types of protein—actin of the I band and myosin of the A band—interdigitate to produce a shortening of the fibre length (Huxley and Taylor, 1958; Huxley, 1963).

A closer look at the Z line using electronmicroscopy reveals that it is really a transverse aqueous channel connecting the cell membrane with the interior of the fibre. The mouth of this system lies on the surface where it merges with the cell

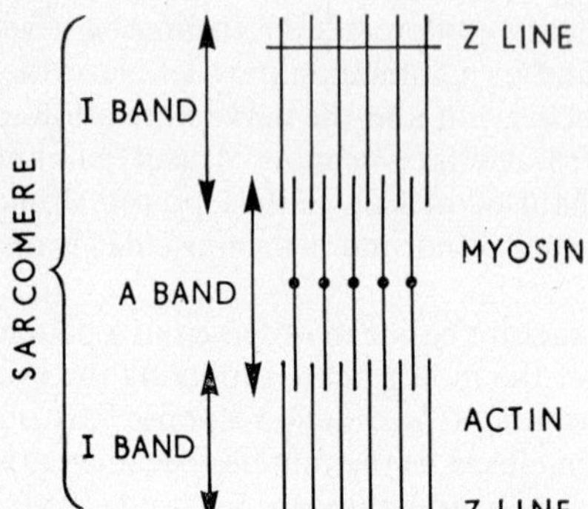

29/Fig. 11.—Diagram of a sarcomere showing the action of the I band and the myosin of the A band.

membrane and is open to the extracellular medium (Page, 1968). This channel is called the transverse tubular or "T" system (Fig. 12*a* and *b*). On passing to the interior it comes very close to another aqueous channel system—the sarcoplasmic reticulum.

The "T" system and the sarcoplasmic reticulum system do not actually join but in certain areas they lie in very close proximity. The sarcoplasmic reticulum is a much larger system and runs vertically between two Z bands.

Thus, when a motor end-plate becomes depolarised the excitatory disturbance is believed to spread into the interior of the fibre along the "T" system (Huxley and Taylor, 1958). Here it comes into contact with the terminal sacs of the sarcoplasmic reticulum (Fig. 13). There is considerable evidence to support the view that the tubules of this system act as an intracellular store for calcium ions which are released on depolarisation. The resulting rise in calcium ion concentration of the sarcoplasm stimulates the activity of the enzyme ATPase, thereby initiating the breakdown of the stored adenosine triphosphate to release energy and produce a contraction (Weber *et al.*, 1964). Relaxation occurs when the calcium ions are re-accumulated within the sarcoplasmic reticulum by the means of a calcium pump (Page, 1968). This process is repeated again and again as the contraction wave spreads along the length of the fibre.

Heat, Energy and Oxidative Phosphorylation in Muscle

The method of producing heat and energy in muscle is a complex one involving a series of reductions and oxidations within the respiratory chain. At each stage in the chain a certain amount of heat and energy is produced (Fig. 14). At three stages this energy is made available for the oxidative phosphorylation of adenosine diphosphate (ADP) to form adenosine triphosphate (ATP) with the help of the enzyme adenosine triphosphatase (ATPase) which is associated with the respiratory chain.

The process could be presented as follows:

(*a*) *Within the mitochondrium:*

$$\underset{\text{from respiratory chain}}{\text{Energy}} + \text{ADP} + \text{P} \xrightarrow[\text{ATPase in respiratory chain}]{} \text{ATP } (= \text{stored energy})$$

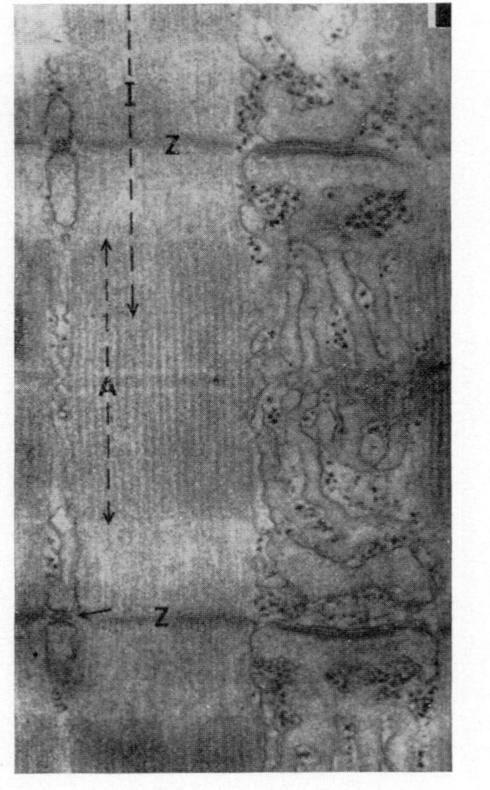

29/FIG. 12(*a*).—Electronmicroscopic section of frog's muscle fibre showing the A and I bands.

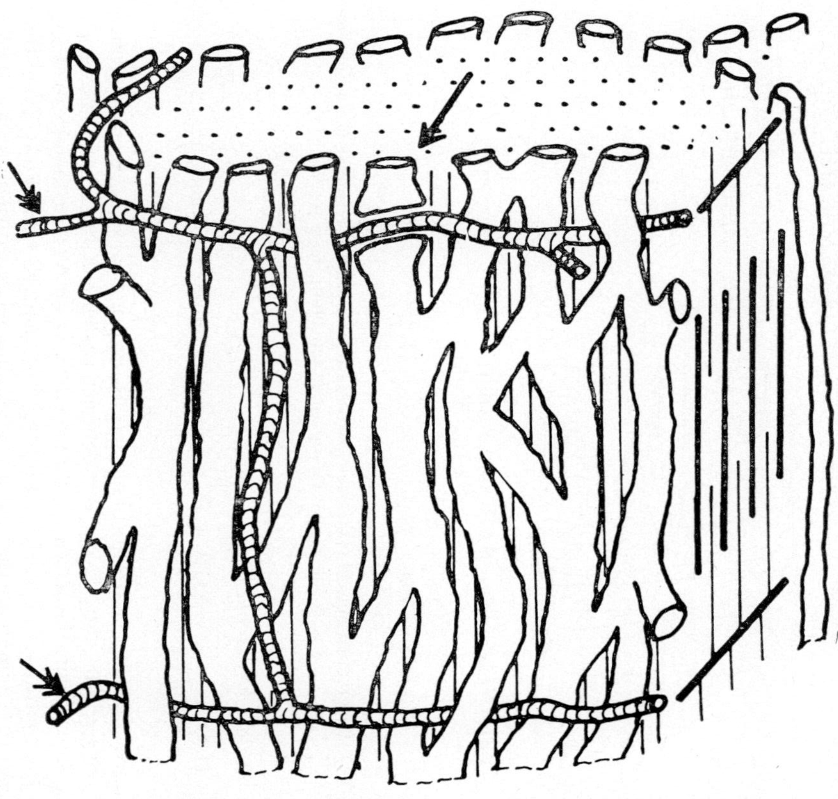

29/FIG. 12(*b*).—Diagram of the 'T' system showing the transverse tubular system.

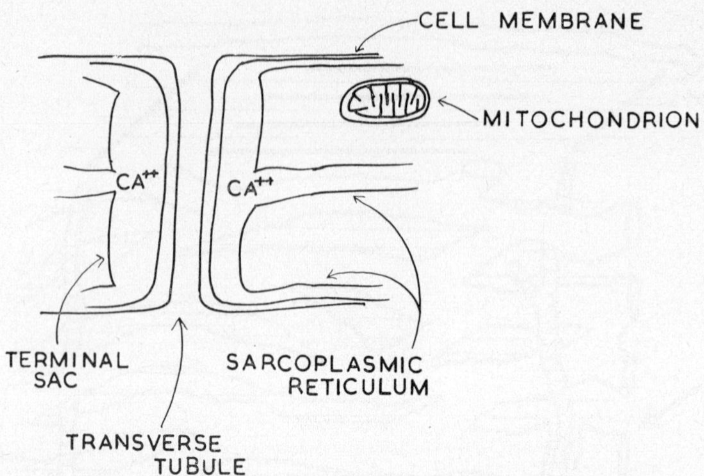

29/Fig. 13.—Diagram of muscle cell system showing relationship of terminal sac, transverse tubule and sarcoplasmic reticulum.

(*b*) *Within the cytoplasm:*

$$\text{ATP} + \text{H}_2\text{O} \xrightarrow[\text{with myosin}]{\text{ATPase associated}} \text{ADP} + \text{P} + \text{Energy of muscle contraction}$$

In muscle, adenosine triphosphate acts as the principal store of energy which can be released on contraction. As mentioned earlier calcium ions in muscle are believed to stimulate the activity of the enzyme myosin ATPase thereby releasing energy for contraction. It has also been shown (Snodgrass and Piras, 1966) that an excess of calcium ions can cause an uncoupling of oxidative phosphorylation. The most likely effect of this mechanism is that the calcium ions depress the activity of the enzyme ATPase in the respiratory chain. This results in a fall in the level of ATP in the cytoplasm and a rise in the concentration of ADP in the mitochondrion whilst the energy of the respiratory chain is released as heat. In these unusual circumstances it is theoretically possible to release vast amounts of heat very rapidly. Another interesting observation is that ATP not only acts as a store of muscle energy but it also causes relaxation of the muscle fibre. Thus, in the event of uncoupling of oxidative phosphorylation the fall in ATP level causes the muscle fibre to become stiff as is witnessed in rigor mortis.

Creatinine phosphate is another high energy store that is available as a reserve for the production of ATP with the aid of the enzyme creatinine phosphokinase viz.

$$\text{Creatinine P} + \text{ADP} \underset{\text{Creatinine phosphokinase}}{\rightleftharpoons} \text{ATP} + \text{Creatinine}$$

In most myopathies or cases of cell destruction a raised level of the creatinine phosphokinase can be detected.

In recent years these facts have assumed particular significance to anaesthetists since the recognition of the syndrome of malignant hyperpyrexia (see p. 924).

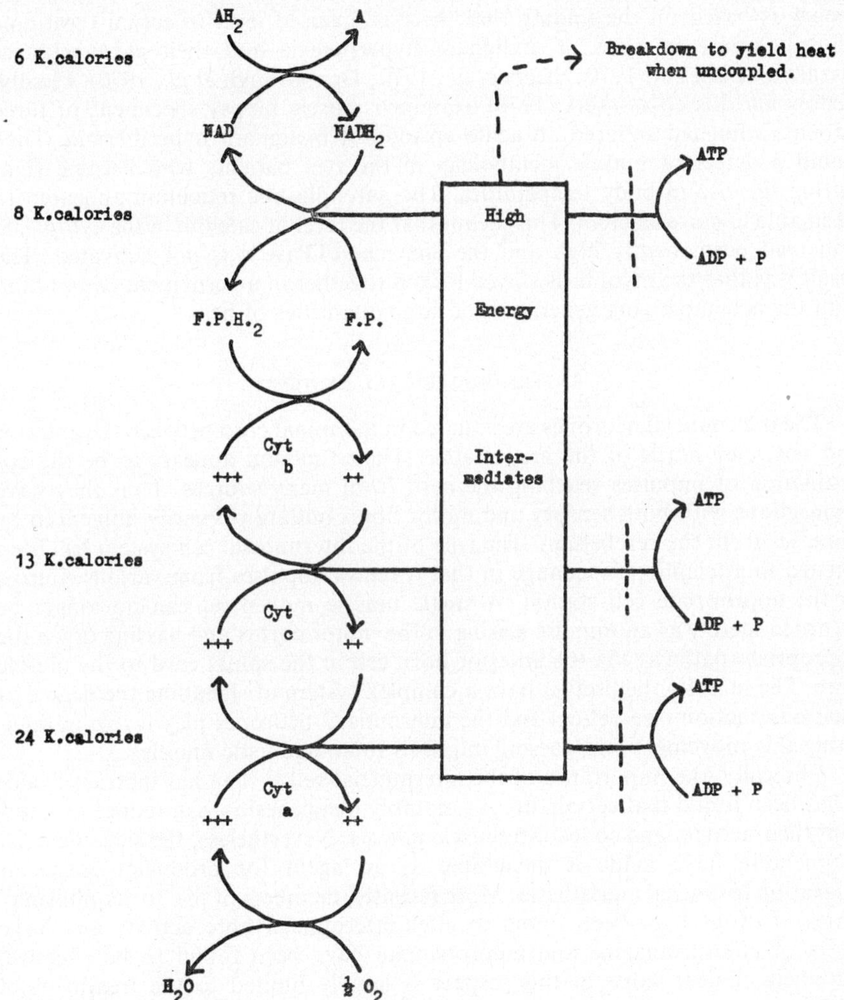

29/Fig. 14—Respiratory chain and oxidative phosphorylation. Note on the left of the diagram there is a steady production of heat at each stage of the chain. The intermediate compound provides the energy for oxidative phosphorylation. The dotted line shows the effect of uncoupling.

The aetiology of this condition is still far from clear. However, there are, at present, several theories. First, that it is associated with uncoupling of oxidative phosphorylation in genetically susceptible people. Only certain agents used in anaesthesia such as halothane and suxamethonium are believed to be capable of triggering off this peculiar response. Experimentally these agents can be shown to produce a dramatic rise in body temperature in the Landrace pig (Harrison *et al.*, 1969) but evidence for the actual presence of uncoupling of oxidative phosphorylation in these circumstances is still lacking. The second theory is based on the finding that there is a raised level of serum creatinine phosphokinase in cases of malignant hyperpyrexia and their close relatives (Isaacs and Barlow, 1970; Steers *et al.*, 1970; Denborough *et al.*, 1970). Finally, Kalow and his co-workers (1970) examined muscle biopsy specimens of three patients who had suffered an acute episode of malignant hyperthermia. They found a defect of muscle metabolism in the two patients who became rigid during the rise in body temperature. The sarcoplasmic reticulum appeared to be unable to store calcium. This meant that the level of calcium in the cytoplasm remained permanently high and the enzyme ATPase was not activated. The result was that the myofibrils stayed locked together in a permanent contraction with the accompanying generation of large quantities of heat.

Internuncial Cell System

The internuncial neurones are situated in the spinal cord between the anterior and posterior horns of the grey matter. Their function appears to be the co-ordination of impulses reaching the cord from many sources. Thus they have connections with both sensory and motor fibres but are primarily influenced by impulses from the cerebellum. The role of the internuncial cell system has been likened to a telephone exchange in that it relays impulses from various sources to the appropriate cell station. A single muscle movement can no longer be regarded merely as an impulse arising in the motor cortex and passing down the appropriate pathway via the anterior horn cell in the spinal cord to the muscle fibre. The muscles themselves have a complex system of signalling the degree of their contraction (see below) and the internuncial neurones play a role in regulating this movement and passing impulses to antagonistic muscles.

Clinically, the importance of the internuncial cell system has increased since it has been found that certain drugs—notably mephenesin—can reduce or interrupt their activity and so lead to muscle paresis. Nevertheless, the side-effects of mephenesin have made it unsuitable as an agent for producing muscular relaxation in clinical anaesthesia. More recently, members of the "tranquillising" series of drugs have been found to alter internuncial fibre activity and large doses of chlorpromazine and meprobamate have been found to be effective, but their clinical value in this respect is largely limited to the treatment of tetanus.

Muscle Spindles and the Small Fibre System

The motor pathway from the anterior horn cell down to the neuromuscular junction on the skeletal muscle fibre is now familiar to all (Fig. 15). Conduction along this route is rapid as the size of the fibre (α efferent) is large, i.e. 14 μ in diameter. Closer scrutiny of this nerve fibre reveals that besides these large fibres there are smaller ones—γ efferent fibres measuring some 4 μ in diameter—which when traced peripherally are found to end in a special structure—the *muscle spindle* (Fig. 16).

The simple act of picking up a pencil from a table not only employs the motor pathway, but afferents reach the spinal cord from the sensory endings in the skin, joints and muscles. In fact, the muscle spindles are the sensory end-organ of the skeletal muscles and are responsible for signalling the degree of

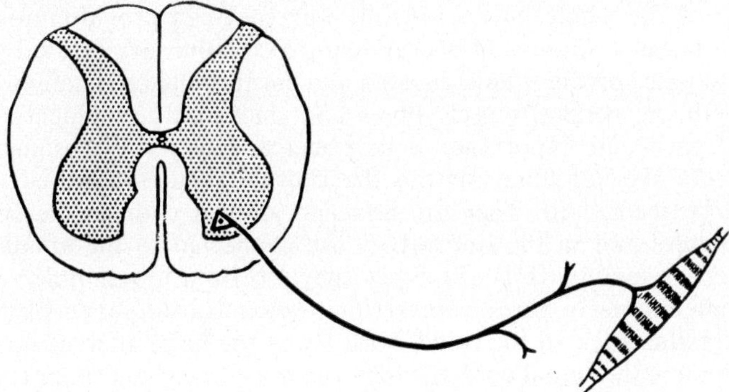

29/FIG. 15.—The motor pathway from the anterior horn cell to the neuromuscular junction

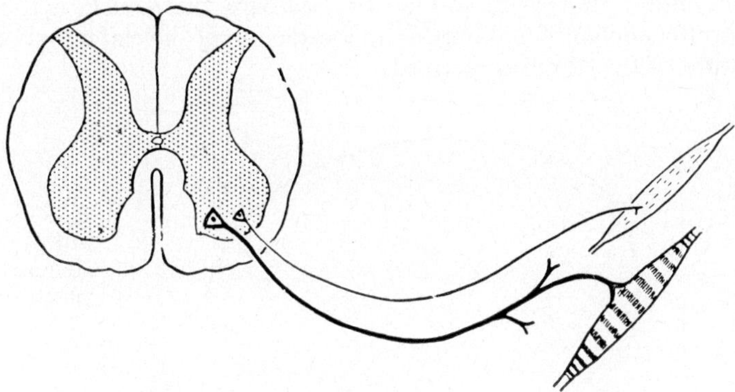

29/FIG. 16.—γ efferent fibres leading to a muscle spindle.

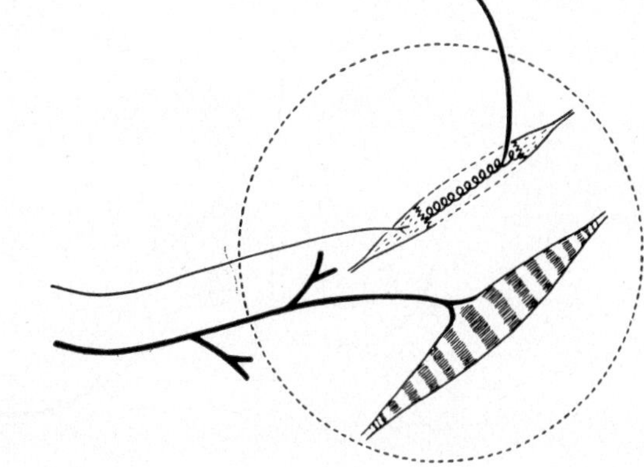

29/FIG. 17.—Intrafusal fibres.

shortening of the whole muscle. In this way they can provide information so that only the exact amount of energy required for the task is used. Histologically, the muscle spindle is an elongated and encapsulated structure which lies in parallel with the skeletal muscle fibres and shares its attachment. This latter point is of particular importance as its principal function is to signal the exact length of the skeletal fibre. Within the capsule small specialised (*intrafusal*) fibres can be recognised. They are attached at their ends to the poles of the muscle spindles and in the centre they are connected to the annulo-spiral or primary sensory ending (Fig. 17). Since they receive a motor innervation from the small efferent nerve fibres, contraction of the intrafusal fibres of the spindles sends a stimulus back to the spinal cord along the large afferent sensory fibre. This fibre enters the spinal cord through the dorsal root and then traverses the grey matter, finally to synapse with the anterior horn cell of the corresponding muscle fibre (Fig. 18).

The small fibre system, therefore, consists of the gamma efferent fibre, the muscle spindle, and the large afferent fibre synapsing with the anterior horn cell of the motor unit. A servo-loop or feed-back mechanism is thus created which can either enhance or dampen the contraction of skeletal muscle according to the nature of the stimulus received.

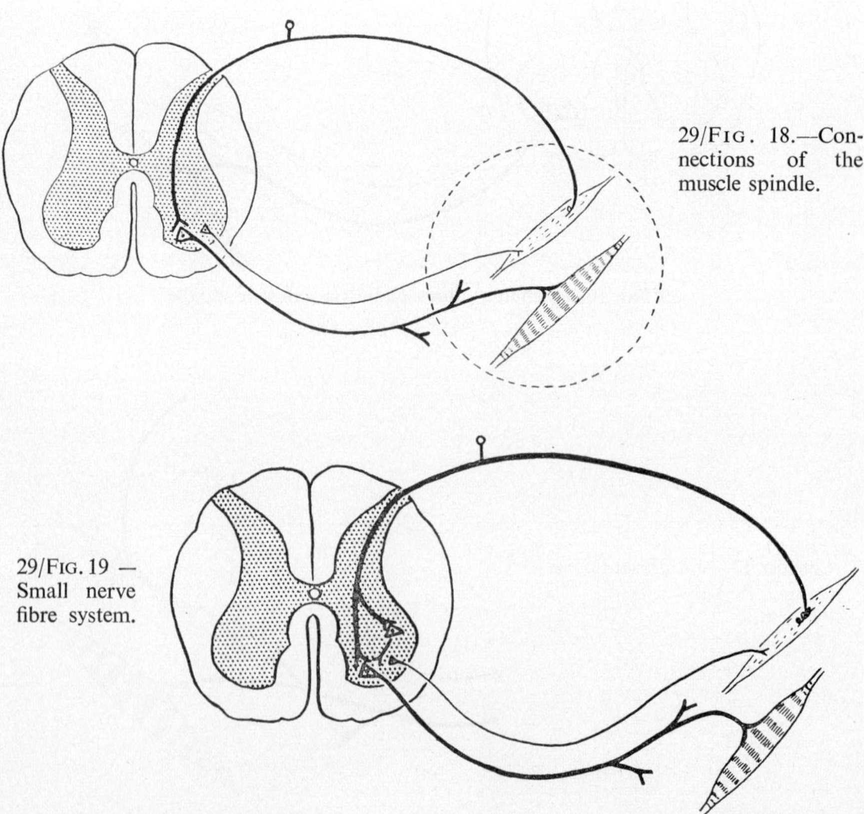

29/FIG. 18.—Connections of the muscle spindle.

29/FIG. 19 — Small nerve fibre system.

Besides the pathways already described, others are also believed to exist. As the large afferent fibre enters the posterior horn of the grey matter it gives off a branch to an internuncial cell which, in turn, synapses with the anterior horn cell of the skeletal muscle fibre (Fig. 19). As the internuncial system is largely under cerebellar control this link introduces a further modifying influence on the sensitivity of the motor cell. Yet another feed-back loop has been described by Renshaw (1941); as the main motor nerve fibre courses through the white matter of the spinal cord a branch loops backwards to synapse with a cell in the anterior horn (Renshaw cell), and in turn this communicates with the large anterior horn cell again (Fig. 20).

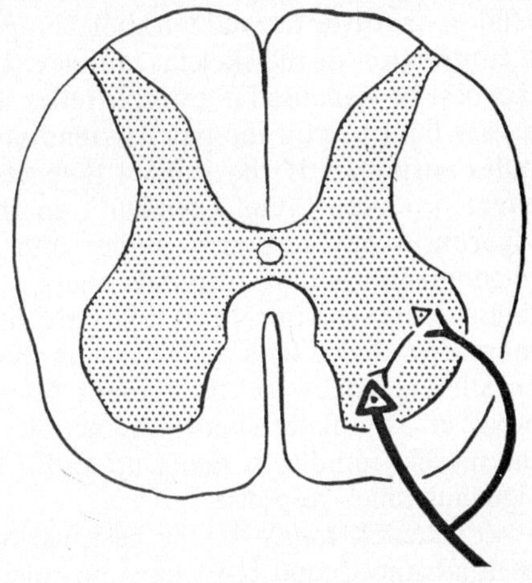

29/Fig. 20.—Renshaw cell.

Clinically the small fibre system has three important functions in relation to muscle activity:

(*a*) *Volitional effort.*—There are two possible motor pathways open to a stimulus arriving at the anterior horn of the spinal cord. First, it may travel along the slow-gamma efferent fibre, stimulate the intrafusal fibres of the muscle spindle to contract and so excite the sensory end-organ to send a stimulus back via the large afferent fibre to the spinal cord. Here it enjoys a number of possible routes before finally reaching the anterior horn cell of the motor unit and stimulating the skeletal muscle fibre into activity. This is probably the normal mechanism of all volitional activity and the various feed-back systems modify the activity according to requirements. Nevertheless, Granit and his associates (1955) have shown that the direct pathway from cortex to skeletal muscle via the anterior horn cell is often used in sudden movements. Hammond and his co-workers (1956) reached the tentative conclusion that the cerebellum (and associated structures) determined whether the small fibre pathway or the direct route was used in a contraction. Furthermore they state that this conception fits with the current notion that "the cerebral cortex decides *what* is to be done and the cerebellum has the job of arranging *how* it is to be carried out".

The importance to the anaesthetist of both these pathways cannot be over-emphasised, because the mechanism of neuromuscular transmission at the muscle spindle is believed to be the same as in skeletal muscle. That is to say, acetylcholine molecules are responsible for exciting intrafusal muscle fibre activity. Neuromuscular block of the small fibre system could lead to a situation where the subject was unable to produce a volitional effort yet electrical stimulation of a main motor nerve would reveal normal contraction of the skeletal muscle fibre. The action of the various muscle relaxants on muscle spindle activity is not yet known, but the available evidence suggests that the interference with activity occurs simultaneously and linearly at both the muscle spindle and the neuromuscular junction.

(*b*) *Reflex activity*.—The elicitation of a reflex, i.e. tapping the appropriate tendon, involves the sudden shortening of the muscle spindles and consequently a contraction of the skeletal muscles. The part played by the small fibre system can best be visualised if a simple reflex like the knee-jerk is studied. For example, a very light tap on the patellar tendon is found to be insufficient to produce a reflex response. If the subject then clasps his fingers together and pulls, the effect produces "reinforcement", so that now a similar light tap produces a vigorous reflex response. Buller and Dornhorst (1957) have explained this phenomenon on the grounds that, at rest, small fibre activity is absent or minimal and the intrafusal fibres are slack. The small shortening of the skeletal muscle produced by a light blow on the patellar tendon is insufficient to initiate an afferent volley up the afferent fibre. Reinforcement (clasping the fingers), however, stimulates small fibre activity throughout the body so the "slack" in the muscle spindles is taken up and a repeat of the patellar tap now produces vigorous reflex response.

(*c*) *Muscle tone*.—In the past, various theories to explain muscle tonus have been advanced, and most have postulated some continuous stream of impulses down the motor nerve to keep the muscle fibres in a state of contraction in order that posture may be maintained. Electromyography, however, has revealed that even in the erect posture many of the main muscles are inactive and a stage may be reached when the individual "balances on his vertebral column". Buller (1956) has described muscle tone as a measure of the sensitivity of the stretch reflex and thus indirectly of small fibre activity. Apart from signalling the exact degree of stretch of the skeletal muscle fibres, this system also appears to record the rate at which the stretch occurs over a given time. The efficiency of the small fibre system can therefore be tested partly by eliciting reflex activity and partly by noting the amount of resistance encountered when a muscle is moved passively through its full range.

REFERENCES

AXELSSON, J., and THESLEFF, S. (1959). A study of supersensitivity in denervated mammalian skeletal muscle. *J. Physiol.* (*Lond.*), **147,** 178.

BIRKS, R., HUXLEY, H. E., and KATZ, B. (1960). The fine structure of the neuromuscular junction of the frog. *J. Physiol.* (*Lond.*), **150,** 134.

BIRKS, R. I., and MACINTOSH, F. C. (1957). Acetylcholine metabolism at nerve-endings. *Brit. med. Bull.*, **13,** 157.

BIRKS, R. I., and MACINTOSH, F. C. (1961). Acetylcholine metabolism of a sympathetic ganglion. *Canad. J. Biochem.*, **39,** 787.

BROWN, G. L., DALE, H. H., and FELDBERG, W. (1936). Reactions of the normal mammalian muscle to acetylcholine and to eserine. *J. Physiol.* (*Lond.*), **87,** 394.

BULLER, A. J. (1956). Muscle tone. *Physiotherapy*, **42,** 203.

BULLER, A. J., and DORNHORST, A. C. (1957). Reinforcement of tendon reflexes. *Lancet*, **2,** 1261.

BURNS, B. D., and PATON, W. D. M. (1951). Depolarization of the motor end-plate by decamethonium and acetylcholine. *J. Physiol.* (*Lond.*), **115,** 41.

Buttle, G. A. H., and Zaimis, E. J. (1949). The action of decamethonium iodide in birds. *J. Pharm. (Lond.)*, **1**, 991.

Chagas, C. (1962). "The fate of curare during curarisation." In: Ciba Foundat. Study Group, No. 12. *Curare and Curare-like Agents*, p. 2. Ed. De Reuck, A. V. S. London: J. & A. Churchill.

Churchill-Davidson, H. C., Christie, T. H., and Wise, R. P. (1960). Dual neuromuscular block in man. *Anesthesiology*, **21**, 144.

Churchill-Davidson, H. C., and Richardson, A. T. (1952). Decamethonium iodide (C.10): some observations on its action using electromyography. *Proc. roy. Soc. Med.*, **45**, 179.

Churchill-Davidson, H. C., and Wise, R. P. (1963). Neuromuscular transmission in the newborn infant. *Anesthesiology*, **24**, 271.

Churchill-Davidson, H. C., and Wise, R. P. (1964). The response of the newborn infant to muscle relaxants. *Canad. Anaesth. Soc. J.*, **11**, 1.

Cohen, E. N., Hood, N., and Golling, R. (1968). Use of whole-body autoradiography for estimation of uptake and distribution of labelled muscle relaxants in the rat. *Anesthesiology*, **29**, 987.

Couteaux, R. (1955). Localisation of cholinesterases at neuromuscular junctions. *Int. Rev. Cytol.*, **4**, 335.

Couteaux, R. (1958). Morphological and cytochemical observations on the post-synaptic membrane at motor end-plates and ganglionic synapses. *Exp. Cell. Res. Suppl.*, **5**, 294.

Dale, H. H., Feldberg, W., and Vogt, M. (1936). Release of acetylcholine at voluntary motor nerve endings. *J. Physiol. (Lond.)*, **86**, 353.

del Castillo, J., and Engbaek, L. (1954). The nature of the neuromuscular block produced by magnesium. *J. Physiol. (Lond.)*, **124**, 370.

del Castillo, J., and Katz, B. (1955). On the localization of acetylcholine receptors. *J. Physiol. (Lond.)*, **128**, 157.

del Castillo, J., and Katz, B. (1956). Biophysical aspects of neuromuscular transmission. *Progr. Biophysics and Biophys. Chem.*, **6**, 122.

Denborough, M. A., Forster, J. F. A., Hudson, M. C., Carter, N. G., and Zapf, P. (1970). Biochemical changes in malignant hyperpyrexia. *Lancet*, **1**, 1137.

Desmedt, J. E. (1966). Presynaptic mechanisms in myasthenia gravis. *Ann. N.Y. Acad. Sci.*, **135**, 209.

Elmquist, D., Hofmann, W. W., Kugelberg, J., and Quastel, D. M. J. (1964). An electrophysiological investigation of neuromuscular transmission in myasthenia gravis. *J. Physiol. (Lond.)*, **174**, 417.

Feldberg, W. (1945). Synthesis of acetylcholine by tissue of the central nervous system. *J. Physiol. (Lond.)*, **103**, 367.

Gill, W. E. (1965). Drug receptor interactions. *Progr. medicinal Chem.*, **4**, 39.

Granit, R., Holmgren, B., and Merton, P. A. (1955). The two routes for excitation of muscle and their subservience to the cerebellum. *J. Physiol. (Lond.)*, **130**, 213.

Hammond, P. H., Merton, P. A., and Sutton, G. G. (1956). Nervous gradation of muscular contraction. *Brit. med. Bull.*, **12**, 214.

Harrison, G. G., Saunders, S. J., Biebuyck, J. F., Hickman, R., Dent, D. M., Terblanche, J., and Weaver, V. (1969). Anaesthetic induced malignant hyperpyrexia, and a method for its production. *Brit. J. Anaesth.*, **41**, 844.

Hodgkin, A. L. (1951). The ionic basis of electrical activity in nerve and muscle. *Biol. Rev.*, **26**, 339.

Huxley, A. F. (1963). Electron microscope studies on the structure of natural and synthetic protein filaments from striated muscle. *J. Mol. Biol.*, **7**, 281.

HUXLEY, A. F., and TAYLOR, R. E. (1958). Local activation of striated muscle fibres. *J. Physiol.* (*Lond.*), **144**, 426.

ISAACS, H., and BARLOW, M. B. (1970). Malignant hyperpyrexia during anaesthesia: possible association with subclinical myopathy. *Brit. med. J.*, **1**, 275.

JENDEN, D. J., KAMIJO, K., and TAYLOR, D. B. (1951). The action of decamethonium (C. 10) on the isolated rabbit lumbrical muscle. *J. Pharmacol. exp. Ther.*, **103,** 348.

KALOW, W., BRITT, B. A., TERREAU, M. E., and HOIST, C. (1970). Metabolic error of muscle metabolism after recovery from malignant hyperthermia. *Lancet*, **2,** 895.

KATZ, B. (1966). *Nerve, Muscle and Synapse*. New York: McGraw-Hill.

KATZ, B., and MILEDI, R. (1964). Localisation of calcium action at the nerve muscle junction. *J. Physiol.* (*Lond.*), **171**, 10–12 PP.

KATZ, B., and MILEDI, R. (1965). The effect of calcium on acetylcholine release from motor nerve terminals. *Proc. roy. Soc. B.*, **161,** 496.

KATZ, R. L., WOLF, C. E., and PAPPER, E. M. (1963). The non-depolarising blocking action of succinylcholine in man. *Anesthesiology*, **24,** 784.

KEYNES, R. D. (1949). Movements of radio-active ions in resting and stimulated nerve. *Arch. Sci. physiol.*, **3,** 165.

KRRYEVIĆ, K., and MITCHELL, J. F. (1961). The release of acetylcholine in the isolated rat diaphragm. *J. Physiol.* (*Lond.*), **155,** 246.

MACLAGAN, J. (1962). A comparison of the responses of the tenuissimus muscle to neuromuscular blocking drugs *in vivo* and *in vitro*. *Brit. J. Pharmacol.*, **18,** 204.

MARSHALL, M. (1964). Action of suxamethonium on ptosis due to third nerve palsy. *Brit. med. J.*, **2,** 1116.

MASLAND, R. L., and WIGTON, R. S. (1950). Nerve activity accompanying fasciculation produced by prostigmin. *J. Neurophysiol.*, **3,** 269.

MERTON, P. A. (1956). Problems of muscular fatigue. *Brit. med. Bull.*, **12,** 219.

NASTUK, W. L. (1954). Relation between extracellular Na^+ and the depolarizing action of $acetylcholine^+$ on the end-plate membrane. *Fed. Proc.*, **13,** 104.

NASTUK, W. L. (1967). Activation and inactivation of muscle post-junctional receptors. *Fed. Proc.*, **26,** 1639.

PAGE, S. (1968). Structure of the sarcoplasmic reticulum in vertebrate muscle. *Brit. med. Bull.*, **24,** 170.

RENSHAW, B. (1941). Influence of discharge of motoneurones upon excitation of neighboring motoneurones. *J. Neurophysiol.*, **4,** 167.

ROBERTSON, J. D. (1956). The ultrastructure of a reptilian myoneural junction. *J. biophys. biochem. Cytol.*, **2,** 381.

SNODGRASS, P. J., and PIRAS, M. M. (1966). Effects of halothane on rat liver mitochondria. *Biochemistry*, **5,** 1140.

STEERS, A. J. W., TALLACK, A. J., and THOMPSON, D. E. A. (1970). Fulminating hyperpyrexia during anaesthesia in a member of a myopathic family. *Brit. med. J.*, **2,** 341.

TAYLOR, D. B. (1959). The mechanism of action of muscle relaxants and their antagonists. *Anesthesiology*, **20,** 439.

TAYLOR, D. B. (1962). "Influence of curare on uptake and release of a neuromuscular blocking agent labelled with iodine-131." In: Ciba Foundation Study Group No. 12. *Curare and Curare-like agents*, p. 21. Ed. De Reuck, A.V.S. London: J. & A. Churchill.

THESLEFF, S. (1955). The mode of neuromuscular block caused by acetylcholine, nicotine, decamethonium and succinylcholine. *Acta physiol. scand.*, **34,** 218.

WASER, P. G. (1960). The cholinergic receptor. *J. Pharm. Pharmacol.*, **12,** 577.

WASER, P. G. (1962). In: *Curare and Curare-like Agents*, p. 50. (Ciba Foundation Study Group No. 12). Ed. De Reuck, A.V.S. London: J. & A. Churchill.

WASER, P. G. (1970). On receptors in the postsynaptic membrane of the motor endplate. *Ciba Foundation Symposium on Molecular Properties of Drug Receptors*, p. 59. Ed. Porter, R., and O'Connor, M. London: J. & A. Churchill.

WEBER, A., HERZ, R., and REISS, I. (1964). The regulation of myofibrillar activity by calcium. *Proc. roy. Soc. B.*, **160,** 489.

ZACKS, S. I., and BLUMBERG, J. M. (1961). Observations on the fine structure and cytochemistry of mouse and human intercostal neuromuscular junctions. *J. biophys. biochem. Cytol.*, **10,** 517.

ZAIMIS, E. J. (1951). The action of decamethonium on normal and denervated mammalian muscle. *J. Physiol.* (*Lond.*), **112,** 176.

ZAIMIS, E. J. (1952) Motor end-plate differences as a determining factor in the mode of action of neuromuscular blocking substances. *Nature* (*Lond.*), **170,** 617.

Chapter 30

NEUROMUSCULAR BLOCK

Forms of Neuromuscular Block

There are two principal ways of producing neuromuscular block.

First, it may simply be a prolongation of the normal depolarisation process that arises at the motor end-plate in the presence of acetylcholine. In a normal person the effects of acetylcholine persist for only a fraction of a second, but after depolarisation has taken place there is theoretically a transient interval during which the muscle fibre will no longer respond to a stimulus arriving via the nerve fibre. In short, a state of *depolarisation block* is present. Decamethonium and suxamethonium are typical examples of drugs that act in this manner.

Secondly, *d*-tubocurarine and allied drugs can prevent the passage of an impulse from nerve to muscle, though the latter will still respond to a direct stimulus. *d*-Tubocurarine is believed to have an affinity for the protein molecules of the motor end-plate, but it does not excite the muscle fibre before causing a state of temporary neuromuscular block. This type is termed *non-depolarisation* block, or competitive inhibition. The nomenclature implies that the molecules of curare are in a loose conjugation with the protein molecules of the end-plate without any chemical reaction. Later these bonds can be parted as easily as they were joined. The liberation and destruction of acetylcholine molecules on the arrival of a nerve stimulus at the neuromuscular junction continues as before, the presence of the *d*-tubocurarine molecules merely raising the threshold required to excite the muscle fibre. In other words, it requires more pressure on the trigger before the shot is fired. The anti-cholinesterase drugs prevent the premature destruction of acetylcholine and permit its concentration in the end-plate region to rise, so that—provided the dose of *d*-tubocurarine is not excessive—the acetylcholine can now reach the end-plate and excite the muscle fibre into activity.

There is another type of neuromuscular block that has great clinical significance. This is termed dual or biphasic or desensitisation block and refers to a type of block that may arise following the administration of any depolarising relaxant drug. Normally, a single injection of a depolarising drug leads to a block with all the characteristics of *depolarisation.* If this dose is repeated again and again, the block gradually undergoes a change until finally it shows many of the characteristics of *non-depolarisation*. The change is always from depolarisation to non-depolarisation and never in the reverse direction. It is always encountered sooner or later if repeated doses of any depolarising drug are used in man. The exact time relationship and the mechanism are still uncertain (see p. 824 *et seq.*).

Other variants of neuromuscular blockade have also been described. A *mixed* block refers to the situation where the patient has been given both a depolarising and a non-depolarising type of drug; theoretically the situation might be described as pharmacological chaos. Essentially, some of the motor end-plates are under the influence of one drug whilst the remainder are affected by the other drug.

A *non-acetylcholine* block is a term used to refer to those rare types of blockade in which there is some interference with the synthesis, transport or the release of acetylcholine. Hemicholinium is believed to inhibit either the synthesis or the transport of acetylcholine and is used widely in pharmacological experimentation although, as yet, it has no clinical significance. Procaine, botulinus toxin and a deficiency of calcium, on the other hand, are believed to affect the release of acetylcholine as also do an excess of magnesium and potassium.

The term *non-competitive* neuromuscular block has been used to describe the unusual mechanism responsible for the interruption of transmission after administration of the relaxant dioxahexadecane ("Prestonal") which is discussed below. Furthermore, the *anti-cholinesterase* drugs are also capable of neuromuscular block through a multitude of actions, principally through the accumulation of acetylcholine molecules, but they also have an important depolarisation action in their own right.

30/TABLE 1

TYPES OF NEUROMUSCULAR BLOCK IN MAN

Name	*Cause*
1. Depolarisation	Decamethonium Suxamethonium.
2. Non-depolarisation	*d*-Tubocurarine Gallamine.
3. Dual (biphasic)	Following a depolarising drug only.
4. Mixed	Any combination of 1 and 2.
5. Non-acetylcholine (*a*) Release	Procaine, botulinus, calcium deficiency, excess potassium and magnesium.
(*b*) Synthesis	Hemicholinium.
6. Anti-cholinesterase	Neostigmine and edrophonium.
7. Non-competitive	Dioxahexadecane ("Prestonal").

Additional Forms of Neuromuscular Block

Linssen (1961) has made an extensive study of the action of the various muscle-relaxant drugs in animals. He concluded that the process was even more complex than that already described and proposed various additions to the recognised types of neuromuscular block. One drug of particular interest was dioxahexadecane ("Prestonal"). This agent was first introduced into clinical anaesthesia by Frey (1956) as a short-acting muscle relaxant. However, it enjoyed only a short spate of popularity due to its side-effects of histamine release and vagal blockade. At the same time, there was considerable speculation as to whether or not the neuromuscular block produced by this drug could be reversed by anti-cholinesterase drugs.

In normal circumstances a depolarising and a non-depolarising drug are mutually antagonistic. Theoretically, if the block is pure and the correct dose can be selected then the antagonistic drug can be used to restore neuromuscular transmission. Though such a perfect balance cannot be easily demonstrated in clinical practice, it is at least possible to show a partial antagonism between *d*-tubocurarine and suxamethonium. Linssen (1961), however, found that dioxahexadecane not only enhanced the neuromuscular blocking properties of curare but also those of the depolarising drugs. This resulted in a situation in which this new relaxant was capable of neuromuscular block in its own right yet it could also enhance the blockade of the two principal types of muscle relaxant.

Further investigation of dioxahexadecane revealed that when injected into the newly-hatched chick it produced a flaccid paralysis similar to that with *d*-tubocurarine, but when given to the cat the block was *not* reversible by anticholinesterase drugs (e.g. neostigmine). It appeared, therefore, that on the basis of this evidence dioxahexadecane could no longer be classified satisfactorily under the accepted forms of neuromuscular block.

In an attempt to clarify this situation, Linssen (1961) put forward a new hypothesis. It is generally conceded that acetylcholine molecules have their own specific receptors. It is postulated that when these are stimulated they excite an "effector receptor" before the muscle fibre is fired into activity. This effector receptor is interposed between the acetylcholine receptor and the muscle membrane so that block of this receptor can still prevent neuromuscular transmission. Dioxahexadecane is presumed to act at this stage (Fig. 1).

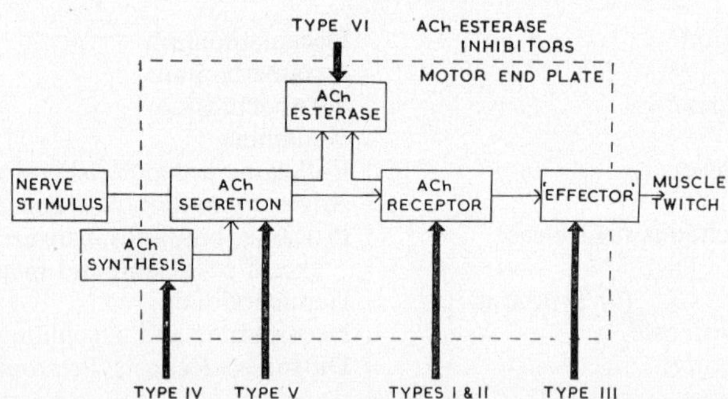

30/FIG. 1.—The various types of neuromuscular block (after Linssen, 1961).

These effector receptors have been termed "non-competitive" on the basis that they are not specific for acetylcholine yet their occupation by a drug such as dioxahexadecane is still capable of producing neuromuscular block.

Benzoquinonium hydrochloride ("Mytolon") is another interesting relaxant drug. Introduced by Cavallito and his colleagues (1950), it again enjoyed only a brief span of clinical popularity. The clinical picture was often confusing. The mode of action of this drug is uncertain but it is believed to be twofold. First, it produced a non-depolarising type of block, and secondly, it was a potent inhibitor of acetylcholine esterase (Linssen, 1961). In short, it combined a non-depolarising relaxant action with its own built-in antidote. It is hardly surprising that this situation led to its own difficulties!

Non-acetylcholine Block

Even during the resting state, small quantities of acetylcholine are released at the nerve terminals, and these ions give rise to small end-plate potentials which are insufficient to depolarise the muscle membrane. Many local analgesics—particularly procaine—are believed directly to suppress the release of acetylcholine and thus cause muscle weakness and paralysis (Harvey, 1939). Other substances which have this property are botulinus toxin (from *Clostridium botulinum*), severe calcium deficiency (Harvey and MacIntosh, 1940), excessive doses of phosphate (Brown and Dias, 1947) and magnesium (Paton, 1956).

The *hemicholinium* group of compounds are quaternary bases which are highly toxic. Though they are not used in clinical practice, their mode of action has excited considerable pharmacological interest. When administered to an animal they ultimately produce complete respiratory paralysis, but this is delayed in onset and can be prevented by the administration of choline. MacIntosh *et al.* (1958) have concluded that these compounds interfere with acetylcholine synthesis by impeding the transport of choline to its site of acetylation.

Mixed Block

The muscles of respiration are normally amongst the first to recover full activity after the injection of a relaxant drug. Electromyographic recordings taken from any peripheral muscle can demonstrate that despite adequate respiratory activity a high degree of neuromuscular block still persists. If, at this point, a further relaxant drug of a different type is given, theoretically some of the motor units will be under the influence of one drug and some affected by the other. A mixed type of neuromuscular block is present.

The practice of mixing the various types of relaxant drug is rarely essential and best avoided. Nevertheless, if the clinical requirements demand such mixing, then it is essential that the anaesthetist should satisfy himself that the muscles of respiration, at least, have fully recovered from the effects of the first drug before the next one is given. Failure to do this may lead to a complex situation if the patient responds in a prolonged manner to either drug.

Measurement of Neuromuscular Block

In the past the action of the various muscle relaxants has been investigated mainly in animals and these findings have often been erroneously assumed to be applicable to man. Unfortunately, there is no single species that responds to these drugs in exactly the same manner as man. This has led to considerable confusion in the literature.

The earliest attempts to study the effects of these drugs in man were based on clinical observations, grip-strength measurements in conscious volunteers, and tidal volume studies in the anaesthetised patient. None of these methods proved entirely satisfactory. First, the pitfalls of clinical observations are known to all. Second, grip-strength recordings are always subject to volitional effort on the part of the individual, and most untrained volunteers have difficulty in making a maximum possible effort under the influence of these drugs. Finally, tidal volume measurements have been widely used in anaesthetised patients; yet many other drugs, such as narcotics, hypnotics, or even inhalational anaesthetic agents, can all depress the tidal volume but are not muscle relaxants. Tidal volume measurements, therefore, can never be considered a satisfactory method of monitoring neuromuscular transmission. Clinically, it has often been wrongly assumed that the muscle relaxants were responsible for respiratory depression at the end of an operation. The danger of this assumption cannot be emphasised too strongly. Such a suggestion can only be satisfactorily upheld if it is demonstrated that neuromuscular transmission is depressed.

There is only one satisfactory method of studying neuromuscular transmission—namely, stimulation of any peripheral motor nerve and observing or measuring the response of the corresponding muscle. The electric current used must be of sufficient intensity to excite all the nerve fibres in the bundle, i.e. it must be supramaximal. Once a stimulus has been propagated down a nerve fibre then, on the basis of the "all or none" law, every one of the corresponding muscle fibres must contract if there is no impairment of neuromuscular transmission.

The principal methods of measuring neuromuscular transmission are outlined below:

(*a*) *Volitional measurements.*—It has already been mentioned above that the value of such measurements is limited. They have, however, proved useful as a guide to laboratory investigations and particularly if repeated comparative measurements are to be made in the same individual. The instrument commonly used is the *recording ergograph* (Fig. 2). The subject squeezes a hand-bulb with a maximum effort at regular intervals. The results are displayed with a pen-recorder. The effect of a particular dose of a relaxant drug or the degree of paresis due to a pathological state can be assessed.

(*b*) *Involuntary measurement.*—Such a technique does not require the co-operation of the patient and therefore is more suitable for use in the unconscious patient. Furthermore, as a supramaximal electrical stimulus can be used, the measurements are more reliable. The resulting contraction of the muscle fibres can be measured either mechanically or electrically. Measurement of mechanical contraction is easier but has the small disadvantage of the inertia of the apparatus, e.g. the strain-gauge. The electrical response of the contracting muscle fibres requires more complex apparatus but gives a greater degree of accuracy. Such recordings, however, are often difficult to obtain in the operating room, where electrical interference is common.

Mechanical method.—Either the hand or the foot muscles can be used. The foot caliper is illustrated in Fig. 3. Cutaneous electrodes are placed either over the medial popliteal nerve or the motor point of the tibialis muscle. A supramaximal stimulus causes the foot to dorsiflex and the mechanical force of each depression is measured with a strain-gauge and a suitable recorder. A similar type of apparatus can be used to measure the movements of the thumb.

Electrical method.—The technique is based on the application of a supramaximal stimulus to a motor nerve and recording the electrical potential generated by a group of muscle fibres all contracting synchronously, i.e. electromyography.

The upper limb is particularly useful in the anaesthetised patient because it is nearly always possible to obtain access to an extended arm in most surgical operations. For measurements the fingers and arm are bound to a splint to

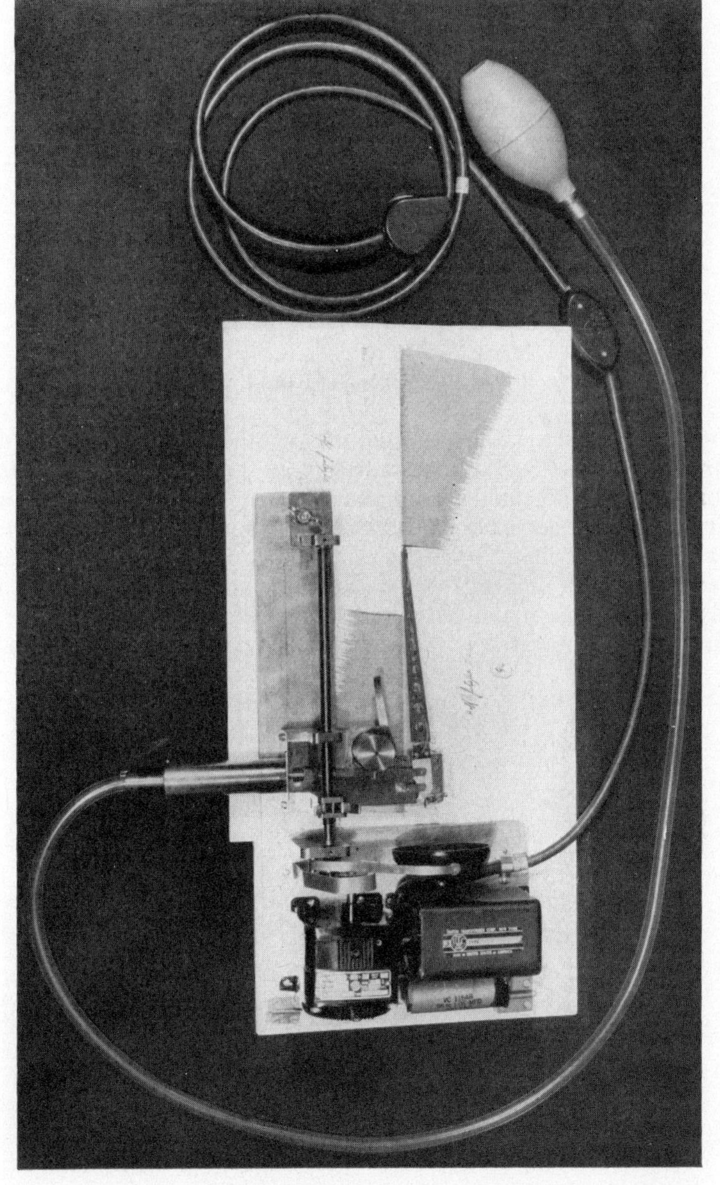

30/Fig. 2.—The recording ergograph.

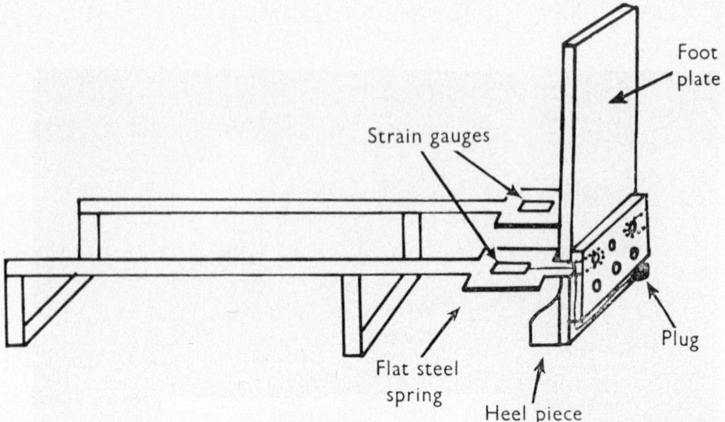

30/FIG. 3.—Diagram of foot caliper.

prevent movement and the contraction of the hypothenar muscles is recorded on the electromyograph (Fig. 4). On stimulation of the nerve fibre (i.e. ulnar), a full motor unit action potential is produced. That is to say, all the 150–300 muscle fibres supplied by that nerve fibre are compelled to contract synchronously. Each of these contractions helps to build the action potential. If the surface electrodes are correctly placed, a number of biphasic motor unit action potentials are recorded as a single large summated potential on the electromyograph.

A normal action potential of the hypothenar muscles in response to a single

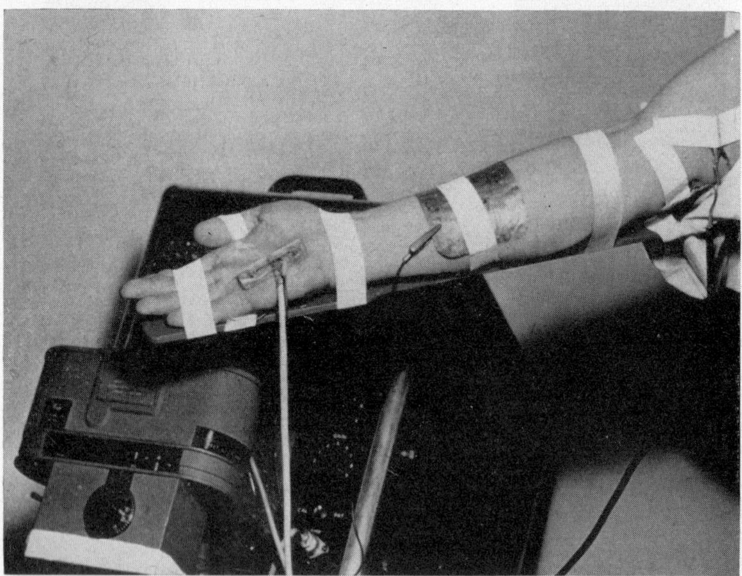

30/FIG. 4.—The electromyographic apparatus arranged for recording from the hypothenar muscles.

supramaximal twitch stimulus of the ulnar nerve is shown in Fig. 5. The stimulus artefact (represented as a small deflection prior to the action potential) represents the administration of the electrical current to the nerve. The time interval between the stimulus artefact and the beginning of the action potential represents the time taken for the stimulus to pass down the nerve fibre and across to the motor end-plate. If the stimulus is administered at two different points along a nerve fibre (e.g. at the elbow and wrist) the difference in the time interval in this case is due to transmission down the nerve between these points.

Under normal physiological conditions a subject can send stimuli down a motor nerve at a rate varying from 20 to 50 per second, depending on the amount of effort expended (Fig. 6). It is impossible to send a single twitch stimulus or a rate as slow as 10 per second without recourse to artificial stimulation.

Regardless of the rate of stimulation (i.e. from 1 to 50 per second), if normal neuromuscular transmission is present then the height of successive action potentials should be well sustained. That is to say, both the height and the shape of the potential will remain virtually unaltered. The size of the action potential is

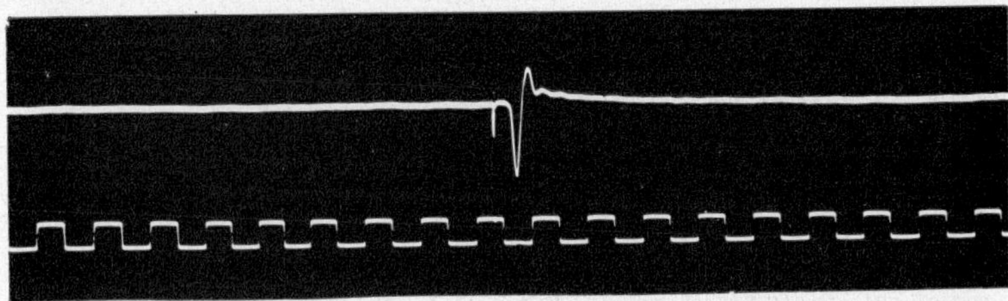

30/FIG. 5.—A normal action potential (twitch stimulus). The small downward depression before the origin of the complete action potential is the artefact caused by the electrical stimulus.

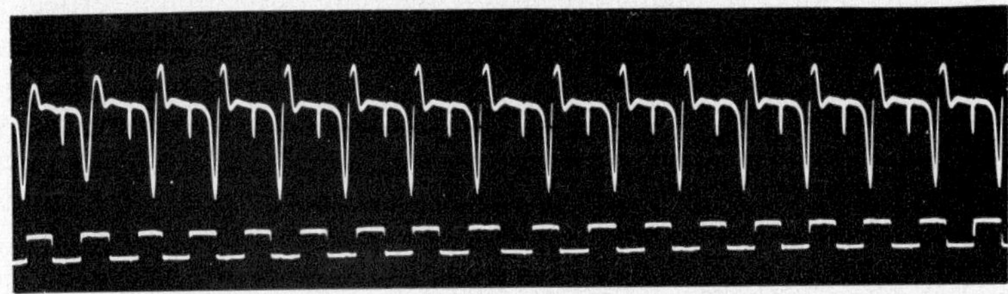

30/FIG. 6.—Normal action potentials (tetanic stimulation).

always slightly greater at tetanic, as opposed to twitch, rates of nerve stimulation. Furthermore, a rate of 50 per second can be maintained in a normal adult for at least twenty seconds before the first signs of fatigue become apparent.

The height of the action potential (or more correctly, the surface area contained within its boundaries) is directly related to the number of muscle fibres that are functioning. Thus, as a muscle relaxant is administered so the height (or area) of the action potential is diminished until finally only the base-line remains when complete paralysis is present.

There are certain other features of abnormal neuromuscular transmission that have already been discussed in Chapter 29, namely post-tetanic potentiation, post-tetanic exhaustion and Wedensky inhibition.

(*a*) "*Fade*" *of successive potentials* (Wedensky inhibition).—This "fade" of successive stimuli is characteristic of a non-depolarisation block, though the explanation of its mechanism is complex. It is clearly related to a change in the threshold of excitation for certain groups of fibres. Essentially, Wedensky inhibition is a term applied to a partial block which transmits slow impulses but fails to transmit high frequency or fast rates of nerve stimulation. This effect is seen in the presence of very small doses of a non-depolarising drug. In clinical practice, however, the decrement of the "fade" will be observed to be similar at both slow and fast rates (see Non-depolarisation block, Fig. 11).

(*b*) *Post-tetanic potentiation.*—This signifies an improvement in neuromuscular transmission *after* a period of tetanic stimulation. It has been defined as a condition where the magnitude or height of the twitch response after 5 seconds of tetanic stimulation is two or more times greater than the last twitch prior to tetanus (Churchill-Davidson and Katz, 1966). It is never seen in the presence of normal neuromuscular transmission, but is always observed in a classical non-depolarisation block (see Fig. 11). It is also seen in those patients with a dual block and in some cases of myasthenia gravis. It is always associated with a "fade" of successive impulses on tetanic stimulation.

The Pattern of Neuromuscular Block

One of the principal features of neuromuscular block is the constant sequence of events as each muscle group becomes involved. This cycle or pattern holds true with minor variations for both depolarising (e.g. decamethonium) and non-depolarising (e.g. *d*-tubocurarine) drugs. These effects can only be observed or recorded satisfactorily if graduated doses are given to a conscious subject. Within thirty seconds to one minute there is a sudden onset of blurring of vision which is rapidly followed by diplopia as the small muscles of the eye become involved. The diplopia is usually horizontal and only rarely in the vertical plane. Next, both eyelids droop (ptosis), but unless extremely heavy dosage has been used this is usually only partial. Following this there is a feeling of weakness or stiffness in the jaw muscles; the exact sensation experienced will depend on the relaxant used. If a depolarising (decamethonium) type of drug is used a peculiar feeling of tightness develops in the jaw muscles and spreads later to the calf muscles: at the same time fasciculations or "twitchings" can be felt in the upper trunk muscles and these gradually spread outwards to involve the lower trunk and limb muscles. With suxamethonium the fasciculations are more rapid in onset and certainly more vigorous. With *d*-tubocurarine, muscle spasm or twitches are never seen. Even though only two minutes may now have passed since the start of the injection, the eye muscles are already starting to improve slowly, but at the same time the muscles of the trunk and then the limbs begin to show signs of involvement. The delay in onset of paresis of the limb muscles is greater with decamethonium than with *d*-tubocurarine and minimal with suxamethonium, but much will depend on the concentration and rate of injection of the substance.

As the dose of relaxant is increased so it becomes possible to paralyse the bulbar muscles whilst still maintaining a reasonable tidal volume of respiration. Nevertheless it must be emphasised that paresis of the swallowing and phonatory muscles in normal subjects is always closely associated with a marked diminution in vital capacity and sometimes a reduction in the minute volume. Once, therefore, the signs of dysphagia and dysphonia are present it is unwise to administer any further relaxant to a conscious subject without artificial ventilation. With all the long-acting muscle relaxants, e.g. *d*-tubocurarine, pancuronium and gallamine, it is a very simple matter, however, to reach a stage of paresis at which the subject is unable to move his arms or legs yet has an unaffected tidal volume. But measurement of vital capacity will reveal a severe reduction. The fact that it is possible to produce almost complete paralysis of the limbs, and yet preserve adequate ventilation, is of importance to the clinical anaesthetist. Such a technique combined with light anaesthesia is suitable for many operations on the extremities.

If too large a dose of relaxant is used the subject may suddenly experience an abrupt cessation of inspiration when it is only half completed. This sensation of "cut-off" is extremely unpleasant and usually leads to panic, but it can quickly be dispelled by manual ventilation. In such a severe degree of weakness there is a danger that inability to swallow secretions or keep the tongue from the back of the throat might lead to respiratory obstruction. It is essential, therefore, that the subject is positioned in such a manner that a free airway is maintained.

Electromyographic Findings

Apart from the muscle weakness experienced by the patient it is possible to trace the onset and recovery of the neuromuscular block by electromyography. Almost any site in the body can be used, particularly if both the motor nerve and the muscles it supplies are readily accessible. Before the introduction of the relaxant the nerve is stimulated and an action potential recorded from the muscle (Fig. 7). As paralysis sets in so the height of the action potential falls as the various motor units drop out, until finally there is no sign at all of electrical activity—in other words, all the muscle fibres in that region are paralysed. Similarly, as recovery takes place, so the height of the action potential grows, until finally it exactly corresponds with the original control figure. This type of measurement or observation can be carried out either with the patient conscious or under anaesthesia; if the latter is used it should be remembered that the thiopentone, nitrous oxide and oxygen sequence is the best method available as it is not believed to have any significant effect on neuromuscular transmission.

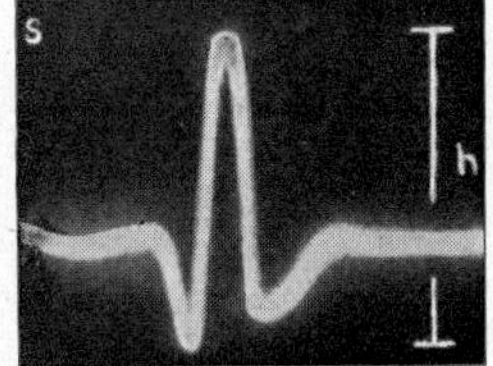

30/FIG. 7.—Action potential of the hypothenar muscles on stimulation of the ulnar nerve. S denotes stimulus artefact, and h the height of the potential.

Recovery

Recovery from the action of the muscle relaxants depends upon a number of factors, the most important of which is the blood supply of the muscle under consideration. Nevertheless, the sequence of events on recovery is almost a mirror image of that on paralysis. That is to say, the respiratory muscles are the first to recover completely, then the bulbar musculature, and finally the trunk and limb muscles. The only muscles which appear to be an exception to this rule are those involved in pathological conditions (e.g. myasthenia gravis).

Possible Reasons for the Sequence of Muscle Paralysis

The causes of the consistency in the pattern of block are not easy to determine, as many factors may be involved, but the main ones to be considered are:

(*a*) *Anatomical position.*—If a muscle is situated and supplied by arterial branches which arise from the early part of the aorta it stands to reason that those which receive the drug first will be affected before those which receive it last. That this fact is important can best be illustrated by observing a patient receiving suxamethonium. Visible fasciculations can first be seen in the eyelids soon after injection and then traced to the trunk muscles and finally, after a considerable delay, can be seen in the hands and feet. This observation, however, does not preclude that some variation in sensitivity of the muscle fibres may also play a part.

(*b*) *Size of the motor unit.*—More specialised tasks, such as vision or fine movements, require the presence of small motor units, whereas cruder movements such as those involved in posture can be carried out satisfactorily by much larger motor units. It has been suggested that the smaller or finer motor units are more susceptible to the muscle relaxants than their more basic colleagues. However, fine movements of the hand appear to be affected in almost equal degree, in both timing and intensity, to such simple movements as grip strength.

(*c*) *Variations in blood supply.*—Apart from the anatomical distribution referred to above, the blood flow to muscles also depends on a number of factors, including vasodilator and vasoconstrictor tone, temperature and metabolites. This matter is discussed in greater detail below (see "Factors altering the duration or degree of neuromuscular block").

(*d*) *Variations in sensitivity of muscles* (*red and white*).—Soon after the introduction into clinical medicine of the methonium compounds it was noted that some muscle groups in animals appeared to be more sensitive to the drug than others (Paton and Zaimis, 1949). Thus, after a given dose of relaxant, some muscles would be in a stage of excitation whilst others were paralysed. This variation in sensitivity appeared to have a constant anatomical association and the only difference between the two groups was the colour of the muscles after total exsanguination. After a total bleed some muscles were found to be "white" and others "red". In the cat, "white" muscles are more sensitive to decamethonium than "red", or, conversely, "red" muscles are more resistant than "white". The response of both these groups of muscles to *d*-tubocurarine is the same. The presence of "red" and "white" muscle in man has never been fully investigated but it is believed that the diaphragm, jaw and calf muscles are examples of the "red" variety. If this were so, then the explanation of the jaw and calf stiffness, together with the resistance of the diaphragm muscles to paralysis might be more easily explained.

Differentiation of Neuromuscular Block

The various characteristics of the two principal types of neuromuscular block—depolarisation and non-depolarisation—are fortunately so different that they can easily be distinguished. This differentiation has important clinical bearings because it enables the anaesthetist to diagnose the exact type of neuromuscular block that is present, even if he does not know the agent used. Principally it is made on four counts:

1. The presence or absence of spontaneous *fasciculations*. These may be observed or recorded electromyographically from an appropriate muscle.
2. The response of the muscle fibre to both *fast* (*tetanic*) and *slow* (*twitch*) rates of nerve stimulation.
3. The presence or absence of *post-tetanic potentiation.*
4. The response to the administration of an anti-cholinesterase drug.

Depolarisation Block (Figs. 8–10)

This type of neuromuscular block follows the administration of acetylcholine (lasting a fraction of a second), suxamethonium (2–4 minutes) and decamethonium (lasting about 20 minutes or more). The four main characteristics of this type of block are:

1. *Fasciculations* can be observed or recorded in muscle just prior to the onset of paralysis. They are particularly well seen after the rapid administration of suxamethonium.

2. Both *fast* (*tetanic*) and *slow* (*twitch*) rates of nerve stimulation are well *sustained.* This statement requires further clarification. Some "fade" or Wedensky inhibition can be observed during a depolarisation block. It is only seen when fast rates are used and when present will be accompanied by post-tetanic potentiation. It is almost always observed during the very early stages of recovery from complete paralysis, but by the time 50 per cent recovery has been achieved the typical signs of a well-sustained response at both twitch and tetanic rates of stimulation are present. If the patient is inhaling halothane then the "fade" at tetanic rates of stimulation is more marked (de Jong and Freund, 1967).

To observe the signs of the block correctly it is necessary to test neuromuscular transmission in the manner demonstrated above. In other words, the sequence of events of nerve stimulation should be *twitch-tetanus-twitch.*

3. *Post-tetanic potentiation* is absent. It will be observed in Fig. 8 that the height of the muscle response to twitch or slow nerve stimulation is the same after a period of fast (tetanic) nerve stimulation as it was before.

4. *Anti-cholinesterase drugs* either produce no effect or *increase* the neuromuscular block. These drugs have an action on the neuromuscular junction tending to potentiate a depolarisation block. Edrophonium ("Tensilon") 10 mg. is sometimes used as a diagnostic agent in the presence of a dual block (see p. 829).

The effect of first a depolarising drug and then the combination of a depolarising drug with an anti-cholinesterase is illustrated in Fig. 9. It will be observed that the classical signs of a depolarisation block are present. The

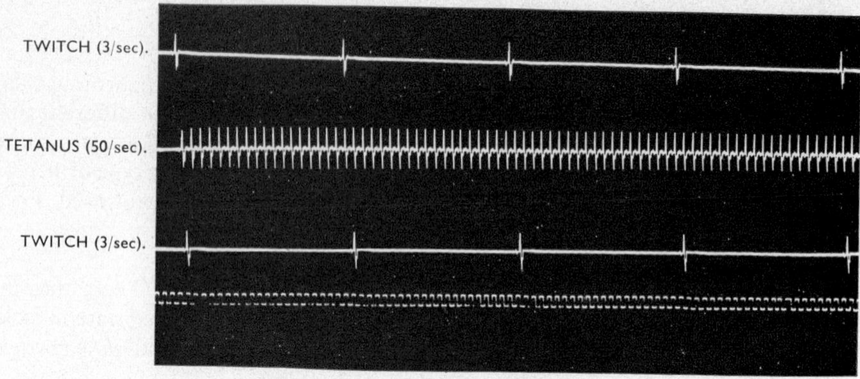

30/FIG. 8.—Depolarisation block.

decamethonium has produced about 95 per cent paralysis of the muscle fibres. Only a minimal change can be observed on the administration of an anti-cholinesterase, though there is some slight increase in the neuromuscular block.

Clinical significance.—These electromyographic changes can also be ob-

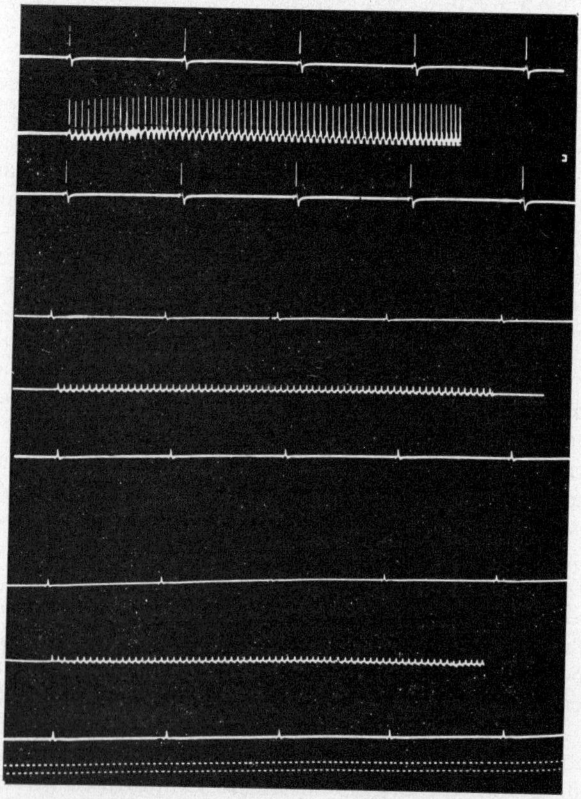

A. NORMAL NEUROMUSCULAR TRANSMISSION

CONTROL

B. DEPOLARISATION BLOCK

AFTER 2·5 mg. DECAMETHONIUM

C. EFFECT OF ANTI-CHOLINESTERASE THERAPY

AFTER 2·5 mg. DECAMETHONIUM + 2·5 mg. NEOSTIGMINE

30/FIG. 9.—Depolarisation block and the effect of neostigmine.

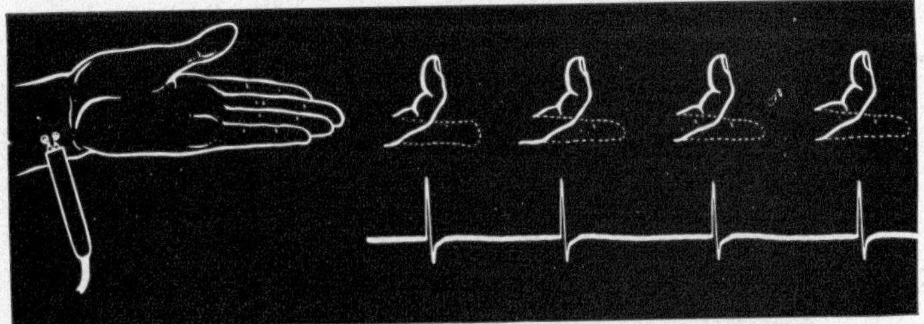

30/FIG. 10.—Depolarisation block. Movements of the fingers on peripheral nerve stimulation correlated with the electromyographic response.

served clinically as movements of the fingers. A simple nerve-stimulator is all that is required and there is no necessity for complex electromyographic equipment. If the ulnar nerve is stimulated either at the wrist or in the ulnar groove at the elbow, the fingers will be seen to take on the characteristic "main en griffe" position each time the stimulus is administered. The main deflexion appears in the 5th and 4th fingers and the hypothenar muscles, but the other muscles of the hand (particularly the thenar muscles) are also often involved.

Clinically, two features of a depolarisation block can be particularly well demonstrated provided total paralysis is not present. As previously mentioned, some "fade" and post-tetanic potentiation may be present in the early stages of recovery and during the inhalation of halothane. Once 50 per cent recovery has been achieved both twitch and tetanus are well sustained. However, in contrast with a non-depolarisation block the slow twitch rates (i.e. 2–5 per second) are always well sustained at any stage of the recovery period. Also, in a non-depolarisation block even the twitch rates show a "fade" or Wedensky inhibition.

1. Successive stimuli are *well-sustained* with both fast and slow rates of nerve stimulation.

2. There is *no* post-tetanic potentiation.

If a short-acting anti-cholinesterase drug (e.g. 10 mg. edrophonium) is given intravenously, a momentary increase in the paresis may be observed. Such therapy, however, is entirely unnecessary (and may even be harmful) if the other signs of a depolarisation block have already been observed.

Non-depolarisation Block (Figs. 11–13)

This type of block normally follows the administration of *d*-tubocurarine chloride, gallamine triethiodide and similar agents.

In direct contrast with the features described for a depolarisation block above, the signs of a non-depolarisation block are as follows:

1. *No fasciculations.*—There is a complete absence of muscle-fibre activity prior to the onset of paralysis.

2. The presence of "*fade*" of successive stimuli on both fast (tetanic) and slow (twitch) rates of nerve stimulation (Fig. 11).

3. The presence of *post-tetanic potentiation* (see above).

4. Improvement of neuromuscular transmission by anti-cholinesterase drugs (see below).

Clinical significance.—The signs of a non-depolarisation block can easily be recognised with the aid of a peripheral nerve stimulator. Stimulation of a motor

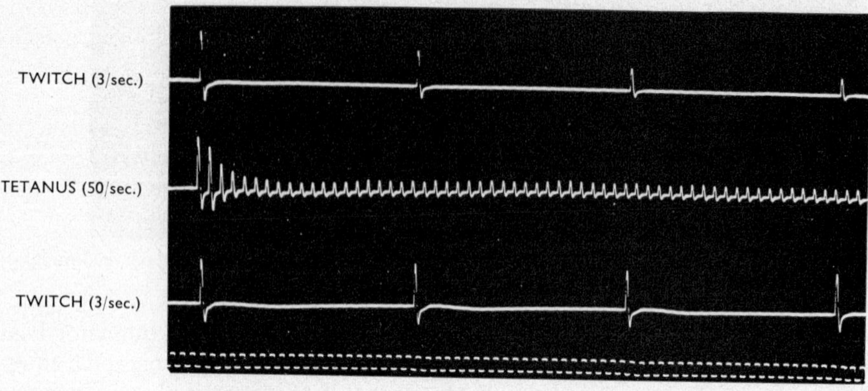

30/FIG. 11.—Non-depolarisation block.

nerve reveals the characteristic "*fade*" and "*post-tetanic potentiation*". These are best observed in the movements of the fingers. As the mechanical movements of the fingers are directly related to the electrical response, the interpretation of these results is virtually interchangeable. Sometimes it is easier to detect the presence of fade and potentiation by "feeling" the movements of the fingers rather than simply observing them. The sense of touch is often more delicate than

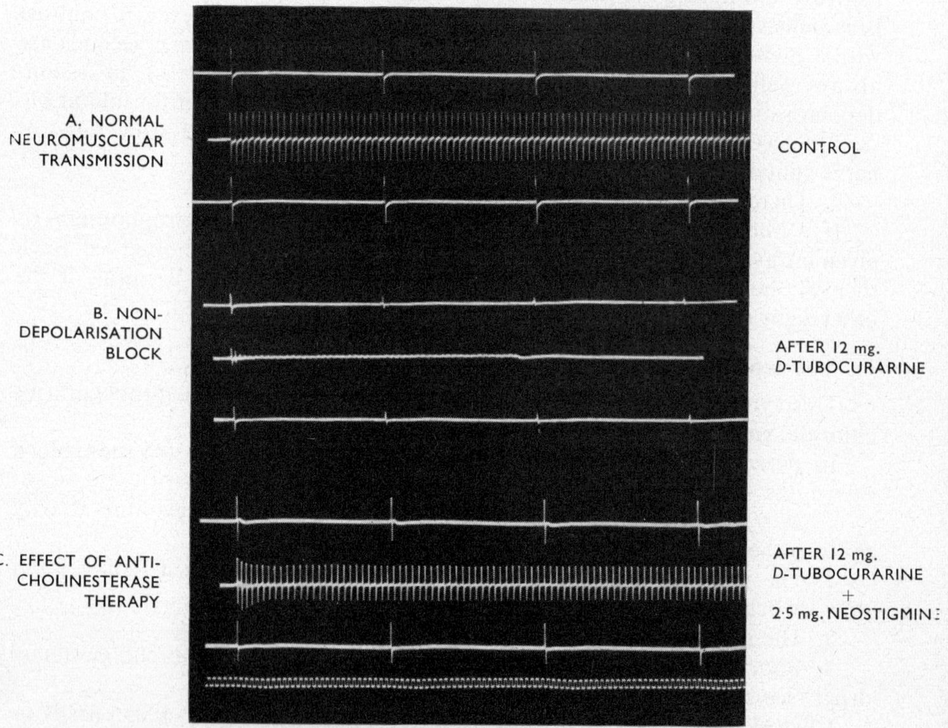

30/FIG. 12.—Non-depolarisation block and the effect of neostigmine.

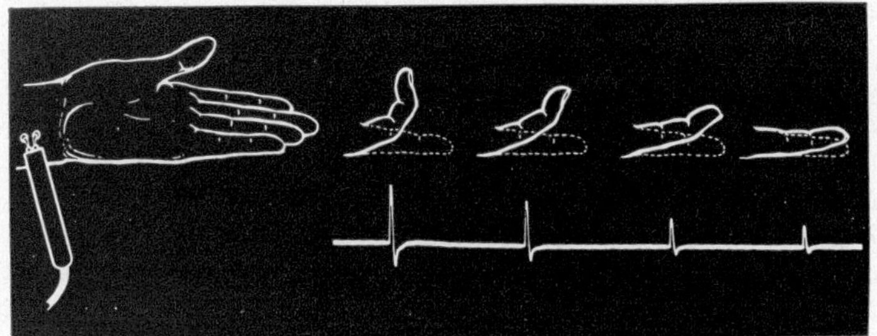

30/Fig. 13.—Non-depolarisation block. Movements of the fingers on peripheral nerve stimulation correlated with the electromyographic response.

vision in this respect. The "fade" of successive stimuli occurs maximally in the first four stimuli whether the rate be fast or slow. In a severe non-depolarisation block the initial contraction may be so short-lived during tetanic stimulation that it is unobserved by the eye yet perceived by touch. To demonstrate post-tetanic potentiation, the actual period of tetanic stimulation should be at least five seconds; at the termination about two seconds should be allowed to elapse before returning to a slow, or twitch, rate of stimulation. In an average case some facilitation can be observed for about thirty seconds after the end of the tetanic stimulation, but this duration depends on many factors such as the rate of tetanus, the duration of the tetanus, and the rate of twitch stimulation. However, it rarely persists more than one minute.

From the clinical aspect, therefore, the anaesthetist (with the aid of a nerve-stimulator) can gauge at the end of every case in which a relaxant has been given an approximate estimate of the degree of neuromuscular block; he can also observe and titrate the effect of anti-cholinesterase therapy. For example, if both "fade" and "potentiation" are present, then this is a clear indication for such therapy, whereas it is unnecessary if they are absent and neuromuscular transmission has recovered. This titration of the clinical effect is particularly useful in cardiac cases, small children, and the severely ill, where it is desired to obtain the maximum benefit of neuromuscular transmission with the minimum quantity of drugs. Finally, with careful observation of the characteristic movements of the fingers on both slow and fast nerve stimulation, then the precise type of neuromuscular block that is present can be diagnosed (Fig. 14).

Comment on the reversibility of *d*-tubocurarine paresis.—Electromyographically it has been observed that it is difficult completely to reverse the neuromuscular block produced by *d*-tubocurarine unless either the dose of relaxant is very low, the time interval between relaxant and antagonist is very long, or the dose of neostigmine is very high. In clinical practice, when a full paralysant dose of *d*-tubocurarine has been used (i.e. 25–30 mg. in an average adult) then 100 per cent normal neuromuscular transmission is difficult to obtain rapidly unless a long interval has elapsed before the anti-cholinesterase is given. However such perfection is seldom required since by the time neuromuscular transmission in the hand muscles has recovered to 25 per cent of normal, the respiratory muscles have recovered sufficiently for normal ventilation. For this reason the hand muscles act as a very useful guide in the diagnosis of hyperventilation or apnoea (see below). It is important to emphasise that anti-cholinesterase drugs (e.g. neostigmine) are only effective provided the motor end-plates have *not* been completely saturated with *d*-tubocurarine. *The skill in the administration of* d-*tubocurarine lies in finding the optimum dose of the relaxant that will just produce ideal conditions for surgery yet which is easily reversible by an anti-cholinesterase drug a few moments later.*

Fortunately, as the duration of action of neostigmine exceeds that of *d*-tubocurarine, the danger of recurarisation is minimal. Nevertheless, this is certainly not true if edrophonium ("Tensilon") is used, because in these circumstances recurarisation frequently occurs. The whole process may be likened to a patient climbing the stairs. Neostigmine will carry him steadily towards the top. Edrophonium will cause him to take five steps upwards, but this is soon followed by four steps backwards. Although some improvement is registered, the end-result will depend on how near the top of the stairs the patient was before the antidote was given.

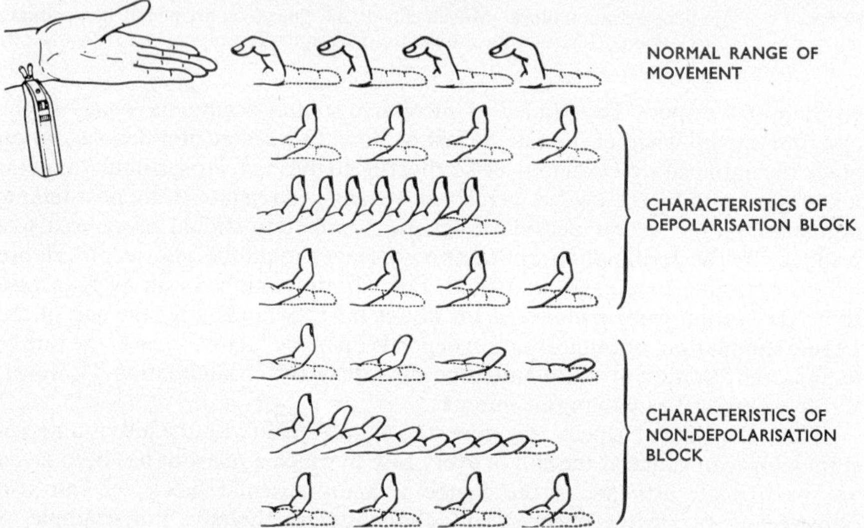

30/FIG. 14.—Finger movements with nerve stimulation.

There still remains one important type of neuromuscular block that is commonly encountered in clinical practice—namely, dual block.

Dual Block (Phase II or Desensitisation)

One of the most interesting developments in the theory of neuromuscular transmission is the finding that the depolarising drugs, e.g. decamethonium and suxamethonium, do not always behave exactly as predicted. In order to understand the background to this new conception, it is necessary to trace the evidence in both animal and human experiments from the introduction of the methonium compounds into clinical medicine.

Investigation in animals.—By 1950 it had been firmly established that decamethonium acted by depolarising the muscle fibre in a small area in the region of the motor end-plate (Brown *et al.*, 1949). Later, this led to the assumption that both decamethonium and suxamethonium produced their neuromuscular block by pure depolarisation in all mammals (Paton and Zaimis, 1952). It had, however, been noted that the response of different muscle groups in the cat to depolarising drugs varied widely, and this difference was thought to be related to the colour of the muscle groups following exsanguination—namely red or white muscle. Thus, the soleus muscle (an example of the "red" kind) is resistant to the depolarising action of decamethonium whereas the tibialis muscle (an example of the "white" kind) is comparatively sensitive (Table 2).

30/TABLE 2

COMPARISON OF THE EFFECT OF DECAMETHONIUM ON THE TIBIALIS AND SOLEUS MUSCLES OF THE CAT

Soleus—Red muscle—Resistant to decamethonium.
Tibialis—White muscle—Sensitive to decamethonium.

At this stage it was generally believed that the depolarising drugs acted by simple depolarisation in all mammals, including man. Nearly all the discrepancies in the response to decamethonium could be explained on the basis of variations in sensitivity between the different muscle groups. This simple conception was shattered, however, when Jenden and his colleagues (1951) observed an altered response in the rabbit and Zaimis (1952) went on to show that a remarkable difference in the response of decamethonium existed amongst the various species. For, although the motor end-plates of the cat might respond to decamethonium by pure depolarisation, it was clear that in the dog, monkey and rabbit a very different type of response occurred. In the case of these latter animals the first injection of decamethonium produced a neuromuscular block with all the signs of pure depolarisation, but second and subsequent injections showed a changing picture until the evidence suggested the block had changed to a non-depolarising type. In short, the block first showed signs of depolarisation and then altered to one of non-depolarisation where it could be antagonised or reversed by the injection of an anti-cholinesterase. A "dual" type of neuromuscular block was present.

There were two further important points about this species variation (Zaimis, 1952). First, although decamethonium produced depolarisation in the cat, if a compound with a slightly longer polymethylene chain was used (i.e. tridecamethonium, or C.13) then the response in the cat was of the dual type. This suggested that simply producing a slight alteration in the molecular structure could change the type of response of the motor end-plate. A dual type of neuromuscular block could theoretically arise from either an alteration of the structure of the molecule injected or from a change in the way in which the motor end-plate responded to the molecule. The second observation clearly demonstrated the dual nature of this type of neuromuscular block. Buttle and Zaimis (1949) had convincingly demonstrated that *d*-tubocurarine, when injected into birds, produced a flaccid paralysis, but that decamethonium led to a spastic paralysis. In reality this latter condition is a *contracture* with rigid extension of the limbs and retraction of the head. When tridecamethonium was used in place of decamethonium a characteristic picture developed. First the animal went into a contracture (signifying depolarisation) and then gradually relaxed until finally a full flaccid paralysis could be recognised.

To summarise, Fig. 15 emphasises the wide range of sensitivity to decamethonium throughout the animal kingdom. Despite this, there is also a large variation in the sensitivity of the different muscle groups in the same animal.

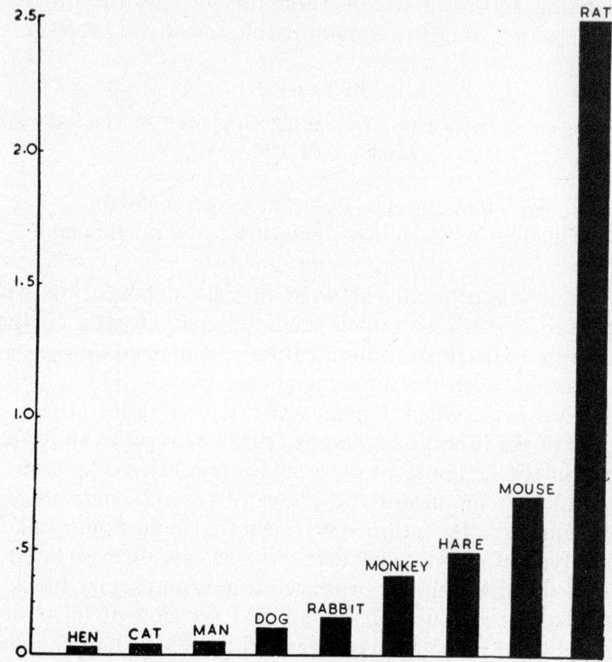

30/Fig. 15.—The sensitivity of various species to decamethonium, as illustrated by the dose in mg./kg. required to produce complete or almost complete neuromuscular block.

In the cat decamethonium acts by pure depolarisation, but in the monkey, dog and rabbit a dual type of neuromuscular block arises. It is essential, therefore, that any statement of the action of the relaxant drugs attributed to man must first have been verified in the human subject.

Clinical interpretation.—A dual block always ultimately occurs after repeated doses of a depolarising drug in man. Only rarely is the presence of this block of any clinical importance. Typically, the administration of a depolarising drug is at first followed by all the signs of a depolarisation block. With repeated doses, gradually some of the signs of a non-depolarisation block occur during the recovery phase. If suxamethonium is used this may be only for a fleeting moment at first, but then slowly the period of "fade and potentiation" becomes more obvious. Ultimately, if repeated doses continue to be given, a stage is reached where the signs of a full dual block are obvious and recovery of normal neuromuscular transmission is slow.

The five stages in the development of a dual block have been described (Churchill-Davidson *et al.*, 1960) as follows:

1. *Depolarisation stage.*—A typical depolarisation block with maintenance of both fast (tetanic) and slow (twitch) rates of nerve stimulation is present when observed at the stage of 50 per cent recovery of neuromuscular transmission. Anti-cholinesterase drugs potentiate the block.

2. *Tachyphylaxis stage.*—The same dose repeated again and again leads to a *diminishing* response. To gain the original response it is necessary to *increase* the dose.

3. *Stage of Wedensky inhibition.*—There is a "fade" of successive potentials to fast rates of nerve stimulation only. Twitch stimulation remains unaltered.

4. *Stage of "fade and potentiation."*—As the dual block develops, so this becomes more and more obvious. The administration of an anti-cholinesterase drug at this point will improve all those fibres exhibiting "fade and potentiation."

5. *Non-depolarisation stage.*—All the classical signs of a non-depolarisation block are present. There is marked "fade and potentiation" and the initial twitch response is high, showing that a large percentage of the muscle fibres are now exhibiting a dual block. The administration of an anti-cholinesterase drug leads to a dramatic improvement in neuromuscular transmission.

An example of the first, fourth and fifth stages of a dual block is given in Fig. 16.

A similar situation can develop if an infusion of suxamethonium is used. In Fig. 17 the twitch response following 50 mg. of suxamethonium is compared with that after 1500 mg. The typical "fade" of a non-depolarisation block is clearly demonstrated.

Dose-relationship of Dual Block

It has already been stated that the repeated administration of a depolarising drug in man will ultimately lead to the signs of a dual block. The process of this change is a gradual one and therefore there is always a long period where the picture is confusion. Churchill-Davidson and his co-workers (1960) found that a dose of at least 0·5 g. of suxamethonium was needed in a group of normal patients (anaesthetised with thiopentone, nitrous oxide and oxygen) to establish a full dual block which could be dramatically reversed by neostigmine. Katz and his colleagues (1963*b*) using a variety of anaesthetic agents, found that the earliest signs of a non-depolarising block were reached after a dose of only 2·2 to 3·0 mg./kg. This represents a total dose of as little as 154 to 210 mg. of suxamethonium in an average 70 kg. patient. Crul and his associates (1966) in a study of the onset of dual block after suxamethonium confirmed that it was both *dose* and *time* dependent. However, by using very small doses they were able to produce the signs of dual block with as little as 0·6 mg./kg. De Jong and Freund (1967) went one stage further and claimed that a depolarisation of Phase I block never occurred in man, but this was probably because their patients had received a considerable dose of halothane. The discrepancy of these results, which is merely one of degree, may lie in the interpretation of the degree of development of dual block, or in the different methods of dose administration. It has already been mentioned that the signs of a dual block can often be observed for a few minutes during the recovery phase. Nevertheless, normal neuromuscular transmission

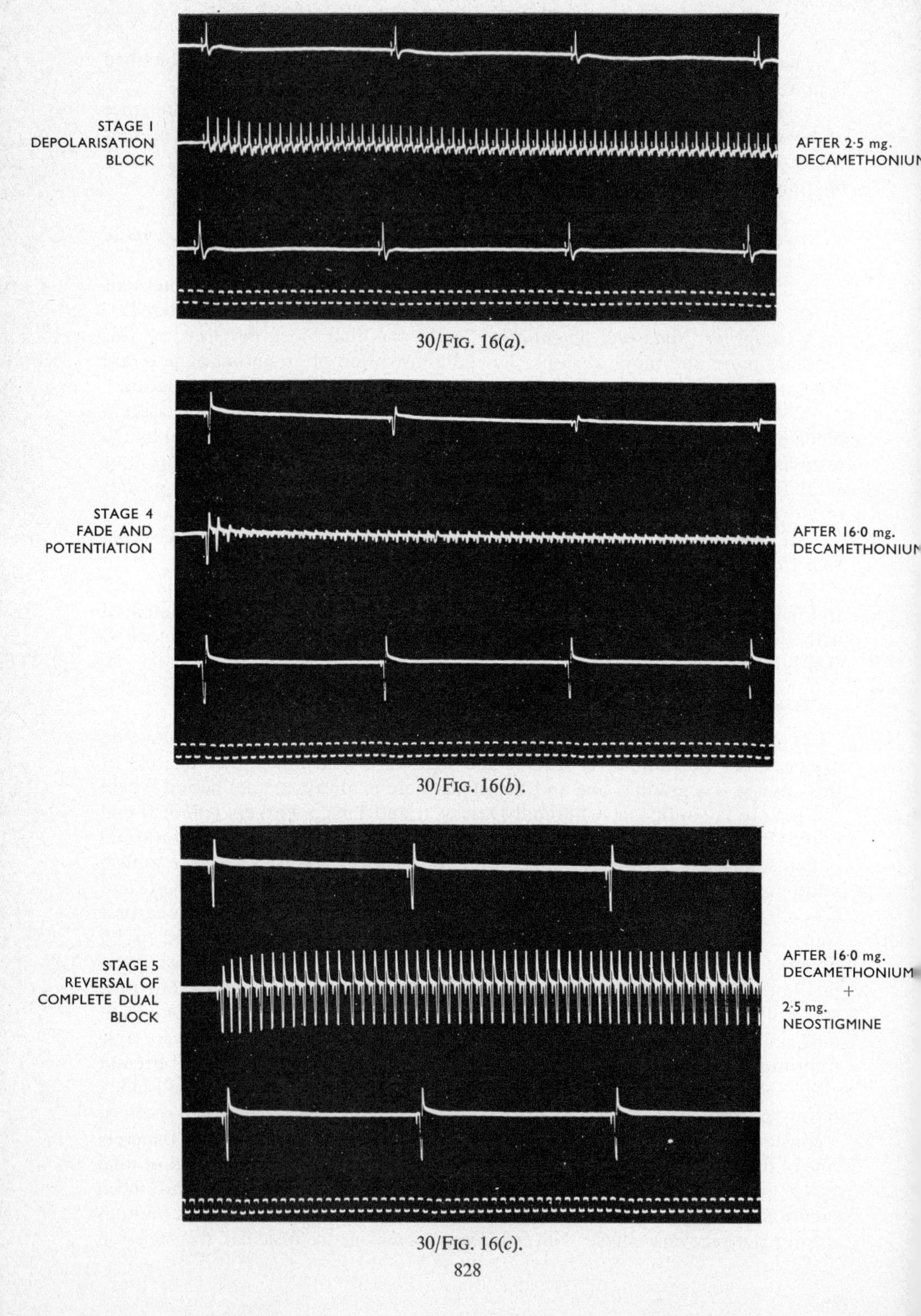

30/Fig. 16(*a*).

30/Fig. 16(*b*).

30/Fig. 16(*c*).

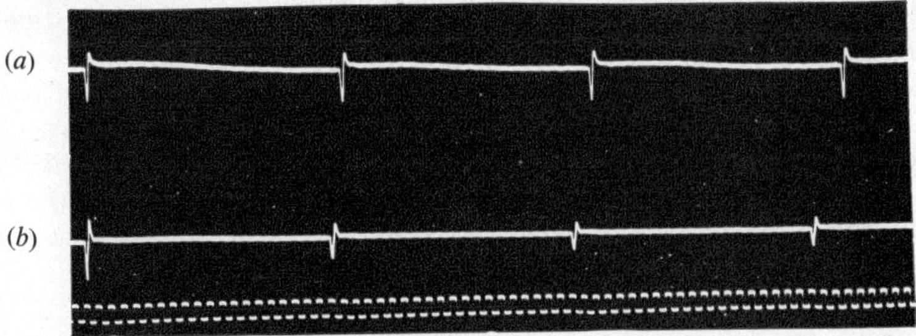

30/FIG. 17.—Effect of infusion of suxamethonium on the twitch response of the hypothenar muscles. (*a*) After 50 mg. (*b*) After 1500 mg.

returns in a matter of minutes. It is only when the signs of a full dual block are firmly established that the recovery of neuromuscular transmission is seriously delayed and the problem assumes clinical importance. This stage is not often reached in normal man with a dose less than 0·5 g. suxamethonium.

Incidence of Dual Block

Essentially there are two occasions in clinical practice when the signs of a dual block may be observed. First, when large doses of a depolarising drug are used (as mentioned above). Secondly, following a small dose of suxamethonium (50–100 mg.) in a patient who has an atypical form of cholinesterase enzyme in his plasma; in this event the suxamethonium is not hydrolysed in the blood stream but continues to circulate for many minutes or hours like a constant infusion. In these circumstances, a dual block is often observed as the patient is emerging from the paresis.

Treatment of Dual Block

The fact that a fully-established dual block can readily be reversed by an anti-cholinesterase drug is now proven. However, Vickers (1963) has pointed out the difficulties that may be encountered in the indiscriminate use of anti-cholinesterase drugs. There are numerous clinical reports of the successful reversal of a dual block in clinical practice: nevertheless, there are also a number of instances when the administration of an anti-cholinesterase drug in an attempt to reverse a dual block has merely increased and prolonged the paralysis (Harper, 1952; Abrams and Ginsberg, 1960; Vickers, 1963).

In considering whether or not one should use anti-cholinesterase drugs in an attempt to reverse a dual block there are a number of points to be taken into account. Experimental evidence has shown that the recovery time from both a depolarisation and a dual block is the same (Katz and Katz, 1967). It has also been demonstrated that the reversibility of an experimental dual block depends mainly on the concentration of the depolarising drug in the circulation (Gissen *et al.*, 1966). When the concentration is high the block cannot be reversed, whilst when it is low recovery can be established.

In clinical practice the anaesthetist using a suxamethonium infusion is likely to monitor neuromuscular transmission with a peripheral nerve stimulator. This avoids total paralysis and prevents an overdose. If, however, no nerve stimulator is used then it is very easy to infuse suxamethonium at a rate faster than it is hydrolysed, so leading to a large accumulation in the circulation.

It is known that a fully established dual block (like a non-depolarisation block) can be reversed by an anti-cholinesterase. Equally it is known that if suxamethonium is still circulating, then the injection of an anti-cholinesterase will slow down any hydrolysis even further and may even augment the block. The fact that some patients are made worse by the anti-cholinesterase suggests that some of the motor end-plates are still in a state of depolarisation and have not yet undergone this change of desensitisation.

There are two courses of action open to the anaesthetist confronted by this problem. First, he can continue to ventilate the lungs and wait patiently for the return of normal neuromuscular transmission. This is the wisest and safest course to adopt. Secondly, he can try to establish the state of the dual block. Using a peripheral nerve stimulator, if a fully established dual block is present, he should be able to observe all the classical signs with both fade of successive stimuli and post-tetanic potentiation. A well-established dual block will show a fade of successive responses even at a slow twitch rate of stimulation (i.e. 3–5/second). If there are signs of a gradual improvement in neuromuscular transmission this suggests that the blood level of suxamethonium is low. Some indication of the possible value of anti-cholinesterases can be gained from observing the effect of post-tetanic potentiation. Anti-cholinesterase therapy tends to restore neuromuscular transmission to the same level as that seen momentarily with post-tetanic potentiation. If, therefore, it is absent or only very small, then no advantage will be gained.

The main factors to be taken into consideration are: (1) that at least 30 minutes have elapsed since the last injection of suxamethonium; (2) that some signs of recovery of neuromuscular transmission have occurred; (3) that a fully established dual block, i.e. fade at slow rates of stimulation as well as during tetanic rates, is present; (4) that there is recovery of at least one-third of the muscle fibres, as observed in the hand muscles. Under these conditions an anti-cholinesterase will improve neuromuscular transmission. However, unless the anaesthetist is thoroughly familiar with various signs of neuromuscular transmission and the use of the peripheral nerve-stimulator, it is wiser practice to refrain from the use of anti-cholinesterase drugs in this type of block. Patience and good ventilation will always receive their just reward!

Factors Altering the Duration or Degree of Neuromuscular Block

The use of the muscle relaxants has now become firmly established as an integral part of modern anaesthesia. It is not surprising, therefore, that their use is sometimes blamed for the failure of the patient to breathe adequately at the end of an operation. Often the muscle relaxants are unjustly convicted when the real blame lies with the administrator for failing accurately to assess the requirements of a particular patient. Occasionally, however, a number of cases are reported in which the relaxants appear to be incriminated. Each time this occurs a new theory is born, often with the minimum of experimental evidence.

The various factors which are known or believed to affect either the degree or duration of neuromuscular block are reviewed below.

Blood Flow

Undoubtedly the single most important factor influencing the duration of neuromuscular block is the blood supply to the muscles. Churchill-Davidson and Richardson (1952) have demonstrated the clinical importance of this finding in a series of simple experiments in conscious volunteers. The duration of action of a relaxant is usually studied with measurements of volitional activity, but electromyography can also be used for the resting limb. The advantage of the conscious subject is that volitional and electromyographic measurements can be compared directly and also each arm can act as a control for its opposite number.

The duration of a given dose of relaxant can be studied under varying conditions of blood flow to the limb. One arm is continuously exercised whilst the other remains passive. The exercised arm rapidly becomes weak and equally rapidly recovers; in contrast, the resting arm takes longer to reach a state of paresis, but once this is attained it remains in a weak state for a very prolonged period (Fig. 18). At the end of this time a small bout of exercise will rapidly

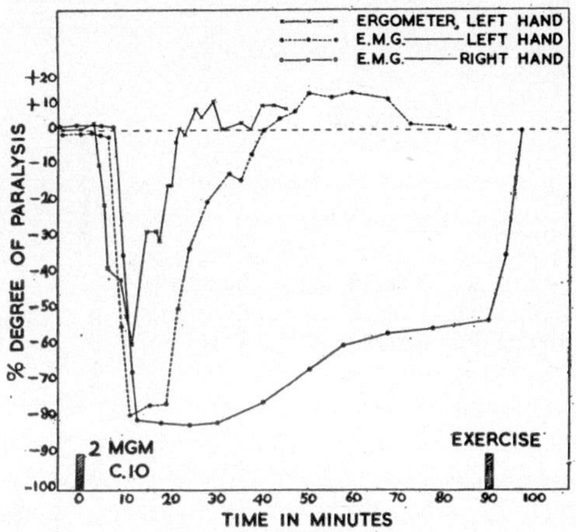

30/Fig. 18.—Comparison of the duration of paralysis from the administration of 2 mg. of decamethonium in resting limb (right) and exercising limb (left).

re-establish normal activity. This effect occurs irrespective of the type of relaxant used.

Again, variations in skin temperature are known to be reflected in changes in the underlying muscle blood flow. If one arm is heated and the other cooled, the warm arm (after a depolarising drug) will show a short duration of paresis whereas the cold arm will remain weak for an indefinite period (Fig. 19). Similar effects can also be obtained by increasing the blood flow with a sympathetic nerve block (Fig. 20). Whether a similar effect occurs in the presence of a non-depolarising drug is not known.

Feldman and Tyrrell (1970), in a classically simple experiment, have drawn attention to the different rates of recovery of a depolarisation as opposed to a non-depolarisation block. A small dose of each relaxant is injected into an isolated limb (tourniquet) in a conscious subject. On restoration of normal blood flow the depolarisation block recovers almost instantly as the plasma level is reduced. However, the recovery of the non-depolarisation block is slow and progressive. The authors believe this is due to a specific grip or attachment of the *d*-tubocurarine molecule to its receptor which is lacking in the case of a depolarising drug, so that recovery now becomes independent of the plasma concentration (see Plasma Concentration, p. 836).

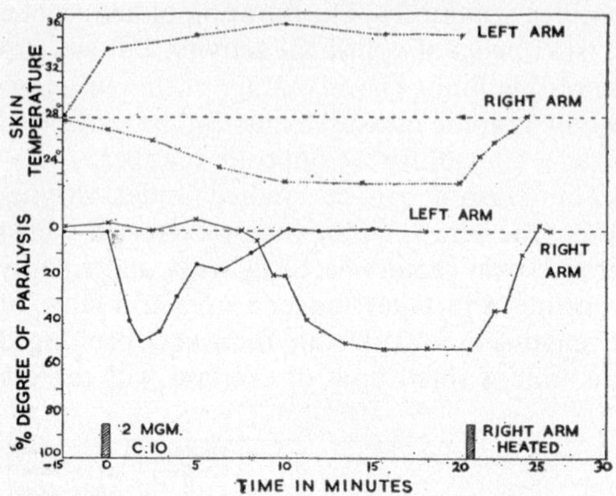

30/Fig. 19.—The effect of variations of temperature on the duration of paralysis following decamethonium (skin temperature recorded).

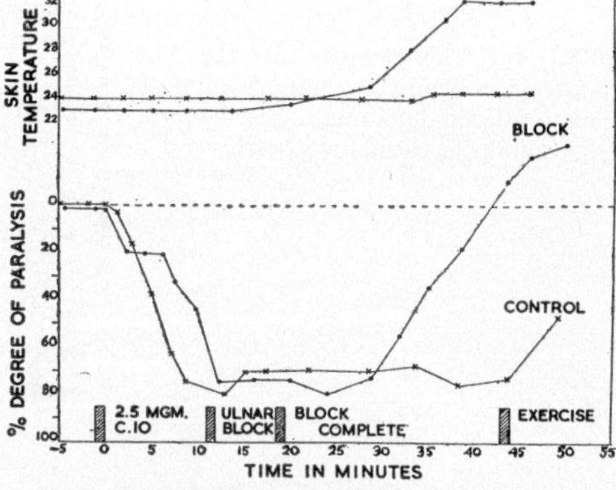

30/Fig. 20.—The effect of an ulnar nerve (sympathetic) block on paralysis following decamethonium.

All these results emphasise the tremendous importance of the blood flow in controlling the duration of action of a muscle relaxant. Often such drugs as gallamine and *d*-tubocurarine are regarded as lasting only 20–30 minutes. Such an impression is based mainly on studies made either on conscious volunteers or in fit young patients. Nevertheless, in an elderly patient, or more particularly in one with a serious illness, the duration of neuromuscular block may persist for many hours. Each individual patient would seem to have an optimum dose for paralysis; if further doses are given at intervals a stage is ultimately reached where the "receptors" appear to be saturated and the paresis persists for many hours. In the young with a vigorous blood flow this is rarely a problem, because the blood flow empties the specific receptors and redistributes the relaxant to neutral inactive receptors. In the aged or the sick where cardiac output and peripheral blood flow are reduced, this mechanism is curtailed and will prolong the duration of action of the muscle relaxants.

Body Temperature

Bigland and her colleagues (1958) have demonstrated in both cats and dogs that the duration and degree of neuromuscular block can be strongly influenced by lowering the body temperature. Hypothermia increases both the magnitude and the duration of the depolarisation block. With both decamethonium and suxamethonium a fall in body temperature of 5° C was sufficient to produce a fourfold prolongation in the period of paralysis. These effects were strictly related to the body temperature and were completely reversed by rewarming. In contrast, hypothermia reduced the degree of block produced by *d*-tubocurarine but had no effect on its duration (Table 3).

The clinical application of these findings has been confirmed in man (Zaimis *et al.*, 1958; Cannard and Zaimis, 1959). However, hypothermia *per se* is probably seldom responsible for a marked prolongation of paralysis, presumably because such patients seldom require large doses of relaxant drugs in the cold state. Once the first few degrees fall in body temperature has been attained the requirements both for anaesthetic and relaxant drugs become correspondingly less. Such drugs are usually required at the beginning of an anaesthetic when the body temperature is around normal; theoretically, although the cold may potentiate or antagonise the action of these drugs, on rewarming the degree of neuromuscular block should return to normal. Fortunately, the block produced by *d*-tubocurarine and gallamine has been found to be readily reversible at a body temperature of 30°–31° C. Nevertheless, the possibility that hypothermia may influence the neuromuscular block must always be borne in mind, particularly in small infants where an unrecognised fall in body temperature may sometimes occur.

30/TABLE 3

THE EFFECT OF HYPOTHERMIA ON THE ACTION OF CERTAIN MUSCLE RELAXANTS IN ANIMALS

Relaxant	*Effect of hypothermia on the neuromuscular block*	
	Duration	*Degree*
Decamethonium . . Suxamethonium	Prolonged +	Increased
d-Tubocurarine . .	No action	Lessened

Carbon Dioxide and the pH of Blood

Dundee (1952) suggested that hyperventilation reduced the dose of muscle relaxant required for abdominal surgery. This led Payne (1958) to study the influence of carbon dioxide and changes in the pH of blood on the neuromuscular-blocking action of the relaxant drugs in the cat. His results proved confusing in that carbon dioxide opposed the action of suxamethonium, decamethonium and gallamine but enhanced that of *d*-tubocurarine. Recently, Katz and his colleagues (1963*a*) re-examined the same problem. They noted that carbon dioxide alone (i.e. in the absence of relaxant drugs) was capable of reducing the twitch response. Furthermore, sodium bicarbonate and THAM were also capable of blocking neuromuscular transmission in their own right. A review of the available literature merely emphasised the variety of results that have been reported (Kalow, 1954; Payne, 1960; Gamstorp and Vinnars, 1961). However, using sodium *carbonate* (which had no effect on neuromuscular transmission yet raised the pH), they found that an induced alkalosis potentiated the neuromuscular block produced by dimethyl tubocurarine, gallamine and suxamethonium yet antagonised the block of *d*-tubocurarine and decamethonium.

Utting (1963), working with dogs, found that the plasma level of *d*-tubocurarine varied with the pH of blood—increasing during acidaemia and falling during alkalaemia. Baraka (1964) in a study in man found that a swing of pH towards the acid side (whether metabolic or respiratory) was associated with a rise in the plasma level of *d*-tubocurarine and also a prolongation of neuromuscular block: on the other hand, a respiratory alkalosis resulted in a fall in the plasma level together with a rapid recovery. The explanation of this phenomenon is at present uncertain but it is suggested that the fluctuations in pH may alter the ionisation of the two hydroxyl groups in the *d*-tubocurarine molecule, thus increasing or decreasing its attachment to the end-plate receptor.

This important finding has focused attention on yet another factor—the pH of blood—which has been found to influence both the duration and the degree of paralysis produced by a relaxant drug. The precise reason for this variation in response is not clear but it could be associated with a change in the amount of the drug circulating in an ionised as opposed to unionised form. Most of the non-depolarising relaxant drugs are believed to be capable of some binding with plasma proteins. This attachment is loose and easily reversible. Once bound, the concentration of the relaxant drug available for the motor end-plate is reduced so that alterations in blood pH could affect the degree of paresis by varying the quantity of the drug carried in the plasma in bound form. Clinically, it is now generally accepted that the action of *d*-tubocurarine is *increased* by acidosis and *decreased* by alkalosis, though under experimental conditions such changes do not prevent the ultimate recovery of neuromuscular transmission (Bridenbaugh *et al.*, 1966) (Fig. 21*a* and *b*). It must be remembered, however, that the conditions of the circulation in a normal volunteer are clearly different from those found in the acute emergency, so that it is still possible that the pH of blood could alter duration of action under these conditions.

The findings with gallamine are the reverse of those quoted for *d*-tubocurarine (Walts *et al.*, 1967). Thus the block is *decreased* by acidosis and increased by alkalosis. In clinical practice these observations probably play a very small role in determining the total degree or duration of action of the relaxant drug and are certainly at variance with the original observation that hyperventilation reduced the dose of muscle relaxant required for abdominal surgery. The explanation for this broad generalisation must be sought elsewhere.

To summarise, the peculiar findings of the alteration in response to both the degree and duration of paresis with *d*-tubocurarine and gallamine remain

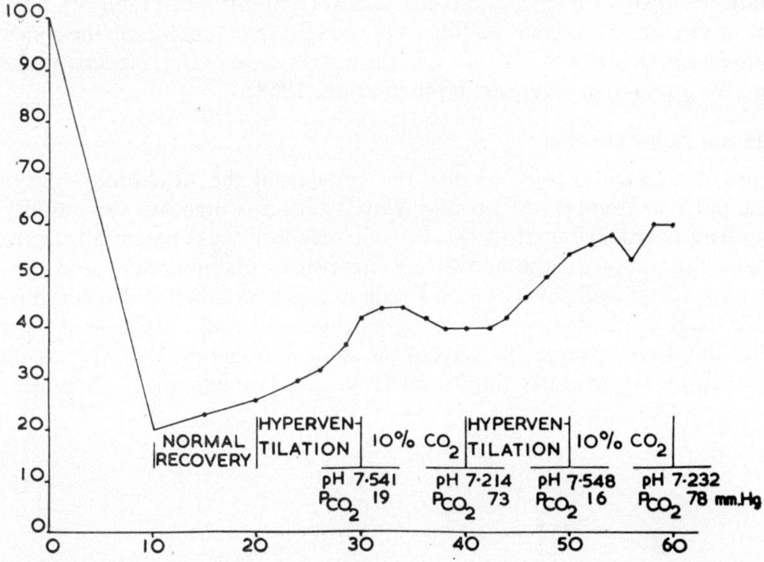

30/FIG. 21(*a*).—Effect of altering the P_{CO_2} on the rate of recovery from muscle paresis following *d*-tubocurarine.

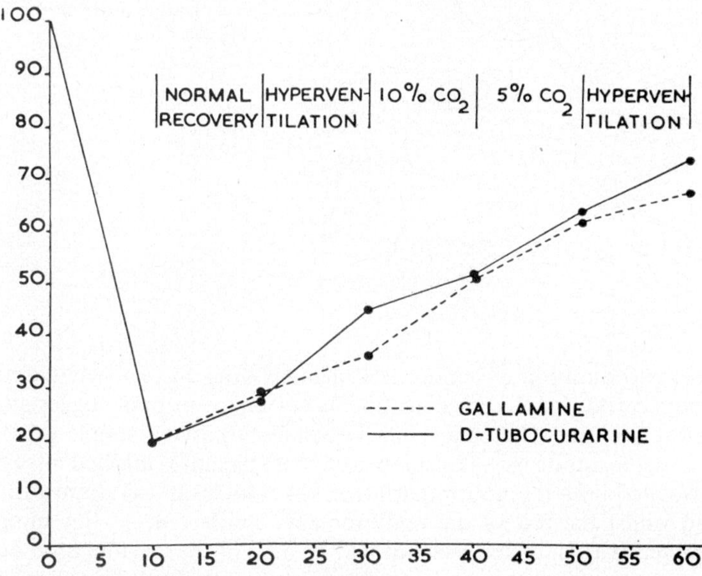

30/FIG. 21(*b*).—Averaged values for effect of hyperventilation and CO_2 on 12 patients receiving gallamine or *d*-tubocurarine. The abscissa represents time in minutes and the ordinate, per cent of control action potential.

puzzling. As always on such occasions, there is a multitude of theories, including alterations in ionisation and binding to plasma proteins, changes in the concentration of serum calcium and alteration in the distribution of the respective relaxants to inactive and active receptors (Cohen *et al.*, 1968).

Plasma Concentration

Once a relaxant is injected into the circulation the distribution follows a specific pattern. At first, the plasma concentration is high but this rapidly falls as the drug is redistributed to the various receptor sites. Essentially, there are two types of receptor—the active (e.g. neuromuscular junction) and the non-active (e.g. vessel wall, spleen, etc.) Using radioactive labelled drugs it has been possible to study the distribution of these drugs in animals. The role of the active receptor in taking up large amounts of the drug, and thereby reducing the plasma concentration, is obviously important (Fig. 22). It might seem, therefore, that

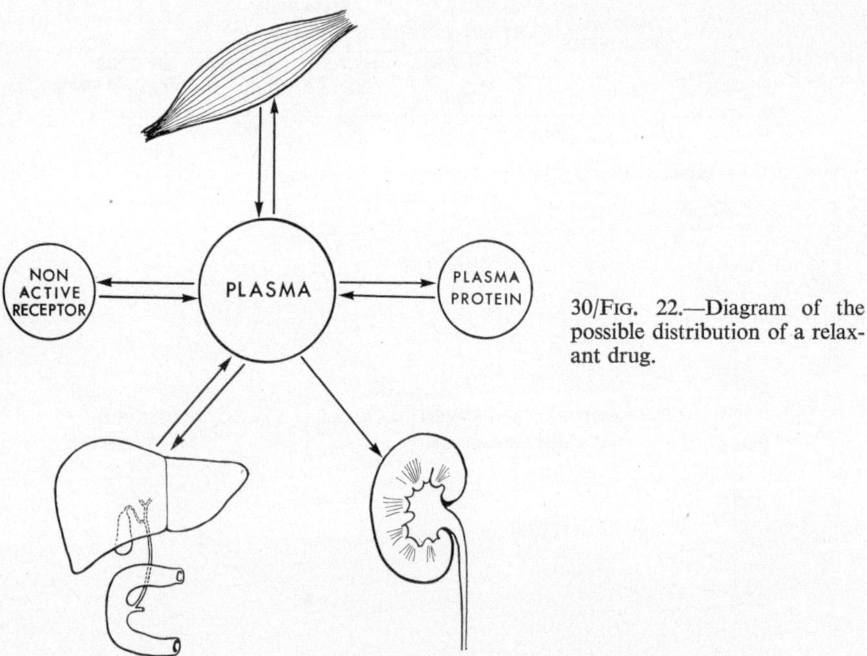

30/Fig. 22.—Diagram of the possible distribution of a relaxant drug.

the degree and duration of action of a relaxant drug was entirely based on the plasma concentration. Recent experimental evidence in man suggests that this is not entirely correct. Feldman and Tyrrell (1970) used a simple experimental method to demonstrate this. If a small dose of a relaxant is injected intravenously into an isolated limb (i.e. tourniquet) then the muscles in that limb will become paralysed whilst the rest of the body remains unaffected. At this moment the plasma concentration of the relaxant will be high in the isolated limb but it will be zero in the remainder of the body. On release of the cuff the plasma entering the isolated limb would be expected to so dilute the concentration of relaxant at the end-plate that instant recovery might be anticipated. However, this is not the case with the non-depolarising drugs (Fig. 23). Decamethonium, a depolarising relaxant, shows an immediate wash-out and recovery, whilst *d*-tubocurarine shows a typical slow recovery which is so familiar in clinical practice. These results suggest that plasma concentration is not responsible for the duration

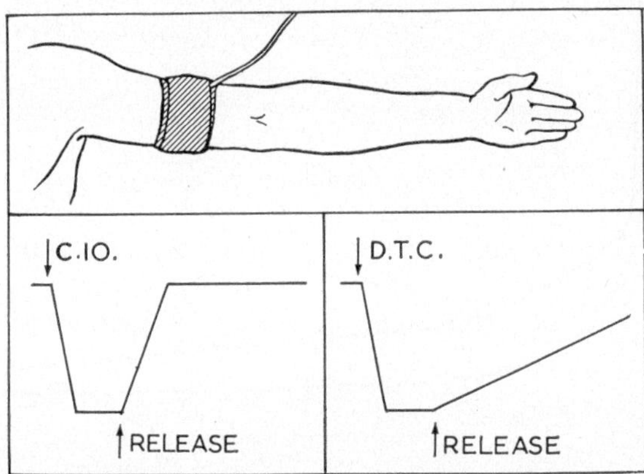

30/Fig. 23.—Diagram showing rapid recovery of decamethonium (C.10) as opposed to the slow recovery of *d*-tubocurarine after release of the cuff. An injection of a small dose of relaxant is made into the isolated limb thus ensuring that the plasma concentration in the remainder of the body is zero (Feldman and Tyrell, 1970).

of action of a relaxant and that other factors, such as the grip of the relaxant molecule for the receptor site, may well play a part.

Renal Excretion

All the muscle relaxants with the exception of suxamethonium are at least partially excreted in the urine. Originally, gallamine was the only relaxant believed to be excreted in entirety by the renal tract. Mushin and his colleagues (1949) recovered 30–100 per cent of the original dose from the urine of rabbits within two hours of its administration.

Until recently the metabolism of *d*-tubocurarine was surrounded by mystery. The studies of Cohen and his colleagues (1967) have now clearly shown that the vast bulk (80 per cent of the injected dose) is excreted unchanged by the kidneys. A further fraction (5 per cent) passes through the biliary system to the bowels. This latter pathway plays an insignificant role when renal function is normal but it assumes great importance during renal failure because much larger proportions (up to 40 per cent) can now leave the circulation by this route (Fig. 24*a* and *b*). Gallamine does not possess this alternative pathway of metabolism.

Clinically, a number of reports have indicated a close correlation between poor renal excretion and a prolonged response to the muscle relaxants (Fairley, 1950; Montgomery and Bennett-Jones, 1956; Feldman and Levi, 1963). As might be expected, there are more instances involving gallamine than *d*-tubocurarine. Furthermore, in a study of patients undergoing bilateral nephrectomy prior to renal transplantation, Churchill-Davidson and his associates (1967) noted the paralysis of *d*-tubocurarine followed a normal pattern of recovery

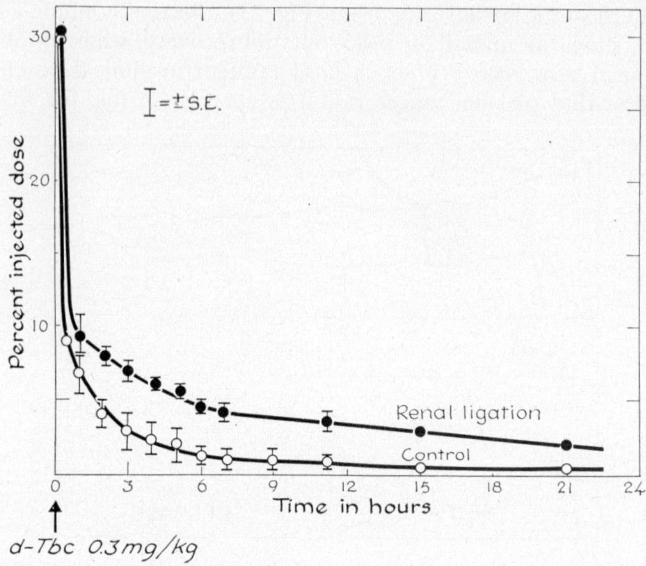

30/Fig. 24(*a*).—Plasma concentration of *d*-tubocurarine-H^3 in control dogs and in those with bilateral renal ligation. Note the raised plasma level in the presence of renal ligation.

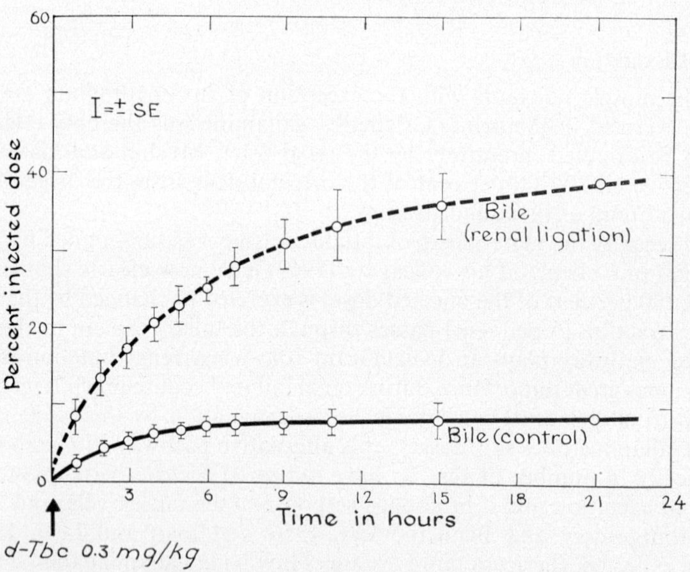

30/Fig. 24(*b*).—Recovery of *d*-tubocurarine-H^3 in the bile in control dogs and in those with bilateral renal ligation. Note the tremendous increase in biliary excretion in the presence of renal ligation.

whereas there was evidence of a very prolonged response in one patient who received gallamine. There is as yet insufficient evidence about the extent of the excretion of pancuronium through the biliary system to warrant its use in the presence of renal failure.

It is clear, therefore, that in the presence of poor renal function *d*-tubocurarine is a much safer relaxant drug than gallamine which relies entirely on the renal system for its elimination from the body. If, however, the liver and biliary system are also damaged—as is often the case in the presence of a hepato-renal syndrome—then all these relaxant drugs are best avoided.

Antibiotics

In 1950, Molitor and Graessle studied the toxicity of streptomycin and observed that the survival rate of their animals was increased if artificial respiration was used. This evidence suggested some action of the drug at the neuromuscular junction. In 1957, Brazil and Corrado took the matter one stage further and demonstrated that streptomycin produced a neuromuscular block in both dogs and pigeons. This block was partially reversed by neostigmine but calcium chloride proved even more effective. In the following year Pittinger and Long (1958) showed that ether potentiated the neuromuscular block of neomycin and this could be antagonised by neostigmine.

It was not long before the full clinical significance of this work was appreciated. Reports were soon forthcoming of accidental deaths associated with anaesthetic and antibiotic drugs. Sabawala and Dillon (1959), using isolated muscle specimens, demonstrated that many of the antibiotic agents were really quite potent neuromuscular blocking drugs. Streptomycin and neomycin appeared to produce a non-depolarising block which could be potentiated by ether and *d*-tubocurarine yet reversed by neostigmine. On the other hand kanamycin and polymyxin B appeared to be weak depolarising drugs.

Markalous (1962) analysed the clinical effect of neomycin sulphate in a group of patients and found that 1·0 g. of neomycin given intraperitoneally was sufficient to reduce appreciably the minute volume. In fact, nearly one-half required artificial respiration after this dose. Nevertheless, if 1·0 g. of neomycin was mixed with 20 ml. of low molecular weight dextran sulphate this mixture did not appear to produce respiratory depression.

To summarise, from the clinical and experimental data available there is little doubt that large doses of streptomycin, dihydrostreptomycin, neomycin, polymyxin B, colomycin, viomycin and paromycin all have significant neuromuscular blocking properties. There is less certainty about kanamycin, bacitracin and tetracycline. However, until all these agents have been completely absolved it is a wise clinical practice to regard all the antibiotics (with the exception of the penicillins) as weak neuromuscular blocking agents. It is quite possible that large doses of these drugs alone in children or the seriously ill patient may limit respiratory activity: in the presence of anaesthetic agents their activity becomes doubly important.

Experiments in animals suggest that in many instances neostigmine will antagonise this block. However, calcium chloride in small doses (200–500 mg.) appears to be the drug of choice for reversing not only the neuromuscular blockade but also the hypotension caused by streptomycin in animals (Pandey *et al.*,

1964). In clinical practice, however, a satisfactory compromise has been found in the insertion of a small intraperitoneal catheter at the time of operation and the administration of the antibiotic a few hours later when all the effects of the anaesthetic drugs have passed.

Tranquillisers

Another example of the interaction of drugs with the muscle relaxants is the recent finding that diazepam increases the duration of block produced by gallamine and shortens that of suxamethonium (Feldman and Crawley, 1970). The inference is that diazepam will probably be found to prolong and increase the action of all non-depolarising drugs as it is believed to reduce the liberation of acetylcholine molecules at the nerve ending in a similar fashion to that of the antibiotics.

Potentiation by other Drugs

Many other agents used in general or local anaesthesia are capable of enhancing neuromuscular blockade. For example, Karis and his co-workers (1967) have shown that both ether and halothane block neuromuscular transmission principally by reducing the sensitivity of the *post-junctional* membrane to acetylcholine. On the other hand, quinidine is believed to potentiate neuromuscular block largely by a pre-synaptic action similar to that of local analgesic drugs (Miller *et al.*, 1967). This concept is disputed by Usubiaga (1968*a*) who believes the principal action of quinidine is on the muscle fibre itself.

The beta blockers have also been shown to have an action at the neuromuscular junction (Wislicki and Rosenblum, 1967; Usubiaga, 1968*b*). Again, this group of drugs is believed to have a pre-synaptic action interfering with the liberation of acetylcholine.

Age

For some years past the response of the newborn infant to the relaxant drugs has always been regarded as different from that of the average adult patient. Jackson Rees (1959) went so far as to suggest that the neonate responded to the muscle relaxants like a patient with myasthenia gravis. Support for this suggestion arose from the observation that suxamethonium did not produce fasciculations in the newborn. Furthermore, neonates appeared to be "resistant" to the depolarising drug and "sensitive" to the non-depolarisers, as in myasthenia (see p. 912).

In a clinical study, Bush and Stead (1962) observed the dose of *d*-tubocurarine required to produce "adequate control of ventilation and satisfactory operating conditions" in a large series of newborn infants undergoing surgery. They concluded that only during the first ten days of life did the neonate show some "sensitivity" to *d*-tubocurarine.

Neuromuscular Transmission in the Newborn

Using an electromyographic technique, Churchill-Davidson and Wise (1963; 1964) reported that neuromuscular transmission in the newborn appeared comparable with that in the adult except for the presence of post-tetanic exhaustion (see p. 790). This is not observed in normal adults but is sometimes seen in patients with myasthenia gravis. In the newborn it occurred primarily in premature infants and during the first two weeks of life.

Using a dose based on body weight, these workers found that neonates were resistant to the depolarising drugs but they did not observe any clear-cut sensitivity to the non-depolarising drugs. Furthermore they found that neuromuscular block produced by the depolarising drugs had some of the typical features of a dual or Phase II block in that both fade and potentiation were observed and neuromuscular transmission was improved by an anti-cholinesterase drug (Figs. 25 and 26).

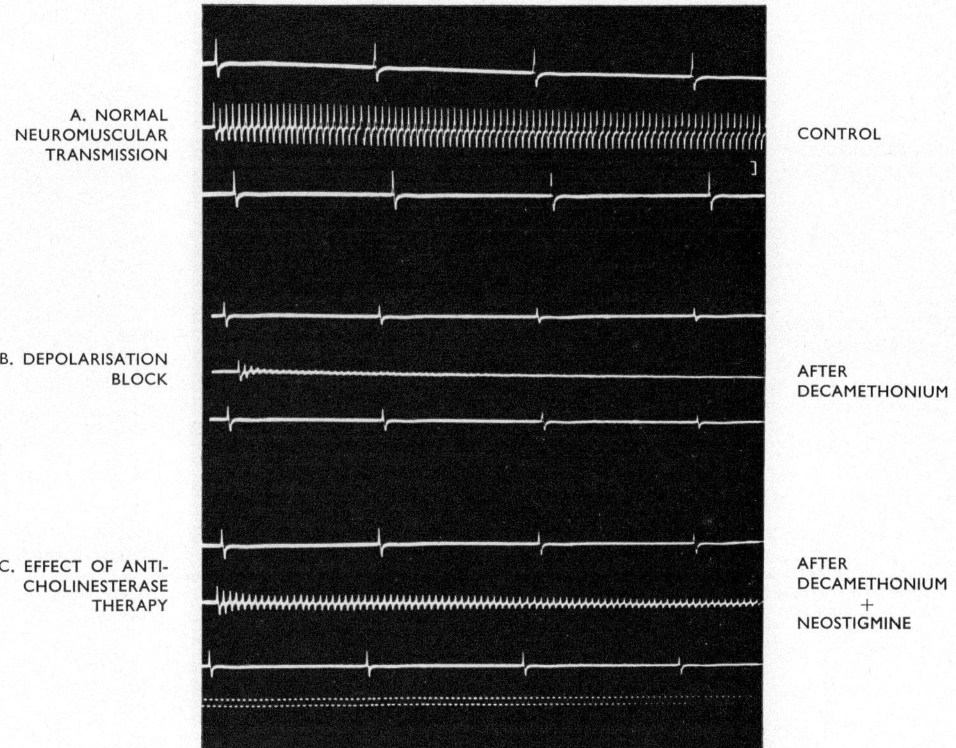

30/Fig. 25.—Signs of dual block following decamethonium in a neonate.

Walts and Dillon (1969) carried out a similar study with one important difference. Instead of selecting their dose on a body weight basis, they used one determined by body surface area. Their results were significantly different. Neither neonates nor adults showed much difference in the degree or duration of action of suxamethonium, but neonates proved 2 to 3 times more sensitive to *d*-tubocurarine than adults. They pointed out, however, that had they based their selected dose on body weight rather than body surface area, the results would then have been very different.

It is safe to assume that the neonate responds to a depolarising relaxant in a similar way to the adult, but will show "sensitivity" to (i.e. will need less of) non-depolarising drugs. A dose selected by body surface area requirements is more accurate than that based on body weight.

Clinical Significance

The neonatal neuromuscular transmission possesses many features which differentiate it from that seen in the adult. Clinically, fasciculations are rarely seen with depolarising drugs. Furthermore, though these infants have a plasma cholinesterase level on the low side of normal, they require relatively large amounts of these drugs to produce paresis.

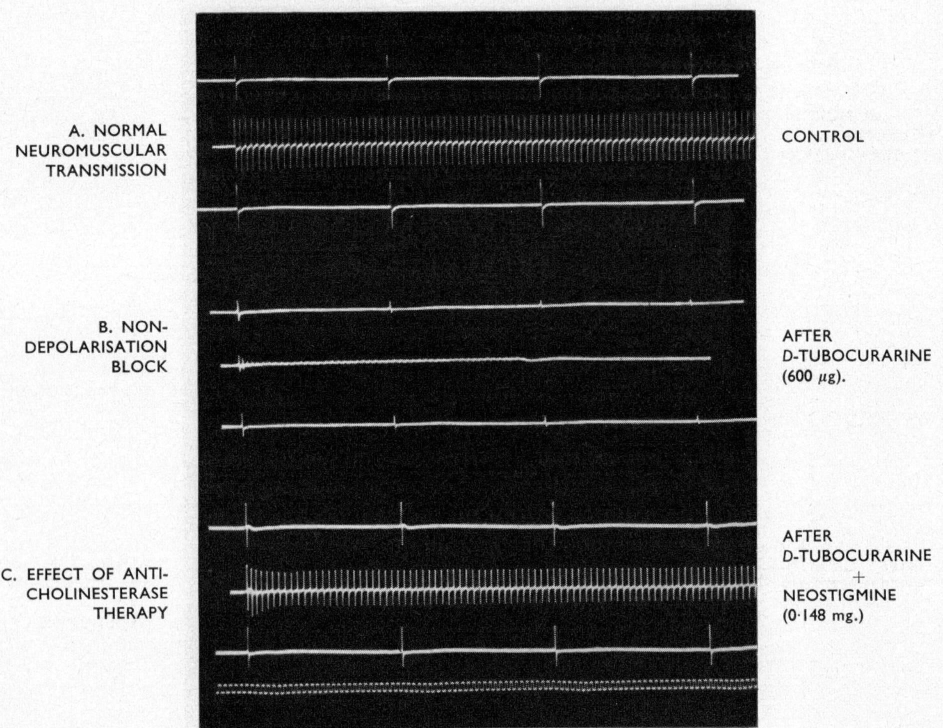

30/Fig. 26.—Signs of a non-depolarisation block in a neonate.

Electromyographic studies have revealed that the premature infant and the neonate respond to a depolarising drug by a dual block. Under clinical conditions in operations lasting only a short time (i.e. about 1 hour), the slightly prolonged recovery time from a dual block as opposed to a purely depolarisation block is rarely noticed. However, if large doses are given over a long period the possibility of a delayed recovery time increases. The younger the infant, the earlier this change is likely to be observed.

The non-depolarising drugs appear to act normally in the neonate. Provided an excessive dose is not used, an anti-cholinesterase drug will reverse the neuromuscular block.

Adequate dilution of the neuromuscular blocking drug is the single most important factor in the administration of relaxant drugs to the newborn. A body weight basis is often chosen for comparison, but it must be remembered that the muscle mass of an infant represents a much smaller proportion of the total body weight than in an adult. Muscle mass is about 20 per cent of body weight at birth, increasing to 33 per cent in early adolescence (Long and Bachman, 1967). The dilution chosen must be related to the fluid requirements of the patient; in clinical practice a dilution of 100 μg. (0·1 mg.)/ml. is often found satisfactory. Although on occasions it may be necessary to use a slightly stronger solution for the initial dose, subsequent doses should always be in a very dilute concentration.

Nightingale and his associates (1966) studied the effects of a suxamethonium infusion on neuromuscular activity at differing age levels in infants and young children. They found that the younger the child the more suxamethonium (on a mg./kg. basis) was required to achieve a comparable degree of paresis. As children grew older so this "resistance" to the paralysing action of suxamethonium became less.

Anti-cholinesterase drugs can also be used safely in this class of patients provided the same principles are applied as in adults (see p. 904). The actual injection using the intravenous route must always be given *very slowly* over a period of ten minutes. The ratio of neostigmine methyl sulphate to atropine sulphate is the same as that used for adults, namely—2·5 mg. neostigmine + 1·0 mg. atropine. This solution is then diluted ten or twenty times before it is used for administration. The total dose used may be calculated on a body weight basis. However, the most satisfactory method for selecting the correct dose of anti-cholinesterase in both infants and children is with the aid of a peripheral nerve stimulator. In the presence of a non-depolarising type of block there will be signs of both "fade" and "post-tetanic potentiation": as the anti-cholinesterase drug is given these signs will disappear and neuromuscular transmission will improve. When there is no further improvement in transmission the administration of the anti-cholinesterase drug is suspended.

REFERENCES

ABRAMS, M. W., and GINSBERG, H. (1960). Prolonged apnoea following the use of suxamethonium. *Anaesthesia*, **15**, 265.

BARAKA, A. (1964). The influence of carbon dioxide on the neuromuscular block caused by tubocurarine chloride in the human subject. *Brit. J. Anaesth.*, **36**, 272.

BIGLAND, B., GOETZEE, B., MACLAGAN, J., and ZAIMIS, E. (1958). The effect of lowered muscle temperature on the action of neuromuscular blocking drugs. *J. Physiol. (Lond.)*, **141**, 425.

BRAZIL, O. V., and CORRADO, A. P. (1957). Curariform action of streptomycin. *J. Pharmacol. exp. Ther.*, **120**, 452.

BRIDENBAUGH, P. O., CHURCHILL-DAVIDSON, H. C., and CHURCHER, M. D. (1966). Effects of carbon dioxide on actions of *d*-tubocurarine and gallamine. *Curr. Res. Anesth.*, **45**, 804.

Brown, G. L., and Dias, M .V. (1947). A acão do fosfato sobre a transmissão neuromuscular na rã. *Ann. Acad. bras.*, **19**, 359.

Brown, G. L., Paton, W. D. M., and Dias, M. V. (1949). The depression of the demarcation potential of cat's tibialis by bistrimethylammonium decane diiodide (C.10). *J. Physiol.* (*Lond.*), **109**, 15P.

Bush, G. H., and Stead, A. L. (1962). The use of *d*-tubocurarine in neonatal anaesthesia. *Brit. J. Anaesth.*, **34**, 721.

Buttle, G. A. H., and Zaimis, E. J. (1949). The action of decamethonium iodide in birds. *J. Pharm.* (*Lond.*), **1**, 991.

Cannard, T. H., and Zaimis, E. J. (1959). The effect of lowered muscle temperature on the action of neuromuscular blocking drugs in man. *J. Physiol.* (*Lond.*), **149**, 112.

Cavallito, C. J., Coria, A. E., and Hoppé, J. O. (1950). Amino and ammonium alkylaminobenzoquinones as curarimimetic agents. *J. Amer. chem. Soc.*, **72**, 2661.

Churchill-Davidson, H. C., Christie, T. H., and Wise, R. P. (1960). Dual neuromuscular block in man. *Anesthesiology*, **21**, 144.

Churchill-Davidson, H. C., and Katz, R. L. (1966). Dual, phase II or desensitization block? *Anesthesiology*, **27**, 536.

Churchill-Davidson, H. C., and Richardson, A. T. (1952). Decamethonium iodide (C.10): Some observations on its action using electromyography. *Proc. roy. Soc. Med.*, **45**, 179.

Churchill-Davidson, H. C., Way, W. L., and De Jong, R. H. (1967). The muscle relaxants and renal excretion. *Anesthesiology*, **28**, 540.

Churchill-Davidson, H. C., and Wise, R. P. (1963). Neuromuscular transmission in the newborn infant. *Anesthesiology*, **24**, 271.

Churchill-Davidson, H. C., and Wise, R. P. (1964). The response of the newborn infant to muscle relaxants. *Canad. Anaesth. Soc. J.*, **11**, 1.

Cohen, E. N., Brewer, H. W., and Smith, D. (1967). The metabolism and elimination of *d*-tubocurarine-H^3. *Anesthesiology*, **28**, 309.

Cohen, E. N., Hood, N., and Golling, R. (1968). Use of whole-body autoradiography for the determination of uptake and distribution of labelled muscle relaxants in the rat. *Anesthesiology*, **29**, 987.

Crul, J. F., Long, G. J., Brunner, E. A., and Coolen, J. M. W. (1966). The changing pattern of neuromuscular blockade caused by succinylcholine in man. *Anesthesiology*, **27**, 729.

De Jong, R. H., and Freund, F. G. (1967). Characteristics of the neuromuscular block with succinylcholine and decamethonium in man. *Anesthesiology*, **28**, 583.

Dundee, J. W. (1952). Influence of controlled respiration on dosage of thiopentone and *d*-tubocurarine chloride required for abdominal surgery. *Brit. med. J.*, **2**, 893.

Fairley, H. B. (1950). Prolonged intercostal paralysis due to a relaxant. *Brit. med. J.*, **2**, 986.

Feldman, S. A., and Crawley, B. F. (1970). Interaction of diazepam with the muscle-relaxant drugs. *Brit. med. J.*, **2**, 336.

Feldman, S. A., and Levi, J. A. (1963). Prolonged paresis following gallamine. *Brit. J. Anaesth.*, **35**, 804.

Feldman, S. A., and Tyrrell, M. F. (1970). A new theory of determination of action of the muscle relaxants. *Proc. roy. Soc. Med.*, **63**, 692.

Frey, R. (1956). "A short-acting muscle relaxant: Prestonal (G 25178). Preliminary report". *Proc. World Congr. Anesthesiologists, Scheveningen, September* 1955. Minneapolis: Burgess Publishing Co.

Gamstorp, I., and Vinnars, E. (1961). Studies in neuromuscular transmission; influence of changes in blood pH and carbon dioxide tension on the effect of tubocurarine and dimethyl tubocurarine. *Acta physiol. scand.*, **53**, 160.

GISSEN, A. J., KATZ, R. L., KARIS, J. H., and PAPPER, E. M. (1966). Neuromuscular block in man during prolonged arterial infusion with succinylcholine. *Anesthesiology*, **27**, 242.

HARPER, J. K. (1952). Prolonged respiratory paralysis after succinylcholine (correspondence). *Brit. med. J.*, **1**, 866.

HARVEY, A. M. (1939). Action of procaine on neuromuscular transmission. *Bull. Johns Hopk. Hosp.*, **65**, 223.

HARVEY, A. M., and MACINTOSH, R. C. (1940). Calcium and synaptic transmission in a sympathetic ganglion. *J. Physiol. (Lond.)*, **97**, 408.

JENDEN, D. J., KAMIJO, K., TAYLOR, D. B. (1951). The action of decamethonium (C.10) on the isolated rabbit lumbrical muscle. *J. Pharmacol. exp. Ther.*, **103**, 348.

KALOW, W. (1954). Influence of pH in ionisation and biological activity of *d*-tubocurarine. *J. Pharmacol. exp. Ther.*, **110**, 443.

KARIS, H. J., GISSEN, A. J., and NASTUK, W. L. (1967). The effect of volatile anesthetic agents on neuromuscular transmission. *Anesthesiology*, **28**, 128.

KATZ, R. L., and KATZ, G .J. (1967). "Clinical use of muscle relaxants". In: *Advances in Anesthesiology: Muscle Relaxants*, Chap, VI, p. 9. Eds. L. C. Mark and E. M. Papper. New York: Hoeber.

KATZ, R. L., NGAI, S. H., and PAPPER, E. M. (1963*a*). The effect of alkalosis on the action of the neuromuscular blocking agents. *Anesthesiology*, **24**, 18.

KATZ, R. L., WOLF, C. E., and PAPPER, E. M. (1963*b*). The nondepolarizing neuromuscular blocking action of succinylcholine in man. *Anesthesiology*, **24**, 784.

LINSSEN, H. G. (1961). *Curariform Drugs*. Nijmegen: Thoben.

LONG, G., and BACHMAN, L. (1967). Neuromuscular blockade by *d*-tubocurarine in children. *Anesthesiology*, **28**, 723.

MACINTOSH, F. C., BIRKS, R. I., and SASTRY, P. B. (1958). Mode of action of an inhibitor of acetylcholine synthesis. *Neurology (Minneap.)*, **8**, Suppl. I, 90.

MARKALOUS, P. (1962). Respiration and the intraperitoneal application of neomycin and meolymphin. *Anaesthesia*, **17**, 427.

MILLER, R. C., WAY, W. L., and KATZUNG, B. G. (1967). The potentiation of neuromuscular blocking agents by quinidine. *Anesthesiology*, **28**, 1036.

MOLITOR, H., and GRAESSLE, O. E. (1950). Pharmacology and toxicology of antibiotics. *Pharmacol. Rev.*, **2**, 1.

MONTGOMERY, J. B., and BENNETT-JONES, N. (1956). Gallamine triethiodide and renal disease. *Lancet*, **2**, 1243.

MUSHIN, W. W., WIEN, R., MASON, D. F. J., and LANGSTON, G. T. (1949). Curare-like actions of tri(diethylaminoethoxy)benzene triethiodide. *Lancet*, **1**, 726.

NIGHTINGALE, D. A., GLASS, A. G., and BACHMAN, L. (1966). Neuromuscular blockade by succinylcholine in children. *Anesthesiology*, **27**, 736.

PANDEY, K., KUMAR, S., and BADALA, R. P. (1964). Neuromuscular blocking and hypotensive actions of streptomycin and their reversal. *Brit. J. Anaesth.*, **36**, 19.

PATON, W. D. M. (1956). *Proceedings of the Conference on the Myoneural Junction.* (Sponsored by Columbia University Division of Anesthesiology and Burroughs Wellcome & Co., U.S.A.) November 4th and 5th, 1955. New York City, N.Y.

PATON, W. D. M., and ZAIMIS, E. J. (1949). Pharmacological actions of polymethylene bistrimethylammonium salts. *Brit. J. Pharmacol.*, **4**, 381.

PATON, W. D. M., and ZAIMIS, E. J. (1952). Methonium compounds. *Pharmacol. Rev.*, **4**, 219.

PAYNE, J. P. (1958). Influence of carbon dioxide on the neuromuscular blocking activity of relaxant drugs in the cat. *Brit. J. Anaesth.*, **30**, 206.

Payne, J. P. (1960). The influence of changes in blood pH on the neuromuscular blocking properties of tubocurarine and dimethyl tubocurarine in the cat. *Acta anaesth. scand.*, **4,** 83.

Pittinger, C. B., and Long, J. P. (1958). Neuromuscular blocking action of neomycin sulfate. *Antibiot. & Chemother.*, **8,** 198.

Rees, G. J. (1959). In: *General Anaesthesia*, Vol. 2. Eds. F. T. Evans and T. C. Gray. London: Butterworth & Co.

Sabawala, P. B., and Dillon, J. B. (1959). The action of some antibiotics on the human intercostal nerve-muscle complex. *Anesthesiology*, **20,** 659.

Usubiaga, J. E. (1968*a*). Potentiation of muscle relaxants by quinidine. *Anesthesiology*, **29,** 1068.

Usubiaga, J. E. (1968*b*). Neuromuscular effects of beta-adrenergic blockers and their interaction with other drugs. *Anesthesiology*, **29,** 484.

Utting, J. (1963). pH as a factor influencing plasma concentrations of *d*-tubocurarine. *Brit. J. Anaesth.*, **35,** 706.

Vickers, M. D. A. (1963). The mismanagement of suxamethonium apnoea. *Brit. J. Anaesth.*, **35,** 260.

Walts, L. F., and Dillon, J. B. (1969). The response of newborns to succinylcholine and *d*-tubocurarine. *Anesthesiology*, **31,** 35.

Walts, L. F., Lebowitz, M., and Dillon, J. B. (1967). The effects of ventilation on the action of tubocurarine and gallamine. *Brit. J. Anaesth.*, **39,** 845.

Wislicki, L., and Rosenblum, I. (1967). Effects of propranolol on the action of neuromuscular blocking drugs. *Brit. J. Anaesth.*, **39,** 939.

Zaimis, E. J. (1952). Motor end-plate differences as a determining factor in the mode of action of neuromuscular blocking substances. *Nature* (*Lond.*), **170,** 617.

Zaimis, E. J. (1953). Motor end-plate differences as a determining factor in the mode of action of neuromuscular blocking substances. *J. Physiol.* (*Lond.*), **122,** 238.

Zaimis, E. J., Cannard, T. H., and Price, H. L. (1958). Effects of lowered muscle temperature on neuromuscular blockade in man. *Science*, **128,** 34.

Chapter 31

NEUROMUSCULAR BLOCKING DRUGS

Chemical Structure

One of the most fascinating contributions to medicine in recent years has been the progress made in relating the chemical structure of a drug to its possible site and mode of action. The muscle relaxants represent a supreme example of the success in this field and this structure-action relationship has been admirably reviewed by Bovet (1951) and Barlow (1955).

The most important single feature of the relaxant drugs is the presence of a quaternary ammonium group—i.e. four carbon radicals attached to one N atom.

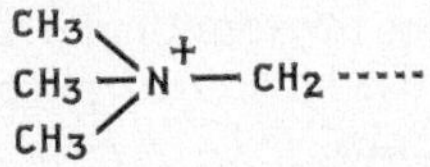

$$(CH_3)_3\overset{+}{N}-CH_2 \cdots\cdots$$

It would be untrue to say, however, that the presence of at least one of these groups was obligatory for muscular relaxation, for erythroidine—a natural alkaloid from *Erythrina Americana* (Folkers and Major, 1937)—contains only a tertiary ammonium group yet is capable of producing neuromuscular block.

The immense advantages to clinical anaesthesia that followed the introduction of the alkaloid *d*-tubocurarine were rapidly appreciated and pharmacologists soon started to search for a drug with similar neuromuscular blocking properties that could be produced synthetically in the laboratory. A close study of the *d*-tubocurarine molecule revealed two interesting features. First, it contained two quaternary ammonium groups, each of which was like acetylcholine:

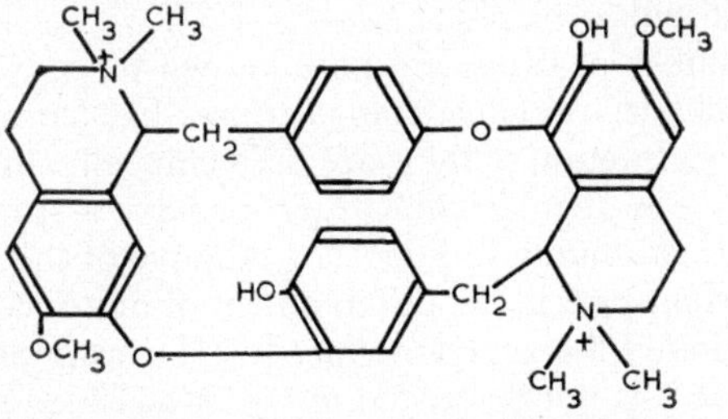

Chemical structure of *d*-tubocurarine (after Barlow, 1955)

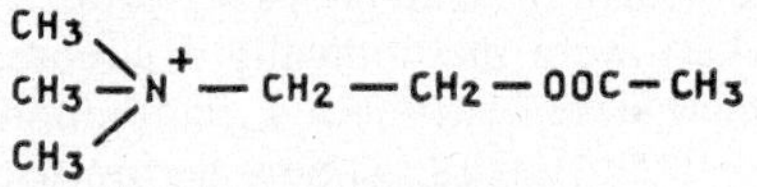

$$(CH_3)_3\overset{+}{N}-CH_2-CH_2-OOC-CH_3$$

Acetylcholine

Secondly, despite its rather complex molecular structure the quaternary ammonium groups were linked through a 10-atom chain. Any synthetic compound, therefore, that contained these two features offered a real chance of success. Decamethonium proved to be just such a drug:

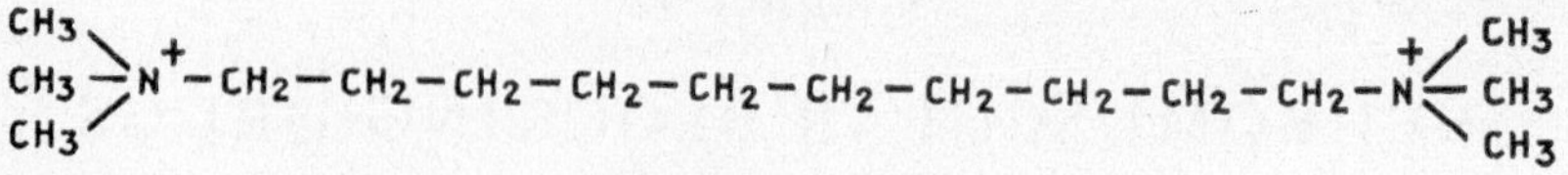

$$\begin{matrix} CH_3 \\ CH_3 \\ CH_3 \end{matrix}\!\!>\overset{+}{N}-CH_2-CH_2-CH_2-CH_2-CH_2-CH_2-CH_2-CH_2-CH_2-CH_2-\overset{+}{N}\!\!<\!\!\begin{matrix} CH_3 \\ CH_3 \\ CH_3 \end{matrix}$$

Decamethonium

The methonium series revealed an excellent example of how minor modifications in the length of the chain were reflected in a great alteration of activity. The neuromuscular blocking properties were greatest when 10 carbon atoms separated the two quaternary ammonium groups but this action was still easily recognisable in compounds with 9–13 carbon atoms in the chain. Tridecamethonium (C.13) possessed in the young chick the interesting capacity to produce a dual type of neuromuscular block rather than one of pure depolarisation like decamethonium, but its mode of action in man is not known.

Attempts to build molecular models of *d*-tubocurarine (Kimura *et al.*, 1948) revealed that the actual distance apart of the two quaternary ammonium groups was important for reproducing neuromuscular blocking activity. Thus all the relaxants in common clinical use have their nitrogen group separated by a distance of about 15 Ångström units.

Summary

The composition and molecular structure of the relaxant drugs bears a strict relationship to their site and mode of action. Each drug may be likened to a key, while the receptors of the motor end-plate are the lock. If the key contains the two necessary quaternary ammonium groups, and these are separated by the correct distance (15 Ångström units), then the door of muscle excitation can be locked or opened at will.

A very large number of drugs are now known to be capable of producing neuromuscular blockade, ranging from atropine-like compounds to the new steroid variety. Only a fraction of these are used clinically. In this discussion only those drugs which are in regular clinical use or have a special importance will be mentioned. Decamethonium iodide is an example of the latter because it has played a very important part in the development of our understanding of neuromuscular transmission. Like acetylcholine, it is an example of a depolarising relaxant, but because it is not destroyed *in vivo* it has been widely used by both physiologists and pharmacologists.

DECAMETHONIUM IODIDE

History

In the same year Barlow and Ing (1948) and Paton and Zaimis (1948) independently described the neuromuscular blocking properties of decamethonium. The latter pair of workers were methodically examining the pharmacological properties of the polymethylene-bistrimethyl ammonium compounds and they found that one member of this series, namely decamethonium (C.10), with ten CH_2 molecules in the chain, was remarkably effective as a muscle relaxant in animals. Later Organe and his colleagues (1949) reported on the effect of this drug on conscious subjects and in clinical anaesthesia.

Physical and Chemical Properties

Decamethonium is a white crystalline powder.

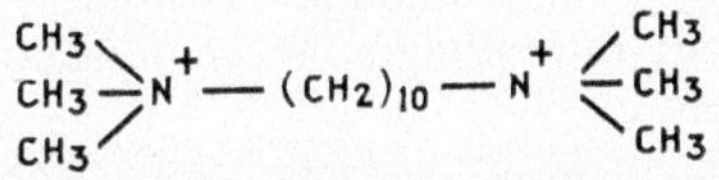

$$(CH_3)_3\overset{+}{N}-(CH_2)_{10}-\overset{+}{N}(CH_3)_3$$

Decamethylene 1:10 bistrimethylammonium.

It is soluble in water, neutral in solution, and relatively stable. It is odourless and non-irritant to the tissues and blood vessels, and is not destroyed by plasma cholinesterase.

Pharmacological Actions

Mode of action.—The action of decamethonium in man is believed to be similar to that of acetylcholine in that it produces depolarisation of the end-plate region. Gissen and Nastuk (1968) found that the action of decamethonium is limited to the post-synaptic membrane of the neuromuscular junction. The neural action potential recorded at the nerve-ending was unaffected by the drug and direct stimulation of the muscle fibre in the presence of neuromuscular block still elicited a contraction. On this evidence they concluded that decamethonium causes post-synaptic membrane receptor activation which was later followed by desensitisation (see Chapter 29).

Cardiovascular system.—Decamethonium has no action on the myocardium (Prime and Gray, 1952). Given intra-arterially in minute doses it leads to muscle weakness without any severe pain. There have been no reports of venous thrombosis following intravenous decamethonium.

Central nervous system.—Within the range of doses used in clinical practice there is no evidence of any action on the spinal cord, brain or autonomic ganglia. Heavy doses in animals have been shown to produce a weak ganglion-depressant action. Ellis and his colleagues (1952) have suggested that decamethonium may depress the spontaneous activity of the respiratory centre.

Fasciculations and muscle pains.—Decamethonium causes widespread fasciculations of muscle in man, but these are not as marked as after suxamethonium. Soon after its intravenous injection a "tight feeling" develops in the masseter muscles of the jaw and in the posterior muscles of the calf. This is an aching type of pain which may persist for several hours.

Histamine release.—Decamethonium liberates only small quantities of histamine and has about half the activity in this respect of *d*-tubocurarine (Sniper, 1952).

Placental barrier.—Decamethonium has been found not to cross the placental barrier in the guinea-pig and rabbit (Young, 1949), but there is no evidence available for man.

Distribution

The distribution of decamethonium throughout the body following an intravenous injection has been beautifully demonstrated by the autoradiograph technique of Cohen and his collaborators (1968). They showed that decamethonium does not cross either the blood-brain barrier or the placental barrier to reach the foetus (Fig. 1). Considerable quantities, however, could be observed in the cardiac muscle though (as mentioned below) no cardiac action has so far been demonstrated. Only a small amount was found in the liver. There is no doubt that this whole-body autoradiograph technique offers an excellent manner

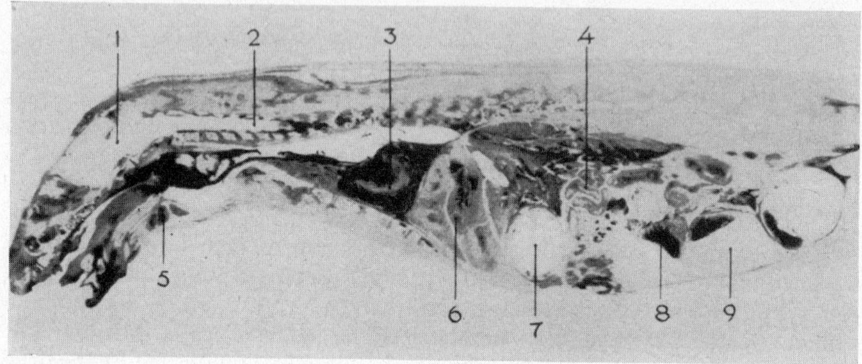

31/FIG. 1.—Autoradiograph of rat sacrificed 15 minutes after intravenous injection of 0.15 mg./kg. decamethonium. 1, brain; 2, spinal cord; 3, heart; 4, intestine; 5, salivary gland; 6, liver; 7, stomach; 8, placenta; 9, foetus.

of comparing the metabolism of the various relaxant drugs. Nevertheless, the presence of a drug at a particular receptor site does not necessarily indicate that it produces any activity in this area as there are numerous non-active receptor sites in the body.

Detoxication and Excretion

There is no evidence available either in animals or man that decamethonium undergoes any form of breakdown *in vivo*. The excretion rate in animals is slow and persists for many hours after a complete recovery of muscle power has been attained; 80–90 per cent of the total dose injected has been recovered unchanged in the urine over a 24-hour period (Paton and Zaimis, 1952). In man, 40 per cent has been recovered unchanged over a three-hour period following a single injection (Churchill-Davidson and Richardson, 1953). As the renal tract is the principal, and possibly the only, route of excretion or detoxication, severe renal damage or hypotension could theoretically produce a prolonged action of the drug. Clinically, however, there is no evidence available to suggest that the duration of action of decamethonium is related to renal function.

Recent evidence has cast some doubt on the concept of decamethonium being excreted entirely unchanged in the urine. Giovanella and his colleagues (1961) have employed a radioisotope technique to estimate quantitatively the amount of C^{14} labelled decamethonium in rats. Following administration of the drug they noted that the blood level displayed two well-distinguished peaks. The first occurred at the time of the injection and the second at a variable interval depending on the dose. The interesting observation is that this secondary rise in the blood level occurred at a moment when the paralysis was just wearing off. The authors concluded that it was due to outpouring of inactivated decamethonium from the muscles. Waser (1962) supports the view that some decamethonium is metabolised *in vivo* from a quaternary to a tertiary compound.

Administration

The intravenous route is the only satisfactory method of giving decamethonium in clinical practice. Thirty to forty seconds after the initial injection the conscious patient notices a difficulty or blurring of vision followed gradually by a generalised weakness which spreads to involve the trunk and limb muscles. In the anaesthetised patient, perfect conditions for endotracheal intubation may not arise until two to three minutes have elapsed.

Dosage.—A dose of 2·25 to 2·50 mg. of decamethonium will produce almost complete paralysis of the limb musculature in the average patient. A dose of 3·0 to 4·0 mg. is necessary for intubation.

Duration of action.—The time taken to return to complete recovery after 95 per cent paresis of the grip-strength is approximately 15–20 minutes in the conscious subject. The conditions of measurement, however, are not comparable to those in the anaesthetised subject, for electromyographic recordings have shown that the duration of action bears a close relationship to the muscle blood flow (see "Factors altering the duration or degree of neuromuscular block," Chapter 30, p. 830).

Antagonists

The depolarisation block produced by decamethonium is difficult to reverse and for this reason a satisfactory clinical antidote is still lacking. Certain drugs, however, will reduce the degree and duration of the neuromuscular block.

1. *Hexamethonium* (C.6) and *pentamethonium* (C.5), although better known as ganglion-blocking drugs, were, at one time, considered to be satisfactory antagonists to decamethonium. There is, however, no experimental evidence available to prove that the neuromuscular block is reversed by these drugs. Theoretically, their mode of action in the presence of decamethonium was believed to be through substrate competition; in other words, their lack of neuromuscular blocking activity combined with their specific affinity for the motor end-plate region helped to "dilute" the concentration of the active decamethonium molecules. Part of any apparent signs of improvement in the neuromuscular block after one of these drugs might be due to an increased blood flow through the muscle due to their ganglion-blocking action.

2. *d-Tubocurarine* in small doses is a theoretical antidote to the depolarising activity of decamethonium. In practice the assessment of the correct dose-relationship makes this suggestion impracticable and merely results in a change in the type rather than the degree of the neuromuscular block. B.W. 49–204 is a satisfactory antagonist to decamethonium in animal experimentation and this compound is known to have weak curare-like activity (de Beer, 1958); there is no report available on its use in man.

Neostigmine and edrophonium cause either no change or an increase in the degree of neuromuscular block. As both these drugs are capable of producing depolarisation in their own right it is difficult to assess whether this action arises from depolarisation or from inhibition of cholinesterase activity. Repeated doses of decamethonium lead to a "dual" type of neuromuscular block and in this case, the effect of neostigmine and edrophonium is to act as an antidote to the neuromuscular block.

SUXAMETHONIUM (SUCCINYLDICHOLINE; DIACETYLCHOLINE)

History

In 1906 Reid Hunt and Taveau first described the pharmacological action of suxamethonium, but though they studied its effect on blood pressure they failed to observe that it caused neuromuscular block, because they were using a previously curarised animal. Glick (1941) demonstrated that the hydrolysis rate was high and that it was broken down by cholinesterase in horse serum. Bovet and his colleagues (1949) in Italy, and Phillips (1949) in the United States, both independently described the neuromuscular blocking properties of suxamethonium. In the same year Bovet-Nitti showed that this substance was broken down by cholinesterases and this hydrolysis could be inhibited by eserine. In the following year Castillo and de Beer (1950) confirmed these findings in animal experiments. The drug was first used in man as a neuromuscular blocking agent by Thesleff at the Karolinska Institute in Stockholm (1951), and by Brucke and his associates (1951) and Mayrhofer and Hassfurther (1951) in Austria. Scurr (1951) and Bourne and his colleagues (1952) described its use in Great Britain, and Foldes and his associates (1952) introduced it in the United States.

Physical and Chemical Properties

Suxamethonium is a synthetic quaternary ammonium compound. It is a

$$(CH_3)_3\overset{+}{N}(Cl^-)-CH_2-CH_2-OOC-CH_2-CH_2-COO-CH_2-CH_2-\overset{+}{N}(Cl^-)(CH_3)_3$$

Suxamethonium chloride

white crystalline substance with a melting point of 150° C. It is relatively unstable and may deteriorate in solution if kept in a warm cupboard. Fraser (1954) has shown that it is unstable in alkaline solution (pH 9·3) and can lose 50 per cent of its activity in 3 hours under such conditions. Owing to its instability it was originally marketed combined with various halogens as the chloride, iodide and bromide. Some manufacturers preferred only to produce it in powder form, but later experience has shown that provided it is not kept for too long in a warm atmosphere the chloride in solution is satisfactory for clinical use.

Pharmacological Actions

Mode of action.—Suxamethonium is believed to act like acetylcholine in man and to bring about a depolarisation type of neuromuscular block. If repeated doses are used the block gradually undergoes a change from one of depolarisation to one showing many of the signs of non-depolarisation (see Dual Block, p. 824).

Cardiovascular system.—Leigh and his colleagues (1957) first demonstrated that suxamethonium produced a slowing of the heart rate in children. Little attention was paid to this finding until it was demonstrated in adults that the bradycardia was often associated with an arrhythmia and sometimes a brief period of "cardiac arrest" (Martin, 1958; Bullough, 1959; Lupprian and Churchill-Davidson, 1960). Though the bradycardia of suxamethonium is seen on the first injection in young infants, it is only seen on the second and subsequent injections in the adult (Fig. 2). This failure to produce a specific response on

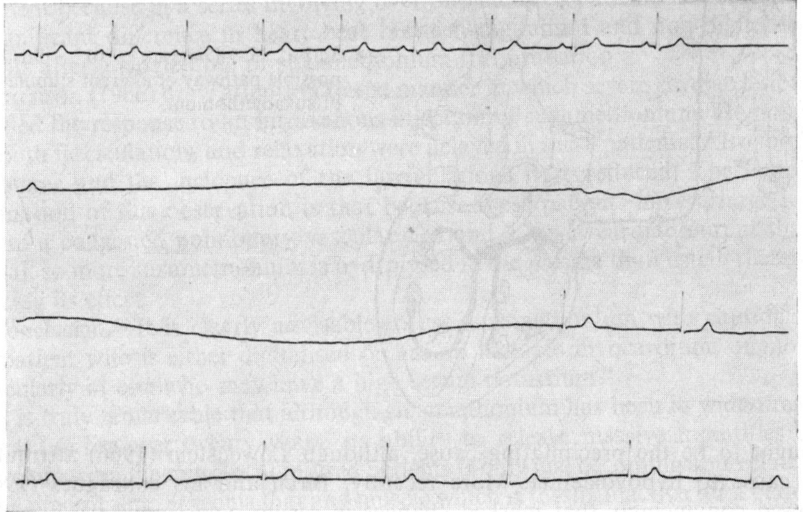

31/FIG. 2.—Example of the bradycardia seen on the administration of a second dose of suxamethonium.

the first injection yet to do so on the second and third is a most interesting feature of the response, because it is a rare event in pharmacology (possibly a unique one). Mathias and Evans-Prosser (1970) have shown that the time-interval between the first and second dose is critical, so that the optimum time for producing a bradycardia is a five-minute interval between the two injections. The precise mechanism of this bradycardia is still not clear. The most likely theories are that it is due either to a direct stimulatory action of the suxamethonium on the myocardium or to stimulation of afferent vagal receptors (e.g. pressor and chemoreceptors) (Fig. 3). The fact that a wide variety of agents such as atropine, the ganglion-blocking group of drugs, and the non-depolarising relaxant agents all block this response to suxamethonium suggests that the latter pathway may be responsible.

The clinical significance of these observations lies in the danger of using suxamethonium in the presence of an irritable myocardium. There are three separate occasions when dangerous arrhythmias including cardiac arrest have been reported. Belin and Karleen (1966) noted that patients receiving suxamethonium for dressing of burns around the sixth week after injury were particularly liable to develop a severe arrhythmia. A high level of serum potassium was

31/TABLE 1
NUMBER OF TIMES MUSCLE-PARALYSING DOSE MUST BE EXCEEDED IN ORDER TO PRODUCE AUTONOMIC BLOCK OF THE INFERIOR MESENTERIC GANGLION OF THE CAT

d-tubocurarine	1– 3
Gallamine	25– 30
Decamethonium	65–100
Suxamethonium	650–700

(after Thesleff, 1952)

Skeletal muscle.—The mode of action of suxamethonium has already been discussed (see above). There is a wide variation in response to depolarising drugs throughout the animal kingdom. For example, the mouse, rat and rabbit are relatively more resistant to these drugs than either man or the cat (Thesleff, 1952). Similarly, in each species there is a wide variation in the response of different muscle-groups. As in almost all these species the diaphragmatic muscle is one of the last to be affected, such terms as "sparing of respiration" have come into being. In man the exact reason why the diaphragm should be the last muscle to be paralysed and usually the first to recover is still unknown, but it may be due either to the rich circulation this muscle possesses or to some intrinsic property of the muscle—e.g. the presence of "red muscle fibres" which are more resistant to depolarisation than white muscle.

The role of suxamethonium and neonatal neuromuscular transmission is discussed on p. 840, and in relation to the release of potassium on p. 853.

Walts and Dillon (1967) compared the intravenous and intramuscular route of administration of suxamethonium on the duration of paralysis. Using comparable doses they found the paresis lasted approximately twice as long when the intramuscular route was used. The intramuscular route is sometimes used in infants because of the simplicity of administration but it allows less immediate control over the paralysis. Also, it must be remembered that the formation of a dual block is both dose- and time-dependent, so that for a given dose of suxamethonium this change is more likely to be observed when the intramuscular, as opposed to the intravenous, route is used.

Fasciculations and muscle pains.—Suxamethonium causes marked fasciculations of the muscles. These contractions frequently lead to muscle pains which are usually noticed by the patient on the day after the operation—particularly when the operative procedure is minor, and therefore does not keep the patient in bed or produce pain itself. The precise mechanism leading to the production of muscle pains is obscure, but Rack and Westbury (1966) observed a high incidence of irreversible changes in the muscle spindles of cats when large doses of succinylcholine were used. It is possible, therefore, that these pains may be due to mechanical damage to these muscle spindles. (See also Chapter 29, p. 793.)

In ambulant patients the incidence of these pains is about 60–70 per cent whereas if the patient is confined to bed after the injection the incidence drops to 10 per cent or less (Churchill-Davidson, 1954; Morris and Dunn, 1957; Foster, 1960; Lamoreaux and Urbach, 1960). At one time it was suggested that the incidence of these pains was less when suxethonium, as opposed to suxamethonium, was used. This has now been shown to be untrue (Parbrook and Pierce, 1960; Burtles, 1961).

These muscle pains are only rarely observed in young children and the aged. Bush and Roth (1961) have pointed out that in children aged 5–14 years the incidence is only 10 per cent, whereas it falls to 3 per cent if the age group of 5–9 years is studied.

Various methods have been tried to eliminate or modify the incidence of these pains. The only satisfactory method is to administer a small dose of a non-depolarising drug (i.e. 3 mg. *d*-tubocurarine or 20 mg. gallamine) at least four minutes before the suxamethonium is given. As the two types of block are antagonistic, however, this frequently reduces the effectiveness of the succinylcholine. Furthermore, as this practice may occasionally be accompanied by a prolonged reaction it cannot be recommended for routine clinical use.

Action on the eye.—The action of suxamethonium on the extra- and intra-ocular muscles is both interesting and complex. The matter has assumed some importance because the anaesthetist frequently uses this drug in anaesthesia for ophthalmic surgery.

Early reports suggested that the rise in intra-ocular tension brought about by suxamethonium is capable of expelling vitreous from the inner chamber of the open eye (Dillon *et al.*, 1957; Lincoff *et al.*, 1957). Katz and Eakins (1969) reviewed all the evidence and in the light of their own work concluded that suxamethonium was capable of increasing intra-ocular tension not only by a contraction of the extra-orbital musculature but also by contracting the intra-orbital smooth muscle. They also pointed out that if suxamethonium produced a rise in systemic pressure then this also would tend to increase intra-ocular tension.

Hess and Pilar (1963) drew attention to two distinct systems of neuromuscular transmission that can be found in the extra-ocular muscles. First, there is the *twitch* system characterised by muscle fibres with small, well-defined fibrils and supplied by the large efferent nerve fibres. These respond with action potentials similar to those found at other mammalian neuromuscular junctions. Secondly, there is the *tonic* system characterised by muscle fibres with poorly defined fibrils and supplied by small efferent nerve fibres. Stimulation of this system leads to a slow summating contraction—a contracture—as occurs in amphibian and avian muscle.

Katz and Eakins (1969) concluded that the varied response to suxamethonium could be explained on the basis of this double neuromuscular system. They postulated that suxamethonium (like other depolarising drugs) stimulates the tonic system, thereby increasing intra-ocular tension. At the same time it depresses the twitch system, though this plays no part in the overall result. *d*-Tubocurarine, on the other hand, depresses both systems and blocks the stimulating effect of suxamethonium not only on the tonic system of the extra-ocular muscles but also on intra-ocular smooth muscle.

Comment.—It is now fully recognised that suxamethonium can produce a rise in intra-ocular pressure. This might prove harmful in cases of glaucoma (where there is already increased tension) or in cases of detached retina (where a further rise in pressure might increase the damage) or by expelling vitreous humour during open eye surgery. In such instances the use of suxamethonium alone is obviously contra-indicated. The alternative is to use a non-depolarising drug which does not raise intra-ocular-pressure, but a small dose of *d*-tubocurarine (3 mg.) or gallamine (20 mg.) given three minutes before the suxamethonium will block this effect of suxamethonium on the orbital musculature (Miller *et al.*, 1968).

Alimentary system.—In animals no deleterious effect on the contraction of the intestine has been noted, even with large doses. If massive quantities are given which are a long way outside the therapeutic range in man there is some evidence that irregular contractions and a decreased sensitivity to acetylcholine may be produced (Thesleff, 1952). It should be remembered that pseudo-cholinesterase is formed in the liver, and this enzyme is responsible for the breakdown of suxamethonium. In the event of severe liver damage, cachexia, or malnutrition, therefore, an increased duration of action of suxamethonium should be anticipated.

Histamine release.—The release of histamine by suxamethonium is believed to be about one hundredth of the activity of *d*-tubocurarine (Bourne *et al.*, 1952; Davies, 1956). However, Laurie Smith (1957) has drawn attention to the fact that patients can be found in whom the intradermal injection of small doses of suxamethonium (10 mg.) produces a weal and flare of almost identical proportion with that of a small dose of *d*-tubocurarine (2 mg.). Certainly cases of possible bronchospasm have been reported (Fellini *et al.*, 1963), but Jerum and his colleagues (1967) described a case of anaphylaxis with the onset of tachycardia, hypotension, bronchospasm, and pharyngeal and facial oedema in a 26-year-old woman.

Placental transmission.—A method for the study of small concentrations of suxamethonium in serum has been described (Kvisselgaard and Moya, 1961). This technique has been used to study the possible transmission of suxamethonium across the placental barrier in women. It has been established that the placental tissue itself (in homogenate suspension) does not significantly contribute to the hydrolysis of suxamethonium (Moya and Margolies, 1961).

Although suxamethonium was rarely encountered in the blood of the umbilical vein of the infant, it was found that when large *single* doses of 300–500 mg. were administered to the mother then "small but definitely detectable quantities were found in the neonatal circulation" (Moya and Kvisselgaard, 1961). Despite the fact that the pseudo-cholinesterase activity of infants is lower than in adults, these babies did not appear to be affected by the profound paralysis in the mother. This may be due to the fact that the newborn is resistant to the effects of the depolarising drugs (see p. 840). The explanation of why suxamethonium does not cross the placental barrier in significant amounts is obscure. It has a low molecular weight (290) and therefore as a small molecule might be expected to pass. Moya and Kvisselgaard (1961) attempted to explain this paradox on the basis that the placenta is essentially a lipid-rich membrane and suxamethonium has a low fat solubility, which might impede its passage.

Distribution

The distribution of suxamethonium is well illustrated in Fig. 5 which is based on whole body autoradiography in a monkey foetus.

Whole Body Autoradiography; Monkey Foetus (Macaca Mulatta)
SUXAMETHONIUM
Intracordal Injection *in situ*

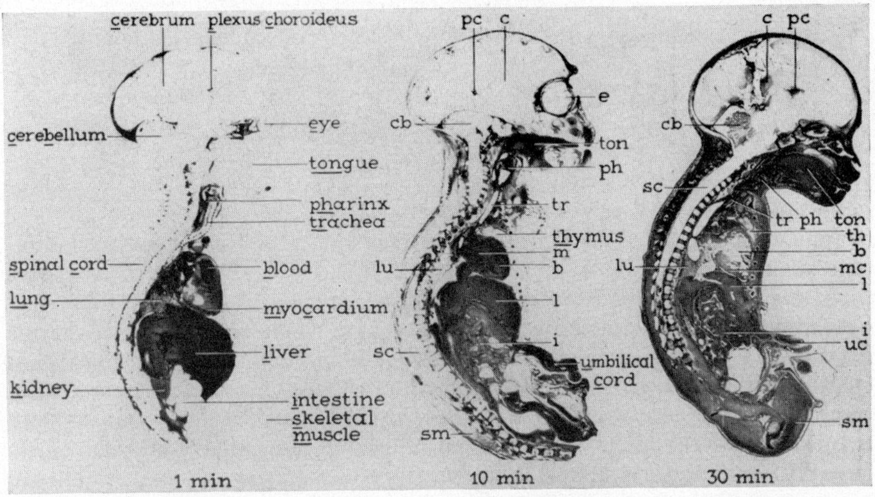

31/Fig. 5.—The distribution of suxamethonium in the monkey foetus (by courtesy of Prof. J. F. Crul).

Detoxication and Excretion

Suxamethonium has held a leading role in clinical anaesthesia principally because of its very short duration of action. Thus, following an intravenous dose it is believed that nearly all the suxamethonium in the plasma has been hydrolysed within one minute of the injection (Pantuck, 1967). This is brought about by rapid enzymatic hydrolysis with pseudo (plasma) cholinesterase. However, other metabolic routes such as redistribution, alkaline hydrolysis and renal excretion may play an important role if enzymatic hydrolysis is impaired.

(*a*) **Enzymatic hydrolysis.**—Pseudo-cholinesterase is a glycoprotein synthesised in the liver and abounds in the plasma. The purpose of its presence in man (other than to destroy suxamethonium) is not yet clear. It must be readily distinguished from another enzyme, true (specific) cholinesterase, which is present in red blood cells and at the neuromuscular junction. This latter enzyme is responsible for the rapid hydrolysis of acetylcholine at the nerve-ending.

The breakdown of succinyldicholine (suxamethonium) takes place in two stages—one rapid and the other slow (Table 2).

1. *Succinyldicholine to succinylmonocholine and choline.*—Within seconds of entering the plasma this process has begun, and is so effective in the normal case that probably not more than 5 per cent of the injected dose reaches the muscles in the periphery. Less than 2 per cent appears in the urine (Foldes and Norton, 1954). The administration of suxamethonium brings about an inhibition of the plasma cholinesterase level, for Doenicke and his colleagues (1968) have been able to demonstrate that this inhibition bears a direct relationship to the duration

31/Table 2

The Breakdown of Suxamethonium (Succinyldicholine)

1st stage:

Succinyldicholine $\xrightarrow[\text{pseudocholinesterase}]{\text{(Rapid)}}$ Succinylmonocholine + Choline

2nd stage:

Succinylmonocholine $\xrightarrow[\text{Specific liver enzyme and pseudocholinesterase}]{\text{(Slow)}}$ Succinic acid + Choline

of apnoea. Spontaneous respiration returned as soon as no further enzyme inhibition was measurable.

2. *Succinylmonocholine to succinic acid and choline.*—This stage is extremely slow and though pseudo-cholinesterase does play some role there is a specific enzyme for hydrolysis of succinylmonocholine found in the liver (Greenway and Quastel, 1955). Though the monocholine derivative is theoretically capable of producing a depolarisation block in its own right, as it only has one-twentieth to one-eightieth the activity of succinyldicholine paresis is unlikely to occur unless large doses of the parent drug have been used (i.e. over 500 mg. of suxamethonium). Foldes and his associates (1954) demonstrated that 5–7 mg./kg. of succinylmonocholine produced good relaxation in an anaesthetised subject lasting 8–12 minutes. This observation was also confirmed by Brennan (1956).

(*b*) **Alkaline hydrolysis.**—This is a non-enzymatic process which in normal circumstances plays only a very small role in the metabolism of suxamethonium. Even in the absence of an enzymatic process it can only play a minor role in shortening the period of paresis, as less than 5 per cent per hour is destroyed by this method (Kalow, 1959). In other words, only 50 per cent of the injected dose would have been broken down in ten hours.

(*c*) **Re-distribution.**—The uptake of suxamethonium at receptor sites (active and non-active) clearly has an important role to play in reducing the concentration in the plasma. The extent to which suxamethonium is bound to protein has yet to be elucidated.

(*d*) **Excretion.**—It has already been mentioned that less than 2 per cent of suxamethonium is excreted unchanged in the urine, but in the absence of enzymatic hydrolysis this percentage might prove to be very much higher. No data is available on this subject.

Plasma Cholinesterase

The enzymatic hydrolysis of suxamethonium in man is now well understood. Nevertheless, cases are occasionally encountered who exhibit a prolonged response to this drug. Originally it was believed that all these could be accounted for on the basis of a diminished production of plasma cholinesterase enzyme by the liver. However, not all these cases appeared to be suffering from malnutrition or liver damage; in fact, some of the apnoeas occurred in very fit, healthy young patients. The puzzle was resolved when Kalow and Davies (1958) discovered that in man there were at least two types of plasma cholinesterase enzyme—a normal and an atypical one. Apparently individuals could lead perfectly normal lives with either one of these enzymes and it was only when they received an injection of suxamethonium that any differentiation could be made. A fit person with the normal plasma cholinesterase enzyme could hydrolyse suxamethonium rapidly, whereas one with the atypical enzyme could not do it at all. The only difference between these two enzymes is one of degree. Both are capable of hydrolysing suxamethonium *in vitro* but only the normal enzyme can do it in clinical conditions where the concentration of suxamethonium is low. Thus, if a patient with the atypical enzyme receives a dose of suxamethonium, the dilution caused by the blood volume rapidly causes a drop in its concentration below the effective level for the atypical esterase. In these circumstances the patient remains paralysed for a long period of time.

A. *Normal pseudo-cholinesterase.*—The enzyme level is normally determined by the Warburg apparatus but this estimation is both difficult and tedious. In clinical practice a simple test paper (incorporating the same principle) has been found satisfactory and reasonably accurate (Churchill-Davidson and Griffiths, 1961). Such methods will give an estimation of the total *amount* of enzyme in the blood but they will not differentiate the *type* of enzyme, i.e. between the normal and the atypical. Fortunately, the patients with only the atypical enzyme in their blood give low values for these tests, but there are a number of patients who have a mixture of some normal esterase and some atypical who merely give values on the low side of normal. For this reason, a low value for pseudo-cholinesterase may be due to two causes (Fig. 6). One is liver damage due to disease and malnutrition; the other is the presence of this atypical enzyme. To differentiate between these two conditions requires a special test.

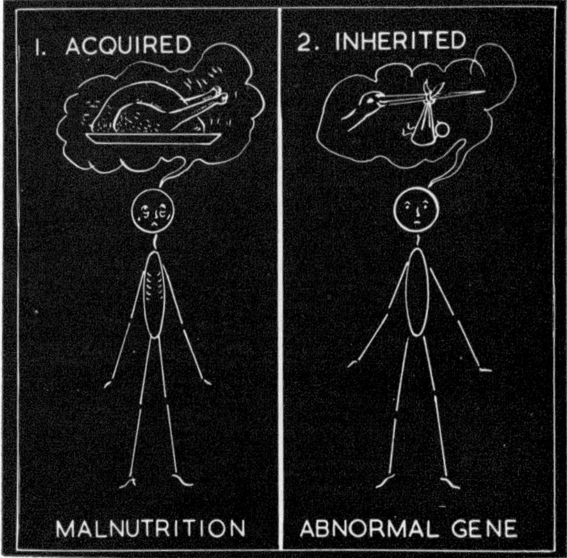

31/Fig. 6.—Illustration of the two causes of reduced plasma cholinesterase enzyme activity.

Kalow and Genest (1957) demonstrated that these two conditions—a low normal pseudo-cholinesterase and the presence of an atypical enzyme—behave differently when a local analgesic agent (dibucaine) is added to the serum.

B. *Atypical cholinesterase enzyme.*—The presence of this enzyme is due to the inheritance of an abnormal gene. An understanding of this process is most easily achieved if the genes for the cholinesterase enzyme are expressed as symbols (Fig. 7).

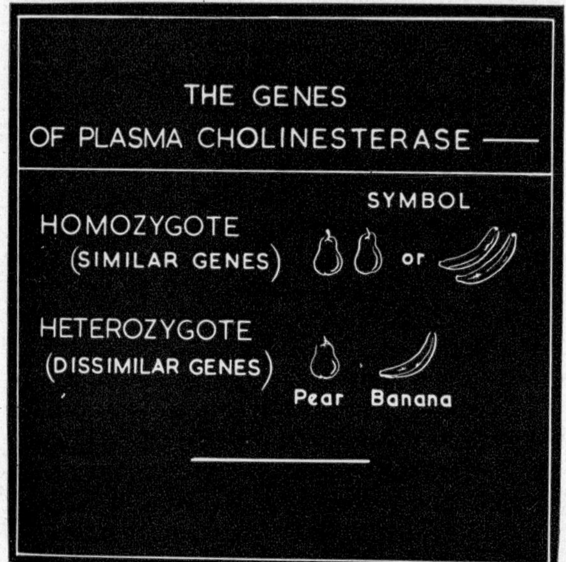

31/Fig. 7.

On the basis of Kalow's studies (1959) the vast majority of the population (96·2 per cent) are normal (i.e. homozygotes or similar genes). These two genes are normal (2 pears). Such people can destroy suxamethonium very rapidly. A small percentage of the population (3·8 per cent) have a mixture, i.e. one normal and one atypical gene. They are described as heterozygotes (dissimilar genes) which are represented below as one pear and one banana. Such persons destroy suxamethonium, but far less efficiently, so that its duration of action may be prolonged to 5–10 minutes. Very rarely (1:2800 people) someone is encountered who has only two atypical genes—i.e. an abnormal homozygote (2 bananas). In clinical practice it is estimated that an abnormally prolonged response to suxamethonium is encountered in 1 out of 2400 cases (Churchill-Davidson, 1961), so that it is probable that the great bulk of "apnoeas" which are met with are due to the presence of an atypical gene.

The manner in which two heterozygotes happen to marry and produce a child with the atypical homozygotic enzyme is illustrated below (Fig. 8).

The dibucaine test.—The basis for this test is to examine the amount of inhibition of a particular serum by dibucaine. If a specimen has a high normal enzyme content then it will be inhibited to a large extent by the dibucaine. This

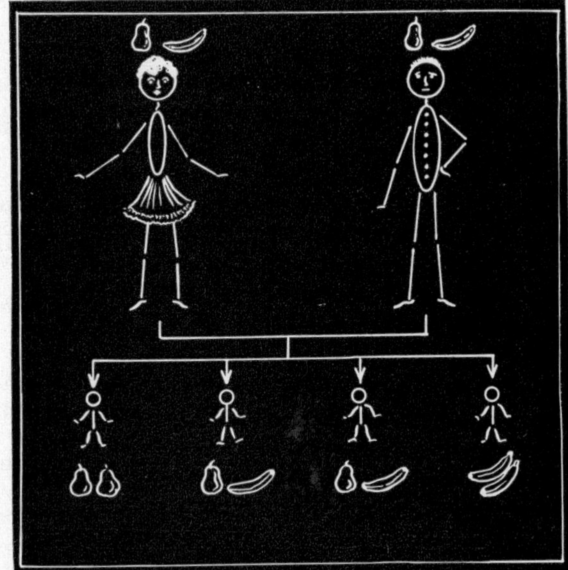

31/FIG. 8.—Diagram of genetic response in the offspring when two heterozygotes marry.

percentage is usually expressed as a number—the Dibucaine number (Table 3).

31/TABLE 3

DIBUCAINE NUMBERS FOR VARIOUS TYPES OF SERA

	Dibucaine Number
A. Normal homozygote (two normal genes) NN	70–85
B. Heterozygote (one normal and one atypical gene) DN	50–65
C. Abnormal homozygote (two abnormal genes) DD	16–25

Smith and Foldes (1968) have pointed out that though it is always easy to differentiate between normal (NN) and abnormal (DD) homozygotes, it is sometimes difficult to be certain of the heterozygote (DN). In order to overcome this difficulty they have suggested using a mixture of procaine and tetracaine rather than dibucaine because this gives a much clearer distinction, e.g.

NN	320–464
ND	152–239
DD	16– 59

Significance of pseudo-cholinesterase and dibucaine test.—Patients with a low dibucaine number also have a low pseudo-cholinesterase, but the converse is not necessarily true. For example, a patient with malnutrition may have a low pseudo-cholinesterase value yet have a normal dibucaine number. In this manner, it is now possible to distinguish between those patients who have a prolonged apnoea due to malnutrition and liver failure and those who have simply inherited an atypical gene. The clinical importance of making this differentiation may seem small but if the process is traced through a family it is possible to forewarn a certain member(s) of that family that a prolonged response to suxamethonium may be anticipated.

The possible results of these two tests (when combined), along with the diagnosis of the result, are presented in Table 4 (Lehmann, 1962).

31/TABLE 4
POSSIBLE RESULTS OF THE COMBINATION OF THE PSEUDO-CHOLINESTERASE ESTIMATION (NORMAL = 60 – 120 UNITS) AND THE DIBUCAINE NUMBER

Ps. ch. esterase in units	*Dibucaine Number % inhibition*	*Diagnosis*	*Genes*
60–120	70–85	Normal homozygote	2 normal
8–59	70–85	Normal homozygote with liver damage	2 normal
26–90	50–65	Heterozygote	1 normal 1 atypical
8–40	50–65	Heterozygote with liver damage	1 normal 1 atypical
8–35	16–25	Atypical homozygote	2 atypical

Other genetic variants.—Further studies on the serum of patients who had a prolonged response to suxamethonium soon revealed certain interesting variations.

1. *Fluoride-resistant variant.*—Harris and Whittaker (1961; 1962) found that sodium fluoride could be used in place of dibucaine. However, they noticed in comparing the results of the two methods that a few patients had a normal-looking dibucaine number yet an abnormally low fluoride number (Table 5). They suggested that here was yet another gene for pseudo-cholinesterase. The homozygote of this fluoride gene was known to give a moderately prolonged response to suxamethonium (Kalow, 1964).

2. *Silent gene.*—Liddell and his colleagues (1962), using the dibucaine test, found evidence for yet another gene. These patients have complete absence of all pseudo-cholinesterase activity. The clinical importance for such patients is that they have a *very* prolonged response to suxamethonium.

Comment.—There would appear to be at least four genes for pseudo-cholinesterase—the normal, the dibucaine resistant, the fluoride resistant, and the silent gene. These can combine to form ten genotypes (Table 6), of which six are associated with markedly increased sensitivity to suxamethonium (Pantuck, 1967). It is estimated that one of these six will appear in every 1500 patients (Kalow, 1964).

In discussing the variants of pseudo-cholinesterase enzymes it must not be forgotten that examples of increased (as opposed to decreased) activity have also been described. For example, an additional enzyme (named C_5) has been identified (Harris *et al.*, 1963). This tends to increase the rate of suxamethonium hydrolysis. Similarly, Neitlich (1966) has described another genetic variant in which the patient showed a great resistance to suxamethonium.

31/TABLE 5

THE VALUES QUOTED BY HARRIS AND WHITTAKER (1961) FOR THE DIBUCAINE AND FLUORIDE NUMBERS IN A STUDY OF 285 PATIENTS

Phenotype		*Dibucaine No.*		*Fluoride No.*	
		Mean	*Standard Deviation*	*Mean*	*Standard Deviation*
Normal Homozygote	"Usual"	80·06	1·56	61·35	3·21
Heterozygote	"Intermediate"	61.93	21·17	47·79	4·48
Abnormal Homozygote	"Atypical"	21·82	2·92	23·14	2·23

31/TABLE 6

HEREDITARY VARIANTS OF PSEUDO-CHOLINESTERASE IN MAN (adapted from Pantuck, 1967)

Genotype	*Incidence*	*Response to suxamethonium*	*Av. Dibucaine No.*	*Av. Fluoride No.*
N–N	96 per cent	Normal	80	60
D–D	1:2,500	Prolonged ++	20	20
S–S	1:100,000	Prolonged +++	0	0
F–F	Rare	Prolonged +	70	30
N–D	1:25	Prolonged	60	45
N–F	?	Prolonged	75	50
N–S	1:200	Prolonged	80	60
D–F	?	Prolonged +	45	35
D–S	1:800	Prolonged ++	20	20
F–S*	?	Prolonged	70	20

N = gene for normal pseudo-cholinesterase
D = gene for dibucaine-resistant variant
F = fluoride-resistant variant
S = silent gene
* Not yet observed

Administration

Suxamethonium is usually administered intravenously, but it can be given intramuscularly or even by the subcutaneous route if the dose is sufficient. If either of the latter routes is used then there is a considerable delay in the onset of paresis and once established it lasts much longer than normal. With the intravenous route the arrival in any group of muscle fibres is heralded by brief but visible twitches or fasciculations, and these are usually first observed in the eyebrow and eyelid muscles, passing later to the shoulder girdle and abdominal musculature, and finally to the hands and feet.

Dosage.—The average single dose in man is 25–75 mg., but when administered by continuous infusion as a 0·1 per cent solution a dose of 20–40 μg/kg./min. will give relaxation of most skeletal musculature, but some assistance to respiration is required. Doses of 50–60 μg/kg./min. and above usually result in complete respiratory paralysis. If total paralysis is produced by continuous infusion there is a considerable danger of administering an overdose, as there are no signs of muscle activity available. It is essential to monitor neuromuscular transmission continuously (see p. 829) whenever an infusion of suxamethonium is used, as this will remove the risk of overdosage.

Duration of action.—A single injection of suxamethonium (25–50 mg.) produces, on average, respiratory paralysis for 2–4 minutes. Doubling the dose does not necessarily double the duration of cessation of respiration. A period of apnoea (in the presence of adequate manual ventilation) lasting longer than ten minutes must be considered as an abnormal response. Electromyography, however, has shown that the recovery of the limb muscles lags far behind that of the respiratory muscles.

Antagonists

Like that of decamethonium, the action of suxamethonium can be opposed by the previous administration of a non-depolarising drug such as *d*-tubocurarine or gallamine; similarly, it can be potentiated by anti-cholinesterase or depolarising drugs whether given before or after the suxamethonium. In clinical practice both hexafluorenium bromide (Foldes *et al.*, 1960) and tetrahydroaminoacridine (Gordh and Wahlin, 1961; MacCaul and Robinson, 1962; Benveniste and Dyrberg, 1962) have been used to potentiate the duration of action of suxamethonium. Both are inhibitors of pseudo-cholinesterase with only weak or absent muscarinic effects, e.g. salivation and bradycardia. The advantage of this combination is claimed to be that it reduces the total amount of suxamethonium required and therefore lowers the incidence of dual block.

Prolonged Response

As has been previously stated, the duration of action of a single dose of suxamethonium (e.g. 50 mg.) is 2–4 minutes in adults, and apnoea lasting longer than ten minutes must be considered abnormal. Often the cause of failure of return of respiration is not related to the relaxant at all but to the sedation, the depression of the respiratory centre or the hyperventilation. The diagnosis of a prolonged response to suxamethonium, therefore, must be made with a peripheral nerve stimulator (Fig. 9). This instrument, when applied to a peripheral nerve, will indicate first the amount of neuromuscular block that is present, and secondly the characteristics of this block—i.e. depolarisation or non-depolarisation. If, after ten minutes of apnoea, the hand muscles are still completely paralysed, then it is safe to assume that this is an abnormal response to suxamethonium. For routine continuous monitoring it is necessary to place needle electrodes under the skin in the vicinity of the ulnar nerve either at the wrist or elbow. Some peripheral nerve stimulators are so arranged that they automatically deliver a single twitch stimulus every 3–5 seconds, thereby enabling the anaesthetist to gauge the depth of paresis and to regulate the suxamethonium infusion. For diagnostic purposes a single application using external electrodes will usually reveal all the information required.

A prolonged response to suxamethonium may occur for three reasons:

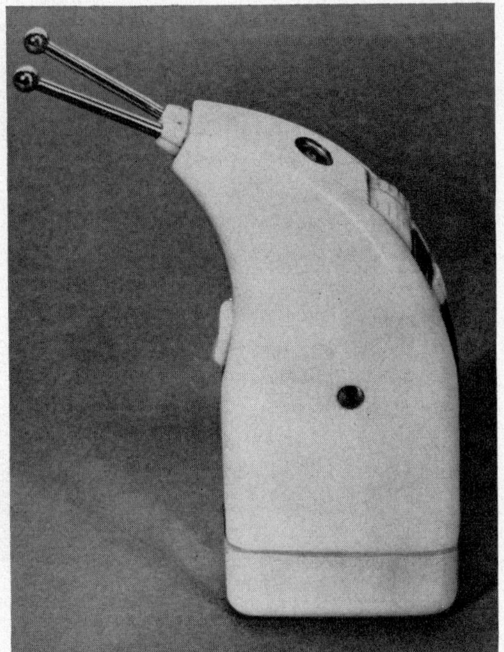

31/Fig. 9(*a*).—A portable peripheral nerve stimulator.

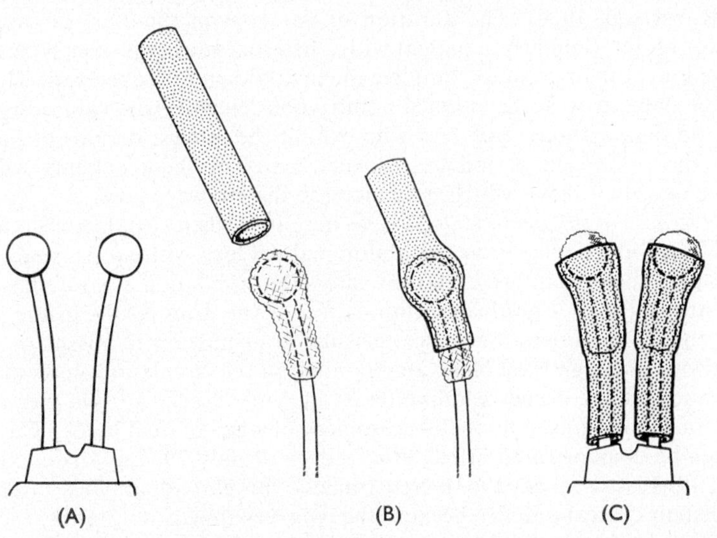

31/Fig. 9(*b*).—Method of improving contact for external skin stimulation. In (B) and (C) a pledget of cotton wool is slipped over the metal electrode (A) and held firmly in place by latex rubber tubing. Before use the cotton wool tip is moistened in a strong salt solution.

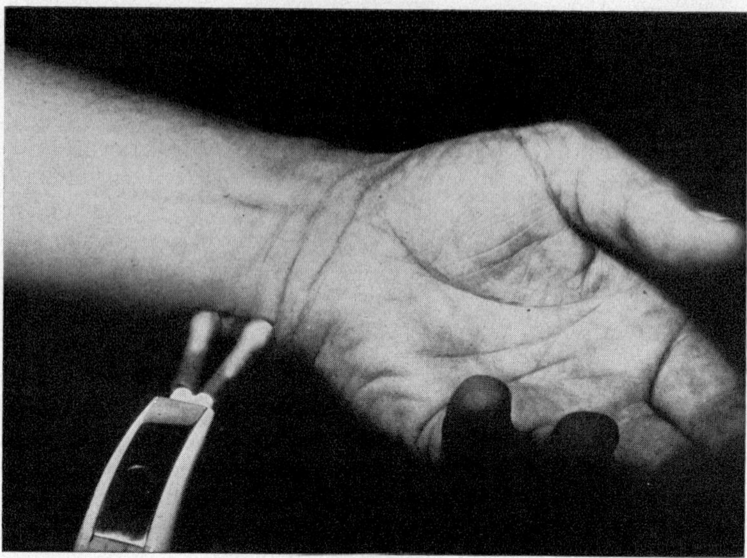

31/FIG. 9(*c*).—Method of applying the peripheral nerve stimulator to the ulnar nerve at the wrist.

1. *Low or atypical pseudo-cholinesterase enzyme activity.*—Patients with a low enzyme activity are most often encountered in severe liver disease, starvation—as in carcinoma of the oesophagus—or in women in late pregnancy (Shnider, 1965; Robertson, 1966). The duration of paralysis in this type of case rarely exceeds ½–1 hour. Similarly, a patient with a heterozygous type of enzyme activity will take longer than usual to complete the breakdown of the relaxant. However, it is those patients with the atypical homozygous enzyme who cannot hydrolyse any of the suxamethonium *in vivo* who exhibit the longest periods of paralysis. During the prolonged period of recovery many of these patients will show evidence of a dual block which may increase the recovery time.

2. *Overdose of suxamethonium.*—This may arise when an intravenous infusion is used to produce relaxation for abdominal surgery without a suitable nerve stimulator. When the infused relaxant enters the circulation at a rate faster than it is destroyed, then a gradual accumulation of the drug results in the plasma. At the end of the operation neuromuscular transmission is absent or returns very slowly. The high level of suxamethonium in the circulation slows down the regeneration of the pseudo-cholinesterase enzyme. Added to this the situation may be further confused by the development of signs of dual block. These signs can often be demonstrated briefly after a dose of only 200 mg. suxamethonium (White, 1963; Katz *et al.*, 1963). Nevertheless, this early dual block rarely poses a problem in clinical practice because the recovery time is not unduly increased. When large doses are used then a prolonged recovery may sometimes be observed clinically.

3. *Long-term anti-cholinesterase therapy.*—The increasing use of anti-cholinesterase drugs in medicine has increased this danger. Such agents are

frequently used to lower intra-ocular tension in cases of glaucoma with ecthiopate iodine. Certain of the cytotoxic agents used in the treatment of cancer also have some anti-cholinesterase action (Wang and Ross, 1963).

Treatment of a prolonged response to suxamethonium.—The fact that the block of suxamethonium changes its characteristic from one of depolarisation to one resembling non-depolarisation (i.e. dual block) is now fully established. The presence of the signs of a non-depolarisation type of block might tempt the unwary to use an anti-cholinesterase to reverse the block. Nevertheless, the term "non-depolarisation" is used in a loose context in this case, because it differs from that produced by *d*-tubocurarine (dtc) in a number of ways. First, unlike the dtc block, the membrane potential does not remain unchanged at the resting level of 60–90 mV. Secondly, there is evidence that suxamethonium penetrates the interior of the muscle fibres (which dtc does not) at about the same time as the non-depolarising element becomes established. Thirdly, and most important, a further dose of suxamethonium antagonises a dtc block but potentiates a dual block.

In clinical practice the use of anti-cholinesterase drugs in the presence of dual block has led to considerable confusion because in some instances it has been successful while in others it has proved disastrous in that the apnoea has been prolonged (Vickers, 1963; Hunter, 1966). The reason depends on the presence or absence of suxamethonium in the circulation (Gissen *et al.*, 1966). If there is no suxamethonium (i.e. it has all been hydrolysed) circulating in the plasma then the neuromuscular block will be reversed. On the other hand, if some is still present then the breakdown process will be slowed down even further. Coupled with this, extra acetylcholine molecules will become available as they are no longer destroyed. Also, large doses of anticholinesterase drugs can act as depolarising agents in their own right. The result is an increase in neuromuscular block.

A dual block will most commonly be encountered on two occasions. First, when a single dose of suxamethonium has been given to a patient who has an atypical type of plasma cholinesterase enzyme. The result is a prolonged apnoea and the signs of a dual block are evident during recovery. The other and more common instance is when an infusion of suxamethonium has been used without adequate monitoring of neuromuscular transmission and the patient has received an overdose. In this case one must assume that normal esterase activity is present, and given time it will hydrolyse any suxamethonium remaining in the plasma.

The treatment of the case with the atypical enzyme is clearly more difficult than that with simple overdose. The administration of an anti-cholinesterase would tend to enhance the block for the reasons given above. A more rational approach would be to try to stimulate urinary excretion of the drug or to attempt to give the patient some normal enzyme. Doenicke and his colleagues (1968) have claimed that even a small dose of purified concentrated human serum esterase (cholase) produces a shortening of the apnoeic period; after a dose of 50 mg. of suxamethonium in normal man the resulting apnoea could be almost entirely neutralised with the esterase dose. If available, therefore, the use of fresh or concentrated enzyme would appear to be indicated, though earlier reports had suggested disappointing results.

tubocurarine in man. They used it to soften the effects of electroconvulsion therapy and from that day onwards the muscle relaxants have played an important part in this treatment. In 1942, Griffiths and Johnson in Montreal introduced curare into anaesthesia, and together they contributed to one of the most spectacular advances in modern surgery. In 1946, Gray and Halton in England presented a series of cases describing the use of *d*-tubocurarine in anaesthesia.

Standardisation

During the early days of the introduction of curare into clinical anaesthesia there were two main types of drug available, which led to a certain amount of confusion in the literature:

(*a*) "Intocostrin" was a trade name in the United States for a total purified extract of *chondodendron tomentosum*. One ml. of this extract is believed to have a paralysing action equivalent to 20 mg. of a standardised preparation of curare. It is clear from the remarks above that some of these relaxant properties might be due to the presence of small amounts of *d*-chondrocurarine as well as *d*-tubocurarine.

(*b*) *d*-Tubocurarine chloride is a purified extract of *chondodendron tomentosum* (Wintersteiner and Dutcher, 1943); 1 ml. of the solution contains 10 mg. of the active principle in the U.K. and 3 mg. in the U.S.A. This substance has now been universally adopted in clinical anaesthesia.

Physical and Chemical Properties*

d-Tubocurarine chloride is a quaternary alkaloid which can be isolated from the roots of the *chondodendron tomentosum*. It contains two phenolic groups and two methoxy groups in its formula. Although the cationic quaternary ammonium groups are believed to be principally responsible for the combination with the anionic end-plate receptor, these phenolic hydroxyl groups may have an important role to play. For, whereas the quaternary ammonium group are completely ionised in the range of pH found in clinical anaesthetic practice, these hydroxyl groups can vary their ionisation in relation to change in pH due

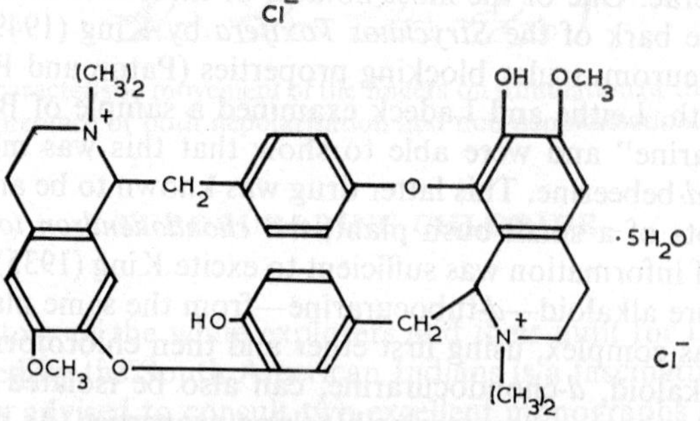

Structure of *d*-tubocurarine chloride

* *Plasma concentration of* d-*tubocurarine.*—A method of measuring the concentration of *d*-tubocurarine in plasma using a spectrophotometer has been described by Elert (1956) and revised by Elert and Cohen (1962) and Utting (1963).

either to respiratory or metabolic causes. Such alterations may influence the duration of action of the relaxant (see Carbon dioxide and the pH of the blood, p. 833).

The crystals are colourless, dextro-rotatory in activity, soluble in saline and to a lesser extent in water. The substance deteriorates on heating for any length of time.

Pharmacological Actions

Mode of action.—*d*-Tubocurarine was the first of a long line of neuromuscular blocking drugs. It acts by non-depolarisation or competitive inhibition. The curare molecule combines with the protein molecule of the end-plate receptor and this denies the acetylcholine molecule access to its normal destination. The characteristics of this type of neuromuscular block have already been discussed in detail (Chapter 30). Briefly, they can be summarised as follows:

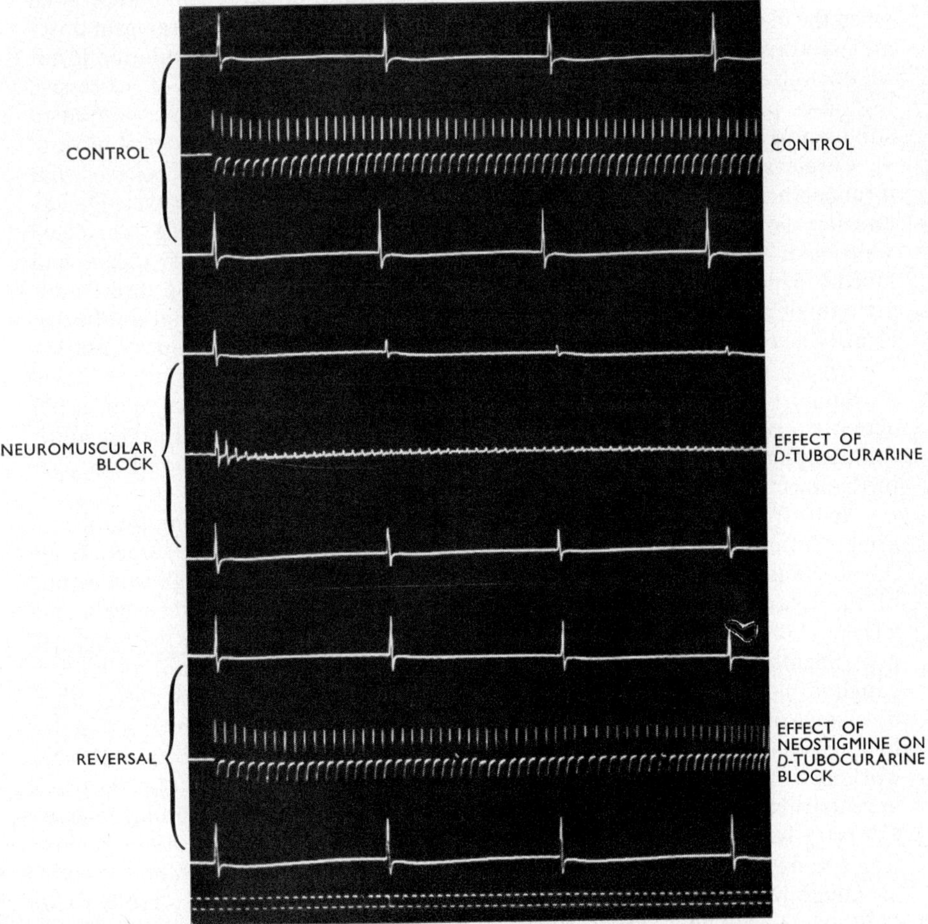

31/Fig. 11.—Electromyograph of classical *d*-tubocurarine neuromuscular block.

1. "Fade" of successive responses to both slow (twitch) and fast (tetanic) rates of nerve stimulation.
2. The presence of post-tetanic potentiation.
3. The above signs are reversed by anti-cholinesterase drugs.

An example of a non-depolarisation block is illustrated (Fig. 11).

Other features of a non-depolarisation block that may sometimes be observed are:

(*a*) Antagonism or reversal of the block by depolarising drugs. This is more theoretical than practical in clinical anaesthesia as it requires a perfect balance of dosage that can seldom be attained.

(*b*) The absence of fasciculations or muscle pains either during or after the injection.

In animal experiments great importance has been attached to the presence of Wedensky inhibition (i.e. the passage of slower rates of nerve stimulation even when the faster rates are blocked). In clinical practice, when full paralysant doses are used this discrepancy between fast and slow rates of nerve stimulation is not so obvious. Whether the rate be fast or slow, the decrement of successive responses occurs mainly with the first four stimuli. Following this, continued stimulation leads to a slight waxing and waning of neuromuscular transmission.

Cardiovascular system.—Until a few years ago it was generally believed that *d*-tubocurarine had virtually no effect on myocardial activity. However, Dowdy and her associates (1965) found that 15–30 mg. of *d*-tubocurarine "corrected ventricular fibrillation in patients in whom all other conventional means had failed". This observation suggested that the relaxant drug had a direct anti-arrhythmic action on the myocardium. These authors also found that *d*-tubocurarine (when injected into the isolated rabbit heart) led to a reduction of contractile tension which resembled quinidine.

Support for the thesis that *d*-tubocurarine may have a direct myocardial action is also given by the work of Cohen and his colleagues with their autoradiographic studies in rats. They observed that, unlike gallamine, a large part of the injected dose could be found in heart muscle (Fig. 12).

Apart from a possible direct inotropic effect on the myocardium, *d*-tubocurarine is often referred to as a ganglion-blocking drug. This arose largely from the observation that some patients developed hypotension following the injection of the relaxant (Thomas, 1957; Bonon and Mapelli, 1960; McDowall and Clarke, 1969). The evidence for actual ganglionic blockade rests with animal experiments and it is extremely effective as such in the cat. In man, all known ganglion-blocking drugs produce a tachycardia yet *d*-tubocurarine causes either no change or a fall in pulse rate. A possible explanation of this dilemma is that the hypotension is due to the release of histamine. Iwatsuki and his associates (1965), working with dogs, demonstrated that *d*-tubocurarine produced a marked decrease in ventricular contractile force which they believed to be due to histamine release. Contrary to the results of earlier workers (Mongar and Whelan, 1953) it now seems more certain that *d*-tubocurarine is capable of raising the blood level of histamine in man (Westgate and Van Bergen, 1962; Salem *et al.*, 1968; Crul, 1970; McDowall and Clarke, 1969) and this could account for the fall in blood pressure observed in some patients.

Finally, Mathias and Evans-Prosser (1970), in a far-ranging study of the bradycardia and arrhythmia produced by suxamethonium, have drawn attention to the fact that only very small doses of *d*-tubocurarine are required to protect the patient against an alteration in either cardiac rate or rhythm. As many other drugs, such as atropine and the ganglion-blockers, are also capable of affording this protection, they have suggested that the most likely site of action for *d*-tubocurarine is on the vagal afferent system. In this way the relaxant is able to protect the heart from afferent stimulation arising in other parts of the body and which otherwise would lead to vagal slowing and possible arrhythmias.

In summary, it now appears to be established that *d*-tubocurarine reduces or abolishes the incidence of arrhythmias. Whether the principal site of this blocking action is at the afferent vagal receptors, on the cardiac ganglion (efferent limb), or on the myocardium itself seems less certain. There is no doubt, however, that the ability of *d*-tubocurarine to liberate significant amounts of histamine has been established.

Central nervous system.—Hersey and his colleagues (1961) used a cross circulation technique in dogs and found that curare produced a depression of the respiratory centre in a dose that approximated closely to that required to produce a peripheral myoneural block in the donor body.

Paton (1959) reviewed much of the evidence for the possible passage of *d*-tubocurarine across the blood-brain barrier and concluded that "although there is little likelihood that these (muscle relaxants) should be able to penetrate the central nervous system . . . a number of conditions such as asphyxia, anaesthesia, dehydration or haemorrhage may weaken the selectiveness of the entry from the blood to the brain." Cohen (1963) tested this hypothesis in dogs and found *d*-tubocurarine—administered to the animal under a variety of adverse conditions—does not pass into the cerebrospinal fluid. Further support to the view that *d*-tubocurarine does not cross the blood-brain barrier is given by the observation (using autoradiography) of the absence of any of the relaxant drug in the brain tissue of curarised rats (Cohen *et al.*, 1968) (see Fig. 12).

Neostigmine-resistant curarisation was a term used by Hunter (1956) to describe cases in which an electrolyte imbalance (often associated with acute intestinal obstruction) was believed to be responsible for a prolonged neuromuscular block that could not be reversed by neostigmine. Despite the passing of nearly fifteen years, evidence is still lacking that a neuromuscular block with the classical signs of a non-depolarisation block was present and that neostigmine failed to improve neuromuscular transmission. It is probable that such cases received an overdose of the relaxant drug and that other factors such as low body temperature, poor muscle blood-flow, and acid-base imbalance all contributed to the degree of block.

Skeletal muscle.—The order of paralysis of muscles following the intravenous injection of *d*-tubocurarine is similar to that with any other muscle relaxant. The eye muscles are the first to be affected and the weakness then rapidly spreads to involve the face and limb musculature before finally reaching the trunk muscles. Fortunately, the bulbar muscles are the last to be affected and for this reason it always is possible to select a dose of *d*-tubocurarine in clinical anaesthesia which will produce complete paralysis of the limb musculature without reducing the respiratory tidal volume. It is not possible, however, to paralyse the abdominal musculature without seriously impairing the function of the respiratory muscles.

Exceptions to this order of muscle paralysis sometimes do occur, but only in rare instances. First, in the presence of generalised myasthenia gravis, where the respiratory muscles are affected by the disease, the administration of *d*-tubocurarine may produce a state of affairs where the patient is apnoeic yet able to signal his distress with his arms. Secondly, in the anaesthetised patient, after large doses of *d*-tubocurarine the muscles of the eyebrow can be seen to move occasionally, although the other muscles in the body still appear to be completely paralysed. The explanation may lie in the theory that the levator palpebrae superioris muscles have a double innervation and that they contain some smooth muscle fibres with a nerve supply from the autonomic system. They would thus remain unaffected by the dose of *d*-tubocurarine used. Some support for this suggestion is given by the occurrence of ptosis after a stellate ganglion block.

Interaction with volatile anaesthetic agents.—In the presence of halothane anaesthesia less *d*-tubocurarine is required to produce the same degree of neuromuscular block (Katz and Gissen, 1967). In other words halothane potentiates the neuromuscular block of a non-depolarising relaxant. The two drugs, however, do not have the same mechanism of action. Halothane interferes with neuromuscular transmission principally by desensitising the post-junctional membrane (Gissen *et al.*, 1966).

Like halothane, ether also potentiates the block produced by *d*-tubocurarine. The mechanism of action is again thought to be due to depression of post-junctional activity but it also appears to have an action slowing the conductivity of both sodium and potassium ions within the muscle fibre (Karis *et al.*, 1966). In an interesting study in man Katz (1966) has demonstrated that ether has a weak neuromuscular blocking action. Nevertheless, he observed that ether depressed the motor activity of the abdominal muscles *before* there was any evidence of paresis in the limb musculature. From this he concluded that under normal clinical conditions the muscle relaxation of ether is mainly attributable to depression of the conduction mechanism in the spinal cord rather than an action at the neuromuscular junction.

Liver and kidneys.—There is no evidence that *d*-tubocurarine has any action on the liver or kidney cells. The kidneys provide the principal route of elimination, with the biliary system in the liver offering an alternative (Cohen *et al.*, 1967). In the event of renal failure the amount excreted through the biliary system is greatly increased. In liver disease larger doses of *d*-tubocurarine than normal may be required (Dundee and Gray, 1953). A possible explanation of the phenomenon is a change in the albumin and globulin content of plasma. In severe liver disease the plasma albumin level falls, but the globulin level rises since this protein is formed in other places than the liver. As a result, protein binding of tubocurarine may be increased.

Uterus and placental barrier.—*d*-Tubocurarine has no detectable action on the smooth muscle of the uterus (Harroun and Fisher, 1949).

Clinically, *d*-tubocurarine does not appear to cross the placental barrier because infants born of curarised mothers do not show any obvious signs of paresis. This clinical impression has been confirmed in animal studies by

Harroun and his colleagues (1947) and Buller and Young (1949). In an investigation of six human patients, Crawford and Gardiner (1956) found that the concentrations of *d*-tubocurarine in the cord blood at delivery were imperceptible, even following a maternal dose as high as 20 mg. Furthermore, Cohen and his co-workers (1953) in a comparative study between the maternal and foetal circulations in patients undergoing Caesarean section, found that although thiopentone crossed the placental barrier *d*-tubocurarine did not. Later studies (Cohen *et al.*, 1968), using autoradiographic techniques in the curarised rat, have confirmed that *d*-tubocurarine does not reach the foetus (Fig. 12). In the light of present knowledge, therefore, *d*-tubocurarine does not cross the placental barrier.

Distribution

This is illustrated in Fig. 12 (Cohen *et al.*, 1968).

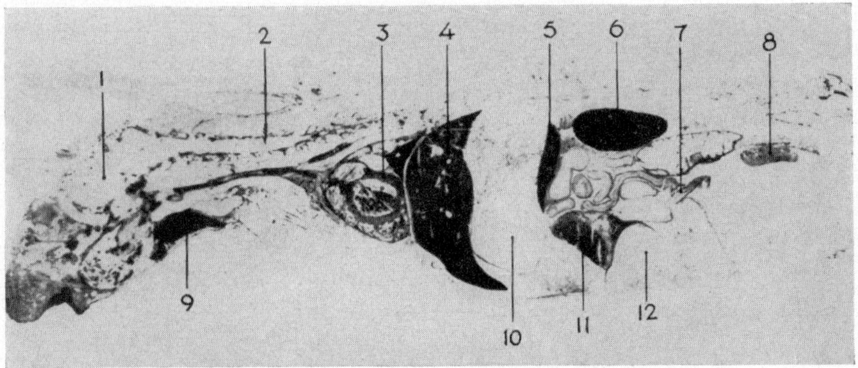

31/Fig. 12.—Autoradiograph of rat sacrificed 15 minutes after intravenous injection of 0·6 mg./kg. *d*-tubocurarine. 1, brain; 2, spinal cord; 3, heart; 4, liver; 5, spleen; 6, kidney; 7, intestine; 8, bladder; 9, salivary gland; 10, stomach; 11, placenta; 12, foetus.

Detoxication and Excretion

Contrary to earlier reports, it is now generally accepted that *d*-tubocurarine is not broken down *in vivo* but is excreted unchanged. The principal route of elimination is the kidney, with the biliary system offering an alternative pathway (Cohen *et al.*, 1968). In the presence of normal renal function, 85 per cent of an injected dose can be recovered in dogs, and of this only 5 per cent leaves the circulation via the biliary tract. On the other hand, in renal failure as much as 15 per cent of the injected dose may leave the body by this route (Fig. 13*a* and *b*).

Recovery of spontaneous respiration is directly related to the level of *d*-tubocurarine in the plasma. This falls, not only due to urinary and biliary elimination but, more importantly, by redistribution. *d*-Tubocurarine is taken up by active and non-active receptors; the active receptors are those found at the neuromuscular junction whilst the non-active ones are spread throughout the body. These receptor sites may be acidic mucopolysaccharides. The widespread distribution is well illustrated in Fig. 12 (Cohen *et al.*, 1968).

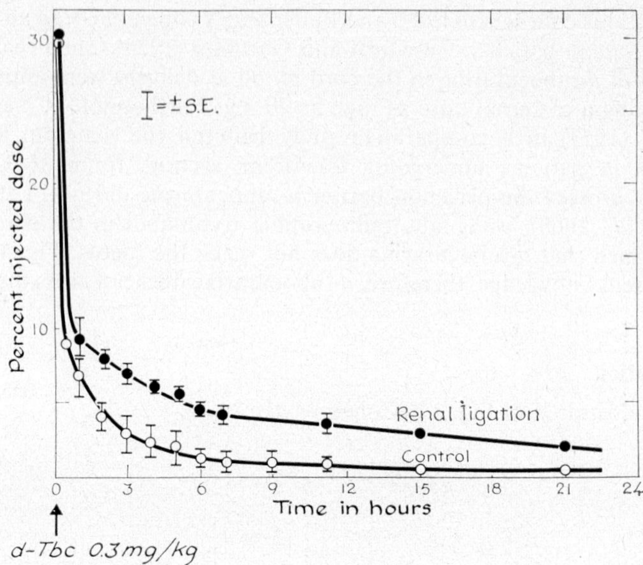

31/FIG. 13(*a*).—Plasma concentration of *d*-tubocurarine-H^3 in control dogs and in those with bilateral renal ligation. Note the raised plasma level in the presence of renal ligation.

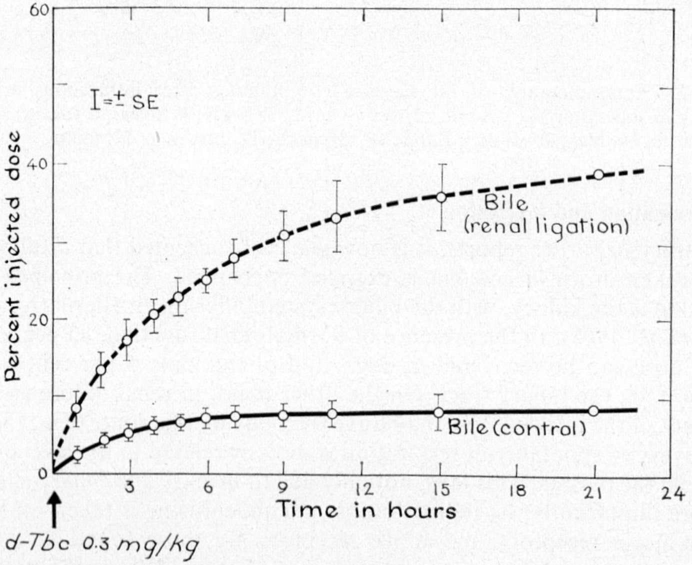

31/FIG. 13(*b*).—Recovery of *d*-tubocurarine-H^3 in the bile in control dogs and in those with bilateral renal ligation. Note the tremendous increase in biliary excretion in the presence of renal ligation.

Administration

Method of administration.—(*a*) *Intravenously.*—This route is most commonly used as it produces maximum relaxation within two to three minutes. Provided the pH of the solution has been suitably adjusted, *d*-tubocurarine can be mixed in the same syringe with thiopentone.

(*b*) *Intramuscularly.*—In the presence of hyaluronidase the paralysant action of intramuscular *d*-tubocurarine is apparent within 2–5 minutes and reaches a maximum in about 5–8 minutes. There is, however, a wide margin of variation in response with this route; consequently the relaxant effect is difficult to control. Clinically, an intramuscular injection is only used in exceptional circumstances when the intravenous route is impracticable.

(*c*) *Orally.*—This route has proved unfavourable as doses at least 50 times greater than those used intravenously are required. Absorption takes place slowly through all mucous surfaces and the gastric juices do not appear to interfere with the passage of the drug, but the main area of absorption is in the small intestine.

(*d*) *Dissolved in oil.*—*d*-Tubocurarine can be dissolved in oil and administered by deep intramuscular injection, so that its duration of action is prolonged. Although used in the past in the treatment of some spastic states, this route is rarely if ever used nowadays. The theory underlying the use of "curare in oil" for patients with spastic paralysis, and also in the treatment of poliomyelitis, lay in the belief that though some muscles were weak or paralysed there were others that were antagonistic to the affected muscles but which remained in a state of spasm; thus weak muscles were hindered in their movements by spasm in their antagonists. Some of this antagonism was believed to be reflex in origin. Theoretically it was argued that *d*-tubocurarine could reduce the spasm of the antagonistic muscles yet leave the already weak muscles unaffected. This is not the case, and the initial benefits claimed were not borne out in clinical practice.

Dosage.—Many attempts have been made to assess the dose of *d*-tubocurarine required on a body-weight basis. There is such a wide margin of response that this is just not possible. For this reason it is better to test each patient individually once he is anaesthetised. This can be done by giving incremental doses until the signs of impending respiratory inadequacy occur. This dose (when combined with controlled respiration) is usually sufficient for abdominal relaxation, though it is inadequate for endotracheal intubation. In the average adult (70 kg.) a dose of 0·1 to 0·2 mg./kg. is required to produce paresis of limb musculature, 0·4 to 0·5 mg./kg. for abdominal relaxation, and 0·5 to 0·6 mg./kg. for endotracheal intubation. General anaesthesia (depending on depth) reduces the dose required.

Duration of action.—The time taken to recover from complete paralysis of the limb musculature is about 20–25 minutes. In the case of conscious subjects this recovery rate is markedly influenced by the blood flow (i.e. the amount of exercise) of the muscles concerned. In clinical practice it is often unnecessary to give a further dose of relaxant following the original paralysing dose until some 40–60 minutes have elapsed. This interval will be influenced by other factors, such as the depth of anaesthesia, the carbon dioxide level of the blood, and the degree of surgical stimulation. When the next dose is required it is rarely necessary to exceed one-fifth of the original amount in order to restore paralysis.

Reversal of *d*-Tubocurarine Paresis (see Chapter 32)

Neostigmine methylsulphate is the anticholinesterase of choice for the reversal of *d*-tubocurarine paresis because it is long-acting and therefore avoids the dangers of recurarisation. It must be combined with atropine to prevent the unpleasant muscarinic side-effects such as salivation, sweating, bradycardia and colic. An important point to remember is that provided the dose of *d*-tubocurarine is not excessive (i.e. paresis is less than 100 per cent) then neostigmine can be administered at any time interval after *d*-tubocurarine and it will be an effective antagonist (Bridenbaugh and Churchill-Davidson, 1968). In other words, a further dose of *d*-tubocurarine can be used to close the peritoneum and it is not necessary to wait another 20–30 minutes before reversal with neostigmine. These authors have also pointed out that often it is necessary to use a dose of neostigmine of more than 2·5 mg. and they recommend a dose of up to 5·0 mg. neostigmine (with 2·0 mg. atropine) for all cases that have received large doses of *d*-tubocurarine. Any increase in dosage above 5·0 mg. is valueless.

Recurarisation

Fortunately, the action of neostigmine outlasts that of *d*-tubocurarine. The dose of neostigmine selected may be insufficient completely to reverse the neuromuscular blockade, but once any progress has been made there is little evidence of any returning paresis. Exceptions to this are possibly found in the return of weakness to the eye muscles in the immediate post-operative period (Hannington-Kiff, 1970) and possible recurarisation in the presence of renal failure.

GALLAMINE TRIETHIODIDE ("FLAXEDIL")

History

Following the introduction of *d*-tubocurarine into clinical anaesthesia, pharmacologists throughout the world sought for synthetic drugs with a similar action. In 1947, Bovet and his co-workers described the muscle relaxant properties of a synthetic product—gallamine triethiodide. The effects of this relaxant in man were first described by Huguenard and Boué (1948) in France and by Mushin and his colleagues (1949) in England.

Physical and Chemical Properties

Gallamine triethiodide is chemically tri-(*β*-diethylaminoethoxy)-benzene triethiodide with the following structural formula:

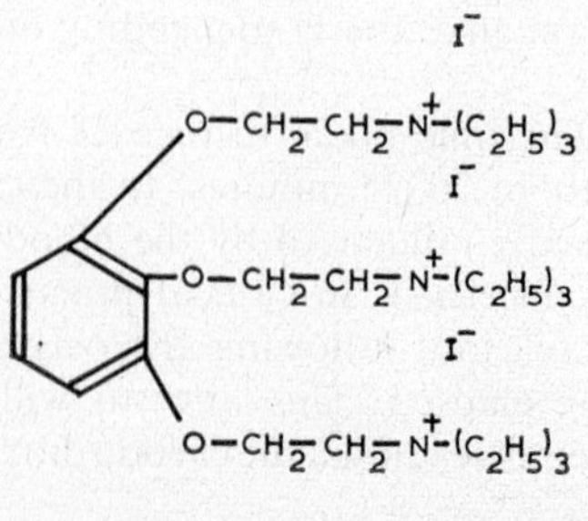

I^-

$O-CH_2-CH_2-\overset{+}{N}-(C_2H_5)_3$

I^-

$O-CH_2-CH_2-\overset{+}{N}-(C_2H_5)_3$

I^-

$O-CH_2-CH_2-\overset{+}{N}-(C_2H_5)_3$

It is a white amorphous powder with a melting point of 145–150° C and a molecular weight of 891. It is non-irritant. Gallamine is prepared synthetically in the laboratory and supplied commercially in a 4 per cent solution containing 40 mg./ml. Ampoules of 80 mg. (2 ml.) and 120 mg. (3 ml.) are available. It is relatively stable and can be mixed with thiopentone.

Pharmacological Actions

Mode of action.—Gallamine triethiodide acts at the neuromuscular junction by non-depolarisation in a similar manner to *d*-tubocurarine.

Cardiovascular system.—Gallamine does not appear to have any direct action on the myocardium although it has been suggested that it reduces the incidence of cardiac arrhythmias under cyclopropane anaesthesia (Riker and Wescoe, 1951). It has a very marked vagal-blocking activity in the doses used in clinical anaesthesia and this factor is particularly useful in combination with halothane, a drug which tends to stimulate this nerve. The action of gallamine on the parasympathetic system was not recognised in the early animal experiments using cats, but was described in man by Doughty and Wylie (1951). These authors noted that it occurred within 1–1½ minutes of an intravenous injection of the drug and was particularly marked in young people. The degree of tachycardia varied widely but, in over half the patients studied, showed an increase of 20–60 per cent over the control value. The rise in pulse rate is sometimes accompanied by an increase in the systemic blood pressure and cardiac output (Kennedy and Farman, 1968). The tachycardia can be abolished by both cyclopropane and halothane.

Central nervous system.—Like *d*-tubocurarine, there is no clear evidence available to suggest that gallamine has any action on the central nervous system in man. In animals, however, its intrathecal injection can lead to convulsions.

Liver and kidneys.—Gallamine has no direct action on either the liver or kidney. Indirectly, however, it has a weak inhibitory effect on the pseudo-cholinesterase produced by the liver (Vincent and Parant, 1954). Like *d*-tubocurarine it is believed to be excreted in the urine either unchanged or in the form of a labile complex with acidic mucopolysaccharides (Chagas, 1962). Mushin and his colleagues (1949) recovered 30 to 100 per cent of the original dose from the urine of rabbits in the two hours following its administration. Chagas (1962) found up to 80 per cent of the original dose in the urine of dogs within 3–5 hours.

A number of reports have appeared in the literature suggesting that a prolonged paresis may follow the use of gallamine in cases with poor renal function (Fairly, 1950; Montgomery and Bennett-Jones, 1956; Feldman and Levi, 1963). (See p. 837.)

Some support for the suggestion that the duration of action of gallamine triethiodide can be modified by the presence or absence of renal function has recently been observed (Churchill-Davidson, 1965). A patient undergoing bilateral nephrectomy (i.e. with complete absence of renal function) received a paralysing dose of the relaxant drug. Although reversal was achieved with an anti-cholinesterase drug, the signs of recurarisation were clearly visible many hours after the operation.

On the basis of the available evidence it would appear unwise to use gallamine as the relaxant agent in the presence of poor renal function.

Histamine release.—Courvoisier and Ducrot (1948) failed to find any evidence of histamine release in dogs. Mushin and his colleagues (1949), working with the rat diaphragm preparation, found that gallamine liberated 1/5th–1/2 the quantity of histamine as compared with *d*-tubocurarine. Sniper (1952), using the intradermal weal test in human subjects, found that the activity of gallamine in liberating histamine was considerably less than that of *d*-tubocurarine.

Uterus and placental barrier.—There is no evidence available to suggest that gallamine influences the contractions of the pregnant uterus. Crawford (1956) found direct evidence in patients undergoing forceps delivery or Caesarean section that gallamine crossed the placenta "in appreciable concentrations". Although he failed to notice any signs of paresis in the infants, gallamine was easily detectable in the cord serum. Nevertheless, Crawford was unable to find a simple relationship between the concentration of gallamine in the maternal and foetal bloods.

Distribution

The distribution of gallamine throughout the body is illustrated in Fig. 14.

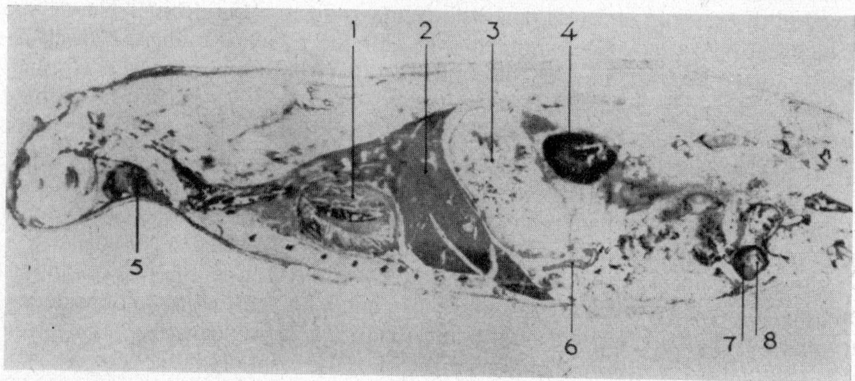

31/FIG. 14.—Autoradiograph of rat sacrificed 15 minutes after intravenous injection of 2.4 mg./kg. gallamine. 1, heart; 2, liver; 3, stomach; 4, kidney; 5, salivary gland; 6, intestine; 7, placenta; 8, foetus (Cohen *et al.*, 1968).

Detoxication and Excretion

Gallamine is not detoxicated *in vivo* but is excreted unchanged in the urine. In the cat, 30–100 per cent of the total dose injected can be recovered from the urine within two hours (Mushin *et al.*, 1949).

Method of Administration

The intravenous route is the only method that has gained widespread popularity in clinical anaesthesia. When injected subcutaneously the activity is about one-quarter that of an intravenous injection (Bovet, 1951).

Dosage.—In the average adult subject 50 mg. is sufficient to produce almost complete paralysis of the limb musculature, yet leaving the respiratory tidal excursion unimpeded. In comparison, 8–9 mg. of *d*-tubocurarine and 2·25–2·5 mg. of decamethonium are required to produce the same effect. A dose of 100–140 mg. of gallamine leads to total cessation of respiration.

Duration of action.—This is believed to be about 15–20 minutes (Mushin *et al.*, 1949) and therefore on a comparative basis is slightly shorter than that of *d*-tubocurarine (20–25 minutes).

Antagonists

Both neostigmine and edrophonium oppose the action of gallamine triethiodide in a similar manner to that described for *d*-tubocurarine.

PANCURONIUM BROMIDE ("PAVULON")

History

Whilst investigating a series of amino-steroids, Hewitt and Savage in 1964 observed that when an acetylcholine-like group was added to these biologically active compounds then some neuromuscular blocking agents were obtained. One such compound—pancuronium bromide—appeared to be a very effective neuromuscular blocking agent without evidence of steroid activity, and the pharmacology has been extensively studied in animals (Bucket and Bonta, 1966; Bucket *et al.*, 1968). It was introduced into clinical anaesthesia by Baird and Reid in 1967.

Physical and Chemical Properties

Pancuronium bromide is chemically 3β, 16β-dipiperidine-5α-androstane-3α, 17β-diol diacetate dimethobromide with the following structural formula:

It is an odourless, white crystalline powder with a bitter taste, which melts at 215° C with decomposition. Pancuronium is a bis-quaternary ammonium salt which is relatively stable and is supplied for clinical purposes in 2 ml. ampoules containing 2 mg./ml.

Pharmacological Action

Mode of action.—Pancuronium acts at the neuromuscular junction in man by non-depolarisation (Baird and Reid, 1967) and has no steroidal activity.

Cardiovascular system.—Pancuronium has little effect on the cardiovascular system. There is no change in pulse rate and the absence of hypotension (compared with *d*-tubocurarine) is particularly noticeable (Baird, 1968; Crul, 1968; Sellick, 1968; McDowall and Clarke, 1969). It has even been suggested that pancuronium may tend to counteract the hypotensive effect of halothane, but there is no experimental evidence to support this thesis. Pancuronium (like *d*-tubocurarine) prevents the bradycardia and arrhythmias produced by the second dose of suxamethonium in man (Mathias and Evans-Prosser, 1970).

Central nervous system.—There is no evidence available in man but it is not believed to cross the blood-brain barrier.

Liver and kidneys.—Pancuronium is, in part, excreted unchanged by the kidneys and it is therefore best avoided in patients with poor renal function. No adverse effects in the presence of severe hepatic disease have been reported.

Histamine release.—A particular advantage claimed for pancuronium is the lack of histamine release. This is believed to account for the absence of both hypotension and bronchospasm following its use.

Uterus and placental barrier.—No evidence is available in man but animal experiments suggest that in normal dosage it does not cross the placental barrier.

Detoxication and Excretion

As mentioned above, pancuronium is believed to be excreted partially unchanged in the urine.

Method of Administration

The intravenous route is used.

Dosage.—Pancuronium has about five times the potency of *d*-tubocurarine. Therefore to produce apnoea a dose of 4–6 mg. will be required in the adult, and if it is used for endotracheal intubation then doses of 8–10 mg. will be required to provide good conditions.

Duration of action.—The paresis would appear to last for about 25–30 minutes and a satisfactory "topping-up dose" is about 1/5 to 1/10 of the original paralysing dose. For simplicity, the duration of action of pancuronium could be described as lying midway between the shorter action of gallamine and the longer duration of *d*-tubocurarine.

Antagonists.—Pancuronium can be easily reversed by neostigmine in the usual manner.

Miscellaneous Group of Muscle Relaxants

The muscle relaxants in common clinical use are suxamethonium, *d*-tubocurarine, gallamine and pancuronium. There are others, apart from decamethonium, which enjoy popularity on a limited scale, and many more which have never seen the light of day outside the laboratory. For the latter the reader must search in a textbook of pharmacology. It is proposed here to describe briefly some of the principal points about a miscellaneous selection of relaxants which have been or still are being used in clinical practice.

Dimethyl Ether of *d*-Tubocurarine (D.M.E.)

History.—This preparation was first described as a methylated derivative of *d*-tubocurarine by King in 1935. It was not until several years later, however, that Collier (1950) described its pharmacological actions in animals. Soon afterwards Wilson and his associates (1950) reported on its use in man.

Physical and chemical properties.—Dimethyl tubocurarine is a stable white substance with a melting point of 236° C. It is commercially available either as the chloride or iodide salt and can be mixed with thiopentone. The structural formula is as follows:

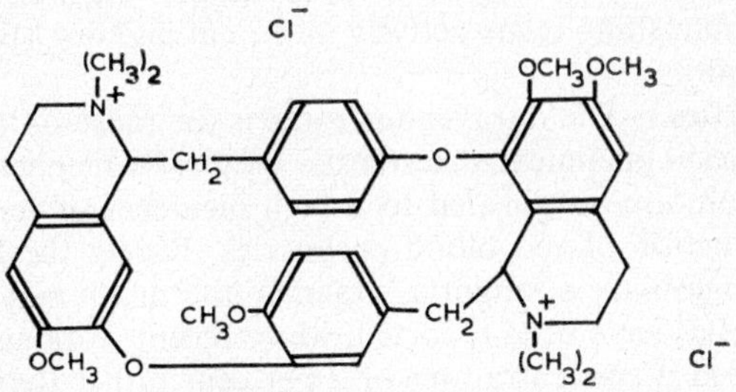

Dimethyl ether of *d*-tubocurarine chloride ($C_{40}H_{48}O_6N_2$)

Mode of action.—This is similar to that of *d*-tubocurarine.

General properties.—Dimethyl tubocurarine is administered intravenously, and as it is 2–2½ times as potent as *d*-tubocurarine, 4 mg. of it are sufficient to produce relaxation of the limb muscles. A dose of 8–10 mg. leads to total paralysis of all muscles including those of respiration. The duration of action is believed to be slightly shorter than that of *d*-tubocurarine, and it is also claimed to have less effect on the autonomic ganglia and to release less histamine (Collier, 1950). Its neuromuscular blocking activity is rapidly reversed by neostigmine and edrophonium.

Despite these possible advantages dimethyl tubocurarine has never gained wide popularity in clinical practice. The principal reason for this is that it possesses no obvious advantages over *d*-tubocurarine. Moreover, Mogey and Trevan (1950) have pointed out that its molecule is so complex that it is difficult to be certain that all batches of the drug possess identical activity.

Mephenesin ("Myanesin", "Tolserol", "Lissaphen")

History.—In 1946, whilst investigating the local analgesic properties of the glycerol ethers, Berger and Bradley discovered one substance—mephenesin—which appeared to have a useful relaxant action. Mallinson (1947) described its use in clinical anaesthesia.

Physical and chemical properties.—Mephenesin is a colourless, odourless, crystalline solid with a melting point of 70–71° C. It has the following chemical structure:

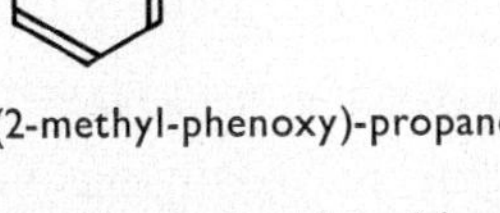

O–CH_2–CHOH–CH_2OH

CH_3

α-*β*-dihydroxy-*γ*-(2-methyl-phenoxy)-propane, or mephenesin.

It is soluble in alcohol and propylene glycol and is supplied in a 10 ml. ampoule as a 10 per cent solution dissolved in an equal volume of propylene glycol and alcohol. It is relatively stable and can be mixed in solution with thiopentone, glucose or saline.

Mode of action.—Mephenesin is believed to act on the internuncial neurones of the spinal cord. These neurones pass between the anterior and posterior horn cell at any segmental level and also connect up neighbouring segments. Reflex pathways involving the spinal cord must pass through the internuncial pathway. It is capable of diminishing reflex activity in the cat and dog (Berger, 1947; Van den Oostende, 1948).

General properties.—The intravenous route is the most suitable for administration of mephenesin in clinical anaesthesia. Originally mephenesin was infused as a 10 per cent solution but this led to a high incidence of venous thrombosis, and also to destruction of red blood corpuscles. Rarely the latter may be so severe that haemoglobinuria, oliguria, uraemia and death may ensue. In fact a number of fatal cases have been reported. More recent work suggests that these risks can be avoided if concentrations of 2 per cent rather than 10 per cent are used.

The intramuscular route has proved useful in the treatment of tetanus, but owing to the irritant properties of the injected material it should always be given by deep intramuscular injection.

The oral route may also be used but absorption from the alimentary tract is slow. The principal danger of oral mephenesin is that since the drug acts as a local analgesic to the larynx and pharynx, and thus desensitises the mucous membrane, it increases the risks of aspiration into the respiratory tract. Added to this, mephenesin is dissolved in high concentrations of alcohol, so that, when large quantities are consumed, the patient may show signs of intoxication.

The rectal route has been used to administer mephenesin, but again the high percentages of propylene glycol and alcohol tend to irritate the mucosa and lead to proctitis.

Mephenesin is partly detoxicated in the liver by conjugation with glycuronic acid and partly excreted unchanged by the kidneys. If it is injected intravenously the major proportion can be recovered within the hour.

Apart from a complex action on the internuncial cell system which is shared by many of the "tranquillising" group of drugs, mephenesin has no depressant effect on the level of consciousness or on the cardiovascular system as a whole. It does not release histamine. This drug enjoyed a brief period of popularity in clinical anaesthesia because it was believed that full abdominal relaxation could be produced without depressing normal respiratory activity. Theoretically, it was argued that although mephenesin blocked transmission to the spinal nerves, it had no action on phrenic nerve activity so that the diaphragmatic movement could continue unabated. In practice, however, abdominal relaxation was rarely satisfactory with mephenesin, and this fact, coupled with the high incidence of complications that followed its use, soon led to its virtual abandonment in clinical anaesthesia. It has also been used for the treatment of tetanus.

Hexamethylene Carbaminoylcholine Bromide ("Imbretil")

History.—In a study of the polymethylene bis-carbaminoylcholine compounds Klupp and his associates (1953) found that one of the synthetic compounds with six methylene groups in the chain proved to be the most active as a relaxant. Brücke and Reis (1954) reported on its use in man.

Physical and chemical properties.—It is a white crystalline powder which is easily soluble in water. The melting point is 172°–176° C. The chemical structure is as follows:

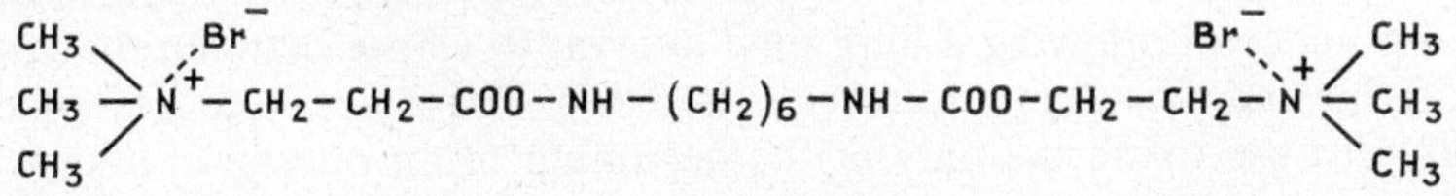

$$(CH_3)_3\overset{+}{N}(Br^-)-CH_2-CH_2-COO-NH-(CH_2)_6-NH-COO-CH_2-CH_2-\overset{+}{N}(Br^-)(CH_3)_3$$

Mode of action.—The evidence in animals and the original work in man suggested that this drug produced a dual response at the neuromuscular junction. Nevertheless, electromyography shows that in man it acts by depolarisation block following a single injection (Christie and Churchill-Davidson, 1958).

General properties.—Hexamethylene carbaminoylcholine is best given intravenously. Fasciculations throughout the body and cramp-like pains in the calves are a common feature of its use. A dose of 1·0–1·5 mg. causes complete paralysis of the peripheral muscles in the average subject, and 2·5 mg. causes apnoea lasting about twenty to twenty-five minutes. In animals 50 per cent of the drug is excreted unchanged within two hours of the injection and 75 per cent within 6–8 hours (Brücke *et al.*, 1954).

It has no detectable action on the central nervous or cardiovascular systems and does not lead to histamine release. It is believed to cross the placental barrier (Brücke and Reis, 1954).

Neostigmine is said to antagonise the neuromuscular blocking action of this compound, but this finding has not been confirmed in man except after sufficient doses of hexamethylene carbaminoylcholine have been given to produce a dual block (Christie and Churchill-Davidson, 1958).

C-Toxiferine I (Toxiferine)

History.—One of the many alkaloids isolated from calabash curare that has neuromuscular blocking properties is C-Toxiferine I. The pharmacological properties of the purified alkaloid were first investigated by Waser (1959) and it was introduced into clinical anaesthesia in Europe by Frey and Seeger (1961) and in the United States by Foldes and his colleagues (1961).

Physical and chemical properties.—Toxiferine is $C_{40}H_{46}Cl_2N_4O_2$ and has a molecular weight of 685·7. Like most relaxants, it is a bis-quaternary ammonium compound, but in solution it is unstable and breaks down to two symmetrical mono-quaternary moieties. For this reason it is available in powder form and prepared just prior to use. It is the most potent relaxant drug available in clinical practice, with the longest duration of action.

Mode of action.—It is a non-depolarising drug which can be reversed by anti-cholinesterase drugs.

General properties.—Toxiferine in doses of 2–3 mg. in an average adult produces profound and prolonged neuromuscular block. The duration of action is some 2–3 times longer than that of *d*-tubocurarine. Because it is so potent it is believed to be relatively free of any side-effects such as histamine release or ganglion-blocking activity.

Despite these possible advantages, the use of toxiferine in clinical practice is difficult unless it can be predicted with certainty that complete paralysis will be required for at least 1–1½ hours. Though normally the neuromuscular block produced by toxiferine is readily reversible by anti-cholinesterase drugs it is easy to administer an overdose which does not respond. Hence the insistence in clinical practice of allowing a long time interval to elapse between the last dose of toxiferine and the attempt to reverse its action. For this reason, it is sometimes advisable to use toxiferine only at the beginning of an operation and to use a shorter-acting drug such as *d*-tubocurarine to supplement the relaxation at a later stage.

The main value of this drug would appear to lie in the treatment of such a disease as tetanus where prolonged muscular relaxation with the absence of circulatory effects is so important.

Diallyl-nor-Toxiferine ("Alloferin")

This compound is a derivation of C-Toxiferine I and was introduced into clinical anaesthesia by Hugin and Kissling (1961). It has twice the potency of *d*-tubocurarine and the same duration of action. The original claim that it did not produce a fall in systemic pressure has been discounted. The incidence of hypotension is similar to that with *d*-tubocurarine (Hunter, 1964; Baraka, 1967).

Clinical Use of the Neuromuscular Blocking Drugs

Indications for a Relaxant

The specific indications for a muscle relaxant in anaesthesia fall into three categories:

1. To relax the muscles for surgical access, and for anaesthetic and investigation procedures.
2. To facilitate the control of respiration.
3. To limit the amount of general anaesthetic when relaxation itself is not the prime requisite.

The first two of these are self-explanatory and, with suggestions for the choice of relaxant, receive more detailed discussion in the various clinical sections of the text where anaesthetic procedure is mentioned. The third, although to some extent part of the other two, needs amplification. By dividing anaesthesia into the three components of narcosis, analgesia and muscle relaxation (Gray, 1954), an attempt can be made to control reflex activity on a more specific basis than can be done with a single anaesthetic agent, and particular drugs chosen to block each sub-division. But—haemorrhage and chemical depression apart—our knowledge of the basic cause of deterioration in the condition of a patient during surgery is so incomplete that such a simple division is no more than a suggested guide. Indeed clinical opinion is divided between those anaesthetists who consider that provided the patient is unconscious, and all motor response to surgical stimuli abolished by adequate paralysis, nothing is to be gained by adding other agents, and those who argue that in such a state deeper anaesthesia or analgesia may be needed to suppress sensory or autonomic activity. Few anaesthetists, however, doubt that the judicious use of a muscle relaxant by diminishing the need for deep anaesthesia can avoid most of the detrimental effects of chemical depression.

Choice of Relaxant

Suxamethonium, *d*-tubocurarine, gallamine and pancuronium are the relaxant drugs most commonly used in this country. Personal preference, suitably modified by experience and a knowledge of the pharmacology of each drug, must be the final arbiter when making a choice. However, as a general rule a short-acting relaxant is used for short procedures and a long-acting one for those lasting more that 15–20 minutes. For this reason suxamethonium is principally used for intubation of the trachea, endoscopies, electro-convulsive therapy, and the setting of fractures. In more prolonged operations the choice will very often depend on whether halothane is to be the principal anaesthetic agent or not. If it is, then the vagal-blocking activity of gallamine makes this drug a particularly suitable choice. On the other hand, if bleeding during the operation is a major consideration then the mild hypotension produced by the combination of halothane and *d*-tubocurarine may make this selection preferable. In vascular surgery and poor risk cases pancuronium is very often selected because it is the drug least likely to lower the blood pressure or change cardiac rate.

In recent years, *d*-tubocurarine has largely replaced suxamethonium in paediatric anaesthesia because it has been found reliable, easily reversible, and avoids the complications of possibly overloading the circulation with a continuous infusion or obtaining a dual block (see p. 840). Nevertheless, suxamethonium is still the relaxant of choice for Caesarean section because it does not cross the placental barrier in clinical doses.

Suxamethonium has certain well-known disadvantages, namely severe muscle pains in ambulant patients, the raising of intra-ocular pressure and the alteration of cardiac rate and rhythm in hypertensive patients or in those receiving multiple doses. All these disadvantages can be prevented or made only minimal if a small dose of a non-depolarising drug (e.g. 5 mg. *d*-tubocurarine) is given two minutes before the suxamethonium. Because these two drugs are antagonistic, it is necessary to increase the dose of suxamethonium slightly (e.g. 75 instead of 50 mg.) in order to achieve the same degree and duration of paralysis.

Mixing of Relaxants

Theoretical considerations suggest that it is unwise to use drugs of differing actions at the neuromuscular junction on the same patient on the same occasion, and there is some practical support for this view as evidenced in the number of bizarre and occasionally long-lasting sequelae following the practice reported in the literature. Yet accumulated clinical experience lends support to the contention that with a proper appreciation of the risks involved and avoidance of certain pitfalls (see below), drugs such as suxamethonium and *d*-tubocurarine can be given with safety to the same patient for a single operation. Needless to say, this practice should not be adopted unless it has a sound clinical indication. For example, it may be desirable to produce total paralysis with suxamethonium, so that the best possible conditions are achieved for intubation of the trachea, and yet to obtain relaxation throughout the subsequent operation with *d*-tubocurarine. Provided the effects of the suxamethonium—as judged clinically from respiratory activity or as demonstrated with a peripheral nerve stimulator—have worn off, there does not seem to be any good reason for supposing that the administration of *d*-tubocurarine will now lead to an abnormal response. The theoretical argument that following a single dose of suxamethonium the neuromuscular junction remains abnormal for a far longer period than is suggested by the clinical state of the patient, does not in our view prejudice this practice. The use of suxamethonium at the termination of an operation to secure full relaxation, say for peritoneal closure, and following a non-depolarising agent, is more problematical. The precise manner in which the motor end-plate responds to suxamethonium under these conditions is unknown. To some extent it may act as an antidote to the residue of the non-depolarising drug, and this action would be helpful. On the other hand, it is equally possible that it might enhance the underlying non-depolarisation block, particularly if it had been used at the beginning of operation to facilitate intubation. A danger arises later when the operation is completed and evidence of muscle paralysis remains. Neostigmine can now only be administered with safety provided the suxamethonium and its breakdown products are ineffective; if they are not, there will be a real risk of prolonged paralysis or paresis. In practice, therefore, it is wisest to avoid suxamethonium in this situation, although the use of approximately 50 to 100 mg. for a patient who has some spontaneous respiration is likely to be safe, provided neostigmine is not given or reserved until respiration has again returned to at least its pre-suxamethonium activity.

Test Dose of Relaxants

The painful contractions associated with the administration of suxamethonium to a conscious patient contra-indicate a test dose of this drug.

A test dose of *d*-tubocurarine (5 mg.) or gallamine (20–30 mg.) prior to the induction of anaesthesia is advocated by some anaesthetists, but it is of doubtful value since the interpretation of its actions on the muscles is so difficult (see Chapter 33). Moreover, the slight degree of paralysis that it produces in a normal but conscious patient is unpleasant. A clinical history of muscle weakness is the best indication that caution must be exercised in the use of these drugs. A more practical method of assessing the response of a particular patient to a muscle relaxant is to anaesthetise him, establish spontaneous respiration, and then give the relaxant in divided doses until the first signs of respiratory paresis are evident. If controlled respiration is now established the dose necessary for abdominal relaxation will have been achieved.

Complications Following the Use of Relaxants

Major complications caused by muscle relaxants are more often than not due to their misuse rather than to any peculiarity in their action. The side-effects of both *d*-tubocurarine and gallamine, however, must be remembered since these may be responsible for some complications in unduly sensitive or physically handicapped patients. Inadequate ventilation, residual paralysis sufficient to enhance or cause difficulty with the airway, and the removal or depression of protective glottic reflexes in the presence of foreign material are the principal causes of mortality and morbidity. The bizarre and occasionally prolonged periods of apnoea that follow the use of relaxants, or injudicious mixtures of them with or without an antidote, should not of themselves lead to death unless artificial respiration is inadequately carried out, or the patient is already moribund.

Dosage

It is quite impossible to be dogmatic about the dose of a muscle relaxant since this depends not only on the physical build of a patient, the normality of his neuromuscular transmission, the presence or absence of certain diseases which affect the metabolism and excretion of these drugs and the anaesthetic agents used, but also on the requirements of the anaesthetist. The approximately equivalent doses of the principal relaxants that will produce complete paralysis of grip-strength in a normal adult are given in Table 7.

31/TABLE 7

COMPARATIVE DOSES OF THE PRINCIPAL MUSCLE RELAXANTS

	Intravenous dose required to produce complete paralysis of grip-strength	*Duration of time until 75 per cent recovery*
d-Tubocurarine . . .	8 mg.	20–25 minutes
Gallamine . . .	50 mg.	15–20 minutes
Suxamethonium . .	10–15 mg.	2–3 minutes
Decamethonium . .	2·5 mg.	20 minutes
Pancuronium . . .	1·5 mg.	20 minutes

Regional Use of Muscle Relaxants

In selected cases requiring limb surgery, muscle paresis has been achieved by injecting the relaxant intravenously after a tourniquet has been applied (Torda and Klonymus, 1966). The recommended doses and dilutions are given below:

	Volume of Diluent (ml.)	*Dose (mg.)* d-*Tubocurarine*	*Gallamine*	*Suxamethonium*
Upper limb	30	1·5	10·0	4·0
Lower limb	50	3·0	20·0	6·0

A similar technique using smaller doses has been advocated as a test for myasthenia gravis (Foldes, 1970).

REFERENCES

BAIRD, W. L. M. (1968). Some clinical experiences with a new neuromuscular blocking drug—pancuronium bromide (Pavulon NA97). *Irish. J. Med.*, 7th series, **1,** 559.

BAIRD, W. L. M., and REID, A. M. (1967). The neuromuscular blocking properties of a new steroid compound, pancuronium bromide. *Brit. J. Anaesth.*, **39,** 775.

BARAKA, A. (1967). A comparative study between diallyl-nor-toxiferine and tubocurarine. *Brit. J. Anaesth.*, **39,** 624.

BARLOW, R. B. (1955). *Introduction to Chemical Pharmacology*. London: Methuen & Co.

BARLOW, R. B., and ING, H. R. (1948). Curare-like action of polymethylene bis quaternary ammonium salts. *Nature* (*Lond.*), **161,** 718.

BELIN, R. P., and KARLEEN, C. I. (1966). Cardiac arrest in the burned patient following succinyldicholine administration. *Anesthesiology*, **27,** 516.

BENNET, A. E., MCINTYRE, A. R., and BENNETT, A. L. (1940). Pharmacologic and clinical investigations with crude curare. *J. Amer. med. Ass.*, **114,** 1791.

BENVENISTE, D., and DYRBERG, V. (1962). Tetrahydroaminoacridine. Clinical use of a cholinesterase inhibitor in conjunction with succinylcholine. *Acta anaesth. scand.*, **6,** 1.

BERGER, F. M. (1947). The mode of action of myanesin. *Brit. J. Pharmacol.*, **2,** 242.

BERGER, F. M., and BRADLEY, W. (1946). The pharmacological properties of α:β dihydroxy-γ-(2-methylphenoxy) propane (Myanesin). *Brit. J. Pharmacol.*, **1,** 265.

BIRCH, A. A., MITCHELL, G. D., PLAYFORD, G. A., and LANG, C. A. (1969). Changes in serum potassium response to succinylcholine following trauma. *J. Amer. med. Ass.*, **210,** 490.

BOEHM, R. (1886). *Chemische Studien über das Curare*. Leipzig.

BOEHM, R. (1895). Das sudamerikanische Pfeilgift. *Abhandl. d. kgl. sachs. Gesselsch. d. Wiss.*, **22,** 199.

BOEHM, R. (1897). Ueber Curare und Curare Alkaloide. *Arch. d. Pharmakol.*, **235,** 660.

BONO, F., and MAPELLI, A. (1960). The effect of *d*-tubocurarine chloride on arterial pressure during general anaesthesia. *Minerva anest.*, **26,** 29.

BOURNE, J. G., COLLIER, H. O. J., and SOMERS, G. F. (1952). Succinylcholine (succinoylcholine) muscle-relaxant of short action. *Lancet*, **1,** 1225.

BOVET, D. (1951). Some aspects of the relationship between chemical constitution and curare-like activity. *Ann. N.Y. Acad. Sci.*, **54,** 407.

BOVET, D., BOVET-NITTI, F., GUARINO, S., LONGO, V. G., and MAROTTA, M. (1949). Proprieta farmacodinamiche di alcuni derivati della succinilcolina dotati di azione curarica. *R.C. 1st sup. Sanità*, **12,** 106.

BOVET, D., DEPIERRE, F., and DE LESTRANGE, Y. (1947). Propriétés curarisantes des éthers phénoliques à fonctions ammonium quaternaires. *C.R. Acad. Sci.* (*Paris*), **225,** 74.

BOVET-NITTI, F. (1949). Degradazione di Alcune sostanze curanzzanti per Azione di Colinesterasi. *R.C. 1st sup. Sanità*, **12,** 138.

BRENNAN, H. J. (1956). Dual action of suxamethonium chloride. *Brit. J. Anaesth.*, **28,** 159.

BRIDENBAUGH, P. O., and CHURCHILL-DAVIDSON, H. C. (1968). Response to tubocurarine chloride and its reversal by neostigmine methylsulfate in man. *J. Amer. med. Ass.*, **203,** 541.

BRODIE, B. C. (1851). "Physiological Researches". Note C. p. 142. Quoted in: *Curare: Its History and Usage*, p. 34, by K. Bryn Thomas. London: Pitman Medical Publishing Co.

BRÜCKE, H., GINZEL, K. H., KLUPP, H., PFAFFENSCHLAGER, F., and WERNER, G. (1951). Bis-cholinester von Dicarbonsäuren als Muskelrelaxantien in der Narkose. *Wien. klin. Wschr.*, **63,** 464.

BRÜCKE, H., KLUPP, H., and KRAUPP, O. (1954). Pharmakologische Eigenschaften des Hexamethylenbiscarbaminoyl-choline (Imbretil) und anderer verwandter Polymethylenbiscarbaminoylcholine. *Wien. klin. Wschr.*, **66,** 260.

BRÜCKE, H., and REIS, H. (1954). Ueber ein hochwirksames Muskelrelaxans aus der Reihe der Polymethylen-dicarbaminol-cholinester. *Wien. klin. Wschr.*, **104,** 283.

BUCKETT, W. R., and BONTA, I. L. (1966). Pharmacological studies with NA97 (2β, 16β Dipiperidine-5α-androstane-3α, 17β-diol diecetate dimethobromide). *Fed. Proc.*, **25,** 718.

BUCKETT, W. R., MARJORIBANKS, C. E. B., MARWICK, F. A., and MORTON, M. B. (1968). The pharmacology of pancuronium bromide (Org. NA–97), a new potent steroidal neuromuscular blocking agent. *Brit. J. Pharmacol.*, **32,** 671.

BULLER, A. J., and YOUNG, I. M. (1949). The action of *d*-tubocurarine chloride on foetal neuromuscular transmission and the placental transfer of this drug in the rabbit. *J. Physiol.* (*Lond.*), **109,** 412.

BULLOUGH, J. (1959). Intermittent suxamethonium injections. *Brit. med. J.*, **1,** 786.

BURTLES, R. (1961). Muscle pains after suxamethonium and suxethonium. *Brit. J. Anaesth.*, **33,** 147.

BUSH, G. H., and ROTH, F. (1961). Muscle pains after suxamethonium chloride in children. *Brit. J. Anaesth.*, **33,** 151.

CASTILLO, J. C., and DE BEER, E. J. (1950). Neuromuscular blocking action of succinylcholine (Diacetylcholine). *J. Pharmacol. exp. Ther.*, **97,** 458.

CHRISTIE, T. H., and CHURCHILL-DAVIDSON, H. C. (1958). Personal communication.

CHURCHILL-DAVIDSON, H. C. (1954). Suxamethonium (succinylcholine) and muscle pains. *Brit. med. J.*, **1,** 74.

CHURCHILL-DAVIDSON, H. C. (1961). The changing pattern of neuromuscular block. *Canad. Anaesth. Soc. J.*, **8,** 91.

CHURCHILL-DAVIDSON, H. C., and GRIFFITHS, W. J. (1961). Simple test-paper method for the clinical determination of plasma pseudocholinesterase. *Brit. med. J.*, **2,** 994.

CHURCHILL-DAVIDSON, H. C., and KATZ, R. L. (1966). Dual, phase II or desensitization block? *Anesthesiology*, **27,** 536.

CHURCHILL-DAVIDSON, H. C., and RICHARDSON, A. T. (1953). Neuromuscular transmission in myasthenia gravis. *J. Physiol.* (*Lond.*), **122,** 252.

COHEN, E. N. (1963). Blood-brain barrier to *d*-tubocurarine. *J. Pharmacol. exp. Ther.*, **141,** 356.

COHEN, E. N., BREWER, H. W., and SMITH, D. (1967). The metabolism and elimination of *d*-tubocurarine-H^3. *Anesthesiology*, **28,** 309.

COHEN, E. N., HOOD, N., and GOLLING, R. (1968). Use of whole-body autoradiography for determination of uptake and distribution of labeled muscle relaxants in the rat. *Anesthesiology*, **29,** 987.

COHEN, E. N., PAULSON, W. J., WALL, J., and ELERT, B. (1953). Thiopental, curare, and nitrous oxide anesthesia for Cesarian section with studies on placental transmission. *Surg. Gynec. Obstet.*, **97,** 456.

COLLIER, H. O. J. (1950). Pharmacology of D-O, O-Dimethyl tubocurarine iodide in relation to its clinical use. *Brit. med. J.*, **1,** 1293.

COURVOISIER, S., and DUCROT, R. (1948). Sur l'effet histaminoide de la *d*-tubocurarine et des curares de synthèse. *C.R. Soc. Biol.* (*Paris*), **142,** 1209.

CRAWFORD, J. S. (1956). Some aspects of obstetric anaesthesia. *Brit. J. Anaesth*, **28.**, 146.

CRAWFORD, J. S., and GARDINER, J. E. (1956). Some aspects of obstetric anaesthesia. The use of relaxant drugs. *Brit. J. Anaesth.*, **28,** 154.

CRUL, J. F. (1970). Studies on new steroid relaxants. *Progress in Anaesthesiology* (Proc. 4th World Congr. Anaesthesiol., Sept. 1968). Amsterdam: Excerpta Medica.

DAVIES, J. I. (1956). Untoward reactions to succinylcholine. *Canad. Anaesth. Soc. J.*, **3,** 11.

DE BEER, E. J. (1958). Personal communication.

DILLON, J. B., SABAWALA, P., TAYLOR, D. B., and GUNTER, R. (1957). Action of succinylcholine on extra-ocular muscles and intra-ocular pressure. *Anesthesiology*, **18,** 44.

DOENICKE, A., SCHMIDINGER, ST., and KRUMEY, I. (1968). Suxamethonium and serum cholinesterase. Comparative studies *in vitro* and *in vivo* on the catabolism of suxamethonium. *Brit. J. Anaesth.*, **40,** 834.

DOUBEK, K., KLEIJN, E.v.d., and CRUL, J. F. (1970). Personal communication.

DOUGHTY, A. G., and WYLIE, W. D. (1951). An assessment of Flaxedil (gallamine triethiodide, B.P.). *Proc. roy. Soc. Med.*, **44,** 375.

DOWDY, E. G., DUGGAR, P. N., and FABIAN, L. W. (1965). Effect of neuromuscular blocking agents on isolated digitalised mammalian hearts. *Curr. Res. Anesth.*, **44,** 608.

DOWDY, E. G., and FABIAN, L. W. (1963). Ventricular arrhythmias induced by succinylcholine in digitalised patients. *Curr. Res. Anesth.*, **42,** 501.

DUNDEE, J. W., and GRAY, T. C. (1953). Resistance to *d*-tubocurarine chloride in the presence of liver damage. *Lancet*, **2,** 16.

DUTCHER, J. (1951). Curare and anti-curare drugs. *Ann. N.Y. Acad. Sci.*, **54,** 326.

ELERT, B. (1956). A new ultraviolet spectrophotometric method for the determination of *d*-tubocurarine chloride in plasma. *Amer. J. med. Technol.*, **22,** 331.

ELERT, B. T., and COHEN, E. N. (1962). A micro spectrophotometric method for the analysis of minute concentrations of *d*-tubocurarine chloride in plasma. *Amer. J. med. Technol.*, **28,** 125.

ELLIS, C. H., NORTON, S., and MORGAN, W. V. (1952). Central depression by drugs which block neuromuscular transmission. *Fed. Proc.*, **11,** 42.

FAIRLEY, H. B. (1950). Prolonged intercostal paralysis due to a relaxant. *Brit. med. J.*, **2,** 986.

FELDMAN, S. A., and LEVI, J. A. (1963). Prolonged paresis following gallamine. *Brit. J. Anaesth.*, **35,** 804.

FELLINI, A. A., BERNSTEIN, R. L., and ZAUDER, H. L. (1963). Bronchospasm due to suxamethonium. *Brit. J. Anaesth.*, **35,** 657.

FOLDES, F. F. (1970). Regional intravenous neuromuscular block: a new diagnostic and experimental tool. *Progress in Anaesthesiology* (Proc. 4th World Congr. Anaesthesiol., Sept. 1968). Amsterdam: Excerpta Medica.

FOLDES, F. F., MCNALL, P. G., and BIRCH, J. H. (1954). The neuromuscular activity of succinylmonocholine iodide in anaesthetized man. *Brit. med. J.*, **1,** 967.

FOLDES, F. F., MCNALL, P. G., and BORREGO-HINOJOSA, J M. (1952). Succinylcholine: a new approach to muscular relaxation in anesthesiology. *New Engl. J. Med.*, **247,** 596.

FOLDES, F. F., MOLLOY, R. E., ZSIGMOND, E. K., and ZWARTZ, J. A. (1960). Hexafluorenium: its anti-cholinesterase and neuromuscular activity. *J. Pharmacol. exp. Ther.*, **129,** 400.

FOLDES, F. F., and NORTON, S. (1954). The urinary excretion of succinyldicholine and succinylmonocholine in man. *Brit. J. Pharmacol.*, **9,** 385.

FOLDES, F. F., WOLFSON, B., and SOKOLL, M. (1961). The use of toxiferine for the production of surgical relaxation. *Anesthesiology*, **22,** 93.

FOLKERS, K., and MAJOR, R. T. (1937). Isolation of erythroidine, an alkaloid of curare action. *J. Amer. chem. Soc.*, **59,** 1580.

FOSTER, C. A. (1960). Muscle pains that follow administration of suxamethonium. *Brit. med. J.*, **2,** 24.

FOSTER, P. A. (1956). Potassium depletion and the central action of curare. *Brit. J. Anaesth.*, **28,** 488.

FREY, R., and SEEGER, R. (1961). Experimental and clinical experience with toxiferine (alkaloid of calabash curare). *Canad. Anaesth. Soc. J.*, **8,** 99.

GIOVANELLA, G., MANNI, C., MAZZONI, P., and MORICCA, G. (1961). Experimental studies on the fate of decamethonium. *Canad. Anaesth. Soc. J.*, **8,** 458.

GISSEN, A. J., KATZ, R. L., KARIS, J. H., and PAPPER, E. M. (1966). Neuromuscular block in man during prolonged arterial infusion with succinylcholine. *Anesthesiology*, **27,** 242.

GISSEN, A. J., and NASTUK, W. L. (1968). The mechanism of action of decamethonium. *Anesthesiology*, **29**, 197.

GLICK, D. (1941). Some additional observations on specificity of cholinesterase. *J. biol. Chem.*, **137**, 357.

GORDH, T., and WAHLIN, A. (1961). Potentiation of the neuromuscular effect of succinylcholine by tetrahydro-amino-acridine. *Acta anaesth. scand.*, **5**, 55.

GRAY, T. C. (1954). Disintegration of the nervous system. *Ann. roy. Coll. Surg. Engl.*, **15**, 402.

GRAY, T. C., and HALTON, J. (1946). A milestone in anaesthesia? (*d*-tubocurarine chloride). *Proc. roy. Soc. Med.*, **39**, 400.

GREENWAY, R. M., and QUASTEL, J. H. (1955). Hydrolysis of succinylmonocholine by liver esterase. *Proc. Soc. exp. Biol.* (*N.Y.*), **90**, 72.

GRIFFITH, H. R., and JOHNSON, G. E. (1942). The use of curare in general anesthesia. *Anesthesiology*, **3**, 418.

HALL, L. W., WOOLF, N., BRADLEY, J. W. P., and JOLLY, D. W. (1966). Unusual reaction to succinylcholine. *Brit. med. J.*, **2**, 1305.

HANNINGTON-KIFF, J. G. (1970). Residual post-operative paralysis. *Proc. roy. Soc. Med.*, **63**, 73.

HARRIS, H., HOPKINSON, D. A., ROBSON, E. B., and WHITTAKER, M. (1963). Genetical studies on a new variant of serum cholinesterase detected by electrophoresis. *Ann. hum. Genet.*, **26**, 359.

HARRIS, H., and WHITTAKER, M. (1961). Differential inhibition of human serum cholinesterase with fluoride: recognition of two new phenotypes. *Nature* (*Lond.*), **191**, 496.

HARRISON, G. G. (1966). The effect of cardiac lesions on the action of suxamethonium. *Anaesthesia*, **21**, 28.

HARROUN, P., BECKERT, F., and FISHER, C. W. (1947). The physiologic effects of curare and its use as adjunct to anesthesia. *Surg. Gynec. Obstet.*, **84**, 491.

HARROUN, P., and FISHER, C. W. (1949). The physiological effects of curare, its failure to pass the placental membrane or inhibit uterine contractions. *Surg. Gynec. Obstet.*, **89**, 73.

HERSEY, L. W., GOWDEY, C. W., and SPOEREL, W. (1961). The central effects of five muscle relaxants. *Canad. Anaesth. Soc. J.*, **8**, 335.

HESS, A., and PILAR, G. (1963). Slow fibres in the extraocular muscles of the cat. *J. Physiol.* (*Lond.*), **169**, 780.

HEYMANS, C., VERBEKE, R., and VOTOVA, Z. (1948). Symptomes cholinergiques et substitilé à l'acetylchima. *Arch. int. Pharmacodyn.*, **77**, 486.

HÜGIN, W., and KISSLING, P. (1961). Preliminary reports on a new short-acting relaxant of the depolarisation-inhibiting type, Ro 4–38161. *Schweiz. med. Wschr.*, **91**, 445.

HUGUENARD, P., and BOUÉ, A. (1948). Un nouvel ortho-curare français de synthèse, le 3697 R.P. *Rapport à la Soc. d'Anesthésie de Paris*, Seance du 17.

HUNT, R., and TAVEAU, R. (1906). On physiological action of certain choline derivatives and new methods for detecting choline. *Brit. med. J.*, **2**, 1788.

HUNTER, A. R. (1956). Neostigmine resistant curarization. *Brit. med. J.*, **2**, 919.

HUNTER, A. R. (1964). Diallyl toxiferine. *Brit. J. Anaesth.*, **36**, 466.

HUNTER, A. R. (1966). Suxamethonium apnoea. *Anaesthesia*, **21**, 325.

IWATSUKI, K., YUAS, T., and KATAOKA, Y. (1965). Effects of muscle relaxants on ventricular contractile force in dogs. *Tohoku J. exp. Med.*, **86**, 93.

JERUM, G., WHITTINGHAM, S., and WILSON, P. (1967). Anaphylaxis to suxamethonium. *Brit. J. Anaesth.*, **39**, 73.

KALOW, W. (1959). The distribution, destruction and elimination of muscle relaxants. *Anesthesiology*, **20**, 505.

Kalow, W. (1964). Pharmacogenetics and anesthesia. *Anesthesiology*, **25**, 377.

Kalow, W., and Davies, R. O. (1958). The activity of various esterase inhibitors towards atypical human serum cholinesterase. *Biochem. Pharmacol.*, **1**, 183.

Kalow, W., and Genest, K. (1957). A method for the detection of atypical forms of human serum cholinesterase; determination of dibucaine numbers. *Canad. J. Biochem.*, **35**, 339.

Karis, J. H., Gissen, A. J., and Nastuk, W. L. (1966). Mode of action of diethyl ether in blocking neuromuscular transmission. *Anesthesiology*, **27**, 42.

Katz, R. L. (1966). Neuromuscular effects of diethyl ether and its interaction with succinylcholine and *d*-tubocurarine. *Anesthesiology*, **27**, 52.

Katz, R. L., and Eakins, K. E. (1969). The actions of neuromuscular blocking agents on extraocular muscle and intraocular pressure. *Proc. roy. Soc. Med.*, **62**, 1217.

Katz, R. L., and Gissen, A. J. (1967). Neuromuscular and electromyographic effects of halothane and its interaction with *d*-tubocurarine in man. *Anesthesiology*, **28**, 564.

Katz, R. L., Wolf, C. E., and Papper, E. M. (1963). The nondepolarizing neuromuscular blocking action of succinylcholine in man. *Anesthesiology*, **24**, 784.

Kennedy, B. R., and Farman, J. V. (1968). Cardiovascular effects of gallamine triethiodide in man. *Brit. J. Anaesth.* **40**, 773.

Kimura, K. K., Unna, K. R., and Pfeiffer, C. C. (1948). Diatropine derivatives as proof *d*-tubocurarine is a blocking moiety containing twin atropine-acetylcholine prosthetic groups. *J. Pharmacol. exp. Ther.*, **95**, 149.

King, H. (1935). Curare. *Nature* (*Lond.*), **135**, 469.

King, K. (1949). Curare alkaloids X. Some alkaloids of *strychnos toxifera*. *J. chem. Soc.*, **4**, 3263.

Klupp, H., Kraupp, O., Stormann, H., and Stumpf, Ch. (1953). Über die pharmakologischen Eigenschaften einiger Polymethylen-Dicarbaminsäure-Bischolinester. *Arch. int. Pharmacoydn.*, **96**, 161.

Kuhne, W. (1862). *Über die peripherischen Endergon der motorischen Nerven*. Leipzig: Engelmann.

Kvisselgaard, N., and Moya, F. (1961). Estimation of succinylcholine blood levels. *Acta anaesth. scand.*, **5**, 1.

Lamoreaux, L. R. and Urbach, K. F. (1960). Incidence and prevention of muscle pain following the administration of succinylcholine. *Anesthesiology*, **21**, 394.

Lehmann, H. (1962). Personal communication.

Leigh, M. D., McCoy, D. D., Belton, M. K., and Lewis, G. B. (1957). Bradycardia following intravenous administration of succinylcholine chloride to infants and children. *Anesthesiology*, **18**, 698.

Liddell, J., Lehmann, H., and Silk, E. (1962). A silent pseudocholinesterase gene. *Nature* (*Lond.*), **193**, 561.

Lincoff, H. A., Breinin, G. M., and De Voe, A. G. (1967). The effect of succinylcholine on the extraocular muscles. *Amer. J. Ophthal.*, **43**, 440.

Lowenstein, E. (1966). Succinylcholine administration in the burned patient. *Anesthesiology*, **27**, 494.

Lupprian, K. G., and Churchill-Davidson, H. C. (1960). Effect of suxamethonium on cardiac rhythm. *Brit. med. J.*, **2**, 1774.

McCaul, K., and Robinson, G. D. (1962). Suxamethonium "extension" by tetrahydroaminoacrine. *Brit. J. Anaesth.*, **34**, 536.

McDowall, S. A., and Clarke, R. S. J. (1969). A clinical comparison of pancuronium with *d*-tubocurarine. *Anaesthesia*, **24**, 581.

Mallinson, F. B. (1947). A new synthetic curarizing agent in anaesthesia. *Lancet*, **1**, 98.

Martin, H. V. (1958). Paper read at an International Symposium in Venice on Curare and Curare-like Drugs.

MATHIAS, J. A., and EVANS-PROSSER, C. D. G. (1970). An investigation into the site of action of suxamethonium on cardiac rhythm. *Progress in Anaesthesiology* (Proc. 4th World Congr. Anaesthesiol., Sept. 1968). Amsterdam: Excerpta Medica.

MAYRHOFER, O., and HASSFURTHER, M. (1951). Kurzwirkende Muskelerschlaffungsmittel. *Wien. klin. Wschr.*, **47,** 885.

MILLER, R. D., WAY, W. L., and HICKEY, R. F. (1968). Inhibition of succinylcholine-induced increased intra-ocular pressure by non-depolarising muscle relaxants. *Anesthesiology*, **29,** 123.

MOGEY, G. A., and TREVAN, D. W. (1950). *D*-tubocurarine salts and derivatives. *Brit. med. J.*, **2,** 216.

MONGAR, J. L., and WHELAN, R. F. (1953). Histamine release by adrenaline and *d*-tubocurarine in the human subject. *J. Physiol.* (*Lond.*), **120,** 146.

MONTGOMERY, J. B., and BENNETT-JONES, N. (1956). Gallamine triethiodide and renal disease. *Lancet*, **2,** 1243.

MORRIS, D. D. B., and DUNN, C. H. (1957). Suxamethonium chloride administration and post-operative muscle pain. *Brit. med. J.*, **1,** 383.

MOYA, F., and KVISSELGAARD, N. (1961). The placental transmission of succinylcholine. *Anesthesiology*, **22,** 1.

MOYA, F., and MARGOLIES, A. B. (1961). Hydrolysis of succinylcholine by placental homogenates. *Anesthesiology*, **22,** 11.

MUSHIN, W. W., WIEN, R., MASON, D. F. J., and LANGSTON, G. T. (1949). Curare-like actions of tri-(diethylaminoethoxy)-benzine triethyliodide. *Lancet*, **1,** 726.

NEITLICH, H. W. (1966). Increased plasma cholinesterase activity and succinylcholine resistance. A genetic variant. *J. clin. Invest.*, **45,** 380.

ORGANE, G. S. W., PATON, W. D. M., and ZAIMIS, E. J. (1949). Preliminary trial of bistrimethylammonium decane and pentane di-iodide (C.10 and C.5) in man. *Lancet*, **1,** 21.

PANTUCK, E. J. (1967). Genetic aspect of neuromuscular blockade. In: *Advances in Anesthesiology: Muscle Relaxants*, Chap. 5, p. 63. New York: Hoeber.

PAPPER, E. M. (1968). Personal communication.

PARBROOK, G. D., and PIERCE, G. F. M. (1960). Comparison of post-operative pain and stiffness between suxamethonium and suxethonium. *Brit. med. J.*, **2,** 579.

PATON, W. D. M. (1959). The effects of muscle relaxants other than muscular relaxation. *Anesthesiology*, **20,** 453.

PATON, W. D. M., and PERRY, W. L. M. (1951). The pharmacology of the toxiferenes. *Brit. J. Pharmacol.*, **6,** 299.

PATON, W. D. M., and ZAIMIS, E. J. (1948). Clinical potentialities of certain bisquaternary salts causing neuromuscular and ganglionic block. *Nature* (*Lond.*), **162,** 810.

PATON, W. D. M., and ZAIMIS, E. J. (1952). Methonium compounds. *Pharmacol. Rev.*, **4,** 219.

PEREZ, H. R. (1970). Cardiac arrhythmia after succinylcholine. *Curr. Res. Anesth.*, **49,** 33.

PHILLIPS, A. P. (1949). Synthetic curare substitutes from aliphatic dicarboxylic acid amino-ethyl esters. *J. Amer. chem. Soc.*, **71,** 3264.

PRIME, F. J., and GRAY, T. C. (1952). The effect of certain anaesthetic and relaxant agents on circulatory dynamics. *Brit. J. Anaesth.*, **24,** 101.

RACK, P. M. H., and WESTBURY, D. R. (1966). The effect of suxamethonium and acetylcholine on the behaviour of cat muscle spindles during dynamic stretching and during fusimotor stimulation. *J. Physiol.* (*Lond.*), **186,** 698.

REES, G. J. (1958). Neonatal anaesthesia. *Brit. med. Bull.*, **14,** 38.

RIKER, W. F., Jnr., and WESCOE, W. C. (1951). Pharmacology of Flaxedil, with observations on certain analogs. *Ann. N.Y. Acad. Sci.*, **54,** 373.

ROBERTSON, G. S. (1966). Serum cholinesterase deficiency. II. Pregnancy. *Brit. J. Anaesth.*, **38,** 361.

SALEM, M. R., KIM, Y., and EL ETR, A. A. (1968). Histamine release following intravenous injection of *d*-tubocurarine. *Anesthesiology*, **29,** 380.

SCURR, C. F. (1951). A relaxant of very brief action. *Brit. med. J.*, **2,** 831.

SELLICK, B. A. (1970). Clinical experience of a new muscle relaxant—pancuronium bromide. *Progress in Anaesthesiology* (Proc. 4th World Congr. Anaesthesiol., Sept. 1968). Amsterdam: Excerpta Medica.

SHNIDER, S. M. (1965). Serum cholinesterase activity during pregnancy, labour and the puerperium. *Anesthesiology*, **26,** 335.

SMITH, J. C., and FOLDES, F. F. (1968). An improved method for the recognition of atypical plasma cholinesterase. *Anesthesiology*, **29,** 211.

SMITH, N. L. (1957). Histamine release by suxamethonium. *Anaesthesia*, **12,** 293.

SNIPER, W. (1952). The estimation and comparison of histamine release by muscle relaxants in man. *Brit. J. Anaesth.*, **24,** 232.

SPÄTH, E., LEITHE, W., and LADECK, F. (1928). Curare alkaloids. I. Constitution of curine. *Ber. dtsch. chem. Ges.*, **61,** 1698.

THESLEFF, S. (1951). Pharmacologic and clinical experiments with o.o. succinycholine iodide. *Nord. med.*, **46,** 1045.

THESLEFF, S. (1952). The pharmacological properties of succinylcholine iodide. *Acta physiol. scand.*, **26,** 103.

THOMAS, E. T. (1957). The effect of *d*-tubocurarine chloride on the blood pressure of anaesthetised patients. *Lancet*, **2,** 772.

TOBEY, R. E. (1970). Paraplegia, succinylcholine and cardiac arrest. *Anesthesiology*, **32,** 359.

TORDA, T. A. G., and KLONYMUS, D. H. (1966). The regional use of muscle relaxants. *Anesthesiology*, **27,** 689.

UTTING, J. (1963). pH as a factor determining plasma concentration of *d*-tubocurarine. *Brit. J. Anaesth.*, **35,** 706.

VAN DEN OOSTENDE, A. (1948). Sur la pharmacologie de différentes substances curarisantes. *Arch. int. Pharmacodyn.*, **75,** 419.

VICKERS, M. D. A. (1963). The mismanagement of suxamethonium apnoea. *Brit. J. Anaesth.*, **35,** 260.

VINCENT, D., and PARANT, M. (1954). Action des alcoloides des curares sur les cholinestérases. *Bull. Soc. Chim. biol. (Paris)*, **36,** 405.

WALTS, L. F., and DILLON, J. B. (1967). Clinical studies on succinylcholine chloride. *Anesthesiology*, **28,** 372.

WANG, R. I. H., and ROSS, C. A. (1963). Prolonged apnoea following succinylcholine in cancer patients receiving AB–132. *Anesthesiology*, **24,** 363.

WASER, P. G. (1959). In: *Curare and Curare-like Agents*. Eds. Bovet, D., Bovet-Nitti, F., and Marini-Bettolo, G. B. Amsterdam: Elsevier.

WASER, P. G. (1962). In: *Curare and Curare-like Agents*. (Ciba Foundation Study Group No. 12). Ed. de Reuck, A. V. S. London: J. & A. Churchill.

WESTGATE, H. D., and VAN BERGEN, F. H. (1962). Changes in histamine blood levels following *d*-tubocurarine administration. *Canad. Anaesth. Soc. J.*, **9,** 497.

WHITE, D. C. (1963). Dual block after intermittent succinylcholine. *Brit. J. Anaesth.*, **35,** 305.

WILSON, H. B., GORDON, H. E., and RAFFAN, A. W. (1950). Dimethyl ether of *d*-tubocurarine iodide as a curarising agent in anaesthesia for thoracic surgery. *Brit. med. J.*, **1,** 1296.

WINTERSTEINER, O., and DUTCHER, J. D. (1943). Curare alkaloids *chondodendron tomentosum*. *Science*, **97,** 467.

YOUNG, I. M. (1949). The action of decamethonium iodide (C. 10) on foetal neuromuscular transmission and its transfer across the placenta. *J. Physiol.* (*Lond.*), **109,** 31P.

ZAIMIS, E. J. (1962). "Experimental hazards and artefacts in the study of neuromuscular blocking drugs." In: *Curare and Curare-like Agents* (Ciba Foundation Study Group No. 12.) Ed. de Reuck, A.V.S. London: J. & A. Churchill.

FURTHER READING

BRYN THOMAS, K. (1964). *Curare. Its History and Usage.* London: Pitman Medical Publishing Co.

MCINTYRE, A. R. (1947). *Curare, its History, Nature and Clinical Use.* Chicago: Univ. Chicago Press.

Chapter 32

CHOLINESTERASES AND ANTI-CHOLINESTERASES

CHOLINESTERASES

It is generally agreed that the cholinesterases play a very important part in normal neuromuscular transmission, for there is clear evidence that this enzyme is responsible for the rapid breakdown of acetylcholine to choline and acetic acid. Some observers, however, question whether the speed of activity in tetanic nerve stimulation could ever be accounted for on a purely molecular basis. However, the distance that the acetylcholine molecule has to travel is extremely short (1 μ) and the speed at which it is broken down by cholinesterase is phenomenal (1/500th of a second). This time may be compared with the apparently slower process of repolarising the muscle membrane after a contraction has taken place—namely 1/250th of a second. In consequence any objection to the chemical theory of neuromuscular transmission on these grounds is highly improbable.

During a period of quiescence the enzyme *choline acetylase* (present inside the nerve fibre) is responsible for the synthesis of acetylcholine. Acetylcholine molecules are then sorted in the matrix of the nerve-ending as freely revolving packets or "quanta". Outside the nerve fibre in the surrounding tissue fluids are found the cholinesterase enzymes. These are distributed widely throughout the body but the highest concentrations are to be found in brain, nerve and muscle. The experiments of Marnay and Nachmansohn (1938), however, have shown that the concentration of cholinesterase enzyme at the myoneural junction is many thousand times greater than that to be found in other parts of the muscle.

Essentially, there are two distinct types of cholinesterase enzymes and the difference is largely based on their site of origin. *Pseudo* or *plasma* cholinesterase is to be found in the serum and in the pancreatic tissue. The normal values in the plasma vary from 40 to 100 units* depending on the method of estimation used. The pseudocholinesterase level is one of a number of tests of liver function and low figures are a prominent cause of prolonged apnoea after the use of suxamethonium. *True* or *specific* cholinesterase is found mainly in the red blood corpuscles, the neuromuscular junction, and the brain. The distinction between these two enzymes is not clear except that pseudo-cholinesterase is capable of

* *Electrometric Method of Michel* (1949).

An indirect method of measuring cholinesterase based on the fall in pH of a barbitone/phosphate buffered system due to the acid produced.

Normal Values:	*Lower Limit*	*Upper Limit*
Red Blood Corpuscles.	51	100
Plasma . . .	40	100
Whole Blood . .	80	129

Aldridge and Davies (1952).

hydrolysing certain non-choline esters (e.g. tributyrin) whereas the activity of true cholinesterase is confined to the choline esters only. Pseudo-cholinesterase is also relatively insensitive to eserine and responds readily to di-fluorophosphate (DFP), but its action in destroying acetylcholine is at its best when the concentration of acetylcholine is high. True cholinesterase is also inhibited by DFP but in contrast the hydrolytic activity of the true esterase is greatest when the concentration of acetylcholine is low.

ANTI-CHOLINESTERASES

As their name implies, all these compounds block the activity of both types of cholinesterase enzyme in varying degrees.

Mode of action.—The principal activity of anti-cholinesterase drugs is to depress the cholinesterase enzyme – both pseudo and true – thus permitting the concentration of acetylcholine molecules to rise. There are, however, other effects of these drugs that must be mentioned. They are capable of acting as depolarising drugs in their own right if sufficiently large doses are used. This effect may be seen as paresis in man if doses of 3·75 to 5·0 mg. of neostigmine are given intravenously in the absence of any *d*-tubocurarine. The presence of even the smallest quantity of the latter drug will normally prevent this in clinical practice. Also these drugs may have an action on the nerve-ending, aiding the release of acetylcholine either directly (Katz, 1967), or through the medium of an increased concentration of acetylcholine (Feldman and Tyrell, 1970). Finally, they may help to dislodge *d*-tubocurarine from its attachment to the receptor site (Katz, 1967). Of all these actions, only the anti cholinesterase effect is of any great clinical importance.

Acetylcholine has a very widespread activity in the body, affecting not only peripheral autonomic ganglia, smooth muscle (including myocardium) and secretory glands, but also skeletal muscle. So various are these actions that they are usually sub-divided into two main groups. First, the *nicotine-like* activity accounting for the action at the neuromuscular junction and also at the autonomic ganglia. Secondly, the *muscarine-like* action which accounts for the effect on the myocardium, bowel, bladder, pupil, and secretory glands (Table 1). Atropine sulphate opposes the muscarinic actions of acetylcholine and therefore

32/TABLE 1

ACTIONS OF ACETYLCHOLINE

Muscarinic effects	*Nicotinic effects*
1. Myocardium = bradycardia. 2. Gut = contraction. 3. Bronchioles = constriction. 4. Pupil = contraction. 5. Salivary glands = mucus ++. 6. Sweat glands = stimulated. 7. Bladder = contracted.	1. Autonomic ganglia stimulated. 2. Skeletal muscle stimulated.
Opposed by atropine sulphate.	

is the drug of choice in the treatment of nerve-gas casualties where the most important lesion is usually spasm of the smooth muscle of the bronchioles. The anti-cholinesterases stimulate both the muscarinic and the nicotinic actions of acetylcholine. If, however, they are combined with a large dose of atropine (1–2 mg.) then only the nicotinic action is revealed and the muscarinic side-effects are reduced or prevented.

Blaber and Bowman (1963) have investigated the action of the anti-cholinesterase drugs and conclude that three distinct sites of activity can be illustrated. These are:—

1. *Depression of acetylcholinesterase activity.*—This increases the amount of acetylcholine available at the motor end-plate.

2. *Action on the pre-junctional nerve-ending.*—The anti-cholinesterase drugs hasten the release of acetylcholine from the nerve-ending. Thus when high rates of nerve stimulation are used, the stores of acetylcholine are rapidly exhausted and neuromuscular transmission fails. However, these stores are sufficient for slow rates of nerve stimulation.

3. *Action on the post-junctional motor end-plate.*—This is one of simple depolarisation.

Neostigmine Methyl Sulphate ("Prostigmin")

This is a white crystalline powder, odourless and soluble in water. The formula is:

$$(CH_3)_3\overset{+}{N}-C_6H_4-O-\overset{O}{\overset{\|}{C}}-N(CH_3)_2 \quad SO_4CH_3^-$$

The fate of neostigmine in the body is interesting, for though a large proportion of the injected material can be accounted for by direct contact with the enzyme cholinesterase, a small proportion is excreted by glomerular filtration in the kidneys and a similar proportion destroyed by the liver. When taken orally the gastro-intestinal tract appears to possess powerful destructive properties for neostigmine, as none survives long enough to reach the faeces, yet only one-thirtieth of the ingested material ever reaches the general circulation (Goldstein *et al.*, 1949).

Fasciculations.—When neostigmine is given intravenously to a conscious subject, fasciculations may be seen or experienced by the individual. These are random firings-off of motor units brought about partly by the accumulation of the packets or quanta of acetylcholine at the end-plate, but also by the direct depolarising action of the neostigmine on an end-plate with anti-dromic excitation of the remainder of the motor unit. Massive doses of neostigmine cause severe and widespread fasciculations which on some occasions may involve a whole limb in a vigorous unco-ordinated twitch. This type of response is usually the prelude to neuromuscular block with failure of respiration. Coupled with the muscarinic symptoms (see below) the whole goes to make up a condition sometimes described as a "*cholinergic crisis*". It is rarely seen in normal subjects except after the ingestion of large quantities of anti-cholinesterase drugs. It may follow poisoning with DFP or other allied compounds sometimes used in the chemical industry. It is most commonly seen in patients with myasthenia gravis who have received excessive parenteral dosage of neostigmine.

Neostigmine and autonomic ganglia.—Neostigmine can reverse the hypotension produced by hexamethonium in dogs (Hilton, 1961) and in cats (Mason, 1962). It is generally believed that neostigmine is capable of stimulating the autonomic ganglia in animals. No evidence is available for man.

Neostigmine and the heart rate.—The fact that neostigmine stimulates the vagus and slows the heart rate is well established. For this reason it has always been advocated that it should be preceded by atropine. A number of isolated cases of cardiac arrest following the use of neostigmine have been reported but most of these date back to the early days of the use of the muscle relaxants (Macintosh, 1949; Clutton Brock, 1949; Lawson, 1956). Other observations suggest that the atropine may have been responsible. In fact, Eger (1962) states that "the injection of atropine intravenously in the presence of cyclopropane or halothane anaesthesia may produce disastrous arrhythmias.".

In the past it has been common practice to administer atropine sulphate (1·0 mg.) at least two minutes before the commencement of neostigmine therapy. Atropine leads to a rapid rise in the heart rate which is followed a few minutes later by a gradual reduction in the rate as the effect of the neostigmine becomes apparent. At that time, based on the work of Bain and Broadbent (1949), it was believed that the combination of atropine and neostigmine was dangerous because the initial bradycardia due to atropine might summate with that of neostigmine to provide a fatal cardiac arrest. Later it was realised that the slowing of the heart rate produced by atropine was dependent on both the size of the dose and the mode of administration. If atropine is given subcutaneously the slow rate of absorption produces a low blood level and therefore a slowing before the onset of an increase in the pulse rate. On the other hand, if 0·5 mg. or more is injected intravenously then no preliminary bradycardia can be observed since a high blood level is quickly achieved (Morton and Thomas, 1958).

Kemp and Morton (1962) took the matter one stage further and demonstrated that if the atropine and neostigmine were administered together intravenously then no initial slowing of the heart rate was observed. With this combination the action of atropine speeding up the pulse rate was evident in about 25 seconds and reached its peak in 45 seconds. The effect of neostigmine came on much later and the heart rate did not begin to be reduced until at least 100 seconds had passed. The conclusion was reached, therefore, that if atropine and neostigmine are combined together the action of the atropine on the heart rate will always precede that of the neostigmine.

Riding and Robinson (1961) studied the incidence of arrhythmias produced by atropine and neostigmine. They observed that respiratory alkalosis (produced by hyperventilation and carbon dioxide absorption) abolished the onset of cardiac arrhythmias, whereas some irregularity was always found in those cases in which the carbon dioxide level of the blood was allowed to rise above normal. They concluded that the incidence of arrhythmias was directly related to the carbon dioxide level of the blood.

Clinical comment.—Experience over the past twenty years has shown that neostigmine and atropine can be used with safety to reverse a non-depolarising block in man, and that neostigmine and atropine may be combined because the action of the atropine always precedes that of the neostigmine. In clinical practice a ratio of 1·0 mg. of atropine sulphate to 2·5 mg. neostigmine methylsulphate has been found satisfactory. The optimum time to administer this mixture is whilst the patient is still being hyperventilated and the carbon dioxide level of the blood is low. It should, however, never be administered in the presence of a high concentration of halothane or cyclopropane.

Though almost every case that has received a paralysing dose of a non-depolarising drug will probably require reversal of the neuromuscular block, it is now possible to demonstrate the degree of this block with a peripheral nerve-stimulator (see p. 866). If, for example, the hand muscles show adequate recovery of transmission then it can safely be concluded that the respiratory muscles are no longer under the influence of the relaxant drug. Recovery of the respiratory muscles always precedes that of the peripheral hand muscles. The only exception to this rule is when a pathological state exists at the motor end-plate, e.g. myasthenia gravis.

In small children, cardiac cases, and severely ill patients it is advisable to titrate the exact dose of neostigmine and atropine required with the nerve-stimulator. Also, in those patients who have received very large doses of a non-depolarising relaxant over a long period of time, then it is sometimes necessary to exceed a total dose of 2·5 mg. of neostigmine and 1·0 mg. of atropine. However, before further therapy is attempted it is important to verify with the stimulator that the signs of a non-depolarising neuromuscular block are still present.

Baraka (1967) has shown that the degree of reversal of a neuromuscular block depends not only on the plasma level of the relaxant but also on the severity of the block. If a dose of *d*-tubocurarine has been used which is much greater than the blocking dose (i.e. 100 per cent paralysis) then neostigmine will be unable to bring about complete reversal. In clinical practice it is never advisable to exceed a total dose of 2·0 mg. atropine and 5·0 mg. neostigmine, as this is sufficient to depress all cholinesterase enzyme activity severely. Reports have varied on the time of activity of neostigmine but this largely depends on whether the heart rate or skeletal muscle activity is being studied (Gravenstein and Perkins, 1966; Katz and Katz, 1967). Nevertheless, it is generally agreed that an interval of about 1–2 minutes elapses before the first signs are present. The maximum effect at the neuromuscular junction is not reached until about twenty minutes later and it persists for more than one hour.

Though the combination of atropine and neostigmine is now considered safe it is perhaps wiser not to administer the mixture in the presence of a bradycardia. In such an instance atropine alone in dilute solution is sometimes used to raise the pulse rate to around 80 per minute before mixing the remainder of the atropine with 2·5 mg. of neostigmine.

The most important single factor in the administration of neostigmine and atropine is that the mixture should be given *slowly*. In practice, at least five minutes should be taken over the injection. During the next five minutes neuromuscular transmission will gradually begin to improve, but this improvement will continue for at least the next ten minutes. The actual time interval depends principally on the blood flow to the peripheral muscles.

Edrophonium Chloride ("Tensilon")

In a study of the quaternary ammonium compounds analogous to neostigmine the pharmacological activity of edrophonium was revealed. The compound is 3-hydroxy-phenyldimethylethylammonium chloride, a white, odourless and crystalline powder which is readily soluble in water but not in alkali.

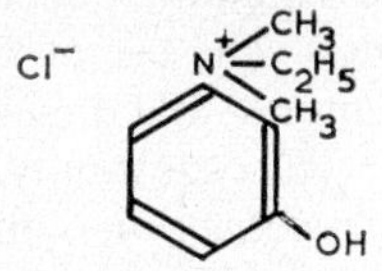

The mode of action of edrophonium has aroused considerable interest, since it was originally believed that it acted mainly by a direct action on the neuromuscular junction similar to that of acetylcholine. Its anti-cholinesterase activity was considered to be very weak (Randall, 1950; Riker and Wescoe, 1950). Subsequently, however, Hobbiger (1952) attacked this concept, and it is now generally accepted that the main action of the drug is an anti-cholinesterase one and that the direct depolarising activity is of secondary importance. The principal reason for this difference of opinion was based on the mode of experimentation. In the early stages *in vitro* experiments suggested that edrophonium had only 1/100–1/400 the anti-cholinesterase activity of neostigmine. However, the use of *in vivo* experiments showed that in fact the anti-cholinesterase activity was in the order of 1/5–1/15 that of neostigmine.

Following the intravenous injection of 10 mg. of edrophonium in a patient partially paralysed with *d*-tubocurarine, a rapid improvement in muscle power occurs between 30–45 seconds after it has been given. The return of muscle power, however, is not maintained, and after a further two to three minutes the original paresis begins to return. The degree of secondary paralysis is rarely as severe as that before the administration of edrophonium. Nevertheless, the fact that the improved muscle power is not maintained is sufficient to prohibit the therapeutic use of this drug. It should be used for diagnostic measures only. In this respect it will be found most useful to diagnose the presence or absence of dual block in a patient suffering from prolonged apnoea following the use of muscle relaxants, or to differentiate between a myasthenic or cholinergic crisis in a patient with myasthenia gravis (see Chapter 33, p. 919).

Pyridostigmin ("Mestinon").—This compound (i.e. the dimethylcarbamic ester of 1-methyl-3-hydroxy-pyridinium bromide) is an analogue of neostigmine and was introduced into medicine for the treatment of cases of myasthenia gravis. Pyridostigmin has about one quarter the potency of neostigmine so that 10 mg. given intravenously are equivalent to 2·5 mg. neostigmine by the same route, but the action of pyridostigmin on the myocardium and the bowel are far less marked.

Brown (1954) investigated the use of this drug in anaesthesia and verified that the muscarinic side-effects are less than with an equivalent dose of neostigmine. He found, however, that about four minutes elapsed before the action at the neuromuscular junction became evident, and also that the drug was generally less reliable than neostigmine.

Other Drugs affecting Neuromuscular Function

Galanthamine hydrobromide ("Nivalin").—This compound is an alkaloid which is extracted from the snowdrop bulb. It is widely used in Bulgaria as an antagonist to non-depolarising relaxants. Galanthamine has about one-tenth the anti-cholinesterase activity of neostigmine but the side-effects on heart rate and salivation are less (Wislicki, 1967). The use of atropine is recommended.

Germine acetate.—Germine mono- and di-acetate are derivatives of the semi-synthetic ester alkaloids of the veratrum family. They are an interesting group of drugs because their principal site of action is on the muscle fibre itself. Germine diacetate is capable of improving neuromuscular transmission in the presence of both a depolarisation and a non-depolarisation block. This is achieved by converting a single muscle action potential into a brief period of tetanic firing by a direct effect on the fibre itself. However, it can have no effect at all if all neuromuscular transmission is blocked by complete paralysis. It would appear to be of possible value in the treatment of myasthenia gravis.

Hexafluorenium.—This is a drug with a variety of interesting actions. It achieved some notoriety in clinical anaesthesia when combined with suxamethonium because it prolonged the latter drug's action, reduced the dose required and therefore lessened the risk of dual block (Foldes *et al.*, 1960). The main action is one of inhibition of pseudo-cholinesterase activity but it also has a specific action on the post-junctional membrane (Nastuk and Karis, 1964). Apart from these actions, it also inhibits true cholinesterase and is a weak non-depolarising agent.

To those accustomed to using suxamethonium for short procedures and *d*-tubocurarine for long procedures, the value of combining hexafluorenium with suxamethonium has never seemed obvious. The combination lacked an adequate antidote. Added to this, there were reports of tachycardia, hypertension, cardiac arrhythmias and fatal bronchospasm (Katz, 1967), so it is hardly surprising that it failed to gain universal popularity.

Tetrahydroaminacrine (T.H.A.).—This drug has also been advocated for combination with suxamethonium. It is a weak anti-cholinesterase but a powerful direct stimulant of the respiratory centre.

Quinidine.—This agent potentiates the neuromuscular block of both the depolarising and the non-depolarising relaxants. In fact, the combination of quinidine and a muscle relaxant has resulted in a case of prolonged apnoea lasting six hours (Way *et al.*, 1967). The most likely explanation of this enhancement of the activity of the muscle relaxants is that the cinchona alkaloids (like the local analgesic agents) depress the release of acetylcholine at the nerve-ending. However, Usubiaga (1968) attacks this thesis and argues that the most likely explanation is a depressant action on the muscle fibre itself.

Clinical Indications for an Antidote to the Muscle Relaxants

The indication for an antidote may arise clinically in the following circumstances (Doughty and Wylie, 1952).

1. To restore full respiratory activity at the end of an operation.
2. To reverse non-depolarisation block after an unexpectedly short operation, e.g. when prolonged surgery is intended but found to be impracticable. In this context it should be remembered that neostigmine is capable of completely reversing the block of *d*-tubocurarine even if it is given only a few minutes after the relaxant, provided that the paralysis is not complete (Bridenbaugh and Churchill-Davidson, 1968).
3. Following a short procedure during which almost complete paralysis of the patient has been necessary with a non-depolarising agent.
4. To abolish paralysis in a patient who has shown an unusual sensitivity to a muscle relaxant, e.g. myasthenia gravis.
5. To abolish the occasional long-lasting mild sequelae of muscle relaxants, e.g. residual paresis short of that which affects respiration.
6. To overcome a dual neuromuscular block in the absence of suxamethonium in the plasma.

To these should be added the use of edrophonium as a diagnostic test as described on pp. 914 and 919.

In clinical practice the only efficient and commonly used antidote to non-depolarising relaxants is neostigmine. The brevity of action of suxamethonium in normal patients obviates the need for an antidote, although an efficient and freely available one would not only be of considerable value for abnormal patients, but also on special occasions when very large total doses of this drug are clinically advisable.

REFERENCES

Aldridge, W. N., and Davies, D. R. (1952). Determination of cholinesterase activity in human blood. *Brit. med. J.*, **1,** 945.

Bain, W. A., and Broadbent, J. L. (1949). Death following neostigmine. *Brit. med. J.*, **1,** 1137.

Baraka, A. (1967). Irreversible tubocurarine neuromuscular block in the human. *Brit. J. Anaesth.*, **39,** 891.

Blaber, L. C., and Bowman, W. C. (1963). Studies on the repetitive discharges evoked in motor-nerve and skeletal muscle after injection of anti-cholinesterase drugs. *Brit. J. Pharmacol.*, **20,** 326.

Bridenbaugh, P. O., and Churchill-Davidson, H. C. (1968). Response to tubocurarine chloride and its reversal by neostigmine methylsulfate in man. *J. Amer. med. Ass.*, **203,** 541.

Brown, A. K. (1954). Pyridostigmin. *Anaesthesia*, **9,** 92.

Clutton Brock, J. (1949). Death following neostigmine. *Brit. med. J.*, **1,** 1007.

Doughty, A. G., and Wylie, W. D. (1952). Antidotes to "true" curarizing agents, including a report on Ro 2–3198 (Tensilon). *Brit. J. Anaesth.*, **24,** 67.

Eger, E. I. (1962). Atropine, scopolamine and related compounds. *Anesthesiology*, **23,** 365.

Feldman, S. A., and Tyrrell, H. F. (1970). A new theory of the termination of action of the muscle relaxants. *Proc. roy. Soc. Med.*, **63,** 692.

Foldes, F. F., Hillmer, N. R., Molloy, R. E., and Monte, A. P. (1960). Potentiation of the neuromuscular effect of succinylcholine by hexafluorenium. *Anesthesiology*, **21,** 50.

GOLDSTEIN, A., KRAYER, O., ROOT, M. A., ACHESON, G. H., and DOHERTY, M. E. (1949). Plasma neostigmine levels and cholinesterase inhibition in dogs and myasthenic patients. *J. Pharmacol. exp. Ther.*, **96,** 56.

GRAVENSTEIN, J. S., and PERKINS, H. M. (1966). The effect of neostigmine, atropine and ephedrine on heart rate in man. *Anesthesiology*, **27,** 298.

HILTON, J. G. (1961). The pressor response to neostigmine after ganglionic blockade. *J. Pharmacol. exp. Ther.*, **132,** 23.

HOBBIGER, F. (1952). The mechanism of anticurare action of certain neostigmine analogues. *Brit. J. Pharmacol.*, **7,** 223.

KATZ, R. L. (1967). Neuromuscular effects of *d*-tubocurarine, edrophonium and neostigmine in man. *Anesthesiology*, **28,** 327.

KATZ, R. L., and KATZ, G. J. (1967). Clinical use of muscle relaxants. In: *Advances in Anesthesiology—Muscle Relaxants*, Chap. 6. Ed. by L. C. Mark and E. M. Papper. New York: Hoeber.

KEMP, S. W., and MORTON, H. J. V. (1962). The effect of atropine and neostigmine on the pulse rates of anaesthetised patients. *Anaesthesia*, **17,** 170.

LAWSON, J. I. (1956). Cardiac arrest following the administration of neostigmine. *Brit. J. Anaesth.*, **28,** 336.

MACINTOSH, R. R. (1949). Death following injection of neostigmine. *Brit. med. J.*, **1,** 852.

MARNAY, A., and NACHMANSOHN, D. (1938). Choline esterase in voluntary muscle. *J. Physiol.* (*Lond.*), **92,** 37.

MASON, D. F. J. (1962). A ganglion stimulating action of neostigmine. *Brit. J. Pharmacol.*, **18,** 76.

MICHEL, H. O. (1949). Electrometric method for determination of RBC's and plasma cholinesterase activity. *J. Lab. clin. Med.*, **34,** 1564.

MORTON, H. J. V., and THOMAS, E. T. (1958). Effect of atropine on the heart rate. *Lancet*, **2,** 1313.

NASTUK, W. L., and KARIS, J. H. (1964). The blocking action of hexafluorenium on neuromuscular transmission and its interaction with succinylcholine. *J. Pharmacol. exp. Ther.*, **144,** 236.

RANDALL, L. O. (1950). Anticurare action of phenolin quaternary ammonium salts. *J. Pharmacol. exp. Ther.*, **100,** 83.

RIDING, J. E., and ROBINSON, J. S. (1961). The safety of neostigmine. *Anaesthesia*, **16,** 346.

RIKER, W. F., Jr., and WESCOE, W. C. (1950). Studies on the inter-relationship of certain cholinergic compounds. V. The significance of the actions of the 3-hydroxy phenyltrimethylammonium ion on neuromuscular function. *J. Pharmacol. exp. Ther.*, **100,** 454.

USUBIAGA, J. E. (1968). Potentiation of muscle relaxants by quinidine. *Anesthesiology*, **29,** 1068.

WAY, W. L., KATZUNG, B. G., and LARSON, C. P. (1967). Recurarisation with quinidine. *J. Amer. med. Ass.*, **200,** 153.

WISLICKI, L. (1967). Nivalin (galanthamine hydrobromide), an additional decurarizing agent: some introductory observations. *Brit. J. Anaesth.*, **39,** 963.

Chapter 33

NEUROLOGICAL DISEASE IN RELATION TO ANAESTHESIA

THE mode of action of various anaesthetic drugs at the motor end-plate and on the spinal cord is gradually becoming elucidated. Nevertheless, at the present time the theories underlying the response of people to these drugs are constantly undergoing change, so that it is hardly surprising that the subject becomes even more confusing when the pathological states of neurological disease are considered. Frequently the anaesthetist is confronted with such a patient undergoing some surgical operation unrelated to his neurological condition. In the majority of patients the response to anaesthetic drugs does not differ from that found in normal subjects; unhappily an abnormal response, particularly to one of the muscle relaxants, is sometimes encountered. This complication most often arises in the presence of undiagnosed myasthenia gravis and, therefore, is considered in detail.

MYASTHENIA GRAVIS

Myasthenia gravis is a chronic disease characterised by variable fatigue and weakness of voluntary muscles which gradually recover with rest. Although loss of reflex activity is not commonly observed, in long-standing cases some wasting of the muscle fibres may be present. The site of this fatigue has long been known to be in the peripheral neuromuscular system and the results of modern research have led to a general acceptance that the abnormality is at the neuromuscular junction.

History

In 1684, Thomas Willis first suggested the existence of such a disease in his book entitled *A Practice of Physick*; he went on to describe in detail the signs in a young woman affected with the disease. Nearly two hundred years later the syndrome again excited great interest when it became known as Erb-Goldflam's disease (Erb, 1879; Goldflam, 1893) and finally received the name of myasthenia gravis pseudo-paralytica from Jolly in 1895; in 1900 this name was modified to myasthenia gravis by Campbell and Bromwell.

Pathological Changes

Two types of thymic enlargement have been described. The commonest is simple hypertrophy of the gland in which lymphorrhages and germ centres are often seen. The second type is a tumour—a thymoma. This may be benign and encapsulated or it may be locally malignant within the thoracic cage. There is a close association between both thymic hyperplasia or tumour and the symptoms of myasthenia gravis, but their presence is by no means certain in every case.

Clinical Features

Little can be added by modern physicians to the early description by Willis and others. Most cases occur in adults of either sex between the ages of 20 and 50, but it has been described in the newborn and in children.

The onset of muscle fatigue is often so insidious that its significance may be missed by both doctor and patient. Occasionally it is precipitated by a severe illness or emotional disturbance. Fatigue of the eyelid muscles (on staring upwards) or of the limb muscle (with elevation of the arms) are sometimes useful in eliciting the early signs of myasthenia. Though the bulbar muscles (i.e. eyelid, facial and swallowing) are the most commonly affected, the signs of the disease can appear in any skeletal muscle throughout the body. Typically, the patient gives a history of fatigue increasing throughout the day with some recovery on awakening in the morning. In long-standing cases some wasting of the muscle fibres can be observed. The progress of the disease fluctuates but often reaches a certain level and then remains static for many years. In the early stages a remission may occur but these are rarely permanent.

Electromyographic Changes

At the end of the last century Jolly was able to demonstrate a difference with electrical stimulation between normal and myasthenic muscle. Classically, the severe myasthenic cannot maintain faradic stimulation of a motor-nerve. The "fade" and post-tetanic potentiation observed are similar to those already described for *d*-tubocurarine, viz. Fig. 1 *a* and *b*.

After a period of post-tetanic facilitation (lasting about 30 seconds) in cases of myasthenia there is a secondary period of post-tetanic exhaustion (see p. 789) which lasts for 20 minutes or more (Desmedt, 1957). This latter phenomenon is not observed in a paralysis due to *d*-tubocurarine chloride.

Unfortunately the classical electromyographic findings cannot be demonstrated in every case of myasthenia. This is probably because they are only observed when the muscles under test are actually showing clinical evidence of myasthenic weakness.

Aetiology of Myasthenia Gravis

The aetiology of myasthenia gravis has fascinated physicians for many years but still remains unknown. The superficial resemblance of this condition to the paresis of curare is known to all, but in the light of present knowledge the old theory of a circulating curare-like substance can no longer be entertained. The three current theories are based on the results of investigations:—

(*a*) *Diminished synthesis or release of acetylcholine*.—This is a pre-junctional theory. It is based on electromyographic recordings made from myasthenic muscle (Desmedt, 1961). The presence of fade of successive responses, post-tetanic potentiation, and post-tetanic exhaustion have been described above. Desmedt pointed out that though post-tetanic exhaustion did not occur in the presence of *d*-tubocurarine in normal muscle, a very similar pattern was observed in the muscle of cats treated with hemicholinium. This drug is believed to inhibit either the synthesis or the release of acetylcholine (see p. 777). On this basis he

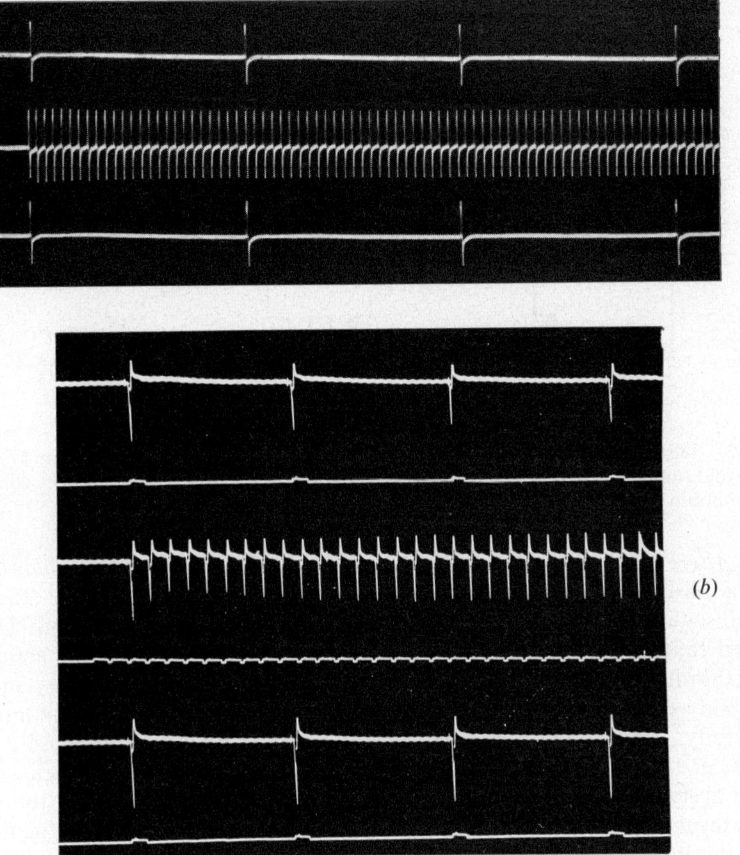

33/FIG. 1.—A comparison of the effects of electrical stimulation in a normal and myasthenic patient.

(*a*) Normal neuromuscular transmission.

(*b*) Myasthenia gravis. Note the "fade" of the twitch and tetanic response, and also the presence of post-tetanic potentiation.

postulated that myasthenia was primarily a failure of the synthesis or release of acetylcholine at the nerve-ending.

Further support for this theory is given by the finding of Dahlback and his colleagues (1961) who investigated isolated specimens (*in vitro*) of both normal and myasthenic muscle with an intracellular micro-electrode. They measured the output of miniature end-plate potentials in both types of muscle and found that it was considerably reduced in cases of myasthenia gravis. Elmquist and his co-workers (1964) took the matter one stage further and demonstrated that the miniature end-plate potentials were diminished to one-fifth of normal (Fig. 2). From further analysis they concluded that the primary fault in myasthenia was a reduction not in the total number of quanta but in the number of *molecules* in each packet.

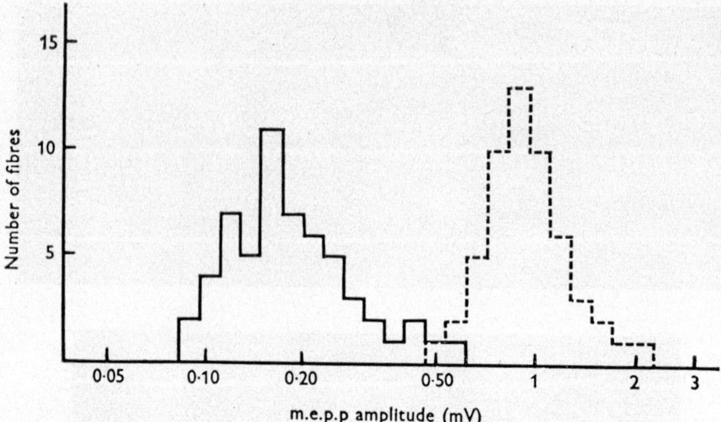

33/Fig. 2.—Distribution of mean miniature end-plate potential amplitudes from 57 myasthenic (solid line) and 54 normal (dotted line) human muscle fibres. All amplitudes corrected to a membrane potential of 85 mv. (From Elmqvist *et al.*, 1964).

(*b*) *Altered response of the motor end-plate.*—This is a post-junctional theory which is based largely on a pharmacological and electromyographic study of neuromuscular transmission. Churchill-Davidson and Richardson (1953) observed that myasthenic patients were resistant to the depolarising action of decamethonium iodide. This resistance can be demonstrated in every muscle of the body even though there are no signs of clinical weakness in the muscles under study. If repeated doses are given this resistance is overcome and a dual response at the motor end-plate is observed. As decamethonium is believed to act like acetylcholine on the post-junctional neuromuscular junction the basic fault in myasthenia was believed to be an alteration in the response of the motor end-plate. In this context it is particularly important to remember two things about the action of decamethonium in a myasthenic patient. First, the finding that all the motor end-plates in the body (whether clinically affected or not) are *resistant* to decamethonium demonstrates clearly that myasthenia gravis is a generalised condition. Some myasthenic patients can receive double or even quadruple the dose of decamethonium which is sufficient to paralyse a normal subject. Secondly, this *resistance* is best demonstrated in the very early or mild case and does not disappear either during a remission or after thymectomy. As it is such an early sign of myasthenia it could well be postulated that amongst the general population there is someone with a marked resistance to decamethonium who at some future date will develop the clinical signs of myasthenia gravis. Such a case has not been described.

The resistance of the myasthenic patient to depolarising drugs is not easily explicable on the basis of a primary pre-junctional lesion. If a gradual reduction of either acetylcholine production or liberation was the principal cause then one might presuppose that the motor end-plate would become more, rather than less, sensitive to acetylcholine in an attempt to compensate for the changing circumstances.

The post-junctional concept is supported by the work of Grob and his colleagues (1955) who used injections of intra-arterial acetylcholine and found that myasthenic muscle reacted differently from the normal subject. Thus, when injected into the brachial artery of a normal patient there was a brief contraction followed by a rapid recovery. But in cases of myasthenia gravis a secondary period of paresis developed which was not so severe but lasted about twenty minutes or more (Fig. 3). This secondary effect alone could be reproduced by the injection of choline, which is a breakdown product of acetylcholine. On this basis they postulated that myasthenia was an alteration of the response of the motor end-plate to either acetylcholine or to the choline formed from its hydrolysis.

(*c*) *Auto-immune response.*—It has been suggested that the physiological function of the thymus is essential for the proper development of lymphoid structures throughout the body. The maximum activity probably occurs during the development of the embryo but it also functions for some time after birth. The principal purpose of the gland is believed to be to ensure that the body can distinguish its own cells from other cells and antigens. This is the basis of the antigen-antibody response and is one of the body's principal protective mechanisms. However, sometimes it functions to the individual's disadvantage as in the case of organ grafting; it is well-known that skin cells can be transplanted from one area to another on the same patient but that this same person cannot normally receive a graft of cells from another donor unless they are identical twins.

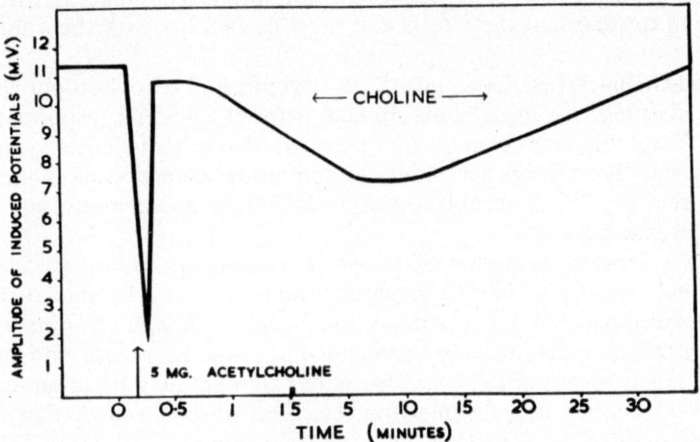

33/Fig. 3.—The intra-arterial injection of acetylcholine in a patient with myasthenia gravis. Note the primary paralysis due to acetylcholine with almost complete recovery, followed rapidly by a secondary phase of prolonged paralysis due to the choline. The second phase of paralysis is reversible by neostigmine, and is not seen in normal neuromuscular transmission.

The development of the auto-immune response is believed to be caused by the thymus gland. On Burnet's hypothesis (1962 *a* and *b*) various mutations occur during early development in the blood cells; it is the responsibility of the thymus gland to destroy or disable these mutations. Once this has been accomplished it no longer has a function to perform so that it gradually atrophies. In myasthenia gravis the body is presumed to lose this ability to be able to distinguish between the different cells, so that antibodies are formed which react with both skeletal and cardiac muscle.

Support for this hypothesis is given by the finding of Nastuk and his associates (1959) who observed an abnormally wide fluctuation in the serum complement activity of myasthenic patients. The level fell with the active phases of the disease and rose during remission. They believed that in myasthenia gravis the muscle fibre itself becomes antigenic and sets up an antibody reaction. These antibodies then become attached to the muscle membrane and are probably concentrated in the motor end-plate region. This could account for the alteration in structure of this region that is observed on histological examination of the area and also for the defect of neuromuscular transmission.

Summary.—There is now general agreement that the defect in myasthenia gravis is located at the neuromuscular junction. Both the pre- and post-junctional sites would appear to be involved. Current opinion favours the acceptance of a theory based on the auto-immune response but the reason why this phenomenon should suddenly or slowly develop still remains a mystery. It is possible that some infection is responsible (Simpson, 1960).

Tests for Myasthenia Gravis

Mild cases of myasthenia gravis present a difficult problem of diagnosis. It is hardly surprising, therefore, that many drugs have been used at one time or another as tests for the presence of this condition. The anaesthetist is often called upon to carry out these tests and must be familiar with their anticipated result.

1. **Anti-cholinesterase tests.**—Both neostigmine and edrophonium have been widely used as tests for myasthenia. In fact, without a positive response to either of these drugs the physician is powerless to make a diagnosis on physical grounds alone. Both drugs act mainly by inhibiting the action of cholinesterase and thus enabling the concentration of acetylcholine at the motor end-plate to undergo a temporary rise.

(*a*) *Edrophonium*, by virtue of its short duration of action (2–5 minutes) and minimal side-effects, can be given intravenously (dose 10 mg.). It has now largely replaced neostigmine as a diagnostic agent. Although atropine is usually omitted in this test there may be some slowing of the heart rate and increased salivation. In normal subjects fine fascicular tremors may be observed in the eyelids 30–45 seconds after the injection. These are absent in cases of myasthenia gravis.

(*b*) *Neostigmine* can be used intramuscularly in a dose of 1·0–2·0 mg. (often combined with 0·5–1·0 mg. atropine to reduce the side-effects). Some improvement in muscle power should be observed within 10–15 minutes.

For accurate assessment of any increase in muscle strength the ergograph is often used both before and after the drug. A false positive must be avoided by repeating the procedure with a placebo or atropine.

2. ***d*-Tubocurarine test.**—Before attempting any test with a muscle relaxant it is imperative that adequate measures for artificial ventilation are at hand.

Foldes and McNall (1962) recommend the administration of 0·5–1·0 mg. of *d*-tubocurarine chloride at 3-minute intervals up to a total of 4·0 mg. They conclude that when this drug is combined with the ergograph the maximum dose should produce a marked reduction in grip strength or vital capacity in cases of myasthenia gravis.

Rowland and his associates (1961) are more conservative and suggest a maximum dose of 0·016 mg./kg. of *d*-tubocurarine chloride. They found that 84 per cent of myasthenia gravis patients exhibited "sensitivity."

Foldes (1970) has described the value of a regional intravenous injection of 0·2 mg. of *d*-tubocurarine in the diagnosis of myasthenia gravis. In normal patients this dose produced a decrease in grip strength of 10 ± 4 per cent, whereas in myasthenic patients the fall was $67{\cdot}9 \pm 7$ per cent.

Details of technique.—The patient lies on a couch and the muscle-power in the upper limbs is measured by dynamometry, ergography or electromyography. After control measurements a needle is inserted into a vein in each arm. Both limbs are then raised for 1 minute in order to empty the venous channels, after which tourniquets are applied and inflated to 40 mm. Hg above the systolic pressure. 0·2 mg. *d*-tubocurarine diluted in 20 ml. of 0·9 per cent sodium chloride is injected into one arm and the diluent only into the other. The cuffs are kept inflated for five minutes. Two minutes after their release the arms are tested for muscle-power.

Decamethonium.—This drug is believed to act in a similar manner to acetylcholine but has the advantage that it is not destroyed by cholinesterase (Zaimis, 1951; Burns *et al.*, 1949; Burns and Paton, 1951). Its action in myasthenia gravis is, therefore, of particular importance and has been fully described by Churchill-Davidson and Richardson (1953 and 1955).

Essentially, in normal subjects the injection of decamethonium produces a neuromuscular block with all the signs of depolarisation; in cases of myasthenia

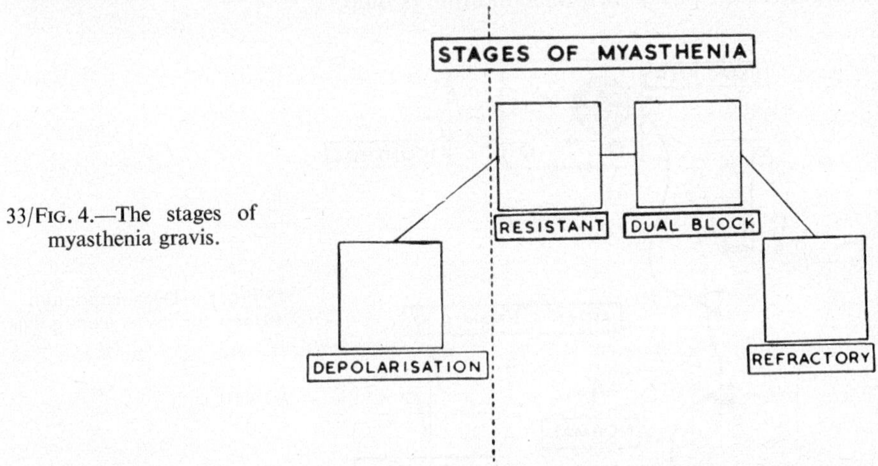

33/Fig. 4.—The stages of myasthenia gravis.

gravis it shows evidence of resistance leading finally to a dual block. Thus fibrillary twitching or fasciculations are common in normal subjects but are rarely observed in cases of myasthenia. The combination of electromyographic techniques with decamethonium and edrophonium has enabled three stages in the development of myasthenia to be identified (Fig. 4).

1. *Stage of resistance.*—In this stage the patient's muscles show no evidence of clinical weakness yet the motor end-plate shows a remarkable tolerance to the paralysing action of decamethonium. Whereas in normal subjects a dose of 2·5 to 3·0 mg. is capable of producing profound paralysis, myasthenic muscle in the stage of resistance can tolerate doses three to four times as great without showing evidence of any weakness. The muscles of myasthenic patients which do not show clinical weakness and function normally are classified as in this stage. The fact that this resistance is so clearly evident in very mild cases of myasthenia makes decamethonium useful as a test in the diagnosis of this condition.

2. *Stage of dual block.*—The onset of this stage is heralded by the appearance of clinical weakness. Decamethonium, acting like a large dose of acetylcholine, produces a dual block which is partially reversible by the injection of an anticholinesterase substance (edrophonium). In contrast, decamethonium in normal subjects leads to a depolarisation type of neuromuscular block; if at this point an anti-cholinesterase drug is given the block either exhibits no change or shows a dramatic increase.

3. *Stage of myopathy* (*or refractoriness*).—After prolonged periods in which the muscle fibre has not contracted due to the persistence of a neuromuscular block, the fibre finally atrophies from disuse. At this point the signs of a myopathy are evident. If a diligent electromyographic search is made, such signs can be found in at least one sixth of all cases of myasthenia gravis: they are more common in long-standing cases.

The evidence available suggests that the natural history of the development of myasthenia goes through the stages in the order that they have been enumerated above. The severity of the disease depends on the number of muscle fibres that are in the dual block and myopathic stages. If most of the fibres are merely in the resistant phase then the condition is mild.

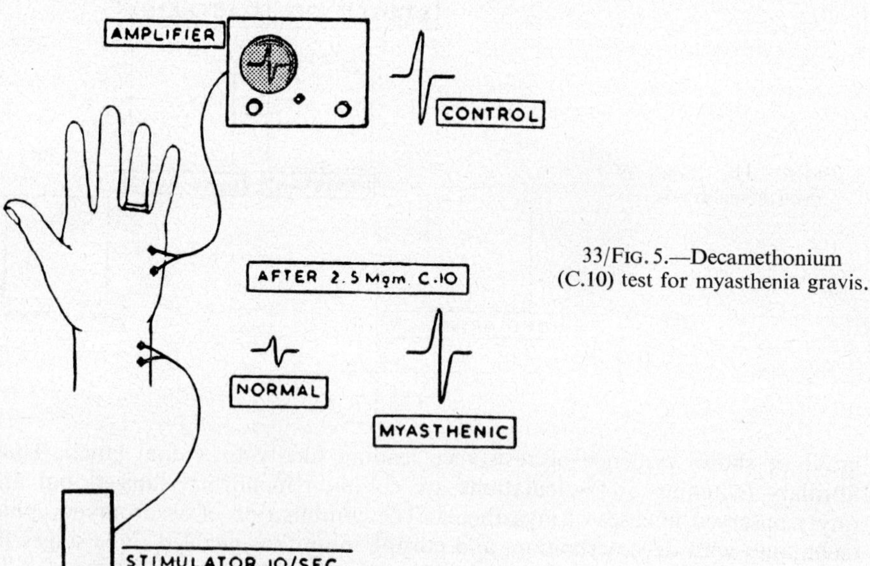

33/Fig. 5.—Decamethonium (C.10) test for myasthenia gravis.

Decamethonium, therefore, may be used as a test for the presence of myasthenia gravis. Details are given below.

DECAMETHONIUM TEST FOR MYASTHENIA GRAVIS (Fig. 5)

The patient is placed on a couch in a position of maximum comfort with the head and shoulders slightly raised. Means of artificial ventilation with oxygen should be discreetly at hand. The muscles of the hypothenar eminence on either hand are selected for examination by electromyography. The ulnar nerve at the wrist or elbow is stimulated supramaximally ten times per second and the height of the resultant action potential is recorded. This is taken as the control value and is expressed as 100 per cent.

The procedure is as follows:

Time	*Operation*	*Total dose of decamethonium*
Zero	1·0 mg. decamethonium injected	1·0 mg.
After 2 minutes	0·5 mg. decamethonium injected	1·5 mg.
After 4 minutes	Height of A.P.* measured. If satisfactory, inject further 0·5 mg. decamethonium	2·0 mg.
After 6 minutes	Height of A.P. measured. If satisfactory, inject further 0·5 mg. decamethonium	2·5 mg.
After 8 minutes	Height of A.P. measured	

* Action potential.

Interpretation of Results

(*a*) *Normal subjects.*—These complain of generalised fasciculations. After 2·5 mg. of decamethonium the height of the action potential has fallen from 100 per cent to 20 per cent or less of the control value. Very occasionally in heavy muscular individuals a total dose of 3·0 mg. is required to depress the action potential completely. Respiration should remain unaffected throughout.

(*b*) *Myasthenic subjects.*—Fasciculations are rarely encountered. Despite the possible increase in the myasthenic weakness the action potential at the wrist remains relatively unaffected. The myasthenic range is 100 per cent to 30 per cent but most cases lie near the control value. If there is a considerable fall then great importance is attached to the response to the injection of edrophonium in the second part of the test. This will reverse the signs of a dual block in myasthenic patients but will potentiate the effect of depolarisation in normal subjects.

In cases of severe generalised myasthenic weakness the injection of decamethonium will merely increase the paresis that is already present. If the bulbar musculature is involved, swallowing and respiration may become embarrassed. The onset of any such signs is a clear indication to stop the administration of decamethonium and test the action of an anti-cholinesterase drug (i.e. edrophonium).

The greatest value of this test lies in the diagnosis of early myasthenia, localised myasthenia or the case that has undergone a complete remission. In such patients the presence of "resistance" to decamethonium enables this drug to be tolerated even better than in normal subjects; it also emphasises a most important point—namely that although myasthenia may seem clinically to be localised to a very small muscle group, in fact the condition is a generalised one which makes every motor end-plate throughout the body respond differently from the normal. Whether this change is inherited or acquired is not known.

Suxamethonium.—Though this relaxant drug acts in a similar manner to decamethonium, its short duration of action coupled with the high initial dosage make it difficult to demonstrate the resistance stage before the onset of a dual neuromuscular block. Thus in myasthenia, suxamethonium brings about a paralysis of muscles through the medium of a dual response, but as it is rapidly destroyed by the enzyme cholinesterase (normal level in myasthenia) the duration of the weakness is only a few minutes. Nevertheless, the recovery does not appear to be either so rapid or so complete as in normal subjects, though the time taken may be shortened by administering an anti-cholinesterase drug.

Muscle biopsy.—Two types of histological abnormality at the motor end-plate have been described (Coërs and Woolf, 1959; Coërs and Desmedt, 1959) using a methylene-blue staining technique. In the first type these changes resemble those commonly observed in other diseases of muscle and consist principally of enlarged end-plates associated with a profuse ramification of nerve fibres. The second type consists of elongated end-plates without side branches which are possibly specific for myasthenia gravis.

MacDermot (1960) investigated cases of myasthenia gravis with a simultaneous muscle biopsy and decamethonium test. She concluded that neural abnormalities could be observed before the appearance of symptoms and these changes were widespread throughout the body even though there was no observable clinical weakness. Despite this observation it appeared that although the changes in myasthenia gravis were characteristic there was insufficient evidence to conclude that they were specific for this disease alone.

Summary

In the majority of cases of myasthenia gravis the edrophonium test reveals a dramatic improvement in neuromuscular transmission. The patient's diagnosis is then finally confirmed by the improvement of muscle strength with anti-cholinesterase therapy. There are some cases, however, in which the response to both the test and therapy are equivocal and it is in these cases that further evidence is sometimes required. If there is generalised weakness then the *d*-tubocurarine test will reveal "sensitivity". On the other hand, if the weakness is limited to one group of muscles (e.g. the eye muscles) then *d*-tubocurarine is of little value because the "sensitivity" reaction is confined largely to those muscles that are already showing evidence of clinical weakness. As the "resistance" to decamethonium is universal throughout the body, this test is the most specific for cases of myasthenia gravis (Churchill-Davidson and Richardson, 1961), but nevertheless is the most complex. It is particularly useful in differentiating an ocular myopathy from ocular myasthenia gravis.

Treatment of Myasthenia Gravis

The anaesthetist may encounter the myasthenic patient unwittingly, in the labour ward, in the course of routine surgery, or for the operation of thymectomy. He may also be called in to advise with the problem of ventilation in a myasthenic or cholinergic crisis; therefore some knowledge of the treatment of myasthenia is essential.

Medical Treatment

Many myasthenic patients are adequately controlled with anti-cholinesterase drugs given by mouth in tablet form. Those most commonly used are:

Neostigmine bromide as a 15 mg. tablet is the most popular. The duration of action rarely exceeds four hours so that from 1–3 tablets are needed at intervals varying from every 2 to 6 hours depending on the severity of the myasthenia. The objective of all therapy is to achieve the maximum benefit of muscle strength pertinent to the patient's requirements with the minimum number of tablets.

Pyridostigmine ("Mestinon") is less potent than neostigmine and the 60 mg. tablet corresponds approximately in activity to 15 mg. of neostigmine. In some patients it is better tolerated than neostigmine with less gastro-intestinal disturbance and a slightly longer duration of action. For this reason it is often used at night.

Ambenonium chloride is used as a 6 mg. tablet which is roughly equivalent to 15 mg. of neostigmine. It is believed to be more rapid in onset, longer acting and with less gastro-intestinal disturbance.

Ephedrine is often combined with these drugs but its value is doubtful. Atropine in the form of tincture of belladonna (5–15 minims) is sometimes used for the treatment of colic. Steroid therapy may exacerbate the myasthenia gravis and therefore should be used with caution in such patients.

The anaesthetist encounters the myasthenic patient under medical care in two particular emergencies.

1. *Myasthenic crisis.*—Often the patient will give a history of a recent pulmonary infection associated with some difficulty in breathing. In a true myasthenic crisis there is dramatic improvement following the administration of an intravenous anti-cholinesterase such as edrophonium (10 mg.). However, in most instances the patient has already increased her normal intake of anti-cholinesterase drugs so that often she is unresponsive to further therapy. The treatment of this condition is control of the airway, suction and adequate ventilation. (See *d*-tubocurarine treatment below.)

2. *Cholinergic crisis.*—This produces very similar symptoms and signs to a myasthenic crisis and although the two are theoretically distinguishable, in practice both myasthenic and cholinergic elements are often present in each case. The diagnosis is made by either no improvement or increased paresis following the injection of 10 mg. edrophonium intravenously. This condition is believed to be due to excessive anti-cholinesterase therapy. However, as both the patient's requirements and the response to an anti-cholinesterase drug may change rapidly in the presence of infection the management becomes extremely complex. Furthermore, whereas some patients may remain stable for years others may become increasingly unresponsive to anti-cholinesterase therapy. Refractoriness to these drugs is one of the basic problems in the treatment of myasthenia patients. It can only be overcome if all such therapy is withdrawn for a period of time. This is the basis for the use of *d*-tubocurarine therapy. The treatment of this condition is the same as for a myasthenic crisis with the exception that no anti-cholinesterase drugs should be used.

***d*-Tubocurarine chloride treatment.**—Despite the increased sensitivity of the myasthenia patient to this drug it has been used as a form of treatment for this condition (Churchill-Davidson and Richardson, 1957). The rationale behind this therapy is based upon the assumption that if the motor end-plate is "rested" by preventing its excitation with acetylcholine, then when activity is resumed the end-plate will have become re-sensitised to the transmitter substance and also to anti-cholinesterase therapy.

Although seldom used today this form of treatment is the basis for the new approach to the management of the myasthenia patient who is refractory to anti-cholinesterase therapy. On most occasions the simple expedient of withdrawing all anti-cholinesterase therapy for 7–10 days, whilst artificially ventilating and feeding the patient, is sufficient to restore sensitivity to these drugs. However, the improvement is usually short-lived, and gradually the refractoriness to anti-cholinesterase therapy returns. In the very severe case or for the patient who tends to "fight the ventilator" then curarisation may be indicated.

Surgical Treatment

A patient with myasthenia gravis may require anaesthesia on a variety of occasions. The principles of management, however, remain the same whatever the operation.

Principles of management.—If possible the patient should be stabilised on oral anti-cholinesterase therapy pre-operatively. The dose selected should not be the same as that used when leading an active life at home but rather should be the amount required by a subject lying at rest in bed. In the past most of the problems in the management of the myasthenia patient for surgery have been created by over-enthusiastic therapy. Anti-cholinesterase drugs may temporarily increase muscle strength but at the same time the production of secretions is also increased. Once stabilised on an oral dose of a suitable drug the patient usually ceases to be affected by the side-effects of colic and increased salivary secretions. Yet, a sudden increase in the dosage will initiate the return of these symptoms. Whenever possible, therefore, the dose of anti-cholinesterase both before and after operation should be administered by mouth and it should be reduced to as small as possible a dose to enable the patient to reach the operating room in comfort. On some occasions with complete bed rest pre-operatively it is possible to withdraw all anti-cholinesterase therapy.

Specific instances in which the myasthenia patient requires anaesthesia for operation may be considered under three different headings.

(*a*) *Incidental general surgery.*—Whenever possible anti-cholinesterase drugs should be administered orally, if necessary through a naso-gastric tube, rather than parenterally. Anaesthesia can be obtained satisfactorily with most agents but halothane has proved particularly useful. If muscle relaxation is not adequate, it can be produced by a local analgesic technique. If the patient requires bowel surgery then control must be by parenteral therapy but this will probably lead to an increase in the secretions in the respiratory tract. In the presence of severe generalised myasthenia and a large abdominal or thoracic incision then the use of prolonged endotracheal intubation or a prophylactic tracheostomy should be seriously considered.

(*b*) *Obstetrics.*—The course of myasthenia gravis in relation to pregnancy is variable. Some patients improve remarkably whilst others become much weaker.

Myasthenia gravis, however, is not an indication for Caesarian section unless there are associated obstetrical reasons. These patients tolerate analgesic drugs well but it should be remembered that the anti-cholinesterase drugs may enhance the effect of the opiates and their analogues (Slaughter *et al.*, 1940). A regional analgesic technique such as pudendal nerve block, epidural or subarachnoid block will provide very satisfactory conditions for delivery. If general anaesthesia is required then ether or cyclopropane are preferable to halothane since at comparable depths of anaesthesia there is less reduction in uterine tone.

Myasthenia gravis in the newborn has been described in two forms—neonatal and congenital myasthenia. In the neonatal variety the mother has myasthenia gravis and the infant has transient symptoms lasting for a few weeks after birth. In the congenital type, on the other hand, the mother is normal but the symptoms in the infant persist. Little is known of the aetiology of this condition but it is possible that the neonatal variety is related to the effects of maternal anti-cholinesterase therapy, whereas the congenital form is an inherited defect of neuromuscular transmission.

(*c*) *Thymectomy.*—The value of this operation in the treatment of myasthenia gravis is still debated but the most successful results have been obtained in females under 40 years of age (Keynes, 1954; Eaton and Claggett, 1955). The particular risks of this operation centre around the problem of the control of secretions due to anti-cholinesterase drugs, the pain in the post-operative period caused by splitting the sternum, the possible complication of bilateral pneumothorax, and the depression of ventilation by analgesic drugs.

Halothane anaesthesia in the presence of controlled respiration (to rest the respiratory muscles during surgery) has proved the most satisfactory agent for general anaesthesia.

In the presence of a severe myasthenia in the pre-operative period then it is advisable to perform an elective tracheostomy at the end of the operation. In this manner the high mortality previously associated with the operation of thymectomy can be eliminated provided adequate means of suction and ventilation are available. Furthermore, the opportunity can be grasped to withdraw all anti-cholinesterase therapy so that the motor end-plates are "re-sensitised" by the time the therapy is renewed.

CARCINOMATOUS NEUROPATHY

Henson and his colleagues (1954) drew attention to the relationship between carcinoma (particularly of the bronchus) and a motor neuropathy. In most cases of advanced carcinoma the cachexia, anaemia and loss of weight are sufficient to produce severe peripheral weakness. However, in true carcinomatous neuropathy the fatiguability is out of all proportion to the severity of the disease. Microscopic examination discloses demyelination of nerve fibres and atrophy of muscle fibres. The response to anti-cholinesterase therapy is poor. The relationship of this condition to the myasthenic syndrome is not clear but carcinomatous neuropathy is much commoner than the myasthenic syndrome and lacks the characteristic electromyographic "growth" of successive tetanic responses which is so essential for diagnosis of the later condition.

MYASTHENIC SYNDROME

In recent years a number of cases have been described suggesting an association between a condition resembling myasthenia gravis and bronchial carcinoma. This relationship was first pointed out by Anderson and his associates (1953) but it was not until four years later that Eaton and Lambert (1957) detailed the specific condition which they termed "myasthenic syndrome".

Although superficially many of the features of the myasthenic syndrome resemble myasthenia gravis, a closer investigation has revealed a wide margin of differentiation. These have been fully described by Wise and Wylie (1964) and are tabulated on p. 923.

The myasthenic syndrome is essentially a condition of peripheral muscle weakness developing in a patient with a bronchial carcinoma. This association is so common that the finding of the characteristic electromyographic response in the absence of obvious evidence of a neoplasm should be sufficient to stimulate an intensive search for its presence.

The specific electromyographic features are illustrated in Fig. 6.

They can be summarised as follows:

1. Low voltage potential on twitch stimulation (Fig. 7).
2. The "fade" of successive responses on twitch stimulation.
3. The "growth" of successive responses on tetanic stimulation.
4. The presence of post-tetanic facilitation.

In a clinical assessment of the effect of relaxant drugs on patients with the myasthenic syndrome Wise (1962) pointed out that these patients were highly sensitive to both the depolarising and the non-depolarising drugs. The presence of the peripheral weakness is always demonstrable in these cases if actually sought by the anaesthetist. However, if the patient has been confined to bed or is suffering from some incapacitating lesion then the presence of a myasthenic syndrome may be missed. The possible presence of this condition should always be borne in mind during the pre-operative examination of the patient for bronchoscopy

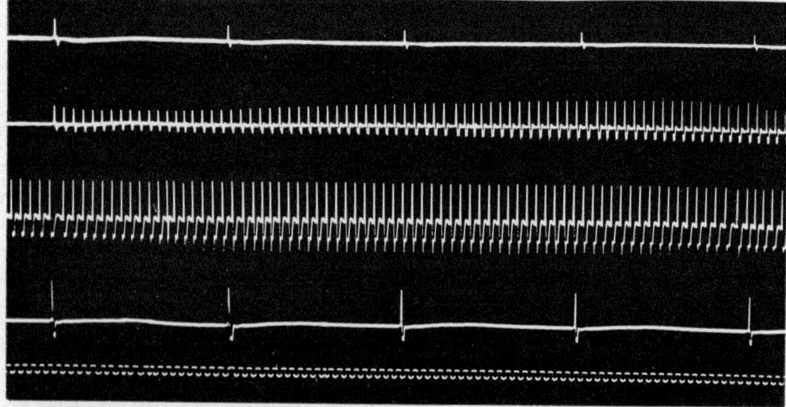

33/Fig. 6.—Electromyographic pattern of myasthenic syndrome. This patient had a proven carcinoma of bronchus.

33/TABLE 1

	Myasthenia gravis	*Myasthenic syndrome*
Sex . . .	Twice as common in women.	Almost entirely men.
Age of onset .	Commonly 20–40 years.	Commonly 50–70 years.
Presenting signs .	Weakness of external ocular, bulbar and facial muscles.	Weakness and fatiguability of proximal limb muscles (legs> arms).
Other signs . .	Weakness of limbs, usually proximal, is a later sign (arms> legs).	Weakness of ocular and bulbar muscles is infrequent.
Other clinical features . .	Fatigue on activity.	Transient increase in strength on activity precedes fatigue.
	Muscle pains uncommon.	Muscle pains common.
	Tendon reflexes normal.	Tendon reflexes reduced or absent.
	Good response to neostigmine.	Poor response to neostigmine.
Response to muscle relaxants . .	Increased sensitivity to non-depolarising relaxants in clinically weak muscles.	Marked sensitivity to non-depolarising relaxants even in muscles relatively unaffected.
	Resistance to depolarising relaxants.	Sensitivity to depolarising relaxants.
Electromyographic features . .	Normal or slightly reduced amplitude of action potentials at slow rates of stimulation.	Very low voltage action potentials at slow rates of stimulation with fade.
	Fade of successive potentials especially on tetanic stimulation.	Marked growth of potentials on tetanic stimulation.
	Post-tetanic potentiation and post-tetanic exhaustion present.	Post-tetanic potentiation present.
Pathologic states	Thymoma in 25 per cent of patients.	Small-celled carcinoma of bronchus always present.
	Motor end-plates abnormally elongated and distal nerves unusually branched.	Non-specific degenerative process of nerve fibres and end-plates.
Prognosis . .	Often good.	Rapid deterioration and death.

under general anaesthesia or a thoracotomy for carcinoma of lung. If this condition is suspected then the diagnosis can easily be confirmed by electromyography. The use of all the muscle relaxants is contra-indicated in the presence of the myasthenic syndrome.

DYSTROPHIA MYOTONICA

Dystrophia myotonica is a familial disease, usually occurring in adult life, characterised by muscle wasting, fatigue, and an inability to relax the muscles

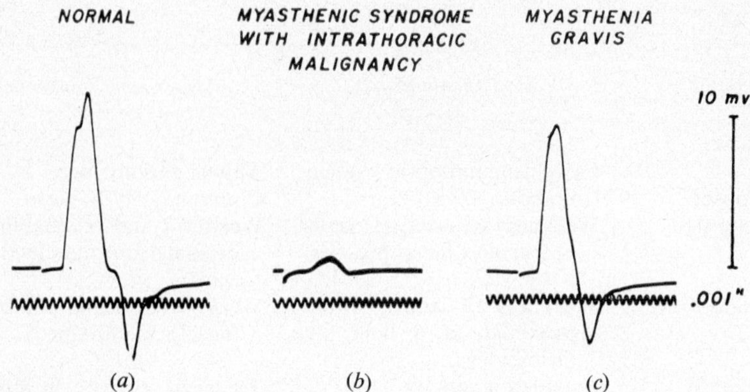

33/FIG. 7.—Illustrates the different height (i.e. voltage) of the action potential in response to a single twitch stimulus in (*a*) normal, (*b*) myasthenic syndrome, (*c*) myasthenia gravis (Lambert-*et al.*, 1961).

after a contraction (myotonia). The myotonia may precede the muscle wasting by many years or may occur independently. The condition is commonly associated with cataract, baldness and testicular atrophy. Occasionally the anaesthetist may be privileged to diagnose the presence of myotonia when the patient "opens and squeezes" his hand before the induction of intravenous anaesthesia.

The abnormality in dystrophia myotonica is believed to be an increase in the sensitivity of the muscle fibre. Brown and Harvey (1939) working with myotonic goats found that the myotonia persisted even after nerve-section and curarisation. Later Geschwind and Simpson (1955) showed in man that neither *d*-tubocurarine nor decamethonium will abolish the myotonia. MacDermot (1961), however, has demonstrated histologically that not only is the muscle fibre itself involved but there is also a defect of the nerve-ending.

Kaufman (1960) investigated the effect of anaesthetic drugs, including the relaxants and thiopentone, in patients with dystrophia myotonica. He observed that thiopentone did not influence neuromuscular transmission. The intense depression of respiration, therefore, that may follow the use of barbiturate or narcotic drugs is probably related to central depression of the respiratory centre in a patient with a limited respiratory reserve.

Both neostigmine and the depolarising drugs (Thiel, 1967) may increase the degree of myotonia whereas *d*-tubocurarine will block neuromuscular transmission without necessarily overcoming the myotonia. Thiel (1967) described a case in which the myotonic episodes were directly attributable to the action of suxamethonium.

Patients with dystrophia myotonica may also have some cardiac or endocrine dysfunction. Regional analgesic techniques are well tolerated. The use of respiratory depressant drugs should be strictly limited. If general anaesthesia is required halothane (which is rapidly eliminated) is most useful.

MALIGNANT HYPERPYREXIA

This newly-discovered syndrome represents one of the most interesting yet baffling conditions associated with anaesthesia. Originally described in North

America (Saidman *et al.*, 1964; Stephen, 1967; Relton *et al.*, 1966; Wilson *et al.*, 1967) it has now been recognised in reports from all over the world.

The paradox of the situation is that in ordinary circumstances the onset of general anaesthesia abolishes the ability of a patient to make heat, so that (unless he can shiver) his body temperature gradually falls to that of his environment (i.e. he becomes poikilothermic). In modern operating theatres with air-conditioning, therefore, it is often difficult to prevent the onset of insidious hypothermia. Yet, in the rare instance of malignant hyperpyrexia, it is possible for the anaesthetised patient to raise his body temperature at the phenomenal rate of 1°C every 5–10 minutes.

Clinical Features

Often the patient is young and healthy, undergoing some relatively minor procedure, and in most cases suxamethonium has been used for intubation. In some of these cases the anaesthetist has observed a stiffness or rigidity of the jaw muscles on intubation, which is usually attributed to an inadequate effect of the muscle relaxant. In malignant hyperpyrexia this rigidity persists and is not abolished by *d*-tubocurarine. In other cases – particularly those who have not received suxamethonium – the induction of anaesthesia is normal and the first untoward signs do not develop until about 30–45 minutes from the start. The anaesthetist may observe a tachycardia, a rise in blood pressure, and an increase in ventilation. A particular feature is a hot, dry skin with flushed facies and ultimately peripheral cyanosis.

All these signs indicate a greatly increased metabolism. This rise in metabolic rate is so great that the normal inspired oxygen concentration is outstripped and the patient gradually becomes hypoxic. Simultaneously, the enormously increased carbon dioxide concentration during expiration often leads to exhaustion of the soda-lime canister. If untreated, the body temperature will continue to rise, the pupils become fixed and dilated, and death ensues due either to cardiac failure or cerebral damage.

Investigations made during the pyrexia have revealed a raised serum potassium level, high carbon dioxide tension, and a grossly acidic pH of the blood (Saidman *et al.*, 1964; Thut and Davenport, 1966; Davies *et al.*, 1969).

Aetiology

As stated above, the cause of this condition is unknown, but the principal theories can be considered under three headings:

1. **Bacteraemia or septicaemia.**—Although the commonest cause of pyrexia in clinical medicine is the presence of bacteria or viruses in the circulation, a very careful examination of samples of blood from patients dying of malignant hyperpyrexia has failed to reveal any such cause (Hogg and Renwick, 1966; Wilson *et al.*, 1967). Similarly, a study of the infusion fluids produced completely negative findings (Papper, 1968 – personal communication). For these reasons it seems unlikely that infection is responsible for malignant hyperpyrexia.

2. **Hereditary metabolic defect.**—In a study of various family histories certain interesting observations have been made. For example, Britt and his colleagues (1969) found a family of 115 people in the Wisconsin area. Twenty of this family

received a general anaesthetic whilst in good health, yet eight of them died. Again, Denborough and his associates (1962) reported another family of 116 people in Australia. Thirty-seven of them received general anaesthesia and ten died. Furthermore, Relton and his co-workers examined four sisters and found that one had died under anaesthesia. The remaining three sisters produced twenty-two children between them, and one half of this number died under general anaesthesia – eight with known hyperpyrexia.

Such figures are so alarming that it is impossible to believe that a hereditary defect is not in some way responsible. Isaacs and Barlow (1970) took the matter a stage further and investigated ninety-nine relatives of a patient who had developed malignant hyperpyrexia. They found that the resting levels of serum creatin phosphokinase and aldolase were raised in a significantly high proportion of their patients. They concluded that the high level of these muscle enzymes was evidence of a subclinical myopathy and that pre-operative estimations might reveal potential sufferers. Further support for the hereditary metabolic defect is given by the observations of Furniss (1970) that hyperpyrexia in association with muscle rigidity occurred predominantly in those patients under the age of twenty. It was argued that a congenital defect would be most likely to be revealed by the young rather than the old.

Support for the hereditary defect theory is also given by the finding that hyperpyrexia occuring during anaesthesia is occasionally observed in pigs. Hall *et al.* (1966) found three pigs from the same litter of the Landrace-Wessex strain who developed hyperpyrexia after an injection of suxamethonium. An even more interesting finding was that of Harrison and his associates (1969) who were working on the problem of liver transplantation in the pig. By chance, they came across the fact that one in every four pigs of the pure Landrace strain would develop rigidity and hyperpyrexia if given an injection of suxamethonium. Furthermore, other anaesthetic agents such as halothane and chloroform could also produce this response, though ether, thiopentone and trichloroethylene would not do so.

Britt and Kalow (1970) reviewed the possible aetiology of this condition and concluded that "the malignant hyperthermia which occurs on the basis of a genetic defect in Landrace pigs is not only clinically identical with the human syndrome but also identical in many of the biochemical features". In a later investigation they reported on the study of muscle biopsy specimens of two patients who had previously undergone an episode of malignant hyperpyrexia accompanied by muscle rigidity. They found that in each instance the calcium uptake in the sarcoplasmic reticulum was low after exposure to halothane. They concluded that the lesion in the rigid type of the condition was due to an inability of the sarcoplasmic reticulum to store calcium. This meant that the concentration of calcium in the cytoplasm remained and the enzyme myosinadeno triphosphatase was not activated in the usual manner. The result was that the myofibrils remained locked together in a persistent contraction. They were unable to suggest the aetiology of those cases in which hyperpyrexia occurred in the absence of muscle rigidity.

One of the more tempting explanations for this remarkable phenomenon is that it is concerned with the uncoupling of the oxidative phosphorylate ion mechanism in muscle cells (see below).

Uncoupling of oxidative phosphorylation.—In normal circumstances when hydrogen passes along the respiratory chain the energy released in the process is coupled with the conversion of adenosine di-phosphate (ADP) to adenosine tri-phosphate (ATP). In this case ATP is acting as a store of energy ready for any future use such as a muscle contraction. This conversion of ADP to ATP is termed oxidative phosphorylation. However, certain chemical agents (e.g. dinitrophenol) can uncouple this process so that hydrogen still passes down the chain but the energy released is no longer able to be stored as ATP. In other words, adenosine di-phosphate is no longer converted to adenosine tri-phosphate, with the result that an enormous amount of energy is released as heat and cannot be stored as adenosine tri-phosphate. Furthermore, the fact that the ATP level is low leads to muscle rigidity.

Szent-Gÿorgyi (1944) in his classical studies of muscle metabolism, demonstrated that rigors or rigidity of muscle was due to a lack of ATP. Thus, it has been suggested that the pyrexia and rigidity of malignant hyperpyrexia could be explained on the basis of certain anaesthetics acting (like dinitrophenol) in producing uncoupling of oxidative phosphorylation in certain patients with a hereditary metabolic defect. In support of this theory, Snodgras and Piras (1966) have shown that both halothane and chloroform are capable of uncoupling of oxidative phosphorylation in rat liver mitochondria.

Pollack and Watson (1971) have drawn attention to the similarity of the condition of hyperpyrexia and muscle rigidity that sometimes follows treatment with a combination of tricyclic antidepressants and monoamine oxidase inhibitors. In this case it has been suggested that the hypermetabolic state is induced by increasing the intracellular concentration of cyclic adenosine monophosphate (AMP). This, therefore, might offer an alternative pathway to the uncoupling of oxidative phosphorylation quoted above.

3. **Drug-induced hyperpyrexia.**—Since the syndrome of malignant hyperpyrexia was first described, there has been a strong tendency to associate the aetiology with either suxamethonium or halothane. The principal reason is that most reported cases had received one of these agents, but this might only reflect on their popularity. The important feature of muscle rigidity has further supported the role of suxamethonium as it could be argued that it was producing a contracture (prolonged muscle shortening) rather than the usual short-lived depolarisation with contraction. Furthermore, as both acetylcholine and neostigmine are known to enhance the myotonia and rigidity of dystrophia myotonica, it is hardly surprising that the possible existence of latent myotonia was suggested.

The evidence against this theory is first, that not all cases of malignant hyperpyrexia have received suxamethonium or halothane. Second, only about half those that do receive these agents develop rigidity at the onset: the remainder only reveal muscle stiffness after an hour or more has elapsed and some not until rigor mortis sets in after death. Last, in only a small number of cases has it been possible to demonstrate evidence of myotonia at post-mortem (Saidman *et al.*, 1964; Papper, personal communication, 1968).

Conclusion

With the limited evidence available, the most likely explanation of malignant hyperpyrexia is that it is a condition induced by certain anaesthetic agents (particularly suxamethonium and halothane) in patients with a hereditary metabolic defect.

Treatment

The rise of body temperature in malignant hyperpyrexia is so rapid that anything less than extreme measures of cooling will prove inadequate. The simplest and most readily available method will probably be surface cooling with ice bags, water, and fans. Once the condition has been diagnosed, the operation must be stopped at the earliest opportunity, the anaesthetic drugs withdrawn, and cooling commenced. Immersion cooling is the most effective method of rapidly reducing body temperature but such facilities are often not readily available. The perfusion of cold fluids in a balloon in the stomach has also proved effective (Papper, 1968).

Whatever method is used, it is the speed and effectiveness that are of paramount importance. For this reason the cooling blanket is often inadequate. Whilst the cooling process is being instituted steps should also be taken to correct the hypoxia, carbon dioxide retention and metabolic acidosis with the appropriate therapy. It must also be remembered that the sudden application of cold to the skin or viscera will lead to vasoconstriction. Unless vasodilatation is brought about the core temperature will rise even faster than would normally be anticipated since the raging furnace within cannot dissipate its heat. If adequate precautions are not taken (such as the careful application of vasodilator drugs) then the myocardium may fail under these conditions.

FAMILIAL PERIODIC PARALYSIS

This is a hereditary condition characterised by recurrent attacks of flaccid paralysis. It is associated with an abnormality of potassium and is of two types:

(*a*) *Hypokalemic form.*—The attacks of paresis are generally associated with a fall in the serum potassium concentration, but there is no critical level for the onset of muscular weakness. These attacks can be induced by the administration of glucose, insulin and epinephrine. During the paresis the muscles will no longer respond to electrical stimulation. Nevertheless, the volume of the muscle fibre increases, suggesting that not only potassium but water enters the fibre during the period of paralysis.

There is no data available of the response of these patients to anaesthetic drugs.

(*b*) *Hyperkalaemic form.*—This is a much rarer form of this condition and is associated with a high serum potassium.

ACUTE INTERMITTENT PORPHYRIA

It has been suggested (Goldberg, 1959) that this condition is caused by the lack of substance X which is responsible for the metabolism of the myelin sheath of nerves. Substance X is normally believed to be present in the liver and the whole process is summarised in Fig. 8.

The absence of the myelin sheath may occur in any nerve throughout the body. The demyelination process, therefore, leads to a widespread variety of

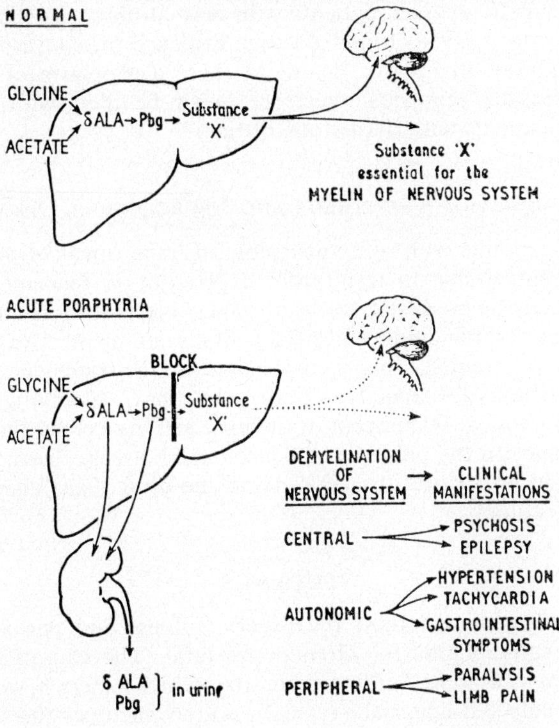

(δ ALA = δ aminolaevulic acid. Pbg. = Porphobilinogen.)

33/FIG. 8.—Diagram to explain a possible mechanism for acute porphyria.

symptoms; these may take the form of psychoses, cardiovascular disturbances or skeletal muscle paralysis. The barbiturate and narcotic drugs are strictly contra-indicated in this condition as they are believed to depress the formation of substance X in the liver.

Cavanagh and Ridley (1967) pointed out that in acute intermittent porphyria there is an increased urinary excretion of δ aminolaevulic acid due to the increased activity of the enzyme δ ALA synthetase. Furthermore, ALA synthetase requires pyridoxal phosphate as a co-factor. Experimentally in rats it can be shown that reducing the pyridoxal phosphate leads to demyelination of the nerves. Therefore, in man in the presence of an abnormal gene acute intermittent porphyria might be due to a fall in pyridoxal phosphate level.

DERMATOMYOSITIS

Certain patients with this disease show a profound peripheral weakness and in some this is associated with an improvement on the administration of an anti-cholinesterase drug. There is also a close relationship between carcinoma and dermatomyositis.

In an investigation of ten patients with dermatomyositis, Churchill-Davidson and Richardson (1958) found positive evidence of a myasthenic response (using decamethonium) in two: in one of these a neoplasm of bronchus was present. The muscle relaxants, therefore, must be used with caution when anaesthetising patients with dermatomyositis.

Summary of Anaesthesia and Neurological Disease

In general, patients with some neurological impairment of muscle function are extremely susceptible to respiratory depressant or relaxant drugs; a fact which could safely be predicted, for in normal subjects the respiratory reserve is such that a considerable number of muscle fibres can be inactive yet the minute volume is well maintained. This is emphasised by the statement, "tidal volume is only 10 per cent of vital capacity in a normal patient," signifying that theoretically it is possible to lose 90 per cent of the fibre activity before diminished ventilation is apparent. In the presence of neurological disease the requirements for anaesthetic drugs are drastically reduced and the dose of any agent used should be selected accordingly.

TETANUS

This disease is characterised by muscle stiffness and paroxysmal spasms which, unless suitably treated, often prove fatal. The causative organism is *Clostridium tetani*, a spore-bearing anaerobe, which enters a wound or small abrasion from infected material—typically soil. Sometimes the site of entry is small and almost insignificant, but from the moment that the bacilli reach the wound the incubation period of the disease begins. This may be as brief as two or three days or as long as three weeks, but the longer the duration of time between infection and the onset of the first symptoms, the more favourable is the ultimate prognosis.

Route of Infection

The bacilli produce an extremely potent toxin which is absorbed by the motor end-plate and gradually passes centripetally to affect the motor nerve cells in the anterior horn of the spinal cord. From the spinal cord the toxin ascends to the bulbar nuclei (Wright, 1954).

Symptoms and Signs

The earliest sign of the onset of tetanus is usually stiffness in the muscles of the jaw which progresses to trismus—hence the name "lockjaw". The masseter muscles are thus the first to become involved but very soon other muscles of the face are affected so that "risus sardonicus" results. The tendon jerks throughout the body become exaggerated as a general increase in muscle tone becomes apparent, until on a sudden stimulation muscle spasm everywhere becomes accentuated resulting in a full scale paroxysm. At this stage there is generally marked opisthotonos, and breathing is hampered. Death may occur suddenly from anoxia due to respiratory difficulties, or after several days as a result of exhaustion.

The spasms of tetanus are very similar to those found in patients with strychnine poisoning but the essential difference lies in their constancy. The muscles of patients with tetanus are in a state of continuous contraction which is accentuated during a paroxysm. Parsons and Hofman (1966) have demonstrated that tetanus toxin lowers the pre-synaptic membrane potential. In strychnine poisoning the muscles are completely relaxed in the intervals between paroxysms.

Prophylaxis

Active immunisation involves the use of a suitably modified tetanus toxoid. This can be given at all times of the year without the risk of allergic or other complications. Tetanus toxoid is often combined with the toxoids of diphtheria and whooping cough as a triple toxoid. Prophylaxis is assured by two doses, the second following the first at an interval of not less than six weeks. Booster doses should be administered at not more than five-yearly intervals.

Anti-tetanic serum, for many years recommended for passive immunisation, is not now recommended for prophylaxis since there is insufficient evidence that it is effective, and its administration is sometimes followed by severe serum sensitivity reactions. It is, however, used for the treatment of tetanus (see below).

Tetanus prophylaxis depends upon the type of wound present, but the following principles are general. The wound, however trivial, must be given an early and thorough toilet with débridement if this is necessary and possible; only clean wounds should be sutured. A course of antibiotic (penicillin or tetracycline) must be administered if the wound is dirty or débridement is not possible. Active immunisation with tetanus toxoid must be started unless the patient is already immunised. A patient is only considered immune when two doses of toxoid have been given within the previous twelve months, or a subsequent booster dose within five years of the injury. If in doubt, it is best to give a booster dose of tetanus toxoid, and if the patient has never been actively immunised every effort must be made to ensure that a second dose is given to complete the course not less than six weeks later.

Treatment (See also Chapter 15)

In recent years anaesthetists have been able to give practical help in the treatment of many patients with tetanus, particularly when the muscles of respiration have been involved. But the many papers in the literature on the subject of treatment testify to the variety of opinions that exists on this subject. Mild cases of tetanus are seldom a problem and can be adequately treated by careful nursing and simple sedation. The onset of paroxysms of muscle spasm calls, however, for more radical treatment. Here the muscle relaxants used to produce total paralysis, combined with artificial respiration, some sedation and careful control of nourishment and the electrolyte balance offer great possibilities (Woolmer and Cates, 1952; Shackleton, 1954; Lassen *et al.*, 1954; Smith *et al.*, 1956; Wilton *et al.*, 1958). But it is certainly not yet established that such treatment is always better than heavy central sedation with a drug such as chlorpromazine. Perhaps the difficulty in standardising the degree of severity of the disease accounts for the differences in opinion. Very severe cases are most probably best treated by full paralysis with a muscle relaxant. Smythe and Bull (1961) have added weight to the argument in favour of the more liberal use of complete paralysis and controlled ventilation. They report that in the years 1951–57 there were 55 cases of tetanus neonatorum which were primarily treated by sedation. The mortality was about 50 per cent. When they adopted tracheostomy and I.P.P.R. in the more serious cases the death rate fell to 11 per cent in the next twenty-five cases. Smythe (1963) has emphasised the importance of total muscle paralysis, regular tracheal suction, and adequate ventilation with regular monitoring of the carbon dioxide level of the blood.

General measures.—Careful and devoted nursing in a quiet and darkened room is essential, and every effort must be made to avoid triggering off paroxysmal spasms. The value of anti-tetanus serum once the disease has become apparent is still debated, but nevertheless it should be given as soon as possible. Provided there is no reaction to a test dose, an intravenous dose of 100,000 units has been recommended. Patel and his colleagues (1963), however, in a series of 3,295 cases of tetanus, found that there was no significant difference in the overall mortality provided a minimum dose of 10,000 units was used. Increasing the dose did not improve the results. Then the wound should be attended to surgically and under general anaesthesia. Penicillin should be administered prophylactically to control secondary infection both in the wound and in the lungs, and other antibiotics prescribed should a particular organism suggest their use.

Sedation.—Although the use of muscle relaxants may still be debated, there is complete agreement that the patient must be adequately sedated throughout the whole period of muscular irritability. Bromethol, thiopentone and paraldehyde have been advocated in the past, particularly when heavy sedation has been indicated. More recently chlorpromazine has found favour and this drug is discussed more fully below. Phenobarbitone or a shorter-acting barbiturate, such as pentobarbitone, is generally satisfactory when other drugs are being used to control the muscle spasm. In severe cases an intravenous infusion of 0·4 per cent thiopentone has been found useful (Jenkins and Luhn, 1962). A sufficient quantity must be given to reduce the patient's awareness of his surroundings, yet to leave the respiratory centre relatively unaffected.

Muscle relaxation.—The muscle relaxants, by blocking activity at the neuromuscular junction, prevent the contraction of the muscle fibres. Because of its duration of action, *d*-tubocurarine has proved the most successful, but suxamethonium has also been advocated. Full paralysis of the body, including the muscles of respiration, must be produced and maintained, tracheostomy performed and intermittent positive-pressure respiration carried out with the aid of a mechanical respirator. For details of the care of patients during long-continued artificial respiration see Chapters 4 and 15. Once tracheostomy has been performed under general anaesthesia, full narcosis is no longer necessary; indeed the maintenance of anaesthesia with nitrous oxide throughout the period of treatment—a matter of weeks for many patients—may be dangerous. Bone marrow depression with an acute aplastic anaemia has been recorded during such treatment (Lassen *et al.*, 1956). It has also been suggested as a concomitant of continuous treatment with large doses of *d*-tubocurarine. Such aplasia might also be due to the effects of prolonged inhalation of a high concentration of oxygen. The evidence to support these theses is scanty and far from conclusive, but since continuous general anaesthesia is unnecessary it should not be practised.

Chlorpromazine has a number of actions of specific value in the treatment of tetanus. It depresses the internuncial neurones of the spinal cord when given in large doses and has an effect on the basal ganglia in the brain. It will abolish the muscle spasm of experimental tetanus in rabbits (Hougs and Andersen, 1954; Kelly and Laurence, 1956). Webster (1962) concludes that chlorpromazine reduces the muscle spasms of tetanus by an action on the reticular system with the aid of the tranquillising effect also reducing the impact of afferent stimuli. Chlorpromazine can be used clinically to control tetanus with some sedative effect but without loss of consciousness and without any clinical impairment of respiratory activity. Laurence and his colleagues (1958) used 100 to 150 mg. of chlorpromazine intramuscularly four- to six-hourly for adult patients and seldom exceeded a total of 1 g. in 24 hours. An intravenous dose of the same size was occasionally used when a spasm urgently needed controlling. For neonates Laurence gave 20–25 mg. approximately four-hourly, using a total of about 220 mg. in 24 hours. These same workers compared a series of patients treated with chlorpromazine with a series treated with barbiturates—adults, phenobarbitone 200 mg. intramuscularly three- to six-hourly or amylobarbitone intramuscularly or intravenously 0·25–1·0 g. for urgent control, neonates phenobarbitone 60 mg. six- to eight-hourly at first and at longer intervals after the first two or three days —and found no statistically significant difference in the outcome of the tetanus. They commented, however, that chlorpromazine is easier to manage than barbiturates since it does not cause loss of consciousness nor noticeable respiratory depression. On the other hand, there is increasing evidence that chlorpromazine alone does not produce sufficient mental sedation to make the patient entirely comfortable, even though it may be controlling the muscle spasm very satisfactorily. It is thus best combined with a small dose of a barbiturate.

Mephenesin—acting as it does on the internuncial neurones of the spinal cord—is theoretically a very valuable drug in the treatment of tetanus and clinically it has been used with success (Parkes, 1954; Docherty, 1955; Webster, 1962). Nevertheless, although it is satisfactory in the treatment of mild and moderate cases, it has three principal disadvantages in the severe case. First, if large quantities of the 10 per cent solution of mephenesin are given intravenously, the patient rapidly develops haemoglobinuria. This complication, which is probably due to the high osmotic pressure of the solution, can be largely avoided by diluting the solution to an isotonic level before administration. Secondly, the solution contains alcohol so that if large quantities are given over a long period, the amount of alcohol consumed must also be taken into account. Thirdly, if the oral route of administration is used, the local analgesic action of the solution on the pharyngeal and laryngeal mucosa may prove sufficiently potent to permit aspiration of fluids into the trachea. Since chlorpromazine is so successful in the management of at least the mild and moderate cases of tetanus, there does not nowadays appear to be any point in using mephenesin.

Nutrition and fluid balance.—In a severe case of tetanus the treatment is likely to continue for at least two weeks. It is important, therefore, to ensure that an adequate fluid and caloric intake is maintained during this period. Intragastric feeding is both easier and preferable to intravenous infusion but carries with it the risk of regurgitation and inhalation of stomach contents. If, however, tracheostomy has been necessary, a cuffed tube will avoid such a complication.

The daily caloric intake should be not less than 2,000 (preferably 2,500) and the total fluid intake should aim at 3·5 litres/diem with a urinary output of not less than 2 litres/diem. If intravenous therapy is used it is advisable to insert either a cannula or a polythene tube into a vein to allow full mobility while nursing the patient.

Discussion

In practice it is the assessment of the progress of the disease that suggests the form of treatment. The clinical picture may change in a matter of hours, let alone days. At the earliest stage, as soon as a tentative diagnosis is made, the administration of a drug such as chlorpromazine would seem reasonable. The dosage must be large and fully adequate to control and prevent paroxysms. In certain cases it may be justifiable to combine this treatment with tracheostomy to avoid laryngeal crises in a patient particularly sensitive to such a complication. At the first sign that full control with chlorpromazine is not possible, a change to muscle relaxants and full paralysis must be made. To delay and risk death from respiratory inadequacy during a paroxysm is dangerous and unnecessary. Although radical treatment has undoubtedly led to a reduction in the mortality from severe tetanus, it is also unfortunately true that some cases die despite adequate control of their muscle spasms. This suggests that toxaemia or some long-lasting effect of the tetanus toxin on the central nervous system still plays a part in the severity of the disease.

REFERENCES

ANDERSON, H. J., CHURCHILL-DAVIDSON, H. C., and RICHARDSON, A. T. (1953). Bronchial neoplasm with myasthenia. Prolonged apnoea after administration of succinylcholine. *Lancet*, **2**, 1291.

BRITT, B. A., and KALOW, W. (1970). Malignant hyperpyrexia: aetiology unknown. *Canad. Anaesth. Soc. J.*, **17**, 316.

BRITT, B. A., LOCHER, W. G., and KALOW, W. (1969). Hereditary aspects of malignant hyperthermia. *Canad. Anaesth. Soc. J.*, **16**, 89.

BROWN, G. L., and HARVEY, A. M. (1939). Congenital myotonia in the goat. *Brain*, **62**, 341.

BURNET, F. M. (1962*a*). Auto-immune disease—experimental and clinical. *Proc. roy. Soc. Med.*, **55**, 619.

BURNET, F. M. (1962*b*). Role of the thymus and related organs in immunity. *Brit. med. J.*, **2**, 807.

BURNS, B. D., and PATON, W. D. M. (1951). Depolarization of the motor end-plate by decamethonium and acetylcholine. *J. Physiol. (Lond.)*, **115**, 41.

BURNS, B. D., PATON, W. D. M., and DIAS, M. V. (1949). Action of decamethonium iodide (C.10) on the demarcation potential of cats' muscle. *Arch. Sci. physiol.*, **3**, 609.

CAMPBELL, H., and BROMWELL, E. (1900). Myasthenia gravis. *Brain*, **23**, 277.

CAVANAGH, J. B., and RIDLEY, A. R. (1967). The nature of the neuropathy complicating acute intermittent porphyria. *Lancet*, **2**, 1023.

CHURCHILL-DAVIDSON, H. C., and RICHARDSON, A. T. (1953). Neuromuscular transmission in myasthenia gravis. *J. Physiol. (Lond.)*, **122**, 252.

Churchill-Davidson, H. C., and Richardson, A. T. (1955). Mestinon in myasthenia gravis. *Lancet*, **1**, 1123.

Churchill-Davidson, H. C., and Richardson, A. T. (1957). Myasthenic crisis. Therapeutic use of *d*-tubocurarine. *Lancet*, **1**, 1221.

Churchill-Davidson, H. C., and Richardson, A. T. (1958). Personal communication.

Churchill-Davidson, H. C., and Richardson, A. T. (1961). "A study of neuromuscular transmission in one hundred cases of myasthenia gravis". *Proceedings 2nd International Symposium on Myasthenia Gravis.* Ed. H. R. Viets. Springfield, Ill.: Charles C. Thomas.

Coërs, C., and Desmedt, J. E. (1959). Nise en evidence d'une malformation caracteristique de la junction neuromusculaire dans la myasthenie. *Acta neurol. belg.*, **59,** 539.

Coërs, C., and Woolf, A. L. (1959). *The Innervation of Muscle*, pp. 101–7 and 134–5. Oxford: Blackwell Scientific Publications.

Dahlback, O., Elmqvist, D., Johns, T. R., Radner, S., and Thesleff, S. (1961). An electrophysiologic study of the neuromuscular junction in myasthenia gravis. *J. Physiol.* (*Lond.*), **156,** 336.

Davies, R. M., Packer, K. J., Titel, J., and Whitmarsh, V. (1969). Case report: malignant hyperpyrexia. *Brit. J. Anaesth.*, **41,** 703.

Denborough, M. A., Forster, J. F. A., Lovell, R. R. H., Maplestone, P. A., and Villiers, J. D. (1962). Anaesthetic deaths in a family. *Brit. J. Anaesth.*, **34,** 395.

Desmedt, J. E. (1957). Nature of the defect of neuromuscular transmission in myasthenic patients; post-tetanic exhaustion. *Nature* (*Lond.*), **179,** 156.

Desmedt, J. E. (1961). "Neuromuscular defect in myasthenia gravis". *Proceedings 2nd International Symposium on Myasthenia Gravis.* Ed. H. R. Viets. Springfield, Ill.: Charles C. Thomas.

Docherty, D. F. (1955). Tetanus treated with intravenous mephenesin. *Lancet*, **1,** 437.

Eaton, L. M., and Claggett, O. T. (1955). Present status of thymectomy in the treatment of myasthenia gravis. *Amer. J. Med.*, **19,** 703.

Eaton, L. M., and Lambert, E. H. (1957). Electromyography and electric stimulation of nerves in diseases of motor unit. Observations on myasthenic syndromes associated with malignant tumours. *J. Amer. med. Ass.*, **163,** 1117.

Elmquist, D., Hofmann, W. W., Kugelberg, J., and Quastel, D. M. J. (1964). An electro-physiological investigation of neuromuscular transmission in myasthenia gravis. *J. Physiol.* (*Lond.*), **174,** 417.

Erb, W. (1879). Ueber einen neuen, wahrscheinlich bulbären Symptomencomplex. *Arch. Psychiat. Nervenkr.*, **9,** 336.

Foldes, F. F. (1970). Regional intravenous neuromuscular block: a new diagnostic and experimental tool. In: *Progress in Anaesthesiology*, p. 425 (Proc. 4th World Congr. Anaesthesiol.). Amsterdam: Excerpta Medica.

Foldes, F. F., and McNall, P. G. (1962). Myasthenia gravis. A guide for anesthesiologists. *Anesthesiology*, **23,** 837.

Furniss, P. (1971). The aetiology of malignant hyperpyrexia. *Proc. roy. Soc. Med.*, **64,** 216.

Geschwind, N., and Simpson, J. A. (1955). Procaine amide in the treatment of myotonia. *Brain*, **78,** 81.

Goldberg, A. (1959). Acute intermittent porphyria. *Quart. J. Med.*, **28,** 1183.

Goldflam, S. (1893). Ueber einen scheinbar heilbaren bulbärparalytischen Symptomencomplex mit Betheiligung der Extremitäten. *Dtsch. Z. Nervenheilk.*, **4,** 312.

Grob, D., Johns, R. J., and Harvey, A. M. (1955). Alterations in neuromuscular transmissions in myasthenia gravis as determined by studies of drug action. *Amer. J. Med.*, **19,** 684.

HALL, L. W., WOOLF, N., BRADLEY, J. W. P., and JOLLY, D. W. (1966). Unusual reaction to succinylcholine. *Brit. med. J.*, **2,** 1305.

HARRISON, G. G., SAUNDERS, S. J., BIEBUYEK, J. F., HICKMAN, R., DENT, D. M., WEAVER, F., and TERBLANCHE, J. (1969). Anaesthetic-induced malignant hyperpyrexia and a method for its prediction. *Brit. J. Anaesth.*, **41,** 844.

HENSON, R. A., RUSSELL, D. S., and WILKINSON, M. (1954). Carcinomatous neuropathy and myopathy. A clinical and pathological study. *Brain*, **77,** 82.

HOGG, S., and RENWICK, W. (1966). Hyperthermia during anaesthesia. *Canad. Anaesth. Soc. J.*, **13,** 429.

HOUGS, W., and ANDERSEN, E. W. (1954). The action of atropine, promethazine and chlorpromazine on experimental local tetanus in cats and rabbits. *Acta pharmacol.* (*Kbh.*), **10,** 227.

ISAACS, H., and BARLOW, M. B. (1970). The genetic background to malignant hyperpyrexia revealed by serum creatine phosphokinase estimations in asymptomatic relatives. *Brit. J. Anaesth.*, **42,** 1077.

JENKINS, M. T., and LUHN, N. R. (1962). Active management of tetanus. *Anesthesiology*, **23,** 690.

JOLLY, F. (1895). Ueber Myasthenia gravis pseudoparalytica. *Berl. klin. Wschr.*, **32,** 1.

KAUFMAN, L. (1960). Anaesthesia in dystrophia myotonica—a review of the hazards of anaesthesia. *Proc. roy. Soc. Med.*, **53,** 183.

KELLY, R. E., and LAURENCE, D. R. (1956). Effect of chlorpromazine on convulsions of experimental and clinical tetanus. *Lancet*, **1,** 118.

KEYNES, G. (1954). Surgery of the thymus gland. Second (and third) thoughts. *Lancet*, **1,** 1197.

LAMBERT, E. H., ROOKE, E. D., EATON, L. M., and HODGSON, C. H. (1961). "Myasthenic syndrome occasionally associated with bronchial neoplasm: neurophysiologic studies". *Proceedings 2nd International Symposium on Myasthenia Gravis*, p. 368. Ed. H. R. Viets, Springfield, Ill.: Charles C. Thomas.

LASSEN, H. C. A., BJØRNEBOE, M., IBSEN, B., and NEUKIRCH, F. (1954). Treatment of tetanus with curarisation, general anaesthesia, and intratracheal positive pressure ventilation. *Lancet*, **2,** 1040.

LASSEN, H. C. A., HENRIKSEN, E., NEUKIRCH, F., and KRISTENSEN, H. S. (1956). Treatment of tetanus. Severe bone marrow depression after prolonged nitrous oxide anaesthesia. *Lancet*, **1,** 527.

LAURENCE, D. R., BERMAN, E., SCRAGG, J. N., and ADAMS, E. B. (1958). A clinical trial of chlorpromazine against barbiturates in tetanus. *Lancet*, **1,** 987.

MACDERMOT, V. (1960). The changes in the motor end-plate in myasthenia gravis. *Brain*, **83,** 24.

MACDERMOT, V. (1961). The histology of the neuromuscular junction in dystrophia myotonica. *Brain*, **84,** 75.

NASTUK, W. L., PLESCIA, O. J., and OSSERMAN, K. E. (1959). Search for a neuromuscular blocking agent in the blood of patients with myasthenia gravis. *Amer. J. Med.*, **26,** 394.

PARKES, C. M. (1954). Mephenesin and gallamine triethiodide in tetanus. *Brit. med. J.*, **2,** 445.

PARSONS, R. L., and HOFMAN, W. W. (1966). Mode of action of tetanus toxin on the neuromuscular junction. *Amer. J. Physiol.*, **210,** 84.

PATEL, J. C., MEHTA, B. C., NANAVATI, B. H., HAZRA, A. K., RAO, S. S., and SWAMINATHAN, C. S. (1963). Role of serum therapy in tetanus. *Lancet*, **1,** 740.

POLLACK, R. A., and WATSON, R. L. (1971). Malignant hyperthermia associated with hypocalcaemia. *Anesthesiology*, **34,** 188.

RELTON, J. E. S., CREIGHTON, R. E., JOHNSTON, A. G., PELTON, D. A., and CONN, A. W.

(1966). Hyperpyrexia in association with anaesthesia in children. *Canad. Anaesth. Soc. J.*, **13,** 419.

ROWLAND, L. P., ARANOW, H., and HOEFER, P. F. A. (1961). "Observations on the curare test in the differential diagnosis of myasthenia gravis". *Proceedings 2nd International Symposium on Myasthenia Gravis.* Ed. H. R. Viets. Springfield, Ill.: Charles C. Thomas.

SAIDMAN, L. J., HAVARD, S. E., and EGER, E. I., II. (1964). Hyperthermia during anesthesia. *J. Amer. med. Ass.*, **190,** 1029.

SHACKLETON, P. (1954). The treatment of tetanus. Role of the anaesthetist. *Lancet*, **2,** 155.

SIMPSON, J. A. (1960). Myasthenia gravis. A new hypothesis. *Scot. med. J.*, **5,** 419.

SLAUGHTER, D., PARSONS, J. C., and MUNAL, H. D. (1940). New clinical aspects of the analgesic action of morphine. *J. Amer. med. Ass.*, **115,** 2058.

SMITH, A. C., HILL, E. E., and HOPSON, J. A. (1956). Treatment of severe tetanus with *d*-tubocurarine chloride and intermittent positive pressure respiration. *Lancet*, **2,** 550.

SMYTHE, P. M. (1963). Studies on neonatal tetanus and on pulmonary compliance of the totally relaxed infant. *Brit. med. J.*, **1,** 565.

SMYTHE, P. M., and BULL, A. B. (1961). Treatment of tetanus, with special reference to tracheotomy. *Brit. med. J.*, **2,** 732.

SNODGRAS, P. J., and PIRAS, M. M. (1966). Effect of halothane on rat liver mitochondria. *Biochemistry (Wash.)*, **5,** 1140.

STEPHEN, C. R. (1967). Fulminant hyperthermia during anesthesia and surgery. *J. Amer. med. Ass.*, **202,** 221.

SZENT-GŸORGYI, A. (1944). Studies on muscle. *Acta physiol. scand.*, **9,** Suppl. XXV.

THIEL, R. E. (1967). The myotonic response to suxamethonium. *Brit. J. Anaesth.*, **39,** 815.

THUT, W. H., and DAVENPORT, H. T. (1966). Hyperpyrexia associated with succinylcholine induced muscle rigidity: a case report. *Canad. Anaesth. Soc. J.*, **13,** 425.

WEBSTER, R. A. (1962). Site of action of chlorpromazine and mephenesin in experimental tetanus. *Brit. J. Pharmacol.*, **18,** 150.

WILLIS, T. (1684). *A Practice of Physick*, p. 167. London.

WILSON, R. D., DENT, T. E., TRABER, D. L., MCCOY, N. R., and ALLEN, C. R. (1967). Malignant hyperpyrexia with anesthesia. *J. Amer. med. Ass.*, **202,** 183.

WILTON, T. N. P., SLEIGH, B. E., and CHANDLER, C. C. D. (1958). Tetanus. *Lancet*, **1,** 940.

WISE, R. P. (1962). A myasthenic syndrome complicating bronchial carcinoma. *Anaesthesia*, **17,** 488.

WISE, R. P., and WYLIE, W. D. (1964). "The thymus gland. Its implications in clinical anesthetic practice." *Clinical Anesthesia: Anesthesia for Patients with Endocrine Disease*, Chapter II. Ed. M. T. Jenkins. Philadelphia: Davis & Co.

WOOLMER, R., and CATES, J. E. (1952). Succinylcholine in the treatment of tetanus. *Lancet*, **2,** 808.

WRIGHT, G. P. (1954). Tetanus. *Brit. med. Bull.*, **10,** 59.

ZAIMIS, E. J. (1951). The action of decamethonium on normal and denervated mammalian muscle. *J. Physiol. (Lond.)*, **112,** 176.

Chapter 34

GENERAL PHARMACOLOGICAL PRINCIPLES

by
S. E. Smith

The logical use of drugs depends on knowledge not only of what effects they exert on tissues but also of how these effects are produced and influenced by the disposal of the drugs concerned. In this chapter the general principles of drug action and disposal are discussed with special, though not exclusive, reference to drugs used in anaesthesia. No mention is made of inhalational anaesthetics in the disposal of which some special factors are involved; these are considered in Chapter 7. Stress is placed on the simple physical laws which determine the ways in which drugs reach their target cells, exert their effects, interact with substances of physiological importance or with other drugs and are then removed from their site of action and from the body. The actions of individual agents are discussed only in relation to the general principles concerned. For details of such actions the reader is referred to the special chapters dealing with particular groups of drugs.

Broad aspects of general pharmacology are divided here into 8 main sections:

1. Drug action on receptors
2. The passage of drugs across membranes
3. Drug concentrations in plasma
4. Protein binding
5. Drug administration
6. Drug metabolism
7. Excretion
8. Variations in response

There is, however, much overlap in the principles involved and such a division is used only for convenience.

Drug interactions may occur clinically in a number of ways; these are considered in the appropriate sections.

DRUG ACTION ON RECEPTORS

Drugs exert many different effects on different tissues. These effects are, however, specific to a greater or lesser extent in that different drugs have different effects. Living cells must therefore possess special sites of drug action, the properties of which are to react with drugs of a specific nature and to initiate a chain of events leading to the pharmacological effect. Such sites of action are receptors. So far, the nature of the receptor remains obscure; it has never been seen nor its structure identified. In some cases receptors have been counted and their surface area measured. One type has been found in association with a lipoprotein complex (Woolley and Gommi, 1964), which is not surprising in view of the location of the receptor concerned on a cell membrane. To a great extent, however, the receptor remains a concept, useful for explaining how drugs act both qualitatively and quantitatively. Recent work in this field has been the subject of a symposium (Porter and O'Connor, 1970).

Drug-receptor interactions.—The attachment of drug to receptor has been the focus of much attention. Studies of the relative effects exerted by closely related drugs have shown that it involves physical bonding by a number of forces, ionic, van der Waal, hydrogen bonding and others. The extent to which each of these contributes to the drug-receptor attraction varies from one drug to another and from one receptor to another. The number of bonds involved is usually multiple and their steric arrangement critical. It is well known, for example, that L-noradrenaline exerts many times the pressor effect of D-noradrenaline, presumably because the three-point attachment of the former is more favourable than that of the latter. Bonding arrangements have been most deeply studied for cholinergic (Waser, 1961) and adrenergic (Belleau, 1963) receptors, for which optimal drug dimensions have been calculated. The relationship between receptor structure and bonding is the subject of a recent review (Ehrenpreis *et al.*, 1969).

Drugs which stimulate receptors are agonists; those which block them are antagonists. Drugs such as nicotine and decamethonium which have both actions are referred to as partial agonists.

Quantitative aspects of drug-receptor interaction were first studied by Clark (1937), who proposed that stimulant drugs occupied receptors and that the tissue response was proportional to the number occupied. He showed that the shape of the dose-response curve could be predicted from the law of mass action in a manner similar to that proposed by Michaelis and Menten (1913) for the

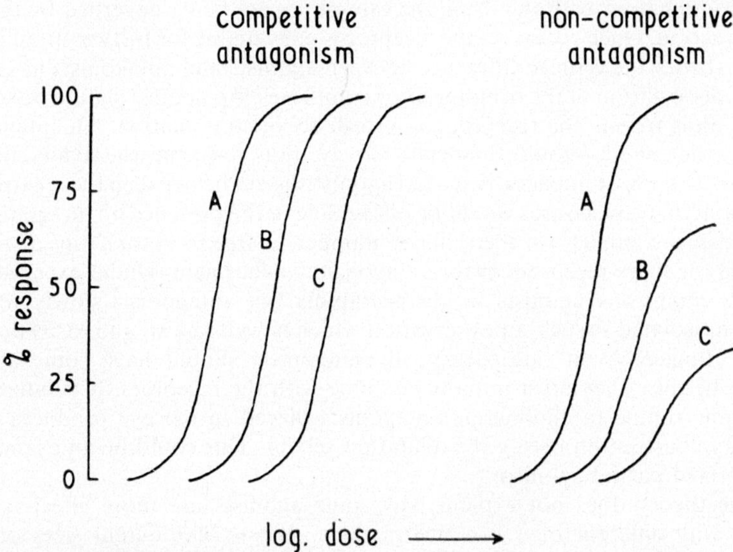

34/FIG. 1.—Theoretical log. dose-response curves for drug action. Competitive antagonists shift the curve to the right. Non-competitive antagonists alter the slope and maximal response. A = response without antagonist, B and C with increasing doses of antagonist.

behaviour of enzymes. The effect of an antagonist could be shown theoretically and in practice to modify the action of the agonist in a way which shifted the log.dose-response curve to the right without altering its shape (Fig. 1). This is competitive antagonism, seen clinically in a number of situations: atropine or tubocurarine acting against acetylcholine, phentolamine against noradrenaline, propranolol against adrenaline and nalorphine under some circumstances against morphine or pethidine. It is so called because the agonist and the antagonist compete for the same receptor.

Clark's occupation theory is not entirely satisfactory for several reasons. First, one must assume that two types of receptor occupation are possible: one for agonists which exerts an effect, another for antagonists which does not do so. Secondly, how is it possible to achieve maximal agonist responses when many receptors are occupied by antagonist molecules? In Fig. 1 the curves reach the same height even though there is antagonist present. One must assume either that the agonist displaces the antagonist from the receptor or alternatively that there is a plentiful supply of extra receptors ("spare" receptors as proposed by Stephenson, 1956) which are not needed for a maximum response. The former explanation is untrue; agonist does not displace antagonist. In anaesthetic practice, partial curarisation can be overcome by administering edrophonium, but when the edrophonium effect wears off one is left with just as much curarisation as if the edrophonium had never been given. Thirdly, how can one account for the action of partial agonists like nicotine and decamethonium which both stimulate and block receptors?

An alternative "rate" theory has been proposed by Paton (1960, 1961) which goes a long way towards overcoming these and other objections. The assumption here is that receptors are stimulated not by occupancy but momentarily by the act of combination with the drug, the rate of impact being governed by the law of mass action. Once occupied, the receptor is unavailable for further stimulation. On this theory the critical difference between agonists and antagonists lies in the rates of dissociation of the drug-receptor complexes. An agonist should dissociate rapidly, thus freeing the receptor for a fresh act of combination. An antagonist, on the other hand, should dissociate slowly, thus reducing the availability of receptors to agonist impacts. A partial agonist should lie between these extremes. Maximum tissue responses would be obtainable in the presence of antagonists by higher rates of impact on the reduced number of free receptors, thus obviating the need for spare receptors or for antagonist displacement. Under experimental *in vitro* conditions agonists would be rapidly but antagonists slowly washed out from isolated tissues, an observation which is well known and easily demonstrable. Logically, on rate theory all antagonists should have some agonist activity because they must initially combine with the receptors. It is interesting that homatropine (a cholinergic antagonist) placed in the eye produces slight pupillary constriction before the dilatation sets in. This could be an example of the expected partial agonism.

Rate theory does not explain why some agonists are more effective than others, why different ones produce maximal effects of different sizes or why log.dose-response curves for the same receptor are not parallel for all agonists. Evidently drugs have other intrinsic properties which influence the effects they induce on the receptor containing tissue.

The action of competitive antagonists serves to verify predictions implied in drug receptor interaction theory. Other types of antagonism are also demonstrable at the tissue site. Non-competitive antagonism is shown under some conditions by phenoxybenzamine. It decreases the maximal effect of alpha adrenergic stimulants and flattens the log.dose-response curve (Fig. 1). Physiological antagonism is that which occurs when two drugs have opposite actions without real interference.

For a number of reasons it is useful to have measures of potency and specificity of drug antagonists acting on particular receptors. This is achieved by the measurement of pA_x, the negative decimal logarithm of the molar concentration of the antagonist required to reduce the potency of a specified agonist x-fold after contact for a stated time (Schild, 1957). Drugs with powerful antagonist potency therefore have high pA_x values, those with weak potency low ones. For example, against histamine's action on guinea-pig ileum mepyramine has a pA_2 of about 9·4 for 14 minutes contact; i.e. $10^{-9 \cdot 4}$M mepyramine reduces the action of histamine two-fold. This and other values are given in Table 1.

34/TABLE 1

pA_2 VALUES OF DRUG ANTAGONISTS ON GUINEA-PIG ILEUM FOR 14 MINUTES CONTACT (from Schild, 1947).

Antagonist	*Against histamine*	*Against acetylcholine*
mepyramine	9·4	4·8
atropine	5·7	8·6
pethidine	6·2	5·8

Such measurements indicate the considerable specificities of mepyramine (40,000 times greater against histamine than against acetylcholine) and atropine (1,000 times vice versa) and the negligible specificity of pethidine as antagonists. One can deduce from these results the obvious clinical implications that mepyramine is a useful antihistamine but a useless anticholinergic, that atropine has the opposite properties and that pethidine is both antihistaminic and anticholinergic.

When two drugs of similar action (either agonistic or antagonistic) act together, synergistically, the resultant effect is the sum of the individual components. If the log.dose-response curves are steep this summation can result in a surprisingly large effect which is often though erroneously referred to as potentiation. It is well known, for example, that combinations of barbiturates with alcohol can produce dangerous cerebral depression, as can combinations of most central depressant drugs. The effects are the result of summation and not potentiation, the latter of which implies that the total is more than the sum of its components. Potentiation occurs almost exclusively when one drug alters the metabolism or the excretion of the other; this topic is discussed later.

Occurrences of antagonism, summation and potentiation in experimental and clinical situations are often difficult to distinguish. One useful method is the construction of isobols (Loewe, 1957), lines, analogous to isobars or isotherms on a map, joining points of equal pharmacological effect in graphs of doses of drug mixtures. Examples are shown in Fig. 2. Drug mixtures, such as barbiturates and alcohol, showing summation produce a straight-line isobol, such that combinations of two half doses produce the same effects as one whole dose (Smith and Herxheimer, 1969). In many instances, one half dose alone may

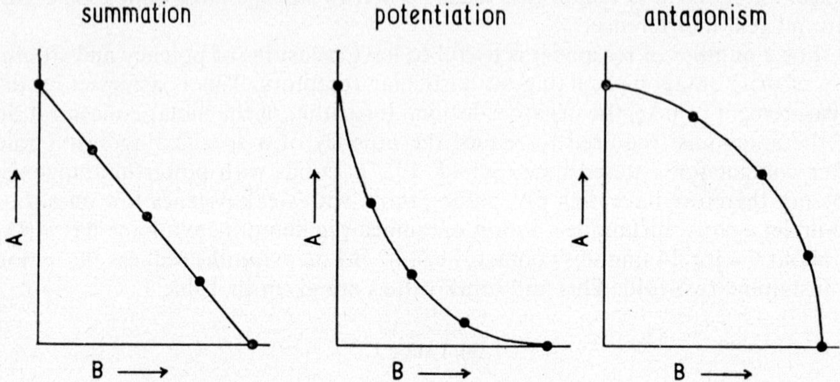

34/FIG. 2.—Theoretical isobols of drug interaction. Combined dose diagrams of equi-effective drug pairs show summation, potentiation and antagonism.

have no measurable action whatsoever (reference the steepness of the log.dose-response curve above); hence the confusion with potentiation. Deviation from the straight line indicates that the drugs interact so that greater or lesser doses are required to produce the defined pharmacological effect.

THE PASSAGE OF DRUGS ACROSS MEMBRANES

The effect of a drug at its site of action in body tissues is dependent on its presence at critical concentration at that site. To achieve this, the drug must be absorbed from its site of administration and be distributed in the body in a suitable manner, such absorption and distribution being dependent on the ability of the drug to cross cellular membrane barriers. Because the physical properties of cell membranes are similar in different parts of the body, the factors involved in absorption and distribution into different tissues are also similar.

Drugs can cross cell membranes in three ways: by diffusion, by penetration through membrane pores and by means of active transport (Christensen, 1962).

Diffusion

Many drugs used in anaesthetic and general practice are weak bases or acids which in solution are ionised to variable extents depending on the ease or difficulty with which they accept or donate protons. Conventionally this is expressed as the pK_a, the negative logarithm of the acidic dissociation constant, analogous to pH. In solution the degree of ionisation is also affected by the pH. Thus:

$$\text{for acids— } pK_a - pH = \log\frac{C_u}{C_i}$$

$$\text{for bases—} pK_a - pH = \log\frac{C_i}{C_u}$$

where C_i and C_u are the concentrations of the ionised and unionised forms respectively. The pK_a values of some important compounds are illustrated in Fig. 3.

The importance of these factors in drug absorption and distribution is that in the unionised (undissociated) form drugs have lipid solubility and are therefore able to diffuse across cell membranes, whereas in the ionised (dissociated) form they have no lipid solubility and therefore cannot diffuse across. Drugs such as barbiturates, phenothiazines and narcotic analgesics which have pK_a values close to physiological pH are about 50 per cent ionised in the body and, having reasonable lipid solubility, are therefore well absorbed from the gastro-intestinal tract, cross the blood-brain and placental barriers and are reabsorbed

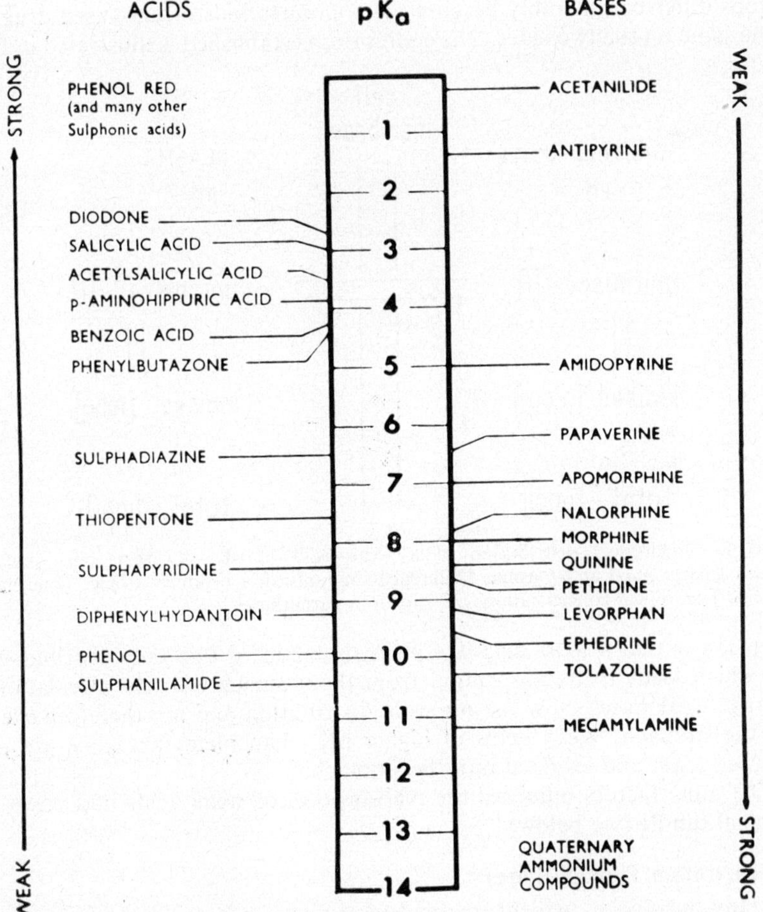

34/FIG. 3.—pK_a values of acids and bases (Brodie, 1964).

in the renal tubule. By contrast, quaternary ammonium compounds like tubocurarine and suxamethonium which are fully ionised at physiological pH have no lipid solubility and are therefore not absorbed from the gastro-intestinal tract, do not cross the blood-brain or placental barriers and are not reabsorbed in the renal tubule. They can, however, cross capillary walls and do therefore penetrate the extracellular spaces where they act.

Transfer of a drug by diffusion across a cell membrane proceeds at a rate which is proportional to its concentration. In theory this rate is unlimited and it requires no metabolic energy. The amount of drug absorbed from the gastro-intestinal tract is therefore a direct function of the dose administered; the amount that penetrates into the brain, the foetus or any other organ is a direct function of the concentration of the drug free in solution in the plasma.

Surprisingly diffusion can set up concentration gradients such that one tissue may contain much more drug than another. If there is a marked pH difference across the membrane such as exists across the gastric mucosa, total drug concentrations differ considerably because the concentrations of unionised drug must be the same on the two sides. The equilibrium established is illustrated in Fig. 4,

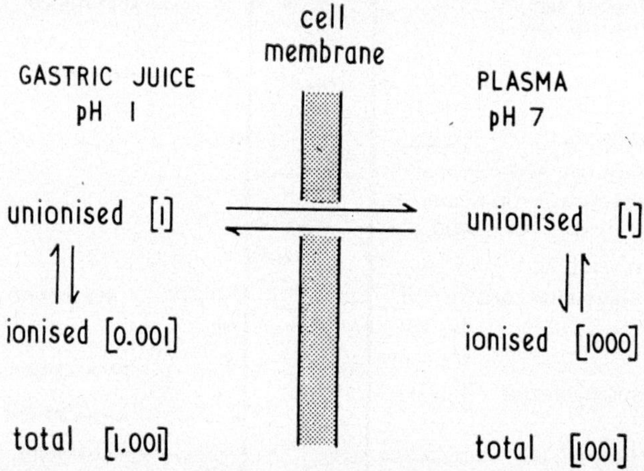

34/Fig. 4.—Theoretical distribution of a weak acid of pK_a 4·5 (e.g. phenylbutazone) between gastric juice and plasma. Differences in ionisation produce a large concentration gradient. Theoretical concentrations are shown in parentheses.

which shows that a weak acid like phenylbutazone is unevenly distributed in a way which leads to its absorption from the stomach into the circulation. By contrast, weak bases show the opposite distribution and are therefore excreted into the stomach. Weak acids of higher pK_a than phenylbutazone are partly absorbed from and excreted into the stomach.

The same factors influence the reabsorption of weak acids and bases from the renal tubule (see below).

Penetration Through Pores

Many substances which are lipid-insoluble can enter cells and penetrate membrane barriers. Such substances as water and urea do so by filtration through pores in the cell membrane. Their movement occurs by diffusion and no energy is required, though the rate is usually slow because the pores occupy only a minute fraction of the cell surface (perhaps 0·2 per cent). Inorganic ions penetrate in the same way, though the rate of their movement is limited further by the polarisation of the membrane surface. Lipid-soluble substances may be absorbed from the gastro-intestinal tract in this manner by solution in chylomicrons.

Active Transport

Many physiological substances and a few drugs are transferred across cell membranes by specialised transport systems. Such systems are thought to involve the use of carriers whose function is to combine reversibly with the substance at one surface of the membrane, transfer it to the opposite surface and release it there. Considerable concentration gradients may be set up and the process is energy-dependent, rate limited and susceptible to blockade by metabolic inhibitors. Special transport systems exist for sugars, amino-acids, inorganic ions and neurohumoral transmitters such as noradrenaline, 5-hydroxytryptamine and gamma-aminobutyric acid. Some synthetic sympathomimetic amines are carried into nerve-endings in the same manner by use of the noradrenaline carrier.

Many drugs in common use are powerful inhibitors of these transport systems and their pharmacological actions are dependent on this property. Cocaine, for example, owes its sympathomimetic action to its ability to inhibit re-uptake of noradrenaline back into nerve-endings (Iversen, 1967). Imipramine is a powerful inhibitor of 5-hydroxytryptamine uptake by platelets (Stacey, 1961); its anti-depressant effect may result from the same action in the brain. The antithyroid action of potassium perchlorate depends on its ability to antagonise thyroid iodide transport.

DRUG CONCENTRATIONS IN PLASMA

The drug concentration at its site of action is a function of its concentration in plasma. In turn the plasma concentration is influenced by the rates of drug absorption, distribution to various tissues, metabolism and excretion and the extent to which the drug is bound to plasma protein (see below). The dynamic equilibrium established is influenced also by the extent to which the drug is ionised in each body fluid. A scheme of distribution is illustrated in Fig. 5. From measurements of drug and metabolite concentrations in plasma and urine, time courses of distribution have been simulated with the help of analogue or digital computers (Wiegand and Sanders, 1964; Beckett and Tucker, 1968). Such simulations enable predictions to be made of durations of drug action and the rates at which drugs are metabolised or excreted. The rate at which a drug is disposed of is often referred to as the half-life, the time taken for its concentration in plasma to drop to a half.

Concentrations of drugs which are not significantly bound to plasma protein decay by a simple exponential whereby the concentration C at time t can be represented by the equation:

$$C = A.e^{-\beta t}$$

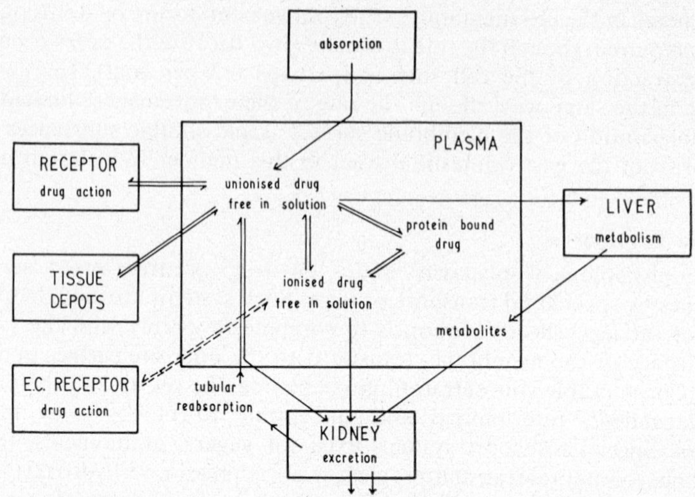

34/FIG. 5.—Distribution of drugs in the body. E.C. receptor = extracellular receptor.

where A and β are constants. This provides a straight line on a log. concentration/time graph and gives a measure of the half-life of the drug in the plasma. Concentrations of many drugs, however, do not decay in this manner, usually because they are markedly bound to plasma or tissue protein. Such binding slows the rate of drug elimination and thus curves the lower part of the line. Plasma concentrations of thiopentone and buthalitone (Kane and Smith, 1959), shown in Fig. 6, are typical of this type of curve. It can be represented by the

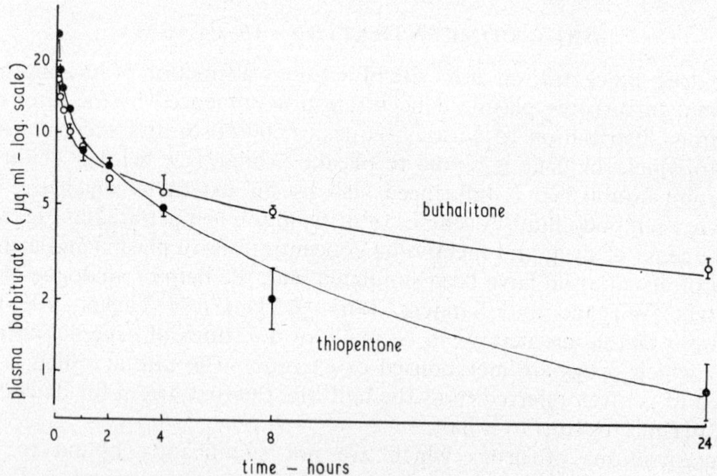

34/FIG. 6.—Plasma concentrations of thiopentone and buthalitone in healthy male subjects following administration of 11 mg./kg. i.v. Lines drawn are best fits for the equation $C = A \cdot t^{-\alpha} \cdot e^{-\beta t}$. (For details, see text). (Adopted from Kane and Smith, 1959).

sum of a number of exponential components, an approximation to which is given by the equation:

$$C = A.t.^{-\alpha}e^{-\beta t}$$

where A, α and β are constants (Anderson *et al.*, 1967). This equation fits the illustrated data closely.

The intensity of drug effect is a direct function of its concentration at the receptor site which may be intra- or extracellular. Such a concentration is influenced not only by the plasma concentration but also by local drug binding to the receptor or to other tissue components and by local ionisation. Plasma concentrations, therefore, give only an indirect indication of the pharmacologically active concentrations at the site of drug action.

PROTEIN BINDING

In the circulation many drugs are bound to plasma proteins, largely to albumin. The extent of binding varies from one drug to another and it is dependent on the drug concentration. The subject was extensively reviewed by Goldstein in 1949. The nature of the binding process is complex and probably involves a number of binding sites of variable specificity. Some of these involve van der Waal bonding, some ionic attractions and others lipophilic affinities. The latter probably account for the binding of barbiturate molecules and explain the fact that it is the ultra-short-acting drugs in the group (the most lipid-soluble) which are most highly bound. Other sites are specific for acidic drugs such as sulphonamides and coumarin anticoagulants.

The extent to which any drug is bound is influenced by its concentration, very high concentrations tending to swamp the binding sites and lower the proportion of bound drug. A rapid increase in effect and toxicity would be expected above this level. It is difficult, however, to predict the exact behaviour because at high concentrations subsidiary binding mechanisms may come into play. For example, thiopentone may then be bound in both its ionised and un-ionised forms. At low concentrations very high proportions of circulating drugs may be bound: thiopentone about 85–90 per cent, digitoxin 95 per cent and warfarin 98 per cent. Among such drugs there remain only small proportions available for diffusion to the tissues where the drugs exert their pharmacological actions, are metabolically degraded or filtered by the kidneys. Extensive binding therefore has the effects of limiting potency and prolonging duration of action. Bound drug is thought to be pharmacologically inactive, though the bound fraction is in a state of dynamic equilibrium with that free in solution and can therefore exert effects once it is released.

Protein binding may vary in different individuals. It is diminished by low circulating albumin levels such as occur in liver disease and malnutrition. Patients with severe liver disease are therefore intolerant of drugs which are usually highly bound because much larger proportions of the drugs circulate free in solution in plasma and are available for diffusion into the tissues. Binding of particular drugs may also be reduced by the presence of other drugs which compete for the same binding sites; this induces true potentiation. Clinically such interactions occur most obviously with acidic drugs such as sulphonamides, penicillins, salicylates, coumarin anticoagulants, sulphonylureas, phenylbutazone and methotrexate. In some instances interactions produced by concurrent administration of two or more of these drugs may be of minor importance. If they include sulphonylureas such as tolbutamide or anticoagulants such as warfarin, however, unexpected and often dangerous potentiation may occur. For further discussion of this subject the reader is referred to a recent survey by Prescott (1969).

Tissue proteins may also bind drugs. Barbiturates in particular are bound to homogenates of most tissues including brain (Goldbaum and Smith, 1954), the extent corresponding roughly with the distribution of these drugs *in vivo*. It is not clear how this influences the effects of such drugs at their sites of action. Some drugs have affinities for particular tissue proteins which influence their distributions in other ways. Antimony, for example, and probably other heavy metals are largely and rapidly bound by the liver because of its content of protein thiol groups (Smith, 1969). Clinically this has the effect of reducing plasma concentrations of the metals to very low levels in a short time, whereas concentrations in the liver may remain high for several weeks.

DRUG ADMINISTRATION

Intravenous

In anaesthetic practice many drugs are administered intravenously. Concentrations of these drugs in the plasma and indirectly in the tissues rise almost instantaneously to a maximum and the time to onset of drug effect is reduced to a minimum. Mixing of the drug solution with the whole circulating plasma volume is relatively slow, however, and is not achieved for several circulation times. Until mixing has occurred, therefore, some blood contains much more drug than the remainder, this effect being most marked immediately following the drug's administration. The difference is exaggerated further if the injection is given quickly and reduced if it is given slowly. After rapid injection a bolus of drug solution of high concentration may travel in the circulation almost unmixed for long enough to exert a powerful drug action; if the total amount of drug administered is mixed completely by slow injection no effect may result. This "slug effect" was described by Paton (1960) and is illustrated in Fig. 7.

In clinical practice such slug effects have a profound influence on drug action. They explain, for instance, why a rapid injection of a small dose of an intravenous anaesthetic exerts a brief but powerful effect, whereas a slowly injected much larger dose has no effect at all. In patients with heart failure, of course, the time to onset of drug effect is greatly increased because of the slow circulation.

Measurements of plasma concentrations of intravenously administered drugs within 5 minutes or so of administration are therefore of doubtful value. They may produce higher or lower levels depending on the phase of mixing.

Intramuscular, Subcutaneous and Intraperitoneal

Following drug administration by these routes, absorption into the circulation occurs depending on the physico-chemical properties of the drug, the extent to which the drug solution spreads in the tissue and the state of the local circulation. Insoluble forms of drugs such as procaine penicillin and depot preparations of insulin are only slowly absorbed because solution must first occur. Given intraperitoneally, drugs are very rapidly absorbed because of rapid spread of solution over the absorptive surface and the highly vascular nature of that surface. Intramuscular and subcutaneous routes allow slower absorption because of reduced spread and blood supplies in these regions. The rates are therefore

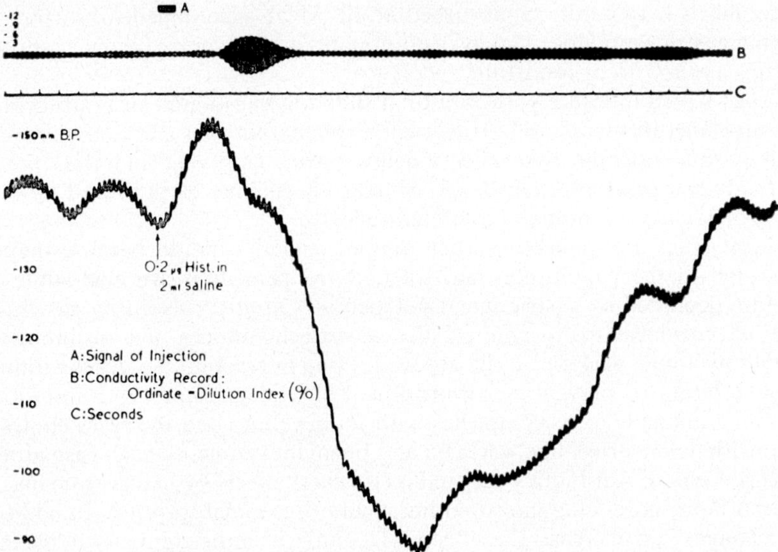

34/Fig. 7.—Slug effect of rapid i.v. administration of histamine 0·2 μg. in 2 ml. saline in an anaesthetised cat. Upper tracing: conductivity of carotid arterial blood gives a measure of drug concentration. Lower tracing: arterial blood pressure. The drug effect follows the slug but wanes in spite of a rising drug concentration with recirculation (Paton, 1960).

further slowed if the regional blood supply is reduced as in states of shock or the addition of vasoconstrictors to the drug solutions. The times to peak plasma concentrations, and indirectly to drug effects elsewhere, are therefore progressively prolonged.

Oral

Absorption of drugs from the gastro-intestinal tract is influenced by the factors mentioned above and also by some special factors. Most rapid and effective absorption occurs at either end, from the oral and the rectal mucosae following local administration. Such mucosae are highly vascular and, provided the drug is lipid soluble, allow rapid transfer of the drug into the circulation. More importantly, such routes allow drug passage directly to the systemic circulation and not into the portal circulation, thus avoiding the immediate effect of the liver which in many cases inactivates drugs by metabolism. Such drugs as glyceryl trinitrate or isoprenaline, given sublingually, exert systemic actions within 2 minutes. When swallowed, these drugs have no effect at all.

When swallowed, some drugs, mostly weak acids, can be absorbed from the stomach if they are largely unionised at the pH of the stomach contents (see above). Such absorption is prevented if the subject has consumed antacids in a quantity sufficient to raise the intragastric pH significantly. Most drugs, however, are absorbed from the small intestine because the pH of the intestinal contents is suitable and because the absorptive surface area of the intestinal mucosa is enormously increased by the presence of villi. Absorption is limited by the presence of food in the lumen such that some drugs taken after, rather than before, meals may hardly be absorbed at all. Meals also impede absorption by delaying gastric emptying. Malabsorption states may of course hinder absorption of drugs as they do of foodstuffs.

Drugs which interfere with intestinal function can inhibit drug absorption. Thus atropine-like drugs and drugs such as phenothiazines and antidepressants which produce atropine-like effects delay gastric emptying and thus prevent intestinal absorption of other drugs. Similar effects may be produced by shock states when gastric motility is inhibited reflexly.

Many drugs are ineffective when administered by mouth because they are inactivated in the gastro-intestinal tract. Some penicillins are acid-labile and therefore degraded by gastric juice; polypeptides are hydrolysed by gastric and intestinal enzymes; many amines such as catecholamines and histamine are oxidised by amine oxidases in the gut wall. Drug interaction can occur within the lumen, limiting or preventing absorption. Thus, magnesium- and aluminium-containing antacids form complexes with tetracyclines and the resin cholestyramine with acidic drugs like warfarin and phenylbutazone. In each case absorption is prevented. Antibiotics may indirectly exert effects by inducing changes in bacterial flora, producing intestinal hurry and thus malabsorption. In addition, such changes can increase the effects of coumarin anticoagulants if bacterial production of vitamin K (with which the anticoagulants compete) is reduced.

Inhalation

See Chapter 7.

DRUG METABOLISM

Most drugs are chemically altered in the body by metabolism, usually in the liver. For detailed reactions of particular drugs the reader is referred to the appropriate chapters. A number of general processes are involved:

Oxidation

Oxidising or hydroxylating enzymes are responsible for the degradation and inactivation of many drugs. The processes, which require triphosphopyridine nucleotide and oxygen, may involve oxidation, dealkylation, deamination, ring or side-chain hydroxylation and sulphoxide formation. Drugs which are affected by oxidative reactions include barbiturates and thiobarbiturates, ethanol, phenothiazines, sympathomimetic and other amines, analgesics and antidepressants.

Reduction

Reduction is important for only a small number of drugs and the alcoholic products which result are usually further oxidised, often quite rapidly. Adrenaline and noradrenaline are partly excreted as reduced products (phenylglycols) and chloral derivatives are reduced to yield the active metabolite trichloroethanol.

Hydrolysis

Hydrolytic splitting is responsible for the destruction of a number of compounds such as cardiac glycosides, anthracene purgatives, procaine and choline esters. Drugs such as procaine and suxamethonium are hydrolysed by plasma butyryl (pseudo) cholinesterase as well as in the liver.

Conjugation

Synthetic processes in the liver are responsible for the formation of conjugates, particularly glucuronides and sulphates. Catecholamines, phenols, steroids, chloral derivatives and tribromoethanol are all partly excreted in this form. Aromatic acids may be conjugated with glycine and some amines such as sulphonamides and histamine by acetylation.

The processes of metabolic transformation in the liver and elsewhere have the physico-chemical effect of making drugs less lipid soluble. For this reason the metabolites are more readily excreted by the kidney and are usually less potent. Potency may be only partly lost in any one metabolic stage and total inactivation thus often depends on more than one stage. For example, heroin (diacetylmorphine) is degraded partly to morphine which has approximately half the potency. Thiobarbiturates are converted in part to their equivalent oxybarbiturates with similar result. In some cases metabolism activates the drug with the opposite effect that the metabolite is more potent than its precursor. Thus phenacetin is converted into paracetamol, cascara into emodin and methyldopa into methyl-noradrenaline; all these conversions result in greater activity.

The metabolism of drugs in the liver occurs largely in the microsomes, the enzymes of which are located in the smooth-surfaced endoplasmic reticulum. Liver damage induced by acute or chronic disease suppresses the activity of these enzymes and induces intolerance to drugs which are normally inactivated by them. Thus patients with cirrhosis or hepatic secondary carcinomatous deposits show exaggerated and prolonged effects to compounds like ethanol, barbiturates and opiates.

Microsomal enzymes can also be affected by drugs. Administration of the experimental compound SKF 525A or of monoamine oxidase inhibitors inhibits the enzymes so that drug metabolism is slowed. Thus monoamine oxidase inhibitors render the patient intolerant not only of sympathomimetic amines which are metabolised by monoamine oxidase but also of drugs which are degraded in microsomes, amphetamine, pethidine, ethanol, phenothiazines and most hypnotics. Drugs can also have the opposite effect. Administration of barbiturates, dicophane (DDT) and some other compounds causes enzyme induction; there is proliferation of the endoplasmic reticulum, increased enzyme formation and resultant accelerated drug metabolism. Patients under this influence become tolerant of drugs which are metabolised by these enzymes. Pharmacological aspects have been reviewed by Conney (1967) and clinical aspects by Burns and Conney (1965) and Prescott (1969).

The clinical implications of enzyme induction are still under investigation. In many instances a two- or three-fold increase in drug metabolism is probably of little consequence. In two fields, however, important interactions can result with unfortunate effects if the patient stops taking the inducing drug (e.g. a barbiturate). The two fields concern the use of coumarin anticoagulants and oral hypoglycaemic agents, most of which are inactivated by microsomal enzymes. The danger is likely to arise in patients who are stabilised on these drugs while in hospital (during which time they often take barbiturates) and then leave hospital (stopping the barbiturates) and continue on the same daily dosage. The inducing effect of the barbiturate wears off in about 2–3 weeks and the original dosage of anticoagulant or hypoglycaemic agent becomes too great. Enzyme induction by phenobarbitone has recently been employed successfully to lower serum bilirubin concentrations in the newborn (Trolle, 1968).

EXCRETION

Drugs and their metabolites are excreted from the body largely by the kidney. Some compounds, however, appear in the faeces, either because they are incompletely absorbed after oral administration or because they are excreted into the intestine via the bile. The purgative phenolphthalein and many antibiotics are re-cycled in this way with resultant prolongation of their actions. Some ions such as bromides, iodides and lithium are also secreted by mucous membranes and by sweat glands.

Disposal by the kidney depends on a balance of three processes:

Glomerular Filtration

Drug free in solution in plasma enters the renal tubular lumen by filtration, protein-bound drug being retained unless albuminuria is present. The glomerular filtrate therefore contains drug or metabolite at the same concentration as is present free in the plasma.

Tubular Reabsorption

During its passage down the tubule, the filtrate is reduced in volume by the removal of sodium, chloride and water, so that drug or metabolite concentration increases progressively to a very high level. Under the concentration gradient thus established between tubular fluid and blood stream the drug may then diffuse passively back into the circulation, limiting its excretion. Only un-ionised drug can cross the tubular cell membrane, however, with the result that the reabsorption of weak acids and bases is strongly pH dependent. This provides the basis for alteration of the urinary pH in cases of drug poisoning. In poisoning by weak acids like barbiturates and salicylates, alkalinisation of the urine with citrates or bicarbonate increases ionisation, limits reabsorption and therefore increases their excretion in the urine *Per contra*, the same effect is produced in poisoning by weak bases such as amphetamines and phenothiazines by acidification of the urine with ammonium chloride. The effectiveness of such manoeuvres is dependent on effective increases in the ionised fraction of the drugs in the urine. Drugs which are totally ionised, even at the extremes of urinary pH, are not reabsorbed at all. Thus drugs such as decamethonium and neostigmine, which are quaternary ammonium compounds and fully ionised, are relatively rapidly eliminated by the kidney.

Tubular reabsorption is diminished if the flow of urine is increased because tubular fluid becomes concentrated to a lesser degree and the drug gradient across the tubular cell membrane is reduced. Thus forced diuresis increases the elimination of many drugs in proportion to the urine flow.

Tubular Secretion

A number of compounds, mostly organic acids, are actively secreted by the tubular cells into the urine. The elimination of such compounds such as penicillins and sulphonamides is thereby accelerated. A few weak bases are also secreted actively but it is doubtful whether the process is important quantitatively.

Tubular secretion is susceptible to inhibition by drugs. Thus probenecid which antagonises the secretion of organic acids has been used to delay the elimination of penicillins. Probenecid, salicylates and phenylbutazone also antagonise active tubular reabsorption of urates; hence their use in the treatment of gout.

The elimination of drugs by the kidney may be retarded in renal insufficiency, largely because of the reduced glomerular filtration rate. Though this is not usually of clinical significance, with a few drugs it is important if they are liable to produce toxic effects at only moderately increased blood concentrations. Such drugs as streptomycin and kanamycin may accumulate in these circumstances to produce labyrinthine and auditory damage. Monitoring blood concentrations provides the only safeguard.

VARIATIONS IN RESPONSE

Healthy normal individuals vary in their response to drugs. This variation is quantitative and sometimes qualitative. It can occur because of differences in receptor sensitivity or because of variations in drug metabolism. It is at least partly under genetic control though how much this affects the clinical situation is not clear. Pharmacogenetics is the subject of a monograph by Kalow (1962).

Some response variations due to differences in receptor sensitivity are known. Thus people with blue eyes are more sensitive to the local actions of sympathomimetic amines than are people with brown eyes. Paxson (1932) recorded

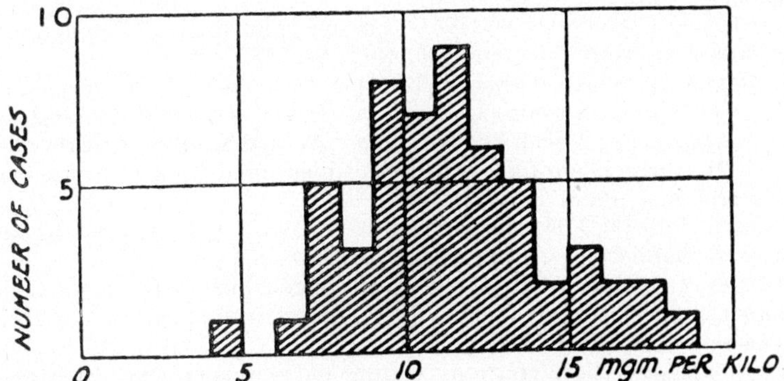

34/Fig. 8.—Frequency distribution of dose of sodium amylobarbitone needed to induce suitable anaesthetic conditions for forceps delivery in 55 subjects. (Paxson, 1932).

similar variations in sensitivity by measuring the dose of sodium amylobarbitone needed in the presence of nitrous oxide to induce suitable anaesthetic conditions for forceps delivery. His results are illustrated as a frequency distribution of doses in Fig. 8. The subjects' requirements varied about 4-fold. A qualitative variation in response to drugs is shown by the reactions to barbiturates of patients with porphyria.

Much interest has centred recently on genetically-determined individual variations in drug metabolism. For the anaesthetist the most important of these are the variations in suxamethonium metabolism caused by atypical varieties of plasma butyryl (pseudo) cholinesterase (see Chapter 31). These varieties are determined by the presence or absence of particular genes. Similar factors affect the metabolism of isoniazid and sulphadimidine by acetylation in the liver. The rate of drug metabolism is also affected by multiple genes which influence the quantity of enzyme present. Information derived from twin studies has shown that inheritance greatly influences the half-lives of dicoumarol, antipyrine and phenylbutazone (Vesell and Page, 1968) and steady-state blood concentrations of nortriptyline (Alexanderson *et al.*, 1969). Inheritance, therefore, appears to play an important part in determining rates of drug inactivation. It remains to be seen whether receptor sensitivity is similarly affected.

REFERENCES

Alexanderson, B., Evans, D. A. P., and Sjöqvist, F. (1969). Steady-state plasma levels of nortriptyline in twins: influence of genetic factors and drug therapy. *Brit. med. J.*, **4,** 764.

Anderson, J., Tomlinson, R. W. S., Osborn, S. B., and Wise, M. E. (1967). Radiocalcium turnover in man. *Lancet*, **1,** 930.

Beckett, A. H., and Tucker, G. T. (1968). Application of the analogue computer to pharmacokinetic and biopharmaceutical studies with amphetamine-type compounds. *J. Pharm. Pharmacol.*, **20,** 174.

Belleau, B. (1963). An analysis of drug receptor interactions. *Proc. First International Pharmacological Meeting*, **7,** 75.

Brodie, B. B. (1964). In: *Absorption and Distribution of Drugs.* Ed. by T. B. Binns. Edinburgh: E. & S. Livingstone.

Burns, J. J., and Conney, A. H. (1965). Enzyme stimulation and inhibition in the metabolism of drugs. *Proc. roy. Soc. Med.*, **58,** 955.

Christensen, H. N. (1962). *Biological Transport.* New York: W. A. Benjamin.

Clark, A. J. (1937). General pharmacology. In: *Heffter's Handbuch der experimentellen Pharmakologie*, Erg. Vol. 4. Ed. by Heubner, W. and Schüller, T. Berlin: Springer.

Conney, A. H. (1967). Pharmacological implications of microsomal enzyme induction. *Pharmacol. Rev.*, **19,** 317.

Ehrenpreis, S., Fleisch, J. H., and Mittag, T. W. (1969). Approaches to the molecular nature of pharmacological receptors. *Pharmacol. Rev.*, **21,** 131.

Goldbaum, L. R., and Smith, P. K. (1954). The interaction of barbiturates with serum albumin and its possible relation to their disposition and pharmacological actions. *J. Pharmacol. exp. Ther.*, **111,** 197.

Goldstein, A. (1949). The interactions of drugs and plasma proteins. *Pharmacol. Rev.*, **1,** 102.

Iversen, L. L. (1967). *The Uptake and Storage of Noradrenaline in Sympathetic Nerves.* London: Cambridge Univ. Press.

KALOW, W. (1962). *Pharmacogenetics: Heredity and the Response to Drugs*. Philadelphia: W. B. Saunders.

KANE, P. O., and SMITH, S. E. (1959). Thiopentone and buthalitone: the relationship between depth of anaesthesia, plasma concentration and plasma protein binding. *Brit. J. Pharmacol.*, **14,** 261.

LOEWE, S. (1957). Antagonisms and antagonists. *Pharmacol. Rev.*, **9,** 237.

MICHAELIS, L., and MENTEN, M. L. (1913). Die Kinetik des Invertinwirkung. *Biochem. Z.*, **49,** 333.

PATON, W. D. M. (1960). The principles of drug action. *Proc. roy. Soc. Med.*, **53,** 815.

PATON, W. D. M. (1961). A theory of drug action based on the rate of drug-receptor combination. *Proc. roy. Soc., B,* **154,** 21.

PAXSON, N. F. (1932). Obstetrical anesthesia and analgesia with sodium iso-amylethyl barbiturate and nitrous oxideoxygen: results in obstetrical practice. *Curr. Res. Anesth.*, **11,** 116.

PORTER, R., and O'CONNOR, M., Eds. (1970). *Molecular Properties of Drug Receptors* (Ciba Foundation Symposium). London: J. & A Churchill.

PRESCOTT, L. F. (1969). Pharmacokinetic drug interactions. *Lancet*, **2,** 1239.

SCHILD, H. O. (1947). pA, a new scale for the measurement of drug antagonism. *Brit. J. Pharmacol.*, **2,** 189.

SCHILD, H. O. (1957). Drug antagonism and pA_x. *Pharmacol. Rev.*, **9,** 242.

SMITH, S. E. (1969). Uptake of antimony potassium tartrate by mouse liver slices. *Brit. J. Pharmacol.*, **37,** 476.

SMITH, S. E., and HERXHEIMER, A. (1969). Toxicity of ethanol-barbiturate mixtures. *J. Pharm. Pharmacol.*, **21,** 869.

STACEY, R. S. (1961). Uptake of 5-hydroxytryptamine by platelets. *Brit. J. Pharmacol.*, **16,** 284.

STEPHENSON, R. P. (1956). A modification of receptor theory. *Brit. J. Pharmacol.*, **11,** 379.

TROLLE, D. (1968). Decrease of total serum-bilirubin concentration in newborn infants after phenobarbitone treatment. *Lancet*, **2,** 705.

VESELL, E. S., and PAGE, J. G. (1968). Genetic control of dicoumarol levels in man. *J. clin. Invest.*, **47,** 2657.

WASER, P. (1961). Chemistry and pharmacology of muscarine, muscarone and some related compounds. *Pharmacol. Rev.*, **13,** 465.

WIEGAND, R. G., and SANDERS, P. G. (1964). Calculation of kinetic constants from blood levels of drugs. *J. Pharmacol. exp. Ther.*, **146,** 271.

WOOLLEY, D. W., and GOMMI, B. W. (1964). Serotonin receptors: V selective destruction by neuraminidase plus EDTA and reactivation with tissue lipids. *Nature (Lond.)*, **202,** 1074.

Chapter 35

SEDATIVE AND HYPNOTIC DRUGS

Normal Sleep

ALTHOUGH sleep is a well-known phenomenon which is easy to define in broad terms, its scientific explanation is difficult. It is associated with a number of changes in body function: a reduction in awareness culminating in unconsciousness, progressive relaxation of body musculature, slight hypotension, bradycardia and reduction of the metabolic rate. The exact origin of sleep in the brain is not fully understood but probably arises in an integrated system involving ascending and descending pathways in the reticular formation, the cerebral cortex, intralaminary nuclei of the thalamus, caudate nucleus, posterior hypothalamus and anterior third of the pons. There appears to be no sleep centre as such, though electrical stimulation of certain parts of the reticular formation induces sleep in animals.

Different depths of sleep can be distinguished by the ease or difficulty with which the subject can be awakened and these have been correlated with electroencephalographic changes (Loomis *et al.*, 1938). Five levels were distinguished: from A (drowsiness) to E (deep sleep). The deepest level occurs only for brief periods, usually early in the night. These types of sleep are usually referred to as orthodox or "slow wave" sleep. The normal person spends approximately one-quarter of the night in paradoxical or "rapid eye movement" (REM) sleep, this type being characterised by fast cortical electrical activity, greater reductions in skeletal muscle tone and rapid movement of the eyes. REM sleep is associated with dreaming (Aserinsky and Kleitman, 1953). The changes in electroencephalographic and electromyographic patterns during the two types of sleep are shown in Fig. 1.

Total deprivation of sleep for 100 hours or more induces psychotic changes, sometimes involving hallucinations and delusions. Specific deprivation of REM sleep for much shorter periods induces anxiety and irritability, difficulties with memory and coordination and increased appetite (Dement and Fisher, 1963). Such deprivation is followed by compensatory increases of REM sleep during the following nights (Dement and Fisher, 1963).

The Effects of Drugs on Sleep

Hypnotic and anaesthetic agents induce sleep by mechanisms which are as yet poorly understood but which probably involve suppression of both cortical and subcortical activity. Progressive anaesthesia is associated with widespread inhibition, manifest by the absence of neuronal discharge. Electroencephalographic patterns change with the depth of anaesthesia (see Chapter 22). During deep anaesthesia REM periods are absent, but in light anaesthesia they are often present and dreaming is common. The content of such dreams is usually highly emotional and often of a sexual nature, the latter being one reason why a chaper-

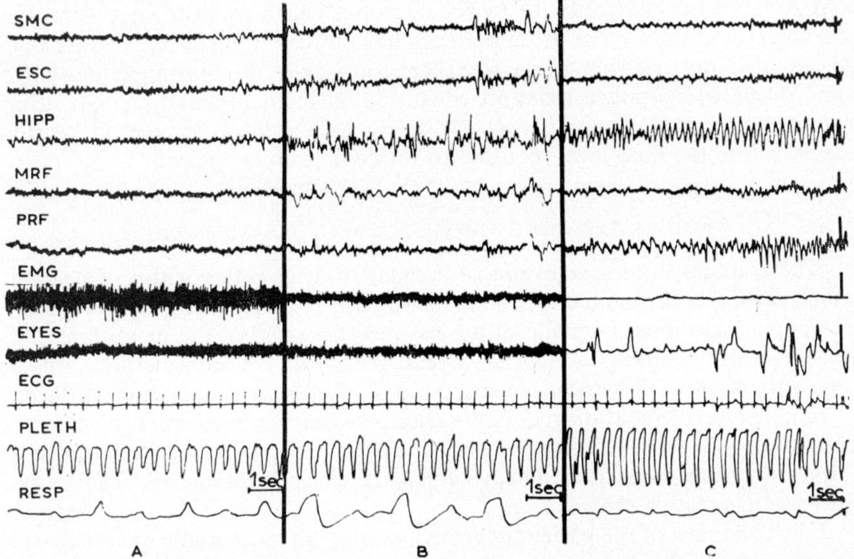

35/Fig. 1.—Polygraphic aspects of the two states of sleep. (A) Wakefulness: Fast cortical and subcortical activity. (B) Slow sleep: Cortical and subcortical spindles and slow waves. Persistence of nuchal EMG activity (EMG). No eye movements (EYES). (C) P.S.: Fast cortical activity similar to (A). Regular θ-activity in the ventral hippocampus (HIPP). Phasic activity in the pontine reticular formation (PRF). Complete disappearance of nuchal EMG activity and rapid eye movements. Changes in respiratory activity (RESP) and the plethysmographic index (PLETH). SMC = sensorimotor cortex; ESC = ectosylvian cortex. MRF = midbrain reticular formation. Scale: 1 sec; 50μV.

one is so essential when minor operations are being performed under solely gaseous anaesthetics.

All the commonly employed hypnotic agents (barbiturates, meprobamate, methaqualone and benzodiazepines) lessen the incidence and shorten the periods of REM sleep (Oswald, 1968), thus prolonging periods of orthodox sleep. With repeated administration recovery of REM sleep occurs, after which withdrawal of the drug precipitates massive compensatory increases of REM periods. Such observations probably explain why patients so often complain of sleeping badly the first night or two after stopping treatment with hypnotics and why so many become habituated to such drugs. Antidepressant drugs and narcotics usually have similar effects but major tranquillisers like reserpine and phenothiazine derivatives may increase REM sleep and shorten the latent period before its onset. Of particular interest are some recent findings that these and other drugs may influence dream content as well as duration (Kramer *et al.*, 1966).

SEDATIVES AND HYPNOTICS

A sedative is a remedy that allays excitement, an hypnotic a drug that induces sleep: neither of these groups of drugs has any direct effect on the sensation of pain. When administered to a patient in pain they may, by depression of inhibitions, produce restlessness and make management more difficult. Pain can be controlled by the analgesics, or by the narcotics which produce sleep as well as relieving pain. Since most of these drugs have different effects depending upon dosage, it is not possible to classify them too rigidly. For instance, most hypnotic drugs will produce sedation when administered in small enough doses; but the converse does not necessarily apply, as a sedative may produce side-effects before the dose level required to produce sleep is reached.

Factors Affecting the Response to Sedative Drugs

The response to a given dose of a sedative drug varies within wide limits which depend in the main on the state of the patient. When prescribing a sedative an appreciation must be made of the desired effect and of the condition of the patient—this is often difficult to assess accurately. A consideration of the following points will help to obviate the risk of gross over- or under-dosage.

The degree of sedation required varies between the production of calmness and a sleep at least deep enough so that the patient has no recollection of leaving the ward or the prick of an intravenous needle. Anaesthesia may also be produced with sedative drugs.

The condition of the patient depends not only on measurable quantities such as age and weight, but also on factors such as muscularity, obesity, general fitness and previous medication with alcohol or narcotics.

There is doubt as to whether the sedatives and narcotics do actually depress the basal metabolic rate but reflex irritability varies in proportion to metabolism, so that consideration of the changes in metabolic rate is a guide to the likely effect of a given dose of sedative.

The effect of age.—The metabolic rate, which is low at birth, rises sharply until the sixth year. It then falls, and after a rise at puberty, it is back to the same value in the twentieth year as it was at the end of the first year of life. Thereafter the metabolic rate steadily declines until in old age it has returned to the same figure as in the first few weeks of life.

The effect of body weight.—Where precision of effect is required, the doses of drugs are best related to the weight of the patient, before making the necessary adjustments for the other factors. But here again allowance must be made, and the dose reduced for excess fat—or water as in patients with ascites and oedema—or increased for patients who are unusually muscular.

The effect of emotion.—The state of reflex irritability depends mainly on the emotional condition of the patient. A placid individual needs less in the way of sedatives than one in whom the nervous system is in a state of hyperactivity.

The effect of metabolic diseases.—Where the basal metabolic rate is altered by a disease such as hyperthyroidism, the action of a given dose of sedative is likely to be less evident and of briefer duration than in a normal subject. Conversely where the metabolic rate is depressed the action of sedatives is profound and prolonged.

The effect of previous medication with alcohol or narcotics.—Long-continued use of these agents produces tolerance to the psychic effects of sedatives, and larger doses may be required; but due to possible disturbances of metabolism already existing—particularly in the liver—sedatives may have a prolonged action and any depression of respiration and the circulation, which are the most important side-effects of these drugs, may be accentuated. In these circumstances a small dose given in plenty of time, so that the position can be reassessed and a further dose given if required, is the best policy.

The effect of the presence of pain.—Since drugs of this group have few if any analgesic properties, they should not be given to those who are in pain, because by removing the higher cortical functions they tend to allow the patient to over-react and produce restlessness. This may then be difficult to control with analgesics or narcotics without producing dangerous depression. The addition of a simple analgesic such as acetylsalicylic acid to a sedative will often make all the difference, and avoid the need for a narcotic. When long-acting sedatives are required pre-operatively it is important that they should be given early enough to allow most of their effect to wear off by the end of the operation, in order to avoid restlessness later.

The general fitness of the patient.—This is the most difficult factor to assess, especially for the inexperienced, and yet is the most vital because in those who are ill the margin of safety is narrow and the required dose may be extremely small. In all cases of doubt as to the fitness of the patient caution must be exercised. A dose which is thought to be too small is first given and when this has had time to act, which will vary with the drug and the route of administration, an assessment of the effect produced can be made and a further dose of the same or another drug added. Small repeated doses are safer than large doses at longer time-intervals. Patients who are ill frequently require very small quantities of a sedative to produce sleep, and these patients, who are least able to withstand any added insults, can all too easily have their respiration or circulation grossly depressed. It is often wiser not to use any pre-operative sedatives in the very ill, thus avoiding relative overdosage. Relative overdosage can cause respiratory depression which in turn allows respiratory obstruction to occur easily, and this may pass quietly into respiratory failure.

Classification of Sedative and Hypnotic Drugs

These drugs may be classified into four main groups:

1. Ethane derivatives.
   - Paraldehyde.
   - Ethyl alcohol.
   - Chloral hydrate and derivatives.
   - Bromethol.
2. Barbiturates.
3. Non-barbiturate hypnotics and sedatives.
4. Tranquillisers (see Chapter 36).

Many non-barbiturate hypnotics are used as tranquillisers, and some tranquillisers as hypnotics or sedatives. The distinction between the two is largely inappropriate.

ETHANE DERIVATIVES

Paraldehyde $(CH_3CHO)_3$

Paraldehyde was discovered by Wiedenbusch in 1829 and introduced into medicine by Cervello in 1882.

Preparation.—

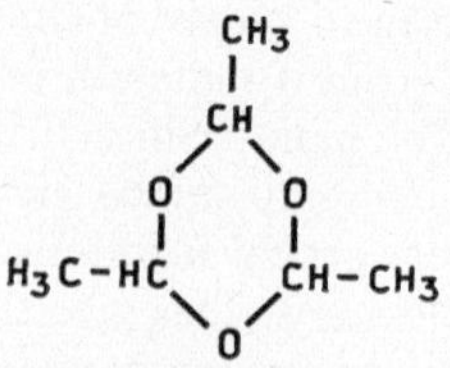

```
           CH3
           |
           CH
          /  \
         O    O
         |    |
   H3C-HC      CH-CH3
          \  /
           O
```

Paraldehyde

Paraldehyde is formed by the polymerization of three molecules of acetaldehyde in the presence of a trace of concentrated sulphuric acid.

Physical properties.—Paraldehyde is a colourless, inflammable liquid, boiling point 122° C, with a pungent odour and an unpleasant burning taste. The solubility in water is only one part in eight at 25° C but it is very soluble in lipoid solvents.

Paraldehyde decomposes in the presence of light, air, or acids to acetaldehyde, and should therefore be kept in dark, well-stoppered bottles.

Pharmacological actions.—Paraldehyde is a mild hypnotic, but occasionally produces excitation. Habituation may follow its use but is very infrequent.

It has a wide margin of safety and produces sleep in ten to fifteen minutes after the administration of the usual oral dose of 2 to 8 ml.

Paraldehyde produces similar changes to the barbiturates in the EEG of resting man. In therapeutic doses it does not cause cardiac or respiratory depression, but with gross overdosage it may cause death from respiratory failure and cardiovascular depression.

The metabolic fate of paraldehyde in man is not definitely known, but in patients with liver disease the duration of hypnosis is greatly prolonged, and it is thought that about 80 per cent of the paraldehyde administered is destroyed in the liver, the rest being excreted by the lungs unchanged. Soon after a dose has been given, paraldehyde can be smelt in the breath, where its continued excretion can be discerned for many hours. This smell is unnoticed by the patient. A trace is excreted by the kidneys in man, but bilateral nephrectomy in animals does not alter the duration of hypnosis.

Clinical uses.—Paraldehyde can be administered by mouth, by rectum, and by intramuscular or intravenous injection. It is rapidly absorbed and produces sleep lasting six to eight hours, within ten to fifteen minutes of its administration.

By mouth the dose is 2 to 8 ml. which is administered in the proportion of 4 ml. to 40 ml. of water—at which strength it is completely soluble—to avoid the burning taste and gastric irritation.

By rectum it is administered in a dose of 0·5 ml./kg. body weight to a maximum of 40 ml., diluted with ten times its volume of physiological saline.

When rectal paraldehyde is being administered prior to surgery it should be given at least two hours before the time of operation to ensure that the patient is asleep and to avoid prolonged post-operative recovery. If a half to two-thirds the normal rectal dose is given two hours before operation and is followed by an injection of morphine 10 mg. and hyoscine 0·4 mg. even fit adults are unlikely to remember being brought to the theatre and there is no post-operative restlessness.

By intramuscular injection the dose is 2 to 8 ml. Paraldehyde is self-sterilizing so that it can be drawn straight from the bottle before injection. The dose by intravenous injection is from 2 to 8 ml. This should be given slowly to avoid a coughing spasm, but should one occur, the rate of injection must be further slowed when the spasm will soon pass. The duration of hypnosis following intravenous administration of paraldehyde is not prolonged, and there is little or no depression of respiration or of the circulation.

The advantages of paraldehyde are its safety and the absence of cardiac or respiratory depression, which make it particularly useful in the elderly. Its disadvantages are its taste, gastric irritation, and its excretion in the breath, although this is not complained of by the patient. It is particularly useful in controlling manic states and post-operatively where sleep is required without depression, as in neurosurgery.

Ethyl Alcohol (Ethanol) (C_2H_5OH)

Alcohol is a substance of more social than medical value, although a "night-cap" is a very useful hypnotic for the elderly. Its interest to the anaesthetist lies in its history and in its value for dealing with patients who are used to large quantities of it and who are therefore likely to be tolerant to the anaesthetic drugs. Alcohol was one of the first substances used to relieve pain: the giving of spirits in large quantities to patients prior to operations before 1847 is well-known. Although it may well have produced amnesia, the patients required to be restrained, since they were usually still in the so-called "excitement stage" of anaesthesia.

When a patient who is tolerant to alcohol has his normal quota withheld prior to anaesthesia, he may well be resistant, particularly when only nitrous oxide is available, as may be the case in the out-patient department. For such a person, the usual amount of alcohol, or even a little more—provided it can be given sufficiently far ahead to avoid the danger of aspiration from vomiting—may be helpful prior to anaesthesia.

Alcohol can be used as a sedative and source of calories by giving it well diluted intravenously, 1 g. of alcohol liberating approximately 7 calories. Fifty ml. of pure 95 per cent ethyl alcohol should be added to 1 litre of saline, or 5 per cent dextrose in water, and administered at a rate of not more than 60 drops per minute. It is oxidised at a constant rate of 10 ml. per hour, so that once the required state has been produced the rate of infusion should not exceed this figure. This procedure is particularly useful in the aged.

Chloral Hydrate ($CCl_3 . CH(OH)_2$)

Chloral hydrate was first prepared by Liebig in 1832 by passing gaseous chlorine into ethyl alcohol, a method by which it is still prepared. The chemistry was described by Dumas in 1834 and it was introduced as a hypnotic by Liebreich (1869).

Preparation.—$2C_2H_5OH + O_2 \rightarrow 2CH_3CHO + 2H_2O$

$$CH_3.CHO + 3Cl_2 \rightarrow CCl_3.CHO + 3HCl$$
$$CCl_3.CHO + H_2O \rightarrow CCl_3.CH(OH)_2.$$

Physical properties.—Chloral hydrate is a colourless non-deliquescent crystalline substance with a pungent odour and a strongly bitter taste. It is freely soluble in water and alcohol, and 1 in 3 of chloroform.

Pharmacological actions.—Chloral hydrate is a sedative and hypnotic. In the usual dosage—0·7 to 2 g.—sedation occurs in ten to fifteen minutes and is followed by sleep in about half an hour. The sleep is quiet and deep, but the patient can be easily aroused, and it lasts five to eight hours. Usually there are no after-effects and "hangover" is rarely seen. The EEG in resting man is depressed in a manner similar to that produced by the barbiturates, but in a less pronounced way.

Larger doses cause a prolonged and deeper sleep and may obtund pain. With doses of 6 g. or more, complete anaesthesia may occur, and with it dangerous respiratory depression.

With the usual hypnotic doses little more depression of respiration or the blood pressure occurs than in normal sleep. Cardiac depression is not seen with normal doses but does occur with large ones.

Chloral hydrate is rapidly absorbed from the gastro-intestinal tract but it is irritant to the stomach. It is mainly reduced to trichloroethanol, which is responsible for its hypnotic effect. Some of this substance is then combined in the liver with glucuronic acid to form trichloroethanol glucuronide (urochloralic acid) which is not a hypnotic. Trichloroethanol glucuronide is then excreted in the urine, from which it can be recovered as white, silky, colourless needle-shaped crystals with a melting point of 142° C. In solution these reduce alkaline copper and therefore when in excess can be mistaken for glucose.

Clinical use.—Chloral hydrate is given in a dose of 0·3 to 2 g. well diluted and with a suitable flavouring such as orange, to avoid gastric irritation and to mask the bitter taste. It is a non-cumulative, safe, and useful hypnotic and should be used more often than it is, especially when depression of respiration and a "hangover" effect are contra-indicated. In view of its long action, should chloral hydrate be used for premedication it must be given at least two hours before operation. Penhearow (1957) recommends the use of chloral hydrate as a pre-operative sedative for children. He gives approximately 50 mg./kg. body weight.

Other preparations of chloral hydrate, its complexes or derivatives, are available. They have less gastric irritant effect and are therefore preferable for routine use (King *et al.*, 1958), particularly in elderly patients (Exton-Smith *et al.*, 1963). The most important of these are:

Approved name	*Trade name*	*Tablet size*
chloral betaine	"Somilan"	0·87 g.
dichloralphenazone	"Welldorm"	0·15 g., 0·6 g.
triclofos	"Tricloryl"	0·5 g.

These and other compounds such as chloralformamide, chlorhexadol, penthrichloral and petrichloral are all metabolised in the intestine and liver to form trichloroethanol, on which their hypnotic action depends.

Bromethol (Tribromethanol; "Avertin") (CBr_3CH_2OH)

Bromethol was discovered by Eicholtz in 1917 and was first clinically employed by Butzengeiger in 1926 (Butzengeiger, 1927).

Preparation.—It is prepared by reducing tribromacetaldehyde (bromal) with the aid of aluminium ethoxide in absolute alcohol in an atmosphere of nitrogen. The resultant is then treated with aqueous sulphuric acid and the drug separated.

Physical properties.—Bromethol is a white crystalline powder with a slight aromatic odour and taste. It melts at 80°C. It is sparingly soluble in water (1 part in 35) but very soluble in amylene hydrate.

Stability.—Bromethol is unstable and is decomposed by heat, light and air to hydrobromic acid and dibromo-acetaldehyde.

$$\underset{\text{Bromethol}}{CBr_3CH_2OH} \rightarrow \underset{\text{Dibrominyl alcohol}}{CBr_2CHOH} \quad \underset{\text{Hydrobromic acid}}{+ HBr}$$

$$CBr_2CHOH \rightarrow \underset{\text{dibromo-acetaldehyde}}{CHBr_2CHO}$$

It is therefore supplied in dark bottles, as a solution of 1 g. of bromethol in 1 ml. of amylene hydrate (methyl butanol), itself a weak hypnotic.

Pharmacological actions.—Following the rectal administration of an adequate dose of bromethol, sleep occurs in five to fifteen minutes. Excitement is never seen. The maximal effect occurs in from twenty to thirty minutes and the patient wakes up in from one and a half to three hours when the blood concentration has fallen to 2 or 3 mg. per cent. Skeletal muscular relaxation is only partial with safe doses.

Bromethol usually causes a fall of blood pressure varying from 15 to 40 mm. Hg, lasting five to fifteen minutes, but in patients with hypertension the fall may be marked. It is caused mainly by depression of the vasomotor centre and partly by a direct action on the myocardium and blood vessels. The direct depressant action on the myocardium is negligible with normal dose levels. ECG changes are minor and perfusion experiments have shown that bromethol is only one-sixteenth as toxic as chloroform to the mammalian heart. Respiration is depressed, the tidal and minute volumes being decreased by about 20 per cent of normal.

The rate of absorption of bromethol from the rectum is very variable; usually 50 per cent of the dose is absorbed in the first ten minutes, 80 per cent in twenty minutes and 95 per cent after 25 minutes. On reaching the liver the drug combines with glucuronic acid to form tribromethanol glucuronide (urobromalic acid). This substance is excreted by the kidneys in about 2 hours. Since bromethol may aggravate hepatic and renal disease, it is contra-indicated when they are present.

Method of administration and dosage.—Bromethol is administered by rectum. A cleansing enema should have been given the previous night and a freshly prepared solution is run in slowly, taking three to five minutes, about thirty minutes before the time of operation. The patient should be placed in a slight head-down tilt to aid retention of the fluid in the rectum. In children the buttocks should also be strapped or held firmly in apposition for a few minutes to prevent leakage.

The dose is calculated according to the patient's weight, the amount per kg. being adjusted in relation to the state of the patient. The normal dose is 100 mg./kg. but for a particularly robust and healthy young adult or a thyrotoxic patient 110–120 mg./kg. may be required, while for the obese and sick the dose should be reduced to 60 mg./kg. Children are more tolerant of the effect of the drug and so they should be given a dose of 110–120 mg./kg. The dose so calculated is dissolved in approximately 40 times its volume of physiological saline which has been heated to 40° C—above 40° C tribromoethyl alcohol is decomposed—and shaken vigorously. The pH of the solution is tested with Congo Red; if a blue or violet colour appears the solution contains hydrobromic acid, showing that decomposition has occurred, and must not be used.

Clinical uses.—There are nowadays few indications for the administration of bromethol in clinical anaesthesia, but the drug is still used for the treatment of eclampsia. It is also sometimes useful for sedation for cardiac catheterisation.

THE BARBITURATE DRUGS

Barbituric acid was first synthesised by Conrad and Guthzeit in 1882. The 5:5′-diethyl derivative was introduced into medicine as a hypnotic by Carl Fischer and von Mering. Since this time innumerable derivatives have been synthesised and many have been introduced into medicine as hypnotics or anti-convulsants.

Preparation and Chemistry of Barbiturate Drugs

Barbituric acid is prepared from chloroacetic acid by reacting it with sodium cyanide to form cyanacetic acid. This is then boiled with alkali and converted to malonic acid and ammonia. The malonic acid thus formed is converted to diethyl malonate, which reacts with urea in the presence of alcohol and sodium ethylate to form barbituric acid and ethyl alcohol.

The substituted derivatives are obtained by using the substituted derivatives of malonic acid.

$$\mathrm{H-\underset{\underset{Cl}{|}}{\overset{\overset{H}{|}}{C}}-\overset{\overset{O}{\|}}{C}.OH \;+\; NaCN \longrightarrow H-\underset{\underset{CN}{|}}{\overset{\overset{H}{|}}{C}}-\overset{\overset{O}{\|}}{C}.OH \;+\; NaCl}$$

Chloroacetic acid — Sodium cyanide — Cyanacetic acid

$$\mathrm{CN-CH_2.COOH \;+\; 2H_2O \longrightarrow H_2C\left\langle\begin{matrix}\overset{\overset{O}{\|}}{C}.OH\\ \underset{\underset{O}{\|}}{C}.OH\end{matrix}\right. \;+\; NH_3}$$

Cyanacetic acid — Malonic acid

$$\mathrm{H_2-C\left\langle\begin{matrix}\overset{\overset{O}{\|}}{C}-O-C_2H_5\\ \underset{\underset{O}{\|}}{C}-O-C_2H_5\end{matrix}\right. \;+\; \begin{matrix}NH_2\\ \quad\rangle C{=}O\\ NH_2\end{matrix} \longrightarrow H_2C\left\langle\begin{matrix}\overset{\overset{O}{\|}}{C}-\overset{\overset{H}{|}}{N}\\ \underset{\underset{O}{\|}}{C}-\underset{\underset{H}{|}}{N}\end{matrix}\right\rangle C{=}O}$$

Diethyl malonate — Urea — Barbituric acid

Barbiturates are pyrimidine derivatives which can exist in keto or enol form. The ring numbering used is indicated below:

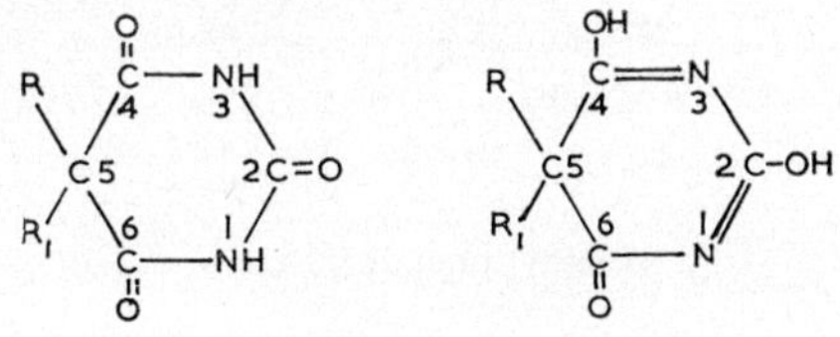

A. Keto form B. Enol form

Barbituric Acid

The barbiturates are a very suitable group of compounds on which to study the correlation between chemical structure and pharmacological activity. As a result of the large number of compounds studied it has been possible to formulate certain principles which enable a forecast to be made of the probable properties of a new derivative with a fair degree of accuracy. Nevertheless, there are some unexplained anomalies, such as the fact that 5 ethyl 5′ (1-3-dimethylbutyl) barbituric acid is a convulsant (Swanson, 1934) and the closely related compound 5 ethyl 5′ (1-methyl butyl) barbituric acid (pentobarbitone) is a hypnotic.

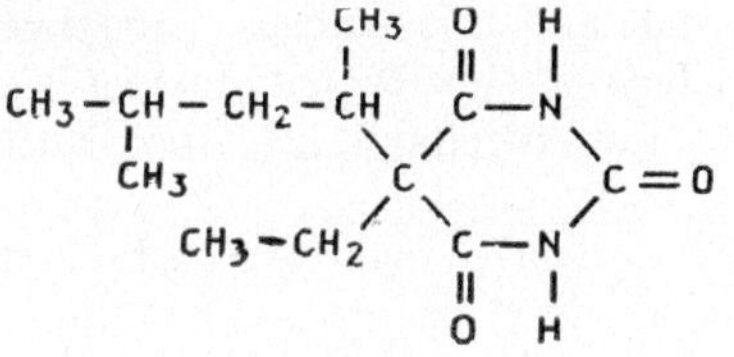

5 ethyl 5′ (1–3 dimethylbutyl) barbituric acid

Convulsant

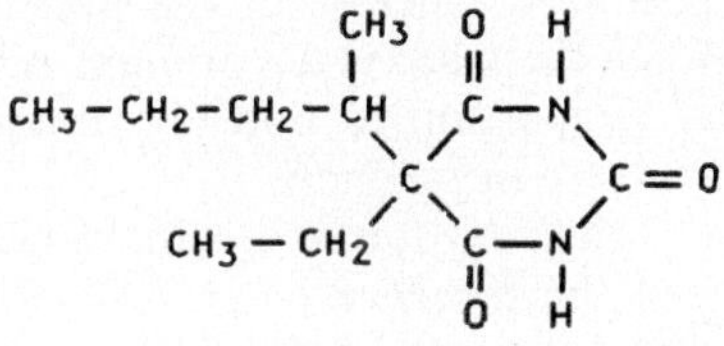

5 ethyl 5′ (1-methyl butyl) barbituric acid

Hypnotic

Variants of Barbituric Acid

There are three main ways of producing variants of barbituric acid:

1. Substitute organic radicals for the hydrogen atoms attached to the number 5 carbon atom.

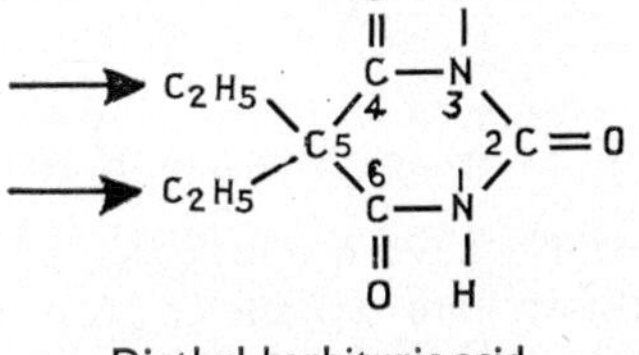

Diethyl barbituric acid

2. Substitute an alkyl radical for the hydrogen atom which is attached to the number 1 nitrogen atom, a process which makes the molecule asymmetric.

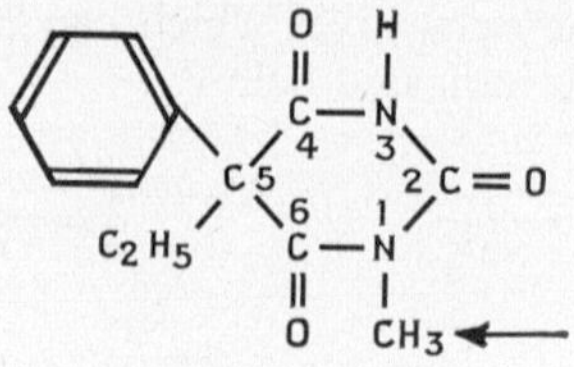

```
                 O   H
                 ‖   |
                 C — N
               / 4   3 \
  (C6H5) —  C5         2 C = O
           /   \ 6   1 /
     C2H5        C — N
                 ‖   |
                 O   CH3 ←
```

Methyl phenobarbitone

3. Substitute a sulphur atom for the oxygen atom attached to the number 2 carbon atom.

```
                      CH3   O   H
                       |    ‖   |
CH3 - CH2 - CH2 - CH        C — N
                      \   / 4   3 \
                       C 5        2 C = S ←
                      /   \ 6   1 /
                 C2H5       C — N
                            ‖   |
                            O   Na
```

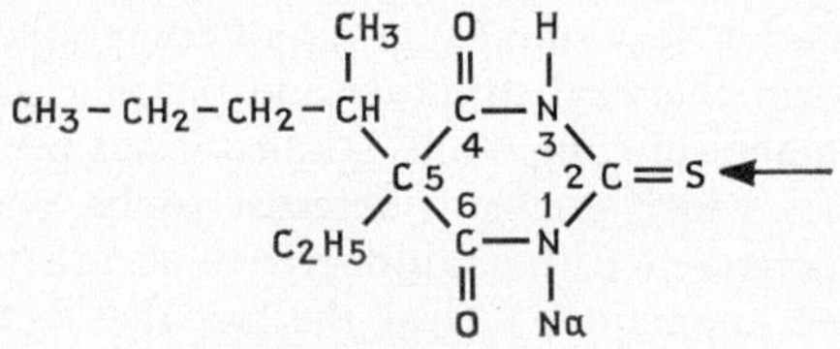

Thiopentone

If the number of carbon atoms in the substituting groups on the number 5 position is increased, the potency is increased, and this reaches a maximum when there are seven or eight carbon atoms. Beyond this, toxicity increases out of proportion to potency. Branching or unsaturated chains lead to a further increase in potency.

The addition of certain radicals makes the derivative inactive as a hypnotic, and the presence of an aromatic nucleus in an alkyl group which is directly attached to the number 5 carbon atom produces compounds with convulsant properties. Direct substitution with a phenyl group confers anticonvulsant activity.

Substitution at the number 1 nitrogen atom by a methyl group leads to increased activity and shortened duration of action with enhanced anticonvulsant properties. Alkyl groups with more carbon atoms produce convulsant properties. Replacement of the oxygen attached to the number 2 carbon atom by a sulphur atom forms thiobarbiturates with increased solubility in lipids, and results in compounds which have a very short duration of action.

Barbituric acid and its derivatives are weak acids and therefore form salts with the alkali metals. Solutions of these salts are alkaline and decompose on keeping.

Pharmacological Actions of the Barbiturate Drugs

Traditionally, barbiturates have usually been classified according to their duration of action, but this system, originally proposed on the basis of animal experiments, does not apply in man when they are used as hypnotics and administered orally (Hinton, 1961; Parsons, 1963). Indeed the duration of action of any one drug is conditioned by the patient's reaction to it rather than by its chemical structure. Although there are individual differences between many of the barbiturate drugs, all except the ultra short-acting ones, as typified by thiopentone, are discussed together in the following sections. Thiopentone and other similar drugs are discussed in greater detail in a separate section (p. 974 *et seq.*).

Central Nervous System

All the sedative barbiturates produce a similar pattern of depression of the nervous system, the extent of which largely depends upon the level of excitability of the patient's nervous system. By choosing a suitable barbiturate, dose and route of administration, any effect can be obtained from mild sedation to deep coma.

Site and mode of action.—The cerebral cortex and the reticular activating system are most sensitive to the barbiturates, the cerebellar, vestibular and spinal systems less so, and the medullary systems least of all. The circulatory and respiratory centres are affected by high concentrations of the barbiturates, but not the vomiting centre. A number of studies using radioisotope methods indicate that the less lipid soluble barbiturates, barbitone and phenobarbitone, are uniformly distributed throughout the central nervous system (Maynert and Van Dyke, 1950; Domek *et al.*, 1960), though early after administration grey matter contains more drug than white matter. Hubbard and Goldbaum (1950) found that thiopentone tends to accumulate in the thalamus and cerebral cortex.

The mechanism of action of barbiturates is unknown and many of the biochemical effects observed may be the result rather than the cause of their general depressant action. Cerebral cell membranes are stabilised, elevation of excitatory threshold occurring. Recovery from excitation is also prolonged. Barbiturates produce metabolic effects *in vitro* (Aldridge, 1962), inhibiting oxidative phosphorylation and activating adenosine triphosphatase. The active concentrations are similar to concentrations found in the brains of barbiturate-treated animals, suggesting that these effects may be exerted *in vivo*. The link between these observations and the hypnotic action, however, remains obscure.

Hypnotic effect.—This varies from mild impairment of performance of simple tasks to sleep. Depression of the cortex produces impairment of function and with high enough dosage sleep occurs in from twenty to sixty minutes. This sleep is similar to physiological sleep, and usually dreamless. After awakening, depression of function can still be detected for some hours and the EEG does not return to normal for up to 48 hours. Goodnow and his colleagues (1951) showed that there was altered function up to 14 hours after 100 mg. pentobarbitone by mouth. Following some of the barbiturates, these effects are felt by the patient as a "hangover," but Hinton (1961) found that this also occurred after placebo medication.

Analgesic effect.—Unlike analgesic drugs such as the opium derivatives or the salicylates, the barbiturates do not have much effect on the pain threshold except in doses which affect the level of consciousness. Beecher (1951) and Keats and Beecher (1950) have shown that post-operative pain is relieved in 50 per cent of cases with an intravenous injection of 60 to 90 mg. of pentobarbitone sodium, in 20 per cent by a placebo, and in 80 per cent by 8 mg. of morphine. But in the presence of severe pain it is found that barbiturates have an anti-analgesic action, making the patient restless and difficult to manage, as the control exercised by the higher centres is diminished. This is seen when children who have had heavy premedication with barbiturates—so that psychic trauma is lessened—become restless and difficult to manage post-operatively. When barbiturates are combined with analgesic drugs such as salicylates or codeine, the combination is found to be more effective than the analgesic alone, but the analgesic does not enhance the hypnotic activity of the barbiturate in the absence of pain. There are many such combinations available commercially.

Anticonvulsant effect.—In anaesthetic doses all the sedative barbiturates are capable of inhibiting convulsions to some extent, such as those of tetanus, eclampsia, and epilepsy. They are also used in the treatment of convulsions caused by strychnine, the local analgesic drugs, analeptics—such as lobeline and picrotoxin—and finally those associated with general anaesthesia. Phenobarbitone has a specific anticonvulsant action not found in the others, which is clinically useful in treating epilepsy, particularly grand mal.

Anaesthetic effect.—If large enough doses of barbiturates are given, anaesthesia is produced, the pattern following roughly that seen with the volatile anaesthetics, but as there is no preliminary period of apparent stimulation (*cf* ether) all the vital functions are depressed. The effect on respiration is particularly marked.

The actions of the barbiturates on the brain and spinal cord differ from those produced by the volatile anaesthetics. Barbiturates inhibit spontaneous cortical activity whilst leaving the cortex accessible to afferent stimuli. Ether, however, prevents these afferent stimuli from reaching the cortex. The intrathecal injection of the barbiturates in man causes spinal anaesthesia. The motor paralysis is incomplete and there are troublesome side-effects. These drugs are therefore not suitable for this purpose. In very large doses barbiturates affect peripheral nerves, as they do nerve cells. They increase the threshold for electrical excitation, prolong the absolute and relative refractory periods, and reduce the action potential spike.

The transmission of impulses at sympathetic ganglia is depressed by small doses of barbiturates in cats (Exley, 1954). The most active drugs are butobarbitone and amylobarbitone: the least active are the thiobarbiturates.

Respiratory System

Barbiturates depress respiration by a direct action on the medullary respiratory centre. The depression is proportional to the dose of the barbiturate. The sedation and lessened muscular activity accounts for part of this fall in respiratory minute volume which is mainly brought about by a decreased amplitude of respiration. Cyclobarbitone in a dose of 600 mg. does not depress the response to carbon dioxide below that which occurs in normal sleep, but does depress the response to hypoxia (Harris and Slawson, 1965). Very large doses of barbiturates produce marked respiratory depression—indeed respiratory failure is the usual cause of death from barbiturate poisoning.

Cardiovascular System

Ordinary oral hypnotic doses of the barbiturates have little effect on the circulation. The sedation they produce may cause a slight lowering of the blood pressure and/or pulse rate. Intravenous use of the barbiturates may cause a fall in blood pressure due to depression of the vasomotor centre with consequent peripheral vasodilatation. Large doses of barbiturates affect directly the small blood vessels causing dilatation and increased capillary permeability. Thiopentone is intermediate in this respect between ether and cyclopropane. Barbiturates do not appear to depress the myocardium in man, although Prime and Gray (1952) showed that thiopentone had a markedly depressant effect on the heart-lung preparation of the dog. Barbiturates do not affect cardiac rhythm or sensitise the heart to the effects of adrenaline. They may even protect the heart against arrhythmias produced by such drugs as adrenaline or cyclopropane (Meek and Seevers, 1934; Robbins *et al.*, 1939; Dance *et al.*, 1956). The haemodynamic effects of short-acting barbiturates are the subject of a recent review (Conway and Ellis, 1969).

In dogs pentobarbitone has been shown to cause a striking leucopenia (20 per cent of the pre-anaesthetic figure) and to increase the coagulation time, while decreasing the prothrombin time (Graca and Garst, 1957). Megaloblastic anaemia has been reported in man due to the prolonged use of amylobarbitone and quinalbarbitone (Hobson *et al.*, 1956).

Alimentary Tract

Barbiturates decrease the tone and amplitude of contractions of the gastro-intestinal tract. The mechanism is probably a direct action on the smooth muscle or on the intrinsic ganglionic plexuses. The thiobarbiturates may even increase intestinal tone. The gastric emptying time is little altered by hypnotic doses of the barbiturates but the gastric secretion is depressed.

These findings are of little significance in clinical anaesthesia.

Kidneys

Barbiturates produce no renal damage but anaesthetic doses do temporarily alter renal function.

The urine volume is decreased owing to increased tubular reabsorption of water produced by increased secretion of the pituitary antidiuretic hormone. Any hypotension produced by the barbiturate together with renal vasoconstriction leads to a decreased glomerular filtration rate and renal plasma flow. If the hypotension is prolonged, severe oliguria or anuria may occur. An increase in the blood urea, even in the presence of normal kidneys, has been shown by Dundee and Richards (1954) to lead to prolonged sleeping time, the extent of which can be correlated with the height of the blood urea. This may be of importance in cases of gastro-intestinal haemorrhage with a raised blood urea.

Liver

Therapeutic doses of the barbiturates have no effect on liver function. The liver is the most important organ for the destruction of the barbiturates, although other tissues such as kidney, brain and muscle also destroy the drug; therefore in cases of liver disease the action of barbiturates tends to be prolonged.

Although the role of the liver as the main organ of destruction of the barbiturates has been known for some time, there has been some argument as to the relative part played by other tissues in the breakdown of these drugs. This assumes some importance with the breakdown of thiopentone, since the sleeping time with this drug is not obviously prolonged, unless the liver is very severely damaged or a large part of it removed.

Uterus

The uterus is relatively resistant to the depressant effects of barbiturates and hypnotic doses have not been found to depress uterine contractions in labour, although full anaesthetic doses may decrease the force and frequency of the uterine contractions (Gruber, 1937). The barbiturates pass across the placental barrier easily and can produce marked respiratory depression in the foetus.

Metabolic Effects

Anderson *et al.* (1930) reported that hypnotic doses of barbitone, butobarbitone and cyclobarbitone produced some decrease in oxygen consumption, but that amylobarbitone and phenobarbitone did not do this. Anaesthetic doses of barbiturates produce a marked fall in oxygen consumption. The fall in metabolism and the peripheral vasodilatation with increased skin temperature lead to a fall in the body temperature of one or two degrees Fahrenheit, depending on the environment.

The blood sugar response to the barbiturates varies from one to the other, with the previous diet, the species which is being investigated, and the dose and route of administration. In man hypnotic doses do not alter the blood sugar regularly to any degree and are therefore safe to use in the presence of diabetes mellitus.

Absorption, Metabolism and Excretion of Barbiturate Drugs

The barbiturates are readily absorbed from the intestines, the rate being slower for the longer-acting drugs. They are also easily absorbed from the rectum or from subcutaneous and intramuscular injection, but where deep anaesthesia is required it is better that they should be administered intravenously, when the rate of injection can be controlled to produce just the effect desired—remembering always the dangers of too rapid intravenous injection and the dangers of extravenous injection.

The distribution of the barbiturates and their metabolism has been reviewed by Richards and Taylor (1956). In the circulation they are adsorbed to variable extents on plasma protein (see Chapter 34). In spite of this they diffuse rapidly out of the blood stream and are taken up by all tissues. This leads to a rapid fall in blood concentration which may be below that in some of the tissues at this stage. The liver and the muscles account for most of the bulk that is withdrawn from the blood. The body fat, which has a poor blood supply, takes some time to absorb most barbiturates. Shideman and his colleagues (1953) found that in man the maximum localisation of thiopentone in fat occurs in $1\frac{1}{2}$ to $2\frac{1}{2}$ hours. Brodie and his colleagues (1950) found that fat has little affinity for pentobarbitone. When equilibration between the barbiturate in the tissues and in the blood occurs, at a varying time depending on the dose and route of administration, the fall in blood concentration is slowed and is a measure of the rate of metabolism of the drug. As the level falls in the blood and the brain, a

35/TABLE 1

THE BARBITURATES

Name	Duration of Action	Chemistry	Dose	Fate
Barbitone B.P. Barbital U.S.P. "Medinal" "Veronal"	Long	Diethyl barbituric acid	0·3–0·6 g.	Mostly excreted unchanged in urine in 5–7 days
Phenobarbitone B.P. Phenobarbital U.S.P. "Luminal" "Gardenal"	Long	Ethyl phenyl barbituric acid	0·03–0·12 g.	Mostly destroyed
Butobarbitone B.P.C. "Neonal" "Soneryl"	Intermediate	Ethyl-n. butyl barbituric acid	0·06–0·12 g.	Partly excreted Partly destroyed
Allobarbitone B.P.C. "Dial"	Intermediate	Di-allyl barbituric acid	0·03–0·18 g.	Partly excreted Partly destroyed
Amylobarbitone B.P.C. "Amytal"	Intermediate	Ethyl *iso*-amyl barbituric acid	0·1–0·6 g.	Mostly destroyed
Cyclobarbitone B.P.C. "Phanodorn" "Phanodorm"	Short	Ethyl *cyclo*-hexenyl barbituric acid	0·2–0·4 g.	Destroyed and excreted
Pentobarbitone B.P. Pentobarbital U.S.P. "Nembutal"	Short	Ethyl methyl butyl barbituric acid	0·1–0·3 g.	Mainly destroyed
Quinalbarbitone B.P. "Seconal"	Short	Allyl.*sec*.amyl barbituric acid	0·05–0·2 g.	Mainly destroyed

Some of the trade names apply to the sodium salts of these drugs. In practice the only difference between the acid and its sodium salt is the greater solubility, and therefore the more rapid absorption, of the latter.

level is reached below which the animal wakes up. It is the rapid removal from the blood which accounts for the brief action of the so-called "ultra-short-acting" barbiturates, and not a rapid breakdown. After some time the breakdown of thiopentone is only 15 per cent per hour.

The breakdown and excretion of barbiturates varies so much with the individual drugs that it is described later when these are discussed.

Prolongation of the action of barbiturates.—Anything that hinders the passage of the barbiturate from the plasma to the tissues will tend to prolong the period of narcosis. It was shown by Adriani (1939) that the duration of barbiturate narcosis was prolonged in animals pre-treated with sulphonamides, but further work has shown that this phenomenon is outside the clinical range unless sulphonamides are given to the point of cyanosis (Lundy and Adams,

1942). The fact that sulphonamides, like barbiturates, are extensively bound to plasma protein suggests that the effects observed may have resulted from interference at binding sites. Disulfiram ("Antabuse") has been used in the hope of prolonging narcosis, and some reports that this is possible have appeared, but Jepson and Korner (1952) showed that those who were treated with this drug did not sleep longer than those untreated. Other metabolic inhibitors that have been tried include dinitro-orthocresol, dimercaprol, dehydroascorbic acid, and cysteine-cystine, but the results have been variable and inconclusive.

The antihistamines appear to alter the permeability of the blood-brain barrier, for the level of barbiturate in the brain is always higher following medication with the antihistaminic drugs (Lightstone and Nelson, 1954). The effect of chlorpromazine and other phenothiazine derivatives in "potentiating" the effects of barbiturates appears to be additive (Dundee, 1954), as does the synergism with the muscle relaxant mephenesin (Berger and Lynes, 1955).

Certain compounds related to atropine, SKF-525A (α-diethyl aminoethyl diphenylpropylacetate), P-19 (Abbott) (diethylaminoethyl α-diphenyl-propionate) and compound 18947 (Lilly) (2,4-dichloro 6 phenyl-phenoxyethyl diethylamine) have a prolonging action upon barbiturate anaesthesia, but have no significant central nervous system action when given alone, even in high dosage. They appear to interfere with the metabolic degradation of the barbiturates. Similar effects have been seen with certain drugs possessing clinical anti-Parkinson activity, such as trihexyphenidyl and atropine. Various other drugs and procedures, such as the injection of dextrose and potassium chloride, have been shown to prolong barbiturate narcosis but in the absence of accurate plasma and tissue concentrations it is difficult to be sure that they are not effects produced by osmotic and permeability changes.

Certain metabolic effects alter the response to the barbiturates; extreme inanition, anaemia or other severe metabolic derangements lead to a prolongation of barbiturate narcosis. Vitamin deficiency of the B group, particularly niacin, and vitamin C deficiency also prolong the actions of those barbiturates which are metabolised in the body.

Tolerance and Addiction to Barbiturate Drugs

Tolerance—that is, a reduced response to a given dose—occurs following long-continued medication with the barbiturates, but the dose that is fatal does not appear to rise to a similar extent.* Isbell and his colleagues (Isbell, 1950) have shown, as the Germans have believed for years, that the barbiturates can cause true addiction. Unlike that most commonly associated with the opium derivatives, barbiturate addiction, however, almost always has its origin in medical treatment.

Barbiturate Drugs

Barbitone ("Veronal"), when given in a dose of 300 to 600 mg. produces sleep in about half an hour, and this lasts six to eight hours. It is excreted over 5–7 days, 65–80 per cent of it unchanged in the urine. Twenty per cent is removed

* Tolerance probably results from increased metabolism in the liver as a result of microsomal enzyme induction (Burns and Conney, 1965).

in 24 hours. It may produce skin reactions and is likely to accumulate when repeated doses are given.

Barbitone sodium ("Medinal") has the same properties and the same dosage as barbitone, but is absorbed more rapidly.

Phenobarbitone is more powerful than barbitone, the dose being 30 to 120 mg. Two-thirds of the dose is cleared from the body in 24 hours. It is broken down in the body mainly by the liver and only 10–40 per cent is excreted unchanged in the urine.

Phenobarbitone has the strongest anticonvulsant properties of the barbiturates. It is used as an anticonvulsant or as a long-term sedative.

Amylobarbitone ("Amytal") is a white powder with a bitter taste which is only slightly soluble in water. The dose is 60 to 180 mg. Its actions are similar to those of barbitone but the sleep it produces lasts four to six hours. Amylobarbitone is excreted more rapidly than barbitone and is therefore less likely to produce cumulation It is largely destroyed by the liver. Three to eight per cent can be recovered from the urine following oral administration.

Amylobarbitone sodium ("Sodium Amytal") is very soluble in water. The dose is 60 to 180 mg. Sleep occurs more rapidly (under half an hour) than with the parent substance and its action is shorter—3 to 5 hours. As a basal narcotic it can be administered intravenously as a 5 per cent solution at the rate of 1 ml. per minute to a maximum of 1 g., but its use for this purpose has been superseded by the ultra-short acting compounds. It was used in obstetrics but found to cause unmanageable restlessness.

Butobarbitone ("Soneryl"), another member of the group, is partly metabolised and partly excreted unchanged. The dose is 100 to 200 mg. It is slightly longer acting than amylobarbitone.

Pentobarbitone sodium ("Nembutal") is a white, odourless, crystalline powder and is very soluble in water. The dose is 100 to 200 mg. Its properties are similar to those of amylobarbitone sodium but it produces sleep a little more quickly, and this lasts about 4 hours after 100 mg.

Pentobarbitone sodium can be used intravenously for the induction of anaesthesia, particularly when a longer effect than is achieved from an ultra-short-acting barbiturate such as thiopentone is required. Administered intravenously pentobarbitone is much slower in its action than thiopentone and it should be given as a 5 per cent solution at the rate of 1 ml. per minute until unconsiousness occurs or a maximum of 0·5 g. has been used. This is a tedious technique, so that there is a temptation to give 2 or more ml. rapidly in order to speed the onset of sleep. Rapid injection must be avoided, since with injudicious use profound depression can easily be caused. It is best used after a premedicant dose of morphine or one of the opiate analogues so that the total dose of pentobarbitone is reduced; pre-operative morphine also helps to reduce post-operative pain and restlessness which can be a difficult problem if the greater part of the pentobarbitone has not been excreted at this stage. The use of morphine soon after an operation for which pentobarbitone has been the principal anaesthetic can result in marked respiratory depression.

Pentobarbitone sodium is also commonly used as a pre-operative sedative for small children and can be used orally or rectally (see p. 988).

Quinalbarbitone ("Seconal") is a white odourless, hygroscopic powder which is very soluble in water. The dose is 100 to 200 mg. An oral dose is effective in 15 to 20 minutes, and lasts from 4 to 6 hours. The metabolism and excretion of quinalbarbitone are thought to be similar to that of pentobarbitone. "Tuinal" is a mixture of amylobarbitone sodium and quinalbarbitone sodium. The dose is 100 to 200 mg.

Clinical Use of the Barbiturate Drugs

The barbiturates are used for their property of depressing the central nervous system in order to produce sedation, sleep, or as anticonvulsive agents. Phenobarbitone in 30–60 mg. doses two or three times a day produces good sedation in an adult, or one of the shorter-acting drugs can be used, but with these some patients may complain of drowsiness. Patients differ in their reaction to the various barbiturates, and where one does not suit, another of the same group may be acceptable, though there is no objective evidence of this.

When an anticonvulsant is needed, phenobarbitone is best for prophylaxis, and sodium amylobarbitone, pentobarbitone or thiopentone (see later) by intravenous injection for treatment of the fit. Barbiturates are of value in protecting against the toxic effects of local analgesics and can be given as preoperative medication for this purpose.

For controlling acute manic conditions sodium amylobarbitone or pentobarbitone can be given intramuscularly.

The disadvantages of the barbiturates are the "hangover" effect that follows the use of the longer-acting drugs, respiratory depression, and an occasional toxic skin rash.

Ultra-short-acting Barbiturates

Hexobarbitone ("Evipan")

This drug was synthesised by Kropp and Taub, and in 1932 the first clinical reports of its use were presented by Weese and Scharpff. Until the advent of thiopentone three years later, hexobarbitone was by far the most satisfactory intravenous barbiturate. It is a short-acting barbiturate with similar properties to pentobarbitone and quinalbarbitone, and a dose range of from 200 to 400 mg.

Physical properties.—Hexobarbitone soluble is sodium N-methyl-5-cyclohexenyl-5′methyl barbiturate.

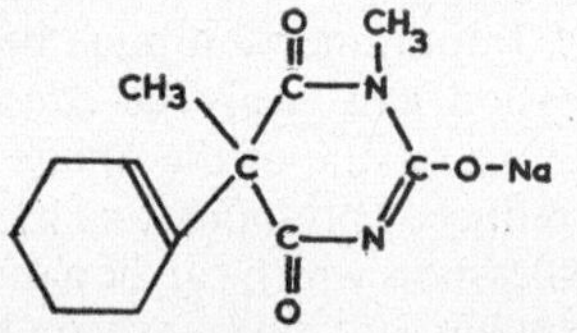

It is a white crystalline powder with a bitter taste, which is readily soluble in water. The melting point of the free acid is 143–145° C.

Pharmacological actions.—Hexobarbitone produces depression of the central nervous system in a similar pattern to other barbiturates, but even at deep levels of anaesthesia spontaneous muscular movements occur. These may not only affect the limbs but cause a shudder of the whole body. Premedication with opiates and the administration of nitrous oxide with oxygen will reduce the incidence of these tremors but does not completely abolish them. Volpitto (1951) found that side-effects following intubation (such as bronchial spasm) were much less after hexobarbitone than after thiopentone or thiamylal. Adriani and Rovenstine (1943), using excised bronchi and bronchioles from rat, dog and man, showed that hexobarbitone produced less bronchial and bronchiolar constriction than thiopentone, but more than pentobarbitone. This difference between hexobarbitone and thiopentone was confirmed in guinea-pigs by Mayrhofer (1954). Hexobarbitone is largely destroyed in the body (Bush *et al.*, 1953).

Clinical uses.—Hexobarbitone is less irritant to the tissues than thiopentone and therefore has been recommended in circumstances where extravenous injection is a distinct possibility—such as in convulsions. It is normally given intravenously as a 10 per cent solution. Approximately 0·3 to 0·4 g. are needed to produce unconsciousness in an average healthy adult. Fundamentally hexobarbitone has no advantages over thiopentone, but it is recommended for patients with a tendency to bronchospasm. The injectable solution is no longer available in the United Kingdom.

Thiopentone ("Intraval", "Pentothal")

Tabern and Volwiler (1935) prepared a large number of thiobarbiturates. They found that substitution by the sulphur atom shortened the period of narcosis compared with that produced by other barbiturates.

In 1934 Lundy (Lundy, 1935) at the Mayo Clinic, and Waters at Madison, Wisconsin, began clinical trials with the compound now known as thiopentone, which is the sulphur analogue of pentobarbitone. Jarman introduced thiopentone into Great Britain in 1935 (Jarman and Abel, 1936). Its property of producing peaceful sleep easily led to its rapid acceptance and the number of cases anaesthetised with thiopentone rose dramatically (Dundee, 1956).

Physical properties.—Thiopentone is a pale yellow, hygroscopic powder with a bitter taste and a slight sulphurous smell. The sodium salt of thiopentone is readily soluble in water but the acid itself much less so. In order to ensure total solution even in the presence of atmospheric carbon dioxide, commercial solutions contain 6 per cent by weight sodium carbonate. The freshly made solution has a pH of 10·6. For the formula see page 966.

Pharmacological actions.—Thiopentone rapidly crosses the blood-brain barrier and the concentration in the cerebrospinal fluid reaches a level almost as high as that of the unbound drug in the plasma. Figure 2 shows how the plasma level falls rapidly for the first 15 minutes and then more slowly. The depth of anaesthesia produced by the intravenous injection of thiopentone depends on its concentration in the blood, but the relationship is not a simple one, for the larger the initial dose the higher the brain concentration or plasma level at which the patient will awake. This has been called acute tolerance, though the fact that a patient will wake sooner from a rapid injection than from a slow one is probably accountable on the basis of the slug theory (see Chapter 34).

Thiopentone produces a progressive depression of the central nervous system. In clinical practice this is produced so rapidly that the usual signs of anaesthesia are of no value. Respiratory depression is marked, and a patient with apnoea may yet react to a surgical stimulus. The response to a surgical stimulus determines to a greater extent than with other agents the clinical signs of anaesthesia. The surgical stimulus may provide the "drive" to respiration and this may lead to fatal respiratory depression when the stimulus is removed.

Thiopentone has no analgesic properties—indeed hypersensitivity to pain and touch may be manifest.

The effect of thiopentone depends greatly on the premedication with analgesic drugs or the supplementation of thiopentone narcosis with analgesia—opiate or nitrous oxide with oxygen. These allow surgical intervention with no response at lower plasma levels of thiopentone and with less respiratory depression.

Cerebral metabolism and blood flow.—Wechsler and his colleagues (1951) showed that there was a significant depression of cerebral utilisation of oxygen in

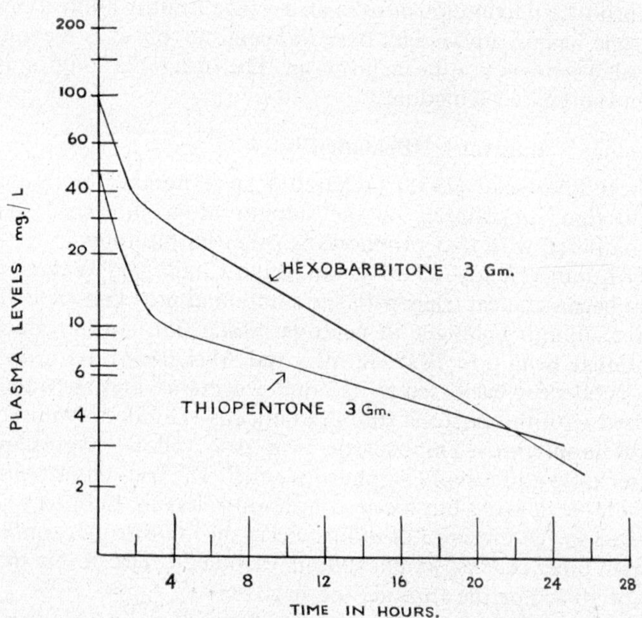

35/Fig. 2.—Comparison of the plasma levels of thiopentone and hexobarbitone.

spite of a blood flow which was normal or a little increased. The blood flow is probably more affected by the carbon dioxide tension in the blood than by the thiopentone.

Respiratory system.—The usual sequence of events when a dose of thiopentone is given slowly is for a few deeper breaths to be taken just prior to the loss of consciousness. There may then be a brief period of apnoea due to the direct effect of the thiopentone on the respiratory centre coinciding with a low carbon dioxide tension from the preceding deep breaths. Respiration returns gradually and then further fades away as more thiopentone is given.

With small doses—i.e. 0·5 g. given in 20 to 25 minutes—respiratory depression is not seen, but following premedication with the opiates respiratory depression is more marked (Helrich *et al.*, 1956).

The laryngeal reflexes are not depressed until the deep levels of thiopentone narcosis are reached, and stimulation, local or remote, may provoke laryngeal spasm at light levels of narcosis. If there is a predisposing cause present—such as a sensitive bronchial tree or stimulation of the larynx by mucus—thiopentone may evoke bronchospasm or laryngospasm, but does not of itself cause these conditions.

Cardiovascular system.—Under light anaesthesia there is widespread dilatation of the muscle and skin vessels but no obvious alteration in the total peripheral resistance (Fieldman *et al.*, 1955). Pauca and Hopkins (1971) showed that the forearm blood flow and vascular resistance were unchanged in unpremedicated volunteers. The increase in peripheral flow (i.e. vasodilatation) is compensated for by constriction of the splanchnic and renal blood vessels so that the blood pressure and cardiac output remain relatively unchanged, In contrast, the rapid induction of deep anaesthesia leads to a fall in cardiac output of 25 per cent or more together with a reduction in the intrathoracic blood volume (Etsten and Li, 1955; Flickinger *et al.*, 1961). These changes are thought to be due to the peripheral vasodilatation causing pooling of the blood in the extremities and a reduction of the venous return to the heart (Eckstein *et al.*, 1961). Thiopentone may also have a direct depressant action on the myocardium (Prime and Grey, 1952), but this has not been demonstrated in man.

Arrhythmias occur in a proportion of cases, and are usually ventricular extrasystoles.

Alimentary tract.—In animals thiopentone produces some depression of intestinal motility, but this soon recovers and has returned to normal when the animal is awake.

Liver and kidneys.—Dundee (1955*b*) considers that doses of over 750 mg. of thiopentone cause liver dysfunction in an appreciable number of patients, but Hugill (1950) notes that hypoxia is the most important factor in the causation of liver damage associated with anaesthesia. The separation of hypoxia from true hepatotoxic effects is extremely difficult in clinical practice.

The effects of thiopentone on the kidneys are secondary to its actions on the circulation, and to the liberation of anti-diuretic hormone that it causes. The urine output during thiopentone anaesthesia is decreased (de Wardener, 1955).

Effect on muscles and myoneural junction.—Thiopentone, in large doses in animals, prolongs the contraction of muscle, whether stimulated directly or indirectly, and there is also evidence of a weak curare-like action at the motor end-plate, but clinically this effect is not as obvious as that caused by ether. Quilliam (1955) showed by examination of the action potential of the posterior gracilis muscle of the rat before and after the intra-arterial injection of thiopentone that its voltage was decreased, its latency increased, and duration prolonged. These facts are consistent with a decreased rate of propagation of the potential on the surface of the muscle. In man there is no evidence that thiopentone in doses up to 1·5 g. affects neuromuscular transmission.

Reproductive system.—In therapeutic doses, thiopentone does not alter the tone of the gravid uterus or the motility of the fallopian tubes. It does not influence utero-tubal spasm. McKechnie and Converse (1955) showed that when 350 mg. of thiopentone was given just prior to delivery, thiopentone was present in the foetus within 45 seconds until in 2–3 minutes its concentration was equal in the maternal and foetal blood, and then fell in both synchronously. Crawford (1956), using 250 mg. thiopentone, produced similar results. McKechnie and Converse could find little correlation between the level of thiopentone in the foetus and the amount of foetal depression—probably because there are so many other factors to be taken into account when considering the causes of foetal depression. Foetal respiration can be depressed by thiopentone, but the degree of depression depends upon the dose of the drug given to the mother and the duration of time that elapses between induction of anaesthesia and delivery of the baby, besides the maturity of the foetus. The available evidence suggests that unless the infant is removed from the uterus within 4 to 5 minutes of an intravenous injection of a small, sleep dose (0·15 to 0·25 g.) of thiopentone, the blood level of a mature, healthy foetus will have fallen to such a degree that it is unlikely to be significant in preventing the onset of respiration.

Blood sugar.—Thiopentone has no effect on the blood sugar (Dundee and Todd, 1958).

Distribution, Metabolism and Excretion

Price (1960) traced the distribution of thiopentone in the body following a single dose administered intravenously. After one minute the blood had given up 90 per cent of the dose to the central nervous system, heart, liver and other well-perfused viscera. During the next thirty minutes other aqueous tissues acquired 80 per cent of the thiopentone leaving these viscera, and fatty tissues received the remainder. The rate at which thiopentone leaves the central nervous system depends upon the rate at which poorly perfused aqueous tissues take it up, and this depends on their blood flow. Fat is so poorly perfused that it cannot concentrate thiopentone to any great extent until the central nervous system has lost 90 per cent of its peak content. After some hours, however, fat depots may contain quite large amounts of the drug. This has a profound effect on the distribution of subsequent doses, causing a greatly increased clinical effect.

Thiopentone is practically completely metabolised in the body, only about 0·3 per cent of an administered dose being excreted in the urine unchanged (Brodie, 1952). Shideman *et al.* (1953) found in dogs that the true rate of metabolism is 6 per cent of the total dose administered per hour. Recent work suggests that in man the rate of metabolism is faster —16 to 24 per cent per hour (Rahn *et al.*, 1969).

The liver is the main site of the metabolism of thiopentone. This was demonstrated in mice and rats by Shideman and his co-workers (1947). Dundee (1952*a*) showed in man that the hepatic dysfunction produced by chloroform anaesthesia prolonged the recovery time from the injection of 1·0–1·5 g. thiopentone.

In vitro experiments show that slices of kidney tissue inactivate thiopentone to a similar extent to liver slices. Brain slices have some activity, but muscle slices none.

Clinical use.—Thiopentone can be used for several purposes—to induce anaesthesia, as a sole anaesthetic, as the principal anaesthetic but supplemented by other drugs, in conjunction with regional analgesia, to relieve acute convulsive states of differing aetiology, and to produce simple sedation.

Thiopentone leads to a rapid and pleasant loss of consciousness that can be produced with the minimum of apparatus. Herein lie its greatest advantages and its dangers—a fatal overdose is very easily administered. The safety of thiopentone—and indeed of all intravenous anaesthetics—is largely dependent upon the skill of the administrator in assessing, both before and during anaesthesia, the requirements of the patient. Although in theory there is probably a dose that is small enough to be safe for any patient and yet produce a desired effect, there are occasions when it may be wise not to use thiopentone, or at least to give it with particular care and with special precautions. These are:

1. *General.*—Out-patients who are unaccompanied should never be given thiopentone because there is frequently a stage of euphoria following the return of consciousness. In this stage, the patient is in no fit state to look after himself or to take responsible action.

   Children are unsuitable for the administration of thiopentone as the sole or principal anaesthetic agent, since they need relatively large doses to produce a satisfactory depression of reflex activity. Provided venepuncture can be accomplished easily and painlessly, thiopentone is, however, an excellent induction agent for children.
2. *Respiratory disease.*—When the adequacy of the airway is in doubt, thiopentone must be used, if at all, with extreme caution (see Chapter 11). Factors which may affect the airway during induction, such as vomiting or bleeding, suggest either a special technique for the use of thiopentone or its avoidance (see Chapters 10 and 47). Thiopentone may be contra-indicated for an asthmatic patient, as it can lead to an aggravation of the condition.
3. *Cardiac and circulatory disease.*—The benefits of a smooth and pleasant induction with thiopentone must be balanced against the deleterious effects of vasomotor and respiratory depression. In fixed output cardiac diseases, such as mitral stenosis and constrictive pericarditis, vasodilatation and consequent hypotension—particularly if acute—may lead to cardiac arrest. Similarly in "shock" states, in which the blood pressure is maintained by peripheral vasoconstriction, the vasodilatation produced by even a small dose of thiopentone can prove fatal. Such conditions do not necessarily contra-indicate the use of thiopentone, unless the administrator is inexperienced and unable to assess the severity of the disease.
4. *Other diseases.*—For patients in whom coma is imminent due to diseases such as severe hepatic dysfunction, uraemia or uncontrolled diabetes, or due to over-sedation with drugs, thiopentone is either best avoided or used in minimal dosage so that recovery from its effect is rapid. Thiopentone is contra-indicated in the presence of the rare disease porphyria, since it may lead to fatal respiratory paralysis, and should be used with caution for patients with Addison's disease, in whom its action may be unduly prolonged (Dundee, 1951). Abnormal respiratory depression may follow the use of thiopentone in dystrophia myotonica (Dundee, 1952*b*).

Untreated myxoedematous patients are sensitive to most anaesthetics, thiopentone amongst them.

Administration.—Thiopentone should not be used as a stronger solution than 5 per cent, i.e. 1·0 g. in 20 ml., and for most purposes it is best used as a 2·5 per cent solution—i.e. 0·5 g. in 20 ml. Solutions should be freshly made, although they keep for a week in a refrigerator. Bottles of solution should be shaken before use to ensure adequate mixing.

The advantages of the weaker solution are that it is less likely to cause harm if placed extravenously or intra-arterially and it is more difficult to give a large dose rapidly.

Intravenous.—A vein should be chosen and palpated before the application of the tourniquet, which should not be applied so tightly as to occlude the arterial inflow to the arm.

When the needle is firmly in the vein and the tourniquet completely released, 2 ml. of thiopentone is injected with a pause after this so that an inadvertent intra-arterial injection may become manifest. Should this have occurred, the patient will complain of a severe burning sensation in the hand (see below). The estimated dose is given at a rate and in an amount that must depend upon the state of the patient and the purpose for which the thiopentone is being given. It may range from as little as 0·05 g. for the induction of anaesthesia in a severely ill patient to 1·0 g. as the sole anaesthetic for a fit adult. It is best to use the smallest effective dose, and to supplement this with more flexible and potent anaesthetic agents rather than to administer large doses of thiopentone.

Rectal.—The rectal administration of thiopentone is useful in children to produce basal narcosis, particularly for such procedures as a minor operation, cardiac catheterisation and lumbar puncture. It is unsuitable where a rapid return of reflexes is required immediately after the operation. If the expected stimulation is great then supplementation should be started before the operation to prevent such reactions as laryngeal spasm.

The usual dose is 45 mg./kg. body weight given as a 2·5 per cent or 5 per cent solution.

Atropine should be given 1 hour before the thiopentone and the patient should have had nothing by mouth for at least five hours. Sleep comes on within 5 to 15 minutes and the maximum effect lasts for another 20 to 30 minutes, consciousness usually beginning to return one hour after the dose has been given.

Since the volume of thiopentone solution needed for rectal instillation is small it is more likely to be retained than the larger quantities of such drugs as paraldehyde or tribromoethyl alcohol.

Thiopentone can also be given rectally as a suppository (see p. 989).

Local complications of thiopentone injections.—Any intravenous injection carries a slight risk of introducing infection, causing a haematoma or losing the broken part of a needle. Cleanliness and efficient sterilisation of syringe and needle are essential to avoid the risk of cross-infection, particularly of infective hepatitis. The incidence of haematomata can be lessened by early release of the tourniquet and the application of pressure to the site of venepuncture while the needle is being removed and for an adequate period of time afterwards. In thin patients, particularly the elderly, pressure should be maintained for three minutes, and elevation of the arm above the level of the heart is a valuable manoeuvre.

Needles break most commonly at the junction of the shaft with the hub (Fig. 3) and they should never be inserted as far as this, so that should one unfortunately break the shaft can be grasped and removed. To avoid trouble, the arm should be gently but firmly held so that at the slightest movement the

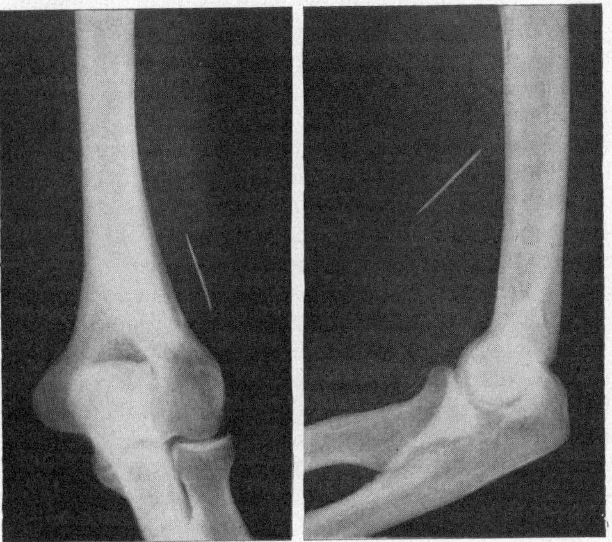

35/FIG. 3.–Broken needle following intravenous thiopentone injection.

grip can be tightened. Movement is more likely to occur in the young and in unpremedicated patients. If a needle breaks, the arm must be held still and if the shaft cannot be grasped and removed, surgical removal with X-ray localisation of the needle must be undertaken. Even with immediate fixation of the arm it is surprising how far the needle may have travelled.

Solutions of thiopentone are alkaline and therefore irritant to the tissues. If enough of the solution is placed extravenously it may cause necrosis of the subcutaneous tissue with an ulcer. If the injection is attempted on the medial side of the antecubital fossa—a site that is not recommended—damage to the median nerve may occur: this is suggested by a shooting pain down the arm and movement of the hand or wrist (Pask and Robson, 1954) (see also Chapter 45, p. 1263).

Intra-arterial injection.—The incidence of this complication, which may have extremely severe sequelae for the patient, is unknown. Cohen (1948) suggests it is 1:55,000, but Dundee (1956) considers that it is probably 1:3,500. The number of permanent sequelae that follow intra-arterial injection is also unknown. Most of the reports of permanent damage refer to those that follow the use of a 10 per cent solution, but 6 out of 16 patients in whom a 5 per cent solution had been injected had permanent sequelae (Dundee, 1956). No permanent sequelae have been reported following the use of a 2·5 per cent solution of thiopentone.

Intra-arterial injection occurs when insufficient attention is paid to the vessel chosen for puncture and to the initial response to a very small quantity of thiopentone. Absence of arterial pulsation may make difficult the normal differentiation between artery and vein, and this may be caused by excessive tourniquet pressure and even by bracing back the shoulders or rotating the neck in some patients. In about 10 per cent of people the ulnar artery may lie superficially beneath the skin on the medial side of the antecubital fossa, and in this position can easily be mistaken for a vein. All in all it is wisest not to select a vein in the antecubital fossa region—at least on its medial side—for the injection of thiopentone, but to choose one on the outer aspect of the forearm, and to administer a 2·5 per cent solution.

Puncture of an arterial wall is usually painless, but the injection of 2 ml. of solution into the vessel nearly always causes pain of a burning character which is radiated to the hand. Following the injection, spasm of the artery occurs and the pulse at the wrist may disappear. The immediate effect is probably due to the local release of noradrenaline in or near the vessel wall (Burn and Hobbs, 1959). Waters (1966) has shown that arterial obstruction can be caused by crystallisation of the drug at the normal pH of plasma, due to the limited solubility of the un-ionised form of thiopentone. In a proportion of patients thrombosis takes place in the artery or its distal terminations. Blanching, and perhas, cyanosis and gangrene of the distal part of the limb are therefore likely to result. Cohen (1948) suggested that thrombosis is a more dangerous factor than arterial spasm, and this view has been substantiated by the experimental work of Kinmonth and Shepard (1959). They found that intra-arterial thiopentone damaged the endothelial and subendothelial tissues of the vessels, and that benign solutions buffered to the same pH (10·6) as thiopentone did not. Arterial spasm, apart from the first 30 seconds after injection, played a small part, and the damage was caused by thrombosis.

The end result depends not only on the efficacy of treatment but on many factors such as the volume and strength of the thiopentone injected and the state of the artery and circulation at the time. There is no scientific proof to support the theory that the stronger the solution the more likely are there to be permanent sequelae. But, as stated above, the facts suggest this to be the case. Cohen (1948) has shown that 4–5 ml. of 35 per cent diodone can be injected intra-arterially before pain is felt in an arm in which the arterial inflow is obstructed. This volume fills the entire distal arterial tree. Four ml. is also the smallest volume of 10 per cent thiopentone that has been reported as being followed by serious effects. These facts support the recommendation of Macintosh and Heyworth (1943) that the anaesthetist should inject 2 ml. and then wait for a complaint of pain before proceeding with the injection. Only rarely (as in a medico-legal case reported in the *British Medical Journal* in 1951) will there be no pain.

When the accident occurs treatment must be aimed at diluting the thiopentone, overcoming the initial arterial spasm, and preventing thrombosis or extension of the clot. Operative removal of a thrombus may be necessary.

The needle must be kept in the artery—this may be difficult due to the intense pain that the patient feels—and 10 to 20 ml. of 0·5 per cent procaine solution injected to dilute the thiopentone and encourage vasodilatation. When available 40–80 mg. of papaverine in 10–20 ml. of physiological saline is preferable. It is also advisable to inject procaine or papaverine around the artery at the site of injection, and to remove other vasoconstrictor influences by performing a brachial plexus block and putting the patient on a general autonomic blocking agent. When the damage is thought to have progressed to thrombus formation, then operative removal of the clot should be undertaken within six hours of the original injection, as it is doubtful whether muscle can survive more than this period of circulatory arrest.

Stone and Donnelly (1961), reviewing the problem of accidental intra-arterial injection of thiopentone, recommend the following. Light inhalational anaesthesia should be induced quickly to obtain peripheral vasodilatation and pain relief. A brachial plexus block should be performed to ensure continued vascular dilatation in the affected limb, and anticoagulant therapy should be started. Stone and Donnelly suggest a catheter technique for the block, so that it can be continued without the risk of bleeding from successive injections. General anaesthesia can usually be quickly induced since an anaesthetic machine is likely to be to hand, whilst a search for procaine or other vasodilator drug may take time. The surgeon must be informed at once, and a decision made whether to postpone the projected operation or not, depending upon the effectiveness of the treatment for the intra-arterial injection.

Venous thrombosis.—The incidence of venous thrombosis has rarely been reported. The belief is that it is much more common after the use of 5 per cent thiopentone than after the use of 2·5 per cent solution. Hutton and Hall (1957) reported four in a series of two hundred unselected surgical patients after the use of 5 per cent solution. Some patients seem to be predisposed to thrombosis, the complication arising on successive occasions in the same patient and despite especial care to prevent it.

Usually the thrombosis is simple, but occasionally a chemical thrombophlebitis may occur with oedema and tenderness in the neighbourhood of the injected vein and its tributaries. Rest for the affected arm is the best treatment, as the condition settles in about seven to ten days: there is no specific therapy. Dundee (1956) quotes three cases of prolonged oedema in a limb following venous thrombosis after a thiopentone injection. In two of them the blood flow from the limb was hindered and it may have been the prolonged period of the contact of the irritant with the vein wall that caused the spreading thrombosis.

Apart from the discomfort of thrombosis, there is a danger of death of tissue distal to it, but this is only inference from the fact that limbs have had to be amputated following the injection of sclerosing fluids into the deep veins of the leg (Cohen, 1948).

General complications of thiopentone administration.—These are usually due to an overdose of thiopentone having been given. This is often not a "large" dose but one too large for the patient due to an inaccurate assessment of his requirements, or attempting too much with thiopentone as the sole anaesthetic. The complications are mainly due to depression of respiration and the circulation, and have been described under the pharmacological actions of the drug. The frequency with which they lead to death is difficult to assess. Dundee (1956) has collected reports on nearly 200,000 thiopentone administrations of which 0·035 per cent (1:2,870) ended in a fatality directly attributable to the drug. Edwards and his colleagues (1956) placed 107 out of 589 deaths caused by anaesthesia in the category of immediate cardiovascular collapse following the injection of an intravenous barbiturate.

Although thiopentone ranks high amongst other anaesthetic agents and factors as a cause of anaesthetic mortality, considering its countrywide and frequent use, and, moreover, the ease with which an overdose can be given, it may be said with some reservations to be a "safe" drug.

Methohexitone Sodium (Brietal Sodium: Methohexital Sodium)

α-dl-l-methyl-5-allyl 5′-(1 methyl-2-pentynyl) barbiturate sodium salt.

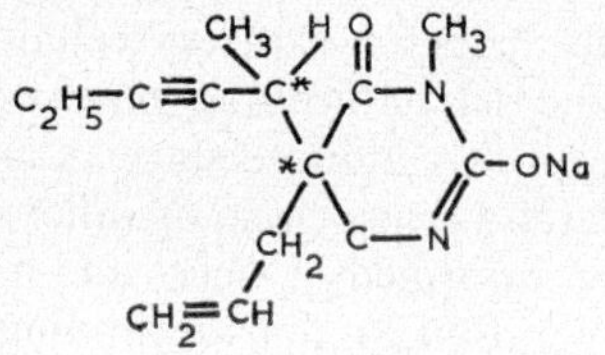

```
          CH3  H  O   CH3
            \ /   ||   |
C2H5-C≡C-C*    C---N
            \ /      \
            *C        C-ONa
            / \      //
         CH2   C---N
         /
    CH2=CH
```

Because there are two asymmetrical carbon atoms, there are four possible isomers of this substance, which can be separated into two pairs: α-dl (high melting point) and β-dl (low melting point). The α-dl pair, which is methohexitone, produce hypnosis without stimulation of skeletal muscle. The mixture of all four isomers is a potent short-acting anaesthetic agent which was found to produce excessive skeletal muscle activity and even convulsions (Taylor and Stoelting, 1960).

Physical properties.—Methohexitone sodium is a white powder. It is readily soluble in water to give a solution of pH 10–11 which is stable at room temperature for six weeks, but has been kept satisfactorily at 5° C for a year (Redish *et al.*, 1958).

Pharmacology.—Taylor and Stoelting (1960) found that methohexitone was twice as potent as thiopentone in five species of animals. In man it was three times as potent and was metabolised three times as fast. Coleman and Green (1960) found the ratio of potency to thiopentone to be 2·8 :1, but Wyant and Chang (1959) had found it was only one-and-a-half times as potent as thiopentone using an 0·2 per cent intravenous infusion of methohexitone and comparing the dose per minute required to maintain satisfactory anaesthesia. The duration of action of methohexitone is shorter than that of thiopentone, therefore it is less cumulative and larger total doses are required to maintain anaesthesia for a long time. The concentration of methohexitone in the plasma is about half that of thiopentone at comparable electro-encephalographic levels of anaesthesia. Methohexitone in the usual clinical doses produces little effect on the blood pressure. When administered during an anaesthetic, it causes a fall of blood pressure of lesser degree and shorter duration than that produced by thiopentone.

Respiratory depression occurs with methohexitone. Wyant and Chang (1959)

* Asymmetrical carbon atoms.

and Taylor and Stoelting (1960) found this on occasions to be greater than that for a similar dose of thiopentone. Coleman and Green (1960) did not see any cases of apnoea in 10,142 patients.

There was no bronchospasm when methohexitone was given to a series of normal and asthmatic patients (Taylor and Stoelting, 1960). Aurup and Hougs (1963) have shown that *in vitro* methohexitone augments acetylcholine-induced bronchospasm to an extent that is midway between that of thiopentone and hexobarbitone. Extravenous injection has been found to lead to a painless erythema needing no treatment, while intra-arterial injection in animals caused gangrene similar to that produced by thiopentone in equal doses (Francis, 1964).

Some muscular twitching may be seen, which rarely is forceful. Hiccups and coughing were reported by Taylor and Stoelting (1960) but not by Coleman and Green (1960). These effects depend on the use and type of premedication. Sleep is longer-lasting in the premedicated patient and there are fewer movements if an analgesic is given (Dundee and Moore, 1961).

Administration.—Methohexitone is supplied as a powder in bottles containing 500 mg. of methohexitone and 30 mg. of anhydrous sodium carbonate, which should be made up as a 1 per cent solution. Solutions of methohexitone should not be mixed with acid solutions or precipitation of the sparingly soluble free acid will occur.

Methohexitone is administered intravenously. Sensations may occur at the site of injection or along the vein; these may be painful, but since they are not remembered afterwards, and thrombophlebitis does not occur, they are of no significance. The patient falls asleep peacefully but more slowly than with thiopentone. The induction dose is approximately 1 mg./kg. body weight, producing sleep lasting two or three minutes from which the patient makes a rapid recovery.

For out-patients requiring dental extractions, Coleman and Green (1960), using approximately 5 mg./stone (0·8mg./1 kg. approx.) of methohexitone, found that 90 per cent of patients were able to leave the dental chair within 6 minutes and 96 per cent were deemed to be safe to go home within half an hour.

Indications.—Methohexitone is recommended for any brief anaesthetic where rapid, complete recovery is required. It is especially useful for out-patients needing electro-convulsive therapy or dental extraction. It has a place in obstetrics, particularly for Caesarean section (Sliom *et al.*, 1962), and as an induction agent in paediatric anaesthesia (Miller and Stoelting, 1963). In the latter instance the dose is 0·5 mg./kg.

Other Ultra-Short-Acting Barbiturate Drugs

There are many of these, but few if any of them are now in clinical use. For the sake of completeness the formulae for these compounds are illustrated here.

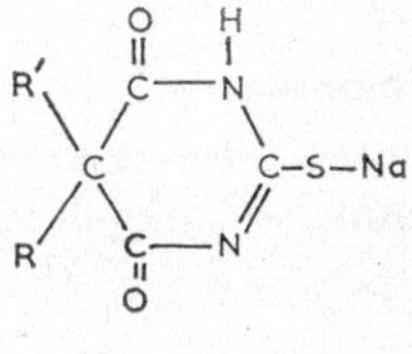

This is the basic thiobarbiturate nucleus. By altering the side chains at R′ and R differing substances are produced. The varying side chains for R′ and R are shown below.

BUTHALITONE

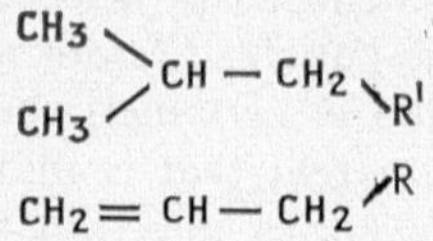

R′: $(CH_3)_2CH-CH_2-$

R: $CH_2=CH-CH_2-$

INACTIN

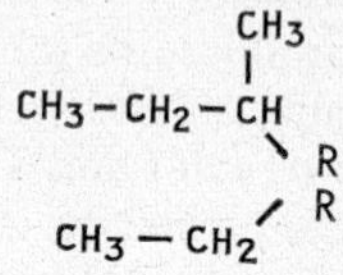

R′: $CH_3-CH_2-CH(CH_3)-$

R: CH_3-CH_2-

METHITURAL

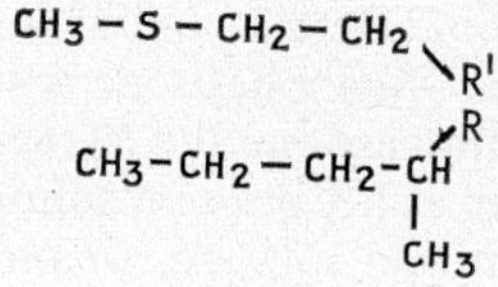

R′: $CH_3-S-CH_2-CH_2-$

R: $CH_3-CH_2-CH_2-CH(CH_3)-$

THIALBARBITONE

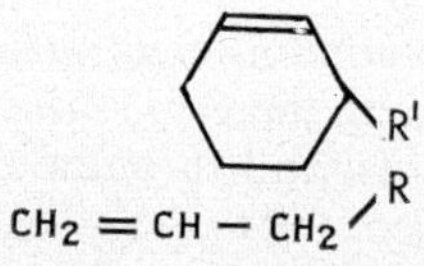

R′: cyclohexenyl

R: $CH_2=CH-CH_2-$

THIAMYLAL

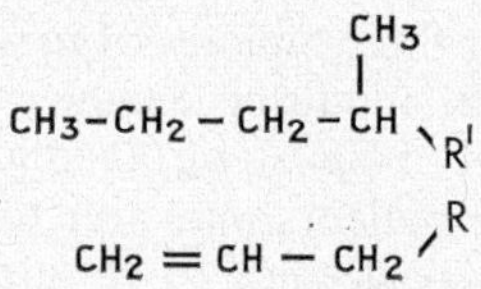

R′: $CH_3-CH_2-CH_2-CH(CH_3)-$

R: $CH_2=CH-CH_2-$

THIONARCEX

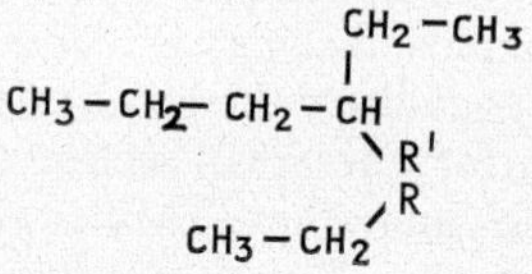

R′: $CH_3-CH_2-CH_2-CH(CH_2-CH_3)-$

R: CH_3-CH_2-

"SPIROTHAL"

R′, R: ring bearing CH_3, CH_3 and C_2H_5

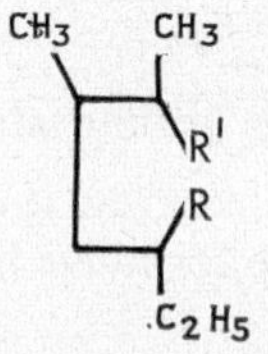

N-methyl and N-ethyl Barbiturates

Many compounds of this type have been synthesised, but some are toxic in that they haemolyse mammalian blood, while others have convulsant properties.

Compound 25398 (Lilly), the sodium salt of 1-methyl, 5-allyl, 5′(1-methyl, 2-pentynyl) barbituric acid (an oxygen barbiturate) was used by Stoelting (1957) and Dobkin and Wyant (1957), who found it three times as potent as thiopentone and that patients recovered more rapidly than after thiopentone, but that it produced greater depression of the cardio-respiratory dynamics.

The destruction of the derivatives was studied in dogs and *in vitro* by Papper and his colleagues (1955), who showed that the brief duration of action of these compounds was due to their greater affinity for fat than was possessed by thiopentone, and not to their rapid breakdown.

Premedication with Barbiturate Drugs

The relief of mental stress and the production of drowsiness and amnesia before an operation are of prime importance. The time of the patient's greatest fear is usually the immediate pre-operative period, while actually waiting in the operating theatre or anaesthetic room. However, the preceding twenty-four hours and the night before the operation are important. In exceptional cases sedation may be necessary for an even longer period while the patient is being prepared for operation.

Phenobarbitone is best used to settle down a worried and frightened patient who is being prepared for operation over some few days. A dosage of 30 or 60 mg. b.d. will prove satisfactory in most cases. Pentobarbitone sodium or quinalbarbitone is valuable for producing a night's rest before the operation, but an intermediate-acting drug, such a butobarbitone, may be needed to keep some patients asleep all night. A dosage of 100 mg. of any of these, given last thing at night, will usually suffice for patients unaccustomed to sedation, whilst 200 mg. will be adequate for those who are more resistant or frightened. This class of barbiturates is also useful for premedication in the immediate pre-operative period as a substitute for opiates or similar drugs, although they may lead to excitement in the post-operative period. This is rarely a manifestation of idiosyncrasy to the particular barbiturate, but is due to the fact that the patient has had no true analgesic—having had no opiate. The dosage of barbiturate given pre-operatively should rarely exceed 200 mg.

For patients suffering from pain before operation, and in whom it is particularly desired to avoid the use of opiates and similar drugs, a combination of barbiturate and simple analgesic, such as acetylsalicylic acid, is usually satisfactory.

Children.—There are no drugs in anaesthesia which combine all the attributes of an ideal pre-operative sedative for children. So much depends upon the particular child, the type of operation, the anaesthetic agents likely to be used, and the immediate post-operative period when reflex activity or full return of consciousness may be essential. Simple sedation alone may be insufficient, and the production of sleep needed, thus necessitating doses of some drugs large enough to border upon the region of undesirable side-effects or a prolonged duration of action spread into the post-operative phase.

In the very young it is often preferable to have the child asleep in bed before the journey to the anaesthetic room is made. The use of sedation, short of sleep, will encourage a helpful frame of mind in a large proportion of these, but unless careful selection is made pre-operatively some will be frightened and considerably upset by the induction of anaesthesia, however skilfully it is performed. Provided sleep can be easily and safely produced by premedication, and provided there are no operative or anaesthetic contra-indications, there seems little reason to deny it in children under seven or eight years of age. Even so, children in older age groups, and some adults on occasion, need similar treatment, and it is most important that their reactions to the unusual circumstances of hospital should be assessed individually. The routine use of drugs is bad in principle—particularly if even a minimum of risk is associated with their administration—and care in the selection of premedication is important so that the whole process of anaesthesia can be made easier, and the risk of a patient being left with unpleasant memories avoided. Quite a lot can be achieved by such simple things as bringing the child to the anaesthetic room in his bed and by the presence of a nurse whom he knows from the ward. Anaesthesia is, however, only a small part of the medical treatment of a patient in hospital, and must not be considered outside the general upsets which are probably far more likely to follow the sudden removal from home influences to those of a hospital.

The post-operative mental state of children after some common otolaryngological operations has been investigated by Eckenhoff (1953), who suggests that 17 per cent of these young patients have a personality change which might be traced to the stay in hospital, the induction of anaesthesia, or the operation. Night terrors, bed-wetting, and untoward fears were the sort of changes noted. Eckenhoff attempts to relate these complications to crying during the induction of anaesthesia, a factor which could be significantly reduced in his series by adequate pre-operative sedation short of sleep, and skill in the administration of the anaesthetic.

In fact skill and kindness are just as important as pre-operative sedation when dealing with small children, who are usually very responsive to a little care and consideration on the part of the anaesthetist. For this reason many combinations of drugs have been advocated at various times, yet it is impossible to say that one is better than another. (See also p. 375.)

Babies and infants up to 18 months of age cannot be included in the above category as they are unlikely to retain any memory of their stay in hospital or of an anaesthetic. It is usually wiser to avoid all depressant drugs and premedicate with atropine only.

Unless in pain, young children rarely need sedation the night before operation, as the need to allay the fear of operation at this stage should not arise if they have been properly handled. Older children, from about 10 to 15 years, are often apprehensive and much can be done by encouragement and simple explanation, but a small dose of a barbiturate may be very helpful. Quinalbarbitone 100 mg. will be satisfactory, but every attempt should be made to judge the dose according to size.

When considering the actual dosage of pre-operative drugs in children, age is a bad guide, since there is marked variability of size at differing ages. Body weight should be the prime consideration.

Short-acting barbiturates.—Quinalbarbitone in a dosage of 7 mg./kg. body weight, or pentobarbitone sodium in a similar dosage, and each with a maximum of 200 mg. will produce satisfactory conditions in most children up to about ten years of age. The younger ones will be asleep, and the older ones at least co-operative. The powder should be removed from the capsules and mixed with jam before being given by mouth. Occasionally it may be impossible to make small children take drugs orally, and in such cases it is helpful to be able to make use of rectal methods. Here pentobarbitone sodium suppositories are satisfactory if they are given two to three hours before the operation is due. The dose is 5 mg./kg. body weight with a maximum of 200 mg.

Prescribing doses above the maximum in older, heavier children does not achieve better sedation but markedly prolongs the action of these drugs. Indeed their principal disadvantage lies in the fact that they are usually effective in some degree post-operatively unless the operation is a very long one. This is a disadvantage since it may mean some reduction in reflex activity with prolonged unconsciousness. Moreover, barbiturates have no analgesic effect, and patients who are in pain while under their effect sometimes become restless and even maniacal, the controlling influence of the higher cortical centres being, as it were, out of action.

Smaller doses of these short-acting barbiturates may be prescribed for children who are out-patients in order to procure some sedation prior to minor operative procedures such as dental extractions. Goulding and his colleagues (1957) carried out a controlled trial in a children's dental out-patient clinic using butobarbitone, methylpentynol, chlorpromazine and a placebo. Judged by their effect on the behaviour of the children, they could not distinguish any of the drugs from the placebo.

Thiopentone.—The rectal injection of thiopentone by the anaesthetist provides a valuable and speedy method for inducing sleep, and has the advantage of a more limited period of action than the medium-acting barbiturates. No sterile precautions are necessary and the powder can be made up in a 5 per cent solution, the dose being assessed on the basis of 45 mg./kg. body weight. When thiopentone is used some method for inflating the child's lungs with oxygen must be to hand, as central depression of the medulla may occur, particularly if the injection is made too quickly. The solution should be given over 10–20 minutes and only until the child is sleeping soundly.

Aladjemoff and her colleagues (1958) have used suppositories of sodium thiopentone in children for the induction of sleep prior to general anaesthesia. They recommend 0·25 g. for children weighing from 6 kg. to 12 kg., and 0·5 g. for those from 12 kg. to 25 kg., and consider that the suppository should be given at least ten to fifteen minutes before the child leaves the ward for the operating theatre. This scaled dosage tends to be too low to produce, at best, more than a brief period of very light sleep unless the children are also sedated with morphine or pethidine—as was the case in Aladjemoff's series. A larger dose, while effective for unsedated children, is less safe.

The use of opiate drugs in premedication is discussed in Chapter 38 and of tranquillisers in Chapter 36.

Barbiturate Poisoning

This may be chronic or acute. Chronic barbiturate poisoning is synonymous with barbiturate addiction. A regular daily dose of 200 mg. of the powerful short-acting barbiturates can probably be taken without harm, but 800 mg. per day will adversely affect performance, and after eight weeks withdrawal symptoms are likely. The average dose taken by the barbiturate addict is 1·5 g. and unless this dose is exceeded severe intoxication is unusual. At any stage an overdose may be taken and then chronic poisoning becomes acute.

Acute Barbiturate Poisoning

Acute barbiturate poisoning is a common means of attempting suicide but may be accidental. In the United States of America—where the barbiturates kill 1,500 people per year—only carbon monoxide exceeds it as the chemical agent of the attempted suicide.

Apart from very rare cases of idiosyncrasy or other complicating factors, five to ten times the full therapeutic dose is required to produce moderate poisoning, while fifteen to twenty times the full therapeutic dose leads to severe poisoning and perhaps death. The fatality rate for all patients with barbiturate poisoning admitted to hospital is about 8 per cent, but for severely poisoned patients rises to 25 per cent. Clemmesen (1954) reported an overall mortality of 1·6 per cent from a special treatment centre in Copenhagen.

Symptoms and signs.—The main effect is depression of the central nervous system which may vary between lethargy and deep coma. Occasionally in the early stages there may be excitement or delirium. Respiration is depressed; the minute volume is decreased but the rate may be slow or rapid—the latter with a very small tidal volume. Cyanosis is common and there may be Cheyne-Stokes respiration. The resulting hypoxia and the direct action of the barbiturate on the circulation causes capillary dilatation and increased permeability. The pulse rate is usually rapid, but the blood pressure may not fall until a late stage of poisoning.

The degree of poisoning can be judged from the amount of reflex activity present, since the pattern of depression produced by the barbiturates is similar to that seen with the anaesthetics. The pupils vary from pin-point, as seen in morphine poisoning, to the large dilated pupils of severe anoxia. If the poisoning is severe the skin is blue, cold, and moist. All bodily functions are depressed. Thus, urine secretion is decreased due to the low blood pressure and the liberation of the anti-diuretic hormone of the pituitary. The body temperature is sometimes low but a rising fever may be present from a secondary pneumonia.

Death, when it occurs early, is usually due to the effects of inadequate respiration due to paralysis of the respiratory centre. At a later stage it is caused by hypostatic pneumonia or pulmonary oedema. Occasionally a fatality results from vasomotor collapse or cerebral oedema; the former is largely secondary to the hypoxia and hypercarbia of inefficient respiration.

Diagnosis.—This depends in part on a knowledge of the circumstances in which the patient was found. Other causes of coma must be excluded and specimens of stomach contents, blood and urine should be obtained for chemical analysis. They may not only assist in the diagnosis but be useful as proof of it for medico-legal reasons. Fortunately the basic treatment of coma is the same whatever its initiator, and should not be delayed while the cause is being looked for.

Treatment.—Clemmesen (1954) evolved in a series of stages a system of treatment that is highly successful. He abandoned gastric washouts in 1942, instituted anti-shock measures in 1946, and laid emphasis on the importance of a clear airway with continuous oxygen therapy in 1947. From 1949 onwards he decreased the use of stimulants until in 1951, following Nilsson's work (Nilsson, 1951), he dispensed with them altogether. Another undoubtedly important step in the reduction of mortality followed the centralisation of all severely poisoned patients in one hospital.

The patient should be carefully nursed, preferably in the lateral position with a slight Trendelenburg tilt to the bed, so that the risk of aspiration of gastric contents is reduced, and pulmonary drainage assisted. Frequent changes of position and percussion of the chest must be carried out. The airway must be closely observed and aspiration of all secretions from the back of the mouth must be repeatedly performed.

Antibiotics should be ordered prophylactically, but when any infection supervenes a specific drug must be chosen after typing the organism. Temperature, pulse, respiration and blood pressure must be carefully observed and recorded. Haemoglobin readings must be taken at regular intervals—at least daily—to check for destruction of red corpuscles, and electrolytes and fluid balances recorded and maintained.

Many patients can be stabilised on this regime, but those who are severely poisoned may need extra help. Hypotension is best treated by the intravenous infusion of blood, but dextran or plasma may be used if the haemoglobin content is high. An endotracheal tube may be necessary to ensure an adequate airway; plastic tubes are preferable. Marked respiratory paresis, or apnoea, will require artificial respiration; a tracheotomy is then best performed. An abnormally low temperature may suggest the need for radiant heat cradles, while a temperature above 102° F (39° C) should be reduced.

Such treatment regimes greatly reduce the mortality of barbiturate poisoning, though deaths occur frequently among severe cases even in special treatment centres. Survival is aided by measures designed to remove barbiturate from the body: forced diuresis, peritoneal dialysis or haemodialysis, of which the last is probably the most effective. An exact comparison between these three is impossible because the allocation of cases to different treatment regimes is usually decided by their severity. Forced diuresis, particularly with alkalinisation of the urine, has been shown to cause considerable loss of drug which loss undoubtedly contributed to the low mortality (less than 2 per cent) of one series of 110 severely poisoned cases (Linton *et al.*, 1967). Drug removal is equally effective with any diuretic agent and is proportional to the diuresis produced (Fig. 4).

In severe cases of poisoning, methods of drug removal should be applied as soon as possible. Lee and Ames (1965) suggest that forced alkaline diuresis is probably adequate for many cases but that haemodialysis should be started thereafter if one of the following criteria is fulfilled:

1. a continued fall of blood pressure,
2. deepening unconsciousness,
3. unobtainable reflexes, or
4. rising plasma barbiturate concentrations.

In such severe cases Matthew and Lawson (1966) have reported a mortality of

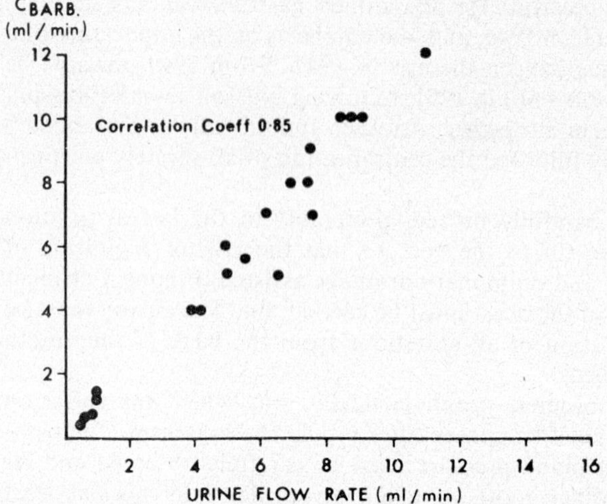

35/Fig. 4. — Butobarbitone clearance and urinary flow-rates.

8·8 per cent (6 of 68 cases) and Setter *et al.* (1966) 12·7 per cent (22 out of 173). In Lee and Ames' (1965) series there were no deaths among 181 patients including 15 who required haemodialysis, in spite of episodes of hypothermia and cardiac arrest.

Non-Barbiturate Hypnotics and Sedatives

The congenital defects produced in babies by the administration of thalidomide to mothers during early pregnancy focused attention on the need to be certain of the safety of new drugs before administering them to patients. These complications also serve to emphasise the safety of established agents.

Several non-barbiturate hypnotics and sedatives are tabulated below. Two that are commonly used—glutethimide and methylpentynol—are described in greater detail.

Gamma Hydroxybutyric Acid

The sodium salt of γ-hydroxybutyric acid (gamma–OH) was introduced into anaesthetic practice by Laborit and his colleagues in France in 1960.

$$\underset{\gamma\text{-hydroxybutyric acid}}{\overset{\mathrm{OH}}{\mathrm{CH_2}}-\mathrm{CH_2}-\mathrm{CH_2}-\overset{\mathrm{OH}}{\mathrm{C}}=\mathrm{O}} \xrightarrow{-\mathrm{H_2O}} \underset{\gamma\text{-butyrolactone}}{\mathrm{CH_2}\diagdown\!\overset{\mathrm{O}}{}\!\diagup\mathrm{C}=\mathrm{O},\ \mathrm{CH_2}-\mathrm{CH_2}}$$

Gamma–OH exists partly in the body as its internal ester γ-butyrolactone and both of these are intermediate products in the metabolism of glucose in normal brain (Fishbein and Bessman, 1964).

Gamma–OH is a hypnotic. When 60–70 mg./kg. is given intravenously sleep occurs in about five minutes and deepens to an unrousable coma which lasts from one and a quarter to one and three-quarters of an hour, after which rapid awakening occurs. Smaller doses may produce a light sleep or even hypomania. It is not analgesic. Clonic movements may occur during induction; these are abolished by small doses of a phenothiazine or a barbiturate and make the induction subjectively more pleasant. Even during the unrousable coma surgical stimuli cause tachycardia, hypertension and sweating.

The electro-encephalographic changes produced by gamma–OH are unique. In man there is no fast activity as seen with the barbiturates, but a steady development of slow, high voltage waves. The disappearance of clinical arousal, which persists after EEG arousal has disappeared, is accompanied by electrical silence punctuated by high frequency bursts similar to K-complexes (Schneider *et al.*, 1963). During light coma there are periods of paradoxical sleep with rapid eye movements and dreaming (Yanagida, 1965). In animals the muscular hypotonia has been shown to be due to depression of the inter-nuncial neurones (Basil *et al.*, 1964).

Cardiovascular effects.—Virtue and his colleagues (1966) investigated the effects of gamma–OH on the cardiovascular system of man in the absence of surgical stimuli. Arterial and central venous pressures were stable, the heart rate slowed and the cardiac output fell to a minimum in 30 minutes. The administration of atropine caused an increase in heart rate, cardiac output and systolic blood pressure and a fall in central venous pressure. Steel (1968), however, found a fall of arterial blood pressure in 60 per cent of patients and a bradycardia even after the administration of atropine. Surgical stimuli produce a sympathomimetic response (vasoconstriction) which leads to a maintenance of a normal or even raised blood pressure. It doubles the survival time of anoxic rabbit hearts (Herold *et al.*, 1961).

Other systems.—In animals respiration is unaffected, but Steel (1968) found a slowing of the respiratory rate and four cases of periodic breathing in man. During labour the frequency and amplitude of the uterine contractions increases and the uterus becomes more sensitive to oxytocic drugs (Alfonsi and Massi, 1964). Gamma–OH produces a rise in blood sugar of 25 mg./100 ml., whilst under similar conditions thiopentone produces a rise of 10 mg./100 ml. Both drugs cause a slight metabolic alkalosis, but it is more marked in those given gamma–OH and persists for the first two post-operative days (Robinson *et al.*, 1968).

During recovery definite mental disturbance may occur; Steel (1968) reported an incidence of 7–8 per cent, but when other drugs such as phenothiazines and analgesics are used as well this complication does not occur (Tunstall, 1968). Gamma–OH has been used for the production of release phenomena in acute anxiety states (du Couedic *et al.*, 1964).

Gamma–OH is an interesting compound but it has not found a useful place in clinical anaesthetic practice.

Glutethimide ("Doriden")

Glutethimide is α-phenyl α-ethylglutarimide

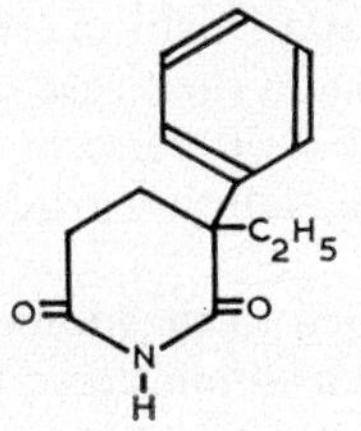

C_2H_5

O O

N

H

Physical properties.—It is a white crystalline powder, relatively insoluble in water and with a molecular weight of 217·3. Its melting point is 83–85° C.

Pharmacological actions.—Glutethimide is a sedative hypnotic with properties similar to phenobarbitone but a shorter action. It has anticonvulsant properties whose intensity lies between those of phenobarbitone and methylpentynol (Gross *et al.*, 1955). It is not depressant to respiration and diminishes oxygen consumption less than phenobarbitone.

Glutethimide 500 mg. has about the same effect as pentobarbitone sodium 100 mg. in normal volunteers (Isaacs, 1957).

Sleep lasts about 8 hours and "hangover" effect is rare, after 500 mg. of the drug. Occasional skin rashes occur. Nausea and mental excitement are reported (Rushbrooke *et al.*, 1956).

Metabolism and excretion.—Orally administered, glutethimide is only

35/Table 2

Various Non-barbiturate Hypnotics and Sedatives

Ethchlorvynol	"Anvynol" "Placidyl" "Serenesil"	250–750 mg.	Lasts 5–6 hours. Detoxified in the liver. Dangerous with alcohol.
Ethinamate	"Valdimate" "Valmid"	500 mg.–2 g.	Lasts 2–4 hours. Completely destroyed in the body.
Glutethimide	"Doriden"	250–500 mg.	
Methaqualone	"Melsedin"	150–300 mg.	150 mg. equipotent with 200 mg. of cyclo- or amylobarbitone.
Methyprylone	"Noludar"	200–400 mg.	400 mg. equipotent with 100 mg. quinalbarbitone.
Methylpentynol	"Oblivon" "Insomnol" "Dormison"	250–500 mg.	
Propiomazine	"Indorm"	20–40 mg.	See under Phenothiazines, p. 1022.

slightly broken down and is mainly excreted in the urine conjugated with glucuronic acid, while about 4 per cent is found as α-phenyl glutarimide.

Clinical uses.—Glutethimide is useful when a patient is sensitive to or intolerant of the barbiturates, but addiction and withdrawal symptoms have been described with it (Johnson and Van Buren, 1962). Overdosage causes results as severe as those due to an excess of barbiturate (Maher *et al.*, 1962). Abbas (1957) found glutethimide to be an effective sedative when administered early in labour, and Burroo and Borromeo (1956) consider that it is preferable to barbiturates or a combination of barbiturates and narcotics as a sedative prior to cystoscopy under local analgesia. Stephen and Duvoisin (1960) consider it an unsatisfactory form of premedication. They based their case on a double blind trial, using 5·0 per cent glutethimide dissolved in 70 per cent polyethylene-glycol-400 and administering it intravenously. This solution produced some haemolysis *in vivo* but not *in vitro*.

Glutethimide is closely related to thalidomide, a drug which is able to produce deformities in a foetus when administered to a woman in the early stages of pregnancy (Smithells, 1962; Rosendal, 1963). There is no evidence that glutethimide might do the same.

Hydroxydione

This steroid derivative is described in Chapter 50.

Ketamine ("Ketalar")

Ketamine, a recently introduced non-barbiturate anaesthetic for intravenous or intramuscular use, is a derivative of phencyclidine.

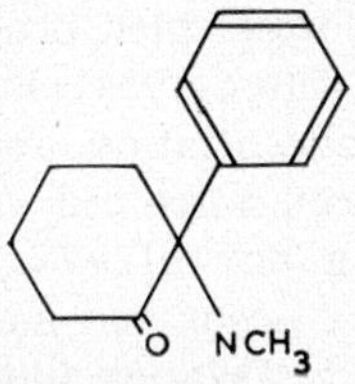

O NCH$_3$

It is available as an aqueous solution of the hydrochloride salt of pH 3·5–5·5 and contains 10 or 50 mg. ketamine base per ml.

Used in doses of 0·5 to 6 mg./kg. body weight it produces rapid onset of anaesthesia with powerful analgesia but only mild transient or no respiratory depression (Langrehr *et al.*, 1967). The anaesthetic state, characterised by marked sensory blockade and minimal effects on the reticular activating and limbic systems, has been termed "dissociative anaesthesia". In a study of about 1,500 administrations at doses of 2–4 mg./kg., Corssen *et al.* (1968) reported that the drug produced surgical anaesthesia lasting 20 to 40 minutes. Moderate hypertension (a rise of more than 25 per cent over resting pressure) occurred in 8·1 per cent of cases and tachycardia (an increase in rate of 50 per cent or more) in 4·3 per cent of cases due to the drug's sympathomimetic action. The opposite effects occurred in fewer than 1 per cent of cases. The drug is therefore contra-indicated in hypertensive subjects.

Ketamine is metabolised by hepatic hydroxylation and has a plasma half-life of two hours. Recovery of consciousness is rapid but complete recovery may take three hours. In the post-anaesthetic state delirium, disturbed dream states and occasional hallucinations occur. These psychotomimetic effects, characteristic of the action of phencyclidine, appear to be commoner in adults than in children (Roberts, 1967; Wilson *et al.*, 1967). To overcome these, either a small dose of a barbiturate is given or—more important—the patient is *completely* undisturbed during the emergence phase. Further assessments of the drug's use are needed but it may have a place in the management of patients for anaesthesia in the sitting position, in whom maintenance of blood pressure is critical, for surgical procedures of short duration in children, and for anaesthesia in difficult situations.

Methylpentynol ("Oblivon", "Dormison")

Methylpentynol (3 methyl pentyne-ol 3), which was first described by Margolin and his associates (1951), is an unsaturated aliphatic carbinol—a higher alcohol—whose structural formula is:

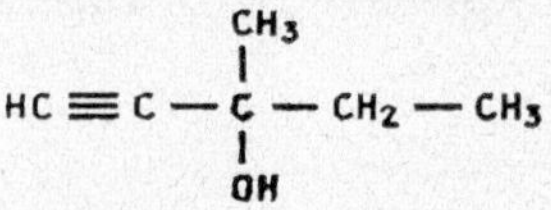

$$HC \equiv C - \underset{\displaystyle OH}{\overset{\displaystyle CH_3}{\underset{|}{\overset{|}{C}}}} - CH_2 - CH_3$$

Physical properties.—Methylpentynol is an oily, volatile liquid with a most unpleasant burning taste.

Pharmacological actions.—Methylpentynol produces alleviation of anxiety and, in some patients, sleep. It acts in a way that is as yet undetermined, but which is not the same as that of ethyl alcohol. Sinton (1954) showed that 1·0 g. of methylpentynol given to normal men produced no signs of intoxication but did diminish nervousness. Trotter (1954) showed that after 0·5 g. of methylpentynol speed of reaction, concentration and co-ordination remained unimpaired and may even have been enhanced. Rowell (1957) reported mental exhilaration for ten hours in a boy of two years who received 0·25 g. of methylpentynol. Side-effects may occur and include dizziness, lightheadedness and deviation of the mood pattern (Marley and Chambers, 1956).

Excessive doses of methylpentynol can produce various nervous manifestations. These vary from confusion-ataxia with slurring of speech and a labile emotional state to diplopia, nystagmus and visual hallucinations (Glatt, 1955). Marley (1955) has reported EEG abnormalities associated with nystagmus ptosis, dysarthria, ataxia, glycosuria and acetonuria following 1 g. of the substance three times a day. Death has followed the administration of 4·5–6·0 g. methylpentynol (Cares *et al.*, 1953), but recovery has followed 8·75 and 10 g. (Lemere, 1952; Brown and Ellis, 1955). On the other hand, prolonged use in animals (Margolin *et al.*, 1951) and in man (Chevalley *et al.*, 1952) has been reported without any toxic effects.

Methylpentynol does not cause any respiratory depression, and does not affect the blood pressure in therapeutic dosage. The pulse rate usually rises slightly. Shaffarzick and Brown (1952) investigated its effect on liver function and reported that two out of six epileptic patients developed a strongly positive cephalic flocculation reaction, while these workers also found that the livers of rats given methylpentynol in their drinking water exhibited a diminution of hepatic cell cytoplasmic basophilia.

Simpson (1954) has shown that methylpentynol does not accumulate in the body.

Clinical uses.—Methylpentynol is made up in capsules, containing 250 mg., and as an elixir containing 250 mg. in 4 ml. The recommended adult dose is 250 mg. ten to fifteen minutes before the time when the effect of the drug is required. Up to 1 g. may be used as a sleeping draught. Its main asset appears to be its power to relieve apprehension, but this result is variable and intoxication occurs occasionally, even with a normal dose. Reports differ on its value as a hypnotic. Chevalley and his colleagues (1952) considered it 90 per cent efficient, whereas Allen and Krongold (1951), administering it to patients with advanced tuberculosis, thought it only 30 per cent efficient.

Gusterson (1955) found methylpentynol as satisfactory as a barbiturate for premedication in children. Both he and Rendell (1954) agree that it does not help the very apprehensive child, but Rendell considers it safer than a barbiturate when post-operative nursing is not of a high standard. The doses recommended by Gusterson are:

> 2 teaspoonsful (500 mg.) of the elixir for children 2–4 years old.
> 3 teaspoonsful (750 mg.) of the elixir for children 4–8 years old.
> 4 teaspoonsful (1 g.) of the elixir for children 8–10 years old.

given 1 hour pre-operatively.

Methylpentynol has not proved as useful as a sedative as was originally hoped. All in all, when a standard effect from a given dose of a drug is required other sedatives are more reliable.

Propanidid ("Epontol", F.B.A. 1420)

This non-barbiturate, ultra-short-acting anaesthetic is a derivative of eugenol.

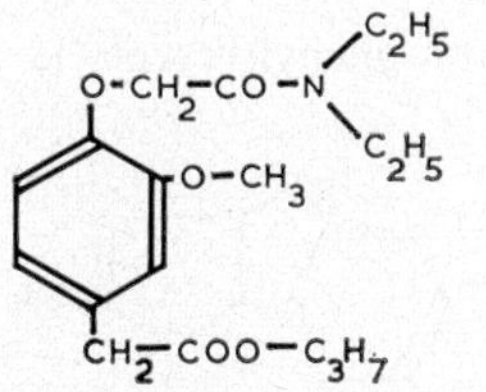

C_2H_5
$O{-}CH_2{-}CO{-}N$
C_2H_5
$O{-}CH_3$
$CH_2{-}COO{-}C_3H_7$

It is a pale yellow oil which, for clinical use, is dissolved in 20 per cent Cremophor El, a non-ionised, surface-active aqueous solution of äthoxylated castor oil, to give a 5 per cent solution of propanidid. This solution is highly viscous but it can be further diluted with an equal volume of physiological saline for easier administration.

It is rapidly metabolised to an anaesthetically inactive acid metabolite by enzymatic splitting of the ester bond, mainly in the liver but also in the blood by pseudo-cholinesterase (Putter, 1965). This rapid breakdown determines the brief duration of anaesthesia.

When 5–6 mg./kg. is administered intravenously over twenty seconds (the recommended rate) the unpremedicated patient is deeply asleep within about thirty seconds. 6 per cent of patients show involuntary muscular movements and 8 and 9 per cent a cough or hiccup. Awakening occurs in four to eight minutes and rational conversation is possible after a further two or three minutes (Wynands *et al.*, 1963). There are no "hangover" effects but phlebitis occurs in 4 per cent, and as a large needle is used for the injection greater care than usual is necessary to prevent haematoma formation.

The blood pressure falls and the pulse rate rises in most patients. The respiratory changes are characteristic (Harnik, 1964), the onset of anaesthesia being accompanied by a period of hyperventilation followed by apnoea which may last up to thirty seconds.

Propanidid prolongs the respiratory effects of suxamethonium because of their common route of metabolism, but the requirements for *d*-tubocurarine are increased (Clarke *et al.*, 1967).

The brevity of its effects means that to prolong anaesthesia either the dose of propanidid must be repeated or other agents administered rapidly to achieve a smooth transition. Premedication helps this but delays recovery.

ANALEPTICS

Could a ready means of shortening barbiturate narcosis be found, it would have two therapeutic applications. First, as a means of treating the many patients suffering from barbiturate overdosage, and secondly, for reversing post-operatively the effects of a therapeutic anaesthetic dose; this would enhance the value of barbiturates in the out-patient department, and in the operating theatre should a rapid return to consciousness be desirable. To date, however, no practical, safe way of shortening barbiturate narcosis has been convincingly demonstrated, and no specific antagonistic drugs exist. Central nervous system stimulants can be used to help overcome respiratory depression but in practice they are not usually very effective. They work by direct and/or reflex chemo-receptor stimulation of the medullary centres.

Amiphenazole ("Daptazole", D.A.P.T.) (see also Chapter 37)

Amiphenazole or diamino-phenylthiazole is 2:4 diamino-5-phenylthiazole hydrochloride:

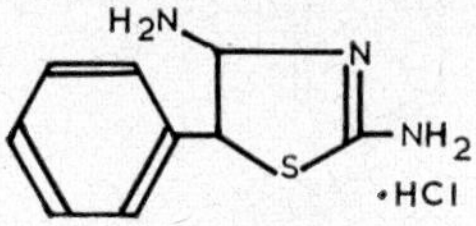

Physical properties.—Amiphenazole is a colourless crystalline compound, readily soluble in water or saline. Solutions of amiphenazole decompose if autoclaved, but 300 mg. of the dry sterilised powder can be easily dissolved in 20 ml. of sterile physiological saline as required: the resulting solution is stable at room temperature for twenty-four hours.

Pharmacological actions.—Amiphenazole is a non-specific respiratory stimulant which antagonises the respiratory depression produced by morphine, heroin, papaveretum and the synthetic analgesics, pethidine and methadone hydrochloride. It usually antagonises the constipation produced by papaveretum, and occasionally the vomiting (Shaw and Shulman, 1955).

In large doses amiphenazole will antagonise the analgesic effects of morphine and leave the patient awake and mentally restless, and may even cause muscular twitching and occasionally vomiting. Amiphenazole has no analgesic properties of its own and has little effect on the blood pressure, but a large dose (75 mg.) intravenously may cause a rise.

Conscious subjects have been given 300 mg. of amiphenazole slowly intravenously with no change in blood pressure, pulse rate, or the electro-encephalogram (McKeogh and Shaw, 1956).

Clinical use.—Amiphenazole has been used as an adjuvant to the treatment of barbiturate poisoning with bemegride (Shulman *et al.*, 1955), but the necessity for its use except in cases with severe respiratory depression is not established.

Amiphenazole has been used in combination with large doses of morphine in the treatment of intractable pain (Shaw and Shulman, 1955; McKeogh and Shaw, 1956).

Hayward-Butt (1957) has described the use of a combination of pethidine, amiphenazole and mepazine (a tranquillising drug) for patients undergoing surgical operations. He considers that satisfactory conditions can frequently be achieved in this manner without resort to anaesthetic agents and without the patient becoming unconscious. He suggests the term "ataralgesia" for the procedure and estimates his drug dosage in terms of units of the mixture—1 unit containing pethidine 100 mg., amiphenazole 25 mg. and mepazine 100 mg. For an average patient 3 units are given intramuscularly forty-five minutes prior to the operation, and further doses of 1 unit or less are added intravenously during the operation when necessary.

Dose.—The drug is available for injection as 15 mg. of powder in ampoules and should be dissolved in 1·5 ml. of sterile water or saline. Tablets of 20 mg. are also made. The dose is 20–60 mg. by injection or by mouth, but a suitable long-term combination with a drug such as morphine can only be found by use on the patient.

Bemegride ("Megimide")

Bemegride is $\beta\beta$-methyl-ethyl glutarimide and it was introduced by Shulman and his associates in 1955 as a specific antagonist to the barbiturates on the basis of structural relationship.

H_5C_2 CH_3

O O

N

H

Physical properties.—Bemegride is a stable crystalline substance. It is supplied as a 0·5 per cent solution which is almost a saturated solution of the drug, so that at low temperatures crystals may be deposited. These will re-dissolve with gentle rewarming.

Pharmacological actions.—Animal experiments suggest that it reduces the period of narcosis with thiopentone and pentobarbitone.

Bemegride has a marked stimulatory action on respiration, and when injected in large doses produces fasciculation or convulsions. Kimura and Richards (quoted by Richards and Taylor, 1956) state that their evidence points to the fact that bemegride is an unspecific central stimulant and convulsant rather than a "specific" barbiturate antagonist. This is also suggested by Louw and Sonne (1956) who investigated the EEG changes after bemegride administration to patients suffering from barbiturate poisoning. They found patterns of universal cortical stimulation in some patients with spikes that appeared before any clinical effect was manifest. Wyke and Frayworth (1957) believe that the site of action of bemegride is on the reticular system of the brain. This system links the cerebral cortex with the reticular nuclei and is thought to be the area that is most affected by the barbiturate drugs. An action at this site would explain the remarkable improvement in reflex activity and respiratory function.

Cass (1956) has demonstrated in rabbits anaesthetised with barbiturates or glutethimide that bemegride can produce in the EEG a return to the patterns of light anaesthesia from those of deep anaesthesia, but he could not produce a similar effect during chloralose, methylpentynol or ether anaesthesia.

Nearly all the clinical evidence suggests that although bemegride can lighten the degree of unconsciousness it cannot shorten the duration of it (Louw and Sonne, 1956; Pedersen, 1956; Wyke, 1957).

Bemegride does not have any effect on the elimination of barbiturates from the body, and its use may be followed by a psychosis resembling that associated with barbiturate withdrawal symptoms (Kjaer-Larsen, 1956).

Clinical uses.—Shulman and his associates (1955) do not recommend that bemegride should be used in the treatment of barbiturate poisoning in an attempt to wake the patient up, but rather to bring him to a "safe state" in which muscle tone and reflex activity are present. This, they say, takes about two hours even from deep coma. There is good clinical evidence that bemegride can help to restore adequate ventilation, and Clemmesen (1956) has confirmed the effectiveness of a mixture of bemegride and amiphenazole on the depressed respiration of severe barbiturate intoxication. But despite these optimistic results the place of bemegride in the treatment of barbiturate poisoning is not yet fully established. Kaufman (1958) does not consider that bemegride is effective as a means of awakening patients after barbiturate anaesthesia.

Dose.—The dose required varies with the depth of coma, but bemegride is usually given as a single intravenous injection of 50 mg. in a 0·5 per cent solution. This dose is then repeated at 3–5 minute intervals until the patient shows signs of rousing. Should reflex activity disappear again after a period of time, further doses must be administered. Twitching, incipient convulsions and perhaps vomiting are indications of overdosage.

Ethamivan. Vanillic Acid Diethylamide ("Vandid")

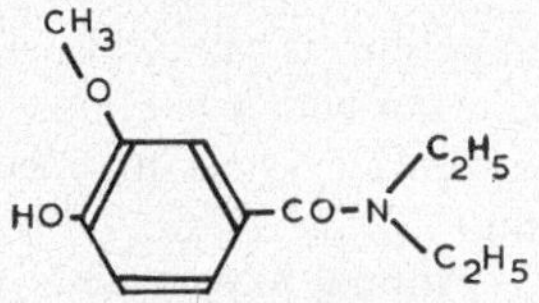

CH_3 O HO CO–N C_2H_5 C_2H_5

Vanillic acid diethylamide is a central respiratory and circulatory stimulant. An intravenous dose of 0·6–2·0 mg. per kg. body weight will produce a rapid increase in the volume of respiration, followed in about a minute by an increase in respiratory and pulse rates with a moderate rise in blood pressure (Auinger *et al.*, 1952). All these effects are, however, of short duration—ten to fifteen minutes.

Leptazol ("Metrazol", "Cardiazol")

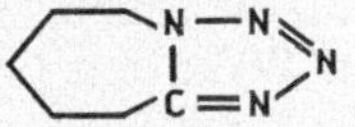

N—N N C=N

Leptazol is a general stimulant of the nervous system, with an action lasting a quarter to half an hour. The dose is 1 ml. of a 10 per cent solution.

Nikethamide ("Coramine", "Anacardone")

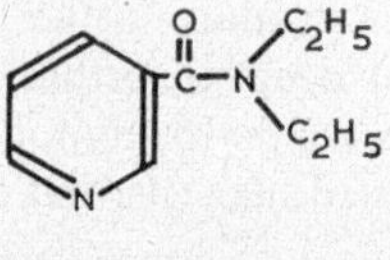

O C–N C_2H_5 C_2H_5 N

Nikethamide is a synthetic substance which is made up as a 25 per cent solution. It stimulates respiration via the chemoreceptors of the carotid body and has a weak vasoconstrictor effect on the peripheral circulation. It has little, if any, effect on the myocardium unless large doses are given, when it raises the output slightly. The action of nikethamide is brief (10–15 minutes) and the dose is 1–2 ml. of the 25 per cent solution given intravenously.

REFERENCES

ABBAS, T. M. (1957). Clinical trial of glutethimide in labour. *Brit. med. J.*, **1,** 563.

ADRIANI, J. (1939). Effects of anesthetic drugs upon rats treated with sulfanilimide. *J. Lab. clin. Med.*, **24,** 1066.

ADRIANI, J., and ROVENSTINE, E. A. (1943). The effect of anesthetic drugs upon bronchi and bronchioles of excised lung tissue. *Anesthesiology*, **4,** 253.

ALADJEMOFF, L., KAPLAN, I., and GETESH, T. (1958). Sodium thiopentone suppositories in paediatric anaesthesia. *Anaesthesia*, **13,** 152.

ALDRIDGE, W. N. (1962). Action of barbiturates upon respiratory enzymes. In: *Enzymes and Drug Action*, p. 155. Ed. Mongar, J. L. and de Reuck, A.V.S. London: J. & A. Churchill.

ALFONSI, P. L., and MASSI, G. B. (1964). Prime esperienze sull'impiego clinico del 4-idrossi-butirrato di sodii in anestesis per l'ostetrecia e la ginecologia. *Minerva anest.*, **30,** 115.

ALLEN, A. W., and KRONGOLD, D. D. (1951). Dormison, a new hypnotic. *Quart. Bull. Sea View Hosp.*, **12,** 61.

ANDERSON, H. H., CHEN, M. Y., and LEXAKE, C. D. (1930). The effects of barbituric acid hypnotics on basal metabolism in humans. *J. Pharmacol. exp. Ther.*, **40,** 215.

ASERINSKY, E., and KLEITMAN, N. (1953). Regularly occurring periods of eye motility and concomitant phenomena during sleep. *Science*, **118,** 273.

AUINGER, W., KAINDL, F., SALZMANN, F., and WEISSEL, W. (1952). Zur Atem- und Kreislauf-wirkung von 3-Methoxy-4-oxy-benzoesäurediä-thylamid. *Wien. Z. inn. Med.*, **33,** 23.

AURUP, R., and HOUGS, W. (1963). Effect of enallynymal natrium (Brietal), enhexymal natrium (Evipan) and thiomebumal natrium (Pentothal) on bronchial muscles. *Acta anaesth. scand.*, **7,** 83.

BASIL, B., BLAIR, A. M. J. N., and HOLMES, S. W. (1964). The action of sodium 4-hydroxybutyrate on spinal reflexes. *Brit. J. Pharmacol.*, **22,** 318.

BEECHER, H. K. (1951). Pain and some factors which modify it. *Anesthesiology*, **12,** 633.

BERGER, F. M., and LYNES, T. E. (1955). Effect of mephenesin on barbiturate anesthesia. *Arch. int. Pharmacodyn.*, **100,** 401.

BRITISH MEDICAL JOURNAL (1951). Medico-Legal Notes, **1,** 707.

BRODIE, B. B. (1952). Physiological disposition and chemical fate of thiobarbiturates in the body. *Fed. Proc.*, **11,** 632.

BRODIE, B. B., MARK, L. C., PAPPER, E. M., LIEF, P. A., BERNSTEIN, E., and ROVENSTINE, E. A. (1950). Fate of thiopental in man and a method for its estimation in biological material. *J. Pharmacol. exp. Ther.*, **98,** 85.

BROWN, I. M., and ELLIS, R. A. (1955). Recovery after overdosage with methylpentynol. *Brit. med. J.*, **1,** 268.

BUCHEL, L., and LEVY, J. (1951). Sur deux nouvelles substances de la série des barbituriques et thiobarbituriques. *Anesth. et Analg.*, **8,** 433.

BUCHEL, L., LEVY, J., and TCHOUBAR, B. (1953). Rapport entre la constitution et l'action dans la série des barbituriques et des thiobarbituriques porteurs de radicaux alcohyles, ramifiés en alpha. *Anesth. et Analg.*, **10,** 343.

BURN, J. H., and HOBBS, R. (1959). Mechanism of arterial spasm following intra-arterial injection of thiopentone. *Lancet*, **1,** 1112.

BURNS, J. J., and CONNEY, A. H. (1965). Enzyme stimulation and inhibition in the metabolism of drugs. *Proc. roy. Soc. Med.*, **58,** 955.

BURROO, H. M., and BORROMEO, V. H. J. (1956). *Alpha*-ethyl-*alpha* phenyl glutarimide (Doriden) as a sedative agent for pre-cystoscopic sedation. *J. Urol.* (*Baltimore*), **76,** 456.

BUSH, M. T., BUTLER, T. C., and DICKISON, H. L. (1953). Metabolic fate of 5(1-*cyclo*-hexen-1-yl) 1,5 dimethylbarbituric acid (Hexobarbital, Evipal) and of 5-(1-*cyclo*-hexen-1-yl) 5-methyl barbituric acid ("nor-Evipal"). *J. Pharmacol. exp. Ther.*, **108,** 104.

BUTZENGEIGER, O. (1927). Klinische Erfahrungen mit Avertin (E 107). *Dtsch. med. Wschr.*, **53,** 712.

CARES, R. M., NEWMAN, B., and MAUCERI, J. C. (1953). Poisoning by methylparafynol (Dormison). Fatal suicidal overdosage of 3-methyl-pentyne-ol-3, a new hypnotic. *Amer. J. clin. Path.*, **23,** 129.

CASS, N. M. (1956). An electro-encephalographic study of the analeptic action of $\beta\beta$-ethyl-methyl glutarimide. *Brit. J. Anaesth.*, **28,** 324.

CERVELLO, V. (1882). Sull 'Azione Fisiologica della Paraldeide e Contributo Allo Studio del Chloralio Idrato. Richerche. *Arch. Sci. med.*, **6,** 177.

CHEVALLEY, J., HEMINWAY, N., MEYER, G., FRANCHAUSER, R., and MCGAVACK, T. H. (1952). A clinical evaluation of methylparafynol as a soporific agent. *N.Y. St. J. Med.*, **52,** 572.

CLARKE, R. S. J., DUNDEE, J. W., and HAMILTON, R. C. (1967). Interactions between induction agents and muscle relaxants. *Anaesthesia*, **22,** 235.

CLEMMESEN, C. (1954). A new line of treatment in barbiturate poisoning. *Acta med. scand.*, **148,** 83.

CLEMMESEN, C. (1956). Effect of megimide and amiphenazole on respiratory paresis. *Lancet*, **2,** 966.

COHEN, S. M. (1948). Accidental intra-arterial injection of drugs. *Lancet*, **2,** 361, 409.

COLEMAN, J., and GREEN, R. A. (1960). Methohexital. A short acting barbiturate. *Anaesthesia*, **15,** 411.

CONWAY, C. M., and ELLIS, D. B. (1969). The haemodynamic effects of short-acting barbiturates. *Brit. J. Anaesth.*, **41,** 534.

CORSSEN, G., MIYASAKA, M., and DOMINO, E. F. (1968). Changing concepts in pain control during surgery: dissociative anaesthesia with CI–581. *Anesth. Analg. Curr. Res.*, **47,** 746.

CRAWFORD, J. S. (1956). Some aspects of obstetric anaesthesia. *Brit. J. Anaesth.*, **28,** 146.

DANCE, C. L., BOOZER, J., NEWMAN, W., and BURSTEIN, C. L. (1956). Electrocardiographic studies during endotracheal intubation. *Anesthesiology*, **17,** 730.

DEMENT, W., and FISHER, C. (1963). Experimental interference with the sleep cycle. *Canad. psychiat. Ass. J.*, **8,** 395.

DE WARDENER, H. E. (1955). Renal circulation during anaesthesia and surgery. *Anaesthesia*, **10,** 18.

DOBKIN, A. B., and WYANT, G. M. (1957). The physiological effects of intravenous anaesthesia on man, *Canad. Anaesth. Soc. J.*, **4,** 295.

DOMEK, N. S., BARLOW, C. F., and ROTH, L. J. (1960). An ontogenetic study of phenobarbital–C^{14} in cat brain. *J. Pharmacol. exp. Ther.*, **130,** 285.

DU COUEDIC, H., DU COUEDIC, A., and VOISSE, M. (1964). Experimental studies of the breakdown of Epontol: Determination of propanidid in human serum. *Brit. J. Anaesth.*, 40, 415.

DUNDEE, J. W. (1951). Thiopentone in Addison's disease. *Brit. J. Anaesth.*, **23,** 167.

DUNDEE, J. W. (1952*a*). Thiopentone narcosis in the presence of hepatic dysfunction. *Brit. J. Anaesth.*, **24,** 81.

DUNDEE, J. W. (1952*b*). Thiopentone in dystrophia myotonia. *Curr. Res. Anesth.*, **31,** 257.

DUNDEE, J. W. (1954). A review of chlorpromazine hydrochloride. *Brit. J. Anaesth.*, **26,** 357.

DUNDEE, J. W. (1955*a*). Cumulative action of four thiobarbiturates with special reference to thiopentone and thiamylal. *Anaesthesia*, **10,** 391.

DUNDEE, J. W. (1955*b*). Thiopentone as a factor in the production of liver dysfunction. *Brit. J. Anaesth.*, **27,** 14.

DUNDEE, J. W. (1956). *Thiopentone and Other Thiobarbiturates.* Edinburgh: E. & S. Livingstone.

DUNDEE, J. W., and MOORE, J. (1961). The effects of premedication with phenothiazine derivatives on the course of methohexitone anaesthesia. *Brit. J. Anaesth.*, **33,** 382.

DUNDEE, J. W., and RICHARDS, R. K. (1954). Effect of azotaemia upon the action of intravenous barbiturate anesthesia. *Anesthesiology*, **15,** 333.

DUNDEE, J. W., and TODD, U. M. (1958). Clinical significance of the effects of thiobarbiturates and adjuvant drugs on blood sugar and glucose tolerance. *Brit. J. Anaesth.*, **30,** 77.

ECKENHOFF, J. E. (1953). Preanesthetic sedation of children. Analysis of the effects for tonsillectomy and adenoidectomy. *A.M.A. Arch. Otolaryng.*, **57,** 441.

ECKSTEIN, J. W., HAMILTON, W. K., and MCCAMMOND, J. M. (1961). The effect of thiopental on peripheral venous tone. *Anesthesiology*, **22,** 525.

EDWARDS, G., MORTON, H. J. V., PASK, E. A., and WYLIE, W. D. (1956). Deaths associated with anaesthesia. A report on 1,000 cases. *Anaesthesia*, **11,** 194.

ETSTEN, B., and LI, T. H. (1955). Haemodynamic changes during thiopental anesthesia in humans. *J. clin. Invest.*, **34,** 500.

EXLEY, K. A. (1954). Depression of autonomic ganglia by barbiturates. *Brit. J. Pharmacol.*, **9,** 170.

EXTON-SMITH, A. N., HODKINSON, H. M., and CROMIE, B. W. (1963). Controlled comparison of four sedative drugs in elderly patients. *Brit. med. J.*, **2,** 1037.

FIELDMAN, E. J., RIDLEY, R. W., and WOOD, E. H. (1955). Hemodynamic studies during thiopental sodium and nitrous oxide anesthesia in humans. *Anesthesiology*, **16,** 473.

FISHBEIN, W. N., and BESSMAN, S. P. (1964). Gamma-hydroxybutyrate in mammalian brain. Reversible oxidation by lactic dehydrogenase. *J. biol. Chem.*, **239,** 357

FLICKINGER, H., FRAIMOW, W., CATHCART, R. T., and NEALON, T. F. (1961). Effect of thiopental induction on cardiac output in man. *Curr. Res. Anesth.*, **40,** 693.

FRANCIS, J. G. (1964). Intra-arterial methohexitone. *Anaesthesia*, **19,** 501.

GLATT, M. M. (1955). Toxic psychosis with neurological features due to methylpentynol. *Lancet*, **2,** 675.

GOODNOW, R. E., BEECHER, H. K., BRAZIER, M. A. B., MOSTELLAR, F., and TAGIURI, R. (1951). Physiological performance following a hypnotic dose of a barbiturate. *J. Pharmacol. exp. Ther.*, **102,** 55.

GOULDING, R., HELLIWELL, P. J., KERR, A. C., and WILKIN, E. M. (1957). Sedation of children as out-patients for dental operations under general anaesthesia. Trial of methylpentynol, butobarbitone and chlorpromazine. *Brit. med. J.*, **1,** 855.

GRACA, J. G., and GARST, E. L. (1957). Early blood changes in dogs following intravenous pentobarbital anesthesia. *Anesthesiology*, **18,** 461.

GROSS, F., TRIPOD, J., and MEIER, R. (1955). Zur pharmakologische Charakteristerung des Schlafmittels Doriden. *Schweiz. med. Wschr.*, **85,** 305.

GRUBER, C. M. (1937). On certain pharmacologic actions of newer barbituric acid compounds. *Amer. J. Obstet. Gynec.*, **33**, 729.

GUSTERSON, F. R. (1955). The management of children undergoing tonsillectomy: premedication with methylpentynol. *Lancet*, **1**, 940.

HARNIK, E. (1964). A study of the biphasic ventilatory effects of propanidid. *Brit. J. Anaesth.*, **36**, 655.

HARRIS, E. A., and SLAWSON, K. B. (1965). The respiratory effects of therapeutic doses of cyclobarbitone, triclofos and ethchlorvynol. *Brit. J. Pharmacol.*, **24**, 214.

HAYWARD-BUTT, J. T. (1957). Ataralgesia. Operations without anaesthesia. *Lancet*, **2**, 972.

HELRICH, M., ECKENHOFF, J. E., JONES, R. E., and ROLPH, W. D. (1956). Influence of opiates on the respiratory response of man to thiopental. *Anesthesiology*, **17**, 459.

HEROLD, M., KARACOFF, O., and CAHN, J. (1961). Research on the prolongation of the function time of the heart by sodium 4-hydroxybutyrate in the curarized mouse. *Agressologie*, **2**, 551.

HINTON, J. M. (1961). The actions of amylobarbitone sodium, butobarbitone and quinalbarbitone sodium upon insomnia and nocturnal restlessness compared in psychiatric patients. *Brit. J. Pharmacol.*, **16**, 82.

HOBSON, Q. J. G., SELWYN, J. G., and MOLLIN, D. L. (1956). Megaloblastic anaemia due to barbiturates. *Lancet*, **2**, 1079.

HUBBARD, T. F., and GOLDBAUM, L. R. (1950). Distribution of thiopental in the central nervous system. *J. Lab. clin. Med.*, **36**, 218.

HUGILL, J. T. (1950). Liver function and anesthesia. *Anesthesiology*, **11**, 567.

HUTTON, A. M., and HALL, J. M. (1957). Incidence of thrombosis following thiopentone. *Anaesthesia*, **12**, 467.

ISAACS, B. (1957). Hypnotic effect of glutethimide. *Lancet*, **1**, 558.

ISBELL, H. (1950). Addiction to barbiturates and the barbiturate abstinence syndrome. *Ann. intern. Med.*, **33**, 108.

JARMAN, R., and ABEL, A. L. (1936). Intravenous anaesthesia with pentothal sodium. *Lancet*, **1**, 422.

JEPSON, N. P., and KORNER, B. (1952). Thiopental anesthesia and antabuse (disulfiram). *Acta pharmacol.* (*Kbh.*), **8**, 418.

JOHNSON, F. A., and VAN BUREN, H. C. (1962). Abstinence syndrome following glutethimide intoxication. *J. Amer. med. Ass.*, **180**, 1024.

KAUFMAN, L. (1958). Clinical impression and clinical trial, with a study of the evaluation of bemegride. *Anaesthesia*, **13**, 43.

KEATS, A. S., and BEECHER, H. K. (1950). Pain relief with hypnotic doses of barbiturates and a hypothesis. *J. Pharmacol. exp. Ther.*, **100**, 1.

KING, R. A., BIERER, I., RICHMOND, P., and WATSON, A. J. (1958). A new form of chloral hydrate. *Lancet*, **1**, 262.

KINMONTH, J. B., and SHEPHERD, R. C. (1959). Accidental injection of thiopentone into arteries. *Brit. med. J.*, **2**, 914.

KJAER-LARSEN, J. (1956). Delirious psychosis and convulsions due to megimide. *Lancet*, **2**, 967.

KRAMER, M., WHITMAN, R. M., BALDRIDGE, B. J., and ORNSTEIN, P. H. (1966). The pharmacology of dreaming. In: *Enzymes in Mental Health*. Ed. Martin, G. J. and Kisch, B. Philadelphia: J. B. Lippincott Co.

LABORIT, H., BUCHARD, F., LABORIT, G., KIND, A., and WEBER, B. (1960). Emploi du 4-hydroxybutyrate de Na en anesthésie et en réanimation. *Agressologie*, **1**, 549.

LANGREHR, D., ALAI, P., ANDJELKOVIĆ, J., and KLUGE, I. (1967). Zur Narkose mit Ketamine (CI 581): Bericht über erste Erfahrungen in 500 Fällen. *Anaesthesist*, **16**, 308.

LEE, H. A., and AMES, A. C. (1965). Haemodialysis in severe barbiturate poisoning. *Brit. med. J.*, **1**, 1217.

LEMERE, F. (1952). Dormison overdosage. *Northw. Med.* (*Seattle*), **51**, 778.

LIEBREICH, O. (1869). *Das Chloralhydrat, ein neues Hypnoticum und Anästheticum.* Berlin.

LIGHTSTONE, H., and NELSON, J. W. (1954). Antihistamine potentiation of pentobarbital anesthesia. *J. Amer. pharm. Ass., sci. Ed.*, **43**, 263.

LINTON, A. L., LUKE, R. G., and BRIGGS, J. D. (1967). Methods of forced diuresis and its application in barbiturate poisoning. *Lancet*, **2**, 377.

LOOMIS, A. L., HARVEY, E. N., and HOBART, G. A. (1938). Distribution of disturbance-patterns in the human EEG with special reference to sleep. *J. Neurophysiol.*, **1**, 413.

LOUW, A., and SONNE, L. M. (1956). Megimide in the treatment of barbituric-acid poisoning. *Lancet*, **2**, 961.

LUNDY, J. S. (1935). Intravenous anesthesia: preliminary report of the use of two new thiobarbiturates. *Proc. Mayo Clin.*, **10**, 536.

LUNDY, J. S., and ADAMS, R. C. (1942). Pentothal sodium intravenous anesthesia. *Army med. dep. Bull.*, **63**, 90.

MACINTOSH, R. R., and HEYWORTH, P. S. A. (1943). Intra-arterial injection of pentothal: a warning. *Lancet*, **2**, 571.

MCKECHNIE, F. B., and CONVERSE, J. G. (1955). Placental transmission of thiopental. *Amer. J. Obstet. Gynec.*, **70**, 639.

MCKEOGH, J., and SHAW, F. H. (1956). Further experience with amiphenazole and morphine in intractable pain. *Brit. med. J.*, **1**, 142.

MAHER, J. F., SCHREINER, G. E., and WESTERVELT, F. B. (1962). Acute glutethimide intoxication. I. Clinical experience (twenty-two patients) compared to acute barbiturate intoxication (sixty-three patients). *Amer. J. Med.*, **33**, 70.

MARGOLIN, S., PERLMAN, P. L., VILLANI, F., and MCGAVACK, T. H. (1951). New class of hypnotics: unsaturated carbinols. *Science*, **114**, 384.

MARLEY, E. (1955). Toxic psychosis with neurological features due to methylpentynol. *Lancet*, **2**, 535.

MARLEY, E., and CHAMBERS, J, S. W. (1956). Toxic effects and side-effects of methylpentynol. *Brit. med. J.*, **2**, 1467.

MATTHEW, H., and LAWSON, A. A. H. (1966). Acute barbiturate poisoning. *Quart. J. Med.*, **35**, 539.

MAYNERT, E. W., and VAN DYKE, H. B. (1950). The absence of localisation of barbital in divisions of the central nervous system. *J. Pharmacol. exp. Ther.*, **98**, 184.

MAYRHOFER, O. H. (1954). Experimentelle Untersuchungen über die Wirkung einiger zu Narkosezwicken gebräuchlicher Barbiturate auf die Bronchialmuskulatur. *Anaesthesist*, **3**, 105.

MEEK, W. J., and SEEVERS, M. H. (1934). Cardiac irregularities produced by ephedrine and protective action of sodium barbital. *J. Pharmacol. exp. Ther.*, **51**, 287.

MILLER, J. R., and STOELTING, V. K. (1963). A preliminary communication on the sleep-producing effects of intramuscular methohexitone sodium in the paediatric patient. *Brit. J. Anaesth.*, **35**, 48.

NILSSON, E. (1951). On treatment of barbiturate poisoning: a modified clinical aspect. *Acta med. scand.*, **139** (Suppl. 253).

OSWALD, I. (1968). Drugs and sleep. *Pharmacol. Rev.*, **20**, 305.

PAPPER, E. M., PETERSON, R. C., BURNS, J. J., BERNSTEIN, E., LIEF, P., and BRODIE, B. B. (1955). Physiological disposition of certain N-alkyl thiobarbiturates. *Anesthesiology*, **16**, 544.

PARSONS, T. W. (1963). Clinical comparison of barbiturates as hypnotics. *Brit. med. J.*, **2**, 1035.

PASK, E. A., and ROBSON, J. G. (1954). Injury to the median nerve. *Anaesthesia*, **9,** 94.

PAUCA, A. L., and HOPKINS, A. M. (1971). Acute effects of halothane, nitrous oxide and thiopentone on the upper limb blood flow. *Brit. J. Anaesth.*, **43,** 326.

PEDERSEN, J. (1956). Arousing effect of megimide and amiphenazole in allypropymal poisoning. *Lancet*, **2,** 965.

PENHEAROW, A. (1957). Paediatric anaesthesia. *Brit. med. J.*, **1,** 644.

PRICE, H. L. (1960). A dynamic concept of the distribution of thiopental in the human body. *Anesthesiology*, **21,** 40.

PRIME, F. J., and GRAY, T. C. (1952). The effect of certain anaesthetic and relaxant agents on circulatory dynamics. *Brit. J. Anaesth.*, **24,** 101.

PUTTER, J. (1965). Uber den firmentativen Abbau des Propanidid. In: *Die intravenose Kurznarkose mit dem neuen Phenoxyersigisaurederivat Propanidid* (*Epontol*), p. 61. Eds. Horatz, K., Frey, R. and Zindler, M. Berlin: Springer-Verlag.

QUILLIAM, J. P. (1955). The action of thiopentone sodium on skeletal muscle. *Brit. J. Pharmacol.*, **10,** 141.

RAHN, E., DAYTON, P. G., and FREDERICKSON, E. L. (1969). Lack of effect of halothane on the metabolism of thiopentone in man. *Brit. J. Anaesth.*, **41,** 503.

REDISH, C. H., VORE, R. E., CHERNIOSH, S. M., and GRUBER, C. M., Jnr. (1958). A comparison of thiopental sodium, methitural sodium and methohexital sodium in oral surgery patients. *Oral Surg.*, **11,** 063.

RENDELL, C. M. (1954). The premedication of children for tonsillectomy. *Brit. med. J.*, **2,** 1397.

RICHARDS, R. K., and TAYLOR, J. D. (1956). Some factors influencing distribution, metabolism and action of barbiturates: a review. *Anesthesiology*, **17,** 414.

ROBBINS, B. H., BAXTER, J. H., Jr., and FITZHUGH, O. G. (1939). Studies of cyclopropane: the use of barbiturates in preventing cardiac irregularities under cyclopropane or morphia and cyclopropane anesthesia. An experimental study. *Ann. Surg.*, **110,** 84.

ROBERTS, F. W. (1967). A new intramuscular anaesthetic for small children. A report of clinical trials of CI–581. *Anaesthesia*, **22,** 23.

ROBINSON, J. S., TOMLIN, P. J., and MORRIS, L. (1968). The metabolic responses following gamma hydroxybutyric acid. *Proc. roy. Soc. Med.*, **61,** 824.

ROSENDAL, T. (1963). Thalidomide and aplasia-hypoplasia of the otic labyrinth. *Lancet*, **1,** 724.

ROWELL, N. R. (1957). Toxic effects of methylpentynol. *Brit. med. J.*, **1,** 164.

RUSHBROOKE, M., WILSON, E. S. B., ACLAND, J. D., and WILSON, G. M. (1956). Clinical trial of "Doriden", a new hypnotic. *Brit. med. J.*, **1,** 139.

SCHNEIDER, J., THOMALSKI, G., TRATMANN, P., SMOLARZ, R., and SABBAGH, R. (1963). The EEG behaviour of humans and animals subjected to the progressive action of sodium 4-hydroxybutyrate. *Agressologie*, **4,** 55.

SETTER, J. G., MAHER, J. F., and SCHREINER, G. E. (1966). Barbiturate intoxication. *Arch. intern. Med.*, **117,** 224.

SHAFFARZICK, R. W., and BROWN, B. J. (1952). Anticonvulsant activity and toxicity of methylparafynol (dormison) and some other alcohols. *Science*, **116,** 663.

SHAW, F. H., and SHULMAN, A. (1955). Treatment of intractable pain with large doses of morphine and diamino phenylthiazole. *Brit. med. J.*, **1,** 1367.

SHIDEMAN, F. E., GOULD, T. C., WINTERS, W. D., PETERSON, R. D., and WILNER, W. K. (1953). The distribution and in vivo rate of metabolism of thiopental. *J. Pharmacol. exp. Ther.*, **107,** 368.

SHIDEMAN, F. E., KELLY, A. R., and ADAMS, B. J. (1947). The role of the liver in the detoxication of thiopental (pentothal) and two other thiobarbiturates. *J. Pharmacol. exp. Ther.*, **91,** 331.

SHULMAN, A., SHAW, F. H., CASS, N. M., and WHYTE, H. M. (1955). A new treatment of barbiturate intoxication. *Brit. med. J.*, **1,** 1238.

SIMPSON, R. G. (1954). Methylpentynol as a hypnotic for old people. *Lancet*, **1,** 883.

SINTON, A. S. R. (1954). Effects of methylpentynol. *Lancet*, **2,** 242.

SLIOM, C. M., FRANKEL, L., and HOLBROOK, R. A. (1962). A comparison between methohexitone and thiopentone as induction agents for Caesarean section anaesthesia. *Brit. J. Anaesth.*, **34,** 316.

SMITHELLS, R. W. (1962). Thalidomide and malformations in Liverpool. *Lancet*, **1,** 1270.

STEEL, G. C. (1968). Clinical application of gamma hydroxybutyric acid as a sleep cover in lumbar epidural block. *Proc. roy. Soc. Med.*, **61,** 825.

STEPHEN, C. R., and DUVOISIN, P. M. (1960). Laboratory and clinical experiences with glutethimide. *Anesthesiology*, **22,** 482.

STOELTING, V. K. (1957). The use of a new intravenous oxygen barbiturate 25398 for intravenous anesthesia. *Curr. Res. Anesth.*, **36,** 49.

STONE, H. H., and DONNELLY, C. C. (1961). The accidental intra-arterial injection of thiopental. *Anesthesiology*, **22,** 995.

SWANSON, E. E. (1934). The present status of the barbiturate problem. *Proc. Soc. exp. Biol. (N.Y.)*, **31,** 963.

TAYLOR, C., and STOELTING, V. K. (1960). Methohexital sodium—a new ultrashort acting barbiturate. *Anesthesiology*, **21,** 29.

TROTTER, P. (1954). The effects of methylpentynol. *Lancet*, **2,** 1302.

TUNSTALL, M. E. (1968). Gamma–OH in anaesthesia for caesarian section. *Proc. roy. Soc. Med.*, **61,** 827.

VIRTUE, R. W., LUND, L. O., BECKWITT, H. J., and VOGEL, J. H. K. (1966). Cardiovascular reactions to gamma hydroxybutyrate in man. *Canad. Anaesth. Soc. J.*, **13,** 119.

VOLPITTO, P. P. (1951). Experiences with ultra-short-acting intravenous barbiturates combined with decamethonium bromide for endotracheal intubation. *Anesthesiology*, **12,** 648.

WATERS, D. J. (1966). Intra-arterial thiopentone. *Anaesthesia*, **21,** 346.

WECHSLER, R. L., DRIPPS, R. D., and KETY, S. S. (1951). Blood flow and oxygen consumption of the human brain during anesthesia produced by thiopental. *Anesthesiology*, **12,** 308.

WEESE, H., and SCHARPFF, W. (1932). Evipan, ein neuartiges Einschlaffmittel. *Dtsch. med. Wschr.*, **2,** 1205.

WILSON, R. D., NICHOLS, R. J., and MCCOY, N. R. (1967). Dissociative anaesthesia with CI–581 in burned children. *Anesth. Analg. Curr. Res.*, **46,** 719.

WYANT, G. M., and CHANG, C. A. (1959). Sodium methohexital: a clinical study. *Canad. Anaesth. Soc. J.*, **6,** 40.

WYKE, B. D. (1957). Electrographic monitoring of anaesthesia (a method for experimental and clinical study of reversal of barbiturate narcosis). *Anaesthesia*, **12,** 373.

WYKE, B. D., and FRAYWORTH, E. (1957). Use of bemegride in terminating barbiturate anaesthesia. *Lancet*, **2,** 1025.

WYNANDS, J. E., and BURFOOT, M. F. (1963). A clinical study of propanidid (F. B.A. 1420). *Canad. Anaesth. Soc. J.*, **12,** 587.

YANAGIDA, H. (1965). Application of sodium gamma-hydroxybutyrate to clinical anesthesia. An evidence of paradoxical phase. *Jap. J. Anesth.*, **14,** 836.

Chapter 36

ANTIHISTAMINES, TRANQUILLISERS, ANTI-EMETICS AND ANTIDEPRESSANTS

ANTIHISTAMINES

THE antihistamine group of drugs is important because, apart from their value in treating conditions associated with the liberation of histamine, some of the compounds have useful side-effects. The related compounds are the phenothiazine derivatives which have such a vogue as tranquillisers.

The antihistamine drugs are defined as those drugs which oppose or prevent the actions of histamine, but which do not produce the opposite pharmacological effects if they are given when no histamine has been released. This definition excludes those drugs whose pharmacological actions are opposed to those of histamine. Therefore, such a drug as adrenaline, which will relax the smooth muscle contraction produced by histamine in the intestine or bronchioles but which produces this relaxation even if there is no histamine present, is not an antihistamine.

These drugs originated from the work of Bovet and his colleagues at the Pasteur Institute in Paris, who in 1937 produced Compound No. 929F which had antihistaminic properties but was too toxic for clinical use.

To understand the value of the antihistaminics a knowledge of the pharmacological actions of histamine is essential.

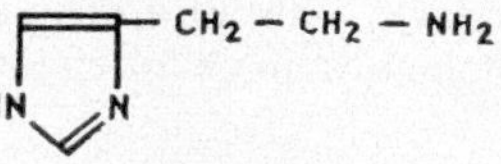

$CH_2 - CH_2 - NH_2$

HN N

Histamine

Actions of histamine.—Histamine produces (1) contraction of smooth muscle which is most marked in the intestines, uterus and bronchioles; (2) a fall of blood pressure in man due to arteriolar and capillary dilatation with increased permeability and a flushed skin (essentially the same as the triple response to stroking of Lewis); (3) increased glandular secretion, particularly of the stomach, where it produces maximal stimulation to the secretion of hydrochloric acid—in fact histamine acid phosphate is used as a test to find out how much hydrochloric acid the stomach can secrete. Pepsin secretion was found to be increased in man (Ashford *et al.*, 1949 *a* and *b*), although this has not been confirmed by other observers. Histamine may also stimulate salivary, pancreatic and intestinal secretions in man, but these effects are more pronounced and easier to study in certain animals. The headache, which occurs after the subcutaneous administration of histamine, commences when the blood pressure has returned to normal and is thought to be due to the stretching of pial and dural arteries (Pickering, 1939).

The antihistaminics antagonise all the above actions of histamine except for the stimulation of secretion of hydrochloric acid by the stomach and possibly also the other secretory actions.

Comparison of Antihistamine Drugs

Since the original work of Bovet was published, many compounds have been synthesised and much comparative work done on the relative merits of these various compounds. A list of compounds is given in Table 1.

36/TABLE 1

ANTIHISTAMINES AND ANTI-EMETICS

Official name	*Trade name*
antazoline	Antistin, Histostab
bromodiphenhydramine	Ambodryl (Bromazine INN)
brompheniramine	Dimotane
buclizine*	Equivert, Longifene, Vibazine
chlorcyclizine	Di-paralene, Histantin
chlorpheniramine	Piriton, Chlor-Trimeton (Chlorphenamine INN)
clemizole	Allercur
cyclizine*	Marzine, Valoid
cyproheptadine	Periactin
dimenhydrinate*	Dramamine
dimethindene	Fenostil
dimethothiazine	Banistyl
diphenhydramine	Benadryl, Histex
diphenylpyraline	Histryl
embramine	Mebryl
isothipendyl	Nilergex, Theruhistin
mebhydrolin	Fabahistin
meclozine	Ancolan
mepyramine	Anthisan, Neo-antergan
methdilazine	Dilosyn
metoclopramide*	Maxolon
phenindamine	Thephorin
pheniramine	Daneral, Trimeton
promethazine	Phenergan
promethazine theoclate*	Avomine
tripelennamine	Pyribenzamine
triprolidine	Actidil, Pro-actidil

* anti-emetics

There are various tests in different species of animals used for this purpose. Although Hawkins and Schild (1951) using human material in the same way that Castillo and de Beer (1947) used guinea-pig tracheal rings, found that the sensitivity of this tissue to histamine and the antihistaminics was of the same order, the relationship of the potency of the different compounds varies with the tests used, and the correlation between the results in animals and those in man are uncertain.

In man using the inhibition of the histamine weal in the skin it has been shown that 25 mg. of promethazine ("Phenergan") was equivalent to 175 mg. of mepyramine (Bain, 1949) and 2·5 mg. of triprolidine.

aching limbs. It is best administered at night because of the drowsiness produced. The other antihistaminics are best administered throughout the day in repeated doses—triprolidine 2·5 mg. phenindamine 25–50 mg., diphenhydramine and tripelennamine 50 mg., mepyramine and antazoline 100 mg.

Uses Associated with Anaesthesia

Promethazine has been used more in this context than the other true antihistaminics because of its marked sedative properties which are unassociated with respiratory depression. It is used as a premedicant, to supplement anaesthesia during operation, and post-operatively.

There have been many reports of its use (Lyon, 1956; Sadove, 1956; Hopkin *et al.*, 1957) and all agree that a dose of 50 mg. given with pethidine 50 or 100 mg. and atropine 0·4 mg. before operation produces a calm patient, sleepy but rousable, and with a normal blood pressure. A dose of 25 mg. is often sufficient. Less thiopentone is required for the induction of anaesthesia than after the more usual premedication of papaveretum and hyoscine; there is a rapid return of reflexes post-operatively and a decreased need for post-operative analgesics for the first twelve hours, with less post-operative nausea and vomiting.

Promethazine appears to be particularly helpful for elderly patients with bronchitis, bronchospasm or emphysema, by preventing such disturbances as bucking, coughing and spasm which often make anaesthetising these patients difficult.

When promethazine is given as premedication it is seldom necessary to give more during the operation, since it has such a long action. Combinations of promethazine, chlorpromazine and pethidine have been used as the "lytic cocktail" in premedication and for neuroleptanalgesia. The combined action of these drugs induces powerful central depression, severe hypotension from widespread vasodilatation and cholinergic blockade. When used as premedication, requirements of anaesthetic agents and post-operative analgesics are greatly reduced but recovery is slow and fluid replacement is critical.

For children there is a syrup of promethazine which is palatable and is given in a dose of 0·50 mg./kg. with atropine; if the child is resistant it can be combined with an equal dose of pethidine.

PSYCHOTROPIC DRUGS

Various terms such as "tranquillisers" or "ataractics" have been loosely applied to a whole group of drugs which have only one property in common—namely an ability to produce "peace of mind". Yet this nebulous term makes it difficult or even impossible to measure or assess their efficacy with any real degree of accuracy, especially as they have little action on normal subjects. No general agreement has yet been reached on a satisfactory classification of this diverse group of drugs, largely because each one has so many actions that it is almost impossible to place them in a select compartment. The following groups of drugs are considered here:

(*a*) Major tranquillisers.
(*b*) Minor tranquillisers.
(*c*) Antidepressants.

The distinction between major and minor tranquillisers is that the former have widespread effects on the central and peripheral autonomic nervous systems and the ability to calm grossly disturbed psychotic patients. Minor tranquillisers have only restricted central action and in practice are useful only in mild anxiety and other reactive states.

MAJOR TRANQUILLISERS

The Rauwolfia Alkaloids

There are about three dozen different alkaloids which have been prepared from *Rauwolfia serpentina* or *canescens*, an apocyanaceous group of plants from Asia. They are used mainly as anti-hypertensive agents, but also for their ataractic properties. They can be administered orally or parenterally. The alkaloids which have been most studied are reserpine and deserpidine.

Metabolism.—Reserpine and deserpidine reduce nervous tension in humans and cause somnolence—the latter effect being not so pronounced in man as in experimental animals.

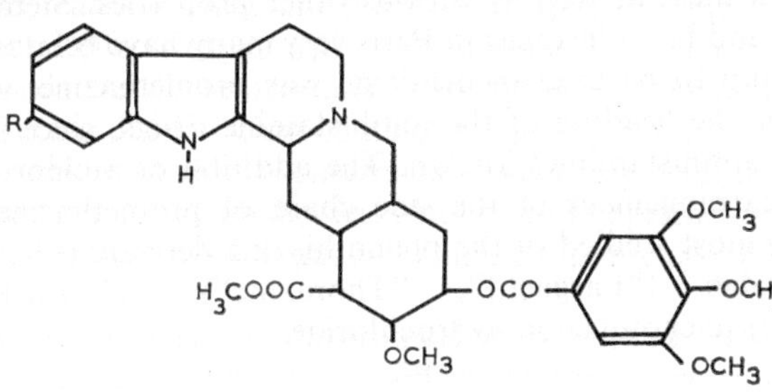

Reserpine R = OCH_3
Deserpidine R = H

Deserpidine causes fewer side-effects—such as anorexia, headaches, bizarre dreams, nausea and vomiting—than reserpine, but it is less regular in its action. Mental depression occurs after long-continued use of either alkaloid.

The sites of action of reserpine in the central nervous system are the hypothalamus and mesodiencephalic alerting system, which consists of the reticular formation and the thalamic diffuse cortical projection. Reserpine stimulates this activating system, whereas chlorpromazine depresses it (Himwich, 1955).

Reserpine and deserpidine have the unusual property of lowering the threshold to electrically induced convulsions and shortening seizure latency: these effects are antagonised by the anticonvulsant drugs. Most tranquillising drugs prolong seizure latency (Slater, 1955).

Reserpine and the other alkaloids induce bradycardia and hypotension (Plummer *et al.*, 1954) as a result largely of their peripheral adrenergic neurone blocking actions. These occur because of disruption of synaptic vesicles in the nerve-endings which depletes these endings of their noradrenaline stores. This is associated with supersensitivity to direct-acting, and insensitivity to indirect-acting, sympathomimetic amines in animals (Burn and Rand, 1958) and man (Gelder and Vane, 1962).

who were on daily doses of chlorpromazine, found that about half showed alteration in the cephalin-flocculation tests, that one third had changes in the total serum protein values and albumin-globulin ratios, and that three developed jaundice. Whether these effects are a primary action on the liver cells or secondary to the hypotension has not been established. Stein and Wright (1956) suggest that chlorpromazine causes increased viscosity of bile, leading to stasis and intrahepatic canalicular obstruction which is indistinguishable from other types of obstructive jaundice. It seems likely that this reaction is allergic in origin (Sherlock, 1964) as it is commoner with second than with first courses of treatment and is not associated with high dosage.

Hyperglycaemia has been noticed, and Courvoisier and her co-workers (1953) found that the hyperglycaemia produced by adrenaline was little affected by chlorpromazine. Moyer and his colleagues (1955) found no evidence of acute renal toxicity or any significant change in renal haemodynamics. Renal blood flow changes in dogs are variable but tend to increase. Sodium and water excretion are slightly increased.

Effects on metabolism.—Decourt (1953) reviews the evidence set out in his many publications, and he suggests that the fundamental activity of chlorpromazine is a reversible inhibition of cellular activity, which he terms "narcobiotic action". He has been able to demonstrate this inhibition—which with higher doses becomes irreversible—in many lowly forms of life. In man, Dobkin and his co-workers (1954) were unable to demonstrate any reduction in oxygen consumption following a dose of 1–2 mg./kg. but they were making sundry other measurements at the same time, which may have interfered with this observation.

Hypothermic action.—Dundee and his colleagues (1954) postulate that it is the prevention of shivering coupled with the peripheral dilatation produced by chlorpromazine that makes it such a powerful hypothermic agent. They consider it superior to the ganglion-blocking agents and the adrenolytic drugs in this respect. Decourt and his co-workers (1953) found that the central temperature of an animal under the influence of chlorpromazine falls, even if the surrounding temperature is high.

Anti-emetic action.—Chlorpromazine is a powerful anti-emetic drug especially against vomiting produced by drugs and by radiation. It appears to act by depressing the vomiting centre.

Anti-shock effect.—Courvoisier and her co-workers (1953) found that, given to a dog immediately after the haemorrhage produced by Wiggers' method, chlorpromazine in a dose of 2 mg./kg. intravenously provided complete protection and a survival time of over 72 hours. Of the non-treated animals 83 per cent died within a few hours. The results in cats were less dramatic. It is postulated that the mechanism of action is its anti-adrenaline action and the maintenance of blood flow through the tissues.

Fate in the body.—Dubost and Pascal (1953) described a method of estimating both free and conjugated chlorpromazine in biological fluids, and gave an account of their findings in the dog and rabbit following the oral and subcutaneous administration of the drug. After large oral doses Dubost and Pascal found 1·7 to 2·5 mg./litre in the blood 24 hours later, but negligible amounts after subcutaneous injection. There was a close correlation between the dose and the blood concentration, irrespective of the route of administration, suggesting that it is well absorbed from the gastro-intestinal tract. This is at variance with the clinical observation that the effects of oral administration are very variable.

Chlorpromazine, like other phenothiazines, is metabolised by two main pathways—(*a*) ring hydroxylation and subsequent conjugation, and (*b*) sulphoxide formation. The large number of resultant metabolites are excreted in both urine and faeces.

Miscellaneous effects.—Chlorpromazine increases the effects of both competitive and depolarising muscle relaxants. Burn (1954) found that skeletal muscle became unresponsive to direct stimulation after 3 mg./kg. of chlorpromazine. This paralysis was delayed in onset and might be preceded by augmentation. Chlorpromazine is two to three times more powerful in this respect than promethazine. Su and Lee (1960) found that in high doses in rat and frog muscles this paralysis could not easily be reversed.

Chlorpromazine has a local analgesic action, but if the concentration of the solution is above 0·1 per cent necrosis of nerves may occur.

Reilly and Tournier (1953) found that chlorpromazine protected 55 per cent of mice from an otherwise fatal dose of the endotoxin of typhoid fever.

Toxicity

Animal studies show wide species variation in the amount of chlorpromazine required to kill. Large intravenous doses produce loss of tone followed by convulsions and death from respiratory arrest. Small areas of congestion may be found in the kidneys, but these are unlike the glomerulitis and lesions of the convoluted tubules, caused by toxic doses of promethazine. Burn (1954) showed that chlorpromazine slowed the rate of growth in rats. Leucopenia has been reported (Anton-Stephens, 1954), but no cases of agranulocytosis have been mentioned in the literature. Large doses of all phenothiazines accumulate with repeated administration and may cause extrapyramidal signs, Parkinsonism, dystonia, dyskinesia and akathisia. These signs disappear on stopping treatment or they can be abated by concurrent administration of anti-Parkinson drugs.

Dermatitis may occur in those who handle the drug constantly, and urticaria and other allergic manifestations have been observed in some patients, but these cleared rapidly after withdrawal of the drug. Other rare sequelae include nausea, anorexia, and epigastric distress.

Acute poisoning from chlorpromazine is rare, but Dilworth and his colleagues (1963) have reported sudden respiratory failure. As well as artificial respiration, they recommend the use of plasma expanders and vasoconstrictors. Of the latter, phenylephrine and noradrenaline are most likely to be effective.

Clinical Uses

Anaesthesia.—Chlorpromazine has been used before, during, and after anaesthesia, but since it has been given in combination with a great variety of drugs the true assessment of its worth in this field is difficult. Laborit and Huguenard in many publications from 1950 onwards have described the complicated technique of "artificial hibernation". In this technique, which is described in *Pratique de l'hibernotherapie en chirurgie et en medicine* (1954), many drugs are used, but lately chlorpromazine has been omitted from these mixtures (Cahn *et al.*, 1954). In this country these methods have been simplified (Smith and Fairer, 1953; Beard, 1954).

The advantages claimed for this technique are that patients are less nervous, little anaesthesia is required—in some cases nothing beyond chlorpromazine, pethidine and promethazine—there is less bleeding, an absence of shock, and less need for post-operative sedatives and analgesics. There is not enough evidence on which to compare the results of this technique with those of orthodox anaesthesia. Chlorpromazine has, however, a place in the premedication of special cases where tranquillity is required without the respiratory depression that follows large doses of morphine. It is valuable prior to thyroidectomy for a patient with thyrotoxicosis that is inadequately controlled by anti-thyroid drugs.

The disadvantages of chlorpromazine are that it causes postural hypotension which may last for up to four hours, and also prolonged depression of reflexes, which may be dangerous.

Administration.—Concentrated solutions of chlorpromazine—and other phenothiazines—are irritant to the tissues, and must therefore be injected intramuscularly. Intravenous injections should be limited to diluted solutions.

Control of vomiting.—Chlorpromazine is a powerful anti-emetic and has been used successfully in vomiting due to such varied causes as carcinomatosis, labyrinthitis, disulfiram ("Antabuse") and alcohol, uraemia, nitrogen mustard, digitalis, hyperemesis gravidarum, acute gastritis and radiotherapy, as well as post-anaesthesia.

The doses used vary from 25 mg. daily to 50 mg. four times a day, but if vomiting is not controlled by two or three injections of 25 to 50 mg. of chlorpromazine it is unwise to push the dosage because of the depression that is produced. A better alternative is to use another phenothiazine, such as perphenazine (dose 5 mg.). Unless the cause of vomiting is known before treatment is begun, the sedation might mask the signs and prevent the diagnosis of a condition which might be serious.

Psychiatry.—Chlorpromazine has proved of value in the symptomatic control of most types of severe psychomotor excitement. Winkelman (1954) summarises his results in 142 patients: "Chlorpromazine . . . is particularly outstanding in that it can reduce a severe anxiety, diminish phobias and obsessions, reverse or modify a paranoid psychosis, quieten manic or extremely agitated patients and make hostile agitated senile patients quiet and easily manageable." Experimentally it antagonises the psychotomimetic effects of lysergide (LSD).

Intractable pain.—Because of its ability to increase the effectiveness of analgesics and its property of producing "pharmacological leucotomy"—a state where pain, although felt, does not distress the patient—chlorpromazine has found a place in the management of patients with intractable pain. Chlorpromazine has no analgesic properties, and therefore is of no value by itself, but in doses of 25 mg. two or three times day it is a useful adjuvant to the analgesics.

Other Phenothiazine Compounds

Many compounds based on the phenothiazine nucleus have been synthesised in an attempt to obtain more specificity without so many or dangerous side-effects and disadvantages. The names, formulae, dosage, side-effects and principal toxic actions of some of them are collected in Table 3. Apart from differences in potency which determine the doses used, the various compounds show little variation in pharmacological activity in practice.

Dundee and his colleagues (1963) found that of thirteen of the phenothiazines clinically used in anaesthesia, pipamazine, pecazine and promethazine were antanalgesic; trifluperazine, perphenazine, thiethylperazine and prochlorperazine were slightly antanalgesic; triflupromazine, chlorpromazine, methotrimeprazine, propiomazine, promazine and trimeprazine were slightly analgesic in ascending order of potency, trimeprazine being about half as potent at 60–90 minutes as 100 mg. pethidine.

Moore (1963) has summarised the properties of nine commonly used phenothiazines. Table 2 is based on this.

36/TABLE 2

	Sedative and Tranquilliser	*Anti-emetic Action*	*Analgesia*	*Side-effects*	
				B.P.	*Dyscrasia*
Promazine 50 mg.	Good	Poor	+	++	—
Chlorpromazine 50 mg.	Good	Good	+	++	—
Triflupromazine 10 mg.	Poor	Good	±	+	—
Promethazine 50 mg.	Fair	Good	—	—	—
Trimeprazine 25 mg.	Very good	—	+	++	—
Propiomazine 20 mg.	Fair	Good	+	—	—
Perphenazine 5 mg.	Poor	Very good	±	+	+
Prochlorperazine 12·5 mg.	Poor	Good	±	+	±
Pecazine 50 mg.	Poor	—	—	—	+

Butyrophenone Derivatives

This group of drugs has actions which are essentially similar to those of the phenothiazines, though their structure is quite different. Important examples are:

droperidol —"Droleptan"
haloperidol —"Serenace"
oxypertine —"Integrin"
trifluperidol—"Triperidol"

They induce mild sedation and tranquillisation in normal and neurotic patients and calm hyperactive psychotics. Their use in anaesthesia has been championed on the European continent but it is not widespread in the U.K. They are employed for premedication and particularly for neuroleptanalgesia (Chapter 38, p. 1107).

They have generalised cerebral depressant actions like the phenothiazines; with chronic use they are probably more likely to cause extrapyramidal upsets. They cause hypotension because of both central and peripheral adrenergic blocking actions and the cerebral depressant actions summate with those of hypnotics, narcotics, analgesics and other tranquillisers. For general anaesthesia, therefore, requirements of all drugs are greatly reduced but, as with phenothiazines, recovery may be very slow.

MINOR TRANQUILLISERS

A number of mild cerebral depressant drugs are in use as sedatives and tranquillisers (Table 4). The most important of these are the benzodiazepines but others are used less frequently. Examples are: hydroxyzine ("Atarax", "Equipose"), meprobamate ("Equanil", "Mepavlon", "Miltown"), methylpentynol ("Oblivon", "Somnesin") and tybamate ("Benvil", "Solacen"). Their depressant effects summate with those of all other cerebral depressant drugs, including anaesthetics. Often repeated claims that these drugs produce a state of calmness without clouding consciousness or reducing the patient's ability to concentrate or coordinate are probably misplaced. In clinical practice, these drugs exert effects which are indistinguishable from those produced by barbiturates.

Benzodiazepines

Four derivatives are at present in common use as minor tranquillisers, hypnotics or anticonvulsants:

chlordiazepoxide—"Librium"
diazepam —"Valium"
nitrazepam —"Mogadon"
oxazepam —"Serenid-D"

Their formulae are indicated in Table 4.

Actions.—All four compounds have general cerebral depressant properties which make them suitable for use as hypnotics and minor tranquillisers, though they do not calm grossly psychotic patients. Chlordiazepoxide and oxazepam are used mostly as tranquillisers and nitrazepam as hypnotic, though the differences in their actions does not warrant this distinction. Chlordiazepoxide markedly reduces the EEG voltage. Diazepam in particular has exaggerated anticonvulsant activity (Randall *et al.*, 1961), probably supraspinal in origin, which makes it a useful agent in the management of tetanus, severe pre-eclamptic toxaemia and upper motor neurone lesions. All four impair concentration and ability to perform skilled tasks and their effects summate with those of other cerebral depressants. Alone, even large doses appear not to depress medullary respiratory and vasomotor centres. These drugs are therefore relatively safe.

Chlordiazepoxide 20–30 mg. t.d.s. has been recommended as useful premedication if given for several days before operation (Inglis and Barrow, 1965).

General pharmacology.—These drugs are absorbed, metabolised and excreted very slowly indeed, disposal taking several days. Daily administration therefore causes cumulation and the effects of overdosage take a long time to pass off. Diazepam is partly metabolised in man to form oxazepam (Schwartz *et al.*, 1965).

Anti-Emetics

About one-third of all patients undergoing anaesthesia and surgery suffer nausea and vomiting afterwards. This may be peripheral or central in origin, the latter arising either from stimulation of the chemoreceptor trigger zone or by activation of labyrinthine reflexes. Anti-emetic drugs act either in the periphery or on the vomiting centre or both. Though anti-emetic drugs often reduce the incidence of post-operative nausea and vomiting, their accurate assessment is very difficult (Riding, 1963). The most useful drugs are antihistamines and phenothiazines, the anti-emetic activity of which are indicated in Table 2.

All writers are agreed that perphenazine is the most potent anti-emetic among the phenothiazines but it does have side-effects. The choice of an anti-emetic depends on circumstances, but Purkis and Ishii (1963) have summarised their criteria for selection of a particular drug. When minimal hypotension and rapid awakening from anaesthesia is important they recommend trifluoperazine; when only small quantities of post-operative narcotic are required they suggest fluopromazine, and when no specific contra-indications to one or other drug exist they consider perphenazine the drug of choice.

Metoclopramide ("Maxolon")

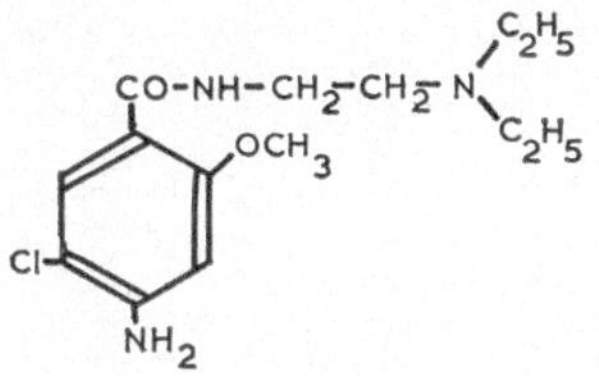

This white crystalline substance, which is freely soluble in water, is an anti-emetic. In doses of 10 mg. t.d.s. it is non-tranquillising. It acts by reducing the sensitivity of both the vomiting centre and the afferent nerves arising in the viscera. It is not effective in vomiting of labyrinthine origin such as travel sickness, vertigo and Menière's disease. Handley (1967) showed that metoclopramide (10 mg. given at the end of the operation) was as effective as perphenazine 5 mg. in preventing post-operative vomiting. Side-effects of prolonged administration of 60 mg. per day include drowsiness, muscle dystonia, diarrhoea and headache.

ANTIDEPRESSANT DRUGS

The Mono-amine Oxidase Inhibitors (MAO inhibitors)

The commonly used drugs of this group are listed in Table 5. Their beneficial effect in the treatment of reactive depression is probably related to the accumulation of brain monoamines (5-hydroxytryptamine, dopamine and noradrenaline) which they cause. Inhibition of monoamine oxidase in the periphery causes

36/TABLE 3

SOME PHENOTHIAZINE COMPOUNDS

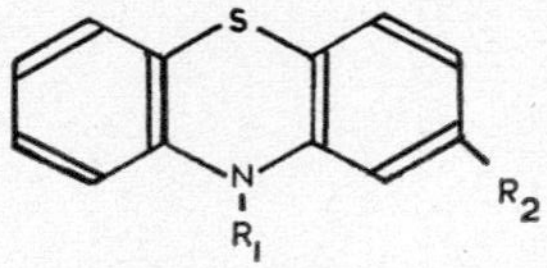

Phenothiazine nucleus

Approved name	*Trade names*	*Formula*	*Dose mg.*	*Side-effects*	*Principal toxic effects*
Dimethylaminopropyl side chain					
Chlorpromazine	Largactil Thorazine	$R_1.CH_2.CH_2.CH_2.N(CH_3)_2HCl$ $R_2.Cl$	25	Drowsiness, hypotension, tachycardia, dry mouth, Parkinsonism, lactation	Jaundice, skin rashes, blood dyscrasia—sometimes fatal
Promazine	Sparine	$R_1.CH_2.CH_2.CH_2.N(CH_3)_2HCl$ $R_2.H$	25	Hypotension, tremor	Agranulocytosis, skin rashes, increased tendency to epileptic fits
Trimeprazine	Vallergan Temaril Panectyl	$R_1.CH_2.CH_2—CH_2N(CH_3)_2$ (with CH_3 on the middle CH_2) $R_2.H$	25		
Fluopromazine	Vespral Vesprin Siquil	$R_1.CH_2.CH_2.CH_2.N(CH_3)_2.HCl$ $R_2.CF_3$	25	Hypotension, dry mouth, lactation, Parkinsonism	
Acepromazine (acetylpromazine)	Notensil	$R_1.CH_2.CH_2.CH_2.N(CH_3)_2HCl$ $R_2.C.O.CH_3$	10	Hypotension, tachycardia	
Propiomazine	Largon Indorm Dorevane	$R_1.CH_2.CH_2—N(CH_3)_2$ (with CH_3 on the second CH_2) $R_2C(=O)—CH_2—CH_3$	20–40	Hypotension rarely, rashes, gastro-intestinal upsets	

Methotrimeprazine	Veractil Levomepromazine	$R_1.CH_2—CH(CH_3)—CH_2N(CH_3)_2HCl$ $R_2—OCH_3$	10	Hypotension, drowsiness	Agranulocytosis
Piperazine side chain					
Prochlorperazine	Compazine Stemetil	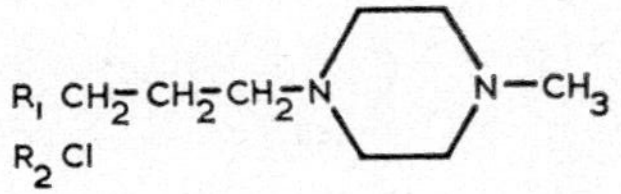 R_1 $CH_2-CH_2-CH_2-N$(piperazine)$N-CH_3$ R_2 Cl	5	Dry mouth, Parkinsonism, motor restlessness	Skin rashes, jaundice, blood dyscrasias
Perphenazine	Fentazin Trilafon	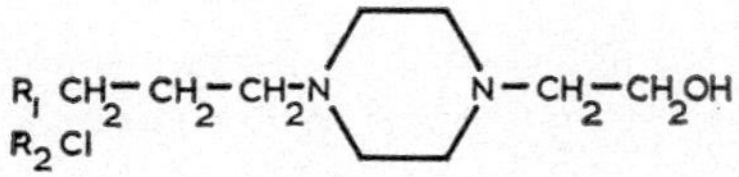 R_1 $CH_2-CH_2-CH_2-N$(piperazine)$N-CH_2-CH_2OH$ R_2 Cl	5	Dry mouth, Parkinsonism dystonic reactions	
Trifluoperazine	Stelazine Eskazine	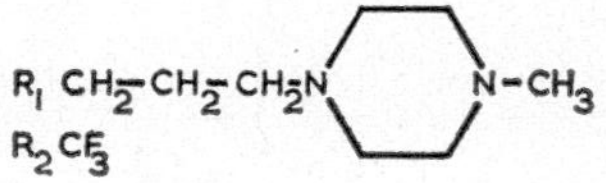 R_1 $CH_2-CH_2-CH_2-N$(piperazine)$N-CH_3$ R_2 CF_3	2	Increased salivation, Parkinsonism	
Fluphenazine	Prolixin Moditen	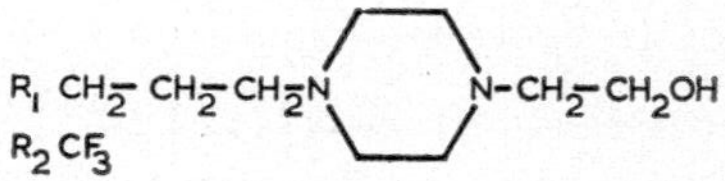 R_1 $CH_2-CH_2-CH_2-N$(piperazine)$N-CH_2-CH_2OH$ R_2 CF_3	1·2	Parkinsonism	
Thiopropazate	Dartalan Dartal	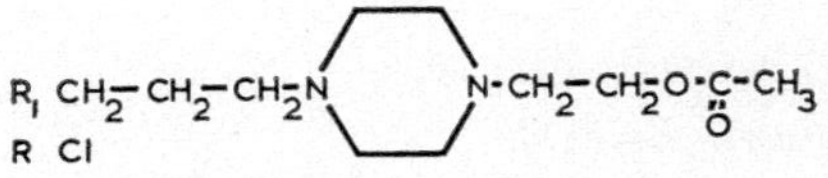 R_1 $CH_2-CH_2-CH_2-N$(piperazine)$N-CH_2-CH_2-O-C(=O)-CH_3$ R Cl	8	Hypotension, Parkinsonism	Jaundice, skin rashes, mildly epileptogenic

36/Table 3 *continued*

Some Phenothiazine Compounds

Approved name	*Trade names*	*Formula*	*Dose mg.*	*Side-effects*	*Principal toxic effects*
Thiethylperazine	Torecan	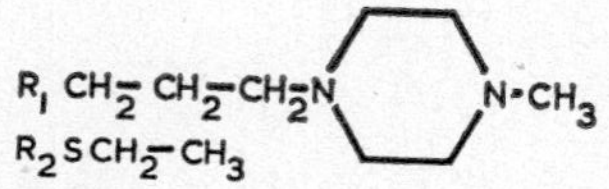 R_1 $CH_2-CH_2-CH_2-N$ (ring) $N\cdot CH_3$ R_2 SCH_2-CH_3	10	Parkinsonism	
Piperidine side chain					
Pecazine	Pacatal Mepazine	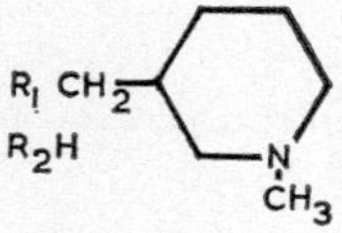 R_1 CH_2- (ring, N–CH_3) R_2 H	25	Hypotension, Parkinsonism, lactation	Agranulocytosis, convulsions, jaundice, dermatitis
Thioridazine	Mellaril	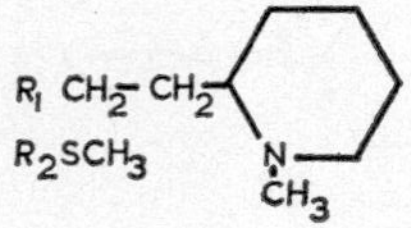 R_1 CH_2-CH_2- (ring, N–CH_3) R_2 SCH_3	20	Dry mouth	Transient leucopenia
Pipamazine	Mornidine	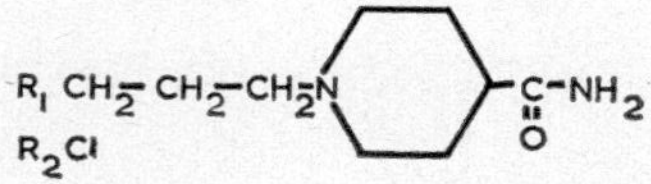 R_1 $CH_2-CH_2-CH_2-N$ (ring) $-C(=O)-NH_2$ R_2 Cl	5		

36/TABLE 4

SOME NON-PHENOTHIAZINE PSYCHOTROPIC DRUGS
(Monoamine-oxidase inhibitors not included)

Approved name	*Trade names*	*Formula*	*Actions*
Chlorprothixene	Taractan Tarason	S; Cl; $=CH-CH_2-CH_2-N(CH_3)_2$	Prolonged sedative action. Strong vasodilator action. Caution is required if used with anaesthesia.
Imipramine	Tofranil	CH_2-CH_2; $N-CH_2-CH_2-CH_2-N(CH_3)_2$	50 per cent prolongation of thiopentone anaesthesia. Elevates mood. Used for treatment of depression.
Amitriptyline	Laroxyl Saroten Tryptizol Elavil	CH_2-CH_2; $=CH-CH_2-CH_2-N(CH_3)_2$	Sedative action. Antidepressant. Vasodilator action but weaker than that of chlorprothixene. No obvious advantages over other drugs.

36/TABLE 4 *continued*

SOME NON-PHENOTHIAZINE PSYCHOTROPIC DRUGS
(Monoamine-oxidase inhibitors not included)

Approved name	*Trade names*	*Formula*	*Actions*
Methyl phenidate	Ritalin Phenidylate	$CH-COOCH_3$; N, H	Stimulant; between caffeine and amphetamine in strength.
Hydroxyzine	Atarax Vistdril	Cl; $CH-N$ $N-CH_2-CH_2-O-CH_2-CH_2OH$	Tranquilliser and moderate antihistaminic.
Azacyclanol	Frenquel	OH; C; NH	Antagonises caffeine and amphetamine. Erases hallucinations produced by lysergide (LSD) and mescaline.

Pipradrol	Meratran	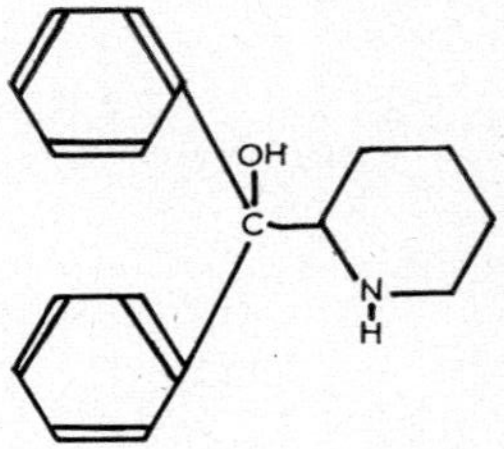	Stimulant.
Meprobamate	Miltown Equanil	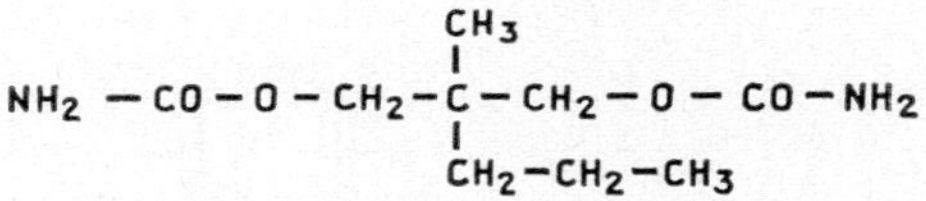 $NH_2-CO-O-CH_2-C(CH_3)(CH_2-CH_2-CH_3)-CH_2-O-CO-NH_2$	Muscle relaxant and anticonvulsant. Taming effect. Depresses interneurones.
Chlordiazepoxide	Librium	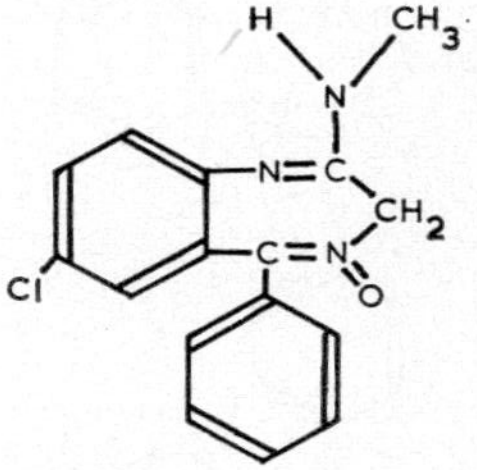	Marked prolongation of thiopentone anaesthesia.
Diazepam	Valium	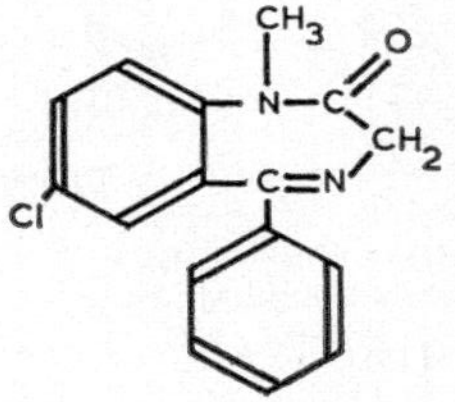	Muscle relaxant; more active than meprobamate. Intravenous analgesic and hypnotic.

36/TABLE 4 *continued*

SOME NON-PHENOTHIAZINE PSYCHOTROPIC DRUGS
(Monoamine-oxidase inhibitors not included)

Approved name	*Trade names*	*Formula*	*Actions*
Nitrazepam	Mogadon	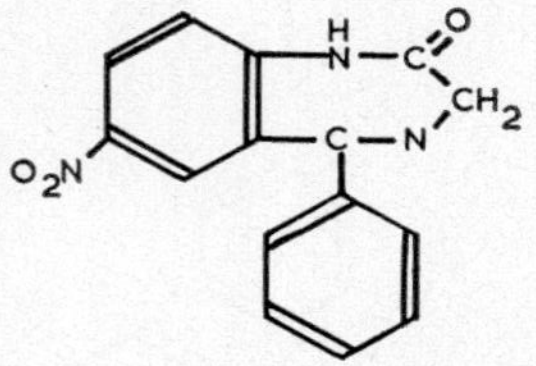	Hypnotic
Oxazepam	Serenid-D	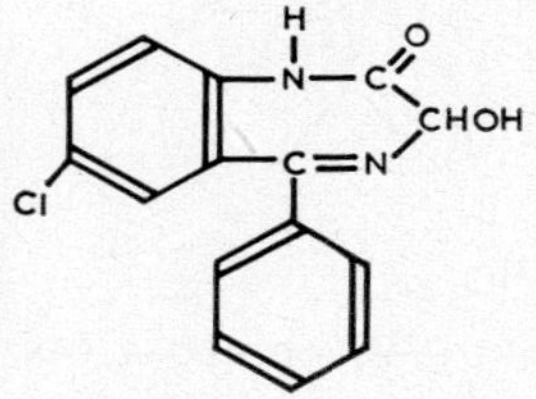	For the control of anxiety

36/Table 5

The Monoamine Oxidase Inhibitors

Approved name:	*Proprietary name:*
iproniazid	Marsilid
pivhydrazine	Tersavid
isocarboxazid	Marplan
phenoxypropazine	Drazine
phenelzine	Nardil
tranylcypromine	Parnate
tranylcypromine with Trifluoperazine	Parstelin
nialamide	Niamid
mebanazine	Actomol
pargyline	Eutonyl
pheniprazine	Cavodil

sympathetic blockade and consequent hypotension, probably due to the formation of octopamine as a false transmitter (Kopin *et al.*, 1965). Severe hypertensive episodes following ingestion of monoamine-containing foods (cheese, Marmite, wine, broad beans) should be treated by alpha-sympathetic blockade with phentolamine or chlorpromazine. Patients under treatment with MAO inhibitors should not be given sympathomimetic vasopressor agents; all will be greatly potentiated.

MAO inhibitors have inhibitory actions also on other enzyme systems, particularly those liver microsomal enzymes responsible for hydroxylation or oxidation of drugs such as barbiturates, alcohol, opiate narcotics, hypnotics and tranquillisers. These drugs are thus potentiated and should be used only in small test doses to assess their effects. Pethidine should probably be avoided altogether, for on occasion hyperpyrexia, restlessness, unconsciousness, hypotension and death have followed its use (see Perks, 1964). If pethidine administration is essential, a small intramuscular test dose of 5 mg. should be given followed by 10 mg. and 20 mg. at hourly intervals if no untoward effect on pulse, blood pressure, respiration or state of consciousness occurs. Thereafter the dose may be increased until normal dosage is achieved without complication. Such a procedure indicates that many patients respond normally (Evans-Prosser, 1968).

There is no evidence that gaseous or volatile anaesthetic agents or neuromuscular blockers are influenced by the administration of MAO inhibitors. The conduct of an anaesthetic may be made more difficult because of the combined hypotensive actions of the antidepressant and anaesthetic agents used. Elective operations under general anaesthesia are probably better postponed for one month, stopping MAO inhibitor treatment if the patient's psychiatric state permits. Stopping antidepressant treatment carries the risk that patients make suicidal attempts. This risk must be balanced against that of anaesthesia in the presence of the drugs.

Tricyclic (Dibenzazepine) Antidepressants

Many compounds of this group are in common use for the treatment of depression, particularly of the endogenous or involutional type. The most important ones are listed in Table 6. These compounds have no inhibitory action against monoamine oxidase or other similar enzymes, their beneficial effect probably resulting from their action in preventing uptake of monoamines by nerve-endings (Glowinski and Axelrod, 1964). Like the MAO inhibitors, they cause mild sympathetic blockade and consequent hypotension. They have also mild parasympathetic blocking (atropine-like) actions. The drugs are metabolised in the liver, partly by N-demethylation. Thus imipramine is converted into desipramine and amitriptyline into nortriptyline. Klerman and Cole (1965) have reviewed the clinical pharmacology of this group of compounds.

No drug or anaesthetic agent is particularly contra-indicated in patients taking these drugs. As with MAO inhibitors, the conduct of an anaesthetic may be made more difficult by the presence of the hypotension, but commonly used analgesics and hypnotics are not potentiated. There is therefore no reason to consider postponing operation if the patient is found to be taking one of these drugs.

36/Table 6

Tricyclic Antidepressants

Approved name	*Proprietary name*
imipramine	Tofranil
desipramine	Pertofran
trimipramine	Surmontil
amitriptyline	Laroxyl, Saroten, Tryptizol
nortriptyline	Allegron, Aventyl
protriptyline	Concordin
amitriptyline with perphenazine	Triptafen

REFERENCES

Anton-Stephens, D. (1954). Preliminary observations on psychiatric uses of chlorpromazine (Largactil). *J. ment. Sci.*, **100**, 543.

Ashford, C. A., Heller, H., and Smart, G. A. (1949*a*). The action of histamine on hydrochloric acid and pepsin secretion in man. *Brit. J. Pharmacol.*, **4**, 153.

Ashford, C. A., Heller, H., and Smart, G. A. (1949*b*). The effect of antihistamine substances on gastric secretion in man. *Brit. J. Pharmacol.*, **4**, 157.

Bain, W. A. (1949). Discussion on antihistamine drugs. *Proc. roy. Soc. Med.*, **42**, 615.

Beard, A. J. W. (1954). Antihistamines in anaesthesia with the use of fewer agents. *Proc. roy. Soc. Med.*, **47**, 407.

Bovet, D., and Staub, A. M. (1937). Action protectrice des éthers phénoliques au cours de l'intoxication histaminique. *C.R. Soc. Biol.* (*Paris*), **124**, 547.

Burn, J. H. (1954). The pharmacology of chlorpromazine and promethazine. *Proc. roy. Soc. Med.*, **47**, 617.

Burn, J. H., and Rand, M. J. (1958). The action of sympathomimetic amines in animals treated with reserpine. *J. Physiol.* (*Lond.*), **144**, 314.

Cahn, J., Dubrasquet, M., Bodiou, J., and Melon, J. M. (1954). Méthodes d'hibernation artificielle: étude expérimentale comparée. *Anesth. et Analg.*, **11**, 141.

Castillo, J. C., and de Beer, E. J. (1947). Tracheal chain; preparation for study of antispasmodics with particular reference to bronchodilator drugs. *J. Pharmacol. exp. Ther.*, **90**, 104.

COAKLEY, C. S., ALPERT, S., and BOLRING, J. S. (1956). Circulatory responses during anesthesia of patients on rauwolfia therapy. *J. Amer. med. Ass.*, **161**, 1143.

COURVOISIER, S., FOURNEL, J., DUCROT, R., KOLSKY, M., and KOETSCHET, P. (1953). Propértiés pharmaco-dynamiques du chlorohydrate de chloro-3(diméthylamino-3-propyl)-10 phénothiazine (4560 R.P.); étude experimentale d'un nouveau corps utilisé dans l'anesthésie potentialisée et dans l'hibernation artificielle. *Arch. int. Pharmacodyn.*, **92**, 305.

DECOURT, P. (1953). Mecanisme de l'action thérapeutique de la chlorpromazine (4560 R.P. ou Largactil). *Thérapie*, **8**, 846.

DECOURT, P. L., BRUNAUD, M., and BRUNAUD, S. (1953). Action d'un narcobiotique (chlorpromazine) sur la température centrale des animaux homéothermes soumis à des températures ambiantes supérieures, égales ou inférieures a leur température centrale normale. *C.R. Soc. Biol.* (*Paris*), **147**, 1605.

DEWS, P. B., and GRAHAM, J. D. P. (1946). The antihistamine substance 2786 R.P. *Brit. J. Pharmacol.*, **1**, 278.

DILWORTH, N. M., DUGDALE, A. E., and HILTON, H. B. (1963). Acute poisoning with chlorpromazine. *Lancet*, **1**, 137.

DOBKIN, A. B., GILBERT, R. G. B., and LAMOUREUX, L. (1954). Physiological effects of chlorpromazine. *Anaesthesia*, **9**, 157.

DUBOST, P., and PASCAL, S. (1953). Dosage du largactil dans les liquides biologiques. Étude du passage dans l'organisme animal. *Ann. pharm. franç.*, **11**, 615.

DUNDEE, J. W., LOVE, W. J., and MOORE, J. (1963). Alterations in response to somatic pain associated with anaesthesia. XV. Further studies with phenothiazine derivatives and similar drugs. *Brit. J. Anaesth.*, **35**, 597.

DUNDEE, J. W., MESHAM, P. R., and SCOTT, W. E. B. (1954). Chlorpromazine and the production of hypothermia. *Anaesthesia*, **9**, 296.

EVANS-PROSSER, C. D. G. (1968). The use of pethidine and morphine in the presence of monoamine oxidase inhibitors. *Brit. J. Anaesth.*, **40**, 279.

FOSTER, C. A., O'MULLANE, E. J., GASKELL, P., and CHURCHILL-DAVIDSON, H. C. (1954). Chlorpromazine. A study of its action on the circulation in man. *Lancet*, **2**, 614.

GAY, L. N., and CARLINER, P. E. (1949). The prevention and treatment of motion sickness. I. Seasickness. *Bull. Johns. Hopk. Hosp.*, **84**, 470.

GELDER, M. G., and VANE, J. R. (1962). Interaction of the effects of tyramine, amphetamine and reserpine in man. *Psychopharmacologia* (*Berl.*), **3**, 231.

GLOWINSKI, J., and AXELROD, J. (1964). Inhibition of uptake of tritiated-noradrenaline in the intact rat brain by imipramine and structurally related compounds. *Nature* (*Lond.*), **204**, 1318.

HALEY, T. J., and HARRIS, D. H. (1949). The effect of topically applied antihistaminic drugs on the mammalian capillary bed. *J. Pharmacol. exp. Ther.*, **95**, 293.

HALPERN, B. N. (1947). Recherches sur une nouvelle série chimique de corps cloués de propriétés antihistaminiques et anti-anaphylactiques: les dérivés de la thiodiphénylamine. *Arch. int. Pharmacodyn.*, **74**, 314.

HANDLEY, A. J. (1967). Metoclopramide in the prevention of post-operative nausea and vomiting. *Brit. J. clin. Pract.*, **21**, 460.

HARANATH, P. S. R. K. (1954). Comparative study of the local and spinal anaesthetic actions of some antihistamines, mepyramine and phenergan with procaine. *Indian J. med. Sci.*, **8**, 547.

HAWKINS, D. F., and SCHILD, H. O. (1951). The action of drugs on isolated human bronchial chains. *Brit. J. Pharmacol.*, **6**, 682.

HEWER, A. J. H., and KEELE, C. A. (1948). A method of testing analgesics in man. *Lancet*, **2**, 683.

HIMWICH, H. E. (1955). Prospects in psychopharmacology. *J. nerv. ment. Dis.*, **122,** 413.

HOPKIN, D. A. B., HURTER, D., and JONES, C. M. (1957). Promethazine and pethidine in anaesthesia. *Anaesthesia*, **12,** 276.

INGLIS, J. MCN., and BARROW, M. E. H. (1965). Premedication—a reassessment. *Proc. roy. Soc. Med.*, **58,** 29.

JASPER, H. H. (1949). Symposium. Thalamocortical relationships: integrative action of thalamic reticular system. *Electroenceph. clin. Neurophysiol.*, **1,** 405.

KLERMAN, G. L., and COLE, J. O. (1965). Clinical pharmacology of imipramine and related antidepressant compounds. *Pharmacol. Rev.*, **17,** 101.

KOPIN, I. J., FISCHER, J. E., MUSACCHIO, J. M., HORST, W. D., and WEISE, V. K. (1965). "False neurochemical transmitters" and the mechanism of sympathetic blockade by monoamine oxidase inhibitors. *J. Pharmacol. exp. Ther.*, **147,** 186.

LABORIT, H. (1950). La phenothiazinyl-éthyldiéthylamine en anesthesia (2987 R.P.). *Presse. méd.*, **58,** 851.

LABORIT, H., and HUGUENARD, P. (1954). *Pratique de l'hibernothérapie en chirurgie et en médicine*. Paris: Masson.

LABORIT, H., and LEGER, L. (1950). Utilisation d'un antihistaminique de synthèse en therapeutique pré, per et post-opératoire. *Presse méd.*, **58,** 492.

LAST, M. R., and LOEW, E. R. (1947). Effect of antihistamine drugs on increased capillary permeability following intradermal injections of histamine, horse serum and other agents in rabbits. *J. Pharmacol. exp. Ther.*, **89,** 81.

LEHMANN, H. E., and HANRAHAN, G. E. (1954). Chlorpromazine: new inhibiting agent for psychomotor excitement and manic states. *A.M.A. Arch. Neurol. Psychiat.*, **71,** 227.

LYON, W. G. G. (1956). Promethazine in burns. *Brit. J. Anaesth.*, **28,** 126.

MAYER, R. L., and KULL, F. C. (1947). Influence of pyribenzamine and antistine upon the action of hyaluronidase. *Proc. Soc. exp. Biol.* (*N.Y.*), **66,** 392.

MELVILLE, K. I. (1954). Observations on the adrenergic blocking and anti-fibrillatory actions of chlorpromazine. *Fed. Proc.*, **13,** 386.

MOORE, J. (1963). Which phenothiazine? *Anaesthesia*, **18,** 108.

MORUZZI, G., and MAGOUN, H. W. (1949). Brainstem reticular formation and activation of EEG. *Electroenceph. clin. Neurophysiol.*, **1,** 455.

MOYER, J. H. (1955). Drug therapy (rauwolfia) of hypertension. Pharmacodynamics of rauwolfia. *A.M.A. Arch. intern. Med.*, **96,** 518.

MOYER, J. H., KENT, B., KNIGHT, R., MORRIS, G., HUGGINS, R., and HANDLEY, C. A. (1954). Laboratory and clinical observations on chlorpromazine (SKF 2601-A): hemodynamic and toxicological studies. *Amer. J. med. Sci.*, **227,** 283.

MOYER, J. H., KINROSS-WRIGHT, V., and FINNEY, R. M. (1955). Chlorpromazine as a therapeutic agent in clinical medicine. *A.M.A. Arch. intern. Med.*, **95,** 202.

PERKS, E. R. (1964). Monoamine oxidase inhibitors. *Anaesthesia*, **19,** 376.

PICKERING, G. W. (1939). Experimental observations on headache. *Brit. med. J.*, **1,** 907.

PLUMMER, A. J., EARL, A., SCHNEIDER, J. A., TRAPOLD, J., and BARRETT, W. (1954). Pharmacology of rauwolfia alkaloids including reserpine. *Ann. N.Y. Acad. Sci.*, **59,** 8.

PURKIS, I. E., and ISHII, M. (1963). The effectiveness of anti-emetic agents: comparison of the anti-emetic activity of trifluopromazine (Vesprin), perphenazine (Trilafon), and trifluoperazine (Stelazine) with that of dimenhydrinate (Gravol) in post-anaesthetic vomiting. *Canad. Anaesth. Soc. J.*, **10,** 539.

RANDALL, L. O., HEISE, G. A., SCHALLEK, W., BAGDON, R. E., BANZIGER, R., BORIS, A., MOE, R. A., and ABRAMS, W. B. (1961). Pharmacological and clinical studies on

Valium, a new psychotherapeutic agent of the benzodiazepine class. *Curr. ther. Res.*, **3,** 405.

REILLY, J., and TOURNIER, P. (1953). The action of chlorpromazine (4560 R.P.) on the toxin in experimental typhoid. *Presse méd.*, **61,** 1031.

RIDING, J. E. (1963). The prevention of postoperative vomiting. *Brit. J. Anaesth.*, **35,** 180.

RINALDI, F., and HIMWICH, H. E. (1955). Drugs affecting psychotic behaviour and function of mesodiencephalic activating system. *Dis. nerv. Syst.*, **16,** 133.

SADOVE, M. S. (1956). Promethazine in surgery. Preliminary report. *J. Amer. med. Ass.*, **62,** 712.

SCHWARTZ, M. A., KOECHLIM, B. A., POSTMA, E., PALMER, S., and KROL, G. (1965). Metabolism of diazepam in rat, dog and man. *J. Pharmacol. exp. Ther.*, **149,** 423.

SHERLOCK, S. (1964). Jaundice due to drugs. *Proc. roy. Soc. Med.*, **57,** 881.

SLATER, I. H. (1955). Pharmacological properties of recanescine: a new sedative alkaloid from *Rauwolfia canescens*. Linn. *Proc. Soc. exp. Biol.* (*N.Y.*), **88,** 293.

SMITH, A., and FAIRER, J. G. (1953). Hibernation in major surgery. *Brit. med. J.*, **2,** 1247.

STEIN, A. A., and WRIGHT, A. W. (1956). Hepatic pathology in jaundice due to chlorpromazine. *J. Amer. med. Ass.*, **161,** 508.

SU, C., and LEE, C. Y. (1960). The mode of neuromuscular blocking action of chlorpromazine. *Brit. J. Pharmacol.*, **15,** 88.

TERZIAN, H. (1952). Studio elettroencefalografico dell' azione centrale del Largactil (4560 R.P.). *Rass. Neurol. veg.*, **9,** 211.

WINKELMAN, N. W., Jnr. (1954). Chlorpromazine in the treatment of neuropsychiatric disorders. *J. Amer. med. Ass.*, **155,** 18.

Chapter 37

PAIN AND THE ANALGESIC DRUGS

Introduction

Pain is one of man's most compelling experiences. It is an unpleasant sensation which only the individual himself can appraise and as such is incapable of a satisfactory objective definition. Sherrington (1906), in his classic work on the central nervous system, has defined pain as "the psychical adjunct to an imperative protective reflex". This concept certainly draws attention to the protective aspect of pain in preventing body injury by noxious stimuli. The burnt fingers of a patient with syringomyelia; or corneal ulceration after division of the fifth cranial nerve bear testimony to this vital aspect of pain sensibility.

This defensive function of pain extends also to disease. The natural inclination to rest an inflamed part not only relieves the pain but also has a beneficial effect on the body's efforts to combat the infection. Similarly, angina pectoris protects the diseased heart from acute myocardial insufficiency due to overexertion.

Leriche (1949) has stressed that on many occasions pain seems pointless and quite often the warning which it affords is inadequate. As he points out, many of the gravest illnesses, such as cancer and heart disease, develop silently and pain only arises when the disease is far advanced, merely making sadder and harder a situation long since lost.

That the ability to experience pain is not essential for the satisfactory adaptation of man to his surroundings is evident from reports on patients with a congenital absence of pain sensation (Ford and Wilkins, 1938; Kunkle and Chapman 1943). As a symptom, pain demands instant relief and is responsible for more patients seeking medical advice than any other cause. Not only is it a distressing experience but if continued it may have a harmful effect on vital organs, leading to impairment of function or even tissue damage (Wolff and Wolf, 1958).

The relief of pain during surgery is the *raison d'être* of anaesthesia. Many anaesthetists have extended the scope of their activities by setting up pain clinics to help alleviate the chronic pain from which some patients suffer.

Nature of Pain Sensation (Theories of Pain)

Although the sensory nature of pain was recognized by the great Greek philosophers, it was conceived more broadly as a moral force with pain and unpleasantness as the natural opposites of virtue and pleasure.

The theory that pain could be produced by intensive stimulation of any sensory organ has been frequently discussed, although by many authors it is accepted as a separate and specific form of sensation. The neuro-anatomical basis of pain sensibility has been unfolded in the past one hundred years, following the discovery of the sensory function of the posterior spinal nerve roots and of the existence of medullary pathways comparatively specialised for pain. The doctrine of specific nerve energies was formulated by Müller in 1840 and implies that the sensation evoked by a stimulus is determined by the particular nerve fibres stimulated and not by the nature of the stimulus. As well as signalling temperature changes, heat and cold may cause pain if the relevant pathways are excited simultaneously. The discovery of separate nerve pathways for specific forms of sensation followed transection experiments on the spinal cord by Schiff (1848) and others. With the introduction by Adrian (1931) of electro-physiological techniques to the study of sensory nerve physiology, a new field was opened for studying the electrical responses in single nerve fibres following their stimulation.

The receptor organs for pain are distributed throughout the body but it is convenient from the clinical aspect to consider pain under different headings. The following classification of pain will be adopted:

Superficial or cutaneous pain. } Somatic pain.
Deep pain (muscles, bones, ligaments, joints, fascia }
Visceral pain.
Referred pain.
Psychogenic or functional pain.

Superficial or Cutaneous Pain

The description of superficial pain will be expanded to include a more general discussion on the physiological mechanisms and neural pathways underlying the reception, conduction and appreciation of painful stimuli.

(i) **Reception of painful stimuli.**—Painful stimuli are detected by a network of non-myelinated or poorly-myelinated nerve fibres which ramify in the superficial, deep or visceral tissues. Pain endings lack specificity and react to a variety of excessive stimuli, all of which pose a threat of tissue damage. Several forms of energy, thermal, mechanical and electrical, as well as chemical stimuli, are all capable of evoking pain.

It is not certain whether these forces cause a direct excitation of the bare nerve endings or whether they produce tissue damage with the secondary release of a pain-producing substance. Hardy and others (1951) found with thermal energy that the onset of pain coincided with the temperature at which alterations of tissue protein began to take place. A release of chemical substances would be anticipated under these conditions. Beecher (1956) rejects this thesis and points out that in man wounds, widespread lacerations and extensive tissue injury can be produced without pain being experienced. He concludes that the level of anxiety is of considerable importance in determining the occurrence of pain.

Wolff and Wolf (1958) consider that in such extensive injuries coagulated serum, oedema and devitalised tissue may shield the pain endings from noxious stimuli. Moreover, damage to nerve terminals and fibres may desensitise traumatised tissue.

A pain-producing substance—probably a polypeptide—has been detected by Armstrong and his co-workers (1957) in inflammatory exudates, and there are a number of substances capable of producing pain on subcutaneous injection or when applied to a blister base (Armstrong *et el.*, 1953). These include histamine, acetylcholine, angiotonin, bradykinin, adenosine triphosphate and serotonin. None of the antagonists of these substances is a useful analgesic, although Graham (1960) has reported favourably on the treatment of migraine headaches with 1-methyl-d-lysergic acid butanolamide, a powerful serotonin blocker.

(ii) **Pain pathways.**—Gasser (1943) has classified nerve fibres by correlating their diameter with the conduction velocity of nerve impulses.The myelinated somatic or A fibres are subdivided into 5 groups.

		Terminology	*Fibre diameter*	*Conduction speed metres per sec.*
Myelinated somatic fibres	A	Alpha	20μ	120
		Beta	↓	↓
		Gamma	↓	↓
		Delta	↓ $(3–4\mu)$	↓ (6–30)→pain fibres
		Epsilon	2μ	5
Myelinated visceral fibres (preganglionic autonomic)	B		$<3\mu$	3–15
Unmyelinated somatic fibres	C		$<2\mu$	0·5–2→pain fibres

Two groups of fibres are responsible for the perception of pain in the epidermis and superficial layers of the dermis. These are the myelinated A-delta fibres and the more slowly conducting unmyelinated C fibres. These latter fibres are the first to be blocked by cocaine but the last to be blocked by asphyxia.

The existence of both a fast and a slow neural pathway for conducting pain impulses to the central nervous system is suggested by the occurrence of double pain sensation or echo pain. This term applies to the twin peaks of pain which may follow a brief painful stimulus to the skin. The more distally the stimulus is applied, the greater the temporal separation of the two pain waves.

From experimental work Landau and Bishop (1953) concluded that C fibre pain had a delayed, burning and persistent character as typified by that associated with inflammation. They considered that sharp pricking pain produced by mechanical or electrical stimulation was transmitted by the delta fibres.

(iii) **Spino-thalamic pathway.**—The cell bodies of the nerve fibres carrying pain impulses are located in the posterior root ganglia. On entering the spinal cord the pain fibres deviate laterally to form the ascending and descending branches of the tract of Lissauer at the tip of the posterior horn. After ascending one to three segments, these fibres synapse in the substantia gelatinosa on the tip of the posterior horn. The axons of the second neurone cross the mid-line in the anterior commissure to form the lateral spino-thalamic tract, which ascends and terminates in the lateral nucleus of the thalamus (Fig. 1). The fibres which arise in the lower parts of the body are displaced laterally by fibres from the upper segments, which thus occupy a medial position in the spino-thalamic tract. This laminar arrangement of the fibres in the tract ensures their precise topographical distribution which is related to body dermatomes and is probably continued to the sensory cortex.

From the thalamus, the third neurone passes through the posterior limb of the internal capsule and is projected to the post-central gyrus of the cerebral cortex.

Pain fibres from the neck and the occipital region of the scalp pass through the 2nd and 3rd cervical nerves. Fibres supplying the face and front of the scalp arise in the cells of the trigeminal ganglion and synapse in the nucleus of the spinal tract of the trigeminal nerve.

(iv) **Reticular system.**—In addition to this classical pain pathway, it has been suggested (Gellhorn, 1953) that collaterals from it are distributed to the ascending reticular system. This multisynaptic pathway relays in the reticular formation of the brain stem and provides an alternative route for pain impulses to bombard a large area of the cerebral cortex. It is believed that stimuli following this pathway activate the cortex and help to maintain consciousness. It is probably a non-specific arousal mechanism, while localisation is a function of the thalamic radiation to the post-central gyrus.

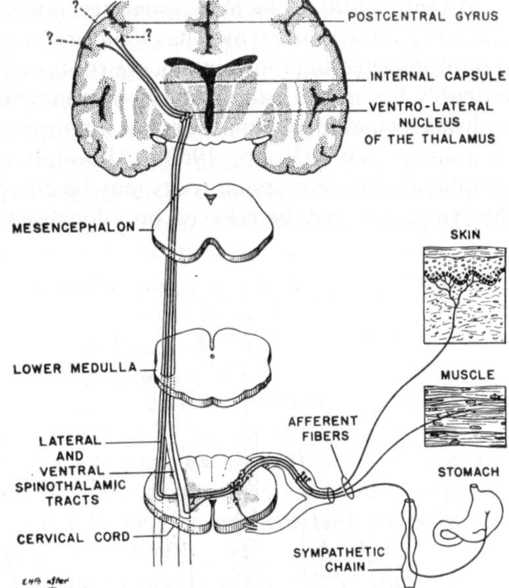

37/FIG. 1.—Pain pathways.

(v) **Dermatomes.**—The cutaneous area supplied by a single posterior nerve root is termed a "dermatome." Knowledge of these is important in determining the nerve roots it is necessary to block when treating superficial pain with local analgesics or when relieving persistent pain with alcohol, phenol or root section. A dermatome chart of the whole body is shown in Fig. 2, every spinal root being represented except C1. The dermatomes are in fact more extensive than those shown on such a chart as there is considerable overlap in the areas supplied by adjacent roots.

(vi) **Thalamus and sensory cortex.**—The dermatomal arrangement of the sensory fibres is maintained in the cortical projection to the post-central gyrus and it is possible to map out a distorted image of the body upon the cortex itself.

The relative importance of the thalamus and the cortex in the perception of pain is still disputed. Head (1920) believed that pain is experienced when nerve impulses arrive in the appropriate part of the thalamus which he regarded as the centre of consciousness for pain. It is known that cortical lesions produce only transient and minimal disturbances of pain appreciation, whereas destruction of the thalamus leads to the abolition of pain sensibility on the opposite side of the body.

Thalamic sensation is crude and poorly localised and the sensory cortex is essential for localising and detecting variations in the intensity of pain. To ascribe sensation to the thalamus and perception to the cortex is to take too narrow a view of a complex functional interrelationship.

ness associated with headaches. These may have an organic basis, as in meningitis, or may be due to the emotional tension accompanying an anxiety state (Holmes and Wolff, 1950).

Visceral Pain

This is transmitted mainly in the sympathetic nerves via the sympathetic chain and the white rami communicantes to the posterior root ganglia, where the cell bodies are situated. The fibres essentially are components of spinal nerves utilising but not relaying in the sympathetic system. The modern tendency is to speak of them as autonomic or visceral afferents. Although the fibres connect with the spinothalamic tract, they are distributed more widely than somatic pain fibres within the cord. This explains why a more extensive cordotomy is generally required for visceral pain. The pain innervation of the viscera is shown in Fig. 3.

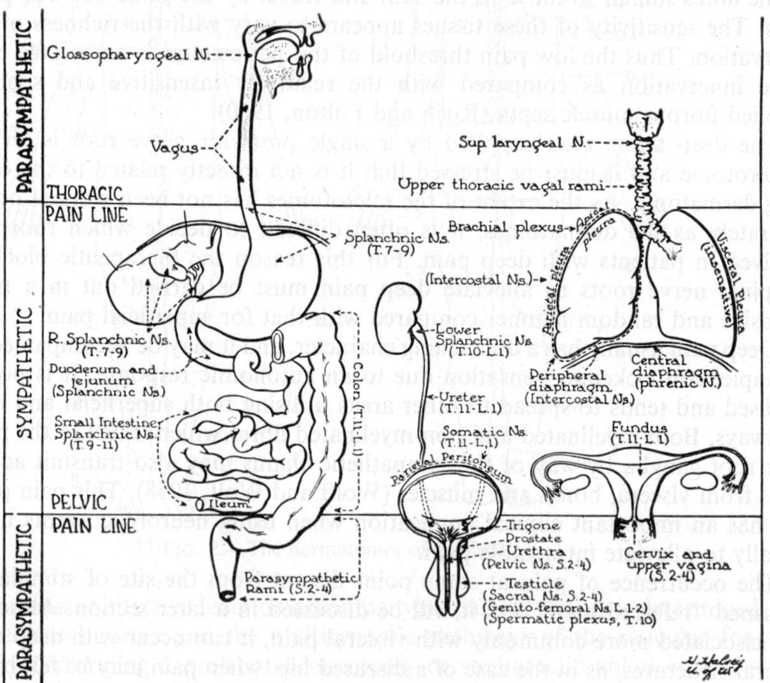

37/Fig. 3.—Pain innervation of the viscera.

Not all visceral pain impulses are conducted by sympathetic nerves. Those from certain pelvic organs such as the bladder neck, prostate, uterine cervix and lower colon travel by the parasympathetic pelvic nerves to the cord. It has also been suggested that some pain fibres from the trachea and oesophagus travel in the vagus nerve.

Viscera have evolved quite different effective stimuli from those which activate cutaneous receptors. It is possible, for example, to handle and even cut and burn viscera under local analgesia without producing pain, although mesenteric traction usually causes discomfort. Pain-producing stimuli include chemical irritants, as in peritonitis, sudden distension of organs and excessive contractions and spasms, especially when associated with changes in the blood supply, as in intestinal obstruction. Normal activity of smooth muscle is painless except when the blood supply is impaired.

Compared with somatic pain, visceral pain is diffuse, less easily localised and often referred. It has a dull, aching character and is often accompanied by a fall in pulse and blood pressure, whereas these usually rise with somatic pain. Muscular rigidity and hyperaesthesia are commonly associated with visceral pain.

Referred Pain

Deep pain, whether visceral or somatic in origin, may be misinterpreted so that it is felt in some part of the body other than the site of stimulation. The reference of cardiac pain to the left arm and diaphragmatic pain to the shoulder are well-known examples of this phenomenon.

Harman (1948) considers that sensation cannot be localised in deep parts of the body that are unperceived by the individual and the existence of which, as in the case of a viscus, he may not be aware. The inability to visualise the site of stimulation creates the need to project the pain to some part of the body where perception is possible. This results in pain being referred to the dermatomes having the same or adjacent segmental innervation as the painful focus itself.

Visceral pain tends to have a characteristic localisation for each organ and it is referred to part rather than the whole of a segment. Pain from abdominal organs, for example, is usually felt anteriorly and not in the dorsal part of the segment. The neurophysiological basis of referred pain probably depends on the convergence of several cutaneous and visceral afferent fibres on the same secondary neurone at some point in the pain pathway. Although this may occur in the thalamus or cortex, it is known that the fibres in the spino-thalamic tract are outnumbered by the pain fibres in the dorsal root, indicating a convergence of fibres at the spinal level (Ruch and Fulton, 1960).

On the basis of previous experience, impulses travelling by a certain tract are interpreted by the brain as arising in a particular cutaneous site. This projection will occur whether the impulses are initiated by cutaneous or visceral receptors. The mechanism is analogous to a shared "party" telephone line. Certain tracts remain "private" and transmit unreferred visceral pain impulses. The muscular rigidity and hyperaesthesia associated with conditions like acute appendicitis are due to the central spread of excitation with the evoking of somatic reflexes and the facilitation of cutaneous impulses which normally would be incapable of producing pain. This facet of referred pain can be removed and the patient's discomfort reduced by infiltrating the hyperaesthetic area with a local analgesic drug.

The therapeutic action of counter-irritants in relieving visceral pain may be in the ability of a strong cutaneous stimulus to crowd out or inhibit visceral impulses from entering the cord in the same segment. The vasodilatation which may be produced in the viscera when a rubefacient is applied to the skin of the corresponding spinal segments is unlikely to produce rapid pain relief.

Anginal pain has been reported in a phantom limb (Cohen and Jones, 1943) so that it is unnecessary for the part actually to exist in order to have pain projected to it by the cerebral cortex. Harman (1951) showed that anginal pain referred to the arm was abolished by a complete brachial plexus block. This made the patient unaware of his arm. The pain persisted, however, with a selective block which achieved analgesia without the loss of touch, position sense and motor power.

The inference from these reports is that the perception of a structure by the cortex is a fundamental requisite for referred pain.

Becher (1950) used an ingenious test in an attempt to localise more accurately the particular dermatomes to which pain was being referred. He injected intradermally 0·2 ml. of a mixture of acetylcholine and neostigmine, two fingerbreadths lateral to the transverse process of each vertebra from T6 to L2. In normal subjects the extent of the erythema in each weal was the same after a given time, whereas in patients with a diseased viscus a larger and more rapidly developing weal appeared in the appropriate dermatomes. This effect was probably due to the enhancement of a sympathetically induced reflex vasodilatation which otherwise would have been undetected.

The viscera and the corresponding segments were as follows:—

Gastric ulcer or carcinoma	T 7–8 left side
Duodenal ulcer	T 7–8 right side
Gallstones	T 8 right side
Renal conditions	T 11 (corresponding side)
Appendicitis	T 11–12 right side
Descending colon	T 12 left side

Hockaday and Whitty (1967) investigated referred sensation by injecting hypertonic saline into the interspinous ligaments of normal subjects. This procedure produced referred deep pain and less commonly skin hyperalgesia and muscle spasm. The site of reference for an individual was constant and reproducible but varied widely within the group of subjects and did not support the idea of a constant segmental reference similar to dermatomes.

Current Concept of the Nature of Pain

In recent years the specificity of sensory perception has been questioned increasingly, especially the psychological assumption that stimulation of pain receptors results in the direct transmission to the brain of impulses which are interpreted as pain. Such a concept has the implication that the sifting of information about a stimulus occurs entirely at the peripheral receptors. Soulairac (1968) considers pain as an affective reaction, dependent not on the nature of the sensory receptors but on the intensity of the impulses transmitted to the central nervous system and on the manner in which they are utilised there.

Pain sensation is one manifestation of a more general reaction or "algic" behaviour and it is often impossible to correlate the sensory phenomenon of pain with the unpleasant affective state that occurs.

The assimilation of sensory pain at the level of consciousness depends on its integration in the central nervous system at different levels of vigilance and on its modification by other sensory information. The first level of vigilance is situated in the mesencephalic (mid-brain) reticular substance (Charpentier, 1968). It does not produce affective awareness but rather an abrupt awakening of the central nervous system and activation of protective homeostatic responses like the startle and flight reactions. The state of alert activates the higher centres, especially the frontal cortex. This first centre of integration is essentially adrenergic in nature and analgesics such as salicylates act at this level by a process of inhibition. The second level of vigilance is in the rhinencephalon and thalamic reticular formation and is responsible for the more specific and affective reactions to pain. This system is activated by strong stimuli and is essentially cholinergic in nature. The potent narcotic analgesics such as morphine and pethidine exert their effect at this level. The third level of integration of pain sensation determines its tempero-spatial analysis and evaluation in regard to the external environment and is located in the frontal cortex. It achieves a co-ordinated response by the animal to the painful stimulus having regard to its cause, strength and its surroundings. The progress of a painful stimulus through the levels of integration is set out in the following scheme (after Charpentier):

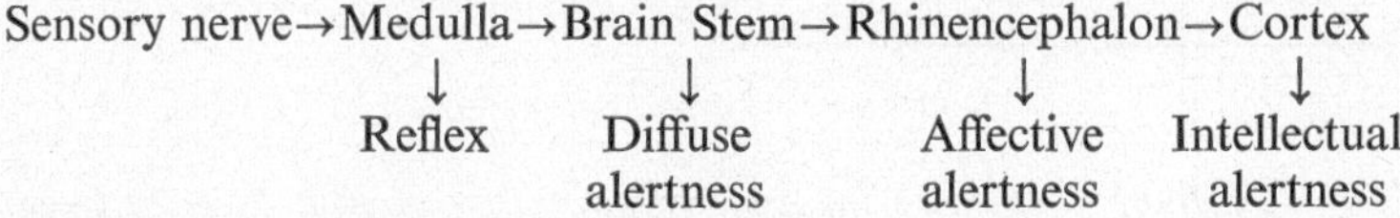

It is only in the two superior levels of integration, where affective regulation is manifest, that pain is transformed to the state of suffering.

Gate Control Theory of Pain

Melzack and Wall (1965 and 1968) have recently proposed a new theory of pain mechanisms, in which it is suggested that the sensory input from the skin is modulated by a gate control system before its eventual perception as pain. The sensory impulses from the skin are distributed to three systems in the spinal cord:—the tracts of the dorsal columns for onward transmission to the brain, the cells of the substantia gelatinosa, and the first central transmission (T) cells in the dorsal horn.

These authors suggest that the substantia gelatinosa acts as a gate control mechanism (see Fig. 4), as it has been shown (Wall, 1962; Mendell and Wall, 1964) that although impulses in large fibres are at first very potent in activating the T cells, their effect is later diminished by an inhibitory process. Impulses transmitted by the small fibres, on the other hand, bring into play an excitory mechanism, which enhances the effect of impulses arriving from the periphery. The nerve impulses which travel continuously to the spinal cord, even when there is no apparent stimulation, are transmitted primarily by the small fibres, and Melzack and Wall propose that they maintain the gate in a comparatively open position. Stimulation of the skin evokes a burst of impulses, in which large fibre activity predominates over that in the small fibres. The T cells are triggered off, but at the same time, due to the inhibitory mechanism, the gate is partly closed. During sustained stimulation, adaptation in the large fibres swings the balance in favour of the small fibre system, so opening the gate and increasing the outflow of impulses from the T cells.

It is also suggested that central influences engendered by emotion or previous

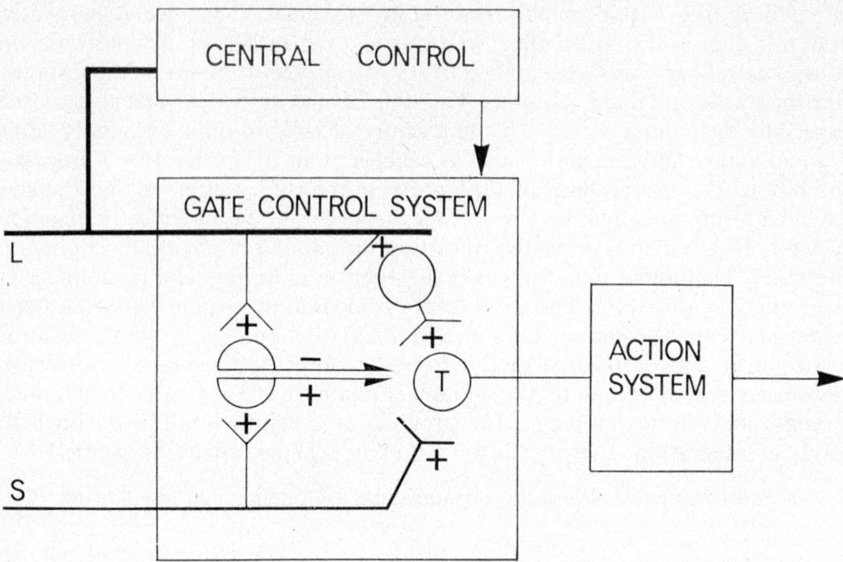

37/FIG. 4.—Diagram to illustrate the gate control theory of pain. L is the large diameter fibres; S is the small diameter fibres; T represents the first central transmission cells.

experience can influence sensory input by means of the gate control mechanism (Hagbarth and Kerr, 1954; Wall, 1967). This effect may be generalized or selective and restricted to a particular part of the body, as for example has been reported in soldiers wounded in battle (Beecher, 1959), who may suffer little pain from their wound but complain vehemently about a careless venepuncture.

This process has been termed the "central control trigger", and it is suggested that it is mediated by the dorsal column system. This carries exact information on the type and location of the stimulus, so altering selective brain mechanisms and also influencing the gate control mechanism by central efferent fibres.

This theory can explain many phenomena of pain, such as that which occurs in alcoholic and diabetic neuropathy and other neuralgias, where there is a selective degeneration of the large fibres. The impaired functioning of the inhibitory mechanism in these circumstances allows the unopposed activity of the small fibres to hold the gate open and so produce severe pain. Trigeminal neuralgia may be explained by such a process, as degenerative changes have been described (Kerr and Miller, 1966) in the large fibres in this condition.

Psychogenic Aspects of Pain

A psychogenic basis for pain can be inferred when no satisfactory organic cause for it can be found, and its distribution does not accord with a known anatomical pattern. These symptoms, which are a manifestation of a psychological disorder, are often described in a characteristic way. A feeling of pressure or of a tight band constricting the head are well-known examples of such a pain. Pains of psychological origin are usually continuous from day to day and involve more than one part of the body but they do not tend to disturb sleep (Merskey,

1968). These patients are prone to self-pity and have an easily aroused resentment, especially concerning previous treatment. The pain may enable the patient to escape some particular situation or duty and may be heralded by symptoms suggestive of an emotional disturbance.

Protracted organic pain frequently leads to exhaustion, while psychogenic pain is often preceded by a phase of exhaustion. Symptoms may occur at the site of previous trauma or infection, the pain persisting and growing in significance as it becomes the focus of the patient's preoccupation and apprehension. Sciatic pain from a prolapsed intervertebral disc may follow this pattern even when there is no question of impending litigation.

From the practical aspect it is important for the anaesthetist to realise that there is a psychological factor to a greater or lesser extent in every patient with whom he has to deal, which can not only cause pain but can also increase its severity. Simple explanation and kindliness can do much to allay the anxiety of an apprehensive patient during a pre-operative ward visit. The relief of post-operative pain by a placebo exemplifies the power of suggestion. Narcotics and sedatives are invaluable during the post-operative period but they are often given too freely when reassurance and skilled nursing could do much to relieve the patient's anxiety and over-reaction to pain.

Certain patients have an abnormal and heightened reaction to pain, so that they suffer more intensely than normal individuals. The hospital atmosphere, together with an attitude of sympathy and firmness from both medical and nursing staff, can do much to help such people. In severe cases psychotherapy may be as important as conventional pain-relieving measures. In any patient suffering from pain, both the somatic and the psychic aspects must be evaluated including the patient's personality and reaction to the present illness.

The anaesthetist should be well-versed in the pharmacological and physical means of relieving pain but will probably need expert psychiatric assistance when dealing with predominantly psychogenic pain. This would involve the use of anti-depressant drugs or E.C.T. for endogenous depression and psychotherapy and sedation in neurotic illnesses. There is no doubt that these patients can suffer as acutely as those with a clear-cut physical cause for their pain and are equally deserving of sympathy and compassion. The acceptance of pain at its face value and the institution of the appropriate treatment should be the underlying principle in cases of doubt, rather than the premature diagnosis of a psychogenic disorder.

Assessment of Pain

When assessing the value of analgesics or techniques aimed at pain relief it is desirable to have some method of clinically estimating the intensity of the pain suffered by the patient. According to Boring (1933) there are four sensory dimensions in consciousness, namely :—quality, intensity, duration, and location. The quality of pain may be described as "burning", "pricking", "aching", "shooting" or "stabbing". Knowledge of the duration of pain is important and whether it is continuous, intermittent, pulsating or exhibiting a wave-like variation in intensity. The site of the pain must be accurately determined, including areas of secondary reference.

Hardy and his co-workers (1947) devised a technique for measuring intensity of skin pain produced by thermal radiation. The limit of discrimination of pain sensibility was measured by determining the smallest change in the stimulus that could be detected. Starting with threshold pain, the stimulus was increased until there was a just noticeable difference in pain intensity. These workers described twenty degrees of pain from zero to ceiling level. Beecher (1959) has stressed the errors which may arise when such experimental pain techniques in man are applied to pathological pain. Assessment of pain intensity will then depend upon the subjective estimation by the patient of his suffering as revealed by a detailed and careful history together with evidence of any autonomic response and an appraisal of the psychological reaction to his pain.

Keele (1948) introduced a useful way of estimating pain when he described the use of a pain chart in the clinical study of pain and the testing of analgesic drugs. The intensity of pain is charted on a graph against time with a space available for each 24 hours of the day. Four grades of pain are defined by Keele :

1. Slight—awareness without distress.
2. Moderate—enough to distract attention from, say, reading or housework.
3. Severe—dominating the field of consciousness, often with reflex visceral accompaniments.
4. Agonising—motor effects such as restlessness occur, or shock ensues.

In practice, three categories of pain suffice and the agony category may be omitted. Each hour, the patient writes on the chart a number corresponding to the intensity of his pain at that time.

A clinical application of this scheme in assaying analgesics was described by Houde (1962) who treated patients with advanced cancer. In his trial the pain relief score ranged from 1, for no pain, to 4, for severe pain. It was possible to build up a pattern of the fluctuations in pain intensity and the efficacy of medications, whether analgesics or placebos.

Assessment of Analgesic Drugs

The appraisal of analgesic drugs is of interest to both pharmacologist and clinician. Their assessment with speed and accuracy is now essential as a result of the flood of new products from the pharmaceutical industry. The assessment of pain is an inseparable concomitant to this field of study which may be tackled basically in three different ways:

1. The relief of experimental pain in human volunteers.
2. The activity of analgesics in preventing or relieving artificially induced pain in experimental animals.
3. The relief of pathological or incisional pain in patients.

Since the value of any analgesic rests ultimately on its ability to relieve pathological pain, Beecher (1962) believes that very often sick man is the only possible final experimental subject.

Experimental Pain in Man

Various types of painful stimuli may be employed in studying pain sense, including mechanical pressure applied to a subcutaneous bony surface or nail bed, a faradic current and radiant heat for skin pain. An alternating current applied to a dental filling produces pain of longer duration. All of these stimuli can be measured quantitatively and reproduced as necessary with an identical intensity. Ischaemic muscle pain from inflation of a sphygmomanometer cuff while the limb is exercised enables deep pain to be studied under standard conditions.

To measure analgesic activity quantitatively it is desirable that there should be a gradation between the stimulation intensity and the dose of analgesic required to relieve the pain. The measurement of pain threshold using both the thermal radiation method and pressure pain from the periosteal tissues of the forehead with a calibrated spring mounted plunger is described by Hardy (1962). In an earlier paper, Hewer and Keele (1948) also describe these various methods and report the effect of twelve different analgesic drugs on ischaemic muscle contraction pain. The doses of each drug necessary to produce the same degree of analgesia can be deduced from these experiments.

The results obtained from these experimental techniques are not necessarily applicable to pathological pain. Beecher (1962) considers that pain has two components (i) the original sensation and (ii) the psychological reaction to the original sensation. He believes that experimentally produced pain is more akin to original sensation, while pathological pain is subject to much more processing as a result of the knowledge of the patient, his previous experiences and the significance of the pain with regard to his present situation. Pathological pain is always relieved by a small dose of morphine to a greater or lesser extent.

Beecher (1959) reported that fifteen groups of workers were unable to demonstrate any reliable relationship between experimental pain threshold in man and even a large dose of morphine. It seems probable that certain analgesics act mainly on the reaction component of pain.

A recent experimental method called the submaximum tourniquet technique (Smith *et al.*, 1966; Beecher, 1968) appears to correspond more closely to pathological pain. Pain was produced by squeezing a hand exerciser twenty times, while the circulation was occluded by a tourniquet round the upper arm. Four grades of pain were designated and under controlled drug and placebo conditions it was found that 10 mg. of morphine intravenously significantly delayed the development of the three higher levels of pain. Precise dose effect curves were constructed using additionally 7·5 mg. and 15 mg. of morphine intravenously. At the three higher pain levels the differences between the three doses were highly significant ($p < 0{\cdot}001$). The larger dose of morphine postponed the onset of pain longer than the smaller dose and the latter delayed it more than the placebo. Beecher considered that with previous experimental methods the end point for threshold pain was not sufficiently definite.

Experimental Pain in Animals

Similar techniques to those described above can be used for the experimental assessment of analgesic drugs in animals. Bonnycastle (1962) described a technique in which a beam of radiant heat focused upon the tails of trained rats caused the animals to flick their tails. This method was sufficiently sensitive to demonstrate the activity of mild drugs like aspirin, as well as that of the morphine group of drugs. The assessment of analgesic drugs by this method was in remarkably close agreement with their evaluation in clinical trials. Since all pain is likely to be meaningful and serious to an animal, experimental pain is equivalent to pathological pain in man (Beecher, 1962). Many of the problems connected with clinical trials, such as patient and observer bias, placebo response and suggestibility, can be discounted in animal experiments. These investigations will undoubtedly retain an important place in the screening of potential analgesic compounds prior to their therapeutic trial in man.

Clinical Assessment

The evaluation of analgesics by clinical studies has much to recommend it and has been the subject of extensive investigations in recent years. It involves the investigation of a large series of patients with pain of moderate severity which may be long-lasting, as in advanced carcinomatosis, or of limited duration, as in the post-operative period. The estimation of drug effects is usually based on the patient's subjective reports, but some workers have preferred the objective observation of the patient's actions and appearance (Steinhaus *et al.*, 1964). Other investigators have used the objective evidence provided by the measurement of vital capacity and peak expiratory flow rates in studying this problem (Masson, 1962*a*; Parkhouse and Holmes, 1963). Beecher and his co-workers have carried out extensive comparisons of analgesic drugs. The papers by Keats and Beecher (1952), Lasagna and Beecher (1954) and the review by Beecher (1957) are recommended for further reading. The trials in the main were carried out in the early post-operative period and the necessity of determining the doses of drugs having an equal analgesic action was emphasised. A dose of morphine of 10 mg. per 70 kg. of body weight was adopted as the standard. Once the equivalent analgesic doses have been determined it is possible to investigate the side-effects which different drugs produce at this analgesic level.

Lasagna and Beecher (1954) showed that there was little difference in the duration and potency of analgesia with 15 mg. of morphine as compared with 10 mg., but at the higher dose in healthy volunteers the incidence of respiratory depression was slightly increased and also that of undesirable side-effects was significantly increased.

Gravenstein and his co-workers (1956) investigated dihydrocodeine (dihydroneopine) bitartrate (D.F. 118) by these methods and concluded that 30 mg. of this drug was slightly inferior to 10 mg. of morphine. Dihydrocodeine did not control severe pain so effectively as morphine, but in patients with moderate pain the two drugs were comparable in effect. Morphine 10 mg. caused a high incidence of nausea and dizziness in thirty normal subjects in a controlled series, whereas none of these side-effects was produced by 30 mg. of dihydrocodeine in the same subjects. The assaying of analgesics by these techniques requires a properly designed experiment to avoid bias of the observer or subject, dissimilarity among patients and differences in the same patient from time to time. The factors to be considered in conducting these trials have been discussed by Gruber (1962). The cross-over method is of value in studying patients with chronic pain. The patients serve as their own controls, as they each receive every drug being studied. This approach may not be satisfactory with pain of short duration as in the post-operative period. Parkhouse and his associates (1961) found that most patients only required one analgesic injection after haemorrhoidectomy or appendicectomy.

The solution of this problem by dividing patients into groups, each receiving one particular drug, may lead to differences among the patients influencing the results. Allocating similar patients to each group may eliminate this bias but the use of large numbers in a series may avoid the necessity of pairing patients.

Double-blind techniques play an essential part in assessing analgesics. They ensure that neither the patient nor the observer knows the dose or whether an analgesic or dummy medication is being given. The usual practice is for the test drugs (placebo and active drugs) to be coded, disguised and administered in a random manner. The code is not revealed until all results are available for analysis.

The administration of dummy (or placebo) tablets and injections plays an important part in clinical trials involving analgesic drugs. The effect of placebos has been well discussed by Beecher (1955) and Wilson (1962). They were shown to produce subjective changes in 35 per cent of a large number of patients. The placebo response is more pronounced in the presence of stress, as shown by the effect being ten times greater on pathological as compared with experimental pain (little stress) (Beecher, 1960). In a clinical trial a dummy tablet can produce pharmacological effects, and the concept that it is inactive is not tenable (Wilson, 1962). The placebo response is enhanced by the doctor-patient relationship at the conscious or subconscious level whenever patients believe their ailments are receiving treatment. Loan and Dundee (1967) consider that it is essential in any study to employ a placebo as it enables the sensitivity of the method to be assessed. If it is impossible to distinguish between the known effective dose of an analgesic and a placebo then the method must be rejected. These authors stress that if the patient is still in pain half an hour after the administration of a placebo then an active preparation must be given.

In a well-conducted evaluation of analgesic drugs in cancer patients with chronic pain, Houde (1962) used a cross-over, double-blind technique. The assessment of drug effect was based on the patient's subjective reports made to one nurse observer who carried out hourly daytime visits to the patients. Pain relief was estimated quantitatively, the figure assigned ranging from 1 for no pain to 4 for severe pain. Additional information that was recorded included site of pain, medication given, side-effects, and whether the patient was comfortable and his pain at least half relieved. Using intramuscular morphine 10 mg. and a saline placebo injection, the latter was found to have an appreciable pain relieving effect which at its peak was only about one-third below that of morphine. Of 67 patients, only just over one-third (37 per cent) were able to distinguish between the two injections in a way that would be anticipated. The placebo response appears to be a common feature among all patients.

Masson (1962*b*) in conducting a trial for pain relief after major abdominal surgery, omitted a cross-over design in favour of a single dose method. The trial established that pethidine 100 mg. was significantly better than saline, but the superiority of pethidine 100 mg. over pethidine 50 mg. and of the latter dose over saline were not statistically significant. The effect of morphine 10 mg. was comparable to that of pethidine 50 mg., but the sensitivity of the trial was not sufficient to differentiate readily between saline and morphine 10 mg.

As the investigator points out, "when one cannot readily distinguish between the effects of 10 mg. morphine and saline, how can one assess an analgesic which has the same effectiveness as 10 mg. morphine?" Doubts must also be cast about the adequacy of post-operative pain relief with the dosage of drugs usually employed.

Parkhouse and Holmes (1963) investigated the best technique for assessing post-operative pain relief when using morphine 10 mg. or saline in a double-blind scheme. The patient made a subjective estimate of his pain while one of the investigators also recorded his assessment of its severity. Other data collected included a measure of the patient's ability to cough, his vital capacity and peak expiratory flow rate. The observer's assessment demonstrated a significant difference between morphine and saline and was more sensitive than the patient's own estimate, which could not achieve this differentiation. The improvement in vital capacity also showed a statistically significant difference between morphine and saline. The measurement of vital capacity only requires a slow expiratory effort, unlike the sharp effort required for peak flow measurement. The latter test did not detect a significant difference between saline and morphine.

The humanitarian aspects of giving inert substances to patients in severe pain must be considered. Once the superiority of pethidine or morphine over a placebo has been established by a clinical trial, then any new drugs can be compared against these.

ANALGESIC DRUGS

Analgesics exert a depressing action on the central nervous system which results in the reduction or abolition of pain sensation without producing loss of consciousness or dangerous side-effects. There are many drugs capable of relieving pain which interrupt the peripheral cause of pain itself. Thus atropine relieves the pain of renal colic by relaxing the smooth muscle spasm of the ureter, while the nitrites relieve anginal pain by relaxing the spasm of the coronary vessels. Migraine may be relieved by ergotamine, which is an effective vaso-constrictor of the meningeal vessels. The pain and swelling of acute gout may be brought under control by giving colchicine, although its mode of action is not clear. Strictly speaking, none of these drugs is an analgesic.

Analgesic drugs may be divided into two main groups:

Potent Analgesics

These are typified by morphine and include its derivatives and the synthetic compounds allied to it. They are outstanding for their effectiveness in relieving severe pain. These drugs are used widely for pre- and post-operative sedation and analgesia, for the control of acute pain due to injury and burns, for a number of acute surgical and medical conditions including vascular occlusion and for the relief of pain in incurable malignant disease.

Morphine is the standard potent analgesic, and acts as a yardstick by which these drugs are measured. Despite its antiquity, it is the most widely used and perhaps the most reliable drug available for the relief of severe pain. It has a number of undesirable side-effects, and for this reason many morphine substitutes have been developed and marketed. The properties of these substitutes are often almost indistinguishable from morphine and any supposed advantages are due to quantitative differences in relative potency.

These are the drugs of addiction, a liability which hitherto has been present in all drugs able to relieve severe pain. Pentazocine is the first drug comparable to morphine in its effectiveness as an analgesic which has minimal addiction liability. Dependence on these drugs appears to be derived from their ability to reduce anxiety and induce a state of detachment in which severe pain becomes acceptable. The effectiveness of these agents depends in fact as much upon the alteration in mood they induce as upon the elevation of the pain threshold. On the basis of their chemical structure these drugs can be divided into three main groups, typified by morphine, methadone and pethidine. Structurally the latter two drugs resemble part of the morphine molecule. Nalorphine, which will antagonise all three drugs, is also structurally akin to morphine and is itself an analgesic. All these drugs probably act on the same site in the brain in a fundamentally similar manner. Subcutaneous or intramuscular injection is the preferred route of administration, as absorption from the alimentary tract tends to be unpredictable. The intravenous route at times is of great value especially for the relief of immediate post-operative pain.

Details of the metabolism of these drugs have been published (Way and Adler, 1960 and 1962). Their potency is partly determined by the structural changes which occur after absorption. The excretion of unaltered drugs plays little part in their inactivation in the body. As the liver is the chief organ for the conjugation of these drugs, an increased sensitivity to them is more likely to occur with hepatic damage than with impaired renal function.

Mild (Non-addictive) Analgesics

This group of drugs, typified by aspirin, is used extensively in the relief of mild pain, either by prescription or self-medication. Aspirin is the most widely used, but mixtures of analgesics, usually incorporating aspirin, are increasingly popular. Very little experimental work has been carried out to investigate the value of such combinations. The individual constituents must be presumed to have a simple additive effect. If the composition of these mixtures is not accurately known, a patient may inadvertently be given a drug to which he is sensitive.

These preparations are exploited commercially on a very large scale, being freely advertised to the general public under proprietary names. Their usefulness should not be underrated and they play an important role in the management of pain, both in and out of hospital. Even for patients with advanced maligant disease they can afford considerable relief and postpone the need for opiates. Analgesics are sometimes combined with other drugs, for example corticosteroids or barbiturates. It is better to give each drug independently in its optimal dose.

The Potent Analgesics

The important alkaloids which are contained in opium are:

Phenanthrene group	Morphine	10 per cent
	Codeine	0·5 per cent
	Thebaine	0·3 per cent

Benzylisoquinoline	Papaverine	1 per cent
	Narcotine	6 per cent

Morphine

Morphine is the most important alkaloid obtained from opium and is the oldest known analgesic, its use dating back to antiquity. Opium is the dried juice which is obtained from the poppy heads of *Papaver somniferum*. There is a curious lack of uniformity in the action of morphine on the central nervous system, in that it depresses certain centres while having a stimulant effect at other sites.

It has a depressant effect on the higher centres of the brain and a therapeutic dose (8–20 mg.) normally produces an inclination to sleep and reduces painful and unpleasant sensations. It is especially effective in combating dull, aching pain, while fear, worry, hunger and fatigue are all diminished. It causes an inability to concentrate and reach decisions and the overall mood is one of euphoria. The removal of apprehension and the feeling of well-being engendered by morphine enhances its value as a premedicant drug.

Spinal reflexes are stimulated by morphine and this paradox of stimulation accompanying depression may lead occasionally to the occurrence of post-operative excitement instead of sedation. Similarly, although most patients become sleepy after small doses of morphine, others remain very wakeful and have no inclination to sleep.

The pain threshold is considerably elevated by morphine. Its analgesic effect rises to a maximum about 90 minutes after injection and lasts about four hours. The tendency to sleep and the development of hypercapnoea both help to elevate the pain threshold, but the powerful effect of morphine upon mood is much more important in the control of pain. The relaxation, dulling of attention and freedom from anxiety which follow the injection of morphine make pain more bearable and acceptable. This effect far outlasts the period during which the pain threshold is raised.

Unlike the mild analgesics, morphine will relieve visceral pain as well as pain originating in muscles and skeletal structures. It is less effective in relieving sharp intermittent pain than a continuous dull ache.

The respiratory centre is depressed, leading to a reduction in the respiratory rate and minute volume. The tidal volume is not necessarily decreased and may even be increased. Carbon dioxide fails to exert its normal stimulant action. The rapid shallow respiratory pattern due to pleuritic pain or the dyspnoea of acute left ventricular failure are both inherently inefficient. Morphine, by slowing the rate and increasing the depth of respiration, considerably enhances the efficiency of ventilation. A further advantage of morphine in cardiac patients is a fall in the metabolic rate of about 15 per cent due to reduced oxygen consumption. The normal physiological deep breaths which occur some 30–35 times an hour are interrupted under the influence of morphine even in doses which do not appear to depress ventilation. This may be a causative factor in the development of post-operative pulmonary atelectasis (Egbert and Bendixen, 1964).

Intravenous morphine, during anaesthesia, exerts its maximal effect on the respiratory rate about three minutes after injection. Respiratory depression is a grave toxic reaction which may develop progressively with continued dosage of the drug, or may occur abruptly without warning. The patient may become comatose, clammy and cyanosed with a respiratory rate as low as three or four a minute. This collapse may be accompanied by a precipitous fall in blood pressure. In acute coronary thrombosis this collapse may be ascribed to the disease rather than to morphine and similarly in the post-operative period, surgical shock and blood loss may be incorrectly blamed. A change in tolerance to morphine may also be a factor. Intense pain seems to antagonise the effect of morphine and patients require much larger doses of the drug. With the easement of pain, tolerance for morphine is diminished and the patient may show signs of overdose. Failure to recognise morphine poisoning may lead to a needless fatality as it can be readily treated with one of the antidotes—nalorphine or levallorphan.

Morphine markedly depresses the cough centre. It also causes the pupils to become constricted to a pin-point size, due to its effect on the parasympathetic part of the oculo-motor nucleus. This effect is probably mediated by a reduction in the inhibitory influence of higher centres. Intra-ocular tension is also raised.

The chemoreceptor emetic trigger zone is stimulated, causing vomiting in about 16 per cent and nausea in about 40 per cent of ambulant patients. These symptoms are commoner in women than in men and are more pronounced in ambulant patients. For this reason morphine is normally given only to those who are confined to bed. Large doses of morphine cause bradycardia by stimulating the vagal centre and also by depressing conduction in the heart. The vasomotor centre is only slightly depressed and toxic doses are required to produce a significant fall in blood pressure. Venous pooling and increased capacitance may occur under the influence of morphine. Cutaneous vasodilatation produces a sensation of warmth in the skin, while sweating and itching sometimes occur.

Morphine inhibits the action of the salivary and other digestive glands. Visceral muscle tone is increased, especially at the pyloric and ileo-colic sphincters. Furthermore, peristalsis throughout the gastric and intestinal musculature is reduced, so causing delay in gastric emptying and constipation. The muscle tone of the biliary ducts is increased and the sphincter of Oddi is contracted, effects which may aggravate the pain of biliary colic. Powerful peristaltic waves may be generated in segments of colon affected by diverticulosis, under the influence of morphine, and the high intrasigmoid pressures so created may cause pronounced distension of the diverticula and an increased risk of perforation (Painter *et al.*, 1965).

Morphine crosses the placental barrier and may lead to difficulty in starting respiration in the newborn infant.

The body gets rid of morphine mostly by excreting it through the kidneys in a conjugated form. About 90 per cent of a dose is removed from the body mostly in a conjugated form, although some free alkaloid is present. Breakdown of the drug only takes place on a limited scale. Conjugation occurs mainly in the liver.

Tolerance, which implies the need to raise the dose in order to maintain the same effect, takes about a fortnight to develop on average doses of the drug. A cross-tolerance develops to other drugs having a similar chemical structure. Tolerance is mainly due to the tissues, and especially the brain, becoming more resistant to its effects and thereby being able to function normally despite the presence of morphine.

poor. It rarely leads to addiction and has little effect on respiration, although it is a useful suppressor of the cough reflex.

By a process of demethylation, codeine is partly converted to morphine in the liver. Analgesia may possibly depend upon the morphine produced in this way rather than the codeine itself. Indeed, it has been suggested that codeine actually antagonises the effect of morphine. This antagonism, together with the limited amount of morphine that is produced, could account for the mediocre performance of codeine as an analgesic (Way and Adler, 1960).

It is a useful drug for alleviating post-operative pain in neurosurgical patients and for post-lumbar puncture headaches. It is commonly prescribed for the treatment of moderate pain, often in combination with mild analgesics such as acetylsalicylic acid and phenacetin.

Codeine is apt to cause constipation, and use is made of this property for controlling non-infective diarrhoea. It is commonly used as an antitussive in the form of a linctus.

The dose when prescribed by itself is 10 to 60 mg. either by mouth or injection.

Tab. Codeine Co. (B.P.) contains 8 mg. of codeine phosphate and 260 mg. each of aspirin and phenacetin.

Heroin (Diamorphine Hydrochloride)

The manufacture and use of this drug is forbidden in the United States of America because of the ease with which addiction can occur. It is still available in the United Kingdom and is even more powerful than morphine as an analgesic, euphoriant, and as a depressant of respiration and the cough reflex. Nausea and vomiting are less common and it does not cause constipation. It is most useful in patients with very severe pain which cannot be controlled with morphine. Its euphoriant effect makes it the most valuable of all drugs in the terminal stages of malignant disease.

The dose is 5 to 10 mg.

Dihydromorphinone ("Dilaudid")

This is a very potent analgesic even in doses which cause little dulling of consciousness. Alimentary side-effects are less marked than with morphine. The usual dose is 2–4 mg. It is effective when given by the oral or rectal routes.

Pethidine (Meperidine U.S.P. "Demerol")

This synthetic drug was introduced in 1939 by Eisleb and Schaumann. At the time they were searching for an antispasmodic drug with atropine-like properties and discovered its analgesic action by chance.

It is ethyl-1-methyl-4 phenyl piperidine-4 carboxylic acid, and structurally is similar to atropine. It is a central depressant with an analgesic action similar to that of morphine but with a shorter duration of effect. About ten times the dose of morphine is required to produce an equianalgesic effect and it is less reliable as a means of relieving really severe pain. Because of its antispasmodic action it is often effective in relieving visceral pain and is commonly used to treat the pain of renal colic. As it does not relax the sphincter of Oddi, however, it is of little value in biliary colic. Unlike morphine, pethidine has no constipating action.

Its respiratory depressant effect is less pronounced and of shorter duration than an equivalent dose of morphine and it does not depress the cough reflex. Pethidine is widely used in obstetrics in the early stages of labour but it crosses the placental barrier and, if given less than three hours before delivery, it may cause respiratory depression in the newborn infant.

The sedative effect of pethidine is mild and it does not cause true amnesia. Patients in pain become less worried and apprehensive after pethidine and it may even induce euphoria. If pain is not present, these effects are less marked and depression may develop.

Pethidine is usually given by intramuscular injection and is supplied in 1 or 2 ml. ampoules containing 50 mg. or 100 mg. Pethidine 100 mg. is equivalent in analgesic potency to 10 mg. of morphine. Infants and children may be given 1·5 mg./kg. of body weight. The action of pethidine by mouth (25 mg. or 50 mg. tablets) is less reliable than by injection but it is useful for ambulant patients because of its mild sedative effect. In an emergency it may be administered intravenously in a 1 per cent solution. This route is also frequently used to supplement nitrous oxide and oxygen anaesthesia. Pethidine is also useful in combating the tachypnoea which may develop during trichloroethylene or halothane anaesthesia. It has a quinidine-like effect on the myocardium which diminishes cardiac irritability and acts as a prophylaxis against ventricular arrhythmias. This action, together with its effect in depressing cardiac and bronchial reflexes, makes it a valuable adjunct during anaesthesia for cardiac and pulmonary surgery.

Side-effects are less common than with morphine but dryness of the mouth, sweating, nausea, vomiting, giddiness, excitement or confusion can all occur. It may cause vasodilatation, hypotension and faintness. Pethidine is a useful alternative to morphine for post-operative analgesia in patients who are known to be upset by the latter drug. As most of it is destroyed in the liver, it must be used with caution in patients with hepatic disease.

Monoamine oxidase inhibitors may cause a dangerous potentiation of morphine and especially of pethidine (Taylor, 1962; Cocks and Passmore-Rowe, 1962). This may result in excitement and hypertension or coma and cardiovascular collapse. To be absolutely safe, a period of three weeks should elapse between stopping a monoamine oxidase inhibitor and the administration of one of these potent analgesics. It has been shown that the excretion of pethidine in the urine is pH dependent (London and Milne, 1962) and as much as 25 per cent is excreted unchanged in the urine if the pH falls below 5. Normally less than 5 per cent of pethidine is eliminated in this way.

Acidification of the urine is a useful therapeutic measure to adopt in pethidine poisoning, especially when it is associated with liver disease or the use of monoamine oxidase inhibitors. This may be achieved by the intravenous infusion over a period of half an hour, of 10 g. of L-arginine hydrochloride dissolved in 500 ml. of 5 per cent dextrose (Wood Smith *et al.*, 1968). Ammonium chloride 1 per cent may be used for the same purpose in the absence of liver disease but arginine is the agent of choice. (See also Chapter 36, p. 1029.)

Long-continued administration of pethidine may lead to addiction. The same restrictions and caution should be adopted as with morphine, especially in the relief of chronic pain.

Other Potent Analgesics

In the following section the main features of the other commonly used potent analgesics are tabulated (Table 1). Many substitutes for morphine have been introduced into clinical practice and new drugs continue to be marketed at frequent intervals. It is usually claimed that these drugs are therapeutically superior to morphine and have fewer of its disadvantages. A reduced incidence of vomiting, constipation, respiratory depression, and especially of addictive properties, are frequently claimed for these drugs. These advantages often fail to be substantiated after their widespread clinical use. The continual proliferation of analgesics, some of which have not been adequately assessed, does not necessarily represent a therapeutic advantage. Most clinicians confine themselves to a limited number of these drugs with which they become thoroughly familiar.

It is certainly useful to be able to switch from morphine to other potent analgesics in chronic painful conditions such as malignant disease. Furthermore, it is often useful to take advantage of some property of a certain drug, albeit the difference from morphine is only marginal. Such an example would be the use of methadone or pethidine to avoid drowsiness. Some patients are able to tolerate one or other of these newer analgesics far better than morphine.

Mild (Non-addicting) Analgesics

Aspirin (Acetylsalicylic Acid)

Dose 0·3 g. to 1·0 g.

This is the best and most widely used of the non-addictive analgesic drugs. It selectively depresses the thalamic centres concerned with the perception of pain. There is evidence that salicylates also alleviate pain peripherally by diminishing local oedema.

Aspirin acts on the heat-regulating centre, setting it at a lower level and so increasing the heat loss in febrile patients. This is achieved by cutaneous vasodilatation and diaphoresis. This drug is of especial value in relieving the aching pains associated with pyrexial illnesses such as influenza. When used at night the reduction in temperature is a useful aid to inducing sleep. Aspirin has no demonstrable effect on mood and may be given safely to patients working at skilled occupations.

It is well tolerated by most individuals but in large doses may cause tinnitus, dizziness, gastric irritation and bleeding from the gastro-intestinal tract, especially in patients with gastric ulcers. Large particles of aspirin can adhere to the gastric rugae and cause erosion and ulceration of the mucosa. This effect can be minimised by always crushing the tablets and taking them with meals.

A soluble form of aspirin containing citric acid, calcium carbonate and saccharin is now commonly prescribed. Such tablets are tolerated more readily and are available under the name of acetylsalicylic acid soluble tablets B.P. A popular trade preparation is "Disprin".

Aspirin may cause skin rashes, pruritus or urticaria in cases of sensitivity or

37/TABLE 1

MORPHINE GROUP

[30 mg.] = Analgesic Equivalent of Morphine 10 mg. (The printed box is empty; the boxed dose in the table below is the analgesic equivalent.)

Drug	Formula	Dose	Side-effects	Comment	Analgesic Efficacy
Dihydrocodeine bitartrate: D.F. 118: "Paracodin"		30–60 mg. oral or parenteral [30 mg.]	Minimal respiratory depression, nausea and vomiting. Mild addicting properties.	Useful substitute for morphine in chronic pain. Ref: SWERDLOW and FOLDES (1958).	Fair–good. Somewhat inferior to morphine.
Dihydrohydroxy-codeinone pectinate: Oxycodone pectinate: "Proladone"		10–20 mg. parenteral. Suppository containing 30 mg. [10 mg.]	Minimal respiratory depression. Low incidence of nausea and vomiting. Addicting.	Pectin molecule causes slow release of alkaloid. Outstanding effect is prolonged action, 6–9 hours. Little sedative effect. Suppositories particularly useful in terminal malignancy. Refs: BRITTAIN (1959); BOYD (1959).	Good.

Drug	*Formula*	*Dose*	*Side-effects*	*Comment*	*Analgesic Efficacy*
Levorphan tartrate: "Dromoran"		2 mg. parenteral. 1·5–3 mg. oral. **2 mg.**	Nausea, vomiting and dizziness similar to morphine but causes less constipation. Addicting.	Little sedative action. Anxiety not relieved. More reliable than morphine by mouth. Long duration of action (6–8 hours). Used for premedication and also as an intravenous supplement for nitrous-oxide–oxygen anaesthesia. Useful in advanced malignant disease, especially for out-patients.	Good. Powerful analgesic.
Methyldihydro-morphinone: "Metopon"		3–6 mg. oral or parenteral. **3 mg.**	Claims for reduced incidence of nausea, vomiting and respiratory depression not substantiated clinically. Addiction and tolerance develop more slowly than with morphine.	More rapid onset of action than morphine. Little sedative effect. Patient remains mentally clear. Unsatisfactory as a premedicant. Effective by mouth. Useful in terminal cancer.	Good. Potent analgesic.
Oxymorphone: "Numorphan"		1–1·5 mg. parenteral. **1·0 mg.**	Respiratory depression more marked than with morphine. Nausea, vomiting and constipation similar to morphine. Addicting	Very similar to dihydromorphinone. More rapidly acting than morphine.	Good.

Drug	*Formula*	*Dose*	*Side-effects*	*Comment*	*Analgesic Efficacy*
Phenazocine: "Prinadol" "Narphen"	CH_2-CH_2; N; CH_3; CH_3; HO	1–3 mg. parenteral. 5 mg. oral. [2 mg.]	Incidence of cardio-vascular depression, nausea and vomiting similar to morphine. Onset of addiction claimed to be slower.	No impairment of consciousness or mental acuity. Onset of action quicker than morphine and duration longer. Used in major and minor surgery, obstetrics and malignancy. Ref: THOMAS (1962); SWERDLOW *et al.* (1964).	Good. Effective analgesic.
Pentazocine "Fortral" "Talwin"	N; $CH_2-CH=C(CH_3)CH_3$; CH_3; CH_3; OH	30–60 mg. parenteral. 50 mg. oral. [40 mg.]	Respiratory and cardiovascular effects similar to morphine but nausea, vomiting and constipation claimed to occur less frequently. Dizziness. Little liability to addiction. Not scheduled as a D.D.A. drug.	Mildly sedative. No euphoria. Mild antagonist of morphine. Cannot be antagonised by nalorphine or levallorphan. Non-specific analeptic such as 30 mg. methyl phenidate (Ritalin) may be used as an antidote (Telford & Keats, 1965). Little cross-tolerance with other narcotics and may precipitate acute withdrawal reactions in narcotic addicts. Used as an alternative to narcotic analgesics in all types of pain. Useful for management of chronic pain where addiction may be a problem. Ref: Cass *et al.* (1964); Telford and Keats (1965).	

PETHIDINE GROUP

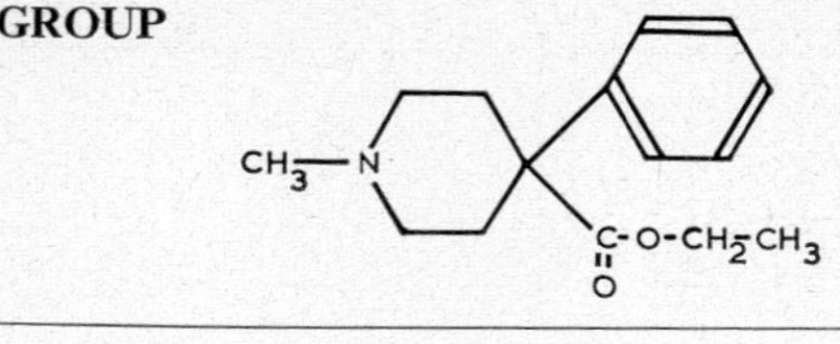

Drug	Formula	Dose	Side-effects	Comment	Analgesic Efficacy
Alphaprodine: "Nisentil"	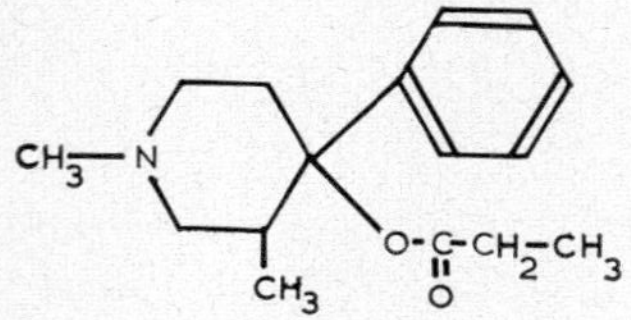	40–60 mg. parenteral or oral. 40 mg.	Respiratory depression, nausea and vomiting less than with pethidine. Addicting.	Little sedative effect or amnesia. More rapid onset than pethidine but shorter duration of action.	Good.

Drug	Formula	Dose	Side-effects	Comment	Analgesic Efficacy
Anileridine: "Alidine" "Leritine"	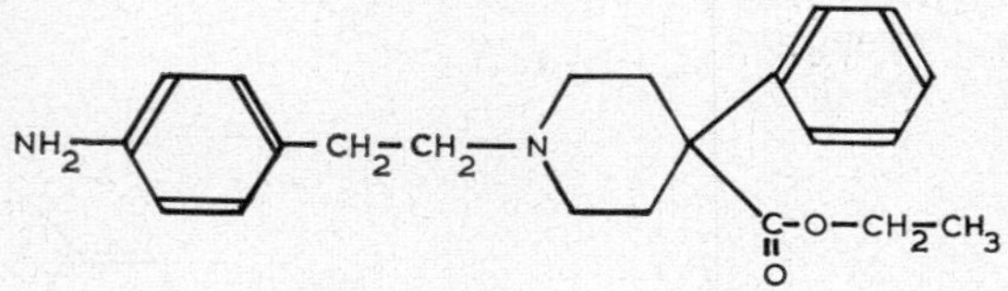	30–60 mg. parenteral or oral. 40 mg.	Respiratory depression. Less tendency to vomiting or constipation. Addiction said to develop more slowly than with morphine or pethidine.	Little sedative effect. Analgesia rapid in onset (10–30 minutes). Duration similar to alphaprodine and shorter than morphine. Antispasmodic. Clinical uses similar to pethidine but unlike the latter it does not liberate histamine. Refs: SWERDLOW (1960); RIFFIN *et al.* (1958).	Good. Intermediate between pethidine and morphine.

Drug	Formula	Dose	Side-effects	Comment	Analgesic Efficacy
Piminodine: "Alvodine"	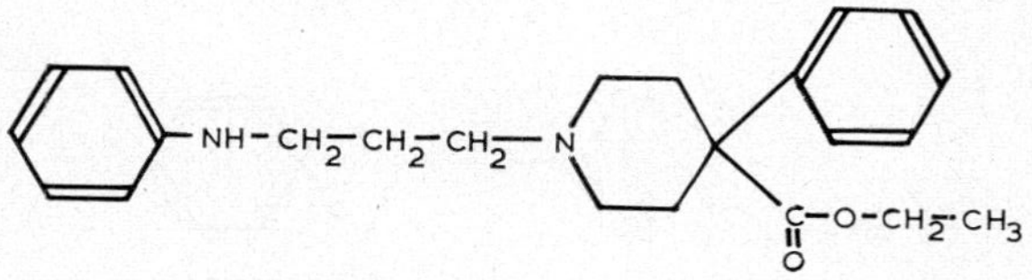 $NH-CH_2-CH_2-CH_2-N$; $C(=O)-O-CH_2-CH_3$	5–10 mg. parenteral. 7·5 mg.	Respiratory depression. Addicting. Reduced incidence claimed for other side-effects.	No drowsiness or euphoria.	Good.

Drug	Formula	Dose	Side-effects	Comment	Analgesic Efficacy
Phenoperidine: "Operidine"	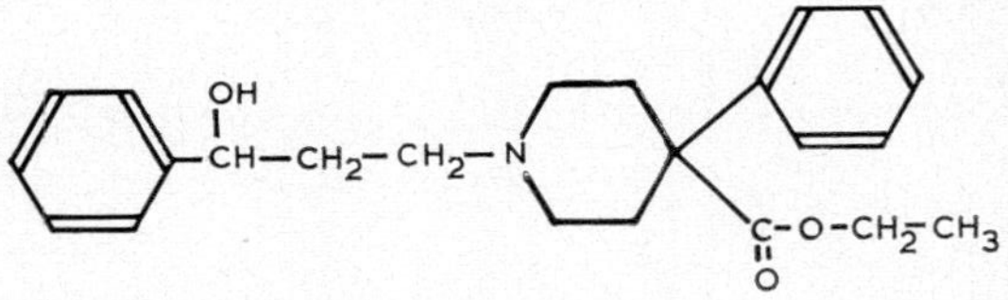 OH; $CH-CH_2-CH_2-N$; $C(=O)-O-CH_2-CH_3$	1–2 mg. parenteral or oral. 2 mg.	Respiratory depression. Addicting. Tendency to vomiting.	Used intravenously to provide analgesia during anaesthesia. An initial dose of 1 mg. with increments of 0·5 mg. every 30 minutes does not depress respiration. Intravenous doses of 2–5 mg. depress respiration and are used when it is desired to control ventilation. Causes little hypotension and has no effect on the diseased heart, so is useful for controlling ventilation after cardiac surgery. Used with a neuroleptic such as droperidol to produce neuroleptanalgesia. Ref: ROLLASON and SUTHERLAND (1963)	Good.

Drug	*Formula*	*Dose*	*Side-effects*	*Comment*	*Analgesic Efficacy*
Fentanyl "Sublimaze"		0·1–0·2 mg. parenteral or oral [0·2 mg.]	Respiratory depression. Hypotension with large doses. Addicting. Bradycardia.	Very potent analgesic. Shorter duration of action than phenoperidine. Developed for use in the technique of neurolept-analgesia. Used intravenously during general anaesthesia in a dose of 0·1–0·2 mg. with spontaneous respiration and a dose of 0·2 to 0·6 mg. for controlled ventilation. Ref: HOLDERNESS *et al.* (1963).	Powerful short-acting analgesic.

Drug	*Formula*	*Dose*	*Side-effects*	*Comment*	*Analgesic Efficacy*
METHADONE GROUP					
Methadone: "Amidone" "Physeptone"		5–10 mg. parenteral or oral. [10 mg.]	Respiratory depression, nausea and vomiting, smooth muscle spasm and constipation. Addicting. Side-effects more severe in ambulatory patients.	Markedly depressant action on the cough reflex and hence very useful as a linctus for intractable cough. Little euphoria. Minimal sedative effect. Less useful than morphine as a premedicant. Effective by mouth. Reliable substitute for morphine in chronic pain. Useful in morphine withdrawal. Tolerance to methadone develops more slowly than with morphine.	Powerful analgesic. Similar potency to morphine.

Drug	Formula	Dose	Side-effects	Comment	Analgesic Efficacy
Dextromoramide: "Palfium"	O ‖ C—N; C; H; C—CH$_2$—N; CH$_3$; O	5–10 mg. parenteral. 2·5–5 mg. oral. 5 mg.	Respiratory depression, nausea and vomiting. Addicting.	Little difference from methadone. Ref: Cope and Jones (1959).	Good.
Dipipanone: "Pipadone"	O ‖ C—CH$_2$—CH$_3$; C; CH$_2$—CH—N; CH$_3$	10–25 mg. parenteral. 25 mg. oral. 25 mg.	Side-effects less frequent than with morphine.	No advantages over methadone. Has sedative effect. Ref: Gillhespy *et al.* (1956).	Good.

allergy and in asthmatics it may precipitate an attack. Large doses may prolong the prothrombin time and cause a haemorrhagic state. Prolonged treatment with salicylates carries a risk of renal damage including renal papillary necrosis, although the danger is considerably enhanced when phenacetin is taken as well.

It is a satisfactory analgesic in relieving pain from deep non-visceral structures such as ligaments, bones, joints and muscles, and especially in pyrexial illnesses, headaches and rheumatic disease. For sustained pain relief it is better to repeat small doses at short intervals as doses larger than 0·6 g. merely prolong the effect and do not afford more effective analgesia. Visceral pain arising from smooth muscle spasm is not effectively controlled by aspirin.

The liberal use of aspirin post-operatively can add much to the patient's comfort and reduce the need for potent analgesics. As a gargle it is very useful after tonsillectomy.

Salicylate poisoning.—Acute salicylate poisoning is a serious problem, especially in children under the age of 4 years, in whom it is the commonest cause of death by poisoning. Salicylates stimulate the respiratory centre, leading to a respiratory alkalosis and a reduction in plasma CO_2 content. At the same time tissue metabolism is stimulated, inducing a metabolic acidosis and an increase in CO_2 production which maintains the hyperventilation.

Metabolic demands are increasingly met by fatty acid catabolism because of the uncoupling effect of salicylates on oxidative phosphorylation and the inhibition of enzymes of intermediary metabolism.

Treatment.—Therapeutic measures include gastric lavage and intravenous fluid therapy to correct dehydration, electrolyte losses and acid base disturbances. These changes can best be managed if repeated blood pH and P_{CO_2} or standard bicarbonate measurements are carried out. The elimination of salicylates may be hastened by the use of a mannitol-induced osmotic diuresis together with alkalinisation of the urine with sodium lactate. Osmotic diuretics are usually contra-indicated in small children because of hyperpyrexia and dehydration.

Rehydration is effected with 5 per cent dextrose solution with the addition of sodium bicarbonate and potassium chloride to correct acidosis and hypokalaemia. Sodium bicarbonate is not indicated unless the arterial blood pH is less than 7·5 and urinary pH less than 7·6. Intravenous calcium may be required to prevent the onset of tetany in the presence of severe alkalosis. In severe intoxication accompanied by renal failure, haemodialysis is the treatment of choice, while in children in the presence of coma and hyperpyrexia, curarisation and artificial ventilation may be indicated (Jackson Rees *et al.*, 1960).

Phenacetin (B.P.)

Dose 0·3 g.–0·6 g.

This drug acts in much the same way and has a similar potency to aspirin. It is generally believed to be less specific for rheumatic pain and is frequently given in combination with aspirin and codeine. The continued use of this drug in large doses may cause methaemoglobinaemia, haemolytic anaemia, renal papillary necrosis or non-obstructive pyelonephritis.

Paracetamol (N acetyl-p-aminophenol: "Panadol")

Dose is 0·5 to 1·0 g.

This is the breakdown product of phenacetin responsible for its analgesic and antipyretic properties. It causes no toxic effects such as methaemoglobinaemia. It is a weaker analgesic than aspirin but it is less irritant to the stomach. It may be used as an alternative to aspirin or phenacetin in the relief of minor aches and pains, especially for patients who cannot tolerate aspirin.

Acetanilide, Phenazone and Amidopyrine

These drugs are classified with phenacetin as analgesics and antipyretics. Their use has largely been given up because of their toxic effects. All three directly depress the myocardium while amidopyrine can cause agranulocytosis.

Phenylbutazone ("Butazolidine")

Dose 200–400 mg. daily.

This drug, which is closely related to amidopyrine, appears to modify experimentally-produced inflammatory reactions. It has analgesic and antipyretic properties and occupies an intermediate position between aspirin and cortisone in relieving pain and tenderness in rheumatoid arthritis.

The main toxic effect is on the bone marrow, causing agranulocytosis, thrombocytopenia or aplastic anaemia. The risk is minimal as long as the daily dose is not more than 400 mg., but regular white cell counts are advisable.

Other toxic effects include diarrhoea, skin rashes, dyspepsia and sodium and water retention. The drug is broken down slowly in the body and its effects persist as long as 72 hours.

Its principal use is in the treatment of chronic arthritis when the pain is not controlled by aspirin and is severe enough to risk the toxic effects of the drug on the bone marrow.

Dextropropoxyphene ("Darvon")

This analgesic drug, which is related to methadone, has been investigated in the U.S.A. It is not an antipyretic and is non-addicting as it has no effect on mood.

The potency of dextropropoxyphene is about the same as that of codeine and the dose is 100 mg. The toxic effects are drowsiness, dizziness, gastro-intestinal disturbances and rashes.

Compound Analgesic Tablets

By far the most popular is Tab. Codeine Co. (B.P.) which contains the following ingredients:

Aspirin	0·26 g.
Phenacetin	0·26 g.
Codeine Phosphate	8 mg.

Although the B.P. dose is 1 or 2 tablets, it is usual to prescribe 2 or 3 tablets for post-operative pain. The very small dose of codeine present in these tablets is of doubtful value. Their analgesic and toxic properties are due almost entirely to the aspirin and the phenacetin. "Veganin" contains the same ingredients in a different proportion.

Tabs. Codeine Co. should be given crushed up to minimise their irritant effect on the stomach. "Codis" is a useful trade preparation which contains soluble aspirin and codeine with phenacetin in a fine suspension. It is well tolerated even by those who are susceptible to aspirin and its solubility increases its speed of absorption.

Tabs. Codeine Co. have a reputation for being more effective than aspirin but this may be entirely a question of dosage, as two of the former contain more analgesic than three aspirin tablets.

Another commonly used compound tablet is acetylsalicylic acid compound tablet (B.P.) more commonly called Tab. A.P.C.:

Aspirin	0·23 g.
Phenacetin	0·16 g.
Caffeine	30 mg.

The caffeine is intended to combat the sedative effect of the other ingredients, so making this tablet particularly suitable for ambulant patients and for use during the day. It is questionable, however, whether this dose of caffeine has any worthwhile stimulant effect.

The relief of pain and insomnia is a common clinical problem so it is not surprising that there are many preparations available containing both an analgesic and a hypnotic. Such remedies are too inflexible and it is better to administer each drug separately so that if a further dose of analgesic only is required, the hypnotic does not have to be given as well.

Antidotes and Antagonists

The high incidence of undesirable side-effects creates a major problem in the use of the potent analgesics. These have been discussed in the previous section dealing with the pharmacology of these drugs and may be conveniently classified as follows:

1. Respiratory. Depression of respiration, especially the rate.
2. Alimentary. Nausea, vomiting and constipation.
3. Addiction.
4. Miscellaneous symptoms. These include drowsiness, anxiety, disorientation, inability to concentrate, dryness of the mouth, blurred vision, nystagmus, itching, flushing, feeling of warmth, shivering and pallor.

These side-effects can be avoided or reduced by cutting down the dosage used or switching to another drug which has fewer or different side-effects. Some patients are able to tolerate one particular drug better than others of this group. It is less certain whether the simultaneous administration of an antagonist and a narcotic analgesic will prevent side-effects while at the same time maintaining adequate analgesia (Telford and Keats, 1961).

The main use of these antagonists is in the treatment of poisoning and overdosage due to narcotic analgesics, in combating unexpected idiosyncrasy to these drugs, and during labour as a prophylaxis against foetal depression. As the morphine antagonists are equally effective against levorphan, pethidine and methadone they are conveniently referred to as the narcotic antagonists.

Narcotic Antagonists

The clinically important drugs which reverse some at least of the effects of the narcotic analgesics are:

1. Nalorphine } true antagonists
2. Levallorphan }
3. Amiphenazole } partial antagonists
4. Tetrahydroaminacrine }

Nalorphine (N-allylnormorphine: "Nalline": "Lethidrone")

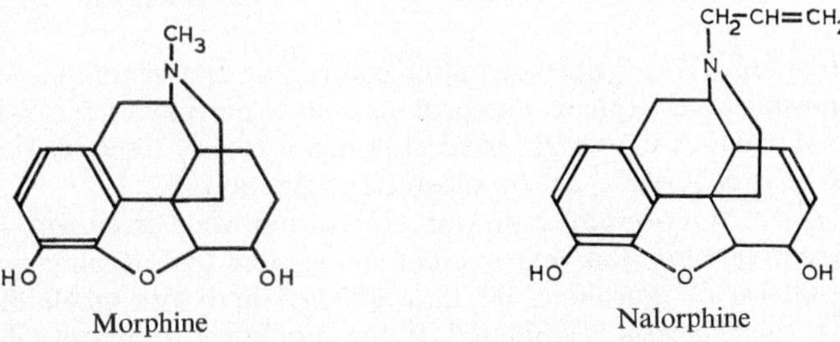

Morphine Nalorphine

This drug probably acts by substrate competition on the receptors that are affected by the opiate drugs. Its actions are similar to those of morphine. When given alone, nalorphine causes respiratory depression but it has little analgesic action. Moderate doses (5 mg.) may also cause miosis, sweating, bradycardia and drowsiness while larger doses may cause dysphagia and even hallucinations (Huggins and Moyer, 1955). When given with morphine or one of the other potent analgesics, it prevents respiratory depression. If respiration is already depressed, however, nalorphine has a marked stimulant effect.

Eckenhoff (1952) found that anaesthetised subjects who had previously received 20–90 mg. of morphine or 200–600 mg. of pethidine, doubled or trebled their respiratory rate after the intravenous injection of 5–10 mg. of nalorphine. Respiratory depression due to barbiturates or anaesthetic gases was unaffected.

The blood pressure of morphine-depressed patients may increase and the depth of coma lighten after the injection of nalorphine, but its influence on analgesia is less predictable. In morphine addicts, nalorphine precipitates an intense withdrawal syndrome with restlessness, tachypnoea, sweating and increased salivary secretions. It can be used in this way as a specific test for addiction.

The use of large doses of narcotics during the first stage of labour predisposes to neonatal respiratory depression. The incidence of this complication in these circumstances can be strikingly reduced by taking advantage of the ability of nalorphine to cross the placental barrier. The mother receives 10 mg. of the drug intravenously about 10 minutes before delivery is anticipated.

Nalorphine is administered intramuscularly or intravenously in doses of 5–10 mg., although in profound narcotic poisoning it may be necessary to use as much as 40 mg. In neonatal asphyxia due to a narcotic crossing the placenta from the mother, 0·2–0·4 mg. of the diluted drug may be injected into the umbilical vein.

Levallorphan Tartrate ("Lorfan")

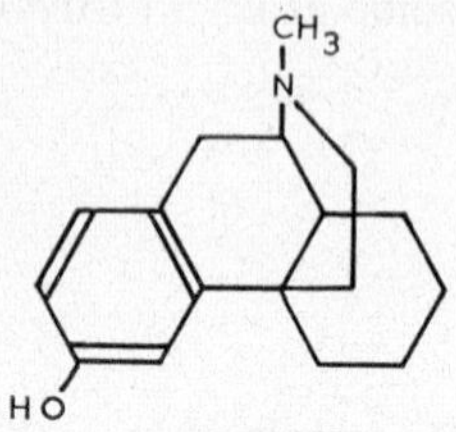

Levorphan 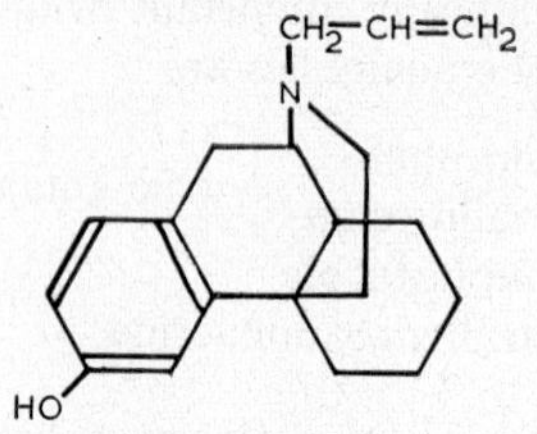 | Levallorphan

This compound was synthesised after nalorphine and bears the same structural relationship to levorphan as nalorphine does to morphine. It is five times as potent as nalorphine on a weight basis although it closely resembles it pharmacologically. It is believed to act by substrate competition.

Levallorphan will prevent respiratory depression when given with morphine and allied compounds and will combat depression that is already present. Other side-effects of morphine are little affected and with small doses it is claimed that the analgesia is unaltered. It does not affect respiratory depression caused by barbiturates or general anaesthetics.

Levallorphan has a longer duration of action than nalorphine in antagonising respiratory depression and moreover it can be given by mouth. It does not appear to have any undesirable side-effects in the doses used clinically. The indications for levallorphan are the same as for nalorphine in combating respiratory depression due to narcotic drugs. The intramuscular or intravenous dose of levallorphan is 1·0–2 mg. In neonatal asphyxia 0·25 mg. can be given into the umbilical vein. Levallorphan has been administered in combination with narcotics in the following proportions:

Morphine 15 mg.	Levallorphan 0·3–0·5 mg.
Pethidine 100 mg.	Levallorphan 1·25 mg.
Levorphan 2 mg.	Levallorphan 0·2–0·3 mg.

Levallorphan crosses the placental barrier and "Pethilorfan" (pethidine 100 mg. with levallorphan 1·25 mg.) has been used extensively in obstetrics in order to reduce the incidence of neonatal asphyxia. The use of narcotic-antagonist mixtures is discussed in the next section.

Narcotic-antagonist Mixtures

The rationale for the use of these mixtures depends on the belief that such a combination in an optimal dose ratio results in reduced side effects, especially respiratory depression, without antagonising the analgesia. This technique was based on animal studies and many articles have been published in an attempt to substantiate the existence of this differential effect in man.

Hossli and Bergmann (1960) showed that the intravenous injection of pethidine (1 mg./kg.) combined with levallorphan in the ratio of 80:1 produced significantly less respiratory depression than pethidine alone. From a study on post-operative pain they concluded that the analgesic effect of pethidine was not reduced by the levallorphan and there was no significant difference in the incidence of side-effects in the two groups. Reports on the use of these mixtures in obstetrics have suggested that the risk of neonatal depression is decreased while adequate maternal analgesia is maintained. Other workers have failed to corroborate the existence of this effect in man and the evidence available has been critically reviewed by Telford and Keats (1961). They point out that in many of the studies, while respiratory depression was measured quantitatively, there was in contrast a striking lack of precision in assessing analgesia.

In order to detect small changes in analgesia it is necessary to employ complicated and time-consuming double-blind techniques, coded drugs and a cross-over procedure to establish adequate controls. These authors are also critical of the use of narcotic-antagonist mixtures to supplement thiopentone-nitrous oxide-oxygen anaesthesia. It has been reported (Foldes and Ergin, 1958) that although the thiopentone (a weak analgesic) requirements were reduced to about one-quarter of the controls, the dose of pethidine or alphaprodine (potent analgesic) increased about five-fold, suggesting that analgesia was antagonised as well as respiratory depression. These reviewers also considered that the studies on the use of narcotic-antagonist mixtures in obstetrics had not proved that the maintenance of adequate analgesia was accompanied by a reduced risk of neonatal depression. The measurement of analgesia did not utilise the necessary controls and double-blind conditions. The higher doses of pethidine necessary for analgesia would also suggest that this effect was being antagonised by the levallorphan. Telford and Keats concluded that there was no pharmacological evidence to justify the belief that the clinical use of narcotic-antagonist mixtures would result in reduced side-effects while maintaining analgesia.

Dundee (1964) reported that a mixture of levallorphan and levorphan in the ratio of 1:10 was clinically unsuitable for the alleviation of intractable pain. A high incidence of side-effects appeared in patients who had been taking drugs of addiction for some time, presumably due to levallorphan-induced abstinence symptoms. If addicting drugs had not previously been taken, the continued use of this mixture led to self-induced withdrawal symptoms after about three weeks.

Amiphenazole (2:4 diamino-5 phenylthiazole hydrochloride, "Daptazole" or D.A.P.T.)

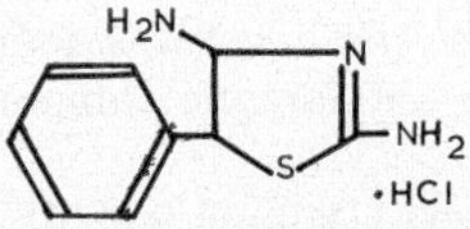

This drug, unlike nalorphine or levallorphan, is chemically unrelated to the opiate drugs. It is a central nervous system stimulant, not a competitive antagonist, and in large doses will cause convulsions. It is claimed that amiphenazole counteracts the side-effects of morphine, including respiratory depression, vomiting and constipation, without interfering with the analgesia.

McKeogh and Shaw (1956) have described the use of a combination of morphine and amiphenazole in the management of intractable pain from terminal carcinoma. It is possible apparently to work up to massive doses of morphine when each injection is accompanied by 25 mg. of amiphenazole, and emphasis is laid on the mental alertness and general feeling of well-being in the patients under treatment. If respiratory depression develops, additional doses of amiphenazole may be given intravenously. It would be desirable to have a carefully controlled double-blind investigation carried out before the value of this technique can be accurately assessed.

Morphine overdose may be treated by the intermittent intravenous injection of amiphenazole 20 mg. up to a total of 200 mg. but it is preferable to employ a specific morphine antagonist.

Ballantine (1957) has reported the successful cure of morphine addiction with amiphenazole.

Tetrahydroaminacrine (T.H.A. "Tacrine")

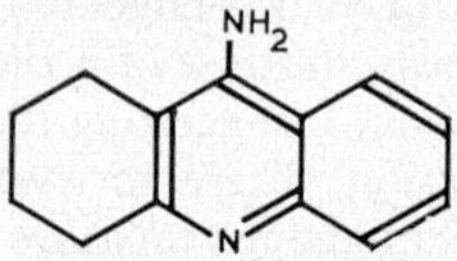

The pharmacology of tetrahydroaminacrine is similar to that of amiphenazole and has been described by Stone *et al.* (1961). It is a central nervous system stimulant, producing convulsions in large doses. As a respiratory stimulant it is claimed to be more reliable than amiphenazole and it has a marked arousal effect on patients after the administration of a barbiturate or a general anaesthetic. It is a potent anticholinesterase and has been advocated for extending the action of suxamethonium and antagonising *d*-tubocurarine. T.H.A. is termed a "partial antagonist" of morphine in that it is claimed to combat the side-effects but not interfere with analgesia. Stone and his co-workers used T.H.A. in combination with morphine to relieve the intractable pain of carcinoma. Morphine was administered in doses of 10–100 mg. four times a day, 10–15 mg. of T.H.A. being given with each injection. Respiratory depression or narcosis did not occur and although tolerance developed the patients did not become addicted and no withdrawal symptoms followed the cessation of morphine.

The advantages claimed for T.H.A. over amiphenazole were its stability in solution which enabled it to be combined with morphine in the same ampoule, its increased reliability as an antinarcotic compound and its non-interference with sleep.

Simpson and his co-workers (1962) in a study on post-operative pain were unable to demonstrate, on statistical analysis, any difference between the pain relief afforded by standard doses of morphine and double doses of morphine combined with T.H.A. Likewise there was no obvious improvement in coughing or movement, but the study did show a significant improvement in the level of consciousness when T.H.A. was used.

It appears that T.H.A. enables patients to receive larger doses of morphine without increased morbidity, but the only benefit that seems to accrue is one of increased alertness and co-operation.

Other Non-analgesic Drugs

There are a number of drugs which may at times be useful in the management of pain either by acting as adjuvants to the analgesics or by combating side-effects of morphine, such as nausea, vomiting, constipation and drowsiness.

Cyclizine Hydrochloride ("Marzine")

This antihistamine, which is relatively free from side-effects, has a strong anti-emetic action. It is a useful drug to give with the potent analgesics to patients prone to nausea and vomiting. Cyclizine should be given prophylactically at the same time as the analgesic, since it will not stop nausea once it has started. Cyclizine lasts for four hours and it may be necessary to give one 50 mg. tablet every four hours even although the analgesic is required less frequently.

Chlorpromazine ("Largactil")

The pharmacology of this interesting drug is discussed elsewhere (Chapter 36) and it is mentioned here for the sake of completeness. It is a central depressant which potentiates the action of the narcotic analgesics so that they can be given in reduced dose. It also has a powerful anti-emetic action.

Perphenazine ("Fentazine")

This is a phenothiazine derivative and is one of the most effective of the anti-emetic drugs. The dose is 2–5 mg. and it can be used to combat the emetic side-effects caused by the potent analgesics. It causes little hypotension and agranulocytosis is rare but extrapyramidal side-effects have been reported.

Promazine ("Sparine")

This drug resembles chlorpromazine but it is less potent. It is a good tranquilliser but it is not so effective as perphenazine as an anti-emetic. The dose is 25–50 mg.

Amphetamine

The hypnotic effect imparted by many of the potent analgesics is at times undesirable. Amphetamine in a dose of 2·5 to 5 mg. not only counteracts this drowsiness but elevates the mood and gives a feeling of well-being. Amphetamine may also potentiate the analgesic action of morphine and mild analgesics such as aspirin. It may impair the appetite and should not be given after midday in case it interferes with sleep.

Hyoscine

This is effective as a sedative in a dose of 0·3 to 0·4 mg. and may be given with a narcotic analgesic to patients in pain who are agitated and restless.

REFERENCES

ADRIAN, E. D. (1931). The messages in sensory nerve fibres and their interpretation. *Proc. roy. Soc. B.*, **109**, 1.

ARMSTRONG, D., DRY, R. M. L., KEELE, C. A., and MARKHAM, J. W. (1953). Observations on chemical excitants of cutaneous pain in man. *J. Physiol.* (*Lond.*), **120**, 326.

ARMSTRONG, D., JEPSON, J. B., KEELE, C. A., and STEWART, J. W. (1957). Pain-producing substance in human inflammatory exudates and plasma. *J. Physiol.* (*Lond.*), **135**, 350.

BALLANTINE, I. D. (1957). Amiphenazole in a case of drug addiction. *Lancet*, **1**, 251.

BECHER, H. (1950). Untersuchung der Head'nchen Zonen mit dem Acetyl-cholin-Prostigmin-Test bei Erkrankung der Bauchorgane. *Neue med. Welt*, **1**, 1343.

BEECHER, H. K. (1955). Powerful placebo? *J. Amer. med. Ass.*, **159**, 1602.

BEECHER, H. K. (1956). Relationship of significance of wound to pain experienced. *J. Amer. med. Ass.*, **161**, 1609.

BEECHER, H. K. (1957). The measurement of pain. *Pharmacol. Rev.*, **9**, 59.

BEECHER, H. K. (1959). *Measurement of subjective responses: quantitative effects of drugs.* New York: Oxford University Press.

BEECHER, H. K. (1960). Increased stress and effectiveness of placebos and "active" drugs. *Science*, **132**, 91.

BEECHER, H. K. (1962). *The Assessment of Pain in Man and Animals* (Proc. Internat. Symp. held under the auspices of UFAW, Middlesex Hosp. Med. School, 1961), p. 168. Ed. by C. A. Keele and R. Smith. Edinburgh: E. & S. Livingstone.

BEECHER, H. K. (1968). *Pain* (Proc. Internat. Symp. on Pain organised by the Lab. of Psychophysiol., Faculty of Sciences, Paris, 1967), p. 201. Ed. by A. Soulairac, A. Cahn and J. Charpentier. New York: Academic Press.

BONNYCASTLE, D. D. (1962). *The Assessment of Pain in Man and Animals* (Proc. Internat. Symp. held under auspices of UFAW, Middlesex Hosp. Med. School, 1961), p. 231. Ed. by C. A. Keele and R. Smith. Edinburgh: E. & S. Livingstone.

BOXING, E. G. (1933). *The Physical Dimensions of Consciousness.* New York: Appleton-Century.

BOYD, R. H. (1959). A clinical trial of dihydro-hydroxycodeinone pectinate. *Anaesthesia*, **14**, 144.

BRADLEY, R. D., SPENCER, G. T., and SEMPLE, S. J. G. (1964). Tracheostomy and artificial ventilation of acute exacerbations of chronic lung disease. *Lancet*, **1**, 854.

BRAIN, R. (1962). *The Assessment of Pain in Man and Animals* (Proc. Internat. Symp. held under auspices of UFAW, Middlesex Hosp. Med. School, 1961), p. 9. Ed. by C. A. Keele and R. Smith. Edinburgh: E. & S. Livingstone.

BRITTAIN, G. J. C. (1959). Dihydrohydroxycodeinone pectinate. *Lancet*, **2**, 544.

CASS, L. J., FREDERICK, W. S., and TEODORO, J. V. J. (1964). Pentazocine as an analgesic. Clinical evaluation. *J. Amer. med. Ass.*, **188**, 112.

CHARPENTIER, J. (1968). *Pain* (Proc. Internat. Symp. on Pain organised by the Lab. of Psychophysiol., Faculty of Sciences, Paris, 1967), p. 171. Ed. by A. Soulairac, A. Cahn and J. Charpentier. New York: Academic Press.

COCKS, D. P., and PASSMORE-ROWE, A. (1962). Dangers of monoamine oxidase inhibitors. *Brit. med. J.*, **2**, 1545.

COHEN, H., and JONES, H. W. (1943). The reference of cardiac pain to a phantom left arm. *Brit. Heart J.*, **5**, 67.

COPE, E., and JONES, P. O. (1959). Relief of post-operative pain. *Brit. med. J.*, **1**, 211.

DUNDEE, J. W. (1964). A clinical trial of a mixture of levorphanol and levallorphan as an oral analgesic. *Brit. J. Anaesth.*, **36**, 486.

ECKENHOFF, J. E. (1952). N-allyl-normorphine: an antagonist to the opiates. *Anesthesiology*, **13**, 242.

EGBERT, L. D., and BENDIXEN, H. H. (1964). Effect of morphine on breathing pattern. A possible factor in atelectasis. *J. Amer. med. Ass.*, **188**, 485.

EISLEB, O., and SCHAUMANN, O. (1939). Dolantin, ein neuartiges Spasmolytikum und Analgetikum (Chemisches und Pharmakologisches). *Dtsch. med. Wschr.*, **65**, 967.

FOLDES, F. F., and ERGIN, K. H. (1958). Levallorphan and meperidine in anaesthesia: study of effects in supplementation of nitrous oxide-oxygen-thiopental sodium anesthesia. *J. Amer. med. Ass.*, **166**, 1453.

FORD, F. R., and WILKINS, L. (1938). Congenital universal insensitiveness to pain. *Bull. Johns Hopk. Hosp.*, **62**, 448.

GASSER, H. S. (1943). Pain producing impulses in peripheral nerves. *Ass. Res. nerv. Dis. Proc.*, **23**, 44.

GELLHORN, E. (1953). *Physiological Foundations of Neurology and Psychiatry*. Minneapolis: Univ. Minnesota Press.

GILLHESPY, R. O., COPE, E., and JONES, P. O. (1956). Dipipanone hydrochloride in the treatment of severe pain. *Brit. med. J.*, **2**, 1094.

GRAHAM, J. R. (1960). Use of a new compound UML-491 (1-methyl-d-lysergic acid butanolamide) in the prevention of various types of headache. *New Engl. J. Med.*, **263**, 1273.

GRAVENSTEIN, J. S., SMITH, G. M., SPHIRE, R. D., ISAACS, J. P., and BEECHER, H. K. (1956). Dihydrocodeine. Further development in the measurement of analgesic power and appraisal of psychologic side-effects of analgesic agents. *New Engl. J. Med.*, **254**, 877.

GRUBER, C. M. (1962). The design of experiments evaluating analgesics. *Anesthesiology*, **23**, 711.

HAGBARTH, K. E., and KERR, D. I. B. (1954). Central influences of spinal afferent conduction. *J. Neurophysiol.*, **17**, 295.

HARDY, J. D. (1962). *The Assessment of Pain in Man and Animals* (Proc. Internat. Symp. held under auspices of UFAW, Middlesex Hosp. Med. School, 1961), p. 170. Ed. by C. A. Keele and R. Smith. Edinburgh: E. & S. Livingstone.

HARDY, J. D., WOLFF, H. G., and GOODELL, H. (1947). Studies on pain: discrimination of differences in intensity of pain stimulus as a basis of scale of pain intensity. *J. clin. Invest.*, **26**, 1152.

HARDY, J. D., GOODELL, H., and WOLFF, H. G. (1951). Influence of skin temperature upon pain threshold as evoked by thermal radiation. *Science*, **114**, 149.

HARMAN, J. B. (1948). The localisation of deep pain. *Brit. med. J.*, **1**, 188.

HARMAN, J. B. (1951). Angina in the analgesic limb. *Brit. med. J.*, **2**, 521.

HEAD, H. (1920). *Studies in Neurology*. London: Oxford University Press.

HEWER, A. J., and KEELE, C. A. (1948). A method of testing analgesics in man. *Lancet*, **2**, 683.

HOCKADAY, J. M., and WHITTY, C. W. M. (1967). Patterns of referred pain in the normal subject. *Brain*, **90**, 481.

HOLDERNESS, M. C., CHASE, P. E., and DRIPPS, R. D. (1963). A narcotic analgesic and a butyrophenone with nitrous oxide for general anesthesia. *Anesthesiology*, **24**, 336.

HOLMES, T. H., and WOLFF, H. G. (1950). Life situations, emotions and backaches. *Ass. Res. nerv. Dis. Proc.*, **29**, 750.

HOSSLI, G., and BERGMANN, G. (1960). A combination of analgesic and antagonist in postoperative pain. *Brit. J. Anaesth.*, **32**, 481.

HOUDE, R. W. (1962). *The Assessment of Pain in Man and Animals* (Proc. Internat, Symp. held under auspices of UFAW, Middlesex Hosp. Med. School, 1961). p. 202. Ed. by C. A. Keele and R. Smith. Edinburgh: E. & S. Livingstone.

HUGGINS, R. A., and MOYER, J. H. (1955). Some effects of n-allylnormorphine on normal subjects and a review of the literature. *Anesthesiology*, **16**, 82.

JACKSON REES, G., STEAD, A. L., and BUSH, G. H. (1960). Salicylate poisoning. *Brit. med. J.*, **2**, 1454.

KEATS, A. S., and BEECHER, K. H. (1952). Analgesic potency and side action liability in man of heptazone WIN 1161-2, 6 methyldihydromorphine, metopon, levo-isomethadone and pentobarbital sodium, as a further effort to refine methods of evaluation of analgesic drugs. *J. Pharmacol. exp. Ther.*, **105**, 109.

KEELE, K. D. (1948). The pain chart. *Lancet*, **2**, 6.

KERR, F. W. L., and MILLER, R. H. (1966). The pathology of trigeminal neuralgia. *Arch. Neurol. (Chic.)*, **15**, 308.

KUNKLE, E. C., and CHAPMAN, W. P. (1943). Insensitivity to pain in man. *Ass. Res. nerv. Dis. Proc.*, **23**, 100.

LANDAU, W. M., and BISHOP, G. H. (1953). Pain from dermal, periosteal and fascial endings and from inflammation; electrophysiological study employing differential nerve blocks. *A.M.A. Arch. Neurol. Psychiat.*, **69**, 490.

LASAGNA, L., and BEECHER, H. K. (1954). The optimal dose of morphine. *J. Amer. med. Ass.*, **156**, 230.

LERICHE, R. (1949). *La Chirurgie de la Douleur*. Paris: Masson et Cie.

LOAN, W. B., and DUNDEE, J. W. (1967). The value of the study of postoperative pain in the assessment of analgesics. *Brit. J. Anaesth.*, **39**, 743.

LONDON, D. R., and MILNE, M. D. (1962). Dangers of monoamine oxidase inhibitors. *Brit. med. J.*, **2**, 1752.

MASSON, A. H. B. (1962*a*). Clinical assessment of analgesic drugs: spirometry trial. *Curr. Res. Anesth.*, **41**, 615.

MASSON, A. H. B. (1962*b*). Clinical assessment of analgesic drugs. *Anaesthesia*, **17**, 411.

MCKEOGH, J., and SHAW, F. H. (1956). Further experiences with amiphenazole and morphine in intractable pain. *Brit. med. J.*, **1**, 142.

MELZACK, R., and WALL, P. D. (1965). Pain mechanisms: a new theory. *Science*, **150**, 971.

MELZACK, R., and WALL, P. D. (1968). Gate control theory of pain. In *Pain* (Proc. Internat. Symp. organised by the Lab. of Psychophysiol., Faculty of Sciences, Paris, 1967), p. 11. Ed. by A. Soulairac, A. Cahn and J. Charpentier. New York: Academic Press.

MENDELL, L. M., and WALL, P. D. (1964). Presynaptic hyperpolarization: a role for fine afferent fibres. *J. Physiol. (Lond.)*, **172**, 274.

MERSKEY, H. (1968). Psychological aspects of pain. *Postgrad. med. J.*, **44**, 297.

MÜLLER, J. (1840). *Handbuch der Physiologie des Menschen*, **2**, 249.

PARKHOUSE, J., and HOLMES, C. M. (1963). Assessing post-operative pain relief. *Proc. roy. Soc. Med.*, **56**, 579.

PAINTER, N. S., TRUELOVE, S. C., ARDRON, G. M., and TUCKEY, M. (1965). Effect of morphine, prostigmine, pethidine and probanthine on the human colon in diverticulosis. *Gut*, **6**, 57.

PARKHOUSE, J., LAMBRECHTS, W., and SIMPSON, B. R. J. (1961). The incidence of post-operative pain. *Brit. J. Anaesth.*, **33**, 345.

RIFFIN, I., WHEATON, H. H., SCHWARZ, B., PREISIG, R., and LANDMAN, M. (1958). Anileridine—an evaluation of its use in anesthesia and in post-operative analgesia. *Curr. Res. Anesth.*, **37**, 154.

ROLLASON, W. N., and SUTHERLAND, J. S. (1963). Phenoperidine (R. 1406). A new analgesic. *Anaesthesia*, **18**, 16.

RUCH, T. C., and FULTON, J. F. (1960). *Medical Physiology and Biophysics*. Philadelphia: W. B. Saunders Co.

SCHIFF, M. (1848). *Lehrbuch der Physiologie, Muskel und Nervenphysiologie*. Schavenburg., Fahr., **1**, 228.

SHERRINGTON, C. (1906). *The Integrative Action of the Central Nervous System.* London: Constable & Co.

SIMPSON, B. R., SEELYE, E., CLAYTON, J. I., and PARKHOUSE, J. (1962). Morphine combined with tetrahydroaminacrine for postoperative pain. *Brit. J. Anaesth.*, **34,** 95.

SMITH, G. M., EGBERT, L. D., MARKOWITZ, R. A., MOSTELLER, F., and BEECHER, H. K. (1966). An experimental pain method sensitive to morphine in man: the submaximal effort tourniquet technique. *J. Pharmacol. exp. Ther.*, **154,** 324.

SOULAIRAC, A. (1968). *Pain* (Proc. Internat. Symp. organised by the Lab. of Psychophysiol., Faculty of Sciences, Paris, 1967), p. 5. Ed. by A. Soulairac, A. Cahn and J. Charpentier. New York: Academic Press.

STEINHAUS, J. E., BEVAN, W., WEBB, S. C., and THOMPSON, W. R. (1964). Evaluation of analgesics by the rating of patient behaviour. *Anesthesiology*, **25,** 64.

STONE, V., MOON, W., and SHAW, F. H. (1961). Treatment of intractable pain with morphine and tetrahydroaminacrine. *Brit. med. J.*, **1,** 471.

SWERDLOW, M. (1960). Anileridine in anesthesia—a clinical trial. *Anesthesiology*, **15,** 280.

SWERDLOW, M., and FOLDES, F. F. (1958). The effects of intravenously administered dihydrocodeine bitartrate in anaesthetised man. *Brit. J. Anaesth.*, **30,** 515.

SWERDLOW, M., STARMER, G., and DAW, R. H. (1964). A comparison of morphine and phenazocine in postoperative pain. *Brit. J. Anaesth.*, **36,** 782.

TAYLOR, D. C. (1962). Alarming reaction to pethidine in patients on phenelzine. *Lancet*, **2,** 401.

TELFORD, J., and KEATS, A. S. (1961). Narcotic–narcotic antagonist mixtures. *Anesthesiology*, **22,** 465.

TELFORD, J., and KEATS, A. S. (1965). Studies of analgesic drugs: antagonism of narcotic antagonist-induced respiratory depression. *Clin. Pharmacol. Ther.*, **6,** 12.

THOMAS, K. B. (1962). Phenazocine ("Narphen") used as an adjunct to anaesthesia. *Brit. J. Anaesth.*, **34,** 336.

WALL, P. D. (1962). The origin of a spinal-cord slow potential. *J. Physiol.* (*Lond.*), **164,** 508.

WALL, P. D. (1967). *J. Physiol.* (*Lond.*), **188,** 403.

WAY, E. L., and ADLER, T. K. (1960). The pharmacologic implications of the fate of morphine and its surrogates. *Pharmacol. Rev.*, **12,** 383.

WAY, E. L., and ADLER, T. K. (1962). The biological disposition of morphine and its surrogates. *Bull. Wld. Hlth. Org.*, **26,** 51.

WILSON, C. W. M. (1962). *The Assessment of Pain in Man and Animals* (Proc. Internat. Symp. held under auspices of UFAW, Middlesex Hosp. Med. School, 1961), p. 213. Ed. by C. A. Keele and R. Smith. Edinburgh: E. & S. Livingstone.

WOLFF, H. G., and WOLF, S. (1958). *Pain.* Springfield, Illinois: Charles C. Thomas.

WOOD SMITH, F. G., STEWART, H. C., and VICKERS, M. D. (1968). *Drugs in Anaesthetic Practice*, p. 138. London: Butterworth & Co.

Chapter 38

THE TREATMENT OF PAIN

THE present chapter is concerned with the practical management of pain as it concerns the anaesthetist and may be considered under the headings of pre- and post-operative pain, and the symptomatic relief of chronic intractable pain which has come to dominate the clinical picture. The last may be due to incurable malignant disease or to some condition such as post-herpetic neuralgia which does not immediately threaten the patient's life. Finally a brief comment is made on neuroleptanalgesia.

PRE-OPERATIVE PAIN

Patients suffering from some painful condition and awaiting surgery should receive the appropriate treatment, whether this necessitates morphine, some less potent analgesic, or merely sedation, rest and reassurance. In the immediate pre-operative period the premedication affords the necessary pain relief and sedation, especially if morphine is used. Pain in the acute surgical emergency presents a more difficult problem. Analgesics should be withheld until a diagnosis has been reached and the course of action determined. Pain then having served its warning purpose, it is justifiable to relieve it with morphine, given intravenously if necessary. Caution must be adopted in the elderly, toxic or shocked patient as a full therapeutic dose of morphine may cause profound collapse.

Patients in pain from acute trauma need and derive great benefit from morphine. A poor peripheral circulation from vasoconstriction may severely limit the absorption of drugs given by subcutaneous injection. The optimal dose of morphine can be given much more safely and rapidly by incremental intravenous injections until the desired effect is achieved. A period of 10–20 minutes should elapse between each injection so that the full effect of each dose can be assessed. Patients in severe pain often need much larger doses of a narcotic than usual because the pain seems to antagonise the depressant effects of these drugs.

Opiate Premedication in Children

Children over the age of five years can be premedicated satisfactorily with morphine or papaveretum in combination with atropine or hyoscine (Anderson, 1960). The effect usually produced is a calm, drowsy, co-operative child with a dry respiratory tract. The intravenous route is undoubtedly the kindest and most pleasant way of inducing anaesthesia in children (Rees, 1960). After an opiate premedication the majority of children will readily accept a venepuncture, particularly if it has been fully explained to them by the anaesthetist in a pre-operative ward visit. Painless venepuncture is facilitated by the opiate-induced venous dilatation and by the use of fine, sharp needles. The induction of anaesthesia in children presents the greatest problem between the ages of 18 months and 5 years. Children of this age group are less amenable to explanations and persuasion, venepuncture is more difficult, and less psychological trauma is caused if they are brought to the anaesthetic room fast asleep. For these premedication is best administered by the oral or rectal route and anaesthesia induced with an inhalational technique. Even in this age group opiate premedication and intravenous induction may be preferred, particularly in co-operative children and prior to cardiac surgery. Opiate premedication has the advantage of considerable latitude in its timing, because of its long duration of action. Precise timing, which is so necessary with barbiturate premedication, is of less importance, and this affords a worthwhile practical advantage in busy wards during a long operating list. Varying dosages of papaveretum and hyoscine have been advocated for premedication in children and in an attempt to determine the optimum amount of this mixture Davies and Doughty (1967) carried out a double blind trial using four different dosage schemes on children undergoing adeno-tonsillectomy. These authors were unable to detect any difference between any of the dosage schemes in the co-operation and behaviour of the children in the anaesthetic room. The highest dosage of papaveretum used in this trial was 0·52 mg./kg. and approximated to the dose recommended by Anderson of 0·6 mg/kg. (0·29 mg./lb.). This dosage, however, was associated with an increase in respiratory depression, post-operative vomiting, violent restlessness and a very dry mouth. It was concluded that there was no justification for using the higher dosages as premedication for children and the lowest of the four dosage schemes in the trial was recommended, namely 0·31 mg./kg. of papaveretum with 0·007 mg./kg. of hyoscine. This represents the adult dose of papaveretum (20 mg.) being given to a 70 kg. child and scaling down the doses proportionately according to body weight.

Post-operative Pain

The incidence of post-operative pain varies with the individual patient's reaction to pain, but is largely governed by the site and nature of the operation. Upper abdominal and intrathoracic operations cause most pain and distress. In a study on the incidence of post-operative pain after general surgical procedures, Parkhouse and his co-workers (1961) found that during the first 48 hours post-operatively, the greatest number of analgesic injections was required by patients after gastric surgery. Much less pain occurs after operations on the head and neck, the extremities, and on the superficial tissues.

Pain may arise from the skin, tendons, bones, muscles or viscera, but from the functional viewpoint may be divided into the dull, aching pain which persists at rest and the severe, sharp pain produced by movement or coughing. The former pain is readily relieved by morphine but the sharp, severe pain which is caused by the contraction of recently incised or injured muscle is much more difficult to obtund. Fear and anxiety may aggravate post-operative suffering by causing rigid muscle contractions in an attempt to splint the operative site. This leads to a self-perpetuating cycle of increased pain, fear, and muscle spasm.

General Analgesics

The powerful effect of the placebo response has been discussed in the previous chapter and must always be borne in mind when prescribing drugs for the easement of post-operative pain. Morphine in a dose of 10 mg. has long been established as the standard drug for this purpose, despite its unpleasant side-effects, especially nausea and vomiting. Papaveretum is preferred by many clinicians because of a belief in its superiority as regards the incidence of side-effects. A dose of 20 mg. is equivalent to 13·3 mg. of morphine sulphate. In the immediate post-operative period, while the patient is still under the close supervision of the anaesthetist in the recovery room, it is often advantageous to give small incremental doses of these drugs intravenously until the desired degree of analgesia has been achieved. For patients who are intolerant of morphine, pethidine, is probably the most widely used alternative drug, and indeed is used as the routine post-operative analgesic by many anaesthetists. The dose of pethidine is 100 mg. and as its duration of action is shorter than that of morphine it may have to be given more frequently. Promethazine in a dose of 25–50 mg. is frequently combined with pethidine both pre- and post-operatively. It affords increased sedation and reduces the incidence of nausea and vomiting (Burtles and Peckett, 1957). Promethazine is one of the drugs which have been described as having an antanalgesic effect – see below (Moore and Dundee, 1961). However, the increased sedation provided by the promethazine does appear to reduce the need for post-operative analgesics.

Chlorpromazine has also been given to potentiate the effects of analgesics both pre- and post-operatively but its undesirable side-effects have led to a decline in its use. It is a valuable drug for patients who are unduly agitated and anxious after operation. The dose of chlorpromazine is usually 25 mg. three times a day. Levorphan ("Dromoran") is an effective long-acting analgesic for post-operative pain but its lack of sedative action may be considered a disadvantage.

Oxycodone pectinate ("Proladone"), in view of its very long action, may enable a more even plane of analgesia to be maintained. Any of the potent analgesics tabulated in the previous chapter may be used to treat post-operative pain, and one drug may suit a particular patient better than another.

Keats (1956) employed a number of the newer analgesics to treat post-operative pain and concluded that equi-analgesic doses of these drugs were accompanied by the same amount of nausea, vomiting and respiratory depression.

Increasing the dosage of analgesics enhances the severity of the side-effects but does not always produce more pain relief. The danger of addiction from the use of potent narcotic drugs in the relief of post-operative pain is small and is no reason for withholding their use. Nevertheless, non-addicting drugs should be substituted as soon as possible. If a series of painful operations is planned, the risk of addiction is increased, and for long-term pain therapy it may be useful to employ the non-addictive drug pentazocine.

The careful use of these pain-relieving drugs in the post-operative period will enable the patient to cough more effectively and to move more freely around the bed. Physiotherapy and breathing exercises should be timed to take place when the analgesia is at its maximum. Such a regime provides a safeguard against respiratory complications and thrombosis. The need of each patient for these drugs must be based on an assessment of his physical and mental state and the nature of the operation. Post-operative sedation must not be regarded as the same set routine for all surgical patients as there is a considerable variation in the therapeutic requirements.

Morphine and allied drugs, although relieving post-operative pain while the patient is lying quietly in bed, are unfortunately not as effective when the patient is coughing vigorously (Simpson and Parkhouse, 1961). The use of larger or more frequent doses of these drugs in an attempt to improve the analgesia can lead to a highly dangerous situation. Respiratory and circulatory depression together with immobility, increased drowsiness and lack of co-operation may contribute materially to post-operative morbidity and may even cost the patient his life. In these circumstances such drugs, instead of preventing, may contribute to the development of respiratory and thrombotic complications. Morphine antagonists and drugs such as tetrahydroaminacrine have been used to prevent these dangers and have been discussed in the previous chapter. There is no convincing evidence to suggest that they have a worthwhile therapeutic effect, and as far as tetrahydroaminacrine is concerned one study showed that the patients were more alert after its use but they did not obviously benefit in other ways (Simpson *et al.*, 1962).

Not all patients require potent analgesics to relieve their pain after major surgical operations. Tabs. codeine co. are extremely useful and may be given freely during the first few days, although they do produce constipation. Even patients who require morphine initially after operation can usually revert to simple remedies such as tabs. codeine co. after the first 48 hours. These tablets are also very useful in relieving the stiffness and discomfort in back and limbs due to the unaccustomed and awkward positions which patients are forced to assume.

Children do not require the same scale of post-operative analgesia as an adult, perhaps because they have less fear of pain. Aspirin or tabs. codeine co. are often sufficient for children post-operatively. For severe pain, children of 12 take the full adult dose of morphine and for smaller children it should be given on a proportionate weight basis. Nepenthe is a traditional way of giving opiates to children by injection (see page 1055).

Antanalgesia

Antanalgesia is the term applied to the action which certain drugs appear to have in lowering the pain threshold. This effect was first described by Clutton-Brock (1960) and is manifest even if an analgesic has been administered previously. Further observations were made by Dundee (1960*b*) who found that small doses of thiopentone produced a transient fall in the pain threshold of patients premedicated with 100 mg. of pethidine. Antanalgesia is in fact experimental confirmation of the clinical observations that sedatives and hypnotics, like barbiturates and chlorpromazine, do not relieve pain unless administered in a dose which is large enough to produce unconsciousness. Smaller doses tend to produce an exaggerated response to pain and are clearly ineffective in relieving post-operative pain.

The post-operative restlessness which occurs so frequently in children who have been premedicated with barbiturates is almost certainly due to persistence of this antanalgesic effect. It is seen typically after painful operations like tonsillectomy and emphasises the advantages of an opiate premedication.

Moreover, thiopentone, which has been used for induction of anaesthesia, may exert an antanalgesic effect in the post-operative period. Low blood levels of thiopentone may persist for long periods and contribute to post-operative pain and restlessness. This effect may necessitate the use of larger doses of analgesics than would otherwise be required.

Local Analgesics

(*a*) **Long-acting drugs.**—Prolonged post-operative pain relief has been achieved by injecting long-acting drugs, especially after proctological procedures. The oily solutions of local analgesics used originally were abandoned because of sloughing and abscess formation at the site of injection. "Efocaine", a non-oily substitute which was subsequently introduced, has also fallen into disfavour following reports of sloughing, post-injection neuritis and transverse myelitis (Bonica, 1953; Clark *et al.*, 1955). These agents in fact cause nerve degeneration. The introduction of local analgesic solutions into the rectus sheath through polythene tubes inserted at operation has been described by Lewis and Thompson (1953). The method is tedious; it increases the risk of wound infection and has never become popular.

(*b*) **Intercostal block.**—Intercostal block has been used to control post-operative somatic pain in the chest or abdomen. It is most effective after superficial operations as it does not block pain fibres from the viscera or peritoneum. The need for repeated multiple injections is the main disadvantage. Bonica (1953) provided analgesia by repeating the injections daily for two to four days. The effect lasted for six to ten hours and the patients were able to breathe deeply and cough more effectively.

(*c*) **Paravertebral block.**—Post-operative analgesia can be produced in any region of the body, except the head, by means of paravertebral block. Unlike intercostal block, it has the advantage of blocking all pain fibres including those from the viscera. It carries the risk of more severe complications including intrathecal injection, pneumothorax and hypotension.

(*d*) **Epidural analgesia.**—Bonica (1953), after a study involving several hundred patients, concluded that continuous epidural analgesia was superior to all other techniques for relieving post-operative pain. Intermittent injections of local analgesic were given through an indwelling catheter. The complete pain relief which resulted from this block permitted more effective coughing and better ventilation. Simpson and his co-workers (1961) employed this technique to control post-operative pain after abdominal surgery. Initially, vinyl catheters were inserted into the lumbar epidural space. The large volume of local analgesic solution injected produced a widespread block which was almost invariably accompanied by hypotension. Subsequently, more selective analgesia was achieved by injecting small volumes of solution through catheters inserted into the mid-thoracic region. Lignocaine in a concentration of 1·5 per cent was the drug of choice, and the volume of solution injected on each occasion ranged from 6 ml. to 14 ml. The injections, which were given under strict aseptic conditions, gave complete analgesia for about 90 minutes and were continued intermittently for the first 2–3 days after operation. With this technique, hypotension ceased to be a major problem. These authors comment on the completeness of the pain relief achieved with epidural blockade, so that patients ceased to be aware of their wounds and were able to breathe deeply and cough more effectively. The procedure is also very successful after thoracotomy and in patients with severe chest injuries. After upper abdominal surgery the vital capacity is reduced to 25–30 per cent of the normal figure and to about 50 per cent after lower abdominal operations. This reduction in vital capacity is probably due to reflex muscle spasm since it does not increase when the pain is relieved with morphine. After epidural blockade there is a significant increase in vital capacity, which returns on average to 85 per cent of the pre-operative level. This form of analgesia is time-consuming, and its value is limited by the short duration of action of the available drugs. Moreover, when the effect wears off there is a sharp end-point, with the rapid return of severe pain.

Bromage (1967) has used epidural analgesia after major surgical operations to enable patients to become ambulant within one hour of leaving the operating theatre. For thoracic epidurals he advocates the "hanging-drop" method with the patient in the sitting position to increase the negative pressure in the epidural space. The long-acting local analgesic bupivacaine is a useful addition to the drugs available for this technique. This procedure is unsuitable for routine use but it is of great value in selected patients with respiratory disease in whom post-operative sputum retention presents a particular problem.

Intravenous Local Analgesia

A number of workers have used intravenous local analgesia to relieve post-operative pain. Pooler (1949) reported on the use of intravenous procaine and de Clive-Lowe *et al.* (1954) on intravenous lignocaine administered during surgery. This technique has never become very popular. Side-effects are not uncommon and it has no particular advantage over morphine. Despite good pain relief, the effect on vital capacity is disappointing.

Inhalational Techniques

The inhalation of known concentrations of trichloroethylene or nitrous oxide may be used to relieve post-operative pain and also for procedures such as changing dressings (Simpson and Parkhouse, 1961). A trial of premixed 25 per cent nitrous oxide in oxygen for relieving post-operative pain was described by Parbrook and Kennedy (1964). After the mixture had been inhaled for fifteen minutes, an improvement in vital capacity could be demonstrated, although it was not as striking as that observed after epidural blockade. Nitrous oxide-oxygen mixtures are of value when narcotic analgesics are contra-indicated or when the analgesia they afford is inadequate, and in patients who are already receiving oxygen therapy (Parbrook, 1967*a*). Because of the risk of leucopenia, long-term nitrous oxide can only be administered for 24 or 48 hours. These gas mixtures may be given with or without air dilution or for a limited number of deep breaths. Parbrook (1967*b*) showed that the inhalation of ten deep breaths of 50 per cent nitrous oxide from a demand valve was equivalent to the continuous inhalation of 25 per cent nitrous oxide for ten minutes. The technique of deep breaths may be of help prior to post-operative breathing exercises.

Discussion

There is usually a progressive reduction in the intensity of post-operative pain and after 48 hours narcotics are no longer required. Pain is the dominant factor in the production of post-operative chest complications and the effective relief of pain after surgery is not merely aimed at making the patient more comfortable but is of vital importance in reducing the incidence and morbidity of such sequelae.

The normal practice in the management of post-operative pain is to prescribe injections of morphine 10–15 mg. at approximately four- to six-hourly intervals depending on the patient's needs. Narcotics must only be given for the relief of pain and not routinely at regular intervals. Pethidine 100 mg. is preferred by some anaesthetists as an alternative analgesic, and after the acute pain has subsided 2–3 tabs. codeine co. may be given as necessary to relieve the patient's residual pain and discomfort.

Morphine does not afford complete relief of the pain produced by vigorous coughing and extradural block has a very useful application in patients who are particularly liable to chest complications.

The need for large doses of narcotics has been questioned by some workers and Roe (1963) in a series of 600 patients was able to reduce the total average dose of morphine to 4 mg. per patient. When narcotics were required by his patients, intravenous morphine was administered in doses of 1–2 mg. at intervals of 10 to 30 minutes until pain and discomfort had been relieved. This striking result was ascribed to psychotherapy given in the form of detailed explanations to the patients before operation. It was explained that pain was the natural sequence of surgery and was not abnormal. The integrity of the wound and its security against the effects of moving and coughing were stressed. Deep breathing and coughing were taught pre-operatively and it was emphasised that early mobility was important in reducing total discomfort.

Egbert and his co-workers (1964), by a similar regime of encouragement and education, were able to reduce the post-operative narcotic requirements by half on days one to five but not on the day of operation itself. These aspects of the patient's reaction to pain are often neglected and they do help to reinforce the benefits which accrue from good nursing and the discipline of a well-run surgical ward under the charge of an efficient and compassionate sister. There are many factors apart from pain which intensify the patient's suffering after operations. These include fatigue, fear, insomnia, together with the discomfort associated with nasogastric tubes, drainage tubes, intravenous infusions and indwelling catheters. Moreover, nausea, vomiting, flatulence or a distended bladder or abdomen may cause more suffering than the pain from the wound (Masson, 1967). Attention to all of these factors and the treatment of the patient as an individual with sympathy and understanding can do much to encourage confidence and reduce the totality of his suffering.

The Management of Chronic or Intractable Pain

Severe intractable pain often presents a most difficult therapeutic problem. Many of the methods which are available for the symptomatic relief of pain are outside the sphere of the anaesthetist and are mentioned here only for the sake of completeness. These measures would include physiotherapy, psychotherapy, hormone therapy for hormone-dependent tumours, chemotherapy (including regional perfusion techniques), deep X-ray therapy, surgery including palliative removal of tumours, amputation of painful useless limbs, adrenalectomy and hypophysectomy for bone secondaries from carcinoma of the breast, cordotomy, leucotomy and rhizotomy.

The following methods will be discussed:

1. Local infiltration.
2. Injection of somatic nerves.
3. Injection of autonomic nerves and ganglia.
4. Intrathecal injection.
5. Epidural injection.
6. Osmolytic neurolysis and hypothermic subarachnoid irrigation.
7. Percutaneous electrical cordotomy.
8. General analgesic drugs and their adjuvants.

1. Local Infiltration

One of the simplest ways of managing intractable pain is to inject a local analgesic solution, such as 0·5 per cent lignocaine, into the painful tissues. In addition to relieving pain locally, this technique may also cause the disappearance of referred pain, muscle spasm and vasomotor disturbances at some distance from the site of injection. Furthermore this secondary relief frequently lasts for a considerable time after the block has worn off. It has been postulated that in certain musculoskeletal disorders "trigger areas" act as a source of constant irritation and set up a vicious circle of impulses which produce the referred pain and other disturbances mentioned above. Local infiltration interrupts this vicious circle and may afford permanent relief of symptoms. This technique is widely used for a variety of disorders such as sprains and strains, painful undisplaced fractures, low back pain, bursitis, tendinitis, arthritis, muscle disorders including myalgia, contusions, torticollis, muscle contractions and "fibrositis". Nowadays injections of hydrocortisone are frequently given for these disorders, either by itself or in combination with a local analgesic. Painful scars following surgery and reflex dystrophies may also be treated successfully by local infiltration. It is often necessary to repeat the infiltration several times at intervals of three days to a week. The period of relief usually increases progressively after each injection.

2. Injection of Somatic Nerves

The injection of a local analgesic drug into a peripheral nerve, or its immediate vicinity, will cause complete analgesia in the area supplied by the nerve for a period of about one hour. In addition to its use in providing analgesia for surgery, it also has an important application for diagnostic purposes and for treating intractable pain. Like local infiltration, pain relief in the distribution of the nerve may persist long after the local analgesic has ceased to act and cutaneous sensation has returned. Post-herpetic neuralgia may be relieved in this way by carrying out a paravertebral block on the appropriate spinal somatic nerve. Repeated nerve blocks may achieve long-lasting relief in this condition, particularly in patients with a short history of neuralgia. The mechanism by which prolonged relief is afforded in this way is not understood, but as mentioned in the previous section it has been suggested that nerve blocks may break up the vicious circle of pain by interrupting the reflexes which initiate or maintain the painful state.

It is not proposed to discuss all the theurapeutic nerve blocks that may be practised. The following list merely sets out examples of conditions in which nerve blocks may be usefully employed. For a full list of the different blocks and the technique of injection, the reader is referred to Bonica's *Management of Pain* (1953) and Moore's *Regional Block* (1965).

(i) Gasserian ganglion block with a local analgesic drug only relieves trigeminal neuralgia for a few hours, but it is an aid to the differential diagnosis of this condition and also allows patients to experience the anaesthesia of the face which would follow permanent relief with alcohol injection or surgery. In recent years phenol has been used as an alternative to alcohol. Very small quantities are injected at a time, the aim being to abolish sensation to pin prick yet retain light touch.

(ii) Bilateral block of the internal larnygeal nerves will relieve the severe pain caused by laryngeal tuberculosis or malignancy.

(iii) Thoracotomies and renal operations are occasionally followed by pain and tenderness which are distributed segmentally and usually appear shortly after the wound has well healed. The aetiology of this post-operative neuralgia is doubtful but may well be due to the involvement of segmental nerves in scar tissue. Intercostal or paravertebral block, repeated at intervals, may prove helpful in such cases.

(iv) Fractured bones. A paravertebral block may help control the pain of fractured ribs, vertebrae or sternum and a superior alveolar or mandibular nerve block that of a fractured jaw. The acute pain and disability of the early stages are relieved and mobility encouraged.

(v) Post-herpetic neuralgia. Repeated nerve blocks with a local analgesic may afford effective pain relief, but often it is necessary to resort to a permanent block with alcohol or phenol, and even then success is not assured. When spinal nerves are involved a paravertebral block can be utilised, but with the trigeminal nerve the affected branches can be injected individually.

(vi) In treating fibrositis and backache, Belam and Dobney (1957) describe the use of paravertebral block of the nerves which correspond with the area of greatest tenderness. These authors emphasise the importance of precise neurological diagnosis and of distinguishing between dermatomes and sclerotomes.

Neurolytic agents—alcohol and phenol.—By injecting agents which destroy the nerve fibres, it is possible to obtain prolonged and even permanent pain relief. This technique is used in patients with severe intractable pain due to malignant disease or conditions like post-herpetic neuralgia which have failed to respond to simpler measures.

Alcohol has been widely used as a neurolytic agent. Bonica (1953) has concluded that with concentrations below 50 per cent only sensory fibres are involved. After an alcohol block the maximum analgesic effect is not apparent for several days. Regeneration of the fibres occurs in time unless the nerve cells are destroyed as well. If superficial nerves are injected, sloughing of the overlying skin may occur. Alcoholic neuritis is a serious complication of this technique and is due to failure to place the alcohol in exactly the right place. This leads to incomplete destruction of the somatic nerve and causes an intense burning pain which may be worse than the original. Absolute alcohol is frequently injected into the Gasserian ganglion for trigeminal neuralgia. A test injection of a small quantity of a local analgesic solution must produce perfect analgesia before the alcohol is given.

In recent years aqueous solutions of phenol (6 per cent) have been used as an alternative to alcohol. It seems to have little effect on tissues adjacent to the nerve and is more effective in blocking sympathetic fibres than somatic fibres. Phenol appears to diffuse less readily than alcohol. It used to be thought that these neurolytic agents destroyed the smaller fibres preferentially before the larger ones but it now seems that alcohol and phenol produce a patchy destruction of all sizes of fibres wherever contact with them occurs. The effect achieved is a quantitative reduction in the barrage of impulses emanating from the painful area rather than any specific qualitative change in the input.

3. Injection of Autonomic Nerves or Ganglia

There are many painful conditions in which the nerve impulses are carried by sympathetic pathways and in consequence sympathetic nerve blocks are among the most frequent that the anaesthetist is called upon to perform.

Vascular disorders.—An injury adjacent to a large vessel causes intense vasospasm which, if unrelieved, may progress to gangrene. Lesser degrees of vasospasm, whether due to trauma or vascular disease, are a frequent cause of pain. Disorders such as embolism, thrombophlebitis, Raynaud's disease, dissecting aneurysms and thromboangiitis obliterans all cause pain by vasospasm which may be relieved by the appropriate sympathetic block. The stellate ganglion may be blocked for disorders of the upper limb and is one of the easiest and most satisfactory blocks to perform. It has been advocated to relieve the vascular spasm caused by the intra-arterial injection of thiopentone and also the spasm after angiography. For circulatory disturbances of the lower limb a lumbar sympathetic block is indicated. When it is desired to interrupt both the somatic and the sympathetic pathways a paravertebral block of the spinal nerves can be carried out.

Reflex sympathetic dystrophies (causalgic states).—This term is applied to a group of conditions all exhibiting a similar symptomatology. This consists of pain, hyperaesthesia, vasomotor disturbances and trophic changes. These conditions may be conveniently classified as follows:

1. *Major reflex dystrophies*

   (*a*) Causalgia—following peripheral nerve lesions.
   (*b*) Phantom limb pain.
   (*c*) Central pain—e.g. thalamic syndrome.

2. *Minor reflex dystrophies*

This group includes many conditions such as the shoulder–hand syndrome (Steinbocker), post-traumatic pain syndrome, Sudeck's atrophy, post-traumatic oedema and the post-frostbite syndrome.

It is believed that in all these conditions a reflex disorder involving the sympathetic nervous system is initiated by local damage. Sympathetic blocks will usually improve and even dramatically cure the pain and vasomotor disturbances associated with these disorders.

Causalgia is a distinct syndrome which develops after a peripheral nerve injury. It consists of a burning pain of varying severity which is exacerbated by minor stimuli, dryness, heat, or emotional disturbances, and relieved by sympathectomy. Doupe and his co-workers (1944) put forward a theory that causalgia is due to fibre interaction or artificial synapses developing at the site of nerve injury. This results in efferent sympathetic impulses being short-circuited at the site of trauma into sensory afferent fibres, whence they return to the spinal cord and are eventually interpreted in the thalamus as pain. At the same time impulses from the artificial synapse can also travel peripherally, causing the release of bradykinin which induces a burning pain distally (Bergan and Conn, 1968). In any particular patient one or other of these processes may predominate but both are abolished by sympathectomy.

Cardiac pain.—Cardiac pain impulses travel via sympathetic fibres through the middle and inferior cervical cardiac nerves and the thoracic cardiac nerves, to reach the upper four or five thoracic sympathetic ganglia and the corresponding posterior spinal nerve roots. These pathways may be interrupted and pain relieved by stellate ganglion block or paravertebral block of the upper four or five thoracic spinal nerves. A left-sided stellate ganglion block is usually sufficient to achieve relief, otherwise the right side must be blocked as well.

Severe incapacitating angina is best managed by surgical interruption of the pain pathways either by posterior rhizotomy or thoracic ganglionectomy. In bad risk cases paravertebral block with alcohol or phenol is the procedure of choice.

Cerebrovascular disease.—Bilateral stellate block produced no alteration in either cerebral blood flow or cerebral vascular resistance in a series of normotensive and hypertensive patients (Scheinburg, 1950). Nevertheless, vasospasm may be an important contributory factor in certain cerebrovascular accidents, typically thrombosis, embolus and haemorrhage, and good results have been claimed from stellate ganglion block following such episodes. Walsh (1956) found that 50 per cent of patients with cerebral thrombosis and hemiplegia could be improved with such treatment, although it may need to be repeated several times. Undoubtedly some patients do improve dramatically after stellate block, with a speed which suggests relief of spasm or increase in collateral blood flow. Assessment of this therapy is made difficult by the spontaneous, rapid and almost complete recovery which can occur after apparently serious cerebral vascular lesions even in the absence of any treatment (Brain, 1956). In a controlled trial on the treatment of cerebral embolus, Carter (1957) concluded that there was no significant difference between the control group of patients and those treated by repeated stellate block. Considerable doubt exists as to the precise value of stellate block in the treatment of these disorders. It should be avoided in patients with acute cerebral haemorrhage because of the risk of increasing the bleeding.

Lungs.—Stellate ganglion block has been advocated in cases of pulmonary embolism and status asthmaticus.

Cancer pain.—Sympathetic pathways are implicated in many cases of cancer pain and sympathetic nerve blocks are often very effective in relieving a large component of the pain associated with inoperable or recurrent malignant disease.

Advanced carcinoma of the breast is often complicated by an uncomfortable oedematous arm and a severe burning pain in the shoulder and brachial plexus. To achieve complete pain relief by injection techniques, it is often necessary to interrupt the somatic pathways with a subarachnoid alcohol or phenol block and the sympathetic pathways with a stellate ganglion block. The use of subarachnoid and epidural techniques to block sympathetic pathways will be discussed in a later section.

Stellate ganglion block is described in Chapter 44. When producing a prolonged block with alcohol the technique is modified to avoid the widespread diffusion of a large volume of solution. The procedure described in Chapter 44 is carried out and a marker is placed on the needle to indicate the depth of the fascial plane where the ganglion is located. The needle is then reinserted so that at the marked depth its tip is 1 cm. below the original position. If a small test dose of lignocaine (1·5 ml.) produces a Horner's syndrome, it can be assumed that the tip of the needle is adjacent to the ganglion and 1·5 ml. of alcohol or phenol can then be slowly injected.

Lumbar sympathetic block.—This procedure will block the sympathetic pathways to the pelvic organs and lower limbs. It has a valuable diagnostic and therapeutic application, especially in vascular disorders of the lower limb, because of its effect in relieving vascular spasm and dilating blood vessels. Mandl's classical technique is described in Chapter 44.

Therapeutic sympathetic blocks may have to be repeated several times and in the case of an arterial embolus in the lower limb it may necessitate a block every day. When a long-term block is required, 6 per cent phenol is probably a more satisfactory agent than alcohol. Before injecting these neurolytic agents, the correct placement of the needle must be verified by producing a block with a small dose of a local analgesic. Since the stellate ganglion and the lumbar sympathetic chain are readily accessible for surgery, the majority of patients requiring permanent interruption of the sympathetic pathways at these sites are submitted to open operation. Chemical sympathectomy may be indicated if the patient is considered a poor risk for surgery.

Coeliac plexus block.—The autonomic fibres innervating the upper abdominal viscera can be interrupted with a coeliac plexus block. Bridenbaugh and his co-workers (1964) described the use of bilateral coeliac plexus block with 40 to 50 ml. of 50 per cent alcohol in 41 patients with intractable pain from advanced carcinoma of the stomach, pancreas, gall-bladder or liver. All these patients, with one exception, were rendered free from pain for periods varying from six weeks to one year. The block is carried out with the patient in the prone position with a pillow under the abdomen. Marks are made at the inferior edge of the 12th thoracic spine and at the lower border of each 12th rib at a distance of 7 cm. from the lumbar spine (Fig. 1). Lines are drawn between these three marks to form a triangle. The coeliac plexus lies at the level of the upper part of the body of the 1st lumbar vertebra, which coincides with the tip of the 12th thoracic spine. A 12 cm. needle is inserted through the mark at the lower border of the 12th rib at an angle of 45 degrees to the skin, and advanced medially and upwards in the direction indicated by the side of the triangle marked on the patient's back. The depth at which the needle makes contact with the body of the 1st lumbar vertebra is noted. After withdrawing the needle, it is reinserted at a

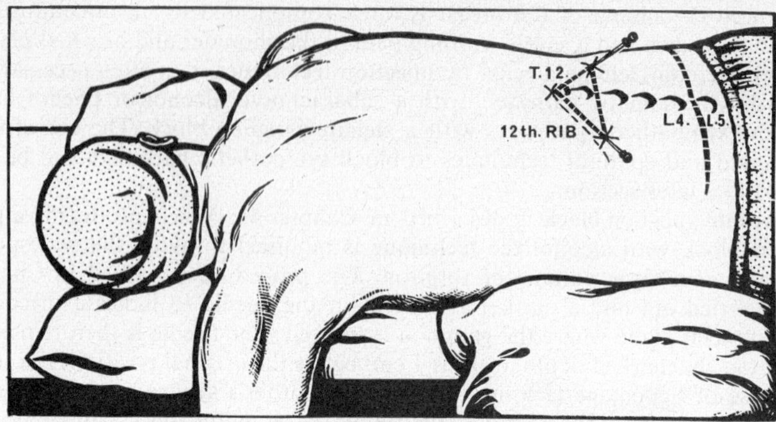

38/Fig. 1.—Coeliac plexus block. The position of the patient and skin markings for needle entries.

slightly steeper angle until it just slips off the body of the vertebra. After advancing the needle a further ½ inch (1·3 cm.), its tip should lie adjacent to the coeliac plexus (Fig. 2). The distance to the plexus from the skin is between 7·6 and 10·2 cm. After a negative aspiration test, 25 ml. of local analgesic solution is injected. These authors used 0·1 per cent tetracaine ("Pontocaine") hydrochloride solution with 1 in 250,000 adrenaline, but 0·5 per cent lignocaine with 1 in 250,000 adrenaline may be used as an alternative. There should be no resistance to the injection of this solution. The other side is similarly blocked and this should produce pain relief for up to eight hours. If the block is successful it is repeated the following day using 25 ml. of 50 per cent alcohol on each side. Initially 1 ml. of alcohol is injected to exclude somatic nerve paraesthesia. If

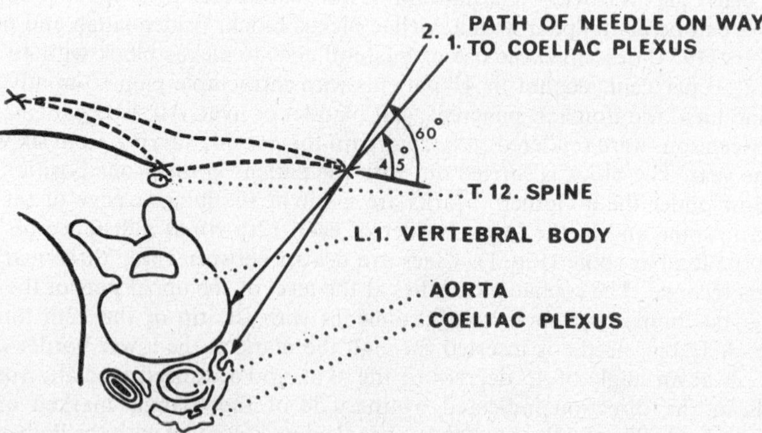

38/Fig. 2.—Coeliac plexus block. Oblique section to show the path of the needle.

the patient complains of a feeling of pressure resembling "a kick in the solar plexus" and of being unable to get his breath, the needle is correctly sited.

A burning sensation lasting about one minute follows the injection of the alcohol. To prevent alcohol affecting the 1st lumbar nerve during withdrawal of the needle, the latter should be cleared by injecting 0·5 ml. of air. The maximum effect from this block is not apparent for several days. Postural hypotension due to widespread interruption of vasomotor fibres may be a problem for a few days, especially in arteriosclerotic subjects. This may be prevented by wrapping the legs in elastic stockings and applying an abdominal binder before the patient gets out of bed.

4. Intrathecal Injections

Spinal analgesia is rarely used therapeutically as a method of interrupting sympathetic pathways, because of the need to repeat it at short intervals. Lumbar sympathetic or epidural block is preferable. The intrathecal route, however, does provide an excellent way of relieving intractable pain, especially that associated with incurable malignant disease. It enables neurolytic agents to be accurately placed so as to denervate localised areas of the body.

Alcohol.—The use of intrathecal alcohol in the management of intractable pain was first introduced by Dogliotti in 1931 and it has since become a widely used and valuable technique. Alcohol is a tissue poison which may cause necrosis if injected into subcutaneous tissues. When injected into the intrathecal space, it acts as a neurolytic agent, destroying nerve fibres wherever it comes into contact with them until it is diluted by the cerebrospinal fluid. Absolute alcohol has a lower specific gravity (0·806) than cerebrospinal fluid (1·007), so that when it is slowly injected intrathecally it acts as a hypobaric solution and forms a layer on top of the cerebrospinal fluid. By careful positioning of the patient it is possible to limit the spread of the alcohol so that it only bathes those dorsal roots whose ganglia it is desired to block. Subarachnoid alcohol block may cause serious complications, so it is obligatory to pay the most careful attention to details of technique and selection of patients.

Selection and assessment of patients.—Because of the risk of complications, this technique is usually reserved for the management of intractable pain in patients with incurable malignant disease. It may at times be justifiable in non-malignant conditions, such as severe long-standing sciatica in a patient considered unfit for laminectomy. A careful history is taken from the patient, particular note being made of the duration, site and character of the pain. It is important to enquire if the patient has any disturbance of bladder or rectal function, as it would probably be aggravated by a block for pelvic or leg pain.

At the clinical examination detailed attention is paid to the nervous system and a note is made of any existing motor or sensory loss, muscle wasting, or alterations in the tendon reflexes. It is important to distinguish between difficulty in walking due to the aggravation of pain and that due to motor weakness.

The distribution of the pain should be plotted on a body dermatome chart. This serves as a guide to the nerve roots that need blocking but it is not accurate for pain arising in sclerotome structures such as bones, ligaments and muscles.

Sympathetic pathways may also be implicated in carcinoma pain, particularly when viscera are involved.

The nature of the proposed treatment must be frankly discussed with the patient. A hopefully optimistic attitude should be adopted rather than a guarantee of success, and the need for a series rather than a single block must be stressed, otherwise the patient may be discouraged if the initial injection does not afford dramatic pain relief. The patient must be warned of possible complications such as numbness, weakness in the legs, and urinary retention. The low incidence of these complications must be pointed out, because if too black a picture is painted the patient may refuse treatment. In the more hopeless case, and especially if the patient is already partially incontinent, less emphasis should be placed on the risk of complications, although they should be fully discussed with a close relative and the reason for the treatment explained.

Most patients require more than one injection for complete relief, especially when the pain originates from a wide area. The response to the initial injection enables the anaesthetist to determine whether his assessment of the involved segments and site of block was correct.

Technique.—It is preferable to carry out the block on an operating table as it enables the patient to be positioned more accurately, but it can be carried out in the patient's bed with appropriately placed pillows. Morphine may be necessary beforehand to enable the patient to lie in the required position, but it is an advantage if the patient has some pain and is able to describe sensory changes during the block.

The patient lies in the lateral position with the painful side uppermost. The body is angulated by breaking the table so as to produce a scoliosis with the maximum curve corresponding to the site of the block. Both the head and legs should be lower than the point of injection. The patient is rolled forward 45 degrees into the semi-prone position so that the sensory posterior roots lie uppermost. Subarachnoid tap is made under strict aseptic conditions, the site of puncture depending on the roots involved. Bonica (1953) argues that it is better to deposit the alcohol at the point of emergence of the affected roots from the spinal cord. The spatial separation of the anterior and posterior roots is at a maximum at this point and, moreover, the expanded origin of the rootlets from the cord is thought to render them more susceptible to the action of the alcohol (Fig. 3). Blocking the roots at their exit through the intervertebral foramina carries an added risk of involving the anterior roots.

In carrying out the block an allowance must be made for the origin of the spinal nerves from the cord being above the level of the corresponding vertebra. It can be calculated as follows:

Cervical region:	Spinal cord segments are one vertebra above the corresponding vertebra.
Upper thoracic region:	Spinal cord segments are two vertebrae above the corresponding vertebra.
Lower thoracic region:	Spinal cord segments are three vertebrae above the corresponding vertebra.
	L 1 segment is opposite T 10 spine.

Using this technique it is unnecessary to do blocks below the T 12–L 1 interspace. The exact segment being blocked becomes apparent during the injection and any necessary adjustment in the level can then be made. Great care must be exercised when inserting the needle in the cervical or thoracic regions, owing to the risk of entering the spinal cord. As the epidural space is approached the stilette is withdrawn and, while slowly advancing the needle, either the hanging drop or the loss of resistance test is used to demonstrate entry into this space. The needle is then very slowly advanced for a further 2 to 3 mm. until its tip just enters the subarachnoid space.

The low pressure in the subarachnoid space may prevent the free flow of cerebrospinal fluid from the hub of the needle during a cervical tap. It is advisable therefore, to exert continuous suction with a syringe at this level so that the

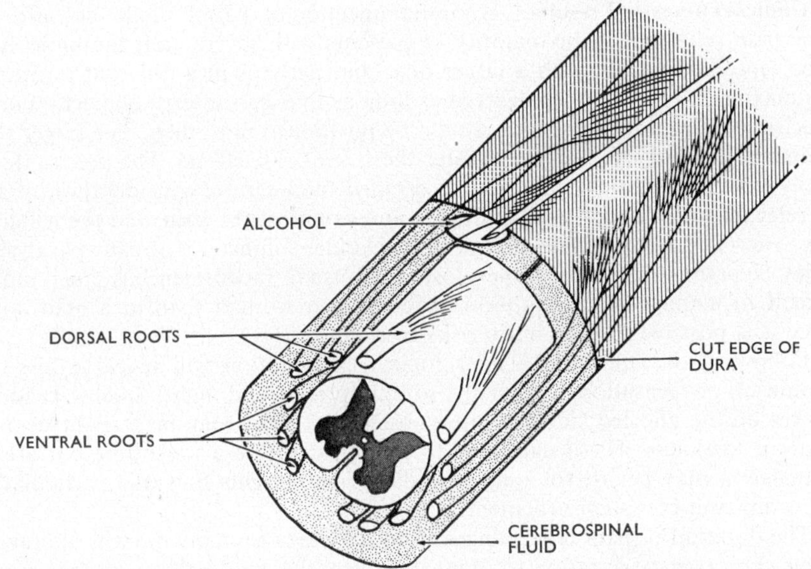

38/FIG. 3.—Intrathecal alcohol block. Diagram of lower thoracic cord region showing method of blocking dorsal roots as they emerge from the spinal cord (see text).

flow of fluid is immediately detected. It is important to position the patient with a slight head-down tilt to avoid spread of the alcohol to the medulla.

Absolute alcohol from a glass ampoule, the outside of which has been sterilised by autoclaving, is used and up to 0·5 ml. is injected as an initial dose. The injection is made very slowly at a rate of about 0·1 ml. per minute in order to localise the effect of the alcohol. The use of a 1 ml. tuberculin syringe facilitates this procedure. Burning paraesthesiae are experienced by the patient and ideally these should be located in the centre of the painful area. By testing sensory and motor functions the extent of the block can be assessed. In the absence of motor impairment, further small increments of alcohol may be injected, but as a general routine not more than 1 ml. should be injected at any one segment. If the paraesthesiae do not coincide with the painful area it may be possible, by tilting the table slightly in the appropriate direction, to float the hypobaric solution on to the involved nerve roots. If the disparity is more than one dermatome, it is preferable to change the position of the needle.

When pain arises from a wide area two or more needles should be inserted at different levels and small volumes of alcohol injected through each needle, rather than trying to produce an extensive block through one. In such cases, and especially when the pain arises from both sides, it may be preferable to carry out these blocks at intervals of a few days. After the injection the patient should lie in the same position for about half an hour to avoid spread of the alcohol and to enable it to be "fixed" to the correct nerve roots.

This technique is unsuitable for out-patients owing to the risks which attend any intrathecal technique. Greenhill (1947), however, considered that it was suitable for use in the patient's own home.

Clinical effects and results.—An initial injection of 0·5 ml. of alcohol affords some pain relief but in the majority of patients with severe pain the block has to be repeated, usually with a larger dose and perhaps in a different position. The maximum relief may be delayed as long as five days after the injection and a decision about a further block should be postponed until then. The larger the volume of alcohol injected, the greater the risk of side-effects. The precise dose in any individual patient can only be decided by a careful consideration of all the relevant factors, such as the severity and extent of the pain, and the willingness to accept the risk of side-effects. If the bladder sphincter is already paralysed it may be permissible to use larger doses than usual. Incontinence is much more difficult to manage as a long-term problem in a woman than in a man, and hence it is possible to take more risks in a man.

Following the injection, a neurological examination will reveal a loss or diminution in sensation, especially to pin pricks and light touch. Tendon reflexes on the affected side are often absent and there may be a slight degree of motor weakness. These signs tend to disappear within a short time but areas of analgesia may persist for long periods. Some patients find this particularly distressing and complain vehemently.

The duration of pain relief ranges from six weeks to many months and even a year. The average duration is about three months, and if the pain does recur a further block can be carried out. Not all suitable patients are relieved by an intrathecal alcohol block. Most reported series have results comparable to those described by Greenhill. In over 100 gynaecological patients with carcinoma he obtained complete relief in 60 per cent and slight improvement in a further 10 per cent.

Complications.—Some side-effects, such as headache and meningismus, are common to both spinal analgesia and subarachnoid alcohol block. The following complications are related to the neurolytic action of alcohol.

Motor paralysis.—This is due to involvement of the anterior roots and is more liable to occur when large volumes of alcohol are injected into the lumbar and lower cervical region. It may also result from bad positioning of the patient.

Bladder paralysis.—The injection of large volumes of alcohol into the lumbar region predisposes to this complication, which is due to involvement of the efferent parasympathetic fibres in the anterior sacral roots. These travel mainly in the second sacral nerve. Interrupting the sensory autonomic fibres, with consequent loss of bladder sensation, may lead to retention with overflow.

Disturbance of bladder function occurs in about 5–10 per cent of cases but the incidence can be reduced by careful attention to technique. Spontaneous improvement usually occurs within a period of weeks or months.

Rectal incontinence.—The aetiology of this complication is the same as bladder paralysis but the incidence is less.

Cutaneous analgesia.—Areas of analgesia may persist for weeks and even months. It is particularly liable to occur when the block has been performed for a non-malignant condition in an otherwise healthy person.

Adhesive pachymeningitis.—Alcohol causes histological changes far beyond the point of injection, indicating that it diffuses widely in the subarachnoid space.

Transverse myelitis and cauda equina syndrome.—The risk of injecting alcohol into the cord can be avoided by ensuring that there is a free flow of cerebrospinal fluid before making the injection.

Phenol.—Alcohol has the disadvantage of diffusing extensively in the subarachnoid space. This rapid diffusion, together with the difficulties of accurately controlling the flow of a hypobaric solution, have led to the search for alternative agents. Maher (1955 and 1957) described a technique for using intrathecal phenol in glycerine to alleviate the pain of incurable cancer. Aqueous phenol is a caustic substance, but when dissolved in glycerine it only diffuses slowly from solution to affect the nerve roots over which it is flowing (Nathan and Scott, 1958). Being a hyperbaric solution (Sp. G. glycerine 1·25: Sp. G. cerebrospinal fluid 1·007) it falls downwards in the subarachnoid space and is easier to control than alcohol. As Maher has pointed out "it is easier to lay a carpet than to paper a ceiling". Maher concluded that 5 per cent phenol in glycerine is the optimal concentration to use as it will abolish pain without affecting other forms of sensation or disturbing motor function. These unwanted effects may result from the use of stronger solutions, while weaker solutions do not afford long-lasting relief. For patients unrelieved with phenol alone a phenol-silver nitrate solution can be used (silver nitrate 0·6 mg. per ml. of 4 per cent phenol in glycerine) (Maher, 1960). This is a more potent agent than phenol by itself but it may cause a meningeal reaction. With improvement in techniques, the need for this solution has decreased. "Myodil" (iophendylate) may also be used as a vehicle for phenol but it tends to protect the nerve roots and the phenol has to be used in a higher concentration (7 to 10 per cent) in order to achieve results comparable with 5 per cent phenol in glycerine.

These new techniques are being used extensively and in many centres phenol has replaced alcohol as the agent of choice in the relief of intractable pain.

Effect of phenol on the nervous system.—The belief that intrathecal phenol has a selective action on the small unmyelinated fibres of the posterior roots is no longer tenable, as a result of a recent study by Smith (1964). She carried out post-mortem studies on the nervous systems of patients who had received intrathecal injections of phenol and also on a control series of spinal cords from patients with malignant disease who had not been given this treatment. The effect of phenol in "Myodil" (iophendylate) on healthy nervous tissue was investigated in cats by means of electrophysiological and histological studies carried out on nerve roots which had been exposed by laminectomy (Nathan *et al.*, 1965). These investigators concluded that initially intrathecal phenol affects a large number of fibres of many roots, acting as a local analgesic. This effect comes on in 50 seconds and lasts about 20 minutes. Some fibres recover completely but others subsequently degenerate, depending on the concentration and duration of application of the phenol. It was concluded that phenol in glycerine or "Myodil" did not affect the spinal cord or posterior root ganglia but acted on the nerve roots, causing indiscriminate degeneration of all fibres, irrespective of their size, wherever it came into contact with them. Although the anterior roots were affected to some extent, the site of action of the solution was predominantly on the posterior roots between the ganglia and the spinal cord. A striking feature in the injected patients was a marked degeneration of nerve fibres in the posterior columns of the spinal cord, secondary to the action of the phenol on the posterior roots. There was no suggestion of any marked meningeal reaction or direct damage to the cord. From these studies it was concluded that the effect of phenol in relieving chronic pain is not achieved by selectively destroying a particular type of nerve fibre (i.e. C fibres) because painful stimuli such as pricking and burning are still appreciated. The explanation is a quantitative rather than a qualitative one, depending on the destruction of a sufficient number of nerve fibres from the affected part of the body. This reduction in the sensory input and the lessening of the opportunity for summation between the opposing large and small fibre systems fits in with the Gate Control Theory of pain of Melzack and Wall (see Chapter 37).

Technique.—The selection of patients and the mapping out of the pain distribution on dermatome charts to determine the nerve roots that require blocking has already been discussed in the section on alcohol subarachnoid block. The needle should be inserted as near as possible to the roots it is desired to block with the phenol. A single injection of 1 ml. of phenol in glycerine will usually block three nerve roots. The majority of patients require more than one injection and additional blocks are carried out at intervals of five days until all pain has been eradicated. With extensive bilateral pain it may be necessary to repeat the injections on three or four occasions.

Although Maher advocates carrying out this treatment at the bedside, the use of an operating table makes it easier to position the patient accurately and to control the flow of the solution after injection. With the patient lying on the painful side, subarachnoid puncture is performed with a 21-gauge needle, care being taken to ensure there is a free flow of cerebrospinal fluid. Rotating the patient posteriorly to an angle of about 30° with the vertical helps to localise the effect of the phenol to the posterior roots. With the bevel of the needle directed downwards, an initial dose of 0·3 ml. of 5 per cent phenol in glycerine is slowly injected. If the needle is correctly sited, the relief of pain is immediate, and is accompanied by a sensation of warmth and paraesthesiae in the distribution of the affected roots. If these sensory symptoms do not coincide precisely with the painful area, the table may be tilted so that the solution flows on to the appropriate nerve roots. Incremental doses each of 0·3 ml. are given at intervals of 5 minutes until the desired effect has been achieved. The "end-point" for stopping the injections is determined by testing sensation immediately before each injection. The object is to diminish or abolish sensation to pinpricks compared with the other side while leaving light touch unaffected.

The patient is kept lying still in the position of the injection for an hour afterwards in order to fix the phenol to the required roots. To minimise the risk of post-lumbar puncture headache, the patient is nursed lying flat in bed for 24 hours.

Details of technique and a guide as to the volume of solution required in each region of the vertebral column are set out below. Most patients suitable for an intrathecal phenol block have pain in the lower part of the body and, in consequence, most injections are carried out in the lumbar or lower thoracic regions.

Sacral region.—A common cause of intractable pain in the perineum and bottom of the coccyx is a recurrence of carcinoma, following an abdomino-perineal excision of the rectum. Subarachnoid puncture at the L5–S1 space is easier to perform with the patient sitting up. He is then made to lie on the most painful side with a 30° head-up tilt. Including the test dose of 0·3 ml., a total of 0·5 to 0·7 ml. of 5 per cent phenol in glycerine is allowed to flow quickly down over the upper sacral roots, which supply the bladder, to form a pool at the bottom of the subarachnoid space. By slowly raising the patient to the vertical it is possible to block the lowermost sacral and coccygeal nerves on both sides. As the phenol does not diffuse through all the sacral roots with this technique, the risk of bladder involvement is much reduced. To block S 2–4 roots usually requires 0·7 ml. and the injection is made with the patient lying with a slight head-up tilt (approximately 20°). If bladder control is normal prior to treatment no disturbance should occur after blocking the sacral roots unilaterally.

Lumbar region.—After a successful lumbar tap, the needle is withdrawn to the edge of the theca so that the injected phenol does not cross the nerve roots which are descending centrally in the cauda equina and emerging at a lower level. The average volume of solution required for this region is 1 ml. and it is given in increments of 0·3 ml. as described above. At times as little as 0·5 ml. of solution is enough to produce the desired effect. If necessary, the table is tilted slightly to localise the effect of the phenol to the appropriate nerve roots. The occurrence of sensory symptoms in the upper leg after the initial injection indicates that the needle has been inserted too far towards the unaffected side, allowing the phenol to trickle over all the roots of the cauda equina. Unless the injection is abandoned the patient may have difficulty in controlling his bladder.

Dorsal region.—Great care must be exercised in carrying out a subarachnoid tap in this region because of the risk of inadvertantly transfixing the spinal cord. A short-bevelled needle is inserted initially into the epidural space, which may be recognised by the loss of resistance or hanging drop techniques. The needle is then advanced a millimetre at a time until cerebrospinal fluid just begins to flow. If the initial dose of 0·3 ml. of 5 per cent phenol in glycerine causes no symptoms in the legs it is safe to give further increments until the pain has been relieved. The volume of solution required in this region is usually 1·5–3·0 ml.

Cervical region.—Because of the danger of phenol flowing into the cranium the patient must be positioned with a head-up tilt of 30° to 40°. The technique adopted is the same as in the thoracic region but as the spinal canal is narrow the needle must be inserted exactly in the mid-line. The results of intrathecal phenol are not so good in the cervical as in other regions, because the solution tends to flow away very quickly and also the cervical nerve roots are much shorter and hence the length available for absorption is less. Maher considers that subdural injections give better results in this area. The technique is to carry out a subarachnoid tap and then withdraw the needle until the cerebrospinal fluid is still just flowing. Reinserting the stilette helps to widen the subdural space prior to injecting 0·5 ml. of 7½ per cent phenol in "Myodil." A honeycomb appearance on the X-ray, caused by the "Myodil" travelling down round the nerve roots, confirms the correct siting of the injection (Maher, 1957). A further injection of 0·5 ml. of 7½ per cent phenol in glycerine is then carried out in order to reach the upper cervical roots.

Preparation of solutions.—Originally it was suggested that these solutions should be freshly made up, but when phenol is dissolved in glycerine and sealed in ampoules it appears to keep without deteriorating. The phenol is dissolved in warm glycerine, filtered through scintered glass, sealed in ampoules and sterilised in a hot air oven. Phenol in "Myodil" must be prepared immediately before use. The outside of the "Myodil" ampoule cannot be sterilised by heat. The contents are drawn up and injected into a sterile ampoule containing phenol crystals.

Intrathecal chlorocresol.—Maher (1963) has suggested using a 1 in 50 solution of chlorocresol in glycerine as an alternative to phenol. Chlorocresol appears to have a delayed effect compared with phenol in glycerine and there are no immediate sensory changes or paraesthesiae. Fewer nerve roots are affected, so that a second injection may be required after three weeks. The higher proportion of successes obtained with chlorocresol may be due to the diffusion affecting a greater length of nerve root.

For rectal, coccygeal and sacrosciatic pain the suggested dose of the solution is 0·5 ml.; for the upper lumbar segments 0·75 ml.; and for the thoracic segments 1·0 ml. This technique appears to be a more effective way of relieving the pain associated with carcinoma of the lung, especially that from a Pancoast tumour.

Factors influencing results of treatment.—Most of the pain caused by cancer is of a constant, unremitting nature. It is carried by the small C fibres and can be eradicated by intrathecal phenol injections. A second type of pain, termed incident pain by Maher, is due to a sudden event such as a fracture or the collapse of a vertebra. This pain is not amenable to treatment by phenol, but as it is evoked by movement it can be relieved by complete rest.

Phenol has both a temporary and a permanent blocking effect (Nathan and Sears, 1960). When injected intrathecally it acts as a local analgesic, relieving all pain within a period of 50 seconds. Recovery takes place gradually after about 20 minutes but a varying number of pain fibres remain permanently damaged, so accounting for the relief of the constant pain in malignancy. Because of this dual effect phenol, unlike alcohol, destroys nerve fibres without causing pain.

Severe pain dominates a patient's whole existence, and if it cannot be relieved by analgesics it may materially shorten his life. Treatment of pain must not be an ordeal for these patients, as the majority have already endured operations and radiotherapy and many do not want anything further done. Good results can only be achieved if patients are referred early for treatment, preferably within two or three months of the pain becoming established. If it is long-standing and has been present for two or three years, the results are bound to be disappointing. Growth of tumour around the nerve roots may have a sheltering effect by preventing the phenol gaining access to them. Successful relief of pain in one part of the body frequently reveals pain in adjacent or more distant regions, which hitherto had been overshadowed by the patient's principal pain.

Long-lasting or even permanent relief can be anticipated if the patient is still pain-free three days after the phenol injection. Failure to obtain relief may be due to too few injections being given to cover adequately all the nerve roots innervating the painful area, or to the needle being inserted at the wrong place.

The return of pain after a period of relief may be due to the spread of tumour to another area or to the occurrence of incident pain.

Results.—The results of treatment depend largely upon the selection of patients and the other factors discussed above. Maher (1960) reported complete relief in 61 (75 per cent) out of 81 cases when intrathecal phenol was used below the level of D 3. Other workers have not achieved such a high success rate. Gordon and Goel (1963) used this technique on 37 patients and reported complete relief in 51 per cent and moderate to good relief in a further 30 per cent of patients. Nathan (1967) reported that 77 per cent of patients obtained relief after cordotomy compared with 54 per cent after phenol injections, but that after phenol motor function in the legs was less affected and the incidence of sphincter trouble was only 12 per cent.

Complications.—The possible complications of this technique are the same as those described in the section on subarachnoid alcohol block. The risk of interfering with the control of bladder or bowel function must always be borne in mind, but by using a meticulous technique the incidence can be kept down to an acceptable level. Temporary difficulty with micturition may occur necessitating the use of an indwelling catheter for a few days or a week.

Intrathecal phenol in the relief of spasticity.—Intrathecal phenol, using either glycerine or "Myodil" as a solvent, has a most useful application in the relief of spasticity and the pain associated with flexor spasms (Kelly and Gautier Smith, 1959; Nathan, 1959). 7·5 per cent–10 per cent phenol in "Myodil" is a suitable solution to use for these patients.

5. Epidural Injection

The success achieved with intrathecal phenol solution has led to the use of these solutions for epidural block. It has been particularly recommended by Maher for non-malignant forms of pain. Finer (1958) used 10 per cent phenol in glycerine epidurally for patients with incurable cancer. He injected 3 ml. of the solution through a Tuohy needle at the L 4–5 space and simultaneously collapsed the dural sac by intrathecal puncture at L 1–2 space. By performing an epidural block with phenol at the D 12–L 1 space it is possible to interrupt sympathetic fibres and hence relieve cancer pain, particularly when it is due to involvement of viscera or blood vessels. Patients with perineal pain due to a carcinoma of the rectum are not always adequately relieved by a somatic block with intrathecal phenol. By performing an epidural block with phenol in glycerine at D 12–L 1 space, such cases can often be rendered pain-free. Doughty (1964) suggested a dose of 5 ml. of 5 per cent phenol in glycerine. If necessary the injection can be repeated after a few days using 7·5 ml. of 7½ per cent or even 10 per cent phenol in glycerine. This block is especially effective in relieving the spasms of burning pain and tenesmus associated with advanced carcinoma of the rectum.

An epidural block may be preferred to an intrathecal one in the cervical or upper thoracic regions for patients with incurable malignant disease, but compared with subarachnoid injections the technique is less precise in localising the solution to the affected nerve root. Moreover, because of the large doses of neurolytic agent used in the epidural approach, accidental dural puncture, if unrecognised, may lead to disastrous neurological damage.

6. **Osmolytic Neurolysis and Hypothermic Subarachnoid Irrigation**

Hitchcock (1967) described a technique for the relief of intractable pain based on the concept of the differential susceptibility of nervous tissue to hypothermia with the unmyelinated C fibres especially sensitive to the effects of cooling.

Further work has led to the belief that the results from this technique were due to the hypertonicity of the solution injected, which in practice was the supernatant liquid obtained from thawing frozen isotonic saline solution (Hitchcock, 1969*a*). Subarachnoid tap was performed in the lateral position at the level of the affected nerve roots and with the painful side underneath. After withdrawing C.S.F. until a subatmospheric pressure was recorded, the table was tilted so that the affected part was below the level of the subarachnoid puncture. 10 ml. of normal physiological saline, cooled to a temperature of 2–4°C in the freezing compartment of a refrigerator, was then injected rapidly into the subarachnoid space and usually afforded complete pain relief within seconds, although some patients complained of unpleasant sacral paraesthesiae for up to one hour afterwards. In the absence of a satisfactory response, further injections were given, a total of 60 ml. being administered on one occasion. In the twelve patients described there was no sensory loss or disturbance of bladder function but the duration of pain relief was variable and at times was only transient.

Hypertonic saline solution has also been used to relieve severe facial pain due to advanced carcinomatosis, by means of a cisternal injection (Hitchcock, 1969*b*). With the patient in the sitting position and the head fully flexed, the cisterna magna was punctured using a large bore lumbar puncture needle. A fine polyethylene catheter was then threaded through the needle into the cisterna magna. After removing the needle and taping the catheter in place, the patient was positioned with the head dependent and lying on the affected side. After rapidly injecting between 8 and 20 ml. of hypertonic saline (7·5 per cent), the catheter was removed. This injection almost invariably caused vertigo, vomiting, tinnitus and facial weakness but these reactions were transient, lasting only a few minutes except in one patient. In the seven patients described, effective pain relief was produced which lasted from 3 to 105 days, while normal sensation seemed to be preserved.

Electrocardiographic changes have been reported during these procedures (McKean and Hitchcock, 1968) which took the form of transient sinus tachycardia or ventricular ectopic beats after lumbar injections and sinus bradycardia in the case of cisternal injections. These changes were ascribed respectively to direct sympathetic and direct vagal stimulation.

This is an interesting addition to the techniques available for the relief of intractable pain and the confirmation of its value in a large series of patients is awaited. It would seem to depend on the use of a hypertonic solution and not from hypothermia as was at first thought. The effect is possibly due to changes in the conductive properties of the nerve roots, irrespective of fibre size. The extent to which it might replace the established techniques using phenol and alcohol cannot be judged at this time.

7. Percutaneous Electrical Cordotomy

Anterolateral cordotomy is the most satisfactory technique for the long-term relief of intractable pain but it involves a major operation, with a variable mortality and morbidity, in patients who may be a poor operative risk.

The development of the technique of percutaneous electrical cordotomy (Mullan *et al.*, 1965; Rosomoff *et al.*, 1965; Lin *et al.*, 1966; Lipton, 1968) has been an important advance in this field, as it affords satisfactory pain relief in patients who may be too ill to submit to open surgical cordotomy. Most patients undergoing this procedure can leave hospital within a few days and may well submit to this type of cordotomy when major surgery would be rejected.

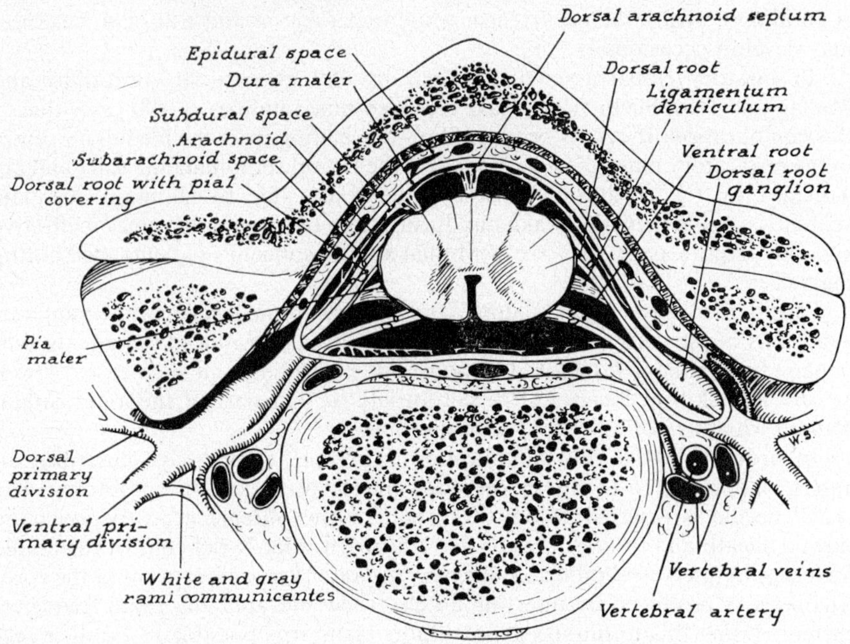

38/FIG. 4.—Cross-section of spinal cord in the spinal canal showing its meningeal coverings and the manner of exit of the spinal nerves (after Rauber).

The technique used by Lipton (1968) is to insert a spinal needle laterally, under X-ray control, between the first and second cervical vertebrae into the subarachnoid space. The aim of the technique is to place the point of the needle in front of the dentate ligament (ligamentum denticulum) (see Fig. 4) which is identified by injecting a mixture of C.S.F. and iophendylate injection B.P.

("Ethiodan"). This emulsion sinks down on to the ligament, which is recognised as a line on the lateral X-ray. An electrode is introduced through the needle and inserted into the anterolateral column of the cord, the depth of penetration being assessed from an antero-posterior film.

If the tip of the electrode is situated too far posteriorly and is lying in the motor tract, stimulation of the cord by passing a current through the electrode causes movement of the limbs or body of the same side (ipsilateral). Movement of the neck of the same side indicates that the electrode tip is placed too far anteriorly and is in the anterior horn cells. With correct positioning there is no movement but there may be paraesthesiae on the opposite (contralateral) side. The anterolateral tract is then coagulated by a radio frequency current to produce analgesia in the contralateral side. With accurate placement of the electrode this analgesia can be localised to one quadrant of the body (body and arm or body and leg).

In fifty-two patients Lipton achieved effective pain relief in 67 per cent and partial relief in 13 per cent.

Percutaneous electrical cordotomy is relatively free from side-effects, although retention of urine may occur, especially after bilateral cordotomy. Headache is an almost invariable occurrence, while hyperalgesia and transient weakness may develop occasionally.

Respiratory embarrassment is a hazard of high cervical cordotomy and Mullan and Hosobuchi (1968) have reported nine fatalities in 400 cases due to this complication. It occurs because fibres descending from the medullary centre to the respiratory muscles lie very close to the lateral spinothalamic tract and are damaged by the cordotomy. These patients are able to maintain adequate ventilation while they are awake but during sleep respiration becomes ineffective and may require assistance. Six of Mullan and Hosobuchi's patients died during their sleep.

This hazard exists when bilateral cordotomies are undertaken in the anterior quadrants of the cord and when unilateral lesions are produced in patients with impaired pulmonary function. Caution must be exercised in such cases as well as care and skill in localising the cordotomy to that part of the anterolateral column which is not essential for respiration.

In order to avoid this complication Lin *et al.* (1966) have described an anterior approach to the lower cervical cord for percutaneous cordotomy. The spinal needle is inserted below the origin of the phrenic nerve between the carotid sheath and the oesophagus and trachea. Under X-ray control the needle traverses an intervertebral disc and enters the anterolateral quadrant of the cord. Analgesia is produced by inserting an electrode and applying radio frequency current. Using this technique these authors claim it is possible to produce segmental analgesia in the thoracic and lumbar regions, sparing the sacral segments and so having a lower incidence of bladder complications. The upper cervical approach, however, probably gives better pain relief.

8. General Analgesic Drugs and their Adjuvants

The narcotic analgesics offer the only hope of pain relief in many advanced cases of malignant disease. The choice and dosage of analgesic depends on a number of factors:

1. Severity and fluctuation of the pain (this can be assessed by keeping a pain chart).
2. Likely duration of the pain or the expectation of life.
3. Effect of drugs already administered.
4. Occurrence of undesirable side-effects.
5. Development of tolerance and addiction.
6. Domestic circumstances of the patient.

The effective use of these drugs entails a careful appraisal of each patient, with special reference to the history and any conditions which aggravate or relieve the pain. Initially, mild analgesics such as aspirin and codeine may be prescribed but most patients eventually require a potent analgesic. The aim of treatment is not merely to relieve pain but to make the patient more contented. There may be other distressing symptoms to alleviate as well, such as cough, dyspnoea, nausea and vomiting, paralysis and mental distress.

The need for sedation must be assessed in each patient. If he is unaware that his pain is caused by malignant disease and is fairly well in himself, so that he can usefully employ his waking hours, sedation is unnecessary and may even be resented. A drug such as methadone is indicated in these circumstances. In the terminal stages of malignancy, when patients are exhausted by pain and suffering, the sedation and euphoria afforded by morphine are invaluable.

Analgesics should be administered orally for as long as possible and when there is a dull, steady background pain they should be given on a fixed time schedule. The aim should be to keep the patient free of pain, rather than treating it when it has occurred. Each dose should be given while the previous one is still exerting its effect. The optimal dose of the drug should be prescribed (Denton and Beecher, 1949) and as tolerance develops the frequency of administration should be increased, rather than the dose. There is often the case for letting a patient have a supply of tablets to take outside the times of the regular drug schedule, if the need arises. Tabs. codeine co., "Panadol," pethidine or methadone are suitable for this purpose. Large doses of analgesics cause a higher incidence of side-effects without affording much additional analgesia (Lasagna and Beecher, 1954). Side-effects, especially the emetic ones, are the limiting factor in analgesic therapy. There is considerable individual susceptibility but they are more common in ambulant patients. Side-effects, such as the sickness caused by pethidine, often persist longer than the analgesia.

It may be necessary to switch to another drug or to use the parenteral route of administration. Constipation may be troublesome with codeine and morphine derivates, as patients do not readily acquire tolerance to this effect. The problems of tolerance and addiction are inescapable when potent analgesics are used over a long period. Tolerance implies a decreasing efficacy of a drug so that larger doses must be given to achieve the same therapeutic effect. Unfortunately, cross-tolerance occurs with these drugs (Dundee, 1960*a*). As tolerance is acquired the patient should be reassured and only a very gradual increase in dose permitted. This is best achieved by shortening the interval between the doses. At a later stage, adjuvant drugs which potentiate the analgesics and combat their side-effects are a valuable aid to treatment.

The fear of addiction should not be a reason for denying potent analgesics to patients in the terminal stage of their illness, when their need of them is greatest. Psychological dependence on these drugs is less likely to occur when they are given for intractable pain and they may be given in large amounts over long periods without necessarily causing addiction. Nathan (1952) has emphasised that these drugs can be readily withdrawn in such patients once their pain has been relieved surgically. Pentazocine represents an important advance in the management of chronic pain as it produces analgesia comparable to that provided by morphine, but without the addiction potential.

The possibility of using nerve blocks or neurosurgical procedures should be considered in all patients with severe pain, as the relief achieved in suitable cases is most gratifying. Moreover, nerve blocks can be repeated several times if the pain returns or extends to other areas.

Potent analgesics should be used freely in the terminal stages when pain is severe. Massive doses of these drugs are often required but the extent to which the patient is kept narcotised must be based on the clinician's knowledge of the patient's personality. Some patients prefer to maintain an awareness of their surroundings and their family until their death. Diamorphine is often the most effective of all drugs to use at this stage.

In chronic medical diseases, such as rheumatoid arthritis, which may last for many years, pain relief should be based on the mild analgesics owing to the high risk of addiction if potent analgesics are employed.

Adjuvants in the relief of pain.—Certain drugs, which may be used to counteract the undesirable side-effects of analgesic drugs, have been discussed in the previous chapter, including the use of narcotic-antagonist mixtures. The present section will be confined mainly to two groups of drugs which can be used to potentiate or influence the effect of the analgesics.

Anticholinesterase drugs.—It has been known for some time that cholinergic drugs such as neostigmine potentiate the effect of morphine both in duration and intensity, although their mode of action is not clear. The use of 0·5 mg. of neostigmine enables the dose or morphine to be cut by half (Slaughter *et al.*, 1940).

Pyridostigmine ("Mestinon") is better tolerated and has a longer duration of action than neostigmine. As well as prolonging the effect of the potent analgesics it also combats their alimentary side-effects. When pyridostigmine 1 mg. was combined with 2 mg. of levorphan, the analgesic effect of the latter drug was increased from 6 to 10 hours (Oehlandt, 1955).

Small doses of neostigmine (0·5 mg.) help to combat the dry mouth which may be caused if phenothiazine derivatives are used as adjuncts to narcotic analgesics.

Phenothiazine derivatives.—Chlorpromazine is a useful adjuvant in the relief of pain as it has been shown to potentiate the potent analgesics (Dundee, 1957*a* and *b*). Patients with advanced malignant disease become more tolerant of their pain if a narcotic analgesic is combined with chlorpromazine, the latter drug being given in a dose of 25 mg. three times a day. The effect on mood is to induce a state of apathy and lethargy akin to that following a leucotomy.

Chlorpromazine is particularly effective for restlessness or when the patient develops overwhelming anxiety. It should be avoided when depression is the main affective response to pain. For out-patients, Dundee found that the best combination of drugs was levorphan with chlorpromazine. With less severe pain, good results are obtained with tabs. codeine co. and chlorpromazine. Side-effects which may occur with chlorpromazine include drowsiness, dryness of the mouth, faintness and loss of appetite, but most of these do not persist.

The most serious complications that can occur with the phenothiazines are jaundice and agranulocytosis. Intrahepatic obstructive jaundice develops in about 1 per cent of patients receiving chlorpromazine (Sherlock, 1962). The jaundice usually comes on within four weeks of commencing the drug but is generally mild and lasts only 1–4 weeks. Other similar drugs which can cause this complication include promazine, prochlorperazine and trifluoperazine. However the anti-emetic action of these and other drugs may be helpful in controlling the sickness produced either by the narcotic analgesics or by the disease itself. The most effective are perphenazine ("Fentazine") (2–5 mg.) and prochlorperazine (5–10 mg.). Methotrimeprazine ("Veractil") is a strong analgesic by itself and Lasagna and De Kornfeld (1961) found it to be almost as effective as morphine. It does cause more sedation and postural hypotension, however, and although it may at times be useful by itself as an analgesic, it provides an excellent adjunct to an opiate.

Other drugs.—There are other sedatives and tranquillisers which may be effectively employed to alleviate the anxiety and suffering of the terminal stages of malignant disease. These include meprobamate ("Equanil"), phenobarbitone, amylobarbitone sodium, and chlordiazepoxide hydrochloride ("Librium").

Alcohol is often very useful for relieving pain and allaying anxiety. Euphoriants such as cocaine, amphetamine, dexamphetamine and cannabis indica (Indian hemp) help by elevating the patient's mood and making the suffering more bearable.

A mixture based on the Brompton Hospital "cocktail" is often invaluable: morphine hydrochloride 15 mg., cocaine hydrochloride 10 mg., gin 4 ml., honey 4 ml., chloroform water to 15 ml. If nausea and vomiting are troublesome prochlorperazine ("Stemetil") syrup (5–10 mg.) may be added, or for extra sedation, chloropromazine syrup (25–50 mg.).

Discussion

Chronic intractable pain often presents a most difficult therapeutic problem. It can be treated in a variety of ways and many factors must be considered in deciding the most appropriate method or combination of methods for the individual patient. Treatment with narcotic analgesics should not begin too soon, especially when the patient's life is not immediately threatened by the condition causing the pain.

Palliative surgery and radiotherapy can afford considerable relief to patients with incurable malignant disease. If these methods fail or pain recurs, a neurosurgical operation may be the procedure of choice, particularly when the patient's physical condition is fairly good and his life expectancy is at least several months. These procedures are also applicable at times to non-fatal conditions. Such an operation may be preceded by a prognostic nerve block. If this is successful, surgical division of the nerve or nerves is indicated (posterior rhizotomy) and may give long-lasting relief. Sensory root section is a very satisfactory way of dealing with trigeminal neuralgia. If precise localisation of pain is impossible in cancer patients, an anterior lateral cordotomy can be carried out, so dividing the spinothalamic tract. Bilateral cordotomy for widespread malignant disease in the pelvis is associated with a high incidence of bladder involvement.

At times it is necessary to attack the pain pathways at an even higher level. Thalamic pain can be relieved by means of stereotaxis and, when the emotional reaction to pain is the major problem, pre-frontal leucotomy may be indicated. At times a course of electro-convulsive therapy is useful for alleviating intractable pain when depression is a prominent feature.

When the patient is unfit for surgery, injection techniques, using neurolytic agents as described in the preceding sections, may give very effective pain relief. They are easily performed, and cause less upset to the patient than the neurosurgical procedures. The introduction of the technique of percutaneous electrical cordotomy has enabled this procedure to be offered to a wider range of patients, who previously may have been considered too ill for a major surgical operation.

Many patients are unsuitable for either nerve blocks or operation and recourse must be had to analgesic drugs at an early stage. Few, if any, patients suffering from intractable pain due to incurable malignant disease, do not require analgesic drugs at some time or other, especially in the terminal stages.

Patients have an individual variation as to the suitability and side-effects of a particular analgesic drug and treatment must be modified accordingly. Each clinician has his own favoured group of analgesics from which to select the drug or mixture of drugs for administration at the optimum dose level.

Pain Clinics

In recent years anaesthetists have taken an increasing interest in the management of patients with chronic pain. This has led to the setting up of pain clinics where patients can be seen and assessed with a view to treatment. As it is impossible for one person to encompass all the techniques and procedures which can be applied to this problem, such a clinic should ideally be under the direction of a radiotherapist, a neurosurgeon, and an anaesthetist, with perhaps a neurologist and a psychiatrist in attendance as well. Most clinics do not conform to this pattern but are run by an anaesthetist who provides symptomatic treatment of pain with nerve blocks and analgesic drugs. Although the majority of patients referred for treatment are suffering from malignant disease, other conditions seen not infrequently include post-herpetic neuralgia and post-operative neuralgia.

A small group of patients, who are referred from time to time, appear to suffer from seemingly intractable pain and yet have no clear-cut aetiological cause. Before dismissing such patients as suffering from psychogenic pain, the possibility of a reflex sympathetic pain should be considered, particularly if it has developed after trauma or surgery.

The complete relief of pain, following the performance of a sympathetic block without an accompanying somatic block, enables the correct diagnosis to be made. A series of sympathetic blocks may lead to a complete cure or it may be necessary to refer the patient for surgical sympathectomy.

The anaesthetist, because of his skill and familiarity with local analgesic techniques, is ideally placed to help these patients. With increasing experience he can achieve worthwhile success in the relief of chronic pain by means of nerve blocks. Simple nerve blocks may be carried out on out-patients but the intrathecal or epidural injection of neurolytic agents should be confined to in-patients. The anaesthetist is at a disadvantage in having no hospital beds of his own, but an arrangement can usually be reached for the clinician referring the patient to provide a bed. Disappointments are not infrequent and relief is often partial or of short duration, but perseverance is rewarded with a worthwhile alleviation of suffering in this group of patients.

The second and equally important function of a pain clinic is to arrange the administration of analgesic drugs to patients who are unsuitable for a block, or who have failed to obtain adequate relief. As an exercise in applied pharmacology, the anaesthetist is able to determine the most suitable analgesic regime for the particular patient, including any adjuvant drugs which may be indicated. The value of pain clinics for conducting controlled trials on new or established drugs is obvious, and anaesthetists have made many important contributions in this field. The extension of the anaesthetist's interests beyond the confines of the operating theatre is a significant and vital trend of current anaesthetic practice. The running of a pain clinic provides abundant clinical interest and a means of affording worthwhile relief to some patients whose suffering might otherwise remain unabated.

Neuroleptics and Neuroleptanalgesia

Neuroleptic drugs such as the butyrophenone derivatives haloperidol and droperidol induce a state of apathy and mental detachment in which the patient is mildly sedated and uncaring about his surroundings. In recent years, a technique has been introduced on the Continent for use in clinical anaesthesia termed "neuroleptanalgesia", which is based on the combination of one of these neuroleptic drugs and an analgesic (Nilsson, 1963). The drugs used in this procedure have been developed by Janssen in Belgium. It is in reality a development of the technique of artificial hibernation based on the lytic cocktail, which was introduced about thirteen years ago. Neuroleptanalgesia differs in the greater emphasis placed upon analgesia and on the stability of the circulatory system.

The narcotic analgesics phenoperidine ("Operidine") and fentanyl (phentanyl) ("Sublimaze") used in this technique are very powerful, the latter being 100 times more potent than morphine, milligram for milligram. Complete general analgesia sufficient for surgical procedures can be achieved with these drugs, without disturbing the circulation or causing marked hypnosis. The analgesia is accompanied by an intense respiratory depression, which in the case of fentanyl is of short duration and disappears before the analgesia. Respiratory depression can be effectively reversed by giving nalorphine in doses of 2 to 10 mg. Rollason and Sutherland (1963) used phenoperidine intravenously in an initial dose of 0·24 mg. per kg. in a series of thirty unpremedicated patients, but found it unsuitable for short surgical procedures such as cystoscopy. Three patients had marked respiratory depression and a further three became apnoeic (total 20 per cent), including one who became unconscious.

In using the technique of neuroleptanalgesia, droperidol 2·5–5 mg. is given intramuscularly 15–45 minutes pre-operatively as a premedication together with fentanyl 0·05–0·1 mg. or phenoperidine 1 mg. This produces a calm patient, free from anxiety or pain, and it should enable procedures such as cardiac catheterisation, air encephalography or burns dressings to be performed without causing distress. Additional doses of the drugs can be given intravenously during the procedure if required. Neuroleptanalgesia has also been reported as affording excellent sedation during the surgical treatment of Parkinsonism, while retaining the patient's full co-operation for three hours or longer (Brown, 1964).

Thomas (1966) reported that neuroleptanalgesia combined with local analgesia provided very satisfactory conditions for intra-ocular surgery. After premedication with 25 or 50 mg. of promethazine he gave a mixture of droperidol 3 mg. and phenoperidine 1 mg. intravenously. Smaller doses of phenoperidine were given to the frail or elderly. During the operation the patients remained placid and there was an absence of coughing, vomiting and fidgeting.

Holderness *et al.* (1963) and Aubry *et al.* (1966) have described the use of these mixtures in combination with nitrous oxide and oxygen for general anaesthesia in a series of 400 patients and 1,000 patients respectively. They used droperidol combined with fentanyl, usually in a 50:1 mixture. This mixture is available as a proprietary preparation called "Thalamonal" or "Innovan", which contains droperidol 2·5 mg. and fentanyl 0·05 mg. in 1 ml. Conventional drugs can be used for premedication and anaesthesia is induced by the intravenous injection of 10–20 mg. of droperidol together with fentanyl followed by the inhalation of nitrous oxide and oxygen to produce unconsciousness. For all but the gravest-risk patients a more rapid loss of consciousness is achieved by injecting a small sleep dose of thiopentone (not more than 100 mg.). Endotracheal intubation, if indicated, is performed after paralysis with suxamethonium or *d*-tubocurarine. For operations not requiring muscular relaxation spontaneous respiration is maintained but the initial dose of fentanyl should not exceed 0·2 mg. or respiration will be unduly depressed. With assisted or controlled respiration, larger initial doses of fentanyl (0·4–0·6 mg.) may be employed and when muscular relaxation is required *d*-tubocurarine is injected. Additional doses of fentanyl of 0·05 mg. are administered if the patient shows signs of lightening of analgesia such as movements or a rise in respiratory rate or blood pressure. Stability of the circulatory system is notable both during and after operation. The alpha-adrenergic blocking effect of droperidol may help prevent the development of shock and animal experiments have shown that it protects against adrenaline-induced arrhythmias. Respiratory depression similar to that seen after other potent narcotics may result from the use of fentanyl but is of shorter duration than with other drugs. The rapid intravenous injection of fentanyl may cause muscular rigidity during anaesthesia and lead to ventilatory insufficiency, but it responds rapidly to small doses of relaxants.

On discontinuing the nitrous oxide at the end of operation, patients rapidly respond to commands, and yet if left to themselves they sleep peacefully oblivious of uncomfortable catheters and suction tubes. The incidence of vomiting is low as droperidol has a potent anti-emetic effect, while in most instances analgesia continues into the post-operative period for several hours. The post-operative state following this technique makes it an ideal choice in patients who are undergoing major oral surgery, such as mandibular osteotomy, in which the jaws are wired together at the end of operation and contrasts with the restlessness which often follows more conventional methods of anaesthesia.

A rare complication of the butyrophenones such as droperidol is the occurrence of extrapyramidal type of movements 24 to 48 hours after administration. They occur most frequently in children or young adults and can be controlled by atropine or anti-Parkinson drugs. Because minor central effects can last for up to 48 hours after the administration of droperidol, patients should be warned not to drive or operate machinery on the day following anaesthesia. As mental depression may be aggravated by droperidol, it should be avoided in depressed patients and care should be taken in patients with hepatic disease.

The value of neuroleptanalgesia in supplementing light general anaesthesia has now been established. The smooth post-operative course, protection against adrenaline-induced arrhythmias, the profound analgesia and minimal hypotension are all desirable features. There are objections, however, to the intravenous injection of mixtures of powerful drugs when there is inadequate human pharmacological data on the individual constituents (Dobkin *et al.*, 1963). Unlike an inhalational agent, there is no way of retrieving them once they have been administered. Nevertheless it has proved a useful technique, especially in geriatric surgery, in patients with haemodynamic disturbances, and those who might require ventilatory assistance in the post-operative period without recourse to tracheostomy. This technique now has an established place in the anaesthetist's armamentarium.

REFERENCES

ANDERSON, S. A. (1960). Premedication of children for surgery. *Brit. J. Anaesth.*, **32,** 125.

AUBRY, U., CARIGNAN, G., CHARETTE, D., KEERI-SZANTO, M., and LAVALLEE, J-P. (1966). Neuroleptanalgesia with fentanyl-droperidol: an appreciation based on more than 1,000 anaesthetics for major surgery. *Canad. Anaesth. Soc. J.*, **13,** 263.

BELAM, O. H., and DOBNEY, G. H. (1957). Persistent pain. Treatment by nerve block. *Anaesthesia*, **12,** 345.

BERGAN, J. J., and CONN, J. (1968). Sympathectomy for pain relief. *Med. Clin. N. Amer.*, **52,** 147.

BONICA, J. J. (1953). *The Management of Pain.* Philadelphia: Lea & Febiger.

BRAIN, R. (1956). Symposium on the treatment of cerebrovascular disease. *Proc. roy. Soc. Med.*, **49,** 164.

BRIDENBAUGH, L. D., MOORE, D. C., and CAMPBELL, D. D. (1964). Management of upper abdominal cancer. *J. Amer. med. Ass.*, **190**, 877.

BROMAGE, P. R. (1967). Extradural analgesia for pain relief. *Brit. J. Anaesth.*, **39,** 721.

BROWN, A. S. (1964). Neuroleptanalgesia for the surgical treatment of Parkinsonism. *Anaesthesia*, **19,** 70.

BURTLES, R., and PECKETT, B. W. (1957). Postoperative vomiting. Some factors affecting its incidence. *Brit. J. Anaesth.*, **29,** 114.

CARTER, A. B. (1957). The immediate treatment of cerebral embolism. *Quart. J. Med.*, **26,** 335.

CLARKE, E., MORRISON, R., and ROBERTS, H. (1955). Spinal cord damage by efocaine. *Lancet*, **1,** 896.

Clutton-Brock, J. (1960). Some pain threshold studies with particular reference to thiopentone. *Anaesthesia*, **15**, 71.

Davies, D. R., and Doughty, A. (1967). Premedication of children with papaveretum-hyoscine. *Brit. J. Anaesth.*, **39**, 638.

de Clive-Lowe, S. G., Gray, P. W. S., and North, J. (1954). Succinylcholine and lignocaine by continuous intravenous drip. *Anaesthesia*, **9**, 96.

Denton, J. E., and Beecher, H. K. (1949). New analgesia: A clinical appraisal of the narcotic power of methadone and its isomers. *J. Amer. med. Ass.*, **141**, 1146.

Dobkin, A. B., Lee, P. K. Y., Byles, P. H., and Israel, J. S. (1963). Neuroleptanalgesics: A comparison of the cardiovascular, respiratory and metabolic effects of Innovan and thiopentone plus methotrimeprazine. *Brit. J. Anaesth.*, **35**, 694.

Dogliotti, A. M. (1931). Traitement des syndromes douloureux de la périphérie par l'alcoolisation sub-arachnoidienne des racines postérieures à leur émergence de la moelle épinière. *Presse méd.*, **39**, 1249.

Doughty, A. G. (1964). Personal communication.

Doupe, J., Cullen, G. H., and Chance, G. Q. (1944). Post-traumatic pain and the causalgic syndrome. *J. Neurol. Neurosurg. Psychiat.*, **7**, 33.

Dundee, J. W. (1957*a*). Chlorpromazine as an adjunct in the relief of chronic pain. *Brit. J. Anaesth.*, **29**, 28.

Dundee, J. W. (1957*b*). Adjuncts in the relief of chronic pain. *Anaesthesia*, **12**, 330.

Dundee, J. W. (1960*a*). A method for assessing the efficacy of oral analgesics: its applications and limitations. *Brit. J. Anaesth.*, **32**, 48.

Dundee, J. W. (1960*b*). Alterations in response to somatic pain associated with anaesthesia. II. The effect of thiopentone and pentobarbitone. *Brit. J. Anaesth.*, **32**, 407.

Egbert, L. D., Battit, G. E., Welch, C. E., and Bartlett, M. K. (1964). Reduction of postoperative pain by encouragement and instruction of patients. *New Engl. J. Med.*, **270**, 825.

Finer, B. (1958). Epidural injection of carbolic acid in incurable cancer. *Lancet*, **2**, 1179.

Gordon, R. A., and Goel, S. B. (1963). Intrathecal phenol block in treatment of intractable pain of malignant disease. *Canad. Anaesth. Soc. J.*, **10**, 357.

Greenhill, J. P. (1947). Sympathectomy and intraspinal alcohol injections for relief of pelvic pain. *Brit. med. J.*, **2**, 859.

Hitchcock, E. (1967). Hypothermic subarachnoid irrigation for intractable pain. *Lancet*, **1**, 1133.

Hitchcock, E. (1969*a*). Hypothermic subarachnoid irrigation. *Lancet*, **1**, 1330.

Hitchcock, E. (1969*b*). Osmolytic neurolysis for intractable facial pain. *Lancet*, **1**, 434.

Holderness, M. C., Chase, P. E., and Dripps, R. D. (1963). A narcotic analgesic and a butyrophenone with nitrous oxide for general anaesthesia. *Anesthesiology*, **24**, 336.

Keats, A. S. (1956). Postoperative pain: research and treatment. *J. chron. Dis.*, **4**, 72.

Kelly, R. E., and Gautier Smith, P. C. (1959). Intrathecal phenol in the treatment of reflex spasms and spasticity. *Lancet*, **2**, 1102.

Lasagna, L., and Beecher, H. K. (1954). Optimal dose of morphine. *J. Amer. med. Ass.*, **156**, 230.

Lasagna, L., and De Kornfeld, T. J. (1961). Methotrimeprazine: a new phenothiazine derivative with analgesic properties. *J. Amer. med. Ass.*, **178**, 887.

Lewis, D. L., and Thompson, W. A. L. (1953). Reduction of postoperative pain. *Brit. med. J.*, **1**, 973.

LIN, P. M., GILDENBERG, P. L., and POLAKOFF, P. P. (1966). An anterior approach to percutaneous lower cervical cordotomy. *J. Neurosurg.*, **25**, 553.

LIPTON, S. (1968). Percutaneous electrical cordotomy in relief of intractable pain. *Brit. med. J.*, **2**, 210.

MCKEAN, M. C., and HITCHCOCK E. (1968). Electrocardiographic changes after intrathecal hypertonic saline solution. *Lancet*, **2**, 1083.

MAHER, R. M. (1955). Relief of pain in incurable cancer. *Lancet*, **1**, 18.

MAHER, R. M. (1957). Neurone selection in relief of pain. Further experiences with intrathecal injections. *Lancet*, **1**, 16.

MAHER, R. M. (1960). Further experiences with intrathecal and subdural phenol. Observations on two forms of pain. *Lancet*, **1**, 895.

MAHER, R. M. (1963). Intrathecal chlorocresol (parachlormetacresol) in the treatment of pain in cancer. *Lancet*, **1**, 965.

MASSON, A. H. B. (1967). The role of analgesic drugs in the treatment of postoperative pain. *Brit. J. Anaesth.*, **39**, 713.

MOORE, D. C. (1965). *Regional Block. A handbook for use in the clinical practice of medicine and surgery*, 4th edit. Springfield, Ill.: Charles C. Thomas.

MOORE, J., and DUNDEE, J. W. (1961). Promethazine. Its influence on the course of thiopentone and methohexital anaesthesia. *Anaesthesia*, **16**, 61.

MULLAN, S., HEKMATPANAH, J., DOBBEN, G., and BECKMAN, F. (1965). Percutaneous, intramedullary cordotomy utilizing the unipolar anodal electrolytic lesion. *J. Neurosurg.*, **22**, 548.

MULLAN, S., and HOSOBUCHI, Y. (1968). Respiratory hazards of high cervical percutaneous cordotomy. *J. Neurosurg.*, **28**, 291.

NATHAN, P. W. (1952). Newer synthetic analgesic drugs. *Brit. med. J.*, **2**, 903.

NATHAN, P. W. (1959). Intrathecal phenol to relieve spasticity in paraplegia. *Lancet*, **2**, 1099.

NATHAN, P. W. (1967). Some aspects of the cancer problem. *Brit. med. J.*, **1**, 168.

NATHAN, P. W., and SCOTT, T. G. (1958). Intrathecal phenol for intractable pain. *Lancet*, **1**, 76.

NATHAN, P. W., and SEARS, T. A. (1960). Effects of phenol on nervous conduction. *J. Physiol.* (*Lond.*), **150**, 565.

NATHAN, P. W., SEARS, T. A., and SMITH, M. C. (1965). Effects of phenol solutions on the nerve roots of the cat: an electrophysiological and histological study. *J. neurol. Sci.*, **2**, 7.

NILSSON, E. (1963). Editorial: Origin and rationale of neurolept-analgesia. *Anesthesiology*, **24**, 267.

OEHLANDT, G. (1955). Klinische Beobachtungen über die Wirkungsverstarkung und verlangerung von Dromoran "Roche" durch Mestinon. *Med. Klin.*, **50**, 2202.

PARBROOK, G. D. (1967*a*). Techniques of inhalational analgesia in the postoperative period. *Brit. J. Anaesth.*, **39**, 730.

PARBROOK, G. D. (1967*b*). Comparison of trichloroethylene and nitrous oxide as analgesics. *Brit. J. Anaesth.*, **39**, 86.

PARBROOK, G. D., and KENNEDY, B. R. (1964). Value of premixed nitrous oxide and oxygen mixtures in the relief of postoperative pain. *Brit. med. J.*, **2**, 1303.

PARKHOUSE, J., LAMBRECHTS, W., and SIMPSON, B. R. J. (1961). The incidence of postoperative pain. *Brit. J. Anaesth.*, **33**, 345.

POOLER, H. E. (1949). Relief of postoperative pain and its influence on vital capacity. *Brit. med. J.*, **2**, 1200.

REES, G. J. (1960). Paediatric anaesthesia. *Brit. J. Anaesth.*, **32**, 132.

ROE, B. B. (1963). Are postoperative narcotics necessary? *Arch. Surg.*, **87**, 912.

and the veins of the vertebrae on the one hand and the cavae on the other. Any factor causing a rise in abdominal or thoracic pressure will not only prevent blood from entering the cavae, but may even cause a retrograde flow from them.

Pearce (1957) has measured the pressure changes in the lower end of the inferior cava when the patient is in the prone position, by means of a catheter attached to a simple water manometer. Pressure on the abdomen sufficient to cause obstruction to the vena cava can cause a rise in pressure of more than 300 mm. of water while even slight compression invariably leads to a rapid increase of 30–40 mm. of water. When the patient is well supported so that the abdominal wall hangs free, low pressures are recorded, although normal contraction of the abdominal muscles during spontaneous respiration leads to a pressure rise of up to 100 mm. of water. To produce optimal results Pearce recommends a well-supported patient who is fully relaxed and having properly controlled respiration without any rise in intrathoracic pressure during the expiratory phase. Undue abdominal compression or respiratory embarrassment can be prevented by placing a wedge-shaped rubber pillow beneath the thorax, with its broad edge just below the level of the acromion processes. Such a wedge effectively maintains the patient in the correct position and gives reasonable freedom for diaphragmatic movement. Further help can be gained by raising the patient's pelvis on supports. The convex bowing of the upper spine of the patient as it curves over the wedge opens up the intervertebral spaces, to the benefit of the surgeon during laminectomy. For laminectomies at the lower end of the spine (lumbar and lower dorsal) this arrangement is not always acceptable to the surgeon as there is a tendency to lordosis, with closing of the intervertebral spaces in the operation site. The lumbar lordosis is accentuated by supporting the pelvis. For these reasons the jack-knife position, with the patient flexed in the prone position over pillows or a "broken" operation table is often preferred, although it tends to embarrass respiration and may lead to marked venous congestion. A modified jack-knife position with the patient raised at the pelvis to free the abdomen has been described (Taylor *et al.*, 1956). These authors agree that with a pelvic support the lumbar lordosis is not undone to the same extent achieved by some other postures, though they consider that the traction exerted by the weight of the legs and trunk as they tend to slide down their respective slopes is beneficial in this respect.

Lateral Position

Another approach to the problem of venous bleeding during laminectomy is to use the lateral position, which enables the patient to be postured with the back flexed. There is little, if any, venous engorgement in this position, provided the surgeon does not need excessive flexion to open up the intervertebral spaces. This can only be achieved by drawing up the thighs with full flexion at the hips, and results in some abdominal compression.

Sitting Position

The sitting or upright position is undoubtedly the most effective method for producing an uncongested operating field for a cervical laminectomy or posterior fossa craniotomy. The patient is placed in a special chair with the head supported anteriorly in a cushioned horse-shoe. An alternative method is to place the patient supine on the operating table, but with the head well over the end and held forward and supported by a wire and caliper which is fixed to the head. The table is set with a pronounced foot-down tilt.

Some Dangers of Posture

Air embolus and severe hypotension are the two dangers associated with these upright positions, although any degree of anti-Trendelenburg tilt is conducive to such potential hazards.

Air embolus.—The incidence of air embolus is difficult to assess and published figures are not available, but it undoubtedly bears a relation to the competence of the surgeon. Furthermore, prompt diagnosis and treatment by both surgeon and anaesthetist sometimes prove surprisingly successful (see Chapter 28). In neurosurgical practice the quantity of air sucked into a vein may be comparatively small, but the site of entry may not be apparent at once. A tear in a venous sinus during the removal of bone is a likely site. Other vulnerable vessels are the suboccipital venous plexus and the mastoid emissarics (Hunter, 1952). Deep breathing or one or two deep respirations following a cough add to the hazard, as they increase the sub-atmospheric pressure which already exists in these veins. Hunter (1960) considers that air embolism is very likely to occur when muscle relaxants and intermittent positive-pressure ventilation are used for a posterior fossa operation in the sitting position and he considers the method unacceptable because effective ventilation, even without a negative phase, reduces the venous pressure above the heart to a dangerously low level. The risk of air embolism can be minimised by maintaining spontaneous breathing and deliberately increasing the venous pressure either by screwing down the expiratory valve until the reservoir bag is distended throughout the respiratory cycle or by pressing on the jugular veins in the neck (Hunter, 1962). If the first method is used, the fresh gas flow should be increased and the valve screwed down from the beginning of the operation until all the bone work is completed and again when the dura is closed until the end of the operation. During this time unremitting attention must be paid to the respiration and cardiovascular stability for which purpose an oesophageal stethoscope and an ECG oscillograph are helpful. At the earliest signs of air embolism treatment must be instituted at once (see p. 764).

Hypotension.—Postural hypotension is more easily detected and tends to be accentuated by the effects of general anaesthesia. Bourne (1957) has drawn attention to the dangers of acute hypotension due to fainting in conscious patients placed in the upright position after surgery. Death may be caused by cardiac asystole, ventricular fibrillation, or brain damage. It seems likely that such episodes may occur during surgery when local analgesia is used, although the essential mechanism may not be recognised. Haemorrhage will increase the hazard. Wolf and Siris (1937) describe three patients who collapsed during operations for division of the sensory roots of the fifth cranial nerve, which were performed under local analgesia in the upright position. In one case the surgeon commented on the complete avascularity of the operation wound and at postmortem all cases showed evidence of changes due to sub-oxygenation.

Fainting is unlikely to occur once general anaesthesia is well established, although it may do so during the induction phase (Bourne, 1957). Loss of blood, particularly in quantities in excess of 1 litre, will cause vasovagal fainting with muscle vasodilatation in conscious patients, but this reaction is prevented by light general anaesthesia (de Wardener *et al.*, 1953). If a patient is placed in the upright position soon after the induction of anaesthesia with a drug such as thiopentone, marked hypotension may occur due to the peripheral effects of vasomotor depression and the consequent sudden venous pooling from the postural change. Furthermore, the addition of thiopentone, or any other drug such as pethidine—which potentiates hypotensive effects—to supplement anaesthesia during the progress of the operation must be made with caution. Even without this vasodilatory effect, the anaesthetised patient in the upright position tends to become hypotensive due to progressive venous pooling, while the level at which the arterial pressure is ultimately maintained depends upon the efficiency of the compensatory processes. As the arterial pressure falls there is a compensatory fall in cerebral vascular resistance (dilatation of cerebral vessels) which helps to maintain a constant cerebral blood flow and therefore normal oxygenation. However, the minimal level of arterial pressure which is compatible with adequate oxygenation of the brain varies from case to case, depending upon the state of the vessels and of the brain itself, the patient's normal blood pressure, and the pressure difference between the heart and the brain. In the upright position it is certainly unwise to allow the systolic pressure of a patient who has a normal circulation to fall below 70–80 mm. Hg. If intracranial pressure is raised this may be too low and the blood pressure must be taken immediately the patient is sat up; if it is too low he must be lain supine at once until it is restored. It is, however, remarkable how well most anaesthetised patients maintain an adequate blood pressure when upright, once they have had time to adapt themselves to the position. Hunter (1952) comments on the stability of the circulation in this position despite moderate blood loss and other depressor influences. Some help towards the prevention of undue hypotention can be gained by firm bandaging of the legs from toes to groins with crêpe bandages and by flexing the patient's thighs and raising his legs (Cheatle and MacKenzie, 1953). Methoxamine (5 to 10 mg.) is usually effective in raising the systolic pressure. The most effective form of therapy is to lower the patient to a more supine position.

The changes in the brain that can be caused by sub-oxygenation have been described elsewhere (see Chapter 45). Here it only needs to be stressed that specific histological changes in the cells are not visible if death takes place within 30 to 36 hours of the period of sub-oxygenation. Post-mortem diagnosis of the cause of sudden death in the operating theatre is rarely satisfactory, and depends far more upon clinical evidence of the sequence of events than upon abnormal pathology.

Discussion

The choice between the upright and prone position usually depends upon the inclinations of the surgeon. Theoretically, better access to a particular part of the brain due to an uncongested and relatively bloodless operation wound enables delicate surgery to be performed with less risk of trauma to surrounding tissue. This is an important factor in neurosurgical work where morbidity and mortality tend anyway to be high when the operation is in an area of the brain which abounds with vital functions. Yet there is insufficient practical evidence that the end results of series of similar operations differ greatly, if at all, when performed in either position by competent surgeons. For this reason it is as well to be certain that the complications specific to a particular position do not mar the ultimate result, and to select a posture which not only suits the surgeon but also the patient.

ANAESTHESIA

The basis of good anaesthesia for neurosurgery can be summarised as a perfect airway, adequate ventilation with minimal expiratory resistance, and a speedy return to consciousness at the end of operation. Intracranial work does not require deep anaesthesia, and indeed the greatest and most frequent stimulus of an entire operation is usually the presence of an endotracheal tube in the trachea. The diathermy is an essential and constant part of neurosurgical technique, so that inflammable anaesthetic agents must only be used as part of a calculated risk. Some surgeons may take upwards of six hours for an operation which is performed by others in under two. To satisfy these several requirements special techniques have been developed, but the differences between them only illustrate the importance that one anaesthetist attaches to some particular aspect of the problem and stress the value of the personal touch. There are few, if any, drugs or techniques which do not in some way adversely affect intracranial or intraspinal mechanics. Such factors can be minimised by careful selection and attention to detail.

Local or General

No single drug or combination of drugs can be considered ideal in the circumstances of neurosurgical anaesthesia. Apart from the skin, fascia, temporal muscle, periosteum and bone of the skull, and certain parts of the basal dura where it is attached to bone, cranial surgery is carried out in an area which is entirely insensitive to pain. The nerves to the skin and fascia also supply the periosteum and bone. They pass through the fascia beneath the skin on a line encircling the skull and drawn approximately from the occipital protuberance to the eyebrows (Pitkin, 1953). Thus local subcutaneous infiltration with a solution of 1 per cent lignocaine produces satisfactory analgesia for burr holes and minor operations. If the incision impinges on the temporal muscle then a deeper infiltration must be made. In terms of pain relief this form of local analgesia is also effective for major craniotomies, and has the advantage of having no adverse effects on intracranial mechanics. Why, then, general anaesthesia?

Local Analgesia

Local analgesia leaves much to be desired in terms of sedation and comfort for the patient, and does nothing to aid the surgeon should the patient be uncooperative or unable to keep perfectly still. Although the mental state of many patients with intracranial disease is confused, the majority are conscious enough to dislike the discomforts of major surgery under local analgesia. The position on the operating table and the need to remain in it, and in a motionless state, for perhaps several hours are effective deterrents. There is a good deal of mental stress associated in the minds of many patients with an operation on the brain, and surgical manipulations in this area, even though painless, evoke indirect sensations, particularly during bone work. Stimulation of brain substance sometimes produces spontaneous motor or sensory activities for the patient, and though these may be valuable under certain circumstances as a guide to the localisation of the surgeon's work, they are unpleasant if repetitive or gross. A patient who is difficult to control because of his disease, or more simply because he or she is unco-operative, cannot be adequately sedated with complete safety, and certainly not as effectively as with a good general anaesthetic. Finally, the duration of action of all known local analgesic drugs is insufficient to cover the length of time that some surgeons take to complete certain operations.

General anaesthesia supplies an answer to all these disadvantages of local analgesia, but it does so at some slight cost. The dangers and disadvantages of general anaesthesia in the hands of inexperienced administrators must be appreciated before criticising those clinics where local methods of analgesia still find favour. So far as the operation of laminectomy is concerned, local infiltration analgesia is far from satisfactory, and either a more complete form, such as an epidural or spinal, must be used, or general anaesthesia preferred.

General Anaesthesia

The airway.—There must be an adequate airway at all times. This can be assured by using a flexible but unkinkable oral endotracheal tube. It must be fitted with a curved wide-bore connection piece. Endotracheal tubes made of latex rubber in which a spiral of thin nylon is incorporated are extremely satisfactory in practice. The connection piece must be pushed right down as far as the first spiral to avoid kinking or narrowing of the tube at this point. The length of the tube must be such that after insertion the shaft of the connection piece within the tube lies between the teeth or gums—so that biting does no harm—and the bevel lies above the carina. This must be checked immediately after intubation and again after final positioning of the head by ensuring that air entry to the left is unimpeded. Unkinkable tubes of this type are made by repeatedly dipping a spiral of nylon into liquid latex. During the setting process the latex fuses in the spaces between each spiral, but when these are set closely together binding may be inadequate. Burns (1956) has shown that heat and the vapour of trichloroethylene can cause bubble-formation in the latex within the interior of the endotracheal tube and that respiratory obstruction is caused. When more widely spaced spirals are used, as in the case in tubes of present manufacture, this complication does not occur.

Since these tubes are straight but flexible they take the natural position of the airway when *in situ*, yet do not exert undue pressure on the glottic structures.

The Oxford pattern of endotracheal tube is also very satisfactory for neurosurgery and has certain advantages over latex armoured tubes (Duckworth, 1962). It is essential to cut a hole in the anterior wall of Oxford tubes close to the bevel, or to cut the bevel itself square across in order to avoid airway obstruction by the posterior wall of the trachea against the bevel when the neck is acutely fixed.

Ventilation.—The importance of adequate ventilation during anaesthesia for all branches of surgery is well known. Incipient carbon dioxide retention—inexcusable in any circumstances—plays havoc with the neurosurgeon's operating field, while a raised expiratory resistance from obstruction, coughing or straining is even more disastrous. The mechanisms at work have been reviewed by Ballantine and Jackson (1954). Resistance to expiration leads to a rise in intrathoracic pressure which in turn obstructs the return of venous blood to the chest. As a result a rise of pressure occurs in the cerebral veins, and also in the vertebral plexus of veins. Increased intra-abdominal pressure from the work of the abdominal muscles during forced expiration contributes by compression of the inferior vena cava to the rise of pressure in the latter, and this rise then accentuates the increasing cerebrospinal fluid pressure. Oxygen lack and carbon dioxide retention act directly to cause cerebral vascular engorgement and enlargement in the size of the brain substance (Kety and Schmidt, 1948). Hypoxia leads to an increase in capillary permeability and probably to an increase in the fluid content of brain cells.

For most operations, particularly when deep anaesthesia is neither necessary nor desirable, muscle paralysis and efficient controlled respiration supply the answer to these problems and this method is now generally recommended for supratentorial intracranial surgery. In operations within the posterior fossa and on the upper cervical cord spontaneous respiration can have special value. It provides an indication—occasionally a life-saving one—of the integrity of the patient's vital functions. Some of the earliest signs of surgical stimulation in certain parts of the brain are made manifest by a change in respiration, and may serve as an indication to the surgeon of potential danger. Furthermore, it is not difficult with care and attention to detail, to maintain satisfactory spontaneous respiration even throughout very lengthy operations. If for any reason spontaneous respiration is unsatisfactory and seems likely to remain so, then it is wiser to take over and control respiration properly, making use of muscle relaxants for this purpose.

There are special advantages in using controlled respiration with muscle relaxants for some neurosurgical operations. The anatomical build of an occasional patient, the state of the lungs of another, or the posture required for the operation may individually or collectively suggest that the best conditions will only be obtained by taking over the patient's ventilation. Irrespective of such indications, brain tension can be reduced when the patient is respired either manually or by a ventilator. Furness (1957) described how effective controlled respiration can be, and considered that a negative phase has a considerable effect on brain tension. Her ideas have been confirmed by others (Mortimer, 1959; Galloon, 1959) though the need for a negative phase is not accepted by everyone (Brown, 1959). Controlled respiration is frequently combined with hyperventilation and there are good reasons for believing that a reduced arterial P_{CO_2} does help to lower the intracranial tension. Rosomoff (1963) considers that, although it may lower cerebrospinal fluid pressure, it never reduces brain volume. The evidence in favour of these techniques is largely based on clinical estimations and it may be that their total value lies in offsetting some of the disadvantages of spontaneous respiration and posture (Rosomoff, 1962), avoiding the need for a volatile anaesthetic and preventing straining (Hunter, 1960). Controlled respiration, particularly with a negative phase, if used for a patient in the sitting position increases the risk of air embolism.

Anaesthetic system.—The type of anaesthetic system is of only slight importance, but it must be designed to avoid rebreathing and to exclude any undue resistance to expiration, It is also convenient to have the anaesthetic trolley some distance from the operation site, and to be able to institute controlled respiration easily and efficiently. Often it is necessary to double the length of the corrugated breathing tubes in which case gas compression and tube expansion make it necessary to increase the minute volume considerably to achieve a given P_{CO_2} (Bushman and Collis, 1967). All methods—semi-closed, one way or non-return valve, "T"-piece, and closed with absorption—have their advocates, and each offers advantages and disadvantages. Personal preference must ultimately decide.

Premedication.—The potential danger of those drugs which cause respiratory depression when given to patients with a raised intracranial pressure is well known. Opiates and their analogues must therefore be prescribed with caution, if at all. Even when there is no apparent contra-indication to using them pre-operatively it must be borne in mind that their action may persist into the post-operative period, particularly when the operation is of relatively short duration. They may reduce reflex activity and the level of consciousness in the post-operative period, while the small and unreactive pupil which follows the administration of opiates is a disadvantage when assessing the state of the patient. Pre-operative sedation is an important factor in the preparation of the patient for any type of anaesthetic, but for intracranial surgery this benefit may have to be foregone. Recent work with diazepam has shown that this drug may be useful for allaying apprehension without the drawbacks of the opiates. It may be given in a dose of 0·15 mg. per kg. up to a maximum of 10 mg. (Marrubini and Tretola, 1965). During maintenance of anaesthesia there is a practical advantage in having an undepressed patient as this allows greater freedom in the use of intravenous drugs. An adequate dose of atropine sulphate should be given subcutaneously about an hour before the induction of anaesthesia.

These arguments do not apply in the case of operations on the spine—indeed opiates are of considerable value in controlling post-operative pain after a laminectomy. However, undue respiratory depression can be a marked disadvantage even during a laminectomy, and this may be accentuated by the position of the patient.

Choice of anaesthetic.—Although adequate anaesthesia can be produced with a single powerful agent such as ether, a combination of drugs has some advantages in overcoming with minimal sequelae the few sensory reflexes that neurosurgical operations and the presence of an endotracheal tube initiate. There has been a general swing away from spontaneous breathing for supratentorial surgery and this has been given added impetus by the work of McDowall and Jennett already referred to. Most neurosurgical anaesthetists give relaxant drugs and use mechanical ventilators to produce moderate reductions in P_{CO_2}. The omission of sedative premedication and the concern for perfect oxygenation inevitably mean that the anaesthetic is conducted close to the level of consciousness. It is therefore often necessary to take other measures to ensure that this level is never reached. Small increments of pethidine are appropriate, or volatile agents may be used. Trichloroethylene or halothane from a calibrated vaporiser in concentrations below 1 per cent are the drugs most commonly used to supplement nitrous oxide. Experience has shown that provided the introduction of these volatile supplements is preceded by a few minutes of hyperventilation and the use—when indicated—of mannitol, the rise in intracranial pressure which they cause need not be taken into account. If grossly raised intracranial pressure is known to be present it is unlikely that any supplement to nitrous oxide will be necessary and volatile anaesthetics should not be introduced until the dura is opened and the brain tension can be assessed.

In posterior fossa surgery a similar technique can be used if the patient is prone, but in the sitting position the case for spontaneous breathing is much stronger.

Intravenous induction of anaesthesia is a blessing to the patient—particularly to those who are unsedated—and if the dose is moderate, less upsetting to intracranial mechanics than a stormy inhalational induction. There may be assets, it is true, in maintaining adequate spontaneous respiration throughout induction and intubation, but they hardly outweigh the intrinsic advantage of a brief period of perfect relaxation from suxamethonium during which laryngoscopy, topical analgesia of the larynx and trachea, and intubation can all be easily performed. However, with this method after the onset of paralysis the patient must be hyperventilated with oxygen. Paradoxically, a minute or so of total paralysis, such as a dose of 75 to 100 mg. of suxamethonium will produce in an average patient, is more useful than a few seconds. Although intubation can be carried out in a matter of seconds, it is convenient to allow time for the topical analgesia to become effective, the trachea to accustom itself to the tube, and the patient to be partly saturated with nitrous oxide from intermittent positive-pressure respiration before reflex activity starts to return. By these means coughing, straining, and carbon dioxide accumulation can be avoided. The short action of suxamethonium provides a quick return of full respiratory activity; indeed, in some patients the nitrous oxide must be supplemented at this stage to avoid bucking on the tube (see below). The principal disadvantage of suxamethonium in this context is the slight though brief rise in arterial pressure that follows its use.

Nitrous oxide alone, except in the presence of paralysis from muscle relaxants, is insufficient to maintain anaesthesia for the whole operation, and more particularly during the first part when the patient is at his fittest and surgical stimulation at its maximum. The skin incision and the movements of the tube in the trachea during the heavy bone work represent the most active stimuli in this respect. As the operation progresses, and provided the position of the head is not suddenly changed, nitrous oxide *alone* usually suffices, although occasional supplementation may be necessary. Intermittent thiopentone or very small doses of pethidine intravenously are helpful adjuncts for the first part of the operation and can be used with safety, particularly when the operation is likely to be a long one.

Pethidine, besides being an effective analgesic, is a useful anti-cholinergic agent. It helps to prevent spasm of the smooth muscle of the trachea and bronchi and depresses the cough reflex. These, and a sedative effect in the post-operative period, can be useful advantages in neurosurgical anaesthesia (Wylie, 1951) and the intravenous route enables them to be attained quickly and with minimal dosage. Pethidine is also a respiratory depressant, but the administration of small doses (10 mg. or less) to an unsedated patient gives plenty of latitude in this respect and is a useful method of smoothing out and controlling an unduly rapid respiratory rate. In certain cases (as indicated above) the risk of marked respiratory depression and its attendant train of physiological intracranial upsets may make it unwise to use pethidine, but such cases are rare. More often this sequence of events is due to injudicial dosage on the part of the anaesthetist.

Pethidine does not affect the pupils and does not lead to nausea or vomiting comparable in degree with that produced by an equivalent amount of morphine. A total dosage of 125 mg. of pethidine need rarely be exceeded for a major craniotomy, even when no other agents than nitrous oxide and the initial induction dose of thiopentone are used. Of this total one might expect to administer somewhere between 50 and 70 per cent during the first part of the operation, which involves raising the bone flap. A much smaller total dosage of pethidine will suffice if a volatile anaesthetic such as halothane is used.

Towards the end of a long operation intravenous supplementation is better avoided, not only because it may prolong the period of post-operative unconsciousness but because at this time it is difficult to give by this route a dose which is effective and yet small enough not to produce some slight respiratory or circulatory change.

Of the inhalational agents the choice is usually between trichloroethylene and halothane. This is one of the few instances in which the balance of advantages favours the selection of trichloroethylene, as effective analgesia is much less likely to be associated with a fall in cerebral perfusion pressure. Nevertheless many experienced anaesthetists prefer halothane and it is a more appropriate agent for babies and small children.

Cerebral Dehydration

The size of the brain can be reduced by substances such as urea or mannitol which cause an abrupt rise in plasma osmotic pressure followed by a brisk osmotic diuresis. Urea is commonly given as a 30 per cent solution in 10 per cent invert sugar (Stubbs and Pennybacker, 1960) and up to 90 g. may be administered on the basis of 1 g. per kg. body weight. But urea, though popular and successful, has several disadvantages. It is contra-indicated in the presence of renal damage, has a markedly irritant effect on tissues when it seeps outside the vein at the site of infusion, can cause changes in the electrocardiograph of the patient (Bering and Avman, 1960) and may lead to some hypovolaemia due to reduction in plasma volume. The most important disadvantage of urea is that is may cause a rebound rise in brain tension (Langfitt, 1961) due to the late diffusion of part of it into the brain substance, and as a result of this a subsequent rise in osmotic pressure and attraction to water.

These disadvantages have led to the use of 20 per cent mannitol, a carbohydrate and diuretic, which has a higher molecular weight than urea and does not cause a rebound phenomenon. It has none of the other disadvantages of urea though it may very occasionally lead to a post-infusion hypovolaemia (Wise and Chater, 1962). To be effective the dose of mannitol should be given in 20 to 30 minutes and fit adults can be given up to 500 ml. of the 20 per cent solution on a 1 g. per kg. body-weight basis. This causes a rapid expansion of plasma volume and any patient in whom this would be undesirable should receive half this dose. Hypertensive patients with evidence of right or left heart failure should not be given osmotic diuretics. The use of mannitol results in a urine volume of 1 to 1½ litres during the following three hours and the patient should either be catheterised or the urine expressed manually; restlessness from an over-distended bladder is particularly undesirable in the recovery period.

Oral glycerol has recently been recommended for the reduction of intracranial tension, cerebral oedema and cerebrospinal fluid pressure (Cantore *et al.* 1964). The advantages of glycerol are simplicity of administration, no rebound phenomena and lack of toxicity—all facts that make this agent advantageous for repeated use, particularly in the pre- and post-operative management of patients with intracranial disease. Given orally, the dose is from 0·5 to 2 g. per kg. body weight, and as much as 5 g. a day has been given to a single patient over several days without troublesome effects. Cantore and his associates recommend making up the estimated dose as a 50 per cent solution with normal saline, and giving it with small quantities of food if possible. When the patient cannot drink spontaneously the glycerol should be given through an oesophageal tube.

Controlled Hypotension

There are few branches of surgery in which so strong a case can be made for induced hypotension, and in which the risks of the ancillary technique can be set against the advantages. At the outset, however, it is important to remember that most intracranial and spinal operations can be performed satisfactorily without it, provided due attention is paid to the essentials of good anaesthesia and posture. Taylor *et al.* (1956) have ceased to use induced hypotension for laminectomy as they consider a well-arranged posture (modified jack-knife) gives as good results with less risk, and theirs is a widely held opinion. But it is often the presence of the tumour which causes congestion during intracranial surgery, so that induced hypotension, which will reduce the swelling, may well lessen the risks of some operations on the brain. Minimal arterial bleeding with no venous ooze materially assists the surgeon to delineate the limits of the disease process and thus to remove it with less risk of damage to normal tissue. Control of haemorrhage may make possible operations which could not otherwise be attempted (Anderson and McKissock, 1953).

A raised intracranial pressure makes exposure at the operation site difficult, since the distended brain tends to bulge out when the dura is opened, and aggravates venous bleeding. A distended brain also necessitates considerable retraction which in turn leads to bruising of tissue. A marked reduction in arterial pressure will help to control these factors.

The site of the lesion determines how effective autonomic blockade will be on intracranial tension (Hewer, 1952). A decrease in vascularity, particularly in normally vascular tumours such as haemangiomata, meningiomata and angiomata, and a reduction in the secretions of the choroid plexus, are of general help, but considerable relief can also be expected in patients with internal hydrocephalus from a block.

Apart from the well-recognised dangers of hypotension (see Chapter 23) there are two, of special importance in neurosurgery, which must be mentioned. Aserman (1953) has described how hypotension leads to retraction of the brain within the cranial cavity and an alteration in its consistency, which he likens to dough. It is then easily compressed, is slow to regain its normal conformity, and is equally slowly replenished with blood. In these circumstances pressure from a brain retractor may be transmitted to comparatively distant parts of the brain, and by impairing their blood supply cause irreversible damage. Aserman calls this "retractor anaemia". He is careful to advise that induced hypotension should only be used for those operations in which retraction is made on brain substance that is ultimately to be excised. Although this may be a sound contra-indication in principle, it is perhaps a little sweeping in practice. Gentle retraction is always advisable, and for operations such as hypophysectomy during which the frontal lobe must be held back for access to the pituitary fossa, induced hypotension is likely to increase the hazards unless the surgeon is careful. In fact for most operations for tumours or cysts of the pituitary, induced hypotension is unnecessary, yet paradoxically it may help the surgeon to remove the normal pituitary completely in patients with secondary carcinomata (Ballantine, 1956). This is of paramount importance, since failure to take away as little as 2 per cent of gland substance can lead to rapid regeneration of the whole and failure of the operation. Thus the risk of retractor anaemia is outweighed by the improved operating field.

The second special danger is reactionary haemorrhage. This is hardly specific to neurosurgical practice, but constitutes a very definite hazard if the surgical and the hypotensive techniques are not balanced. There must be an adequate systolic blood pressure—preferably at normal or near-normal level—before the dura is closed, so that the dangers of a small bleeding point being missed are minimised, and a meticulous surgical technique. By using trimetaphan or homatropinium rather than hexamethonium bromide, the anaesthetist has more scope to alter the patient's blood pressure according to surgical needs. Even so, both these drugs have usually to be combined with posture if a satisfactory degree of hypotension is to be produced in the majority of patients, and there is occasionally some post-operative hypotension, although its duration varies. A controlled pressure can be obtained by the application of negative pressure to the lower limbs with moderate doses of hexamethonium bromide (James *et al.*, 1953). The blood pressure can then be varied at will over a large range and there is minimal post-operative hypotension.

Hypothermia

Hypothermia leads to a fall in cerebral blood flow and cerebrospinal fluid pressure, and to a reduction in brain volume (Rosomoff and Holaday, 1954; Rosomoff and Gilbert, 1955). Access to various parts of the brain is improved, and the surgeon can temporarily occlude a major end-artery. At rectal temperatures of about 30° C Burrows and his colleagues (1956) have been able to clamp the middle cerebral artery for from 4½ to 12¾ minutes without evidence of permanent cerebral damage. The induction of hypothermia will lead to some fall in systemic blood pressure, but not necessarily to very much. The reduction in metabolism that the fall in temperature causes will, however, offer some protection against the potential dangers of induced hypotension. It will also play an important part in reducing or preventing cerebral oedema, which in some neurosurgical procedures is often the ultimate factor leading to death. Hellings (1958) describing her experiences with surface cooling for a large series of patients with ruptured intracranial aneurysms and angiomata, reports that the technique may be used with small risks (no deaths due to it in over 100 patients), when compared with the use of a general anaesthetic alone. She considers that hypothermia can reasonably be used for other intracranial procedures, such as removal of a meningioma, when the improved operating conditions may be of value. It is difficult to be certain of the overall advantages of hypothermia for neurosurgical operations unless there is a specific indication, such as the temporary occlusion of an important vessel. Most of its advantages can be achieved by simpler means, such as controlled respiration with hyperventilation. Even so, if an overall reduction in morbidity and mortality can be shown when hypothermia is provided for operations which would normally be performed under routine general anaesthesia, the disadvantages of the technique should be accepted. The complications of many intracranial operations are still common enough to warrant attempts at improvement—perhaps even on such an empirical basis.

NEURORADIOLOGICAL INVESTIGATION PROCEDURES

The special neuroradiological investigation procedures fall into three groups—air replacement of the cerebrospinal fluid to outline the ventricular system, intraventricular or spinal subarachnoid injection of a radio-opaque dye to outline a tumour or other obstruction to the flow of cerebrospinal fluid, and arterial and venous angiography. All these investigations can be, and indeed frequently are, performed under local analgesia with or without sedation, but some of them—particularly the air-replacement techniques—are often so unpleasant as to warrant complete loss of consciousness. Children and uncooperative adults apart, there is still little unanimity of opinion amongst the doctors concerned about the indications for general anaesthesia for these investigation procedures, and some discussion of its merits and demerits is therefore worth while.

The dangers of the anaesthetic are those common to all anaesthetics and primarily dependent on the competence of the administrator. However, anaesthesia for neurological investigations carries special risks by virtue of the varied postures the patient will need to be placed in, and the effects of the disease on the vital centres. An experienced anaesthetist is essential, and with this assumption and some selection of cases, there is little evidence that general anaesthesia increases the mortality or morbidity associated with these procedures. Indeed Brown (1955) considers that light general anaesthesia is to be preferred to local analgesia for angiography, because it enables the patient's response to the injection of dye to be more simply and quickly assessed. This facilitates quicker treatment of any complications that may occur. However, loss of consciousness does necessitate manhandling the patient at intervals during the investigation to get the correct positions for radiography, which is a distinct disadvantage if staff is very limited. Paradoxically, anaesthesia enables the radiologist concerned to get on with the procedure without undue worry about the personal feelings of the patient—an important advantage when the symptoms caused by the investigation are barely tolerable—and the head can be kept perfectly still while the pictures are taken.

In the final event pleasantness for the patient must be the object of the anaesthetist, and provided this can be achieved without increasing the hazards of the investigation or adding special risks of its own, there are no legitimate reasons for refusing full anaesthesia. Nevertheless an accurate appreciation of the true nature of the symptoms produced by each investigation is essential before recommending general anaesthesia routinely, besides cognisance of the mental state of the patient concerned when the investigation is known to be relatively simple and devoid of unpleasant sequelae.

Most neurological investigations cause only slight discomfort to the average patient, but many patients—particularly if the progress of their suspected disease has not dulled the intellect—are extremely apprehensive.

Sedation and Analgesia in Neuroradiology

The fundamental consideration in management is the presence or absence of raised intracranial pressure. A drowsy patient with papilloedema is not a suitable candidate for any form of sedation.

If apprehension and the unpleasantness of the positioning rather than pain are the main considerations then diazepam 5 to 10 mg. or droperidol 5 mg. intravenously are unlikely to have any unwanted effects on cardiovascular or respiratory function. They are best given by slow intravenous injection immediately before the investigation. If pain is also to be taken into account, phenoperidine may be diluted and given intravenously, 0·25 mg. at a time, while its effect on respiration is very carefully watched. The use of these drugs has very much increased the versatility of sedation and the choice between them and general anaesthesia depends on many factors and is often difficult to make. A consideration of the individual procedures will enable these factors to be better understood.

Ventriculography and Air-encephalography

Ventriculography is the replacement of cerebrospinal fluid in the ventricular system from above and can be likened to the injection of air into a bottle full of fluid after the cork has been removed. Air-encephalography is replacement from below through a lumbar puncture, and by a similar analogy is injection into a bottle with the cork still in place. Thus, potentially, air-encephalography is a more dangerous procedure than ventriculography, as the passage of air into the ventricles may lead to or accentuate cerebral oedema and displace the medulla downwards. For many years the feeling that this sequence of events might occur limited the practice of air-encephalography, and the prospect of danger is still sometimes used as an argument against the production of general anaesthesia during the investigation. Indeed, if the circumstances of the patient's disease are so dire that general anaesthesia—by raising carbon dioxide tension or causing some sub-oxygenation—might accentuate the existing oedema sufficiently to produce a pressure cone, then general anaesthesia should not be induced, but, even more important, air-encephalography should not be performed at all. In such circumstances the injection of air by this method is as likely as general anaesthesia to be fatal. This type of patient is best investigated by ventriculography, and a drainage tube left in one or other lateral ventricle so that cerebrospinal fluid can be taken off at intervals. But even ventriculography may be followed by a central reaction in the brain leading to oedema and rising pressure.

At the present time air-encephalography is more frequently performed than ventriculography because it is a simple non-surgical procedure and the risks referred to are only likely in exceptional cases. These exceptional cases constitute the majority of patients who are submitted to ventriculography.

Ventriculography.—The investigation consists of making two burr holes in the posterior part of the skull, passing a canula into each lateral ventricle, and replacing part of the cerebrospinal fluid in them with air or oxygen. The outlines of the ventricular system are then defined on X-rays taken subsequently.

The patient is placed on the operating table in the supine position with head supported at a high level in a horse-shoe rest so that the occipital protuberance is well displayed.

The whole procedure can be carried out with minimal discomfort in co-operative adults under local infiltration analgesia. Premedication is neither desirable nor usually necessary, and to be effective is often more depressant than full general anaesthesia. The skin and deep tissues of the scalp down to the periosteum are infiltrated in the line of the incision with 1 per cent lignocaine. The dura and brain substance are painless, but the injection of air or oxygen into the lateral ventricles may cause some headache. There are no absolute contra-indications to general anaesthesia for ventriculography—indeed the presence of a burr hole and ventricular drainage is a factor for safety in those patients who have a high intracranial pressure—but in practice the procedure is well tolerated under local analgesia.

Oxygen is best for injection since it is more rapidly absorbed from the ventricular system than air. It is also less likely to cause any reaction and is cleaner than atmospheric air. Oxygen is drawn off from a medical gas cylinder through a sterile connecting rubber tube into a 10 ml. syringe and injected directly from the syringe into the canulae. Oxygen is always preferable to air, although there may be a case for using the latter when prolonged radiographic studies over a day or two are contemplated. There seems to be no good reason for using air—as is the usual practice—for air-encephalography (see below).

The patient must be carefully observed for some hours after ventriculography is completed. Removal of fluid from the ventricle relieves undue intracranial pressure but leaves room for cerebral oedema to accumulate. Even oxygen replacement causes some degree of reaction of this type and this may ultimately be sufficient to produce a rise in both systolic and diastolic blood pressures and respiratory difficulties. Further judicious drainage from the lateral ventricle will then be indicated.

Air (or oxygen) encephalography.— The patient is placed in the sitting position, preferably in a special chair which supports the front of the body and the head, which must be angled forward, and leaves the back free. A lumbar puncture is performed, about 10 ml. of fluid are withdrawn and an equivalent quantity of air or oxygen replaced. It is seldom that the persistence of air is desirable and oxygen is therefore usually to be preferred. Lateral X-rays of the skull are then taken to check that the oxygen is in the subarachnoid space and able to pass up into the ventricular system. This is sometimes difficult to achieve, particularly if a diagnostic lumbar puncture has been performed within the past week or two, since the oxygen then tends to track up in the epidural space.

Once the oxygen has passed into the ventricles a further 20 to 30 ml. of cerebrospinal fluid are withdrawn in 10 ml. quantities and replaced at once by equivalent amounts of oxygen. The X-rays are then taken (Fig. 2). This period may be protracted for as long as one or two hours. It will require movement of the patient, both to the supine and prone positions, to facilitate filling of the entire ventricular system and to ensure adequate pictures from different angles.

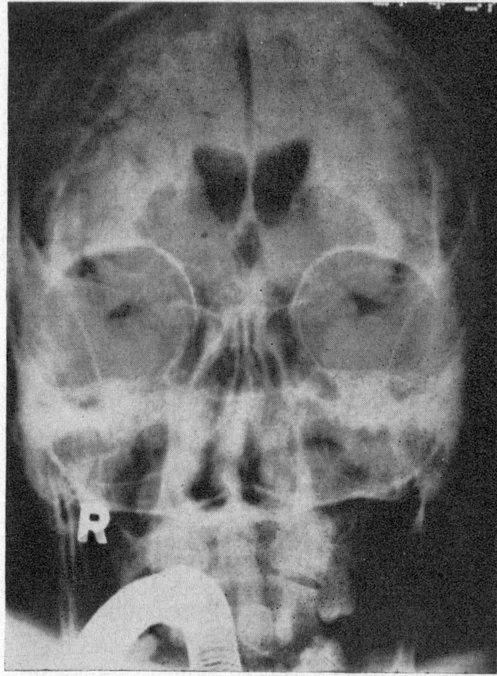

39/Fig. 2.—Normal air-encephalogram.

For an unanaesthetised patient lumbar encephalography is tedious and unpleasant. Nevertheless the difficulties of positioning are less if the patient can co-operate, and provided that he is carefully and skilfully managed the procedure can be made more tolerable.

Management without general anaesthesia.—The legs are bandaged with crêpe bandages as for posterior fossa surgery: an indwelling intravenous needle is inserted and a blood pressure cuff applied. Vasovagal fainting with its attendant nausea can be prevented by injecting 0·6 mg. atropine intravenously immediately the patient is sat up. Diazepam 2·5–7·5 mg. is given and small increments of a vasopressor such as methoxamine if there is any tendency for the blood pressure to fall.

General anaesthesia.—General anaesthesia is essential for children and for adults unable to co-operate. If there is any doubt about tolerance of the procedure under sedation it is better to choose general anaesthesia. The problems are similar to those of posterior fossa surgery and a marked fall of pressure must be looked for and guarded against, particularly after sudden movements or the intravenous injection of anaesthetic drugs. There is also a danger that normal gastric secretions may be aspirated into the respiratory tract should vomiting occur in the upright position, so a cuffed tube must be used and inadequate control of anaesthesia avoided at all times.

General anaesthesia not only eliminates the unpleasantness of the procedure but may also reduce the severity and duration of the headache that follows. Analgesia and sedation should be maintained in the post-anaesthetic stage by suitable drugs, provided they are compatible with the patient's neurological and general condition. The intermittent inhalation of oxygen may be of some benefit in the treatment of the headache when air has been injected (Macintosh *et al.*, 1958).

Myelography and Ventricular Dye Injection

Myelography consists of the injection of a radio-opaque dye into the subarachnoid space, either at the lumbar or the cisternal level, and posturing the patient to allow it to run towards the tumour. Spinal myelography with lumbar injection of the dye should only be managed by general anaesthesia when the patient is unable to co-operate. There is often no objection to the use of sedation, if necessary with opiates, and the very steep head-down tilt in the prone position in a darkened room makes general anaesthesia hazardous. No patient should be managed in total darkness and it is essential that the oxygen rotameter and the reservoir bag are continuously watched.

For ventricular dye injection the same considerations apply as to gas ventriculography and general anaesthesia is usually strongly contra-indicated. "Myodil", which is used as the contrast medium, is an iodinated lipoid with a low specific gravity, more fluid than iodised poppy-seed oil ("Lipiodol") and relatively non-irritant. Injection of a dye to outline the ventricular system necessitates one or two burr holes and the passage of a rubber catheter into one or other lateral ventricle. Although the operation is done in the theatre, the dye is better injected in the X-ray department.

Cerebral Angiography

Carotid arteriography stems from the work of Moniz who in 1926 attempted puncture of this vessel under local analgesia (Moniz, 1940). Percutaneous injection of diodone into the carotid or vertebral artery on one or other side is now commonly performed to delineate the arterial tree of the brain. Aneurysms, vascular tumours or arterial displacement by other tumours may be depicted. Carotid injection will outline most of the vessels above the tentorium, while vertebral injection depicts those below this structure as well as the posterior cerebral artery (Figs. 3-6).

The internal carotid or the vertebral artery is punctured in the neck with the patient lying supine. The needle is kept clear by the continuous slow injection of normal saline, while the patient's head is angled correctly in the X-ray apparatus. The opaque dye is then injected and the pictures are taken. Although the procedure is uncomfortable it is not unbearable with simple local infiltration of the skin, and, provided the operator is adept at the technique and the patient co-operative, general anaesthesia is not essential. Recent work however has caused a re-appraisal of the role of general anaesthesia in this investigation because it has

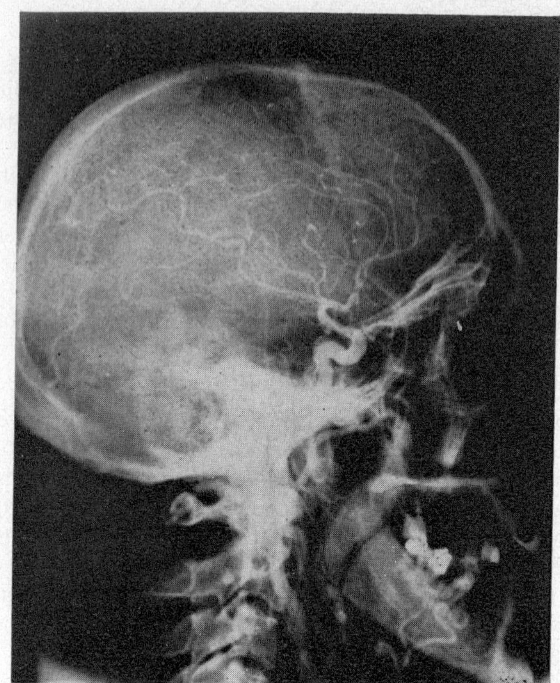

39/FIG. 3.—Normal carotid arteriogram, lateral view.

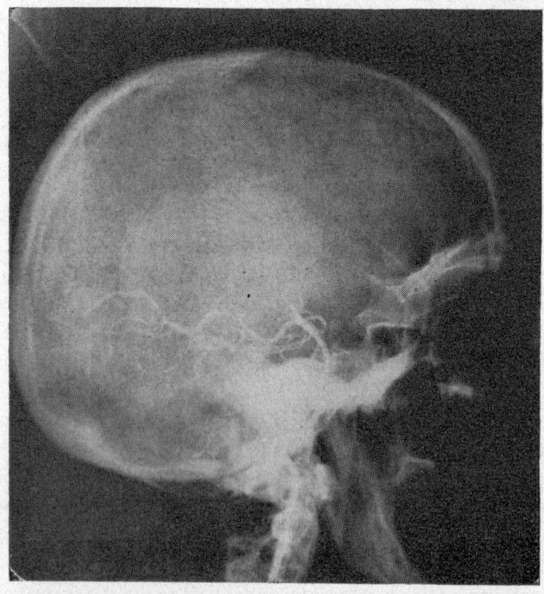

39/FIG. 4.—Normal vertebral arteriogram, lateral view.

shown that lowering of the carbon dioxide tension results in much improved angiograms, particularly in patients with tumours (Samuel *et al.*, 1968; Dallas and Moxon, 1969).

The older technique involving spontaneous breathing and the use of volatile agents has definitely been shown to be much less satisfactory, and relaxation with curare or pancuronium is now the method of choice. Patients with grossly

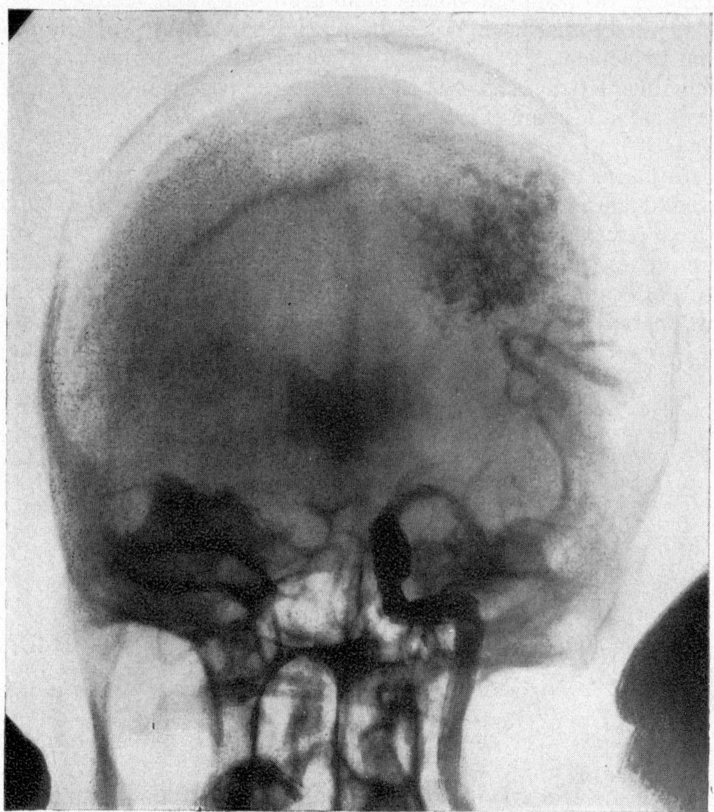

39/Fig. 5 (*a*)

raised intracranial pressure are better managed without anaesthesia, but if this is not possible relaxation and hyperventilation is preferable to the further increase in intracranial pressure which volatile agents and a rise in arterial carbon dioxide tension inevitably cause.

Certain dangers must be noted both in relation to the technique of arterial puncture and to the results of the injection of the radio-opaque dye. In arterio-sclerotic patients, particularly if firm pressure is not applied to the site of arterial puncture for some time after withdrawal of the needle, a haematoma may develop in the neck. When this lies behind the trachea it may cause respiratory embarrassment and necessitate the passage of an endotracheal tube (Fig. 7). Repeated attempts at arterial puncture may cause spasm of the vessel, and this can be offset to some extent by a liberal infiltration of local analgesic solution to which has been added a small quantity of 5 per cent papaverine solution.

The actual injection of dye may lead to various disturbances, but all are fortunately rare. Vomiting and coughing may occur, and marked hypotension may follow generalised vasodilatation (Duncalf and Thompson, 1956). The neurological sequelae recorded include hemiplegia, death from haemorrhage into a tumour or from an intracranial aneurysm, and transient blindness (Geddes, 1952). Temporary hypotension plays a part in the production of some palsies, but an element of vascular spasm and subsequent thrombosis is probably more dangerous. Extravasation of the dye into the neck can cause injury to the cervical sympathetic chain (Dunsmore *et al.*, 1951).

Brown (1955) has recorded a detailed description and discussion of the circulatory disturbance that may occur during or following cerebral angiography under general anaesthesia. When cases of recent spontaneous subarachnoid haemorrhage are submitted to the procedure, an immediate fall of blood pressure sometimes occurs. If the fall is slight, a return to normal usually occurs in a matter of minutes, but if it is severe recovery may take several hours, and supportive therapy may be necessary. Brown considers that hypotension of this

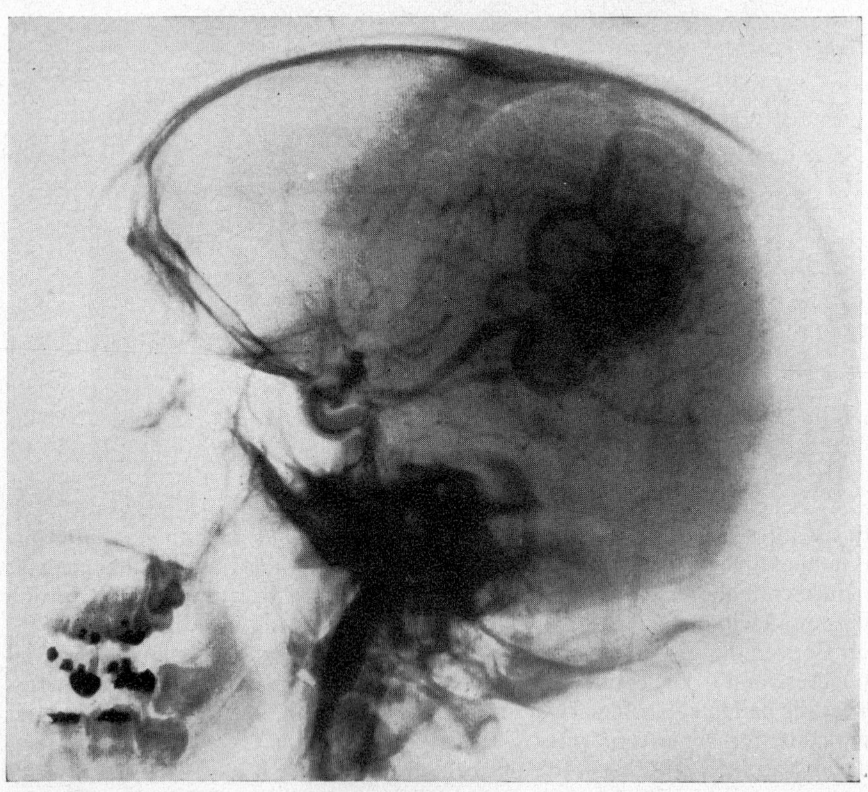

39/FIG. 5 (*b*)

39/FIG. 5. —Carotid arteriogram—haemangioma. (*a*) Antero-posterior, (*b*) Lateral.

type is due to the irritant effect of the dye on vessels which are already hypersensitive because of injury from haemorrhage in their vicinity. The degree of hypotension bears some relation to the site of the haemorrhage, its severity, and the time between its onset and the angiography.

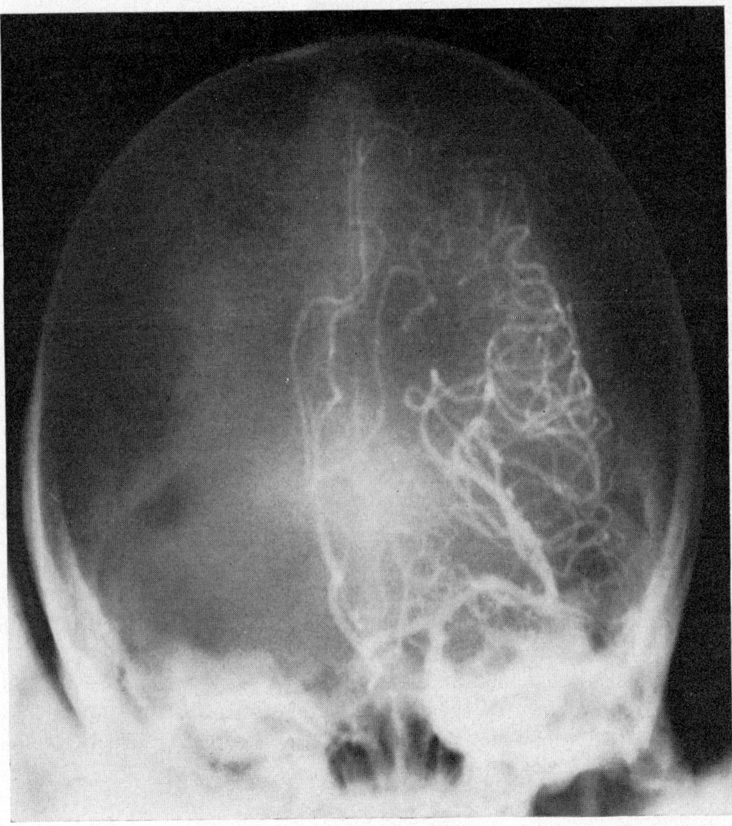

39/FIG. 6.—Subdural haematoma. Antero-posterior carotid arteriogram of a 60-year-old male with a severe head injury, showing lentiform avascular area over the cerebral hemisphere.

BACKGROUND TO ANAESTHETIC PRACTICE IN NEUROSURGERY

If the anaesthetist is to do more than satisfy the immediate aim of technical proficiency in neurosurgical anaesthesia he must have some background knowledge of the patient's disease, the neurosurgical procedure—its aims and the major steps in its performance—and the complications specific to the operation. Technical skill must not, however, be unduly denigrated, for there are few practical sides of anaesthesia in which obsessional attention to detail can be so effective in the final result, and in which a minor disruption can so quickly upset

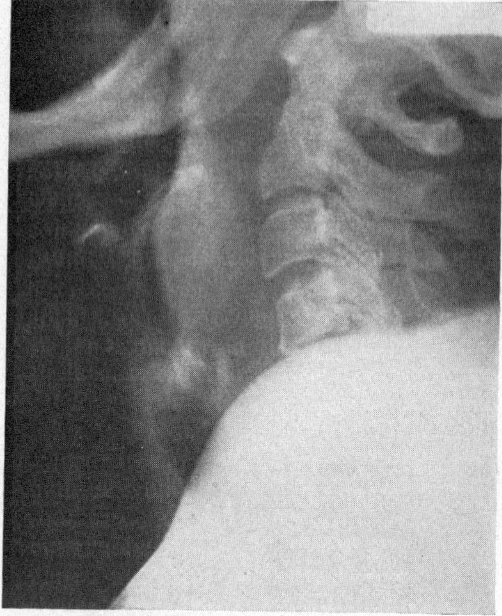

39/FIG. 7.—Haematoma causing tracheal obstruction following carotid arteriography.

the operation field, and perhaps jeopardise the patient's life. Despite the intricate formation of the brain and its connections, surprisingly extensive operations can be performed in its substance without permanent damage to important tissues, and without evoking any localised or generalised response on the part of a lightly anaesthetised patient. There are, however, exceptions, and the implications of these may be of importance.

Not every anaesthetist has the opportunity to work in a neurosurgical unit, so that some amplification of the subject is felt to be justified, even though it often represents an anaesthetist's view of the problem, largely consists of generalisation, and is far from exhaustive.

Circulatory and Respiratory Changes caused by Neurosurgical Operations

Observation of the pulse rate and blood pressure may enable the anaesthetist to warn the surgeon that he is disturbing the vital centres. Those centres which are likely to be damaged or stimulated lie in the floor of the third ventricle and hypothalamus or in the floor of the fourth ventricle near the dorsal portion of the pons and the medulla oblongata (Hunter, 1952). Interference with the hypothalamic centres may take place during an operation on the pituitary, or ones for a suprasellar cyst or for an olfactory groove meningioma—all of which abut on the vital area. Hypotension results and is an indication for the surgeon to stop at once. If the pressure then returns to normal in all probability all will be well, but persistent or severe hypotension suggests a bad prognosis. After irreversible hypothalamic damage the patient does not recover consciousness, but gradually succumbs over twenty-four to forty-eight hours with a rising pulse rate, hypotension and hyperpyrexia.

The centres in the floor of the fourth ventricle are sometimes affected during operations on the brain stem or in its vicinity. The damage may be direct, particularly when a tumour extends into that area, but may also be due to interference with the blood supply from thrombosis or the tearing of small vessels. The centres may also be indirectly affected if the brain stem is rotated during retraction. The alteration in pulse rate and blood pressure which these factors cause are variable, but usually take the form of temporary hypertension and bradycardia. The occurrence of either is an indication that all is not well. A sudden and marked hypertension, even though of brief duration, often portends permanent damage.

Bradycardia and temporary respiratory arrest have been noticed to follow deliberate or accidental stimulation of the uncal gyrus of a temporal lobe (Howland and Papper, 1952). These variations, like the tachycardia and respiratory irregularities which follow stimulation in light anaesthesia of those few intracranial structures with a sensory nerve supply, are not of grave significance, although the anaesthetist must seek for their cause. Persistent and increasing tachycardia usually heralds a rise in intracranial pressure due to obstruction to the flow of cerebrospinal fluid, and is most commonly seen in patients with subtentorial lesions. It is the earliest sign that pressure is building up and a warning that worse may follow in the form of a medullary coning, unless the ventricular pressure is quickly released.

Respiratory arrest may occur during intracranial surgery as a result of indirect interference with the vital centres—usually when tumours are growing in their vicinity—but it is usually temporary. It also occurs as the late result of medullary coning, and may momentarily follow the sudden release of a high intracranial pressure.

Cervical laminectomy for tumour removal may result in injury to the phrenic nerve roots with respiratory embarrassment. Laminectomies are sometimes associated with autonomic reflex activity. The mass reflex which may occur in patients with high spinal traumatic injuries is associated with sweating, bradycardia, and a very high blood pressure and has been noted under anaesthesia (Ciliberti *et al.*, 1954).

Tumours of the Cerebello-pontine Angle

The commonest tumour found in this vicinity is the acoustic neuroma, which arises from the eighth nerve within the internal auditory meatus. Although benign in nature, this tumour is in such close proximity to many cranial nerves and the vital centres of the brain that operative removal is associated with a high mortality and morbidity. Surgical treatment can be roughly divided into two groups. First, total removal, and secondly, intracapsular removal—though in fact part of the capsule is usually removed—but to appreciate the significance of each method certain factors must be considered.

The tumour is solid but usually has a quantity of fluid encapsulated in arachnoid mater around it. Within the internal meatus it is in close contact with the seventh cranial nerve, and, as it grows in size, it encroaches on the fifth, ninth, tenth, eleventh and twelfth cranial nerves, as well as the pons and cerebellum. Therefore total removal of the tumour and capsule may well result in permanent damage to the seventh nerve and enhances the risk of damage to the other nerves. Swallowing is very likely to be uncoordinated in the post-operative period and a plastic naso-gastric tube should be passed at induction. Retraction and operation in that area may also produce effects on the vital centres which lie in the floor of the fourth ventricle either directly or as a result of damage to the blood supply (see above). If the patient survives, total removal constitutes a cure, and a facial palsy can be improved by anastomosing this nerve to the hypoglossal nerve in the neck at a later operation, or by a sling operation designed to support the facial muscles. Neither of these plastic operations is very satisfactory, but the former improves the contour and movement of the face and helps to control a watery eye and mouth dribbling. On the other hand, it leads to hemiatrophy of the tongue. Intracapsular removal, although incomplete, and therefore likely to be followed by recurrence in a matter of years, is less likely to produce damage to adjacent structures, though it can and does do so on occasion. It can be argued, certainly so far as elderly patients are concerned, and particularly if they have coexisting disease in other systems, that an intracapsular removal is perfectly satisfactory treatment and likely to suit the normal expectation of life for such a patient. Choice of operation can also be made to justify a particular posture, since there can be no doubt that perfect access to the cerebello-pontine angle materially assists the surgeon to locate and avoid these important structures. Thus the upright or sitting position is nearly always routinely used by the advocates of total removal, though this in itself probably plays a part in the death of some patients either from air embolus or severe hypotension.

Subarachnoid Haemorrhage

The commonest cause of spontaneous subarachnoid haemorrhage is rupture of an intracranial aneurysm. Other causes are intracranial angiomata, spreading haemorrhage from a burst atheromatous vessel in the brain and, very rarely, certain blood diseases. Although there may be severe hypertension, spontaneous subarachnoid haemorrhage may also occur without evidence of local disease. McKissock (1956) has summarised the position by referring to the results of carotid angiography. On a statistical basis 50–60 of 100 patients admitted to hospital with spontaneous subarachnoid haemorrhage will be found to have an intracranial aneurysm either upon the circle of Willis or one of its major branches, about 10 patients will have an intracranial angioma, and in the remaining patients no vascular lesion will be demonstrated. The distribution and incidence of the major groups of intracranial aneurysms is illustrated in Fig. 8.

Speedy diagnosis is essential, and once cerebral arteriosclerosis and essential hypertension and other systemic diseases have been excluded by clinical methods, cerebral angiography should be carried out. The risk of this investigation causing a further bleed or enhancing the generalised spasm of the cerebral vessels that the original haemorrhage causes, is probably very small, and is in any event usually accepted nowadays. Diagnosis is an urgent matter, since the choice of treatment affects the prognosis. Once more the position has been concisely summarised by McKissock (1956). With medical treatment 50 per cent of patients shown to have an aneurysm will die during the first eight weeks after the first bleed and another 20 per cent will die from recurrent haemorrhage later. With surgical treatment 33·3 per cent of patients with a proven aneurysm will die in the first eight weeks. These figures are for intracranial aneurysms in all situations, and a more impressive case for active therapy can be made when the results of medical and surgical treatment of aneurysms at particular sites are analysed. Even in the most awkward situations surgical treatment more often offers a favourable result than the natural course of the disease (McKissock and

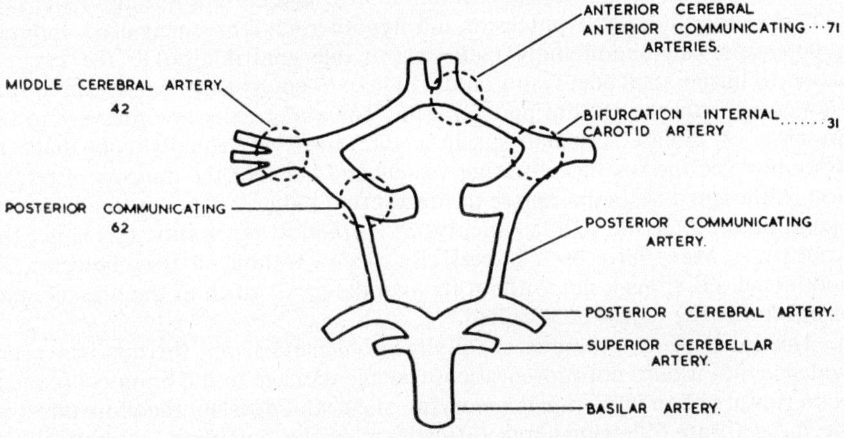

39/FIG. 8.—Diagram of the circle of Willis, showing distribution of major groups of aneurysm in a series of 206 patients.

Walsh, 1956). Although early operation is, therefore, usually recommended when the site of the aneurysm suggests that surgical treatment will be possible, picking the exact time to operate needs consideration. Immediate operation after establishment of the diagnosis is common practice, though this hardly leaves time for any associated vascular spasm in the neighbourhood of the haemorrhage to settle. In any event operation must not be delayed for more than a week as a second bleed commonly occurs on or about the tenth day.

Angiomata have a different natural history. They bleed at longer intervals than aneurysms and a second bleed, even when soon after the first, is not necessarily fatal. On the other hand, they are more often than not amenable to surgical treatment.

Some of the probable changes that take place after rupture of an intracranial aneurysm have been described by Logue (1956). Immediately following the rupture, the vessels in continuity with the aneurysm and near by it go into intense spasm. The spasm has the beneficial effect of reducing the tension of blood in the sac so that the tear shrinks in size and becomes sealed with clot. The spasm has the detrimental effect of producing ischaemia in the area of the brain supplied by the vessels and in about 15 per cent of cases the consequent cerebral oedema raises the intracranial pressure. It seems probable that spasm with its associated cerebral ischaemia and swelling is the cause of death or neurological damage in many cases, although destruction of brain substance plays a major part in some. Logue also stresses the importance of spasm in the small perforating vessels, particularly following rupture of an aneurysm of the anterior cerebral artery. Here the result will be ischaemia in the hypothalamus, basal ganglia and internal capsule, and the retraction necessary for the exposure of the aneurysm at operation is very likely to accentuate the damage.

It is consideration of factors such as these which illustrates the dangers of dogmatising on the virtues of induced hypotension or hypothermia. It is now established that the major advance in the improvement of operating conditions has been the use of controlled ventilation with moderate lowering of the P_{CO_2} so that neither induced hypotension nor hypothermia is routinely used. Induced hypotension can undoubtedly make a valuable contribution to the surgical access to intracranial aneurysms, and will help to control any sudden bleed that may occur from the sac during operation. The abnormally low pressure in the presence of intense vascular spasm could, however, equally contribute to thrombosis of the small perforating vessels and enhance the dangers of retraction. Although it is commonplace to suggest that induced hypotension has made operation on these intracranial aneurysms a practical possibility, this is not the strict truth. Many have been successfully treated without it. It is, however, an undoubted aid, though not without its own dangers, which in the present state of our knowledge must be accepted.

The value of hypothermia is equally problematical but there is increasing evidence that it does not prevent the ischaemic damage to the brain consequent upon rupture of an intracranial aneurysm, and that it does not therefore improve the survival rate following surgical treatment of this condition (Hamby, 1963). McKissock and his colleagues (1965), in a study of aneurysms of the anterior communicating artery, substantiate this view. Good arguments in favour of hypothermia are that it enables the surgeon to occlude temporarily a major end-artery, leads to a reduction in brain bulk, and helps to prevent the onset of cerebral oedema. However, the disadvantages and dangers of hypothermia *per se* must not be overlooked. When it is indicated a body temperature of not less than 30° C is satisfactory, but deep hypothermia to 20° C or less has been used for the surgical repair of intracranial aneurysms (Uihlein *et al.*, 1960; Michenfelder *et al.*, 1963).

Campkin and Dallas (1968) have described a technique for producing total circulatory arrest under hypothermia in the management of aneurysms of the anterior communicating and middle cerebral arteries. The method involves electrical pacing of the heart by an electrode in the right ventricle and occlusion of the ascending aorta with a saline-filled balloon on a catheter introduced through the right femoral artery. It is used only when the size or position of the aneurysm make its surgical occlusion particularly hazardous and the authors claim a reduction in the operative mortality.

Stereotactic Operations

Localised lesions can be produced in the depths of the brain by thermo-coagulation or by freezing with liquid nitrogen. Stereotaxis is the method by which the region to be treated is determined and localised. The technique is commonly used for making lesions of the globus pallidus in patients suffering from Parkinsonism. It is also valuable for the treatment of intractable pain and has recently been used for frontal leucotomy. Local analgesia will suffice but it is not always pleasant for the patient. When general anaesthesia is used it must be so chosen that at certain times during the operative procedure the patient will regain consciousness and co-operate fully with the surgeon. This is particularly important during the stage of stimulation when the area of the brain to be treated is being localised, and while the lesion is being made. Coleman and De Villiers (1964) describe a technique for anaesthesia consisting simply of the continuous intravenous infusion of a 0·1 per cent solution of methohexitone. When tremor or abnormal movements are severe they also use small paretic doses of gallamine triethiodide to induce some reduction in muscle power. No premedication is used, and all sedative drugs are stopped for 24 hours before the operation. By stopping or slowing the drip it it possible to effect a rapid return of full consciousness, or, in an unduly apprehensive subject, a co-operative but sedated patient. An alternative technique is to make use of neuroleptanalgesia which provides sedation and suppression of mental and physical discomfort, but leaves the patient co-operative (Brown, 1964), (see p. 1107).

Leucotomy

This operation is so commonly performed that it merits brief mention, although there are no anaesthetic problems peculiar to it. The mental state of the patient makes general anaesthesia almost mandatory, and occasionally necessitates particular care in the choice of pre-operative sedation and of induction of anaesthesia. The operation consists of division of the white matter below the prefrontal cortex and between this and the basal ganglia. It is modified to suit the particular patient.

Since leucotomy is a "blind" procedure in the sense that the brain is divided by a blunt leucotome through a burr hole, care is taken to avoid haemorrhage. Vessels are pushed out of the way by the instrument. Although it is very uncommon indeed, continuous bleeding into the brain substance is the principal cause of mortality following this operation, so that a congested brain, which might increase this hazard, must be avoided.

At one time and another it has been suggested that acute hypotension may occur during the brain cut, but there does not seem to be any reason why this should happen, and in practice it does not.

Cordotomy (Tractotomy) and Rhizotomy

Cordotomy is a gross but effective method of treating severe pain on either or both sides of the body. It is usually performed for those patients in whom neoplastic disease is the cause of the pain and in whom a reasonable expectation of life seems likely. A successful result enables more general treatment, such as that by opiates, to be stopped, or at least diminished. It is worth noting that patients who have been treated by large doses of opiates prior to a successful cordotomy do not always crave for these drugs when they are stopped. The therapy of genuine pain by large doses of opiates does not apparently invariably lead to addiction.

Cordotomy is always done at the cervical level so that the sense of touch is undisturbed, and a bilateral cut is rarely performed at the same operation, in order to avoid sphincter disturbances. If a bilateral cordotomy is needed then an interval of 6–8 weeks is usually allowed between the two. The approach is as for a laminectomy and the actual cord division is gross enough to be performed under general anaesthesia, although a more accurate assessment of the extent of section can be made if the patient is awake and co-operative. In this country general anaesthesia is commonly used. Simple infiltration is a not very successful method of ensuring good pain relief for laminectomy, though it can be used in combination with light enough anaesthesia to ensure sufficient return of consciousness at the crucial time. Segmental epidural analgesia will provide complete analgesia in the operation site without disturbing the area of pain and thus allowing adequate testing during the operation (Krumperman *et al.*, 1957).

Rhizotomy, or root section, is a precise method of treating pain which can be localised. With the exception of the cranial nerves, it is usual also to cut the nerve roots above and below the one supplying the affected segment, since there is an overlap in the sensory supply from the spinal nerves.

POST-OPERATIVE CARE OF THE NEUROSURGICAL PATIENT

The immediate post-operative period is of considerable importance in neurosurgical practice. After cranial operations it may be difficult to distinguish between the effects of surgery and of anaesthesia—both may make common ground in the production of unconsciousness. In this respect anaesthesia can only be considered perfect when it ceases as soon as the surgeon completes the operation, for then the level of consciousness and the state of reflex activity are true guides to the condition of the patient. Unfortunately neither anaesthesia nor surgery is invariably perfect, and their combined or individual effects sometimes create problems which make the immediate post-operative period of considerable importance.

The sensitive intracranial mechanisms, already disturbed by the surgical procedure, may easily become unbalanced by apparently trivial complications of anaesthesia, and it is no exaggeration to suggest that a brief anoxic episode or a momentary rise in the level of carbon dioxide in the blood might even affect the patient's chance of survival. Either accentuates the element of cerebral oedema that follows all cerebral surgery. Oxygen should be given at this time for the first few hours and if there is any doubt about the adequacy of ventilation the endotracheal tube should be left in place and mechanical ventilation continued. Even successful surgery—successful, that is, by the standard of removing a tumour completely—may be followed by nerve palsies, or more bizarre complications such as vasomotor collapse, hyperpyrexia, and respiratory disorders, all of which cause exceptional difficulties.

Thus the normal hazards of the post-anaesthetic period and the special requirements of the neurosurgical patient are a strong indication for the provision of recovery room space next to the operating theatre, so that both anaesthetist and surgeon can be within sight and sound of the patient at this potentially critical time.

Routine Post-operative Care

Apart from the patient, the most important person in the recovery room is the nurse. The institution of continuous and skilled nursing care after surgery plays a vital part in the reduction of overall morbidity for many cranial operations. This is particularly so when cranial nerve palsies are present, since the dangers associated with partial respiratory obstruction and tracheal aspiration are very real. An adequate airway must be kept at all times, and in doubtful cases it is wiser to leave the endotracheal tube in position until the situation has clarified.

Observation

The nurse must observe and record all essential clinical data at regular intervals—every ten minutes for the first hour or so. Pulse and respiration rates, blood pressure level, the level of consciousness, response to stimuli, fluid intake, drugs given and any other points likely to be of value must be written down. These observations are of paramount importance in assessing the progress of intracranial complications, while differentiation of the effects of anaesthesia from those of surgery is possible only if a record is available to show the general trend of events. Thus the earliest signs of reactionary haemorrhage may be the onset of sleep in a previously sleepy but conscious patient, or a rise in blood pressure in a semi-conscious one.

Posture

As soon as consciousness is regained, and provided the systolic blood pressure is over 100 mm. Hg, patients who have had cranial operations should be brought to a sitting position. Even before this, if the danger of vomiting can be circumvented or appears unlikely—patients can be reflexly normal but cerebrally unconscious—it may be advisable to have the head raised on pillows. The prime object of posture at this early stage is to reduce the twin risks of cerebral oedema and reactionary haemorrhage. However, in the exceptional case it may be wiser to wait several hours before sitting the patient up at all. Occasions of this type occur after removal of a large tumour from the posterior fossa, when the adjacent compressed tissues cannot be expected to fill up the resulting hole straight away. In these circumstances a sudden change in posture could lead to marked movement of the brain stem, due to inadequate compensation for the change in blood pressure, and consequent disturbance of function.

Patients who have had a laminectomy are nursed flat for several days.

At a later stage in the post-operative period posture must also be adjusted to encourage lung drainage, particularly for those patients who remain semi-conscious or suffer from respiratory dysfunctions.

Changes in posture are facilitated by nursing all neurosurgical patients in special beds designed to tilt or rise in various ways with minimal inconvenience to the patient or nursing staff.

Sedation and Analgesia

Patients who have had cranial operations do not usually suffer from acute pain as a result of surgery. They are often restless and occasionally nauseated, particularly after operations in the posterior fossa, but rarely uncomfortable except from headache. The reason for this presumably lies in the insensitiveness of the structures involved, the skin being a notable exception, and the fact that movement of the patient is not, as in most other operative sites, reflected in increased tension in the wound. Laminectomy wounds, however, are very painful and usually require full doses of a potent analgesic such as an opiate or analogue. These agents are never necessary after cranial surgery, and indeed their potency, accentuated by the lack of acute pain, coupled with their well-known side-effects—particularly respiratory depression and pupillary contraction—contra-indicate their use.

The restlessness and headache can be adequately controlled by codein phosphate in a dosage of from 32 to 65 mg., combined if necessary with phenobarbitone 100 to 200 mg. and given intramuscularly. The effectiveness of codein as an analgesic is open to doubt, but as a mild sedative without marked side-effects it is useful in these circumstances. Occasional patients may be so seriously disturbed by the surgery as to become vociferous and in need of restraint. For these, paraldehyde intramuscularly (2–3 ml.) is very effective.

Intravenous Fluids

There is still no general agreement about the exact distribution of water between the cells and the extracellular fluid in the brain. It is however agreed that cerebral oedema, unlike oedema in its more usual manifestations, is due to intracellular accumulation of water particularly in the white matter (Aldridge, 1965). Equilibration of water between blood and brain is very rapid and occurs within a few minutes (Bering, 1952), and it is extremely important not to over-hydrate neurosurgical patients in the immediate post-operative period.

Many patients are able to take fluids by mouth in a matter of hours and if the intravenous infusion has been left running it is very easy to give them more fluid than is desirable. It is wise to restrict the total fluid intake by all routes to 1½–2 litres on the day of operation and on the following day. Temporary diabetes insipidus is not uncommon after operations near the hypothalamus and if a catheter has been passed can be recognized during operation by a sudden increase in urine volume—usually to between 7 and 12 ml./minute. In such cases dextrose/saline (4·3 per cent dextrose in 0·18 per cent saline) should be given 3 hourly in amounts equivalent to the previous 3-hourly urine volume if the patient is unable to drink.

Blood.—The blood loss in neurosurgery is difficult to estimate and impossible to measure accurately during operation. It is essential to insert a large bore intravenous cannula and when heavy losses are expected a second one is a wise precaution. It is preferable to keep the neurosurgical patient slightly oligaemic and extremely undesirable to over-transfuse. Dextran 70 in isotonic saline may be used when the estimated blood loss is considered too small to justify the use of blood.

Cerebral Oedema

Apart from posture, the most effective method of reducing raised intracranial pressure is intravenous mannitol. Its use at induction is described on page 1124. When used post-operatively 500 ml. of 10 per cent mannitol is given in the course of an hour and repeated 12 hourly. During this time the total fluid intake (including the volume of the mannitol solution) is restricted to 2 litres in 24 hours. Such a regime cannot usually be continued safely for more than 48 hours as it will cause progressive depletion of body water. This is indicated by a rise in serum sodium concentration which should not be allowed to exceed 155–160 mEq/l.

Alternative methods of treatment are by repeated lumbar puncture with the withdrawal of small quantities of CSF and the use of oral glycerol.

Reactionary Haemorrhage

Bleeding into the operation site leads to a rise in intracranial pressure which will be manifested by the signs already described, but specific localising signs, such as nerve palsies, which can be accounted for by the pressure of the accumulating blood clot, may also be present.

Treatment is essentially operative to remove the blood and stop the bleeding. Anaesthesia is often not required but an endotracheal tube should be passed with the aid of a relaxant, and adequate ventilation ensured. Once the compression has been relieved, however, anaesthesia will be needed, since consciousness often rapidly returns.

Particular note must be taken of the quantity of blood lost when a craniotomy wound is re-opened, and immediate replacement made should it appear necessary. Despite the constricted space in which the bleeding takes place, a surprisingly large quantity of blood can be lost while re-opening the wound since such an emergency allows no time for meticulous haemostasis until after the clot has been evacuated. Circulatory collapse during reactionary haemorrhage or while re-opening is in part due to central factors, but undoubtedly owes something to blood loss. This simple fact must not be forgotten.

Special Post-operative Care

Operations in the posterior fossa, particularly those for total extirpation of an acoustic neuroma, may be followed by cranial nerve palsies. Following removal of an acoustic tumour, a seventh nerve palsy is not uncommon, but more dangerous in the immediate post-operative period are palsies of the glossopharyngeal and vagus nerves. These may be only temporary and incomplete, but while present swallowing lacks co-ordination, and with laryngeal and glottic sensitivity diminished normal feeding may lead to aspiration into the respiratory tract. For this reason it is a good plan to have a plastic tube of 4 to 6 mm. diameter passed through the nose into the stomach before the operation is started. During the post-operative period all feeds should be given down this tube and great care taken to avoid vomiting or regurgitation, either of which may lead to aspiration. A suction apparatus should be next to the bed at all times. After 48 hours, a small quantity of water should be given to the patient by mouth to test whether swallowing is normal; if it is, the tube should be removed. When there is any likelihood of fifth nerve damage, a tarsorrhaphy should be performed to protect the affected eye.

Patients who remain unconscious or semi-conscious for more than an hour or so after operation should be treated generally in a similar manner, and when they seem likely to remain in such a condition for several days—yet with a prospect of ultimate recovery—a temporary tracheostomy must be considered. Certain complications—pulmonary aspiration lesions or inadequate ventilation—may be considered as indications for tracheostomy, but unconsciousness alone is not, provided competent nursing staff is available.

When gross aspiration of stomach contents into the lungs occurs during a bout of vomiting or regurgitation—a rare complication with adequate supervision and posturing—immediate bronchoscopy with lavage offers a reasonable prospect of removing the material and preventing infection. There are rarely, if ever, any other indications for bronchoscopy in the post-operative treatment of neurosurgical patients, or even for suction through an endotracheal tube. Simple pulmonary complications are best treated by posture and encouragement of normal drainage. If these fail, and the essential cause—such as unconsciousness or semiconsciousness—persists, then a tracheostomy enables efficient suction to be carried out simply and at regular intervals.

Respiratory Failure

This may be the terminal result of a rising intracranial pressure—in which case the essential treatment is that of the cause—of surgical interference, or of the direct effect of the disease process.

Operations on the cervical cord may be attended by bilateral phrenic paralysis, and although intercostal activity may be complete it is unlikely to be sufficient to maintain adequate ventilation, particularly during the immediate post-operative period. In cases of this type assisted or controlled respiration, preferably by a mechanical respirator, should be carried out, and a tracheostomy considered.

Vasomotor Failure

Hypotension is more often central than peripheral in origin. A peculiar type of circulatory collapse, characterised by a low blood pressure, with a slow pulse and dilated peripheral vessels, sometimes occurs after operations in the region of the fourth ventricle. The degree of hypotension is often sufficient to cause unconsciousness. Repeated intramuscular or intravenous doses of methoxamine, 5–10 mg., may be successful in restoring the blood pressure to normal, but more often than not the initial cause is incurable and the condition fatal.

Hyperpyrexia

So often in cranial surgery the post-operative complications are indicative of irreversible lesions in the brain itself, so that treatment, however effective in controlling the measurable signs or symptoms, only very rarely cures the cause. This is particularly true of severe hyperpyrexia, which is more often than not due to thrombosis in the region of the brain stem or thalamus. For such cases the production of hypothermia or the use of drugs such as chlorpromazine is unlikely to be successful—a more simple procedure, such as tepid sponging, is usually just as effective. If, however, the hyperpyrexia is likely to be due to cerebral oedema, then the more active measures may be found helpful.

Pulmonary Oedema

Certain operations in the region of the mid-brain, typically for tumours in the floor of the fourth ventricle, may be followed by pulmonary oedema. Here again postural drainage is the simple treatment of choice, but intubation and mechanical ventilation should be started if it is not quickly brought under control. The use of frusemide in the treatment of pulmonary oedema is mentioned on page 663.

Post-operative problems peculiar to operations on the pituitary are discussed in Chapter 50.

ACUTE HEAD INJURIES

Bryce-Smith (1950) has pointed out the contribution that an anaesthetist may make to the care of patients with acute head injuries. Four factors are likely to be present which may affect the adequacy of the airway when the patient is unconscious. First, there may be severe reflex depression. Not only can the tongue cause obstruction but the cough reflex may be in abeyance. Second, gastric motility is reduced and the likelihood of vomiting or regurgitation is increased. Third, the direct results of injury may affect various parts of the oropharynx, and bleeding or cerebrospinal fluid leaking from a fractured base may add to the difficulties. Fourth, there may be pulmonary oedema of central origin.

For these reasons it is essential that all such patients should be transported and managed in the semi-prone position with a slight head-down tilt if other injuries allow. They are particularly at risk during emergency radiography. If unobstructed breathing cannot be achieved with an oropharyngeal airway, or if the patient is deeply unconscious, a cuffed endotracheal tube should be passed and the stomach contents aspirated through a large bore oesophageal tube. If shock is present it should be treated and its cause sought as it is seldom due to an uncomplicated head injury. As soon as the airway is secure and the blood pressure allows, the head and shoulders should be raised to prevent aggravation of cerebral swelling.

The respiratory gas changes following head injury have been described by Froman (1968). The usual findings are reduced arterial tensions of both oxygen and carbon dioxide, and oxygen should accordingly be added to the inspired air.

If an anaesthetic becomes necessary it will inevitably tend to aggravate damage already caused to the brain and everything possible should be done to minimise this. Blood loss, particularly in children, may be considerable and an "open vein" is essential. If there is any likelihood of a fracture causing a dural tear and cerebrospinal fluid leak, oxygen should be given before induction and inflation with a facemask avoided. Reference has already been made to the increase in intracranial pressure caused by all the non-explosive volatile anaesthetics and the method of choice is a relaxant technique with moderate hyperventilation. It is important to use this method even if the surgery has nothing to do with the treatment of the head injury.

Immediate tracheostomy has tended to give place to a trial period making use of an endotracheal tube. Once the acute phase is over a nasotracheal tube has several advantages and Rees and Owen-Thomas (1966) have described one which is particularly suitable. Such a tube may be left down for 48 to 72 hours during which oxygen-enriched humidified air is given. If secretions form which cannot easily be aspirated the tube must be changed at once. The respiratory blood gas tensions should be closely monitored and if the P_{CO_2} begins to rise or the P_{O_2} cannot be kept above 80–90 mm. Hg ventilation should be taken over. Many patients can be extubated after this trial period and tracheostomy is resorted to only if the airway cannot be kept clear or if sputum retention cannot be overcome.

The long-term care of an unconscious patient necessitates continuous, devoted nursing and special attention to diet, sedation and the prevention of infection. Feeding should whenever possible be by naso-oesophageal tube, the only exception being when intestinal disturbances make an adequate fluid and food intake by this route impracticable. Particular care must be taken to ensure a proper fluid and electrolyte balance and to prevent muscle wasting by providing the correct amount of protein.

REFERENCES

ALDRIDGE, W. N. (1965). The pathology and chemistry of experimental oedema in the brain. *Proc. roy. Soc. Med.*, **58,** 599.

ANDERSON, S., and MCKISSOCK, W. (1953). Controlled hypotension with Arfonad in neurosurgery. *Lancet*, **2,** 754.

ASERMAN, D. (1953). Controlled hypotension in neurosurgery with hexamethonium bromide and procaine amide. *Brit. med. J.*, **1,** 961.

BALLANTINE, R. I. W. (1956). Hypophysectomy. *Anaesthesia*, **11,** 303.

BALLANTINE, R. I. W., and JACKSON, I. (1954). Anaesthesia for neurosurgical operations. *Anaesthesia*, **9,** 4.

BATSON, O. V. (1940). The function of the vertebral veins and their rôle in the spread of metastases. *Ann. Surg.*, **112,** 138.

BERING, E. A. (1952). Water exchange of central nervous system and cerebrospinal fluid. *J. Neurosurg.*, **9,** 275.

BERING, E. A., and AVMAN, N. (1960). The use of hypertonic urea solutions in hypothermia. An experimental study. *J. Neurosurg.*, **17,** 1073.

BOURNE, J. G. (1957). Fainting and cerebral damage. *Lancet*, **2,** 499.

BROWN, A. S. (1955). Circulatory disturbances during cerebral angiography. *Anaesthesia*, **10,** 346.

BROWN, A. S. (1959). Controlled respiration in neurosurgical anaesthesia. *Anaesthesia*, **14,** 207.

BROWN, A. S. (1964). Neuroleptanalgesia for the surgical treatment of Parkinsonism. *Anaesthesia*, **19,** 70.

BRYCE-SMITH, R. (1950). The management of head injuries from the anaesthetist's point of view. *Brit. med. J.*, **2,** 322.

BURNS, T. H. S. (1956). A danger from flexometallic endotracheal tubes. *Brit. med. J.*, **1,** 439.

BURROWS, M. MC., DUNDEE, J. W., FRANCIS, I. LL., LIPTON, S., and SEDZIMIR, C. B. (1956). Hypothermia for neurological operations. *Anaesthesia*, **11,** 4.

BUSHMAN, J. A., and COLLIS, J. M. (1967). The estimation of gas losses in ventilator tubing. *Anaesthesia*, **22,** 664.

CAMPKIN, T. V., and DALLAS, S. H. (1968). Elective surgical arrest in neurosurgical operations. *Brit. J. Anaesth.*, **40,** 527.

CANTORE, G., GUIDETTI, B., and VIRNO, M. (1964). Oral glycerol for the reduction of intracranial pressure. *J. Neurosurg.*, **21,** 278.

CHEATLE, C. A., and MACKENZIE, R. M. (1953). Anaesthesia for cranial surgery in the sitting position. *Anaesthesia*, **8,** 182.

CILIBERTI, B. J., GOLDFEIN, J., and ROVENSTINE, E. A. (1954). Hypertension during anesthesia in patients with spinal cord injuries. *Anesthesiology*, **15,** 273.

COLEMAN, D. J., and DE VILLIERS, J. C. Anaesthesia and stereotactic surgery. *Anaesthesia*, **19,** 60.

DALLAS, S. H., and MOXON, C. P. (1969). Controlled ventilation for cerebral angiography. *Brit. J. Anaesth.*, **41,** 597.

de Wardener, H. E., Miles, B. E., Lee, G. de J., Churchill-Davidson, H. C., Wylie, D., and Sharpey-Schafer, E. P. (1953). Circulatory effects of haemorrhage during prolonged light anaesthesia in man. *Clin. Sci.*, **12,** 175.

Duckworth, S. I. (1962). The Oxford non-kinking endotracheal tube. *Anaesthesia*, **17,** 208.

Duncalf, D., and Thompson, P. W. (1956). Anaesthesia for cardiovascular and neurosurgical radiological investigations. *Brit. J. Anaesth.*, **2,** 450.

Dunsmore, R., Scoville, W. B., and Whitcomb, B. B. (1951). Complications of angiography. *J. Neurosurg.*, **8,** 110.

Fitch, W., Barker, J., McDowall, D. G., and Jennett, W. B. (1969). The effect of methoxyflurane on cerebrospinal fluid pressure in patients with and without intracranial space-occupying lesions. *Brit. J. Anaesth.*, **41,** 564.

Froman, C. (1968). Alterations of respiratory function in patients with severe head injuries. *Brit. J. Anaesth.*, **40,** 354.

Furness, D. N. (1957). Controlled respiration in neurosurgery. *Brit. J. Anaesth.*, **29,** 415.

Galloon, S. (1959). Controlled respiration in neurosurgical anaesthesia. *Anaesthesia*, **14,** 223

Geddes, I. C. (1952). Anaesthesia for cerebral angiography. *Brit. J. Anaesth.*, **24,** 252.

Hamby, W. B. (1963). Intracranial surgery for aneurysm. *J. Neurosurg.*, **20,** 41.

Hellings, P. M. (1958). Controlled hypothermia: recent developments in the use of hypothermia in neurosurgery. *Brit. med. J.*, **2,** 346.

Hewer, A. J. H. (1952). The practical aspects of neurosurgical anaesthesia. *Proc. roy. Soc. Med.*, **45,** 431.

Howland, W. S., and Papper, E. M. (1952). Circulatory changes during anesthesia for neurosurgical operations. *Anesthesiology*, **13,** 343.

Hunter, A. R. (1952). The present position of anaesthesia for neurosurgery. *Proc. roy. Soc. Med.*, **45,** 427.

Hunter, A. R. (1960). Discussion on the value of controlled respiration in neurosurgery. *Proc. roy. Soc. Med.*, **53,** 365.

Hunter, A. R. (1962). Air embolism in the sitting position. *Anaesthesia*, **17,** 467.

James, A., Coulter, R. L., and Saunders, J. W. (1953). Controlled hypotension in neurosurgery. *Lancet*, **1,** 412.

Jennett, W. B., Barker, J., Fitch, W., and McDowall, D. G. (1969). Effect of anaesthesia on intracranial pressure in patients with space-occupying lesions. *Lancet*, **1,** 61.

Kety, S. S., and Schmidt, C. F. (1948). Effects of altered arterial tensions of carbon dioxide and oxygen on cerebral blood flow and cerebral oxygen consumption of normal young men. *J. clin. Invest.*, **27,** 484.

Krumperman, L. W., Murtagh, F., and Wester, M. R. (1957). Epidural block anesthesia for cordotomy. *Anesthesiology*, **18,** 316.

Langfitt, T. W. (1961). Possible mechanisms of action of hypertonic urea in reducing intracranial pressure. *Neurology* (*Minneap.*), **11,** 196.

Logue, V. (1956). Surgery in spontaneous subarachnoid haemorrhage due to intracranial aneurysms. *Brit. med. J.*, **1,** 473.

Macintosh, R. R., Mushin, W. W., and Epstein, H. G. (1958). *Physics for the Anaesthetist*, 2nd edit. Oxford: Blackwell Scientific Publications.

McDowall, D. G., Barker, J., and Jennett, W. B. (1966). Cerebrospinal fluid pressure measurements during anaesthesia. *Anaesthesia*, **21,** 189.

McKissock, W. (1956). Subarachnoid haemorrhage. *Ann. roy. Coll. Surg. Engl.*, **19,** 361.

McKissock, W., Richardson, A., and Walsh, L. (1965). Anterior communicating aneurysms. *Lancet*, **1**, 873.

McKissock, W., and Walsh, L. (1956). Subarachnoid haemorrhage due to intracranial aneurysms. *Brit. med. J.*, **2**, 559.

Marrubini, M. B., and Tretola, L. (1965). Diazepam as a pre-operative tranquillizer in neuro-anaesthesia. *Brit. J. Anaesth.*, **37**, 934.

Michenfelder, J. D., Terry, H. R., Daw, E. F., MacCarty, C. S., and Uihlein, A. (1963). Profound hypothermia in neurosurgery: open-chest versus closed chest techniques. *Anesthesiology*, **24**, 177.

Moniz, E. (1940). *Die Cerebrale Arteriographie und Phlebographie*. Berlin.

Mortimer, P. L. F. (1959). Controlled respiration in neurosurgical anaesthesia. *Anaesthesia*, **14**, 205.

Pearce, D. J. (1957). The role of posture in laminectomy. *Proc. roy. Soc. Med.*, **50**, 109.

Pitkin, G. P. (1953). *Conduction Anesthesia*, 2nd edit. Philadelphia: J. B. Lippincott Co.

Rees, G. J., and Owen-Thomas, J. B. (1966). A technique of pulmonary ventilation with a nasotracheal tube. *Brit. J. Anaesth.*, **38**, 901.

Rosomoff, H. L. (1962). Distribution of intracranial contents after hypertonic urea. *J. Neurosurg.*, **19**, 859.

Rosomoff, H. L. (1963). Distribution of intracranial contents with controlled hyperventilation: implications for neuroanesthesia. *Anesthesiology*, **24**, 640.

Rosomoff, H. L., and Gilbert, R. (1955). Brain volume and cerebrospinal fluid pressure during hypothermia. *Amer. J. Physiol.*, **183**, 19.

Rosomoff, H. L., and Holaday, D. A. (1954). Cerebral blood flow and cerebral oxygen consumption during hypothermia. *Amer. J. Physiol.*, **179**, 85.

Samuel, J. R., Grange, R., and Hawkins, T. D. (1968). Anaesthetic technique for carotid angiography. *Anaesthesia*, **23**, 543.

Stubbs, J., and Pennybacker, J. (1960). Reduction of intracranial pressure with hypertonic urea. *Lancet*, **1**, 1094.

Taylor, A. R., Gleadhill, C. A., Bilsland, W. L., and Murray, P. F. (1956). Posture and anaesthesia for spinal operations with special reference to intervertebral disc surgery. *Brit. J. Anaesth.*, **28**, 213.

Uihlein, A., Theye, R. A., Dawson, B., Terry, H. R., McGoon, D. C., Daw, E. F., and Kirklin, J. W. (1960). The use of profound hypothermia, extracorporeal circulation and total circulatory arrest for an intracranial aneurysm. *Proc. Mayo Clin.*, **35**, 567.

Wise, B. L., and Chater, N. (1962). The value of hypertonic mannitol solution in decreasing brain mass and lowering cerebrospinal-fluid pressure. *J. Neurosurg.*, **19**, 1038.

Wolf, A., and Siris, J. (1937). Acute non-traumatic encephalomalacia complicating neurosurgical operations in the sitting position. *Bull. neurol. Inst. N.Y.*, **6**, 42.

Wylie, W. D. (1951). Some aspects of anaesthesia for neurosurgery, with special reference to pethidine hydrochloride. *G. ital. Anest.*, **17**, 305.

FURTHER READING

McComish, P. B., and Bodley, P. O. (1971). *Anaesthesia for Neurological Surgery*. London: Lloyd-Luke (Medical Books).

Chapter 40

ANAESTHESIA FOR OPHTHALMIC OPERATIONS AND FOR ELECTROCONVULSIVE THERAPY

OPHTHALMIC OPERATIONS

ALTHOUGH an increasing number of ophthalmic operations are performed today under general anaesthesia in preference to local analgesia, the wide variety of drugs available offers a choice of methods which include local analgesia alone, local analgesia with sedation, general anaesthesia alone and general anaesthesia combined with local analgesia.

Traditionally, local analgesia has much to recommend it for this branch of surgery, because the operations performed are usually limited in extent and complete loss of pain can be accomplished fairly easily. But local analgesia has disadvantages and hazards. It is unsatisfactory for unco-operative patients, for children and for those people with disease of the eye which might be accentuated by local analgesia. Rosen (1962) lists three principal hazards. An incomplete block may lead to compression of the globe. If this occurs when the eye is open there will be expulsion of the intra-ocular contents. A retrobulbar haemorrhage produced during local block will cause a tense orbit and compression of the globe, prolapse of the iris, expulsion of the lens and loss of vitreous may all follow. Direct penetration of the optic nerve meninges may involve the optic nerve in trauma.

The main disadvantages of general anaesthesia are the potential complications of coughing and straining and these, though easily prevented by a skilled anaesthetist during anaesthesia, may occur in the post-operative period: there is also perhaps an increased incidence of nausea and vomiting. However these disadvantages can usually be avoided whilst on the positive side a properly selected and well managed general anaesthetic has much to offer to both patient and surgeon. Apart from the patient's personal views, many surgeons prefer general anaesthesia provided the local conditions in the eye can match those of local analgesia, as an unconscious patient makes the whole procedure much easier.

Local Analgesia

Topical.—The installation of 2 per cent cocaine drops provides satisfactory surface analgesia lasting about half an hour. Cocaine dilates the pupil and slightly damages the corneal epithelium; the former contra-indicates its use for cases with glaucoma whilst the latter produces haziness which impedes the surgeon's view of the intracapsular structures. It is a satisfactory agent for cataract operations. Amethocaine 0·5 per cent or 1 per cent is equally effective, lasts longer and neither causes corneal damage nor dilates the pupil, but it is a vasodilator and therefore causes mild conjunctival hyperaemia. Its properties

ELECTRIC CONVULSION THERAPY

No satisfactory explanation of the therapeutic action which may result from the passage of an electric current through the brain has yet been advanced. Electric convulsion therapy is thus entirely empirical, but the passage of time since Cerletti and Bini (1938) first described this method of treatment and the clinical successes in many thousands of patients throughout the world, bear witness to its value. The best results follow its use for states of endogenous depression—these most frequently, but not exclusively, occur in elderly patients—and it is also of value in some manic and stuporose conditions. Variable responses to electric convulsion therapy are very often an indication of unwise selection of patients.

The passage of the electric current results in an immediate loss of consciousness, a tonic convulsion of about 5 seconds duration, and, following this, a clonic convulsion during which regular muscular movements occur for 40 to 50 seconds. Consciousness with confusion returns in about a further 10 minutes, and full mental activity after 40 to 60 minutes. During the period of the convulsion respiration may be inadequate and a brief period of apnoea often follows this phase. Although the patient is fully conscious immediately before the current is passed, amnesia usually covers this period, besides a considerable part of the post-convulsion phase. Insufficient current may fail to precipitate a convulsion but it always produces loss of consciousness.

Patterson and King (1957) postulate two different sequences of events during electric convulsion therapy. First, direct stimulation of the intracranial structures, primarily of the pyramidal tracts at the level of the internal capsule, and of the cranial nerves. Secondly, indirect stimulation as the impulse passes first to the mid-brain and then back to the motor area of the cortex. The first part of the sequence is potentially dangerous in unmodified therapy as it leads to powerful muscular contractions of the whole body; but these can be diminished by placing the electrodes far forward on the head and allowing the current to pass for a very brief duration. The second part of the sequence is described by Patterson and King as a tonic-clonic self-continuing convulsion and the therapeutic process of value.

Unilateral ECT to the non-dominant hemisphere was first proposed in 1957. Its increasing use represents an advance in technique, in that it reduces the incidence and severity of memory disturbance associated with bilateral treatment, while attaining the same therapeutic results (Zinkin and Birtchnell, 1968).

The patient can be partially controlled by covering the body with a blanket or canvas sheet and having this firmly held by several attendants so that some restraint is exerted against excessive movement. This is an incomplete method and for this purpose a very poor second best to the use of anaesthesia with a muscle relaxant. The complications of unmodified ECT are largely fractures, dislocations, and the results of hypoxia. The fractures are often vertebral and of the crush variety, occasionally not producing any symptoms, and indeed not always diagnosed until many months after treatment. Fractures of the upper end of the femur or humerus also occur. Hypoxia can be traced to the excessive demands of an unmodified convulsion—particularly in elderly patients who may have circulatory and respiratory disease—and the period of sub-oxygenation from inadequate ventilation during the convulsive phase.

Provided a competent anaesthetist is present, there can be little reason for refusing to give modified ECT using anaesthesia with relaxants. It is now fully accepted that fully modified ECT does not adversely affect the value of the treatment, but the specific effects of general anaesthesia must be borne in mind. Mental depression increases in frequency with advancing age, so that a considerable number of patients with hypertension and cardiac disease are submitted to treatment. Relative overdose of thiopentone or methohexitone may cause hypotension in these patients whilst mismanagement of respiratory paralysis after suxamethonium is given is also a hazard. Although an occasional prolonged apnoea is to be expected when relaxants are used, there are no reasons why it should be dangerous if a competent anaesthetist is present. It is sometimes difficult to guarantee an empty stomach in psychiatric out-patients, or even in-patients, while on occasion ECT may be an essential form of emergency treatment.

A final factor in favour of general anaesthesia is pleasantness, With it, the immediate preparations of the head and positioning of the electrodes, and most especially the brief period of post-convulsion, can be eliminated from consciousness.

General Anaesthesia

Sedative premedication is usually unnecessary but there is no objection to its use when specially indicated. A short-acting barbiturate is the most satisfactory method for such cases. Atropine sulphate 1·2 mg. must always be given, preferably intravenously either just before or mixed with the barbiturate so that an unpleasant dry mouth is avoided. Dobkin (1958) considers that ECT may occasionally produce a period of cardiac asystole which is normally brief, but could lead to cardiac arrest, and which can only be prevented by a large dose of atropine prior to treatment.

Anaesthesia may be induced with intravenous methohexitone, an average dose being 80–100 mg., and followed immediately by suxamethonium. Methohexitone offers the advantages over thiopentone of a quicker recovery and fewer cardiovascular disturbancs (Woodruff *et al.*, 1968). For the first treatment, the dose of suxamethonium can be assessed on a weight basis or taken as 30–40 mg. It is, however, important to record on the patient's notes both the doses of methohexitone and of suxamethonium given and the patient's response to them and the passage of the current. This enables the necessary adjustments to be made on subsequent occasions. Successful modification should allow slight twitching of the face and limbs, but little more. If no movements occur—because the dose of suxamethonium has been excessive—two signs may be useful as suggestive evidence of the successful passage of a current. The first is the presence of goose-flesh (Edridge, 1952) and the second, failure of the pupils to react when inspected immediately after the stimulus (Thomas and Honan, 1953).

As soon as the patient is paralysed the lungs must be inflated with 100 per cent oxygen for at least one minute: then the electrodes are fastened on to the head, a special prop placed in the mouth, and the current passed. A mouth prop must always be inserted between the upper and lower teeth; this is an essential preliminary because even with relaxants there is usually a response in the muscles of facial expression and of mastication to the effect of the electrical stimulus. It may be direct to the muscle, or possibly the result of a greater preponderance passing into the cranial nerves supplying these muscles than into the pyramidal tracts. In the latter event presumably the relaxant effect is overcome. The actual type of prop and its position must be selected with some care, bearing in mind the situation of any loose or poor teeth.

The current should be about 100 volts and its duration about one-third of a second. Immediately after its passage the patient should again be gently ventilated with oxygen until adequate spontaneous respiration returns. The patient can then be turned on to his side and allowed to rest until fully conscious and orientated, when he can safely be allowed to return home provided he is accompanied.

The return to consciousness is usually quiet if the patients have been properly selected for treatment, but unsuspected neurotics or hysterics may be difficult to control for a short period. The commonest complication of both unmodified and modified treatment is headache.

REFERENCES

ADAMS, A. K., and BARNETT, K. C. (1966). Anaesthesia and intraocular pressure. *Anaesthesia*, **21,** 202.

BREININ, G. M. (1962). *The Electrophysiology of Extraocular Muscle*, p. 1112. Toronto: University of Toronto Press.

BURN, R. A., and KNIGHT, P. (1969). Anaesthesia in ophthalmic surgery. *Brit. J. hosp. Med.*, **2,** 1527.

CERLETTI, V., and BINI, L. (1938). L'ettroshock. *Arch. gen. Neurol. Psichiat.*, **19,** 266.

DOBKIN, A. B. (1958). Cardiac arrest following electroplexy. *Lancet*, **1,** 640.

EDRIDGE, A. (1952). Discussion on new muscle relaxants in electric convulsion therapy. *Proc. roy. Soc. Med.*, **45,** 869.

KATZ, R. L., EAKINS, K. E., and LORD, C. O. (1968). The effects of hexafluorenium in preventing the increase in intraocular pressure produced by succinylcholine. *Anesthesiology*, **29,** 70.

MILLER, R. D., WAY, W. L., and HICKEY, R. F. (1968). Inhibition of succinylcholine-induced increased intraocular pressure by non-depolarising muscle relaxants. *Anesthesiology*, **29,** 123.

MOONIE, G. T., REES, D. I., and ELTON, D. (1964). The oculo-cardiac reflex during strabismus surgery. *Canad. Anaesth. Soc. J.*, **2,** 621.

PANTUCK, E. J. (1966). Ecothiopate iodine eye drops and prolonged response to suxamethonium. *Brit. J. Anaesth.*, **38,** 426.

PATTERSON, A. S., and KING, D. W. (1957). Electric convulsion fractures. *Brit. med. J.*, **1,** 1118.

ROSEN, D. A. (1962). Anaesthesia in ophthalmology. *Canad. Anaesth. Soc. J.*, **9,** 545.

THOMAS, E., and HONAN, B. F. (1953). Electro-convulsive therapy. *Brit. med. J.*, **2,** 97.

WOODRUFF, R. A., JNR., PITTS, F. N., and MCCLURE, J. N., JNR. (1968). The drug modification of E.C.T. I. Methohexital, thiopental and pre-oxygenation. *Arch. gen. Psychiat.*, **18,** 605.

ZINKIN, S., and BIRTCHNELL, J. (1968). Unilateral electro-convulsive therapy: its effect on memory and its therapeutic efficacy. *Brit. J. Psychiat.*, **14,** 973.

Chapter 41

THE PHARMACOLOGY OF LOCAL ANALGESIC DRUGS

by

DR. FELICITY REYNOLDS

A local analgesic drug is one which reversibly blocks nerve conduction beyond the point of application, when applied locally in the appropriate concentration. Many drugs have local analgesic properties, notably quinidine-like anti-arrhythmic drugs, antihistamines and β-adrenergic blockers, but this chapter refers only to those drugs used primarily for local analgesia.

History

For many centuries the inhabitants of the highlands of Peru and Bolivia chewed the leaves of the indigenous shrub *Erythroxylum coca* for the sake of their effects of diminishing fatigue and appetite. These effects are due primarily to the principal alkaloid they contain, namely cocaine. Numbing of the oral mucosa was, of course, merely regarded as a side-effect; it was not until the second half of the nineteenth century that the possible nature of the active substances contained in the plant roused the interest of scientific investigators in Europe. The active principal, cocaine, was first isolated in 1860 by Neimann, who noted its local analgesic effect. It was over a generation, however, before this discovery was exploited. In the 1880's Sigmund Freud studied the physiological effects of cocaine and used it to treat morphine addiction, thereby producing the first cocaine addict in Europe. While Freud was away visiting his fiancée in 1884, a colleague, Karl Köller introduced cocaine as a local analgesic for the eye at an ophthalmological congress, with immediate success. Freud was of course destined to become famous in other ways and so could afford to be magnanimous towards his colleague. Thereafter the field of local analgesics expanded quickly to include infiltration, nerve block and, later, spinal analgesia. Very soon the high systemic toxicity and addictive properties of cocaine stimulated the search for less toxic synthetic substitutes. A number of synthetic local analgesics emerged during this period, of which procaine, introduced by Einhorn in 1905, was the most important. It proved to be a drug with a much lower toxicity than cocaine, but with a short duration of action. Numerous related compounds with few advantages over procaine emerged in the years that followed, but the major advance of the period was probably the production of cinchocaine in Germany in the late 1920's. The next milestone was the introduction of lignocaine in 1948, and among the new drugs that have emerged since, bupivacaine, introduced in the 1960s, probably represents the greatest advance since lignocaine.

Chemistry

The local analgesics in current use have the following basic formula:

Aromatic lipophylic group	—	Intermediate chain (ester: —COO— or amide—NH.CO—)	—	hydrophylic group 2^{ary} or 3^{ary} amine.

Individual formulae are given in Fig. 1.

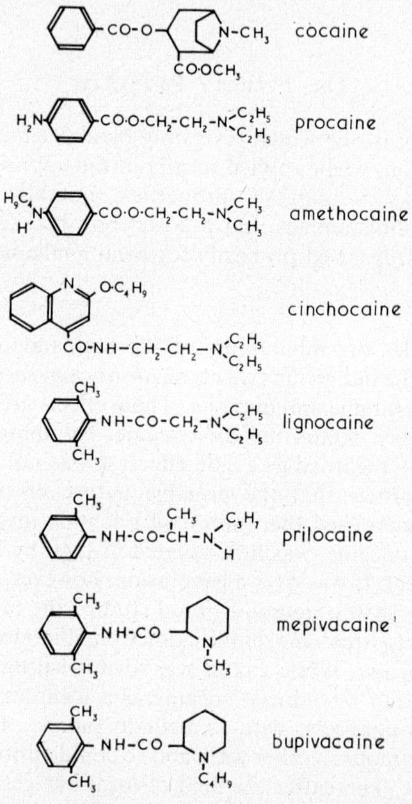

cocaine

procaine

amethocaine

cinchocaine

lignocaine

prilocaine

mepivacaine

bupivacaine

41/Fig. 1.—The structural formulae of local analgesic drugs.

1. *Aromatic group.*—In cocaine the aromatic residue is benzoic acid, in procaine it is para-aminobenzoic acid, and in lignocaine and bupivacaine it is a xylidine.
2. *Intermediate chain.*—Procaine is an example of an ester, while lignocaine is an amide.
3. *Hydrophylic group.*—Prilocaine is the only secondary amine referred to in this chapter: the rest are tertiary amines. In cocaine the moiety containing the amine group is derived from the organic base ecgonine. The tertiary amine in mepivacaine and bupivacaine is incorporated into a piperidine ring.

The amine group confers on the molecule the property of a weak base (or proton acceptor) which can combine with an acid to form a water-soluble salt. This salt ionises in solution and is usually stable.

$$\underset{\text{base}}{R_1R_2R_3N} + HCl \rightleftharpoons \underset{\text{cation}}{R_1R_2R_3N^{+}H} + Cl^{-}$$

The unionised form of the molecule (that is the base) tends on the other hand to be lipid-soluble and consequently can penetrate tissue barriers. The proportions of the two forms of the molecule present in solution depend upon the pK_a of the molecule (see Chapter 34) and on the pH of the environment, and can be calculated from the Henderson-Hasselbalch equation.

A local analgesic for injection is presented as a salt—usually the hydrochloride. The pH of the resulting solution is usually low, as the salt is derived from a strong acid and a weak base. In a more alkaline solution the drug is less stable.

At pH 7·4 a basic drug with a pK_a of 7·86 such as lignocaine is 25 per cent unionised, whereas for a drug with a pK_a of the order of 9 such as procaine only 2·5 per cent is present in this form. At physiological pH, therefore, and at equal total concentrations, the concentration of lignocaine base is ten times that of procaine base.

Nerve Conduction

A nerve fibre consists of a central semi-fluid core, the axoplasm, enclosed in a tube, the cell membrane. The cell membrane is believed to be built up of a bimolecular lipid palisade, bounded inside and out by a monomolecular protein layer. Each fibre of a peripheral nerve is enclosed in a tube of neurilemma, from which it is separated by the myelin sheath, except at the nodes of Ranvier. The myelin sheath, an insulating layer, is absent—or nearly so—in non-medullated nerves. Nerve fibres so encased are collected in bundles within the endoneurium. The perineurium surrounds a collection of bundles, and the epineurium encloses a whole nerve. There is therefore a substantial barrier between a local analgesic drug and its site of action at the nerve cell membrane.

During nerve conduction, changes occur in the *cell membrane*. In the *resting state* there is a potential difference across the cell membrane, inside negative, due to a higher concentration of sodium ions outside than in. The concentration of potassium ions is higher within the cell. The cell membrane is relatively impermeable to sodium ions and the potassium ions therefore tend to be held within the cell by an electrical gradient created by the sodium pump.

Depolarisation phase.—When a nerve is stimulated, partial depolarisation of the membrane is accompanied by a release of calcium ions and leads to a large transient increase in permeability to sodium ions which therefore enter the fibre, resulting in massive depolarisation. Thus, the threshold required to produce the action potential is exceeded, with consequent propagation of the nerve impulse.

During the *neutralisation phase*, potassium ions pass out of the fibre to restore electrical neutrality.

In the *restoration phase* sodium ions return to the outside and potassium ions re-enter the fibre.

In myelinated nerves these changes take place only at the nodes of Ranvier, giving rise to saltatory conduction of the nerve impulse.

Mode of Action

The action of a local analgesic drug is one of membrane stabilisation: the resting potential is maintained but response to stimulation is inhibited. In order to act, the local analgesic must first penetrate the surrounding tissues and the nerve sheath. Only the uncharged form, therefore, can gain access to the cell membrane.

According to the evidence of Ritchie *et al.* (1965), however, the cation is probably the active form of the molecule. This they demonstrated in the following way. They suspended intact and desheathed nerves in bath fluids of different pH values and added different concentrations of lignocaine. By measuring the action potential produced by stimulation of the nerve they were able to find the minimum concentration of lignocaine necessary to produce conduction block in different pH conditions. They showed that while a high pH favoured block by lignocaine of an intact nerve, in a desheathed preparation the optimum pH for the action of lignocaine was neutral. Thus, where little or no penetration was required the lowest effective concentration was one which contained a predominance of the cationic form of the drug.

Nevertheless *in vivo* a certain minimum concentration of the free base must be present in the tissues in order to penetrate and to produce nerve block. This minimum local analgesic concentration depends upon the molecular configuration of the drug, and tends to be related to its lipid-solubility and protein binding characteristics (af Ekenstam, 1966). Thus high potency, high lipid solubility, high acute toxicity, and to an extent long duration of action, are all directly related. A high pK_a, however, tends to reduce the concentration of base present in the tissues, increase the water solubility of the molecule and therefore accelerate its removal from the site of action (Åström, 1966). The production of local vasodilatation by the local analgesic drug itself also accelerates its removal and so shortens its action.

Action of local analgesics on the cell membrane.—Initially they increase the threshold for electrical excitation, reduce the rate of rise of action potential and slow propagation of the impulse; eventually they block conduction completely (Ritchie and Greengard, 1966). They act as membrane stabilisers and inhibit the transient increase in permeability to sodium ions in response to stimulation. A number of theories have attempted to explain the mode of action of local analgesics. Release of calcium ions from the cell membrane precedes membrane depolarisation and local analgesics have been shown to block the release of calcium ions, which may themselves act as membrane stabilisers. It has been postulated that local analgesics interfere with the transport of sodium and potassium or calcium ions across the membrane by forming complexes with the phospholipids which normally act as carriers of the inorganic ions. More recently, the changes have been described differently (af Ekenstam, 1966). The protein layer of the nerve cell membrane may be considered to possess receptor sites which, when stimulated, initiate depolarisation of the membrane by increasing its pore size to allow passage of large hydrated sodium ions. Local analgesics are said to become attached to these receptor sites, rendering them unavailable, so stabilising the membrane, and preventing depolarisation from taking place. This is thus analogous to the action of many drugs such as neuromuscular blockers.

All types of nerve fibres are affected by local analgesic drugs, but small fibres are more readily blocked than large fibres, and non-myelinated than myelinated. Thus pain and temperature are the most sensitive modalities, and somatic motor power the least. Autonomic fibres are also among the more readily blocked, accounting for the early appearance of vasodilatation in the area affected. "Good relaxation"—that is, loss of muscle tone—is produced more readily than motor paralysis, probably due to interruption of the sensory side of the reflex arc.

Pharmacological Effects

The effects of local analgesics may be *local* or *general* (systemic). The *local* effects, occurring only at high concentrations of the drug, are due to the primary action of blocking nerve conduction and are seen in the area of supply of the nerves affected by the block. They are therefore loss of pain and sometimes sensation, vasodilatation (which may cause hypotension if the area of supply is sufficiently large, as in spinal and epidural analgesia) and, if the concentration of local analgesic is sufficiently high, loss of motor power. By definition, a local analgesic drug does not irritate tissues locally or damage nerves permanently. The *systemic* effects occur with absorption from the site of local administration or with systemic administration. They are seen at lower ambient concentrations than the local effects. Thus the so-called analgesic properties of a procaine infusion are due to central sedation and not to any peripheral nerve blocking action. The chief systemic effects of local analgesics are on the heart and the central nervous system, and are believed to be due to membrane stabilisation.

Cardiovascular system.—Local analgesics have a stabilising effect on the cell membrane of cardiac tissue. They tend to depress automaticity in abnormal or damaged fibres and thereby suppress cardiac arrhythmias. Many have quinidine-like effects and may slow the rate of rise of the action potential and increase the effective refractory period of cardiac cells (Singer and Ten Eick, 1969). Some, e.g. procaine, also reduce responsiveness and conduction and effectively depress myocardial contractility, as does quinidine. Local analgesics are effective in the treatment of many non-specific cardiac arrhythmias such as those induced by ischaemia and digitalis, and this property is shared by β-blockers such as propranolol (Morales-Aguilerá and Vaughan Williams, 1965). However, unlike local analgesics in general, propranolol, by virtue of its specific β-blocking action, is also highly effective in suppressing catecholamine- and sympathetically-induced arrhythmias.

The action of lignocaine on the heart appears in man to differ significantly from that of procaine and procainamide (Harrison *et al.*, 1963). This is discussed further in the section on lignocaine (p. 1176).

The effect of local analgesics on vascular smooth muscle varies. While procaine is undoubtedly a vasodilator and cocaine a vasoconstrictor (due to its sympathomimetic effect not shared by other local analgesics) the rest show a varying tendency to cause vasodilatation, depending on the nature of the drug and the state of vasoconstrictor tone. Of the current drugs the one with the most vasoconstrictor action is probably bupivacaine, and the next mepivacaine.

Central nervous system.—The concept of local analgesics as central nervous system stimulants should be eschewed. It dates from the last century when cocaine was the only local analgesic. Cocaine alone has undoubted stimulant effects which are quite unrelated to its local analgesic action. This is stressed because the use of sedatives in the treatment of convulsions after local analgesia may be more dangerous than therapeutic (Steinhaus, 1952). Early central nervous system symptoms may be anxiety and excitement, in which case inhibitory neurones have proved more susceptible than excitatory ones to local analgesic blockade. More often with drugs in current use mild central nervous system involvement is manifested as sedation and disorientation. There may sometimes be restlessness, pins and needles or tremors and twitching, which if severe proceed to convulsions and unconsciousness. Coma may be accompanied by apnoea and cardiovascular collapse, both of which can occur because of medullary depression (Steinhaus, 1957). Convulsions and unconsciousness may occur unheralded in severe intoxication of rapid onset.

Both lignocaine and procaine have been used by intravenous infusion primarily to produce central sedation. The sedative effect of lignocaine absorbed after administration in epidural blockade, for example, is well recognised.

Autonomic nervous system.—A sympathomimetic effect has been attributed to cocaine alone (see under Cocaine, p. 1171). Ganglia: local analgesics are not ganglion blockers in clinical doses and any apparent block produced experimentally at extremely high concentrations is probably due to a stabilising action on the nerve terminals.

Neuromuscular junction.—While local analgesics can certainly block motor nerves if present in sufficient concentration, only procaine has been shown to produce any effect on the neuromuscular junction, probably by a mechanism similar to that on ganglia (see under Procaine, p. 1173).

Hypersensitivity.—Hypersensitivity to local analgesics is not commonly encountered in patients. Repeated skin contact with local analgesics, e.g. in applications to the skin, or among dentists, may occasionally cause dermatitis. Para-aminobenzoic acid, commonly used in sun tan lotions, can give rise to skin sensitivity, in which case cross-sensitivity to procaine administered by any route may produce a rash.

Supersensitivity probably does not occur. The cause of intoxication in reported cases is much more likely to have been overdose, or accidental intravenous administration (see under Systemic Intoxication).

Distribution and Fate

Absorption.—A dose of local analgesic must eventually be absorbed virtually entirely into the systemic circulation. The rate of absorption depends on several factors. The pK_a and lipid solubility of the agent together determine the proportion remaining in the aqueous phase available for rapid removal by the blood, and the proportion taken up by the tissues and therefore only slowly released into the systemic circulation (see also sections on Chemistry and Mode of Action). The vascularity of the tissues influences removal and can be altered by the local analgesic itself and by adrenaline (see below). Absorption of some local analgesics e.g. amethocaine, from mucosal surfaces such as the trachea or an inflamed urethra, can give rise to plasma concentrations akin to those produced by direct intravenous injection (Adriani and Campbell, 1956).

Distribution.—In the plasma, local analgesics become bound to plasma protein to a varying extent, and a proportion enters the red cells. They are rapidly removed from the blood by the tissues. In general, distribution is so rapid and widespread that most of the drug has disappeared from the circulation before mixing in the blood is complete. Local analgesics readily cross lipid barriers such as the blood/brain barrier, and therefore enter the central nervous system.

Placental transfer.—The factors affecting placental transfer of drugs are discussed in Chapter 3. Local analgesic drugs in the unbound and unionised state are sufficiently lipid soluble to cross the placental barrier without difficulty by simple diffusion. Rate of placental transfer of a particular drug therefore depends upon (i) the concentration gradient between maternal and foetal circulation; (ii) the size of the free drug fraction in the plasma, i.e. that not bound to plasma protein or taken up by red cells; (iii) the degree to which the free drug is unionised, depending on its pK_a; and (iv) the lipid solubility of the free unionised fraction (Moya and Thorndike, 1962). In practice a high maternal concentration is the biggest influence on the foetal concentration, and drugs such as mepivacaine which give rise to high maternal levels tend to produce high foetal levels also. The passage of the more potent drugs which are highly bound to plasma protein is slower and is unlikely to produce foetal plasma concentrations equal to the maternal, because foetal proteins bind local analgesics less. In practice neonatal umbilical blood levels of local analgesics are usually below those of the mother at delivery, and a reverse gradient has only been observed with prilocaine and occasionally with mepivacaine. The umbilical venous: maternal venous blood concentration ratios are on average about 0·3 for bupivacaine, 0·55 for lignocaine (Reynolds and Taylor, 1970), 0·7 for mepivacaine (Morishima *et al.*, 1966) and $>$ 1·0 for prilocaine (Epstein *et al.*, 1968). Procaine, highly ionised at physiological pH, will not cross the placenta readily, and tends to be broken down by placental esterases.

Shnider and Way (1968*a*) showed that the neonate appeared to metabolise lignocaine at the same rate as did the mother, and Reynolds and Taylor (1970) found no evidence of foetal accumulation of bupivacaine. Foetal intoxication with local analgesics has been reported but has occurred chiefly in two specific situations, either when the placenta is artificially bypassed by accidental direct injection into the baby's head during attempted caudal block (Sinclair *et al.*, 1965) or during paracervical block, when placental transfer may occasionally be abnormally high. Paracervical block is a risky technique, associated with a 20 per cent incidence of foetal bradycardia (observed by continuous monitoring of the foetal heart; Hellman, 1965). Such foetal bradycardia has been recorded after lignocaine (Nyirjesy *et al.*, 1963), mepivacaine (Hellman, 1965) and bupivacaine (Murphy *et al.*, 1970) and is not seen after caudal injection of the local analgesic or after paracervical injection of saline. The incidence appears to be related to the concentration of the local analgesic and not to the use of adrenaline. The same syndrome probably produces the small but undoubted incidence of intra-uterine death which is associated with abnormally high foetal levels of the drug used. Apart from such peculiar situations, local analgesia is rarely associated with severe foetal or neonatal depression. Neonatal depression, accompanied by high blood concentration of local analgesic, has been reported after prolonged epidural blockade with lignocaine (Shnider and Way, 1968*b*) and mepivacaine (Morishima *et al.*, 1966). Such a case has not yet been reported with bupivacaine.

Metabolism.—With the exception of procaine, local analgesics are chiefly metabolised in the liver. Several pathways are involved. N-dealkylation of the tertiary amine has been shown to take place in a number of local analgesics, producing a more water soluble secondary amine, and in the case of lignocaine for example, rendering it more susceptible to amide hydrolysis (Hollunger, 1960), as is the more rapidly metabolised secondary amine prilocaine (Geddes, 1965). Hydroxylation of the aromatic nucleus is believed to occur in the case of lignocaine, mepivacaine and bupivacaine and produces a more polar compound. Amide and ester hydrolysis probably takes in some cases thereby producing smaller moieties which are rapidly excreted or destroyed. Procaine and to a much lesser extent other esters, can be hydrolysed in the plasma (Kalow, 1952).

Excretion.—While both an ionised drug and the water soluble products of its metabolism are rapidly excreted in the urine, a lipid soluble local analgesic base, having passed into the glomerular filtrate, can be reabsorbed into the blood from the renal tubule (Milne *et al.*, 1958). However, in an acid urine a typical local analgesic will become highly ionised, and its reabsorption inhibited, as the cation cannot pass the tubule cell barrier. However, with high tissue uptake of a local analgesic, excretion is an unimportant means of disposal of the unchanged drug, even when the urine is acid.

Systemic Intoxication

The toxicity of a drug like a barbiturate is simply an extension of its therapeutic action. Such is not necessarily the case with a local analgesic whose therapeutic effect is local, while intoxication is systemic. Although the potency of a local analgesic is directly related to its acute toxicity (Luduena *et al.*, 1958), that is the toxicity measured after rapid administration such as intravenous injection, the occurrence of side-effects during local analgesia is influenced by other factors such as the rate of absorption of the drug into the systemic circulation and by its distribution and fate in the body. There is evidence that the toxicity of a local analgesic drug is not always influenced by the concentration of the solution used (Braid and Scott, 1965), as has been suggested. As the rate of metabolism of a local analgesic can barely affect its duration of action or potency but can affect its chronic toxicity during repeated administration, a rapidly metabolised drug has an advantage.

However, before demanding the ideal local analgesic drug of high potency, slow absorption and rapid metabolism, it must strenuously be pointed out that nowadays most cases of intoxication occur as a result of inadvertent massive intravascular administration, while some are due to considerable overdosage (Sunshine and Fike, 1964). Cases of minor toxicity are commonly due to accidental intravenous injection. Rapid systemic absorption from the inflamed urethra was among the commoner causes of death from local analgesia, before the hazard was realised (Deacock and Simpson, 1964). The dangers of overdosage in the very young and old are now more widely recognised than they were, though such subjects are probably no more sensitive on an mg./kg. basis than others. Widespread field blocks and excessive surface application of local analgesic drugs are out of fashion in Great Britain. Intoxication may still occur with chronic administration, for example during continuous epidural analgesia for post-operative pain or childbirth or during intravenous infusion in the treatment of ventricular arrhythmias. It is in these situations that a local analgesic with a more favourable therapeutic ratio is advantageous.

Systemic intoxication by a local analgesic may be manifest by twitching, convulsions and coma while, if severe, cerebral anoxia may lead to medullary depression, respiratory arrest, cardiovascular collapse and death. Severe intoxication of rapid onset may produce cardiac arrest with alarming rapidity but the primary cause even in this situation is probably medullary depression (see also Pharmacological Effects; Central Nervous System).

Treatment.—If signs of minor central nervous system toxicity occur administration of the local analgesic should be discontinued. In the case of an intravenous infusion, simply stopping it may be sufficient treatment. In more severe cases and after local administration (when absorption cannot be stopped) oxygen should be given. In many cases correcting cerebral anoxia by this means may be all that is necessary. With full convulsions, intravenous suxamethonium and artificial ventilation with oxygen via an endotracheal tube should be given. If convulsions return with recovery from suxamethonium, Moore and Bridenbaugh (1960) suggest that one more dose of suxamethonium should be given, followed if necessary by tubocurarine. Hypotension or circulatory arrest must of course be treated in the usual ways. Barbiturates, e.g. thiopentone, should have no place in the treatment of a condition with so large a component of depression.

Adrenaline

Adrenaline is frequently used with a local analgesic to prolong its action and delay absorption into the circulation, thereby, it is hoped, reducing the incidence of systemic intoxication. However, a common cause of side-effects during local analgesia is accidental intravenous injection. In this situation, adrenaline could be as dangerous as the local analgesic itself. Adrenaline 5 μg./ml. (1:200,000) has been shown to increase the toxicity of local analgesics injected intravenously into mice (Henn and Brattsand, 1966). However, in a total dose of 100–150 μg, which is often used in man, it would seem unlikely to cause trouble. Adrenaline may theoretically increase the likelihood of anterior spinal artery syndrome, a rare complication of epidural analgesia, and if used for digital block may produce gangrene. Thus it is important before using adrenaline with a local analgesic in any situation to take extreme care and to be sure that it will have the beneficial properties attributed to it. When the very short-acting procaine was one of the few safe local analgesics the use of adrenaline for anything but the shortest procedures was justified. It increases the duration of action of lignocaine quite considerably, and when prolonged blockade is required it may reduce the number of repeat doses needed and delay the onset of chronic toxicity and tachyphylaxis. A short-acting vasoconstrictor such as adrenaline, however, cannot be expected to increase the duration of action of a long-acting drug more than fractionally. By delaying and reducing peak absorption it may diminish systemic toxicity, but even this effect is less marked with the newer drugs, which are in some cases mild vasoconstrictors, than it was with older, vasodilator local analgesics. Adrenaline has negligible effect on the duration and toxicity of prilocaine, for example (Braid and Scott, 1965) and little on that of bupivacaine (Reynolds and Taylor, 1971). It is more valuable in highly vascular areas such as the intercostal space and the broad ligament, than in the less vascular epidural space.

For general purposes, adrenaline should not be used with local analgesic solutions in a concentration higher than 5 μg./ml. (1:200,000), while in some cases an even lower concentration may be sufficient. In dentistry, however, adrenaline 12·5 μg./ml. (1:80,000) is still frequently used, though in this situation of course the total dose is small.

Adrenaline Substitutes

Noradrenaline might be thought a more satisfactory drug than adrenaline in this field, because it is a less potent β-receptor stimulant, and therefore less likely to produce cardiac arrhythmias, etc. However, many workers have found it less effective than adrenaline as a vasoconstrictor in local analgesia, and it has not found widespread favour in this field.

Felypressin (Octopressin®), a synthetic polypeptide related to vasopressin, has recently been introduced as an adrenaline-substitute to delay absorption of local analgesic drugs (Åkerman, 1969). It was found to reduce the subcutaneous toxicity of lignocaine, prilocaine, amethocaine and procaine variably but to increase their intravenous toxicity less than did adrenaline. It is marketed with prilocaine for dentistry. Sufficient evidence is not yet available to evaluate felypressin fully.

Hyaluronidase

Hyaluronidase is an enzyme which, when injected with a drug into the tissues, promotes its spread and consequently its absorption into the systemic circulation by breakdown of intercellular ground substance. It is primarily used to promote systemic absorption of drugs or fluids when intravenous injection is not feasible, for example with ergometrine given by midwives, or with subcutaneous fluid and electrolyte administration in infants. It may also be used to promote dispersion and absorption of inadvertently extravascular injections.

It has been used to promote the spread of injected local analgesics. Even with procaine, a drug of poor penetration, it can only be of marginal value because it enhances absorption and renders the addition of adrenaline doubly necessary. Nowadays it has no place in the administration of a correctly placed local analgesic block using a modern drug of adequate penetration. Hyaluronidase itself is not without dangers since inadvertent intravascular administration may lead to a hypersensitivity reaction owing to the presence of small amounts of bovine serum proteins.

Desirable Properties

There can be no such thing as the ideal local analgesic drug because different circumstances require different properties. However, a number of characteristics are usually desirable. The first is good penetration. This tends to promote rapid onset of action, to eliminate patchy analgesia and to make topical application effective if this is required. A local analgesic should not produce local irritation. A safe therapeutic ratio is always necessary and not hard to achieve if the local analgesic is to be used in a single dose for most techniques in current use. In the past, paravertebral and intercostal block for tuberculosis surgery, for example, sometimes necessitated dangerously large doses. In the techniques commonly used at present, such as epidural blockade, it is relatively easy to keep within safe limits of dosage.

For the production of prolonged local analgesia many more properties are required. A long duration in action becomes an advantage for both convenience and safety, and it should be unnecessary to add adrenaline to achieve this. Tachyphylaxis should not occur and slow absorption but rapid metabolism of the drug will tend to improve its therapeutic ratio (see discussion on Systemic Intoxication). Reversibility of action is stipulated by definition.

A local analgesic solution should be able to withstand repeated autoclaving and minor pH changes and should be stable in light and air.

Assessment

Most local analgesics are fairly satisfactory drugs and improvements gained in the manufacture of new drugs are likely only to be marginal. Therefore careful assessment of a new drug is mandatory if it is to be adopted in preference to a well-tried agent.

Local analgesics lend themselves to fairly accurate assessment as it is easier to measure their effects objectively than it is those of systemic analgesics. However, multifarious methods of testing have led to numerous conflicting reports of their relative efficacy and toxicity.

Before the first clinical trials of a new drug take place, extensive preliminary investigations in both animals and man will have established a number of facts. It behoves the clinician about to embark on a clinical study to acquaint himself with the relevant literature.

Laboratory Investigations in Animals and Man (Bülbring and Wajda, 1945; Bianchi, 1956).

Animal studies can be used to compare the acute and cumulative toxicity of drugs by various routes of administration (subcutaneous, intramuscular, intravenous, etc.) and to make a rough assessment of latency, potency and duration of action. The inhibition of the corneal reflex in the rabbit is used to measure surface analgesic activity. Inhibition of reaction to pinprick after intracutaneous injection in the guinea-pig can test infiltration analgesia. Conduction analgesia may be tested by sciatic nerve block in guinea-pig or frog, or by mouse tail root infiltration measuring inhibition of the pain reflex. In man a series of intradermal injections of different concentrations of the new drug, together with

side-effects should be noted. As many data as possible should be recorded in each subject of a clinical trial, and measurements made at the same and sufficiently frequent time intervals.

With regard to toxicity, assessment in man presents a problem. The therapeutic ratio (that is, the ratio of mean toxic dose: mean effective dose) of a single local analgesic drug varies not only with species (owing to great differences in enzyme systems, etc.) but also with route of administration, because of variation in the rate of absorption from different sites. Thus theoretically it should be determined in man for each technique of local analgesic blockade. However, it is to be hoped and expected that after the correct administration of a single dose of a local analgesic by any accepted route the incidence of systemic toxicity will be nil. It is nevertheless essential to judge the margin of safety that may be expected from a drug in any given situation, as for instance with a large dose, an accidental intravenous injection, repeated injection after failed block, or for prolonged analgesia. Such assessment should not be made by trial and error as often happened in the past. It may be judged by measuring blood concentrations of the local analgesic which occur in clinical practice in different situations and comparing these with the blood concentration which gives rise to signs of systemic toxicity during experimental intravenous infusion.

Complete testing of a local analgesic may take a long time if this regime is followed. For many years local analgesia was regarded as a safe alternative to general anaesthesia for surgery in the sick, and only reports of increasing numbers of deaths gave the lie to this idea. Full knowledge of the behaviour of the drug that is used, together with careful attention to technique, should render local analgesia safer than it has proved in the past.

INDIVIDUAL LOCAL ANALGESIC DRUGS

The number of drugs that have been marketed as local analgesics is legion, and only products in current use by anaesthetists, or those of historical importance, are included here. They are presented in chronological order. Numerical data are often misleading, because they may have been calculated from experiments under varying conditions by different workers. However, in the ensuing text, an attempt has been made to supply only such as enable some quantitative comparison of different local analgesic drugs to be made.

Cocaine

Cocaine is an ester of benzoic acid and methylecgonine.

CO-O- N-CH_3 cocaine
COOCH_3

It is a naturally occuring substance, derived from the leaves of the South American shrub *Erythroxylum coca*. The first agent to be employed as a local analgesic, it was introduced into ophthalmology in 1884. It is now little used, owing to its toxicity and addictive properties.

Cocaine has two chief actions:

1. In common with other local analgesics, it blocks nerve conduction by a stabilising action in the cell membrane.
2. Uniquely among local analgesics, it potentiates the effect of sympathetic stimulation and of catecholamines by preventing the re-uptake of noradrenaline etc. into sympathetic nerve endings (see below).

Local analgesic properties.—Cocaine is not a markedly potent or long-acting local analgesic, except in so far as the sympathomimetic vasoconstriction it produces tends to retard its absorption from the site of application. It is, however, about four times as toxic as procaine on intravenous or subcutaneous administration. The therapeutic ratio for clinical use is significantly less than that of most other local analgesics, and it is no longer used for any local analgesia other than surface application. It is active as a surface analgesic, because it penetrates mucous membranes. The vasoconstriction it produces tends to delay its systemic absorption, and furthermore has made it popular for ear, nose and throat work.

The eye.—Cocaine is an effective surface analgesic on the eye, where it also causes vasoconstriction and dilatation of the pupil because of its ability to potentiate sympathetic activity. Dilatation of the pupil may precipitate glaucoma, but may be overcome by an anticholinesterase drug. The cornea may become clouded, pitted and ulcerated as a result of cocaine analgesia. These properties have greatly reduced its popularity in ophthalmology since there are safer alternatives: midriasis may be produced by homatropine and analgesia by a more modern local analgesic.

Autonomic nervous system.—Cocaine enhances the effect of sympathetic stimulation and of injected noradrenaline. Sympathetic activity is normally terminated because transmitter substance is removed from the region of the receptor by its re-uptake into sympathetic nerve endings. Cocaine inhibits this re-uptake process and therefore allows accumulation of transmitter at the receptor site. The marked difference between the effects of cocaine and of other local analgesic drugs is largely a reflection of this property.

Central nervous system.—Cocaine, like other local analgesics, produces convulsions and coma in big doses, but in much lower doses it has a marked stimulant effect like that of amphetamine. It produces excitement, euphoria and generally sociability and talkativeness. It has been a popular drug of addiction. Known as "snow", it used to be taken as snuff but frequently caused ulceration of the nasal mucosa. The advanced addict was apt to become unsociable, hallucinated, and paranoid. Cocaine also diminishes hunger and fatigue. It is probably for these properties that it is consumed in crude form by Peruvian workers, who often give up the habit at low altitudes and are therefore not true addicts. Medullary centres: the vasomotor centre, the respiratory centre and the vomiting centre, may all be stimulated, giving rise to increased vasomotor tone and respiratory rate, and often to vomiting. In severe cocaine intoxication coma, convulsions and depression of these vital centres may cause death.

Body temperature may rise in cocaine intoxication, owing to increased heat production due to muscular overactivity, diminished heat loss because of vasoconstriction, and possibly resetting of the temperature regulating centre.

Cardiovascular system.—The arterial pressure is raised by cocaine, owing to vasoconstriction and to a sympathomimetic effect on the heart. The effect on heart rate is variable, bradycardia due to stimulation of the vagal medullary centre usually giving way to tachycardia of peripheral sympathomimetic origin. Ventricular fibrillation may cause sudden death.

Dosage.—Cocaine hydrochloride is usually employed as a 10 per cent solution for endotracheal spray and other surface application to the nose and throat, and 20 per cent cocaine paste is sometimes employed in the nose. It is hard to believe that such high concentrations are really necessary. The maximum safe dose is often given as 100 mg. but as this would mean only 0·5 ml. of cocaine paste and 1 ml. of cocaine hydrochloride solution, it is often exceeded. The upper safe dose is probably in the region of 2 mg./kg. of cocaine hydrochloride. The LD_{50} for intravenous injection in rats (LD_{50} i.v. rats) has been given as 17·5 mg./kg., that is to say it is considerably less lethal than cinchocaine, amethocaine and bupivacaine, but cocaine produces many an undesirable side-effect before lethality, and its effect is very variable. There is, however, no value in the so-called cocaine sensitivity test, because cocaine has produced more toxicity as a result of simple overdose than any abnormal response, and its addictive tendency should not be overlooked.

PROCAINE

Procaine was synthesised by Einhorn in 1905, as a substitute for cocaine, and though now largely superseded it has enjoyed considerable popularity.

Physico-chemical properties.—Procaine is an ester of para-aminobenzoic acid and diethylaminoethanol:

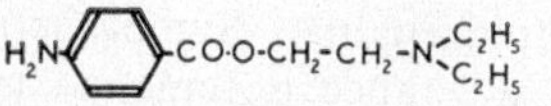

$$H_2N-C_6H_4-CO{\cdot}O-CH_2-CH_2-N{<}^{C_2H_5}_{C_2H_5} \quad \text{procaine}$$

It is not highly lipid soluble; it has a pK_a of about 9·0. Solutions of procaine hydrochloride are unstable and cannot be autoclaved.

Local analgesic properties.—Procaine is a local analgesic of short duration of action and extremely poor penetrative powers. These properties stem from its marked vasodilator activity and its relatively high pK_a, which renders it highly ionised at physiological pH. It is absorbed rapidly into the systemic circulation when injected (see Chemistry p. 1158). It is inactive as a surface analgesic. The potency of a local analgesic is hard to determine because it varies with the route of administration, but for simple nerve block or infiltration analgesia procaine is of lower potency than lignocaine and of much lower penetrative power. A higher concentration is therefore often found necessary, and procaine carries a lower chance of completely successful blockade than does lignocaine. Its duration of action is generally about half that of lignocaine but can be prolonged considerably by the addition of adrenaline, which counteracts the vasodilatation.

Procaine, once in the circulation is hydrolysed by pseudocholinesterase in the plasma and liver to *p*-aminobenzoic acid and diethylaminoethanol. It is therefore effectively of low toxicity. Several drug interactions, however, are possible:

1. Procaine may prolong the effect of suxamethonium by competing with it for the same enzyme.

2. Anticholinesterase drugs may increase the toxicity of procaine.
3. One product of hydrolysis, *p*-aminobenzoic acid, is a potent inhibitor of the bacteriostatic effects of sulphonamides.
4. Diethylaminoethanol potentiates the effect of digitalis and therefore might precipitate intoxication in patients on digitalis-type drugs. Otherwise the products of metabolic degradation are non-toxic.

Central nervous system (see general section).—Procaine has been given by intravenous infusion to produce analgesia. This is a systemic effect, occurring at a much lower extracellular fluid concentration than that required to produce peripheral pain nerve blockade, and is simply a reflection of the central sedation it produces.

Peripheral nervous system.—Procaine has been recorded as producing ganglionic and neuromuscular junction blockade, though only after direct application or close intra-arterial injection of relatively huge doses. There is evidence that it causes presynaptic blockade by preventing release of acetylcholine, but this is probably due to blockade of presynaptic nerve fibres in the normal local analgesic manner. It has been stated that procaine should not be given to patients with myasthenia gravis. A reason for this is that such patients are likely to be taking anticholinesterase drugs, rather than because of any enhancement by procaine of neuromuscular blockade. Neither procaine nor any other local analgesic should be regarded as a ganglionic or neuromuscular blocker in therapeutic doses.

Cardiovascular system.—Procaine was early found to be an effective anti-arrhythmic drug, but procainamide soon replaced it as it has a more specific cardiac effect and is less likely to produce central nervous system toxicity; it is not broken down by pseudocholinesterase and therefore has a more prolonged systemic effect. Both drugs have an anti-arrhythmic effect (see systemic effects of local analgesics, p. 1161) and a vagolytic action causing tachycardia and enhanced AV conduction. Indeed, their actions are very close to those of quinidine. Because conduction is readily depressed, a wide QRS complex may herald ventricular extrasystoles and fibrillation. Asynchronous contraction of ventricular muscle may induce or aggravate a negative inotropic effect, and thus a fall in cardiac output and blood pressure.

Procainamide administered orally, however, has a place in the treatment of supraventricular arrhythmias. The possibility of an increase in ventricular rate during the treatment of atrial fibrillation usually necessitates prior digitalisation to reduce AV conduction; in this field DC defibrillation, where available, has largely taken its place. Procainamide is occasionally used prophylactically against ventricular ectopics and ventricular tachycardia, though a danger of actually producing ventricular extrasystoles makes control difficult.

Dosage.—For extensive subcutaneous infiltration 0·5 per cent procaine hydrochloride with adrenaline has generally been used. For restricted infiltration, such as is required to set up an intravenous infusion or to take blood from a donor, procaine hydrochloride 1 per cent is still a very useful drug, as penetration and prolonged duration are not required and vasodilatation can be useful. Procaine hydrochloride 2 per cent with adrenaline may be used for nerve blocks, though without full confidence because of its poor pen tration.

Procaine hydrochloride crystals are prepared dry in ampoules containing 50–500 mg. for use in spinal analgesia. In this site, good powers of penetration are less important as the nerves are more readily accessible in the subarachnoid space than elsewhere. In the treatment of arrhythmias, procainamide tablets, 250 mg., are usually given at the rate of one to three tablets six-hourly.

The upper limit of safety of a local analgesic depends upon route and rate of administration and also upon individual variation. For procaine it is of the order of 10 mg./kg., provided absorption is reasonably slow. The LD_{50} i.v. rats is 55 mg./kg.

CINCHOCAINE (DIBUCAINE (USP) "NUPERCAINE")

Cinchocaine was synthesised in 1929 and was introduced into clinical practice in the 1930's.

Physico-chemical properties.—It was the first of the amide type of local analgesics. Its aromatic moiety is based on quinoline.

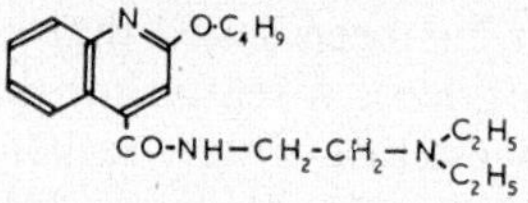

N O-C_4H_9

CO-NH-CH_2-CH_2-N(C_2H_5)(C_2H_5) cinchocaine

It has a pK_a of 8·54 and is very highly lipid soluble. Solutions of cinchocaine hydrochloride are stable and will withstand autoclaving, though if they include glucose the latter may become charred.

Local analgesic properties.—Cinchocaine is the most potent local analgesic in medical use. For infiltration and nerve block, concentrations of one-tenth to one-twentieth those of procaine are required. It is effective as a surface analgesic, having better penetrating powers than procaine. Although more potent than bupivacaine, its duration of action is not as great, as it produces vasodilatation and has a higher pK_a; the addition of adrenaline is therefore useful and limits its absorption. The importance of cinchocaine lies in the pride of place it has held over many years for spinal analgesia. For some time three solutions of cinchocaine were made for this purpose: light (1:1,500 or 0·0$\dot{6}$ per cent), isotonic (1:200 or 0·5 per cent) and heavy (1:200 or 0·5 per cent in 6 per cent glucose). The light spinal technique, involving a subarachnoid injection of a large volume of dilute solution, was associated with chronic adhesive arachnoiditis and other serious neurological sequelae, and should not be used. Spinal analgesia in any form is rarely used in the United Kingdom nowadays, and only the heavy technique is employed. Injecting 1–3 ml. of heavy solution with adrenaline, a duration of 3–4 hours may be expected. Anaesthetists have reason to be grateful to the manufacturers for continuing to supply heavy cinchocaine in response to a demand so limited that there can be no commercial advantage in its production.

Cinchocaine has been used in epidural analgesia, in an 0·1$\dot{6}$ per cent (1:600) solution but it is not satisfactory for this purpose because, although it has a longer action, it has less penetrative power than lignocaine.

The maximum safe dose of cinchocaine is probably about 0·4 mg./kg. This is not an important consideration, however, for spinal analgesia, because the dose is relatively small. The LD_{50} i.v. rats is 2·5 mg./kg.

Other uses of cinchocaine.—Under its USP name, dibucaine, this drug is used in the detection of atypical pseudocholinesterase (see Chapter 31).

AMETHOCAINE (TETRACAINE (USP): "DECICAINE": "PONTOCAINE")

Amethocaine was introduced very soon after cinchocaine.

Physico-chemical properties.—It is a homologue of procaine.

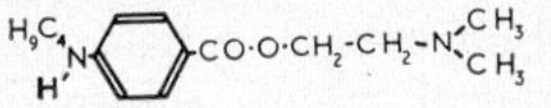

$$\underset{H}{\overset{H_9C_4}{}}\!>\!N\!-\!C_6H_4\!-\!CO\!\cdot\!O\!\cdot\!CH_2\!-\!CH_2\!-\!N\!<\!\begin{matrix}CH_3\\CH_3\end{matrix}\quad \text{amethocaine}$$

It is a highly lipid soluble compound, though less so than cinchocaine. Its pK_a is 8·39. As it is an ester, a solution of amethocaine is unstable and cannot be autoclaved.

Local analgesic properties.—Amethocaine is a potent, long-acting local analgesic, and is a very effective surface analgesic. It is used in a 0·5 per cent concentration in the eye, and a 1 to 2 per cent solution for application to mucous membranes. Amethocaine hydrochloride for injection is usually presented as a dry powder and may be added to lignocaine solution to prolong the action of the latter in nerve blocks and epidural analgesia. It is also used alone, in a 0·25 per cent or occasionally a 0·5 per cent concentration, 15–20 ml., for epidural analgesia, with or without adrenaline, when its duration of action is similar to that of bupivacaine. It appears that 0·5 per cent is no more effective or long acting than 0·25 per cent (Bromage, 1969). Amethocaine has also been used for spinal analgesia.

The LD_{50} i.v. rats is 8 mg./kg. (*cf.* procaine, 55 mg./kg.). However, amethocaine is more slowly broken down in the body than procaine, and as procaine breakdown is thus more likely to keep pace with absorption, amethocaine may be about 10 times as toxic as procaine in clinical use. It is rapidly absorbed from mucous surfaces and has caused a number of fatalities by this and other routes. Nevertheless, the maximum safe dose is probably at least 1 mg./kg.

Both cinchocaine and amethocaine are described as very toxic local analgesics, yet they are frequently ascribed toxicity and potency values such that their therapeutic ratios would be higher than that of procaine (Gray and Geddes, 1954). The reason for this is probably that intravenous toxicity is taken to represent clinical toxicity, which it does not (see Systemic intoxication, p. 1164). Such a calculation would indicate that they were exceptionally safe local analgesics: a moment's reflection suggests that this is not the case, although admittedly many cases of toxicity have occured through their being given in unnecessarily large doses.

LIGNOCAINE (LIDOCAINE (USP): "XYLOCAINE")

Lignocaine was sythesised in 1943 in Sweden, by Löfgren of AB Astra, and it was introduced into clinical practice in 1948. It has numerous advantages over many of its predecessors, and has been popular ever since.

Physico-chemical properties.—Lignocaine is an amide of xylidine.

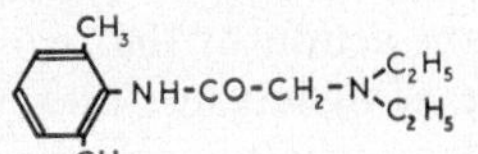

$$(CH_3)_2C_6H_3\!-\!NH\!-\!CO\!-\!CH_2\!-\!N\!<\!\begin{matrix}C_2H_5\\C_2H_5\end{matrix}\quad \text{lignocaine}$$

It has a pK_a of 7·86 and is only moderately lipid soluble. Solutions of lignocaine hydrocloride are extremely stable and will withstand repeated autoclaving.

Local analgesic properties.—Lignocaine is a local analgesic of moderate potency and duration, but of very superior penetrative powers and rapid onset of action. It is effective by all routes of administration and its advent was partly responsible for the increased popularity of epidural analgesia, because its excellent penetration renders blockade by this method highly successful.

It usually causes little local vasodilatation. Adrenaline prolongs the action of lignocaine and also reduces its rate of systemic absorption. Thus the duration of action epidurally is about ¾–1 hour, prolonged up to 2½ hours with adrenaline. With repeated injection, tachyphylaxis often occurs: indeed it may occasionally be practically impossible to produce analgesia after some hours. Adrenaline can reduce but not abolish this feature.

Lignocaine 1 per cent in 10 per cent "Dextraven" has been used by infiltration and intercostal nerve block to produce post-operative analgesia of long duration (Loder, 1960). When used with adrenaline 4 μg/ml., "Dextraven" has been found to prolong the action of lignocaine from 2½ to 10 hours.

The carbonate of lignocaine has remarkable penetrative powers, thus a rapid onset of action and a high incidence of motor block (Bromage and Gertel, 1970).

For surface application lignocaine is very effective, and may be used in solution as a liquid (4 per cent) for spraying or application on wool pledgets, or in a lubricating gel for the urethra (2 per cent) or on instruments, endotracheal tubes and oropharyngeal airways (4 per cent). Absorption of lignocaine from mucosal surfaces, however, is rapid and may give rise to high blood levels unless the dose is carefully controlled. Absorption from the inflamed urethra can take place at a rate equivalent to intravenous injection.

Central nervous system (see general section, p. 1162).—The marked sedative effect of lignocaine slowly absorbed after correct local administration is well recognised during, for example, epidural blockade. It has even been used as an anticonvulsant in the treatment of status epilepticus (Bernard *et al.*, 1955). Lignocaine has been given by intravenous infusion to produce sedation and general analgesia, but if pain relief is required lignocaine is safer and more useful injected to block the appropriate nerve supply, while there are a number of general sedatives less likely to produce convulsions in accidental overdosage.

Cardiovascular system (see general section, p. 1161).—Lignocaine is a useful drug in the treatment of cardiac arrhythmias. It stabilise the membrane of damaged and excitable cells, tending to prevent the generation of automaticity in ectopic foci. In therapeutic doses it has no vagolytic action, and causes no consistent rate change. Responsiveness of myocardial fibres is normal or elevated, and it does not depress conduction in Purkinje tissue (Bigger and Heissenbuttel, 1969). Widening of the QRS complex is not seen and there is usually no apparent myocardial depression. Even an improvement in cardiac output and blood pressure has been observed when it is used in the treatment of cardiac arrhythmias (Harrison *et al.*, 1963). Because of its lack of vagolytic action, it is less useful than quinidine or procainamide in the treatment of supraventricular arrhythmias, in which the myocardial depressant action of the two latter drugs is often of little importance. The great value of lignocaine, however, is in the acute and emergency treatment of ventricular arrhythmias, after myocardial infarction or cardiac surgery. It is also of value in the treatment of digitalis-induced arrhythmias. The lack of depressant effect is valuable in such situations. As the main use of lignocaine is in emergency treatment, it has largely been given intravenously by slugs and infusion. Because an infusion of lignocaine given too fast is dangerous, it requires careful monitoring. There have been attempts in this field to give lignocaine orally, by intramuscular injection or by suppository, in the hope that slow steady absorption would have an effect equivalent to intravenous infusion and would allow lignocaine to be used safely in situations other than the intensive care unit and the theatre. However, there remains a difficulty, because there is a wide individual variation in the resulting systemic levels and, furthermore, the effective concentration is likely in many cases to be near the toxic one—that is to say, the therapeutic ratio approaches unity. So, logically, it will in many instances be impossible to guess at a safe but effective dose of lignocaine, which can therefore only be arrived at by intravenous infusion, at a rate that can be adjusted from minute to minute if need be.

Dosage.—Concentrations of lignocaine hydrochloride of 0·25—0·5 per cent are used for infiltration block. If extensive block is required 0·25 per cent with adrenaline should be used. Up to 40 ml. of 0·5 per cent lignocaine without adrenaline is usually used for intravenous regional analgesia. For paracervical block no more than 1 per cent lignocaine should be used and the same concentration suffices for most nerve blocks. Concentrations of 1·2–2 per cent are used for epidural analgesia. For topical application, 2–4 per cent concentrations are used, for example 2 per cent gel for the urethra, 4 per cent gel or spray for the trachea.

In the treatment of cardiac arrhythmias, 1 mg./kg. is usually given as a slug dose intravenously, followed by an infusion of 1–2 mg./minute. Such a régime gives rise to a short-lived high blood concentration initially, followed by one which may be too low to be effective for an hour or so. Therefore infusion should be rapid at first (e.g. 4 mg./minute for 10 minutes) then gradually slowed down as the tissues begin to take up lignocaine less rapidly. Such an infusion kept up at a steady rate for days is liable to give rise to systemic toxicity.

Intoxication with lignocaine has not been uncommon in the past partly because it has not always been realised that lignocaine may in some circumstances be almost twice as toxic and potent as procaine. Furthermore, misapplication to mucosal surfaces has been a notable cause of death from lignocaine intoxication. Also, it is apt to be cumulative in repeated doses, especially as tachyphylaxis is a conspicuous feature of its repeated local use.

The safe dose limit for lignocaine has been much disputed. After the publication by Deacock and Simpson (1964) of a series of fatalities from lignocaine, the upper safe dose ascribed to lignocaine was 200 mg. plain and 500 mg. with adrenaline. However, this decision failed to take into account differences in weight of patients and different absorption rates from various sites of injection. The maximum safe dose in man is probably about 7 mg./kg.—possibly less than this for plain solutions in vascular areas—while more than this has often been given with impunity with adrenaline into less vascular areas. Toxic symptoms may occur at plasma levels of 3 (Jewitt *et al.*, 1968) to 5 (Foldes *et al.*, 1960) μg/ml. yet such levels are not uncommonly produced by epidural analgesia (Braid and Scott, 1965 and 1966). The LD_{50} i.v. mice is about 30 mg./kg.

Mepivacaine ("Carbocaine": "Scandicaine")

Mepivacaine was synthesised by Bo af Ekenstam of AB Bofors in Sweden (af Ekenstam *et al.*, 1956), as one of a large homologous series. Since its introduction it has been widely used for local analgesia in Scandinavia and the States but has only recently been put on the market in Great Britain.

Physico-chemical properties.—Mepivacaine, like lignocaine, is an amide of xylidine.

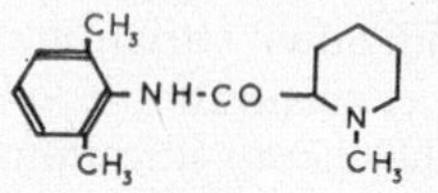

CH_3 — NH-CO — N — CH_3 — CH_3 mepivacaine

Its pK_a is 7·8 and its lipid solubility is of the same order as that of lignocaine. Solutions of mepivacaine are stable and can be autoclaved.

Local analgesic properties.—Mepivacaine is similar to lignocaine as a local analgesic, having in some circumstances a slightly longer duration of action. Its penetrative powers are certainly as good as those of lignocaine, while it causes less vasodilatation. Its duration of action can be increased by the addition of adrenaline. It has been used for all types of analgesia, in doses and concentrations akin to those of lignocaine, and like lignocaine has caused death when used in excessive dosage (Sunshine and Fike, 1964). Experimentally, it has been shown to have slightly lower intravenous toxicity than lignocaine, the LD_{50} i.v. mice being 40 mg./kg. but its subcutaneous toxicity is higher (Henn, 1960). Moreover, it is markedly cumulative when given epidurally (Moore *et al.*, 1968) and gives rise to higher blood levels than does lignocaine. The toxic plasma level may be slightly higher than that of lignocaine (Jorfeldt *et al.*, 1968) but it is readily produced by repeated doses. Therefore for long continued use it is certainly less safe than is lignocaine. It has nevertheless been used extensively in obstetrics in the United States, with reports of foetal intoxication during caudal epidurals, accidental foetal injections and paracervical blocks. Whether any of these troubles can be directly laid at the door of mepivacaine remains debatable, but during caudal and lumbar epidural block there is no doubt that mepivacaine gives rise to relatively higher foetal blood concentrations than do other local analgesics that have been measured (Morishima *et al.*, 1966; Moore *et al.*, 1968; Reynolds, 1971).

Prilocaine ("Citanest": "Propitocaine": L67)

Prilocaine emerged in 1960, shortly after mepivacaine, from the same stable as lignocaine—AB Astra—having been synthesised some years previously by Löfgren.

Physico-chemical properties.—Prilocaine is an amide of *o*-toluidine and is a secondary amine.

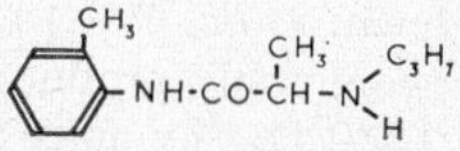

CH_3 — NH-CO-CH(CH_3)-N(C_3H_7)H prilocaine

Its pK_a is 7·89 and it is slightly less lipid-soluble than lignocaine. Solutions of prilocaine are stable and can be autoclaved.

Local analgesic properties.—The potency of prilocaine is of the same order as that of lignocaine; it has good penetrative powers and can be used for all types of local analgesia in concentrations similar to those of lignocaine. Its duration of action is the same as or slightly longer than that of lignocaine, but cannot be increased to anything like the same extent, if at all, by the addition of adrenaline (Bromage, 1965). For dental analgesia, its action is extremely short-lived.

The administration of prilocaine gives rise to much lower blood concentrations than does an equal dose of lignocaine. This is in part accounted for by more rapid metabolism and possibly also by greater tissue uptake (Eriksson, 1966). It is therefore only about two-thirds as toxic as lignocaine after a single dose, and considerably less cumulative. The LD_{50} i.v. mice is about 35 mg./kg. but a small reduction in infusion rate causes a huge increase in LD_{50}, while the subcutaneous LD_{50} is much higher than that of lignocaine.

However, although it may be relatively safe from the point of view of central nervous system toxicity, in large or repeated doses it has one notable disadvantage, in that it induces methaemoglobinaemia (Scott *et al.*, 1964; Adamson and Spoerel, 1966; Hjelm and Holmdahl, 1965). The methaemoglobin level of the normal individual is less than 1 per cent of the total haemoglobin. After 600 mg. of prilocaine it rises to about 5 per cent. The peak concentration produced is directly proportional to the size of the prilocaine dose. The maximum methaemoglobin concentration is normally seen four to six hours after prilocaine administration and declines to normal in about 24 hours. Methaemoglobinaemia can be treated successfully in this situation with methylene blue, 1 mg./kg. Nevertheless, its occurrence may contra-indicate prilocaine in many situations, though a slight, transient rise in methaemoglobin level is harmless to most people.

BUPIVACAINE ("MARCAIN": "MARÇAINE": LAC-43)

Bupivacaine is one of the homologous series synthesised by Bo af Ekenstam to which mepivacaine belongs. First reports of its use were made in 1963 (Telivuo, 1963), since which time it has been used widely in Scandinavia and more recently elsewhere.

Physico-chemical properties.—Bupivacaine is a very highly lipid soluble substance.

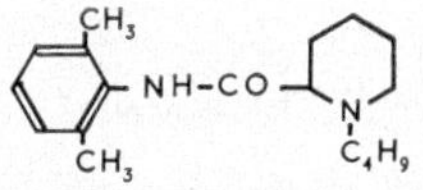

CH_3 / NH-CO / N / C_4H_9 / CH_3 bupivacaine

It has a pK_a of 8·2. Solutions of bupivacaine hydrochloride are stable and can be autoclaved.

Local analgesic properties.—Bupivacaine is three to four times as potent as lignocaine, and considerably longer lasting. It has been used for all manner of nerve blocks, for lumbar and caudal epidurals, and for paracervical block.

The duration of action is similar to that of amethocaine but it is less likely to produce motor block than amethocaine, especially in low concentration. It has become very popular for providing long-lasting analgesia, especially by continuous epidural blockade, when tachyphylaxis is much less likely than with lignocaine, and it appears that safe and effective analgesia can be provided almost indefinitely (Duthie *et al.*, 1968). For the relief of pain in labour its duration of action is from two to four hours, while it has produced post-operative analgesia for more than twelve hours (Telivuo, 1963).

Bupivacaine produces no vasodilatation at the site of injection. The addition of adrenaline has usually been found to increase its duration of action marginally except when small doses of bupivacaine are used, for example in continuous epidural analgesia in obstetrics (Reynolds and Taylor, 1971).

Clinically occurring blood levels of bupivacaine (Reynolds and Taylor 1970) are usually well below those likely to produce toxic symptoms (Jordfeldt *et al.*, 1968) and it is a less cumulative drug than lignocaine, and much less so than mepivacaine (Reynolds, 1971). It is highly bound to plasma protein and does not give rise to high foetal blood concentrations (Reynolds and Taylor, 1970 and 1971).

Dosage.—Concentrations of 0·25—0·5 per cent of bupivacaine are used for epidural analgesia. A concentration of 0·25 per cent has been found by some workers to fail to give complete blockade occasionally, while 0·5 per cent bupivacaine invariably achieves successful analgesia. Others have found 0·25 per cent satisfactory and the lack of motor blockade advantageous (Duthie *et al.*, 1968). It is probably advisable to include adrenaline, 2·5–5·0 μg/ml. (1:400,000–1:200,000) when prolonged continuous blockade is required.

For paracervical block 0·25 per cent bupivacaine may be used (Gudgeon, 1968). A higher concentration than this is more likely to give rise to foetal bradycardia.

With regard to the toxicity of bupivacaine, the original experimental work suggested an acute toxicity five times that of mepivacaine and similar to that of amethocaine. The LD_{50} i.v. mice is 7·8 mg./kg. Cumulative toxicity, however, is reduced relative to these two drugs (Henn and Brattsand, 1966).

In clinical practice bupivacaine is less toxic than amethocaine. The maximum safe dose is of the order of 2 mg./kg. In man, no conspicuous systemic toxicity has been reported after correctly placed and administered bupivacaine for local analgesia. Moreover, because it yields low blood concentrations, accumulates little and has a long duration of action, bupivacaine appears the safest drug available for continuous use. These factors, and the low foetal levels achieved, make it particularly useful during labour.

"Proctocaine" "Efocaine"

Older so-called long-acting local analgesics, Proctocaine and Efocaine, were solutions of procaine, etc., in benzyl alcohol and polyethylene glycol respectively. Analgesia lasting for days, weeks, or indefinitely was due to nerve destruction by the solvent rather than, as was hoped, to slow release of procaine. These agents were therefore highly dangerous and by definition not local analgesics.

REFERENCES

ADAMSON, D. H., and SPOEREL, W. E. (1966). Methaemoglobin levels during continuous epidural analgesia using prilocaine. *Acta anaesth. scand.*, Suppl. **23,** 379.

ADRIANI, J., and CAMPBELL, D. (1956). Fatalities following topical application of local anesthetics to mucous membranes. *J. Amer. med. Ass.*, **162,** 1527.

ÅKERMAN, B. (1969). Effects of felypressin (Octopressin®) on the acute toxicity of local anaesthetics. *Acta pharmacol. (Kbh).*, **27,** 318.

ALBERT, J., and LÖFSTRÖM, B. (1961). Bilateral ulnar nerve blocks for the evaluation of local anaesthetic agents. *Acta anaesth. scand.*, **5,** 99.

ÅSTRÖM, A. (1966). The pharmacological action of local anaesthetics. *Acta anaesth. scand.*, Suppl. **25,** 19.

BERNARD, C. G., BOHN, E., and HOJEBERG, S. (1955). New treatment of status epilepticus: intravenous injections of local anesthetic (lidocaine). *A.M.A. Arch. Neurol. Psychiat.*, **74,** 208.

BIANCHI, C. (1956). A simple new quantitative method for testing local anaesthetics. *Brit. J. Pharmacol.*, **11,** 104.

BIGGER, J. T., and HEISSENBUTTEL, R. H. (1969). The use of procaine amide and lidocaine in the treatment of cardiac arrhythmias. *Progr. cardiovasc. Dis.*, **11,** 515.

BONICA, J. J. (1957). Clinical investigation of local anasthetics. *Anesthesiology*, **18,** 110.

BRAID, D. P., and SCOTT, D. B. (1965). The systemic absorption of local analgesic drugs. *Brit. J. Anaesth.*, **37,** 394.

BRAID, D. P., and SCOTT, D. B. (1966). Dosage of lignocaine in epidural block in relation to toxicity. *Brit. J. Anaesth.*, **38,** 596.

BROMAGE, P. R. (1965). A comparison of the hydrochloride salts of lignocaine and prilocaine for epidural analgesia. *Brit. J. Anaesth.*, **37,** 753.

BROMAGE, P. R. (1969). A comparison of bupivacaine and tetracaine in epidural analgesia for surgery. *Canad. Anaesth. Soc. J.*, **17,** 37.

BROMAGE, P. R., and GERTEL, M. (1970). An evaluation of two new local anaesthetics for major conduction blockade. *Canad. Anaesth. Soc. J.*, **17,** 557.

BÜLBRING, E., and WAJDA, I. (1945). Biological comparison of local anesthetics. *J. Pharmacol. exp. Ther.*, **85,** 78.

DEACOCK, A. R., and SIMPSON, W. T. (1964). Fatal reactions to lignocaine. *Anaesthesia*, **19,** 217.

DUTHIE, A. M., WYMAN, J. B., and LEWIS, G. A. (1968). Bupivacaine in labour. *Anaesthesia*, **23,** 20.

EKBLOM, L., and WIDMAN, B. (1966). A comparison of the properties of LAC 43, prilocaine and mepivacaine in extradural anaesthesia. *Acta anaesth. scand.*, Suppl. **21,** 33.

EKENSTAM, B. af (1966). The effect of the structural variation on the local analgesic properties of the most commonly used groups of substances. *Acta anaesth. scand.*, Suppl. **25,** 10.

EKENSTAM, B. af, EGNÉR, B., ULFENDAHL, H. R., DHUNÉR, K. G., and ALJELUND, O. (1956). Trials with carbocaine: a new local anaesthetic drug. *Brit. J. Anaesth.*, **28,** 503.

EPSTEIN, B. S., BANNERJEE, S. G., and COAKLEY, C. S. (1968). Passage of lidocaine and prilocaine across the placenta. *Curr. Res. Anesth.*, **47,** 223.

ERIKSSON, E. (1966). Prilocaine, an experimental study in man of a new local anaesthetic, with special regards to efficacy, toxicity and excretion. *Acta chir. scand.*, Suppl. **358.**

FOLDES, F. F., MOLLOY, R., MCNALL, P. G., and KOUKAL, L. R. (1960). Comparison of toxicity in intravenously given local anesthetic agents in man. *J. Amer. med. Ass.*, **172,** 1493.

GEDDES, I. C. (1965). Studies of the metabolism of citanest. *Acta anaesth. scand.*, Suppl. **16,** 37.

GRAY, T. C., and GEDDES, I. C. (1954). A review of local anaesthetics. *J. Pharm. Pharmacol.*, **6,** 89.

GUDGEON, D. H. (1968). Paracervical nerve block with bupivacaine 0·25%. *Brit. med. J.*, **2,** 403.

HARRISON, D. C., SPROUSE, J. H., and MORROW, A. G. (1963). Antiarrhythmic properties of lidocaine and procaine amide: clinical and physiologic studies of their cardiovascular effects in man. *Circulation,* **28,** 486.

HELLMAN, L. M. (1965). Electronics in obstetrics and gynaecology. *J. Obstet. Gynaec. Brit. Cwlth.*, **72,** 896.

HENN, F. (1960). Determination of toxicological and pharmacological properties of carbocaine, lidocaine and procaine by means of simultaneous experiments. *Acta anaesth. scand.*, **4,** 125.

HENN, F., and BRATTSAND, R. (1966). Some pharmacological and toxicological properties of a new long-acting local analgesic, LAC–43 (Marcaine®), in comparison with mepivacaine and tetracaine. *Acta anaesth. scand.*, Suppl. **21,** 9.

HJELM, M., and HOLMDAHL, M. H:son (1965). Biochemical effects of aromatic amines. II. Cyanosis, methaemoglobinaemia and Heinz-body formation induced by a local anaesthetic agent (Prilocaine). *Acta anaesth. scand.*, **9,** 99.

HOLLUNGER, B. (1960). On the metabolism of Lidocaine II. The biotransformation of Lidocaine. *Acta pharmacol. (Kbh.)*, **17,** 365.

JEWITT, D. E., KISHON, Y., and THOMAS, M. (1968). Lignocaine in the management of arrhythmias after acute myocardial infarction. *Lancet,* **1,** 266.

JORFELDT, L., LOFSTROM, B., PERNOW, B., PERSSON, B., WAHREN, J., and WIDMAN, B. (1968). The effect of local anaesthetics on the central circulation and respiration in man and dog. *Acta anaesth. scand.*, **12,** 153.

KALOW, W. (1952). Hydrolysis of local anesthetics by human serum cholinesterase. *J. Pharmacol. exp. Ther.*, **104,** 122.

LODER, R. E. (1960). A local anaesthetic solution with longer action. *Lancet,* **2,** 346.

LUDUENA, F. P., HOPPE, J. O., and BORLAND, J. K. (1958). A statistical evaluation of the relationships among local anesthetic activity, irritancy and systemic toxicity. *J. Pharmacol. exp. Ther.*, **126,** 269.

MILNE, M. D., SCRIBNER, B. H., and CRAWFORD, M. A. (1958). Non-ionic diffusion and the excretion of weak acids and bases. *Amer. J. Med.*, **24,** 709.

MOORE, D. C., and BRIDENBAUGH, L. D. (1960). Oxygen: the antidote for systemic toxic reactions from local anesthetic drugs. *J. Amer. med. Ass.*, **174,** 842.

MOORE, D. C., BRIDENBAUGH, L. D., BAGDI, P. A., and BRIDENBAUGH, P. O. (1968). Accumulation of mepivacaine hydrochloride during caudal block. *Anesthesiology,* **29,** 585.

MORALES-AGUILERÁ, A., and VAUGHAN WILLIAMS, E. M. (1965). The effects on cardiac muscle of receptor antagonists in relation to their activity as local anaesthetics. *Brit. J. Pharmacol.*, **24,** 332.

MORISHIMA, H. O., DANIEL, S. S., FINSTER, M., POPPERS, P. J., and JAMES, L. S. (1966). Transmission of mepivacaine across the human placenta. *Anesthesiology,* **27,** 147.

MOYA, F., and THORNDIKE, V. (1962). Passage of drugs across the placenta. *Amer. J. Obstet. Gynec.*, **84,** 1778.

MURPHY, P. J., WRIGHT, J. D., and FITZGERALD, T. B. (1970). Assessment of paracervical nerve block anaesthesia during labour. *Brit. med. J.*, **1,** 526.

NYIRJESY, I., HAWKS, B. L., HERBERT, J. E., HOPWOOD, H. G., and FALLS, H. C. (1963). Hazards of the use of paracervical block anesthesia in obstetrics. *Amer. J. Obstet. Gynec.*, **87,** 231.

REYNOLDS, F. (1971). A comparison of the potential toxicity of bupivacaine, lignocaine and mepivacaine during epidural blockade for surgery. *Brit. J. Anaesth.*, **43,** 567.

REYNOLDS, F., and TAYLOR, G. (1970). Maternal and neonatal concentrations of bupivacaine. A comparison with lignocaine during continuous extradural analgesia. *Anaesthesia*, **25,** 14.

REYNOLDS, F., and TAYLOR, G. (1971). Plasma concentration of bupivacaine during continuous epidural analgesia in labour: the effect of adrenaline. *Brit. J. Anaesth.*, **43,** 436.

RITCHIE, J. M., and GREENGARD, P. (1966). On the mode of action of local anesthetics. *Ann. Rev. Pharmacol.*, **6,** 405.

RITCHIE, J. M., RITCHIE, B., and GREENGARD, P. (1965). The effect of the nerve sheath on the action of local anesthetics. *J. Pharmacol. exp. Ther.*, **150,** 160.

SCOTT, D. B., OWEN, J. A., and RICHMOND, J. (1964). Methaemoglobinaemia due to prilocaine. *Lancet*, **2,** 728.

SHNIDER, S. M., and WAY, E. L. (1968*a*). The kinetics of transfer of lidocaine (Xylocaine®) across the human placenta. *Anesthesiology*, **29,** 944.

SHNIDER, S. M., and WAY, E. L. (1968*b*). Plasma levels of lidocaine (Xylocaine®) in mother and newborn following obstetrical conduction anesthesia. *Anesthesiology*, **29,** 951.

SINCLAIR, J. C., FOX, H. A., LENTZ, J. F., FULD, G. L., and MURPHY, J. (1965). Intoxication of the fetus by a local anesthetic. *New Engl. J. Med.*, **273,** 1173.

SINGER, D. H., and TEN EICK, R. E. (1969). Pharmacology of cardiac arrhythmias. *Progr. cardiovasc. Dis.*, **11,** 488.

STEINHAUS, J. E. (1952). A comparative study of the experimental toxicity of local anesthetic agents. *Anesthesiology*, **13,** 577.

STEINHAUS, J. E. (1957). Local anesthetic toxicity: a pharmacological re-evaluation. *Anesthesiology*, **18,** 275.

SUNSHINE, I., and FIKE, W. W. (1964). Value of thin layer chromatography in two fatal cases of intoxication due to lidocaine and mepivacaine. *New Engl. J. Med.*, **271,** 487.

TELIVUO, L. (1963). A new long-acting local anaesthetic solution for pain relief after thoracotomy. *Ann. Chir. Gynaec. Fenn.*, **52,** 513.

Chapter 42

SPINAL AND EPIDURAL ANALGESIA:
ANATOMY AND PHYSIOLOGY

by

D. D. B. MORRIS

THE ANATOMY OF THE SPINAL COLUMN, SPINAL CANAL, SPINAL CORD AND COVERINGS

THE vertebral column is made up of 33 vertebrae: 7 cervical, 12 thoracic, 5 lumbar, 5 sacral, and 4 coccygeal. A typical vertebra is composed of the following parts (Fig. 1):

1. *The Body*, which is weight-bearing and separated from adjoining vertebral bodies by the intervertebral disc.
2. *The Vertebral Arch*, composed of pedicles and laminae which surround and protect the spinal cord and its coverings.
3. *The Transverse and Spinous Processes*, which give attachment to muscles acting on the vertebral column.
4. *The Superior and Inferior Articular Processes.*

Each pedicle is grooved, especially on the lower surface. These grooves are termed the superior and inferior vertebral notches and together make up the intervertebral foramen for the passage of the spinal nerve. The two laminae meet in the mid-line posteriorly and at the point of fusion arises the spinous process. The transverse process arises at the junction of the pedicle and the lamina.

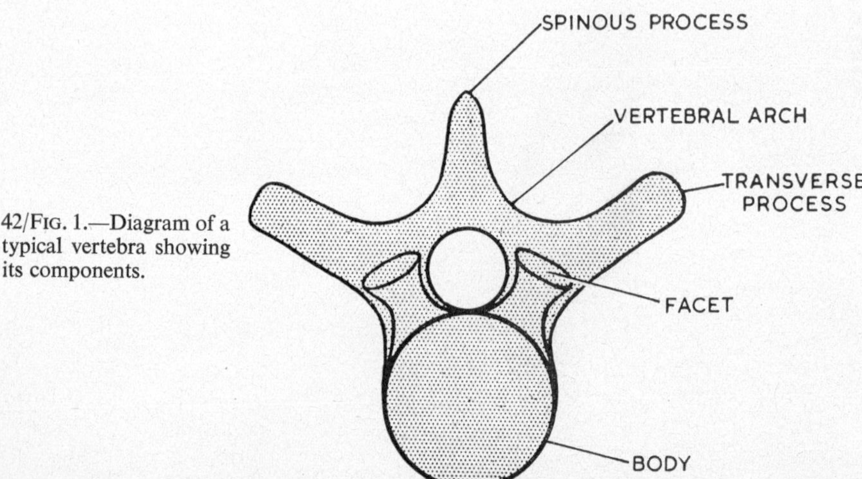

42/FIG. 1.—Diagram of a typical vertebra showing its components.

The vertebral arch, its processes and connecting ligaments are the anatomical parts of greatest interest to the anaesthetist, for it is in this region that the needle is passed to introduce the local analgesic solution. The space enclosed posteriorly by the laminae and spines of adjoining vertebrae is termed the inter-laminar foramen and it is through this that the spinal needle passes to pierce the dura.

Although the lumbar region is the commonest site for the introduction of local analgesic solutions to the spinal or epidural space, the cervical and thoracic regions may in certain circumstances be used and the anaesthetist therefore requires an anatomical knowledge of them.

The Vertebrae

The cervical vertebrae.—The atlas, axis, and seventh cervical vertebra are atypical, but the remaining four vertebrae conform to a common type. These vertebrae have the following characteristics (Fig. 2):

1. The body is broader from side to side than in the antero-posterior diameter, and the upper surface has a raised lip at the back and sides.

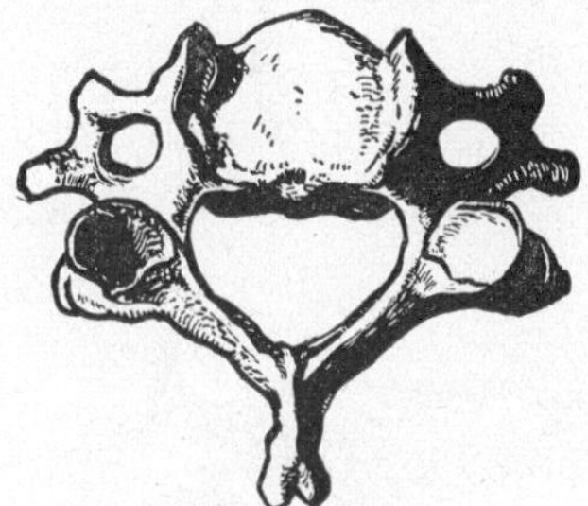

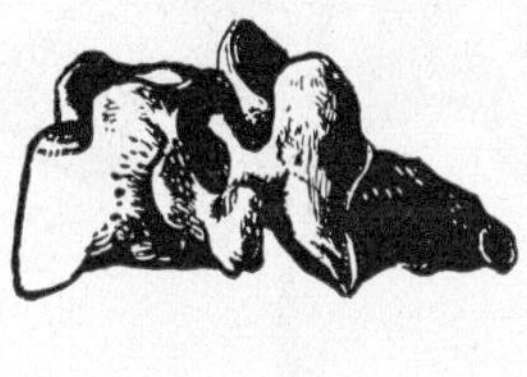

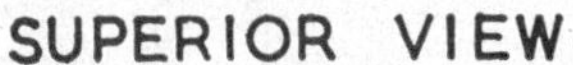

42/FIG. 2.—A typical cervical vertebra.

2. The pedicles arise from the lateral aspect of the body, midway between the upper and lower margins, and as a result the superior and inferior vertebral notches are of equal depth.
3. The laminae are narrow and thin and meet in the mid-line posteriorly to form short bifid spinous processes. The vertebral foramen is triangular as in the lumbar region.
4. The articular processes and facets project laterally from the junction of the pedicles and laminae. The superior articular facet faces upwards, backwards, and slightly medially, while the inferior facet faces downwards and forwards.
5. The transverse processes lie anterior to the articular processes. On the extreme outer portion of the transverse process are the anterior and posterior tubercles connected by the costo-transverse bar which is grooved for the issuing spinal nerve. In the transverse process lies the foramen transversorium through which run the vertebral artery, vein, and sympathetic nerves. The anterior tubercle of C6 is particularly prominent and known as the carotid tubercle, as at this bony point the carotid artery can be compressed against the tubercle.

The thoracic vertebrae.—Only the middle four of the twelve thoracic vertebrae can be regarded as typical. T1–T4 in some measure resemble cervical vertebrae. The upper half of T1 is like a cervical vertebra in that the body turns up at the sides and back, the superior articular processes and facets face upwards and backwards, and the vertebral foramen is triangular and not circular as in the mid-thoracic region. The last four thoracic vertebrae resemble lumbar vertebrae. The lower half of T12 is like a lumbar vertebra in that the body is

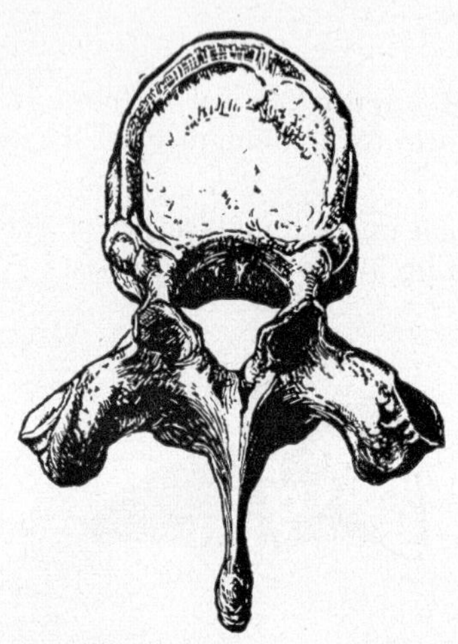

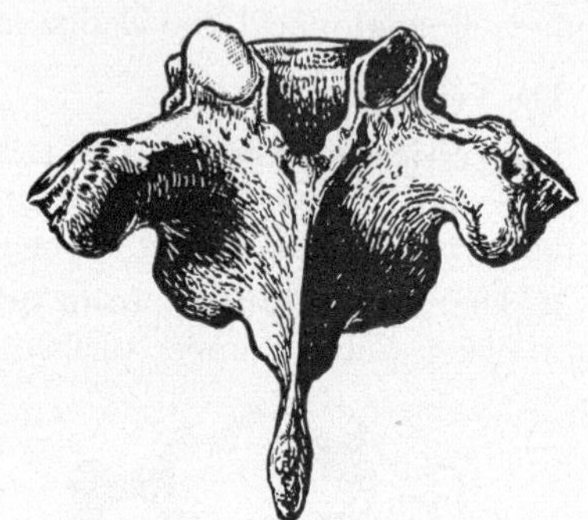

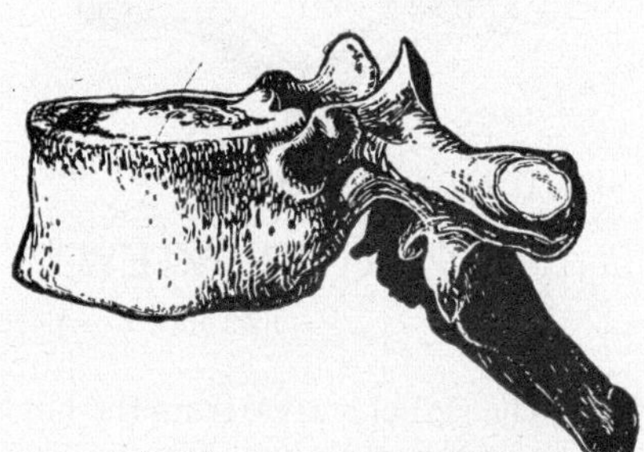

42/FIG. 3.—A thoracic vertebra.

kidney shaped, the inferior articular processes face laterally, and the vertebral foramen is triangular.

The distinctive feature of a thoracic vertebra is that the body bears articular facets for the heads of the ribs. The arrangement of facets is a useful guide to the numerical placing of an individual thoracic vertebra. T1 bears a single facet for the head of the first rib and a demi-facet for the upper part of the head of the second rib. The arrangement of facets is shown in the diagram (Fig. 3).

The bodies of the middle four thoracic vertebrae are heart-shaped. Each body is taller posteriorly than anteriorly and so makes the thoracic curve concave forwards. The bodies of T3–12 show a gradual increase in size proportionate to the increased weight they have to support. The bodies of T5–8 are flattened on the left side by the pressure of the descending aorta.

The spines are of anaesthetic interest because they necessitate oblique placing of an epidural needle in the mid-thoracic region (Fig. 4). The spines of T5–8 are almost vertical and in consequence their tips lie at the level of the body of the vertebra below. The spines of T1 and 2 and of T11 and 12 are almost horizontal, while those of T3 and 4, and of T9 and 10 are somewhat oblique. The articular processes are set almost perpendicularly, the superior facets facing backwards and laterally. The inferior facets face forwards and medially.

The transverse processes are directed backwards and laterally in conformity with the backward sweep of the ribs. The facets are concave for articulation with the tubercles of the ribs.

The cervical enlargement of the cord extends as far as T2 and hence the vertebral canal in the upper two thoracic vertebrae is triangular to accommodate the laterally expanded cord. In the same way the lumbar enlargement beginning at T10 produces a triangular vertebral canal in the last two thoracic vertebrae.

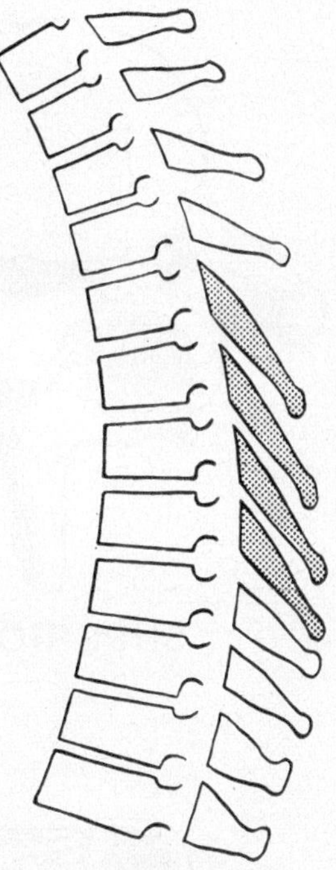

42/Fig. 4.—The inclination of the thoracic vertebral spines.

The lumbar vertebrae.—These are five in number, with large and massive kidney-shaped bodies because of their weight-bearing function, and are distinguished from thoracic and cervical vertebrae by having no foramen in the transverse process and no articular facets for ribs on the vertebral bodies (Fig. 5). The bodies are slightly taller anteriorly than posteriorly and the intervertebral discs are similarly shaped, producing the lumbar curve. The pedicles are directed backwards and laterally as in the cervical region. The superior intervertebral notch is small and the inferior large. The laminae are thick and sloping, as in the thoracic region, and the vertebral foramen is triangular. The spine is a thick oblong plate which projects backwards nearly horizontally. The transverse processes arise from the junction of the pedicles and laminae, those of L1, 2 and 3 increasing in length and those of L4 and 5 becoming shorter. The superior articular processes and facets arise from the pedicles, and face medially, and articulate with the laterally facing inferior articular facet. The fifth lumbar vertebra is characterised by three features: the body is markedly taller in front than behind, the inferior articular process nearly faces forwards, and the transverse process encroaches along the pedicle until it reaches the body.

Important Ligaments of the Vertebral Column

It is essential for the anaesthetist practising spinal and epidural analgesia to have an accurate knowledge of those ligaments in the spine through which the spinal or epidural needle passes. The different sensations of resistance that these ligaments impart to the advancing needle can with practice be appreciated by the operator and are an invaluable aid to successful technique.

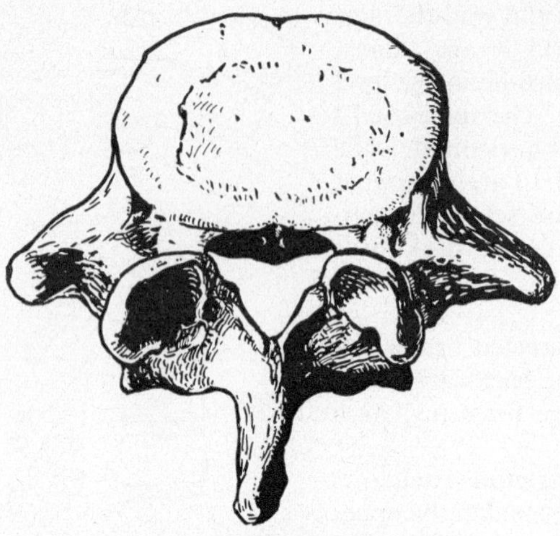

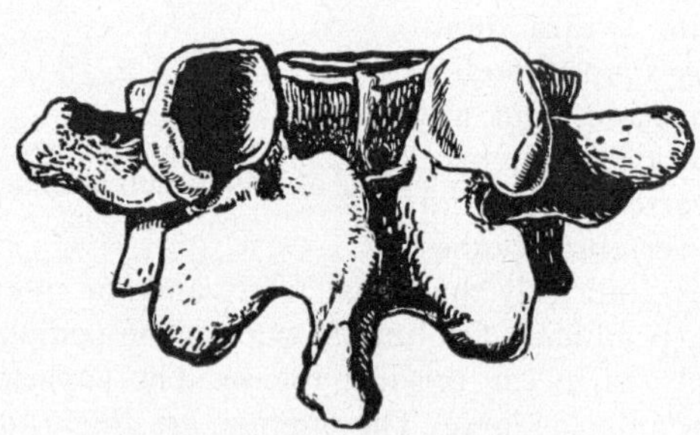

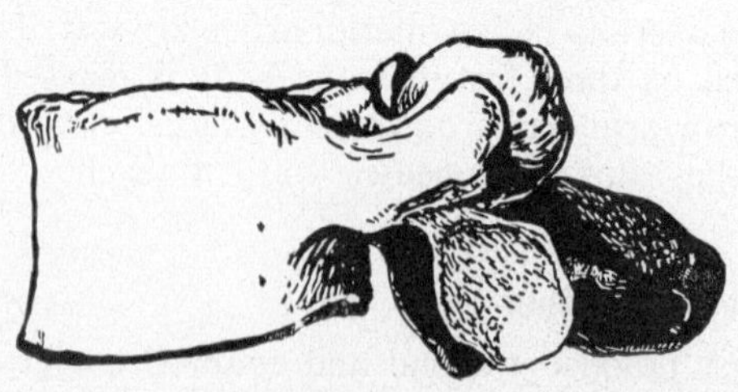

42/FIG. 5.—A lumbar vertebra.

The vertebrae are held together by a series of overlapping ligaments which not only bind together the vertebral column but assist in protecting the spinal cord (Fig. 6).

The anterior longitudinal ligament.—This ligament is more of anatomical than anaesthetic interest. It begins at the axis as a continuation of the atlanto-axial ligament and extends down the entire front of the bodies of the vertebrae to the sacrum, closely attached to the margins of the vertebral bodies. It is thickest in the thoracic and lumbar regions.

The posterior longitudinal ligament.—This ligament begins on the posterior surface of the vertebral body of the axis and extends down through the entire length of the vertebral column, fanning out at the vertebral margins to reinforce the intervertebral discs. The ligament is thinnest in the cervical and lumbar regions. It is possible for this ligament to be pierced by a too-far-advancing lumbar puncture needle, and for damage to the intervertebral disc to result.

The ligamentum flavum.—This ligament is of considerable importance to the anaesthetist and must be described in detail. It is composed entirely of yellow elastic fibres, which account for its name. It is placed on either side of the spinous process and extends laterally to blend with the capsule of the joints between the superior and inferior articular processes. It runs from the anterior and inferior aspects of the lamina above to the posterior and superior aspect of the lamina below. In the mid-line there is a cleft between it and the ligamentum flavum of the opposite side for the passage of veins. A spinal needle accurately placed in the mid-line would only pass through a few thin fibres of the ligamenta flava and impart very little change of resistance to the anaesthetist. In practice, however, the needle is probably always a little off centre and passes through the full thickness of the ligament. The ligamenta flava are thinnest in the cervical region and thickest in the lumbar region, where powerful stresses and strains have to be countered. They are functionally muscle sparers, assisting in the recovery of the erect posture after bending, and in maintaining the erect posture.

Interspinous ligaments.—These ligaments connect adjoining spinous processes from their tips to their roots. They fuse with the supraspinous ligament

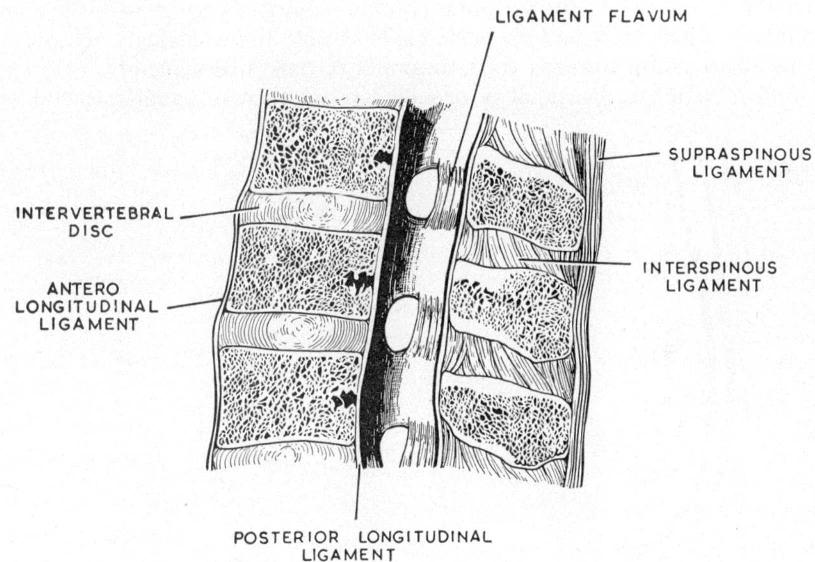

42/Fig. 6.—Important ligaments of the vertebral column.

posteriorly and with the ligamentum flavum anteriorly. In the lumbar region they are wide and dense.

Supraspinous ligament.—This ligament is a continuation of the ligamentum nuchae and joins together the tips of the spinous processes from the seventh cervical vertebra to the sacrum. It increases in thickness from above downwards and is thickest and widest in the lumbar region.

The Intervertebral Discs

These discs are responsible for a quarter of the length of the spinal column, and, functionally, are shock absorbers placed between the vertebral bodies. They are thicker in the cervical and lumbar regions, where they allow of great mobility, than in the thoracic parts of the column. Each disc consists of a peripheral fibrous portion—the annulus fibrosus—and a gelatinous central portion —the nucleus pulposus—which accommodates itself to changes in shape during movement between the vertebrae.

The Spinal Cord and its Coverings

The spinal cord, a direct continuation of the medulla oblongata, begins at the upper border of the atlas and ends at the lower border of the 1st lumbar vertebra. It is 18 inches in length. It is not uncommon for the cord to extend to the second lumbar vertebra, particularly in negro races. Exceptionally the cord can reach the 3rd lumbar vertebra. In order to avoid possible damage to the cord, lumbar puncture should, if possible, be made in the L4–5 interspace. In the new-born child the cord ends at the 3rd lumbar vertebra, and in foetal life the cord extends the entire length of the vertebral canal and the spinal nerves run in a horizontal direction. As the vertebral column elongates with growth the spinal cord does not keep pace and the nerve roots assume an increasingly oblique and downward direction towards their foramina of exit. Consequently, below the 1st lumbar vertebra the canal is occupied by a leash of lumbar, sacral and

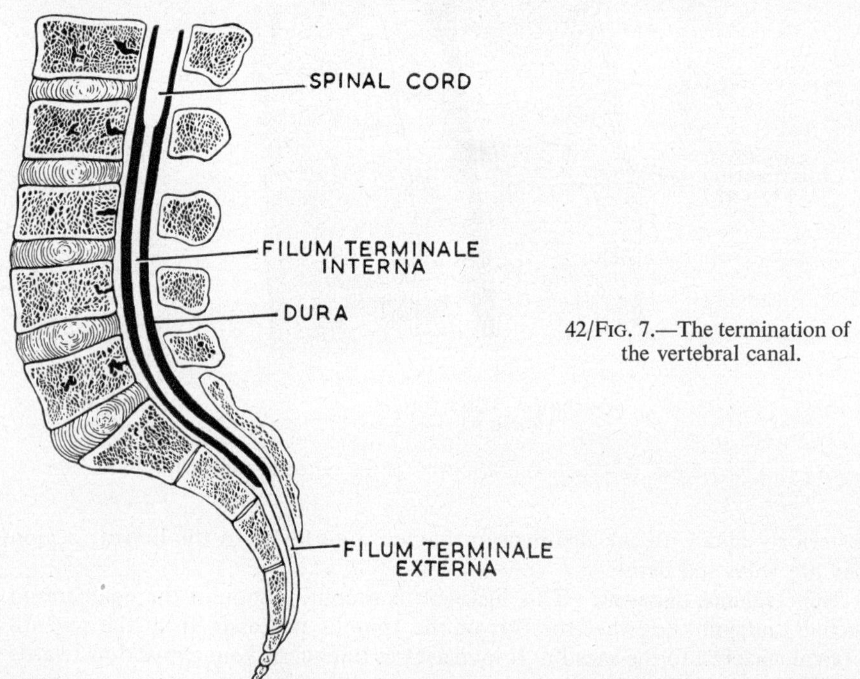

42/Fig. 7.—The termination of the vertebral canal.

coccygeal nerve roots, termed the cauda equina. The difference between the cord level of a given spinal root and the vertebral level has important practical consequences when it is desired to block accurately spinal nerve roots with small volumes of neurolytic agents. Failure to appreciate this point and the choice of the vertebral level rather than the cord level for injection will result in destruction of nerve roots below the desired levels.

From the lower end of the spinal cord extends a thread-like structure known as the filum terminale interna which ends with the dura and the arachnoid mater at the level of the second sacral vertebra (Fig. 7). It pierces the dura and arachnoid and is continued below this level as the filum terminale externa eventually blending with the periosteum on the back of the coccyx. The 31 spinal nerves emerge from the spinal cord in pairs, 8 cervical, 12 thoracic, 5 lumbar, 5 sacral, and one pair of coccygeal nerves. The cord presents two enlargements, cervical and lumbar, corresponding to the nerve supply of the upper and lower limbs. The cervical enlargement extends from C3 to T2 and the lumbar enlargement from T9–12.

The spinal cord is enveloped by three membranes, dura, arachnoid, and pia mater, which are direct continuations of those surrounding the brain.

The spinal dura mater.—In the cranial cavity the dura is arranged in two layers, "periosteal" and "investing", which are firmly adherent except where they split to enclose venous sinuses. The outer periosteal layer is the periosteum of the inner surface of the skull bones which, in the spine, acts as the periosteum lining the spinal canal. The inner or investing layer is continued from the cranium into the spinal canal. Between the two layers in the spinal canal is the extra- or epi-dural space which anatomically would be better termed the *inter-dural* space.

The inner layer of dura is firmly adherent to the margins of the foramen magnum where it blends with the outer or periosteal layer. Hence solutions deposited correctly in the spinal epidural space cannot enter the cranial cavity or produce nerve block higher than the 1st cervical nerves. The inner layer is loosely attached to the posterior longitudinal ligament by fibrous strands anchoring it in place. The epidural space is narrower anteriorly and wider posteriorly where the inner layer of dura is unattached; its greatest width (6 mm.) occurs in the mid-thoracic region.

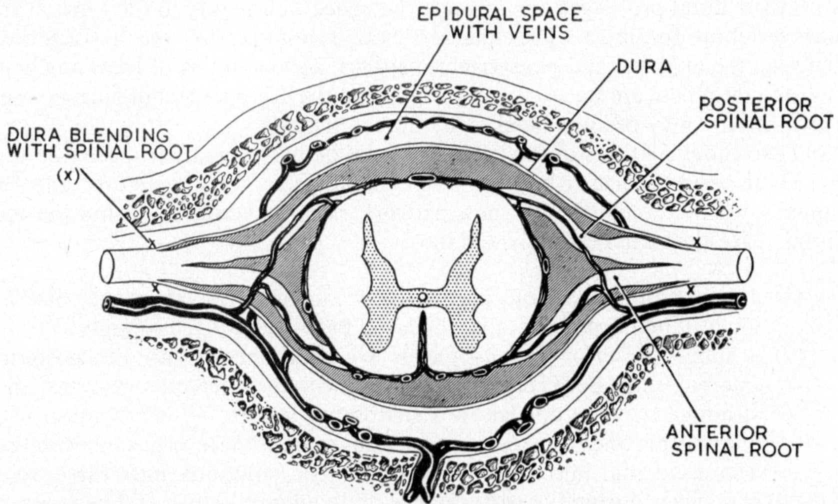

42/FIG. 8—Dural cuffs and the venous plexus of the epidural space.

The anterior and posterior nerve roots issuing from the spinal cord pierce the investing layer of dura and carry tubular prolongations (dural cuffs) which blend with the perineurium of the mixed spinal nerve (Fig. 8).

The investing layer of dura ends as a tube at the 2nd sacral vertebra, and so also does the arachnoid, so that cerebrospinal fluid is not found below this level. The dura ends by giving an investment to the filum terminale externa and blends eventually with the periosteum on the back of the coccyx.

The arachnoid mater.—The spinal arachnoid is a continuation of the cerebral arachnoid. An incomplete and inconstant septum divides the spinal subarachnoid space along the mid-line of the dorsal surface of the cord.

The pia mater.—In the vertebral canal the pia is closely applied to the spinal cord and extends into the anterior median fissure. The blood vessels going to the brain and spinal cord lie in the subarachnoid space before piercing the pia. They carry with them into the brain and spinal cord a double sleeve of meninges; the inner wall of the sleeve is derived from the pia, and the outer from the arachnoid.

In the depths of the brain and spinal cord the perivascular space containing cerebrospinal fluid becomes continuous with the perineural space.

The circulation of cerebrospinal fluid deep into the interstices of the brain may be of considerable significance as regards the route of absorption of local analgesics injected into the subarachnoid space.

The Epidural Space

The formation of the epidural space by the splitting of the two layers of the spinal dura mater has been described. It remains to define the space and its contents anatomically and in greater detail. The space is limited superiorly by the fusion of the two layers of dura at the foramen magnum, and inferiorly by the sacro-coccygeal ligament closing the sacral hiatus. The 31 pairs of spinal nerves with their dural prolongations traverse the space on the way to their exit at the intervertebral foramina. The intervertebral foramina are the passageways between the epidural and paravertebral spaces, and solutions of local analgesic injected into them are free to travel from one to the other, except in old age when the foramina may become blocked by fibrous tissue.

The venous plexuses of the vertebral canal lie in the epidural space (see Fig. 8). These veins receive tributaries from the adjacent bony structures and the spinal cord. Although they form a network running vertically within the epidural space they can be subdivided into:

(1) a pair of anterior venous plexuses which lie on either side of the posterior longitudinal ligament, into which the basivertebral veins empty;

(2) a single posterior venous plexus which connects with the posterior external veins. Both (1) and (2) connect with the intervertebral veins, and, although they are divided into anatomical groups, all interconnect with one another and form a series of venous rings at the level of each vertebra. The accidental injection of local analgesic solutions into these veins may occur during the performance of an epidural block and be responsible for toxic reactions.

In addition to the venous plexuses, branches from the vertebral, ascending cervical, deep cervical, intercostal, lumbar and ilio-lumbar arteries enter the intervertebral foramen and anastomose with one another, chiefly in the lateral parts of the epidural space.

Fatty tissue corresponding in amount with the adiposity of the subject lies between the arteries, veins and nerves in the epidural space.

The Paravertebral Space

The paravertebral space is not defined as such in formal anatomical works. It has, however, been described and defined by the Oxford School (Macintosh and Bryce-Smith, 1962) and their description cannot be bettered (Fig. 9).

The space is wedge-shaped and in the thoracic region is bounded above and below by the heads and necks of adjoining ribs. The posterior wall is formed by the superior costo-transverse ligament running from the lower border of the transverse process above to the upper border of the rib below. The base is formed by the postero-lateral aspect of the body of the vertebra, and the intervertebral foramen and its contents. Medially the space communicates with the epidural space through the intervertebral foramen and laterally at the level of the tips of the transverse processes the apex is continuous with the intercostal space. Anterolaterally the space is limited by the parietal pleura.

Communication between spaces is not possible anteriorly or posteriorly but local analgesic solutions can pass from one space to another medially via the intervertebral foramen and epidural space.

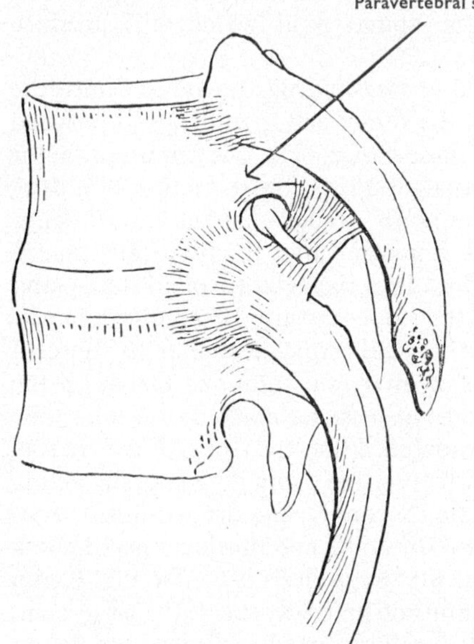

42/Fig. 9.—Diagram to illustrate the boundaries of the paravertebral space (see text).

The Physiology of Spinal and Epidural Analgesia

Following the introduction of a local analgesic solution into the subarachnoid space, pre-ganglionic sympathetic fibres are blocked first. After these autonomic fibres, in order of increasing diameter come fibres transmitting the sensations of temperature, pain, touch, and finally pressure. As outlined in the previous chapter, the order of these effects is a direct consequence of fibre size. The largest fibres are motor and proprioceptive, and these too will be ultimately blocked if the concentration of analgesic drug is high enough. This sequence of events can be observed in the conscious patient during spinal analgesia. When sensory blockade is complete, skeletal muscle movement may still be possible, though this in turn will disappear if the concentration of drug is high enough to affect the larger fibres of the motor roots.

Position sense is the most resistant, and even with complete motor block a patient may be able to give an account of the direction in which his foot is moved. From the purely physiological point of view, the most important effect is the paralysis of sympathetic fibres. Spinal analgesia may be regarded as a chemical sympathectomy, and as a consequence of it a train of physiological events follows which affects, amongst other things, the cardiovascular system—particularly the blood pressure and blood flow to organs such as the brain—the respiratory and gastro-intestinal systems. Similar considerations apply to epidural analgesia.

The site of action of local analgesic drugs in the subarachnoid space is assumed to be on the fibres of the dorsal and ventral roots. At what particular point on the dorsal root is not certain: it could be on the cells of the dorsal root ganglia, their axons, or both. Frumin and his co-workers (1953*a*) have produced evidence that the site of action of minimally effective concentrations of procaine which block sensory but not motor impulses is the dorsal root ganglion. The minimal concentration of procaine in the spinal fluid which will produce sensory blockade is 0·02 mg. per cent.

While the precise site of action of local analgesic drugs introduced into the subarachnoid space is of scientific interest, the site of action of drugs introduced into the epidural space is of even greater importance. The one common factor to all the neurological sequelae of spinal analgesia is the introduction of a drug into the subarachnoid space, and it is commonly argued that the use of drugs epidurally will avoid these neurological sequelae. But if epidurally placed analgesic solutions do diffuse across the dura into the cerebrospinal fluid—and there is now considerable evidence that they do—the use of epidural blocks might be expected to be followed by neurological sequelae similar to those of spinal analgesia. The exact site of action of analgesic solutions placed in the epidural space is, however, still not worked out with certainty. For a long time only two possible sites of action were considered. First, the drug diffuses across the dura into the subarachnoid space and effects a true "spinal" analgesia, acting on either nerve roots or dorsal root ganglia. Secondly, the drug diffuses from the epidural space through the intervertebral foramina and produces nerve block in the paravertebral space. Evidence for the first hypothesis is conflicting. Rudin and his co-workers (1951) in dogs, and Frumin and his co-workers (1953*b*) in man, studied the permeability of the dura to epidurally injected procaine, and found that procaine appeared in the cerebrospinal fluid in significant quantities. In dogs it is possible to recover up to 10 per cent of the dose of the local analgesic placed in the epidural space; four minutes after the injection of 2 per cent procaine the concentration of procaine in the cerebrospinal fluid rises to 0·8 mg.

per cent (minimal effective concentration 0·02 mg. per cent). Using in man the two catheter technique—one in the epidural space and the other in the subarachnoid space—Frumin found that the waxing and waning of clinical analgesia closely followed the concentration of procaine in the cerebrospinal fluid. Skin analgesia was present when the concentration of procaine in the cerebrospinal fluid rose above 0·015 per cent—a figure closely approximating to the known minimal effective concentration of procaine in the cerebrospinal fluid. More recently the problem has again been studied in man by Foldes and his associates (1956) who also used the two catheter technique, but with 2-chloroprocaine as the analgesic. During well-established epidural block, the concentration of this drug in the cerebrospinal fluid was lower than the concentration found later at the moment when the epidural analgesia came to an end. The conclusion to be drawn from Foldes' work is that, at least with 2-chloroprocaine, an analgesic concentration of the drug is not present in the cerebrospinal fluid during effective epidural block.

It is known for certain that epidural solutions do diffuse into the paravertebral space and presumed that they can produce nerve block at this site. Even this concept has its difficulties. Bromage (1954) describes a patient in whom a radio-opaque analgesic solution injected into the epidural space did not spread through the intervertebral foramina of the mid-thoracic region although analgesia was present in this area, and concludes that spread into the paravertebral space is not a prerequisite of successful epidural analgesia.

Bromage (1962*a*), from a statistical study of the spread of analgesic solutions in the epidural space, has advanced a third view on their site of action which, he considers, reconciles all the clinical and experimental evidence available at the moment. It has been shown that in the region of the dural cuffs, where the anterior and posterior nerve roots fuse (see Fig. 8), material up to 0·5μ in size can readily diffuse between the subarachnoid, subdural and epidural spaces. Likewise, extremely small quantities of radioactive substances, introduced without pressure into the sub-perineural spaces of the sciatic nerve, can enter the spinal cord, brain stem, and even the basal ganglia, in significant amounts after a short time. But passage into the cerebrospinal fluid is slow, and does not reach a maximum until 50 or 60 minutes after injection (Brierley and Field, 1948 and 1949; Brierley, 1950; Field, 1951). A comparable time lag was recorded in the experiments of Foldes and his colleagues (1956). The similarity of the time relationships in the two sets of data is very suggestive of a common underlying mechanism. Bromage thus puts the view that analgesic solutions can reach the sub-perineural spaces by diffusion around the capillary and lymphatic channels of the vasa nervorum at and beyond the dural cuff areas. Once inside the endoneural spaces longitudinal capillary networks provide tissue interspaces along which solutions can travel up the spinal roots and into the sub-pial spaces of the cord. From there, diffusion into the cerebrospinal fluid occurs, but only after nerve blockade, and thus analgesia, has occurred.

This concept of neuraxial spread is a most important one, since if it is correct and if the view is taken that some neurological sequelae of spinal analgesia are due to the analgesic drug itself, then it follows that epidural analgesia cannot be regarded as potentially free from the same risks.

Bromage's views are summarised in Fig. 10.

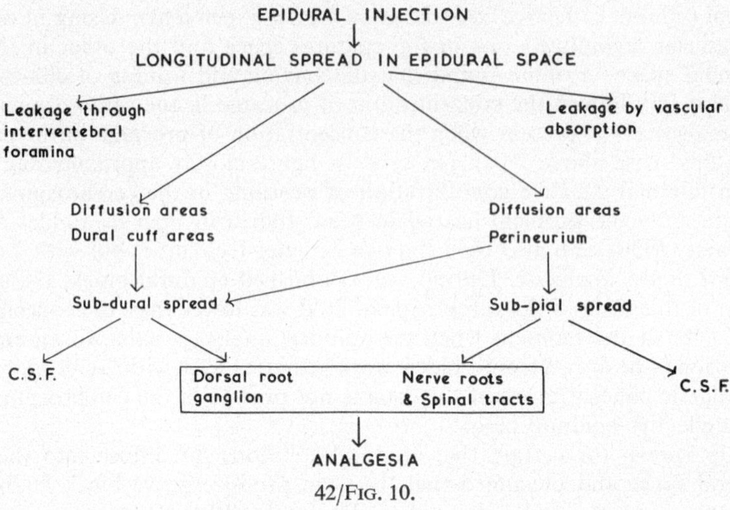

42/FIG. 10.

The amount of drug available to diffuse along the neuraxis will depend on the state of the neural coverings and the physical laws of diffusion. These factors have an important bearing on the height of epidural analgesia and will be discussed later.

Fate of Analgesic Drugs in the Subarachnoid and Epidural Spaces

Following the injection of an analgesic drug into the subarachnoid space, the concentration falls rapidly in the cerebrospinal fluid at the point of injection. The rate of fall is quickest during the first five minutes after injection and is then more gradual. The initial steep fall is due to diffusion of the drug away from the point of injection which is in turn dependent on such factors as the speed of injection, the specific gravity of the analgesic solution, the posture of the patient and the rate of absorption into nerve roots. These factors will shortly be discussed. It is during this period that spinal analgesia is said to become "fixed".

Local analgesic drugs are not destroyed in the cerebrospinal fluid, and so the more gradual decrease in concentration reflects the removal of the drug by vascular absorption. Detoxication ultimately takes place in the liver. Detectable amounts of local analgesic remain in the cerebrospinal fluid during the effective duration of the analgesia and even up to the point where analgesia is waning.

There are three possible mechanisms of absorption.

1. *Absorption through the spinal arachnoid villi.*—Elwan, in 1923, demonstrated cell clusters in the regions where the arachnoid is reflected proximally on to the segmental nerves as they leave the subarachnoid space. Some absorption of spinal analgesic drugs probably occurs through these cells.

2. *Absorption through capillaries.*—Figure 8 shows the numerous vascular channels that lie within the subdural and epidural spaces. Cerebrospinal fluid is probably absorbed by this capillary network. Such a mechanism would therefore play an important part in the removal of drugs from the subarachnoid space.

3. *Absorption through the cranial arachnoid villi into the venous sinuses.*—Absorption undoubtedly takes place in effective amounts before the solution reaches the cranium. Koster and his co-workers (1936 and 1938) have shown in man, by means of serial taps above the lumbar puncture injection, a rapidly decreasing concentration of the drug in the subarachnoid space.

Studies with radio-active dibromo-procaine in animals indicate that the greater portion of an analgesic drug leaves the subarachnoid space by the venous drainage, and a much smaller proportion by the lymphatics (Howarth, 1949).

As might be expected, the use of a vasoconstrictor in conjunction with the local analgesic drug results in considerable prolongation of the duration of analgesia. Bonica and his colleagues (1951) have shown in a large controlled series of subarachnoid blocks that adrenaline and "Neosynephrine" both increase the duration of analgesia by 50 per cent and this has been confirmed by Helrich (1951) and his associates. Ephedrine is far less effective and reliable than the other two drugs.

Absorption of epidural solutions is largely by way of the epidural vessels and is delayed if vasoconstrictors are added. The ultimate clearance of an epidural solution is complex, for it is now appreciated that apart from spreading longitudinally in the epidural space, it also traverses meningeal and perineural barriers to reach the cerebrospinal fluid. Thus it will be cleared to some extent by mechanisms that apply to drugs directly introduced into the cerebrospinal fluid.

Pathological states may also influence clearance of drugs both in the epidural space and the cerebrospinal fluid. Decreased blood flow to the vessels surrounding the subarachnoid space could explain the longer duration of analgesia in arteriosclerotic patients. Similarly, impeded absorption from thickened epidural blood vessels will influence clearance of epidural solutions (see p. 1199). Hypotensive states will also prolong both spinal and epidural analgesia.

Factors Controlling the Height of Spinal Analgesia

The upward passage of an analgesic solution in the subarachnoid space depends upon a number of factors. The following are the most important which control the subsequent level of analgesia:

1. **Specific gravity of the solution.**—Of the many factors which influence the spread of spinal analgesic solutions in the cerebrospinal fluid, gravity is the most important. Spinal analgesic solutions are classed as hyperbaric, isobaric, and hypobaric according to whether their specific gravity is higher, the same, or lower than that of cerebrospinal fluid. The movement of hyperbaric and hypobaric solutions in the C.S.F. depends in turn upon the position of the patient during injection, and any change in position after the injection is completed.

2. **Volume of analgesic solution.**—The greater the volume of solution injected into an area of fixed volume, such as the subarachnoid space, the more extensive is the subsequent spread. The effect of volume is independent of concentration and specific gravity. The extent to which this variable is used in clinical practice will be discussed under the description of spinal analgesic techniques.

3. **Total dose of drug injected.**—In general, the larger the dose of drug injected the longer the duration of the analgesia and the greater the height to which it rises. However, absorption into the venous plexuses of the spinal canal is rapid, and cases have been recorded where the administration of as much as

800 mg. of procaine has not resulted in analgesia above the inguinal region (Burford, 1942). Another explanation of this phenomenon is that spinal analgesic drugs are rapidly taken up by nervous tissue, and then slowly given off and absorbed by the mechanisms previously described.

4. **Speed and force of injection.**—The faster the rate of injection, the higher the level of analgesia obtained. Turbulent currents are set up by rapid injection and these cause spread of the solution. Macintosh (1951) has described experiments with saline-filled "glass spines" and shown that rapid injection with the production of eddies is facilitated by the use of small syringes and large bore needles. With the fine needles now recommended to diminish the incidence and severity of post-lumbar puncture headache it is difficult to inject sufficiently rapidly to set up big enough eddies to spread the drug widely in the cerebrospinal fluid.

5. **Barbotage.**—The term is derived from the French *barboter*—to puddle, to mix. The word "barbotage" was coined by Le Filliotre and the technique was popularised in spinal analgesia by Labat. The basis of the technique is to leave the injecting syringe attached to the spinal needle and make repeated aspirations and injections, thus mixing and dispersing the original dose of local analgesic. The spread of a given dose of an analgesic is closely related to the amount of barbotage used, a much higher level of analgesia resulting from its use.

6. **Site of injection.**—It is of course possible to use any spinal interspace for the introduction of a local analgesic, but in order to avoid possible damage to the spinal cord it is safer to restrict lumbar puncture to the interspaces at L3–4 or L4–5, other variables being then responsible for the ultimate height of the analgesia.

Factors Controlling the Height of Epidural Analgesia

Some of the principles which control the spread of local analgesic solutions in the subarachnoid space also apply to the spread of analgesic solutions in the epidural space.

1. **Site of injection.**—Any interspace of the spine may be used for the injection of the analgesic solution. If it is desired to keep the dose down to the minimum, injection should be made at the level of the spinal segment corresponding to the middle of the area to be blocked. Thus puncture at levels between C7 and T3 has been used for upper thoracic operations, and between T4 and T10 for upper abdominal operations. In general the lumbar region is the easiest route technically and from it the desired level can usually be reached by using an appropriate volume of solution.

2. **Volume of analgesic solution.**—This is a very important factor in the spread of epidural solutions. The larger the volume used the greater the area blocked. The height to which a given volume may rise depends also on the patency of the intervertebral foramina which, as previously explained, are the normal escape route for epidural solutions. In the elderly these foramina tend to become blocked by fibrous tissue and a given volume of solution produces a much greater area of analgesia than in a young person with widely patent intervertebral foramina.

3. **Position of the patient after injection.**—Position is important since epidural solutions flow under the influence of gravity and will diffuse cephalad in the Trendelenburg position and caudally in a patient sitting up.

4. **Speed of injection.**—Rapid injection spreads the solution upwards and downwards in the epidural space. A given volume injected rapidly will produce a more extensive area of analgesia than the same volume injected slowly, though the duration of analgesia will be shorter, since the volume of solution is widely dispersed and more rapidly removed by venous absorption (Bromage, 1954).

5. **Other factors.**—As has been previously outlined, two mechanisms are involved in the ultimate spread of an epidural injection ; these are, longitudinal spread in the epidural space governed by factors 1 to 4, and neuraxial spread. Again it is to Bromage that we owe an understanding of this very important mechanism.

Neuraxial spread itself will depend on the state of the neural coverings and the physical laws of diffusion across these coverings. The important facts here in relation to the epidural space are the potency of the analgesic drug, the area of contact between neural coverings and analgesic drug, the concentration of the analgesic drug, and the duration of contact.

The area of contact will depend on the volume of solution injected and the patency of the intervertebral foramina. The duration of contact will depend on the rate of removal of analgesic drug from the epidural space, which in turn will depend again on the patency of the intervertebral foramina and the physical state of the epidural vessels. Diffusion gradients appear to be very important even in relation to volume, and small volumes of concentrated solutions—4 to 5 per cent lignocaine—can produce widespread blockade. With these small volumes of concentrated solution, longitudinal spread in the epidural space is presumably confined to a few segments, but neuraxial spread is extensive owing to the high concentration gradient.

Bromage (1962*b*) has also drawn attention to the exaggerated spread of epidural analgesia in arteriosclerotic patients. Fifty-six patients who were severely arteriosclerotic reacted to 2 per cent lignocaine as if they had received a solution of 3 per cent, 4 per cent, or 5 per cent. It is probable that the degenerative changes in connective tissue associated with arteriosclerotic disease produce increased permeability of neural coverings, and that thickened epidural vessels reduce the rate of absorption from the epidural space. Furthermore, sclerosis of the vasa nervorum hastens the normal degeneration of myelin sheaths that occurs with increasing age, thus bringing the analgesic solution more readily into contact with the axons of the posterior nerve roots.

This concept of a neuraxial spread that is exaggerated in arteriosclerotic patients provides a rational explanation of some previously unexplained cases of total spinal blockade. A number of patients have been reported in whom identification of the epidural space seemed certain, and from which neither cerebrospinal fluid nor blood could be aspirated, and yet total spinal analgesia resulted from the injection of a comparatively small volume of analgesic solution. In some reported instances total spinal analgesia was delayed for 30 to 40 minutes, or even longer (Morrow, 1959). Severe arteriosclerotic disease is the only common feature of all such cases. For those who take the view that neurological sequelae following spinal epidural analgesia are due to a direct action of the drug, here indeed is supporting evidence.

Thus the spread of an epidural injection of an analgesic solution is the result of a number of complex interrelated factors, with age and pathological processes probably playing an important part. Bromage has aptly stated that our ideas on this subject need to be more sophisticated than hitherto. These factors will be considered further in the discussion of dosage for epidural block.

Circulatory Effects of Spinal and Epidural Analgesia

The fall in blood pressure that accompanies spinal and epidural block is of great practical and theoretical importance. Unfortunately the mechanism of its fall is still controversial, and while study of the literature tends to give the impression that a single factor is at work, a number undoubtedly contribute.

Although it is a good working rule to regard the fall in blood pressure as correlated with the height of the spinal or epidural analgesia and therefore with the number of sympathetic fibres blocked, the situation is really more complicated. Smith and his colleagues (1939) were the first to suggest that the fall in blood pressure under high spinal analgesia is due to a fall in cardiac output and not necessarily a reduction in arteriolar tone consequent upon sympathetic paralysis. They attributed the fall in cardiac output to venous pooling of blood associated with the skeletal muscular relaxation. They also noted in normal individuals a fall in systolic blood pressure, while the diastolic was well maintained despite sympathetic blockade, and attributed this to the inherent tone of the arterioles of the splanchnic viscera and skeletal muscles. This tone is maintained in the presence of sympathetic paralysis.

Rovenstine and his associates (1942), from measurements of cardiac output and arterial blood pressure made upon unoperated human subjects under spinal analgesia to the level of T5 or higher, concluded that the peripheral resistance was maintained at control values, and that there was little if any tonic activity in the thoraco-lumbar sympathetic vasoconstrictor nerves excluding those of the skin, which in any case do not form an important part of the peripheral resistance. They further concluded from their experience that extensive falls in blood pressure in subjects undergoing an operation are the result of decreased venous pressure following opening the peritoneal cavity, and attendant operative procedures. Hypoxia, haemorrhage, and the pressure of packs, may all contribute to a fall in blood pressure.

Pugh and Wyndham (1950) pointed out that in patients with hypertension the fall in blood pressure during a spinal is greater than in normal subjects, and that thoraco-lumbar sympathectomy produces a less constant reduction in blood pressure in hypertensives than does spinal analgesia. They also measured the cardiac output of hypertensive and control subjects under high spinal analgesia and found that the main factor in the fall of blood pressure is a fall in cardiac output without significant change in the peripheral resistance. Their conclusion was that the fall in cardiac output may be due to relaxation of venous tone, and the role of the sympathetic nervous system in the control of blood pressure depends on the control of the veins at least as much as on the control of the arterioles.

The experimental work of Neumann and his associates (1945) sheds a different light on these conflicting findings. They made plethysmographic studies on subjects during spinal analgesia and found vasodilatation in the vessels of the toes, while vasoconstriction was present in those of the fingers. The more extensive the vasoconstriction in the fingers, the less marked the fall in blood pressure. Similar conclusions have been reached by Milwidsky and de Vries (1948). Their work, and that of Neumann, shows how conclusions reached from a failure to demonstrate no change in diastolic pressure and peripheral resistance under spinal analgesia must be judged with caution, as it is possible for a large part of the arteriolar bed to be dilated under the influence of a sympathetic blockade, while the average peripheral resistance remains unchanged due to compensatory vasoconstriction elsewhere.

Greene (1958), after a thoughtful and extensive review of published investigations of the cardiovascular effects of spinal analgesia, regards the fall in blood pressure as primarily the result of pre-ganglionic sympathetic paralysis and secondarily due to changes in cardiac output. The extent of the blood pressure fall is indicative of the relative roles played by changes in peripheral resistance and cardiac output. Minor degrees of arterial hypotension are principally due to changes in peripheral vascular resistance, but if the pressure continues to fall below a certain critical level, then further falls are most frequently due to changes in cardiac output. This critical level is about 90 mm. Hg systolic in a normal patient. The position of the patient during spinal analgesia has an important effect on the cardiac output. A patient with a pre-anaesthetic systolic blood pressure of 120 mm. Hg who is given high spinal analgesia and tipped into the head-down position to maintain the cardiac output will often only have a fall in systolic blood pressure to 100 or 90 mm. Hg. If the same patient is placed horizontal or in the foot-down position, the cardiac output falls due to gravitational pooling of blood, and severe hypotension develops.

Many authorities in the past have claimed that the fall in blood pressure from an epidural block is less than that from a spinal of comparable height (Odom, 1936; Gutierrez, 1939; Dogliotti, 1939; Dawkins, 1945). It is doubtful if this is really so, and Bromage (1951) has produced evidence that the fall in blood pressure bears a linear relationship to the height of the block during epidural analgesia. It must not be forgotten in what is largely a physiological discussion, that psychic factors may also affect the blood pressure under both spinal and epidural analgesia. These may work either way, accentuating or decreasing the expected fall in blood pressure. Taylor and his co-workers (1951) and Taylor and Page (1952) have shown that the isolated brain can act as a pressor organ. Bromage (1954) has pointed out that in a few patients the blood pressure is maintained at normal levels after a moderately high epidural block, but that as soon as light general anaesthesia is induced the mean arterial pressure falls to a level determined by the segmental extent of the block, and rises again immediately the patient awakes.

In conclusion, it is fair to say that a variety of factors contribute to the fall in blood pressure of spinal and epidural block. These are paralysis of the pre-ganglionic sympathetic nerves with arteriolar dilatation and compensatory vasoconstriction elsewhere, a fall in venous return due to vasodilation causing a fall in cardiac output, block of the pre-ganglionic nerve fibres to the adrenal medulla, and psychic influences. To these basic physiological changes must be added the effects of the operation, the position and age of the patient, and the pre-operative circulatory blood volume. The individual importance of each factor will vary considerably under clinical conditions. The responsibility of assessing these various factors, and their relationship to one another, rests with the anaesthetist in his management of the patient.

Respiratory Effects of Spinal and Epidural Analgesia

Spinal analgesia can depress respiration centrally and peripherally. As the drug diffuses upwards in the cerebrospinal fluid, the intercostal nerves become progressively blocked and the diaphragm steadily takes over respiration. If the analgesic reaches the phrenic roots, respiration ceases altogether. This combination of circumstances is only likely to arise when gross errors of dosage and technique have occurred, for, as has already been outlined, the removal of the local analgesic by normal absorption mechanisms and adsorption on to nervous tissue is so rapid that high concentrations of it are unlikely to reach the phrenic roots. In a correctly managed spinal analgesia it is even less likely that an effective concentration of local analgesic could reach the fourth ventricle, though it could occur with gross overdosage and the use of excessive barbotage. Experiments in dogs have shown that the maximum concentration of procaine which could be present in the brain stem region without producing respiratory changes averaged 1·0 per cent with a range of 0·5–1·25 per cent (Vehrs, 1931 and 1934). Koster *et al.* (1938) have shown that in twenty-two patients given 150 mg. procaine in the lumbar subarachnoid space, the maximum concentration reached in the cisterna magna was 0·21 mg. per ml. This concentration was inadequate to produce medullary paralysis under laboratory conditions. Hill and Macdonald (1935) have shown in dogs that the direct application of a local analgesic to the floor of the 4th ventricle produces immediate respiratory paralysis. However, if the animal is adequately oxygenated by artificial respiration, spontaneous respiration begins again after an interval which depends upon the particular local analgesic. Should respiratory and cardiovascular collapse occur despite a correct technique, it is nearly always due to an inadequate circulation in the brain stem as the result of severe hypotension. With an accidental total spinal from an epidural injection, it is possible that the concentration of local analgesic drug may rise sufficiently high to depress the medullary centres directly.

Although both the medulla and the intercostal nerves are susceptible to the action of local analgesics injected into the subarachnoid space, it is noteworthy that surgery of the head and neck has been performed under spinal analgesia. The probable explanation is that the concentration of drug reached high in the subarachnoid space is only sufficient to produce sensory block and therefore spares the motor fibres, and that such concentration of the drug that might be reached in the 4th ventricle is insufficient to depress the respiratory centre. It is obvious that techniques of this type are extremely dangerous and should only be employed in situations where no other form of anaesthesia is available.

Respiratory failure is the great risk of high spinal analgesia when this is required for thoracic and upper abdominal operations. During the critical first few minutes of spinal analgesia when the solution is being "fixed" the anaesthetist should be constantly on the watch for signs of it. These signs are the progressive failure of intercostal respiration, with increasing diaphragmatic activity, reduction of the voice to a whisper, dilatation of the alae nasae, the use of the unparalysed accessory muscles of respiration, and a tracheal tug. The anaesthetist must be prepared to clear the airway, intubate, ventilate the lungs with 100 per cent oxygen, and restore the blood pressure by a combination of the head-down position and the use of vasopressor drugs. The restoration of blood pressure is the primary physiological consideration since most cases of apnoea during spinal analgesia are due to hypotension rather than spread of the analgesic to the brain stem. Should the apnoea be due to phrenic paralysis the same treatment is needed. Speed is vital in treatment as cardiac arrest rapidly follows respiratory arrest in cases of ischaemic medullary paralysis. The term "fixed" implies that the concentration of local analgesic has fallen below the minimum concentration necessary to depress the functional activity of the spinal nerve roots, phrenic roots, and the medullary centres. This dilution is produced by the normal absorptive mechanisms and the uptake of local analgesic by nervous tissue. Once the drug is fixed the patient can be postured to meet the needs of the particular surgical procedure and surgeon, as alterations in position no longer cause changes in the level of analgesia. Fixing normally takes about 5 to 6 minutes.

The mechanism of respiratory failure with epidural analgesia presents a somewhat different picture. It used to be thought that provided the analgesic solution is correctly placed in the epidural space, the highest level to which analgesia can extend is the first cervical nerve, due to the fusion of the two layers of the dura at the foramen magnum. Spread to the fourth ventricle was therefore regarded as impossible unless there was massive intrathecal injection. This view must now be modified in the light of Bromage's concept of "neuraxial" spread within the central nervous system (see p. 1195). However, in most cases the dangers of intercostal and—more important—phrenic paralysis are slight with epidural analgesia provided the correct strength of solution is employed and excessive volumes are not injected, e.g. 1·5 per cent lignocaine gives complete sensory block but leaves the motor side of respiration relatively unimpaired. The use of excessive volumes of 2 per cent lignocaine might well result in intercostal and phrenic paralysis.

Apart from the effects of spinal and epidural analgesia on the respiratory muscles, the effects of autonomic block on the bronchial tree are important. Bromage (1954) has pointed out that it might be expected with the sympathetic blockade present during epidural analgesia that there would be a tendency to bronchial constriction. From his own clinical practice he has, however, observed the reverse situation in which the laboured, forced expirations of the emphysematous subject under general anaesthesia are considerably aided by the introduction of an epidural block. Various explanations of this phenomenon have been discussed by Bromage. Daly and Schweitzer (1951) have shown that vascular hypotension is accompanied by bronchodilatation brought about through baroreceptors in the carotid sinus. The vascular hypotension of epidural block may thus be the underlying cause of the bronchial dilatation. Another possibility is the increased oxygen uptake from the lungs during hypotension. It has been shown that in emphysema there is an opening up of anastomoses between the bronchial and pulmonary arteries, so that the pulmonary pressure becomes abnormally high. The higher the pulmonary pressure the lower is the oxygen uptake from the lung. Hence a falling systemic blood pressure from epidural analgesia in a patient with a patent bronchial-pulmonary artery anastomosis will lead to an increase in oxygen uptake from the lung. The picture is not completely clear, however, because restoration of the blood pressure with vasopressors is not followed by a return of laboured breathing.

These same results might also be expected to follow a fall in blood pressure from spinal analgesia.

Effects of Spinal and Epidural Analgesia on the Gastro-intestinal Tract and Related Structures

Sympathetic blockade, whether from spinal or epidural analgesia, results in a contracted bowel with relaxed sphincters. The contracted bowel is one of the main factors responsible for the popularity with surgeons of spinal and epidural analgesia for abdominal operations. It must be clearly understood that the vagus is not blocked by spinal analgesia so that, in a conscious patient, handling of the viscera may set up stimuli which result in nausea and retching. A separate vagal block is advisable during operations such as gastrectomy under spinal or epidural analgesia alone to prevent these complications.

The spleen enlarges two or three times in high spinal analgesia due to paralysis of the splanchnic nerves.

Bromage (1952) has observed swelling and a change in colour of the liver under high epidural analgesia when the blood pressure falls to about 60 mm. Hg. He attributes this to local tissue hypoxia consequent upon the hypotension.

The Cerebrospinal Fluid

Physical Characteristics and their Relation to Spinal Analgesia

Cerebrospinal fluid (C.S.F.) is a clear, colourless liquid with a slight opalescence due to the presence of globulin. The average volume is usually given as 110–150 ml. Fontecilla and Sépulveda (1920) gave the average volume as 128–130 ml. based on measurements from three accident cases after death. Authorities vary as to the volume of cerebral and spinal C.S.F. Harris (1951) and Evans (1954) state that approximately half (i.e. 60 ml.) is in the brain reservoir, and half in the spinal subarachnoid space. Lee (1953), however, gives a figure of 25 ml. for the volume of spinal cerebrospinal fluid. These variations in figures are, however, of little practical importance.

An important factor determining the spread of drugs in the subarachnoid space is the specific gravity of the drug compared with that of the C.S.F. The exact Sp.G. of C.S.F. is therefore of considerable importance. Macintosh (1951) has drawn attention to the confusion prevailing upon this point, since many authorities quote different figures. Maxson (1938) gives an average between 1·005 and 1·007, Etherington Wilson (1934 and 1943) gives an average figure of 1·004, and Levinson (1929), quoting no fewer than 13 authorities, gives figures of 1·001–1·010. Macintosh discusses this point at great length, pointing out that the Sp.G. of C.S.F. and spinal analgesic drugs that are quoted may relate to different standards; no confusion would exist if workers adhered to the scientific practice of using water at 4° C as the standard when referring to the Sp.G. of any solution. The most accurate report he has been able to find in the literature is that by

Stanford, who arrived at an average figure of 1·0045 at 25° C (C.S.F. temperature) referred to water at 4° C. These figures have been confirmed by Wolman *et al.* (1946).

The Sp.G. of "heavy" cinchocaine ("Nupercaine") 1 in 200 in 6 per cent glucose is 1·023 at 37° C (body temperature). The difference in Sp.G. between this figure and that of C.S.F. is in the second decimal place, so that this solution is certainly hyperbaric.

Cerebrospinal fluid pressure in health varies between 70–180 mm. H_2O in the lateral position to 375–550 mm. H_2O in the vertical position. While there is a positive pressure in the dural envelope, there is a negative pressure in the epidural space. The injection of solutions into the epidural space converts its negative pressure to a positive pressure, which is transmitted to the C.S.F. A conscious patient will often notice a sensation of dizziness during the performance of epidural block, which can be attributed to a transient rise in C.S.F. pressure.

The normal protein content of C.S.F. is 20 mg. per cent (as equal albumin and globulin fractions) and sugar 45–80 mg. per cent. After spinal analgesia there is a rise in both the albumin and globulin content: the albumin level rises until about the 18th day, when it is nearly double the normal level.

REFERENCES

Bonica, J. J., Backup, P. H., and Pratt, W. H. (1951). The use of vaso-constrictors to prolong spinal anesthesia. *Anesthesiology*, **12,** 431.

Brierley, J. B. (1950). The penetration of particulate matter from the cerebrospinal fluid into the spinal ganglia, peripheral nerves, and perivascular spaces of the central nervous system. *J. Neurol. Neurosurg. Psychiat.*, **13,** 203.

Brierley, J. B., and Field, E. J. (1948). The connexions of the spinal sub-arachnoid space with the lymphatic system. *J. Anat.* (*Lond.*), **82,** 153.

Brierley, J. B., and Field, E. J. (1949). The fate of an intraneural injection as demonstrated by the use of radio-active phosphorus. *J. Neurol. Neurosurg. Psychiat.*, **12,** 89.

Bromage, P. R. (1951). Vascular hypotension in 107 cases of epidural analgesia. *Anaesthesia*, **6,** 26.

Bromage, P. R. (1952). Effect of induced vascular hypotension on the liver: alterations in appearance and consistence. *Lancet*, **2,** 10.

Bromage, P. R. (1954). *Spinal Epidural Analgesia.* Edinburgh: E. & S. Livingstone.

Bromage, P. R. (1962*a*). Spread of analgesic solutions in the epidural space and their site of action: a statistical study. *Brit. J. Anaesth.*, **34,** 161.

Bromage, P. R. (1962*b*). Exaggerated spread of epidural analgesia in arteriosclerotic patients. Dosage in relation to biological and chronological ageing. *Brit. med. J.*, **2,** 1634.

Burford, G. E. (1942). The tolerance of humans for procaine injected into the sub-arachnoid space. *Anesthesiology*, **3,** 159.

Daly, M. de B., and Schweitzer, A. (1951). Reflex broncho-motor responses to stimulation of receptors in the region of the carotid sinus and arch of the aorta in the dog and the cat. *J. Physiol.* (*Lond.*), **113,** 442.

Dawkins, C. J. M. (1945). Discussion on extradural block. *Proc. roy. Soc. Med.*, **38,** 302.

DOGLIOTTI, A. M. (1939). *Anesthesia: narcosis, local, regional, spinal.* Chicago: S. B. Debour.

ELWAN, R. (1923). Spinal arachnoid granulations with especial reference to the cerebrospinal fluid. *Bull. Johns Hopk. Hosp.*, **34,** 99.

EVANS, F. T., Ed. (1954). *Modern Practice in Anaesthesia*, 2nd edit. London: Butterworth & Co.

FIELD, E. J. (1951). Observations on the passage of Weed's Prussian Blue mixture along the axis cylinder and inter-fibre fluid of nerves. *J. Neurol. Neurosurg. Psychiat.*, **14,** 11.

FONTECILLA and SÉPULVEDA (1920). *Le liquide céphalo-rachidien.* Paris: Maloine.

FRUMIN, M. J., SCHWARTZ, H., BURNS, J. J., BRODIE, B. B., and PAPPER, E. M. (1953*a*). Sites of sensory blockade during segmental spinal and segmental peridural anesthesia in man. *Anesthesiology*, **14,** 576.

FRUMIN, M. J., SCHWARTZ, H., BURNS, J. J., BRODIE, B. B., and PAPPER, E. M. (1953*b*). The appearance of procaine in the spinal fluid during peridural block in man. *J. Pharmacol. exp. Ther.*, **109,** 102.

GREENE, N. M. (1958). *Physiology of Spinal Anesthesia.* Baltimore: Williams & Wilkins Co.

GUTIERREZ, A. (1939). *Anestesia extradural.* Buenos Aires.

HELRICH, M., PAPPER, E. M., BRODIE, B. B., FINK, M., and ROVENSTINE, E. A. (1951). Effect of sympathomimetic amines on duration of procaine spinal anesthesia. *Anesthesiology*, **12,** 595.

HILL, E. F., and MACDONALD, A. D. (1935). The action of local anesthetics on the respiratory apparatus. *J. Pharmacol. exp. Ther.*, **53,** 454.

HOWARTH, F. (1949). Studies with radio-active spinal anaesthetic. *Brit. J. Pharmacol.*, **4,** 333.

KOSTER, H., SHAPIRO, A., and LEIKENSOHN, A. (1936). Procaine concentrations at the site of injection in subarachnoid anesthesia. *Amer. J. Surg.*, **33,** 245.

KOSTER, H., SHAPIRO, A., and LEIKENSOHN, A. (1938). Concentration of procaine in the cerebro-spinal fluid of the human being after sub-arachnoid injection. *Arch. Surg. (Chicago)*, **37,** 603.

LEE, J. A. (1953). *Synopsis of Anaesthesia*, 3rd edit. Bristol: John Wright & Sons.

LEVINSON, A. (1929). *Cerebrospinal Fluid in Health and in Disease*, 3rd edit. London: Hy. Kimpton.

MACINTOSH, R. R. (1951). *Lumbar Puncture and Spinal Analgesia.* Edinburgh: E. & S. Livingstone.

MACINTOSH, R. R., and BRYCE-SMITH, R. (1962). *Local Analgesia: Abdominal Surgery*, 2nd edit., p. 26. Edinburgh: E. & S. Livingstone.

MAXSON, L. H. (1938). *Spinal Anesthesia.* Philadelphia: J. B. Lippincott Co.

MILWIDSKY, H., and DE VRIES, A. (1948). Regulation of blood pressure during spinal anesthesia: observations on intramuscular pressure and skin temperature. *Anesthesiology*, **9,** 258.

MORROW, W. F. K. (1959). Unexplained spread of epidural anaesthesia. *Brit. J. Anaesth.*, **31,** 359.

NEUMANN, C., FOSTER, A., Jr., and ROVENSTINE, E. A. (1945). The importance of compensatory vasoconstriction in unanesthetized areas in the maintenance of blood pressure during spinal anesthesia. *J. clin. Invest.*, **24,** 345.

ODOM, C. M. (1936). Epidural anesthesia. *Amer. J. Surg.*, **34,** 547.

PUGH, L. G. C., and WYNDHAM, C. L. (1950). The circulatory effects of high spinal anaesthesia in hypertensive and control subjects. *Clin. Sci.*, **9,** 189.

ROVENSTINE, E. A., PAPPER, E. M., and BRADLEY, S. E. (1942). Circulatory adjustments during spinal anesthesia in normal man with special reference to the autonomy of arteriolar tone. *Anesthesiology*, **3,** 421.

RUDIN, D. O., FREMONT-SMITH, K., and BEECHER, H. K. (1951). The permeability of the dura mater to epidural procaine in dogs. *J. appl. Physiol.*, **3,** 388.

SMITH, H. W., ROVENSTINE, E. A., GOLDRING, W., CHASIS, H., and RANGES, H. A. (1939). The effects of spinal anesthesia on the circulation in normal unoperated man with reference to the autonomy of the arterioles and especially those of the renal circulation. *J. clin. Invest.*, **18,** 319.

STANFORD, R. V. (1913). Vergleichende Studien über Cerebrospinal-flüssigkeit bei Geisteskrankheiten. I. Dichte. *Hoppe-Seylers Z. physiol. Chem.*, **86,** 43.

TAYLOR, R. D., PAGE, I. H., and CORCORAN, A. C. (1951). A hormonal neurogenic vasopressor mechanism. *Arch. intern. Med.*, **88,** 1.

TAYLOR, R. D., and PAGE, I. H. (1952). The origin and properties of a cerebral pressor substance (CPS). *Amer. J. Physiol.*, **170,** 321.

VEHRS, G. R. (1931). Heart beat and respiration in total novocaine analgesia. *Northw. Med. (Seattle)*, **30,** 256 & 322.

VEHRS, G. R. (1934). *Spinal Anesthesia. Technic and Clinical Application.* St. Louis : C. V. Mosby Co.

WILSON, W. E. (1934). Intrathecal nerve root block. Some contributions and a new technique. *Brit. J. Anaesth.*, **11,** 43.

WILSON, W. E. (1943). Specific gravity of the cerebrospinal fluid, with special reference to spinal anaesthesia. *Brit. med. J.*, **2,** 165.

WOLMAN, I. J., EVANS, B., and LASKER, S. (1946). The specific gravity of cerebrospinal fluid. A review of methods and the application of a newer micromethod in spinal anesthesia. *Amer. J. clin. Path.*, **16,** Tech. Bull. VII, p. 33.

Chapter 43

SPINAL AND EPIDURAL ANALGESIA: TECHNIQUE AND COMPLICATIONS

by

D. D. B. MORRIS

GENERAL CONSIDERATIONS

THE anaesthetist should always visit patients for whom spinal or epidural analgesia is planned, in order that he may examine the spine for any points of difficulty, and, if general anaesthesia is not also to be used, explain to the patient some important details. A few words about flexion of the spine and lying still during the procedure (particularly important for epidural analgesia) are of great assistance in securing the patient's co-operation at the time of injection. The psychological background to local analgesia cannot be over-emphasised. In units where operations are performed under local analgesia, preparation begins in both the out-patient department and the ward, so that by the time the patient arrives in the theatre most of his fears have been dealt with. For patients who are to remain awake during operation it may be advisable to give a heavy pre-medication, especially if they are likely to be unco-operative or nervous. The value of the pre-operative visit is that all these things can be assessed beforehand.

The choice of drugs for premedication before spinal and epidural analgesia varies widely from one anaesthetist to another. Papaveretum gives very good results and can be safely used in large doses for adults, as much as 40 mg. being administered intramuscularly beforehand and a further 20 mg. slowly intravenously on arrival in the anaesthetic room. Even with doses of this order, a fit male adult may remain awake. Dosage must of course be reduced for elderly and poor risk and for such patients the value of a pre-operative visit to choose premedication to suit the individual is obvious. There is nowadays a very good case to be made for a neuroleptic drug such as droperidol in combination with an analgesic. For elderly and poor risk patients 5 mg. of droperidol with 0·1 mg. of fentanyl one hour before anaesthesia produces tranquillity without hypotension. Young, fit patients require doses of the order of 10 mg. and 0·2 mg. respectively, and these can be safely supplemented by a further intravenous injection of 5–10 mg. of droperidol with 0·05–0·1 mg. of fentanyl according to the patient's response to the initial dose given as premedication. Neuroleptic drugs, producing as they do analgesia for needle pricks and a loss of awareness for surroundings, produce particularly satisfactory conditions for a patient who is to have an operation under block analgesia.

So few operations in this country are performed under local analgesia with the patient awake, that there is a tendency for theatre teams to neglect the elementary points of care of the conscious patient. There should be complete silence in the operating theatre, essential conversations being carried on in whispers. The anaesthetist must be in attendance to answer any questions from the patient and to give encouragement. A surgeon experienced in operating under local analgesia—be it epidural, spinal, or intercostal—handles tissues gently and never clatters instruments or specimens.

Sterilisation

All spinal and epidural sets of equipment should be kept packed in conveniently sized metal drums set aside for the purpose, and autoclaved before use. It is important to stress the danger of inadequate washing of syringes and needles after previous use and before sterilisation, particularly if they have been in contact with any chemical solution. Needles, ampoules, syringes, files and any other equipment should be kept together in a linen pack, and sterile towels, swabs, swab-holding forceps and gallipots for skin cleansing solutions included in the drums. Each anaesthetist will have his own individual ideas on equipment, and everything which might be needed should be included in the drum. It is not uncommon for a sterile technique to break down because some vital piece of equipment is missing and has to be boiled separately before the anaesthetic can proceed. Infection is the one completely preventable complication of spinal and epidural analgesia, so that the anaesthetist practising these techniques should personally take pains to avoid it. Only in this way can a break down of sterile technique, such as occurs when an ampoule is opened with an unsterile file, or a local analgesic solution for the skin weal drawn up from a rubber capped bottle, be prevented.

The anaesthetist should scrub up as for a surgical operation, and wear cap, mask, sterile gown and gloves. The contents of the drum should be laid out on a sterile trolley by an experienced assistant using sterile forceps. The skin should be cleaned with sterile swab-holding forceps, using two lots of 2 per cent iodine in spirit; the use of a coloured antiseptic helps to avoid contamination of the fingers on unsterile skin. The site of the puncture should be surrounded by sterile towels as it is very easy, while palpating bony prominences and concentrating on the introduction of the needle, to dirty the hands against unsterile areas.

The Blood Pressure

The statement is sometimes made that patients under spinal analgesia should not be disturbed by frequent blood pressure recordings, but this seems unwise and unnecessary. The control of the blood pressure under a high spinal or epidural block is vital, and an adequately premedicated and sedated patient does not find repeated recordings disturbing. Unless there is a clear cut indication for using the accompanying hypotension of a spinal or epidural block to limit bleeding, the blood pressure should be kept to near-normal limits by vasopressors (see Chapter 20). Restlessness, due to the accompanying cerebral hypoxia, is often associated with hypotension, and may be mistaken for incomplete analgesia. Should the anaesthetist fail to recognise the true cause of the restlessness, he may be tempted to quieten the patient with a small intravenous dose of thiopentone; such treatment may easily be fatal in the circumstances.

It is therefore a wise precaution always to have ready access to a vein, so that a vasopressor can be given immediately if there is a dramatic fall in blood pressure. A Gordh or Mitchell needle can be conveniently placed in an arm vein before the block is done, and if a fall in blood pressure is likely a vasopressor can be given immediately after the local is injected, and further doses added during operation. As an alternative to a vasopressor, a controlled rapid infusion of dextran 70 has certain advantages. This allows a precise but gradual regulation of blood pressure without the rapid overswing produced by a vasopressor and due to sudden alterations in regional blood flow. This is particularly important in certain types of patient—for example, old men undergoing prostatic operations (Morris and Candy, 1957). This sort of patient, often with associated coronary and cerebrovascular atheroma, must have the blood pressure maintained if cerebral damage from hypotension is to be avoided (see Chapter 23). It is important for the anaesthetist to remember that while managing the level of blood pressure during spinal or epidural block, he is also indirectly controlling the cerebral circulation. It is only in comparatively recent years that anaesthetists have come to realise the morbidity, actual and potential, from falls in cerebral blood flow consequent upon falls in arterial blood pressure. It is true that during widespread sympathetic blockade there is a decrease in cardiovascular resistance, but it is doubtful if this in itself is due to sympathetic paralysis. Studies of cerebral blood flow before and after stellate ganglion block have almost invariably shown that such a procedure has no significant effect on cerebral blood flow (Scheinberg, 1950; Harmel *et al.*, 1949). Precisely how decreases in arterial blood pressure produce decreases in cardiovascular resistance is unexplained. Moreover, there is no direct relationship between arterial pressure and cardiovascular resistance. With ganglion blocking drugs, although falls in blood pressure are associated with decreases in cardiovascular resistance, Morris and his co-workers (1953) have found that resistance decreases much less than blood pressure. Kety has similarly found in patients under differential spinal block that though cardiovascular resistance decreased, it did not do so to the extent that a fall in cerebral blood flow was prevented. Severe arterial hypotension under spinal analgesia is certain to be associated with dangerous decreases in cerebral blood flow (Greene, 1958), and Wyke (1960), in a review of changes in the cerebral circulation during anaesthesia, warns of the dangers of arterial hypotension. Cerebral vasodilatation, even when maximal, will be unable to maintain an adequate blood flow to the brain when the blood pressure has dropped beyond a critical level. As a clinical rule of thumb, it is wise to assume that in the supine position levels of mean arterial blood pressure below 55 mm. Hg are associated with dangerous decreases in cerebral blood flow in normal patients, and should be avoided. In patients with arteriosclerotic changes involving cerebral vessels the blood pressure must be maintained considerably above this level in order to ensure an adequate cerebral blood flow (Shanbrom and Levy, 1957).

Should severe arterial hypotension develop during spinal or epidural analgesia, the table must be tilted head-down immediately, and if this is insufficient to raise the blood pressure to a safe level, a vasopressor drug must be given as well. The tilt increases venous return from the lower limbs and trunk to the right side of the heart, thus raising cardiac output and so the arterial pressure. Reliance alone on head-down tilt should be avoided as too steep a tilt may so increase cerebral venous pressure as to have a deleterious effect on cerebral capillary blood flow. Particular care must be taken to guard against a sudden fall in blood pressure when a patient is moved from the lithotomy position. It is also an important part of spinal and epidural techniques that the blood pressure should be recorded back in the ward and that it should be maintained while the block is wearing off.

Respiration

The anaesthetist must constantly be on the alert for the effects of high epidural and spinal block on the respiration. The effects of hypoxia on the respiratory and cardiac centres of the brain stem consequent upon severe falls in arterial hypotension have already been discussed (p. 1164). The use of the head-down position must again be stressed. The commonest cause of hypoxic paralysis of the brain stem is use of a foot-down tilt in the presence of arterial hypotension. This is the commonest cause of death under spinal or epidural analgesia and is completely preventable with correct management. The anaesthetist must think of the blood pressure and respiration together. Hypoxia from a failing respiration will aggravate hypoxic effects on the brain and heart from severe arterial hypotension. Low blocks present no problem as the intercostal muscles are not affected. With a high spinal block the intercostal muscles are paralysed and only the diaphragm and possibly a few of the upper intercostals remain for ventilation. The Trendelenburg position, abdominal packs and retractors, or the presence of an abdominal mass, ovarian cyst or pregnancy may add to the respiratory difficulties. Macintosh (1957) has strongly emphasised how important it is to give oxygen to these patients. One of the advantages of an epidural block is that satisfactory analgesia and complete relaxation can be obtained without impairing respiration. For example, 1·5 per cent lignocaine will give profound analgesia, excellent relaxation, and leave the respiration relatively unaffected. It must not be supposed, however, that supplementary oxygenation is never necessary during epidural analgesia, since some degree of motor loss may occur even with this strength of solution, though on the whole it is slight. As with spinal analgesia, the effect of posture, abdominal packs and retractors on the respiration must also be taken into account.

Sickness

Nausea may be experienced by the patient under epidural or spinal analgesia, and is due either to a fall in blood pressure or to traction on a hollow viscus during an abdominal operation. The nausea is vagal in origin, and is particularly likely to occur during the operation of gastrectomy, especially when the left and right gastric arteries are tied. The most satisfactory way to prevent it and those conditions with which it is found to be associated, is for the surgeon to do a para-oesophageal vagal block on opening the abdomen.

Hiccup

Hiccup may occur during upper abdominal surgery under spinal or epidural analgesia. Like sickness it may well have its origin in the stimulation of vagal nerve endings, so that local infiltration of these nerves should be carried out.

Supplementary Anaesthesia

Intravenous thiopentone or methohexitone are very useful in small doses for maintaining light sleep during epidural or spinal analgesia. With lignocaine epidural blocks patients tend to become drowsy and only very small quantities of thiopentone or methohexitone are required. When a patient has been tranquillized with droperidol only the minutest quantities should be used, doses about 25 mg. of thiopentone and 10 mg. of methohexitone being sufficient to maintain a light sleep with an active eyelash reflex. If gas and oxygen is added as well, much of the dry field which constitutes one of the principal advantages of operating under epidural analgesia is likely to be lost. A technique of light sleep with thiopentone, nitrous oxide and oxygen plus epidural block and a normal blood pressure will, however, give far superior operating conditions from a bleeding point of view to those produced by a thiopentone, nitrous oxide and oxygen, and relaxant sequence.

Management of the Total Spinal

Accidental massive subarachnoid injection occurring during epidural block should not be regarded as a catastrophe but as a reversible complication. The basis of treatment is twofold—efficient ventilation and oxygenation, and the maintenance of blood pressure by vasopressors. The incidence of this distressing occurence can be reduced to negligible proportions by careful technique, but the means of resuscitation must always be at hand when epidural blocks are being done. The following figures are quoted for the incidence of a total spinal following an epidural injection in the lumbar area:

Moore	0 in 1,700 cases	0·00 per cent
Bonica	1 in 2,290 cases	0·04 per cent
Selva de Assis	2 in 1,000 cases	0·20 per cent
Bromage	1 in 1,000 cases	0·10 per cent

The duration of respiratory paralysis depends on the local analgesic drug used. Gordh (1949) reports a case in which respiratory paralysis lasted 9 hours after the injection of a mixture of cinchocaine and procaine. Gordon Jones (1953) and Stringer (1954) report cases in which paralysis lasted up to 2 hours with 2 per cent lignocaine. de Saram (1956) describes 3 cases, and draws attention to the value of the prophylactic vasopressor given immediately after the injection. Respiratory paralysis and loss of consciousness occurred in these three cases, but the blood pressure did not fall below 100 mm. Hg. In one case where 1·5 per cent lignocaine was used respiration returned in 45 minutes, and in two cases where 1·75 per cent was used, respiration returned in 1 and 1½ hours respectively.

Dawkins (1956*a*) recommends that the operation should not be abandoned when an accidental total spinal has been given.

SPINAL ANALGESIA

Lumbar Puncture

Macintosh (1957) has described and illustrated in great detail the anatomical points concerned in successful lumbar puncture. The chief points to be remembered are:

1. In median puncture the needle passes through the skin, subcutaneous tissue, supraspinous ligament and interspinous ligament, between the ligamentum flava, and then through the epidural space and finally the dura, to enter the subarachnoid space. A successful lumbar puncture will be followed by a free flow of C.S.F., usually at the rate of 1 drop a second. Median puncture is the easiest to use, but if the needle goes off centre it will pass through the dura having pierced one of the ligamentum flavum, since in the lateral parts of the epidural space these and the dura lie adjacent. In elderly osteoarthritic subjects the supraspinous and interspinous ligaments may be fused and heavily calcified, making the introduction of a fine spinal needle extremely difficult. For such patients the lateral approach may be advisable.

2. In lateral puncture the needle passes through the skin, subcutaneous fat, lumbar aponeurosis and lumbar muscles, and then with correct angulation through the ligamentum flavum.

3. The interlaminar foramen is a bony ring formed between two vertebrae, the upper border bounded by the laminae and root of the spine of the vertebra above, the lower border by the laminae and root of the spine of the vertebra below and the sides by the articulation between the superior and inferior facets. The foramen is closed by the ligamentum flavum. An incorrectly angulated spinal needle may impinge on any part of this bony ring. Flexion of the spine increases the diameter of the ring, so that the advancing needle is then less likely to be arrested by the bony margin. The lumbar spines have a slight downward inclination and the needle must be advanced inclined slightly upwards.

The distance from the skin to the epidural space is reasonably constant in the average individual, and any variation is largely dependent on the thickness of the subcutaneous fat. Gutierrez (1939) has found in a series of 3,200 cases that in 80 per cent the distance from the skin to the ligamentum flavum is 1½–2 inches (3·75 to 5 cm.). The author has noted that a mark from the iodine painted on the skin appears on the shaft of an epidural needle that has been in use a few weeks.

In lumbar puncture the differing resistance of the ligaments can often be appreciated—the resistance increasing as the needle enters the ligamentum flavum—and a "give" occurring as the needle enters the epidural space. Sometimes an audible click can be heard as the needle passes through the dura. With the fine spinal needles at present in use, these sensations have become more difficult to appreciate. In epidural work, however, it is almost essential to use a thicker needle (18 S.W.G.) so that the feel of the ligaments can be appreciated. Needles for both spinal and epidural analgesia are illustrated in Figs. 1 and 2.

In some cases there are good reasons for using a Sise spinal needle introducer. For instance, in mid-line puncture when the supraspinous and interspinous ligaments are very tough, the introducer is advanced for about 1 inch down to the ligamentum flavum and then a fine spinal needle (passed through the introducer) has only to pierce the ligamentum flavum and dura.

A Sise introducer probably offers an additional safeguard against infection, since it and the stilette pierce the epidermis so that no part of the spinal needle comes into contact with the skin. Dickson (1944) has found in the centrifugalised deposits of lumbar puncture specimens squamous cells from the skin surface, together with their accompanying staphylococci and occasionally even a little cylindrical fragment of skin punched out by the spinal needle.

An introducer is also of value in an elderly patient whose lumbar vertebrae are fixed in extension, so that the interlaminar foramen is small, necessitating repeated attempts to get the angle just right. It eliminates the need to touch the skin and removes the temptation to touch the shaft of the needle (Macintosh, 1957). The size of the needle has an important bearing on the incidence of postspinal headache (see p. 1233). An introducer makes it possible to use a very fine spinal needle.

Types of Technique

At the time of writing spinal analgesia has almost fallen into disuse in the United Kingdom. As already described (p. 1174) the manufacturers of cinchocaine now only make hyperbaric solutions, and these in response to a very limited service need. A great many techniques have been described, often elaborate in nature and a burden on the memory, and it is not proposed here to include them all but rather to outline a few simple, well-tried methods for the anaesthetist who is called upon to undertake the occasional spinal analgesia.

Hyperbaric solutions.—A very useful technique for ano-rectal operations for haemorrhoids, fissures and the like, and for a bladder neck operation such as transurethral prostatectomy, is to inject at the L4–5 interspace, with the patient sitting up, 0·6–1·0 ml. of heavy cinchocaine (1:200) or heavy amethocaine (1:200). For operations about the anus where only the 4th and 5th sacral roots require to be blocked, 0·6 ml. of solution is sufficient, and for bladder neck operations (S1–5) 1 ml. The patient should be kept sat up for five minutes after the injection while the heavy solution sinks rapidly to the bottom of the dural sac, blocking the necessary sacral nerves. There is little or no fall in blood pressure so that a vasopressor is very seldom required.

For lower abdominal operations such as appendicectomy, prostatectomy and Caesarean section, 1·4–1·8 ml. of solution is injected at the L2–3 interspace with the patient on his side and in a slight but definite head-down tilt. Immediately after the injection the patient is turned on his back. The heavy solution then spreads under the influence of gravity to the 7th or 8th thoracic segment. Mushin (1943) has pointed out that while in the average patient in the lateral position the vertebral column is more or less horizontal, in some women it may incline downwards towards the head because of the width of the pelvis relative to the shoulders, and in some men towards the coccyx because of the width of the shoulder relative to the pelvis. Thus the solution may spread in the wrong direction until the patient is rolled supine and tipped into the correct position. It is therefore best when using a heavy solution for an upper abdominal operation in a man, to tip the table until it is obvious that the vertebral column inclines towards the head. With the spine exactly horizontal the solution may not run high enough when injected at L3–4, the apex of the lumbar curve, and tends to spread down towards the coccyx when the patient is rolled on to his back.

For upper abdominal operations where analgesia to the 4th or 5th thoracic segment is required, 2 ml. of solution are injected at the L2–3 interspace with the patient head-down. The spine should be in about 5 degrees of Trendelenburg position. As before, the solution spreads by gravity, and any excess of unfixed drug pools in the hollow of the thoracic curve, opposite the 4th and 5th nerve roots.

In planning the height to which analgesia is required for a particular operation it is useful to remember the following segmental levels:

Nipple line	T4–5
Xiphisternum . .	T7
Umbilicus . . .	T10
Groin	L1
Perineum . . .	S1–4

For upper abdominal operations analgesia must not only be sufficient to reach the xiphisternum at T7, but also to include the splanchnic nerves (greater splanchnic nerve—T4, 5, 6, 7, 8), since an incomplete block of these makes surgical handling of the omentum and mesentery uncomfortable for a conscious patient. Moreover, as explained on p. 1211, it is advisable to combine the spinal with para-oesophageal block of the vagus.

A point frequently not always appreciated about such lower abdominal operations as abdomino-perineal resection of the rectum is that while the incision may not extend to the costal margin, nevertheless analgesia up to this region is needed, since the surgeon requires to push the lower abdominal contents into the upper abdomen and may want to palpate the liver.

Hypobaric solutions.—Techniques using solutions of local analgesic drugs that have a lower specific gravity than that of C.S.F. are no longer recommended.

Continuous spinal analgesia.—Any place that continuous spinal analgesia may have had in anaesthetic practice has been lost. A technique with such potential morbidity from the introduction of catheters into the subarachnoid space should not be used, particularly when safer alternatives are readily available.

EPIDURAL ANALGESIA

There is a tendency to think of epidural analgesia as a recent development in anaesthesia. This can probably be accounted for by the decline in the popularity of spinals since the late forties and a search for methods with the advantages of the spinal, but without its dangerous sequelae. In point of fact the approach to the epidural space is of some antiquity and as long ago as 1901 the French investigators Sicord and Cathelin described epidural injections through the sacral hiatus. By 1920 the technique had become popular and Zweifel was able to analyse the incidence of fatalities encountered in 4,200 sacral epidural blocks recorded in the literature. Although the interspinous approach to the epidural space had also been demonstrated at the beginning of the century,

Poges (1921) was the first to describe the practical application of lumbar epidural analgesia. Later Dogliotti (1931–33) in Italy popularised the technique, followed by other clinical exponents, Hess (1934), Odom (1936) and Harger *et al.* (1941) in the U.S.A., and Gutierrez (1939) in South America.

The next important development was the adaptation of Tuohy's (1945) catheter technique—developed for continuous spinal analgesia—to epidural analgesia by Curbello (1949).

Methods of Identifying the Epidural Space

The technique of the sacral approach to the epidural space will be discussed later and only the lumbar approach dealt with here. Methods can be regarded as falling into two groups, those dependent on the loss of resistance as the needle pierces the ligamentum flavum and enters the epidural space, and others upon a negative pressure in the epidural space.

The loss of resistance sign.—The basis of the method is to exert continuous pressure on the plunger of a syringe loaded with air or fluid as the needle is advanced through the interspinous ligament and ligamentum flavum, then as the point pierces the ligamentum flavum and enters the epidural space the plunger will surge forward. The interspinous ligament offers only slight resistance to the needle: resistance increases sharply as the ligamentum flavum is reached—in a large man it may be as much as $\frac{1}{3}$ inch (7·2 mm.) thick. The needle should not be allowed to deviate to one side and enter the lumbar muscles, as a false loss of resistance will be obtained and the solution deposited outside the epidural space. The main points in favour of this technique are its essential simplicity, and that it concentrates the attention of the anaesthetist on the feel of the ligaments the whole time, while visual and mechanical aids have a tendency to distract the anaesthetist from the essential feel of the ligaments. Its disadvantage is that it cannot be used for the lateral approach to the epidural space, as the lumbar muscles will not satisfactorily block the point of the needle.

Mechanical aids to the loss of resistance sign.—In general these are not to be recommended. When they work at a demonstration they are dramatic and convincing, but the sense of touch is really the key to successful epidural analgesia. Macintosh's (1953) needle with the spring-loaded stilette is better than Brunner and Ilké's (1949) spring-loaded syringe. The latter is far too heavy in practice, while both it and Macintosh's stilette—as with all mechanical devices—are only reliable if kept in perfect working order. Both these devices of necessity need very large-bore needles, which, if pushed on through the dura cause a large dural hole, so that a post-lumbar puncture headache is likely. For general hospital use a simple needle and syringe is the best.

Macintosh's (1950) balloon technique must be mentioned here. A tiny balloon is attached to the epidural needle, and, when the point of the needle is lying in the interspinous ligament, inflated by injecting air through its thick self-sealing neck. Deflation occurs as soon as the epidural space is entered.

The negative pressure sign.—The existence of a negative pressure in the epidural space is a highly controversial subject and as Bromage (1954) remarks, "much ink has been spilt in the protracted discussion centred around the problem of pressure differences in the epidural space". Briefly there are two main theories. First, a negative pressure is simply created by indentation of the dura by the point of the advancing needle. Janzen (1926) from a careful investigation came to the conclusion that the negative pressure depended on the type of needle used. Blunt needles, which tended to push the dura away for some distance, before piercing it, gave a greater negative pressure than sharp needles, and a needle with a side opening and closed end gave greater negative pressures than an open ended one. He observed that the negative pressure could be increased or decreased by advancing or withdrawing the needle. When using an Odom's indicator (see below) regularly for epidural work the same phenomenon can be observed. A slight advance of the needle sucks in the coloured solution in the capillary tube, and as the hand is taken away the solution flows back. Subsequent workers—Heldt and Moloney (1928) and Eaton (1939)—using a water manometer attached to the epidural needle, demonstrated that the negative pressure increases as the needle advances across the epidural space until the dura is punctured. Odom (1936), however, suggested that a negative pressure was created by flexion of the spine. Dawkins (1954), describing his technique of epidural injection with an Odom's indicator, stated that should localisation of the space take longer than three minutes, the spine should be extended for one minute and then reflexed in order to restore the negative pressure. Macintosh and Mushin (1947) and Bryce-Smith (1950) further investigated the problem and recorded the conclusion that a negative pressure exists in the epidural space and is created by the transmission of the negative intrapleural pressure. Since the epidural space is filled with fat, connective tissue and venous plexuses, the negative pressure is poorly transmitted caudal to the thoracic region. Macintosh (1950) further showed that with his balloon indicator attached to a needle in the epidural space, a cough by the patient would re-inflate the balloon. Dawkins (1963) points out that no experimental proof of this theory has been produced. In his own experience of a series of 1,176 cases using Odom's indicator, a negative pressure was present in 72·8 per cent in the lumbar region, but in only 51·8 per cent in the thoracic region.

The position of the patient may play an important part in the degree of negative pressure present. In a patient sitting up, the diameter of the epidural space might be reduced by bulging of the theca in the lumbar region. Bonniot (1934) has shown that an epidural pressure of −0·5 cm. of water is decreased to −5·0 cm. on tilting the patient 35° head-down, and increased to zero on restoring the patient to the horizontal position.

The hanging drop sign.—This is a very simple technique first described by Gutierrez (1933). The epidural needle is placed in the interspinous ligament, and a drop of fluid deposited on the hub; as the needle enters the epidural space the drop is sucked in.

Odom's indicator.—Odom (1936) described a similar device to that of Gutierrez, the drop of fluid being contained in a small glass capillary tube attached to the needle. As the epidural space is entered there is a movement inwards of the fluid: in some cases it disappears entirely.

Both these methods are positive in about 85 per cent of cases. In the remaining 15 per cent, provided the anaesthetist concentrates on the feel of the ligaments as well as on watching the movements of the capillary tube or drop of liquid, the loss of resistance on entering the epidural space can be noted and a spinal tap prevented despite no movement of the indicator. When both signs—the sense of "give" on piercing the ligamentum flavum and the sucking in of the indicator fluid—occur together, the anaesthetist can be completely certain the epidural space has been correctly identified. The negative-pressure sign has the advantage that it can be used with a lateral approach to the epidural space, since it does not depend on the continuity of ligaments to block the needle point as is the case with the loss of resistance signs.

Other devices.—Several devices have been designed incorporating the principles of loss of resistance and negative pressure combined with a visual aid. Zelenka (1956) described a calibrated curved piece of glass tubing filled with air and water which is attached at one end to the hub of the epidural needle and at the other to a small balloon which exerts a positive pressure. As the needle enters the epidural space the contents of the indicator are sucked and pushed into the epidural space. Dawkins (1957) has modified this device, making it much simpler. The point of an epidural needle with attached Odom's indicator is placed in the interspinous ligament. A small piece of soft rubber tubing, closed at one end, is pushed over the open end of the indicator and around its shaft for about 1 cm. This causes a slight positive pressure which will reinforce the visual indication of a negative pressure in the epidural space. Brooks (1957) has devised an Odom's indicator with a bulb at the end. The whole is filled with air and attached to the epidural needle. The bulb is then warmed by touching with the hand, thus causing a slight positive pressure as the air expands, which is released when the epidural space is entered.

Dawkins (1963) has designed a gravity indicator which utilises the force of gravity to move the indicator. A vertical nylon tube of 3 mm. internal bore is attached at right angles to a mount which plugs into the needle hub, the tube is filled with sterile saline, and a bubble of air is added to provide a meniscus. Dawkins claims a 95 per cent success rate using this device.

Summary.—It matters little that there are so many methods for locating the epidural space, each with its advantages and disadvantages. That there are so many simply underlines the fact that no one method is completely satisfactory and that much depends on the anaesthetist's personal preference. Lightness of control, the author feels, is most important, particularly in the thoracic region where ligaments are less well defined. If special indications exist to warrant puncture in the thoracic region, a light device such as an Odom's indicator, or the gravity indicator of Dawkins (weight only 5 g. as compared with the 42 g. of a 10 c.c. syringe and 5 ml. of saline) are best. All in all, for the most satisfactory results the anaesthetist should stick to a method which suits him best.

Epidural Needles (see Figs. 1*b* and 2)

Any lumbar puncture needle can be used for epidural work, but an unduly fine gauge is not helpful. Special needles such as those designed to magnify the loss of resistance sign (p. 1216) and that of Tuohy for continuous epidural work (p. 1224) are not essential for single dose analgesia. When the epidural space is approached through the sacral hiatus a different pattern is advisable (p. 1229).

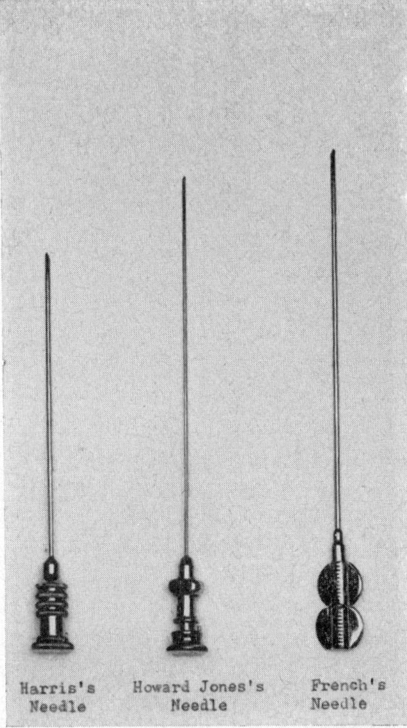

43/FIG. 1(*a*)—
Spinal needles.

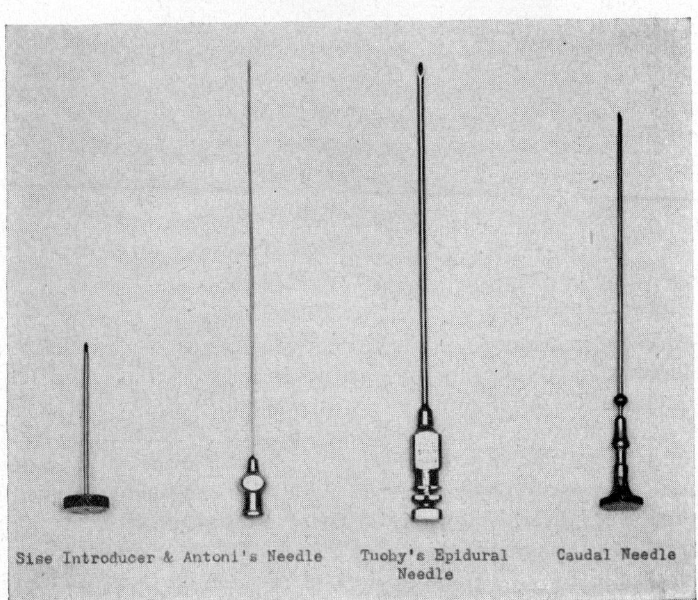

43/FIG. 1(*b*)—Epidural needles.

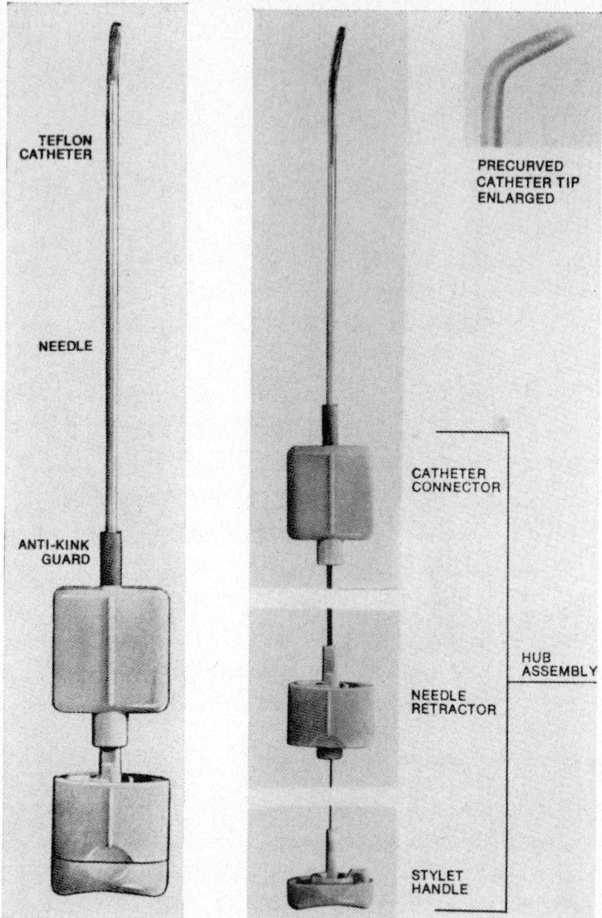

43/Fig. 2.—Disposable continuous epidural unit ("Bardic Henkin Epidural Unit").

The Epidural Injection

While the consequences of epidural infection are possibly less disastrous than those of subarachnoid infection, they are nevertheless serious enough to warrant a scrupulous aseptic technique.

Those for whom an epidural block is indicated will often be unsuitable for general anaesthesia, and it is therefore better for the anaesthetist to develop his technique with conscious patients. Sudden and unexpected movements during the injection are, however, not only irritating but dangerous, and though a co-operative patient can avoid these, an unco-operative one may not. For the latter a general anaesthetic is desirable if it is practicable, but it is well to remember that a patient will often respond actively to a pin prick under light anaesthesia.

Only when the epidural space has been identified with certainty should any injection of analgesic solution be made. Confirmation that the position of the needle is in this space can be made in several ways. If the loss of resistance sign is being used, then at the moment when the syringe is detached, a little fluid may drip back from the hub of the needle. A few drops should be allowed to fall on the bare skin of the anaesthetist's forearm, when injected analgesic solution at room temperature will feel cold while cerebrospinal fluid will be warm. In some cases this drip back is considerable, and it is therefore important that the first few drops are tested, as the analgesic solution rapidly becomes warm after injection. Other confirmatory tests, that can be applied before injection, are aspiration (nothing should return if the needle point lies in the epidural space) and injection of a little air followed once more by aspiration. A helpful sign of a satisfactory position for the needle is the commonly noticed increase in the rate and depth of respiration during epidural injection, which can attributed to the stimulating effect of the cold analgesic solution on the intercostal nerve roots. Finally, when injecting into the epidural space—having been satisfied that the dura is not punctured—the solution runs very freely with no sense of resistance. The sensation is quite characteristic and readily appreciated after a little practice with this technique. If there is the slightest doubt about the situation of the needle, the epidural space should be identified again at a different level, as only in this way can an accidental total spinal be avoided.

A percentage of spinal taps is inevitable in any series of epidural blocks. It is particularly liable to occur in old people with tough ligaments where a good deal of pressure on the advancing needle is required. The "give" of the ligamentum flavum is then very sudden and difficult to arrest. Once spinal tap occurs all attempts to locate the epidural space at that level should stop and another convenient space be used. There is only a remote possibility that the solution spreading in the epidural space will pass through such a dural puncture hole against the C.S.F. pressure. Once a dural tap occurs, however, one of the main advantages of an epidural is lost, because the patient is liable to a post-operative headache—especially with the size of hole made by an epidural needle.

It is difficult to lay down precise rules for avoiding a total spinal. Never inject when in doubt is the best rule, and doubt can only be converted to certainty by practice. Many anaesthetists regard epidural blocks as a formidable undertaking, but the technique is easily learned by anyone with the interest and patience to do so. Injection into the epidural space should be slow, 10 ml. at a time, and the patient carefully observed. Any untoward signs can be detected before a massive intrathecal dose is given should the needle have pierced the dura. This is one of the advantages of doing an epidural block on a conscious patient.

Posture.—Positioning of the patient during injection varies with the operative requirements. For saddle blocks the sitting position can be used if the anaesthetist prefers, or the lateral position with the table tilted into the reverse Trendelenburg. The spread of solution in the epidural space is not so certain as with subarachnoid injection and even in saddle epidural blocks, with the patient sitting up, a fall in blood pressure can occur. It is wise, therefore, to give a vasopressor immediately the injection is completed. For lower abdominal cases the lateral position is used with the spine tilted slightly head down as for hyperbaric spinal solutions. For upper abdominal operations, after the injection has been completed, the patient must be turned on his back and the table tilted into about 15 degrees Trendelenburg position.

Drugs.—Lignocaine is recommended for epidural work. It has a very rapid onset of action, produces complete analgesia and has a reasonable duration of effect. A concentration of 1·5 per cent. does not cause motor paralysis, but effective sensory and autonomic block.

Those factors governing the spread of solutions in the epidural space which have an important bearing on dosage have already been discussed. In general, accurate dosage is difficult to calculate for epidural work because there are so many variables to be reconciled such as the patency of intervertebral foramina, the amount of fat in the epidural space, the degree of atherosclerosis, and the volume, concentration and total mass of drug injected.

The anaesthetist is primarily concerned with producing a spread of analgesia of high quality sufficient to cover the operative area without achieving a toxic blood level and avoiding so extensive a spread as to cause severe and dangerous hypotension. It is this difficulty of accurately determining dosage and height of analgesia which enables critics to state that the hypotension of epidural block is an uncontrolled hypotension, steep falls requiring correction by the rather blunderbuss use of vasopressors. The quality of blockade determines the need for supplementary anaesthesia but it is nearly always inferior to subarachnoid block. More careful attention to dosage may partially resolve some of these problems. Bromage has done extensive and meticulous work to lay down accurate guide lines for dosage. While acknowledging the importance of volume and concentration of local analgesic drug, he places considerable emphasis on the total mass of drug injected in determining the height of analgesia achieved (Bromage *et al.*, 1964). Thus for solutions of lignocaine between 2 and 5 per cent, 35 mg. per spinal segment is required at 20 years of age, decreasing steadily to about 15 mg. per segment at 80.

43/Table 1

Choice of Lignocaine Concentration

Clinical requirements		*Best choice of solution*
Rapid onset		1 per cent Plain 5 per cent Plain 3 per cent + Adrenaline
Surgical analgesia	"One shot" injection	3 per cent + Adrenaline
	Intermittent injections via catheter	1 per cent or 5 per cent plain for initial injection followed by 2 per cent or 3 per cent with Adrenaline
Post-operative and therapeutic analgesia	(*a*) Frequent injections	0·75 — 1 per cent + Adrenaline
	(*b*) Injections at long intervals	2 — 4 per cent + Adrenaline

(Adapted from Bromage *et al.*, 1964)

Concentration does however seem to influence both the time for complete spread of analgesia and factors such as tachyphylaxis during continuous analgesia. Bromage also makes suggestions regarding lignocaine concentrations for varying clinical requirements. His choice of a 3 per cent solution with adrenaline for single injections is interesting, as the experiments show this to be more efficient than the commonly used 2 per cent solution which has one of the longest spreading times of all solutions, an average of 18 minutes.

Bromage thus lays great emphasis on the mass of solute—or put in another way the number of milligrams of drug per segment—in estimating dosage for a given height of analgesia, concentration playing a secondary part to meet varying clinical conditions.

Other workers however lay stress on the influence of volume of solution. Erdemis *et al.* (1965) investigated the behaviour of two solutions, one of 30 ml. of 1 per cent lignocaine, and the other of 10 ml. of a 3 per cent solution. These should give comparable heights of analgesia on the basis of total mass of solute determining height of analgesia. However, they found that the larger volume of weaker solution produced significantly higher levels of analgesia.

For the anaesthetist who does not extensively practise epidural blocks but who wishes to meet the occasional need, the following scheme, using 1·5 per cent lignocaine, will give good results:

1. Upper abdominal operations . 30 ml. of solution injected between L1–2 with the patient in 15–20° Trendelenburg tilt.
2. Lower abdominal operations . 20 ml. of solution injected between L1–2 with the patient in 10° Trendelenburg tilt.
3. Herniae and varicose veins . 20 ml. of solution injected between L1–2 with the patient horizontal.
4. Perineal and bladder neck operations . 15 ml. of solution injected between L2–3 with the patient sitting up.

These volumes can be reduced for elderly and atherosclerotic patients.

Special mention must be made of the need for precise control of dosage in obstetrics, since exaggerated spread is particularly likely at term and during labour. Bromage (1962) has shown that a reduction of dosage of about one-third is required if the risks of hypotension and impaired efficiency of the process of labour are to be avoided.

Continuous Epidural Analgesia

Continuous epidural analgesia dates from the adoption of Tuohy's (1945) catheter technique—developed for continuous spinal analgesia—to epidural analgesia by Curbello (1949). In most clinics at the present time the catheter technique is used only when the length of operation is likely to be greater than the duration of action of a single dose of the analgesic drug. Thus lignocaine is one of the best analgesics for epidural work because of the profound analgesia it produces, but it can only be relied upon to give a maximum of two hours opera-

effective and rendered hypotensive complications insignificant. Vital capacity measurements during the first twenty-four hours after the operation showed an average return to 85 per cent of the pre-operative level. Bromage (1967) has reported on the use of this technique to provide early and immediate ambulation after major abdominal procedures. The patient can be walked around the recovery room within an hour of leaving the operating theatre. For success the technique must provide a narrow band of analgesia sufficient to cover the wound area, and leave the lower limbs unaffected.

A continuous epidural technique has proved useful for patients after thoracotomy, and for those with chest injuries. It also has possibilities in the post-operative management of patients with bronchitis and emphysema. But the technique is exacting and unsuitable for routine use except where the facilities of a post-operative recovery ward or intensive care unit are available.

Crush injury of the chest.—Continuous epidural analgesia is increasingly used in the treatment of chest injuries. The complete relief from pain that it affords reduces paradoxical respiration and allows the patient to clear the lower airways by coughing freely. As a result many patients can be spared a tracheostomy. This value of epidural analgesia is, however, limited to the "mild" case of chest injury or Group I in the classification of Lloyd *et al.* (1965). In this group there are perhaps two or three fractured ribs but the patient is unable to breathe easily or cough because of the pain. Group I patients who also have concomitant chest diseases, such as chronic bronchitis or emphysema, are particularly suitable for epidural analgesia. Patients with moderate or severe chest injuries (Groups II and III of Lloyd *et al.*) usually require tracheostomy and intermittent positive pressure ventilation and because of the number of fractured ribs they are unsuitable for epidural analgesia. The extensive block needed would very likely be followed by marked hypotension, particularly in a patient who has suffered blood loss. Epidural analgesia is worth considering after resuscitation when the bony injury is limited to the lower part of the thoracic cage.

Intractable pain.—Dogliotti and Ciocatto (1953) reported that when a mixed nerve is repeatedly subjected to concentrated solutions of a local analgesic the pain fibres are selectively destroyed. Using 2 per cent lignocaine injected every 3 hours for 72–96 hours, they obtained pain relief lasting over two years in 50 per cent of patients. Other workers have been unable to repeat these results (Bonica *et al.*, 1957). Any long term relief of pain achieved by this method is perhaps due to reorganisation of sensory input at a higher level (Melzack and Wall, 1965). Cases of intractable root pain are better managed by intrathecal injections of neurolytic agents (see Chapter 38).

Sciatic nerve pain.—The use of epidural analgesia for the relief of sciatic pain was reported many years ago (Evans, 1936; Kelman, 1944). Cyriax (1957) advocates it as the conservative treatment of choice for those patients who have a low lumbar disc lesion causing nerve root pressure with neurological signs in the affected leg. More recently, Coomes (1961), from a comparison of the results of treatment by epidural injection with those from rest in bed, has reinforced this view.

Peripheral vascular disease.—A single epidural injection is a convenient way of assessing the likely effects of a subsequent sympathectomy and saves the discomfort of blocking the sympathetic ganglia by several paravertebral injections. The value of epidural analgesia for the treatment of vascular diseases in the lower limbs is described on p. 1231.

Visceral pain.—The severe pain of acute pancreatitis, and the agonising pain of dissecting aneurysm of the aorta, can be successfully relieved by continuous epidural analgesia.

Eclampsia.—The value of epidural block for eclampsia is described on p. 1231.

SACRAL EPIDURAL ANALGESIA

Anatomy of the Sacrum, Sacral Canal and Hiatus

The sacrum represents the fusion of 5 sacral vertebrae. Variations of this fusion are common and have an important bearing on the failure rate of sacral epidural analgesia. Indeed the comparative anatomical constancy of the lumbar compared with the sacral region is a strong argument in favour of using the former approach to the epidural space whenever possible.

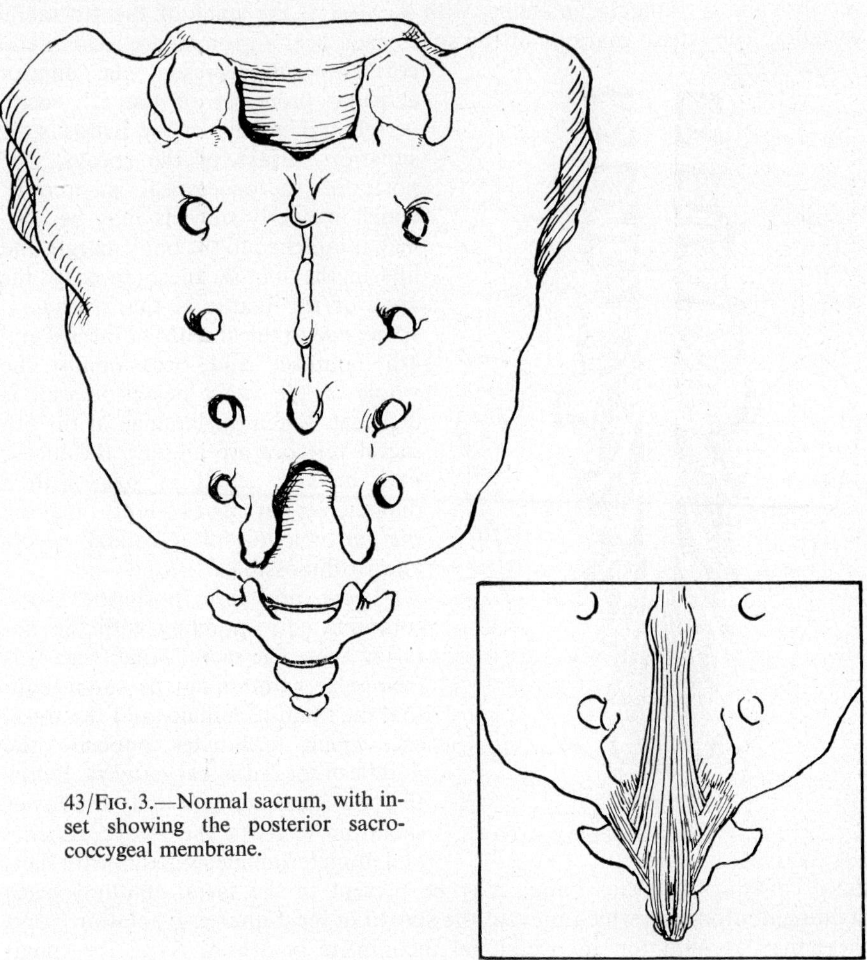

43/FIG. 3.—Normal sacrum, with inset showing the posterior sacrococcygeal membrane.

The sacrum is triangular in shape; the apex, below, articulates with the coccyx, while the base, above, has median and lateral portions. The median part represents the body of the 1st sacral vertebra and articulates with the corresponding surface of the body of the 5th lumbar vertebra. The lateral portions, known as the alae, represent fused costal and transverse elements.

The anterior surface is concave and ridged at the sites of fusion between the five sacral vertebrae. Lateral to the ridges are the large anterior sacral foramina through which the anterior primary rami of the first four sacral nerves pass. Local analgesic solutions injected into the sacral epidural space can pass freely through these foramina, and this is a factor in the unpredictable height to which sacral analgesia may extend.

The posterior surface has the greater interest for the anaesthetist (Fig. 3). It is convex, and in the mid-line runs a bony ridge, the median sacral crest, with three or four rudimentary spinous processes. The sacral hiatus is a deficiency of the posterior wall formed by the failure of fusion of the laminae of the 4th sacral vertebra and is triangular in shape, with its apex at the spine of the 4th sacral vertebra. The lateral margins of the space each bear a prominence—the sacral cornu—which represent the inferior articular processes of the 5th sacral vertebra. The base of the hiatus is the superior surface of the coccyx. The posterior sacrococcygeal membrane, which in elderly subjects may be ossified, is attached to the bony margin and fills in the hiatus. In some cases the apex of the hiatus is the 3rd sacral spine, due to the absence of the 3rd and 4th laminae, and occasionally the whole of the bony posterior wall is deficient. When the laminae of the 5th sacral vertebra are present, the hiatus may be very small in size—with a diameter as narrow as 2 mm.—making the introduction of a caudal needle almost impossible.

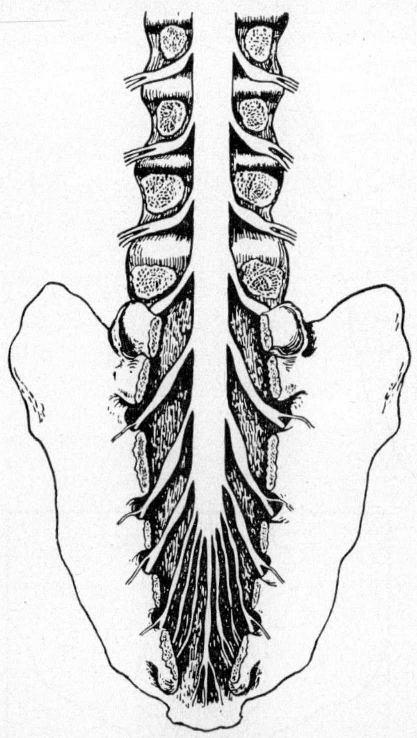

43/Fig. 4.—The sacral canal.

There are four posterior sacral foramina corresponding with the anterior ones. The sacral canal (Fig. 4) is triangular, containing the cauda equina, the filum terminale, and the dural sac which terminates opposite the middle of the 3rd sacral vertebra. Below this the canal contains only the lower sacral nerve roots, the coccygeal nerve and filum terminale, together with their dural coverings. Fibrous bands may be present in the sacral epidural space dividing it into loculi which prevent the spread of local analgesic solutions, and these may account for an occasional incomplete analgesia. As in the spinal epidural space, fatty tissue, varying with the obesity of the subject, and venous plexuses are also present.

Needles

A malleable steel needle (Fig. 1*b*) is best, as this will adapt itself to the curve of the sacrum and will not break. Such needles are likely to come apart where the hub joins the shaft, and for this reason there is placed near the hub a small round enlargement which ensures that a portion of shaft must always stick out of the skin. The length of the shaft, between point and enlargement, should be between 2 or 3 inches (5 and 7·5 cm.). Other types of needle may be used—for example an ordinary spinal needle, a No. 1 intravenous needle, or a No. 17 hypodermic needle. As with spinal epidural analgesia, however, the wider-bore needles give a better feel of the structures they pass through, while a short bevel at the point minimises the risk of puncturing the dura.

For continuous techniques a malleable needle may be left in the sacral canal and serial injections made through it or through plastic tubing attached to the hub. Perhaps a more satisfactory method—as it reduces the risk of needle displacement—is to pass a fine vinyl plastic catheter through the needle into the sacral epidural space and then to remove the needle. Whatever method is chosen the site of entry of the needle or catheter into the skin over the sacral hiatus should be sealed off with collodion solution to avoid infection.

Technique

The block can be done with the patient either in the prone or left lateral position. For obstetric patients in or near labour the latter position is the more convenient. A scrupulous aseptic technique, as described for spinal analgesia, must be observed.

The sacral hiatus is identified by feeling for the sacral cornu with the tip of the index finger; a skin weal of local analgesic solution is then raised over it using a fine needle. In obese patients it is difficult to feel, and in others it may be smaller than normal. When in difficulty Galley (1949) recommends identifying the tip of the coccyx and placing the tip of the index finger over this with the rest of the finger in the intergluteal fold. The hiatus should then coincide in position with the proximal interphalangeal joint. The caudal needle is passed through the skin weal to pierce the sacrococcygeal membrane at right angles to the skin surface. The hub of the needle is then depressed until it is almost in the intergluteal fold parallel to the skin over the sacrum. The needle is then pushed forwards into the sacral canal, taking care that the point does not ascend any higher than a line from the posterior superior iliac spines at which level the subarachnoid space begins.

Aspiration tests for blood and C.S.F. are made. A drop or so of blood is no contra-indication to proceeding with the injection, but if C.S.F. is aspirated the block must be abandoned or converted to spinal analgesia. Free bleeding from the needle hub means that an epidural vein has been pierced and the needle should be withdrawn for 0·5 cm. A test dose is then injected—say 5–8 ml. of solution—and if the patient can move his toes at the end of 5 minutes the needle can be assumed to be safely in the epidural space and the main dose is injected.

In spite of careful technique the needle may pass into sites other than the epidural space: it may miss the sacrococcygeal membrane and pass dorsal to the sacrum. If this is suspected it can be tested for by injecting a few ml. of air and palpating the skin over the tip of the needle for crepitus. The main danger is if the needle slips past the base of the coccyx into the rectum, for should it be withdrawn and then correctly placed in the epidural space, severe infection may occur. Marked resistance to injection, with complaint of backache, suggests the needle point has run beneath the periosteal layer of the sacral canal, and this can be corrected by slightly withdrawing the needle. When the needle is correctly placed in the epidural space the solution should run freely without any sensation of resistance as with lumbar epidural injection. Any feeling of resistance suggests the needle is not correctly placed.

Drugs.—Lignocaine is recommended, as for lumbar epidural work, but bupivacaine is an excellent alternative when a long period of analgesia is required.

Dosage.—The level of analgesia depends on the quantity of solution injected, the speed of injection, and the position of the patient. The average capacity of the sacral canal is 34 ml. in males and 32 ml. in females.

About 20–30 ml. of solution are required for blocks up to L4–5 for operations on the anus, perineum or vagina. About 60 ml. of solution plus a slight Trendelenburg position will give a block up to the umbilicus, and up to 90 ml. of solution are required for high blocks for upper abdominal operations. With these large doses there is a definite risk of toxic reactions so that for an upper abdominal operation, and when it is not necessary to block the sacral nerve roots, the lumbar epidural route should be used to cut down the volume of solution.

Indications for Sacral Epidural Analgesia

Surgical operations.—The main value of this route is for the production of analgesia of the sacral nerves for such procedures as cystoscopy, operations on and near the anus, and gynaecological operations on the vulva and vagina. In obese patients for whom a local block is likely to provide better operating conditions in these regions of the body than a general anaesthetic, the sacral approach to the epidural space may be technically difficult. For such, lumbar epidural analgesia is easier and satisfactory if performed with the patient sitting up to allow the analgesic solution to run down into the sacral canal. For an operation such as abdomino-perineal resection of the rectum in which lumbar and dorsal, as well as sacral, analgesia is required, the sacral route is the logical choice.

Obstetrical analgesia.—The motor and sensory innervation of the whole birth canal lends itself to the use of epidural analgesia for the relief of pain in labour (see Chapter 51). The whole sensory supply to the uterine body, cervix, vagina, perineum and vulva arises from the level of D11 and below, while the motor innervation of the uterine body arises from D10 and above. This arrangement enables pain relief to be provided without affecting the motor supply of the uterine body by an epidural block up to the level of D11.

The use of continuous sacral epidural analgesia has never caught on in this country although recently there have been signs of a revival of interest. It is very popular in the U.S.A. where it was pioneered by Higson. Modern practice now veers towards using the lumbar route for continuous epidural analgesia in labour (see Chapter 52).

Eclampsia.—Bryce-Smith and Williams (1955) have reported that it is difficult to achieve an adequate control of the blood pressure with sacral epidural analgesia in eclampsia. A lumbar epidural block leads to better control of the blood pressure since the dorsal spinal segments can be easily reached by this route. They regard subarachnoid block as the most efficient local technique in this respect, and, considering the risks to mother and foetus of uncontrolled eclampsia, this, in spite of its inherent dangers, is perhaps justified.

Peripheral vascular disease.—Galley (1952) has reported on the value of sacral epidural analgesia in patients with arteriosclerotic gangrene accompanied by severe pain. "Proctocaine" 50 ml. injected into the sacral canal has given up to three months' freedom from pain, with improvement in the blood supply to the limb and rapid demarcation between good and gangrenous skin. Cases of intermittent claudication have shown marked symptomatic improvement on the same treatment. The block of sympathetic fibres produced by a sacral epidural injection of local analgesic has a particular value in the presence of vascular spasm. The prompt treatment by this technique may save a limb endangered by arterial embolism, as it will open up the collateral vessels that are in spasm. A white leg of pregnancy may also respond. Here the deep vein thrombosis is thought to produce a reflex spasm of the small veins and arterioles, resulting in hypoxia and transudation of fluid from the capillaries into the tissue, where it increases the oedema further by pressing on the lymphatics. An early sympathetic block may free the vicious circle, but it usually has to be repeated or maintained over several days for successful treatment.

Diabetic neuropathy.—Galley (1952) claims success in the treatment of the pain of diabetic neuropathy by sacral epidural block with "Proctocaine". The pain of this disease is thought to be due to degenerating fibres, and ceases when the degeneration is complete.

The Complications of Spinal and Epidural Analgesia

Traumatic Results of Subarachnoid and Epidural Puncture

Backache.—This is caused by damage to the supraspinous and interspinous ligaments and the ligamentum flavum through which the spinal or epidural needle passes, and is also occasionally due to damage of an intervertebral disc. With the fine spinal needles in use today backache is very uncommon, but it is the commonest post-analgesia complication of epidural analgesia. Foldes and his associates (1956) have reported an incidence of 3 per cent in 422 cases, using the Tuohy needle and catheter technique. The condition is due to trauma inflicted by the wide-bore needles essential for epidural work.

It seems remarkable that damage to an intervertebral disc can occur, but it undoubtedly can and Dripps and Vandam (1951) report that they have seen gelatinous material drip from a needle which entered the nucleus pulposus in a 14-year-old girl during lumbar puncture. That the disc is pain sensitive is shown by the observations of Wiberg (1949) who, during operations on the lumbar spine under local analgesia, pressed on the disc and produced pain referred to the lumbar-sacral angle. Histological evidence indicates that the ligamentous covering of the disc, the annulus fibrosus, is responsible for this pain. Prolapse of the disc may follow damage to the annulus fibrosus (Everett, 1941). It is possible that the flexion of the spine needed during lumbar puncture increases the pressure in the discs and causes them to bulge into the spinal canal.

Damage to epidural arteries, veins and nerves.—Injury to the epidural plexus of vessels is a common cause of "bloody tap". Bleeding can be severe enough to result in the formation of an epidural haematoma, and if blood reaches the subarachnoid space signs of meningeal irritation will follow. Damage to the epidural vessels is more likely to occur with an epidural catheter technique than with a simple lumbar puncture. Damage to the nerve roots in the epidural space during attempted lumbar puncture can occur if the needle is deviated in a lateral direction, and will be associated with pain in the appropriate distribution.

Damage to the spinal cord and nerve roots in the subarachnoid space.—Although in 94 per cent of cases the cord terminates in the region of the 1st lumbar vertebra, in some cases it may end as low as the 3rd and can be damaged by a lumbar puncture needle inserted above the L3–4 interspace. This applies particularly in infants and young children where the cord terminates relatively lower in the spinal canal than in the adult. Dripps and Vandam (1951) report contact with sensory roots of the cauda equina in 13 per cent of cases in a series of lumbar punctures performed by them.

Headache

There is considerable evidence that most post-spinal headaches are due to a low C.S.F. pressure consequent upon seepage of C.S.F. through the dural puncture hole. Headache can also result from a raised C.S.F. pressure from meningeal irritation or it may herald the onset of infective meningitis. Typical post-spinal headache comes on within an hour or two of the analgesia. It is not, however, generally appreciated that its onset may be delayed for 7–10 days, and may last for weeks or even months, although these protracted headaches are difficult to explain on a simple leakage theory.

Low pressure headache has certain well-defined characteristics. The patient recognises that the headache is different from any other previously experienced and is made worse by sitting up and relieved by lying down or abdominal compression. Pain may spread across the whole frontal area or be localised behind the eyeballs or in the nuchal region. In the latter case it is often accompanied by a stiff neck and is difficult to distinguish from meningeal irritation. Nausea and vomiting not uncommonly accompany the headache and the patient may find difficulty in focusing his eyes on an object. Tinnitus and deafness may occur—these are explicable on the basis of a low C.S.F. pressure resulting in a fall in intralabyrinthine pressure, since the impairment of hearing is for high tones. Dripps and Vandam (1951) mention a case with severe post-lumbar puncture headache and diminution of hearing which improved after raising the C.S.F. pressure by injection of epidural saline. A typical spinal headache can be produced in man by withdrawal of C.S.F. in the upright position and the headache relieved by re-injection (Kunkle *et al.*, 1943; Wolff, 1948). Many observers (Pickering, 1948; Marshall, 1950; Glesne, 1950) have found the C.S.F. pressure to be low or absent in patients with post-spinal headache, and others (Weintraub *et al.*, 1947; Ahearn, 1948; McCord *et al.*, 1951) have shown that epidural injection or abdominal compression, which temporarily raise the C.S.F. pressure, will relieve the headache.

Strong supporting evidence comes from the fact that a dural puncture hole can persist for as long as 14 days after injection (Franksson and Gordh, 1946). Macintosh (1957) also reports that he has seen—at laminectomy—C.S.F. escape through a dural puncture hole made 36 hours previously. Franksson and Gordh in experiments on human beings showed that with a pressure of 100–200 mm. H_2O (or a C.S.F. pressure of about 150 mm. H_2O) a leakage of 0·17 ml./min. of C.S.F. into the epidural space is possible, which in 24 hours would amount to a loss of 240 ml. Anything which is likely to increase the leak through the dura may increase the incidence of headache. Thus, the high incidence of post-spinal headache in obstetric patients can be accounted for by the straining during normal labour and the early ambulation in the puerperium. Similarly, patients with a cough often develop a severe post-spinal headache. Reduction in the size of the dural hole by the use of fine spinal needles significantly reduces the incidence of spinal headache. Dripps and Vandam (1951) have shown from their series that with a 16-gauge needle the incidence of headache was 24 per cent while with a 24-gauge needle it fell to 6 per cent. The latter is the smallest size needle which can in practice be used without the aid of an introducer. Haraldson (1951) reports the use of a needle designed by Sjovall which has a tapering solid point and an orifice about 2 mm. from the actual tip of the point. With this needle the dural fibres are pressed apart without being cut, so that the gap closes on its withdrawal. Haraldson claims that by this method he has reduced the incidence of headache by two-thirds.

The leakage theory is not, however, accepted by all authorities. Harris (1951) points out that the whole volume of C.S.F. is normally replaced 4–6 times daily and seepage of C.S.F. must cease as soon as its pressure in the epidural space equals that in the subarachnoid space. Against this view is the fact that in young people there is free communication between the epidural and paravertebral spaces via the intervertebral foramina; on the other hand, in older people it is possible that Harris's view holds good because the normal escape routes from the epidural space are considerably narrowed by fibrous tissue; moreover the incidence of post-spinal headache is less frequent in the over 40 age group.

If it is to be accepted that the underlying cause of spinal headache is low C.S.F. pressure, the question arises what structures are responsible for the pain. Wolff (1948) and his co-workers have shown that the venous sinuses, basal parts of the dura, and basal dural cerebral arteries are sensitive to pain. Painful stimuli arising from the superior surface of the tentorium cerebelli and above are transmitted via the 5th nerve and referred to the anterior half of the head. Pain from below the tentorium is transmitted by the 9th and 10th cranial nerves and upper three cervical nerves and referred to the posterior half of the head. Traction on all these structures would arise when the normal cushioning effect of C.S.F. is lost; this is the probable reason for the severe headache that occurs after an air-encephalogram, in which a large volume of C.S.F. is removed and replaced by air.

The high incidence—nearly double that of general surgical patients—of spinal headache in obstetric patients calls for further comment. A number of factors contribute. General surgical patients are often confined to bed for a few days after operation. Howe and Chen (1951) in a series of 400 spinals found that the incidence of headache in patients ambulant on the first post-operative day was 42·7 per cent, and in patients not allowed up until the fourth day 4·3 per cent. Analgesics required for post-operative pain of general surgical operations during the first 36–48 hours may mask a mild spinal headache. Fluid balance is carefully attended to in general surgical patients and therefore C.S.F. pressure is not likely to be further lowered from dehydration. This factor is difficult to evaluate since patients in labour are enthusiastically given fluids to drink, but may retain large volumes of fluid in the stomach. Finally, the straining of vaginal deliveries may raise C.S.F. pressure and increase the loss of fluid through the dural puncture hole.

Jarman (1937) stated that the use of intravenous thiopentone immediately before lumbar puncture reduces the incidence of spinal headache. Again, it is difficult to assess the importance of this in relation to so many other factors, but it could be explained on the basis of decreased C.S.F. production and pressure associated with the fall of blood pressure which accompanies thiopentone and spinal analgesia. It is also hard to assess to what extent spinal headache is due or accentuated by psychic factors. Redlich and his associates (1946) assessed the personality traits of 100 patients subjected to lumbar puncture. They used 16- and 22-gauge needles on alternate patients, and concluded that anxiety and emotional factors played little part in the cause of spinal headache.

Although the basic cause of low pressure headache is seepage of C.S.F. through the dural puncture hole, it is not surprising when so many additional factors play a part that the reputed incidence varies on average between 10 and 30 per cent. It must be remembered, too, that there is a definite incidence of headache after general anaesthesia.

High pressure headaches are presumed to be due to the development of an aseptic inflammatory meningeal reaction, perhaps caused by the contamination of the spinal fluid by blood from the epidural space or some irritant in the injected solution. Harris (1951) refers to a series of spinal headaches in a venereal disease department—where diagnostic lumbar punctures are common—which was traced to the presence of minute charred carbon particles in the lumbar puncture needle. In this department the needles were packed for sterilisation with the points in cotton wool pads and then autoclaved. The headaches, which resulted from charring of the cotton wool, did not occur when the substance was eliminated from the process.

Thorsen (1947*a*) attributes 20 per cent of spinal headaches to a raised C.S.F. pressure. It is doubtful, however, whether the raised C.S.F. pressure is itself ultimately responsible for the headache because relief does not always follow a lumbar puncture, even though the result is sometimes magical (Evans, 1954).

Treatment.—The treatment of low pressure headache begins with the prophylactic use of a fine spinal needle and the horizontal position for the first 24 hours post-operatively. Simple measures, such as the maintenance of this posture and the use of mild analgesics like acetyl-salicylic acid and tab. codein. co., are often sufficient for the established headache. Occasionally the headache may be so severe as to warrant more vigorous treatment, which should be directed towards decreasing the dural leak and raising the C.S.F. pressure to compensate for the continual loss of fluid until the puncture hole in the dura heals. Intrathecal or epidural injections of saline will both produce relief of headache (Rice and Dobbs, 1950; McCord *et al.*, 1951). Intrathecal injections may, however, only make a further dural leak, so that the headache is ultimately worse, while both it and the epidural injection are unfortunately only likely to be temporarily successful. For an intractable headache epidural saline with a continuous catheter technique would seem the better method.

Intravenous hypotonic solutions have been recommended with the object of increasing the production of C.S.F. Kreuger (1953) suggests 2·5 per cent dextrose in 0·45 per cent saline, to each 500 ml. of which has been added 100 mg. of nicotinic acid to dilate the vessels of the choroid plexus. A variation of this is to inject pitressin and enforce a daily fluid intake of at least 3 litres for a period of three days. Deutsch (1952) advised intravenous alcohol made up as 5 per cent glucose and 5 per cent alcohol in a litre of water. The alcohol produces euphoria besides dilating the pial vessels and shifting water from the intra- to the extra-cellular space.

High pressure headaches may respond to the dehydrating effect of rectal magnesium sulphate or intravenous hypertonic glucose.

Meningitis

This is the dreaded complication of lumbar puncture, but is completely preventable if a rigid aseptic technique is used. In the opinion of the writer it is surprising that it is not seen more frequently considering the way in which lumbar puncture is often performed in routine hospital practice.

Meningitis can usually be traced to an error of technique, but occasionally occurs in apparently inexplicable circumstances (Davidson, 1947). Clinically it is usually acute in form, but cases of protracted low grade infection of many months' duration have been recorded. The latter do not respond to antibiotics and may perhaps be due to virus infections.

Paralysis of the 6th Cranial Nerve (Abducens)

With the exception of the 3rd (oculomotor), 9th (glossopharyngeal) and 10th (vagus) nerves, paralysis of every cranial nerve has been reported following spinal analgesia, but the abducens is affected in over 90 per cent of cases (Hayman and Wood, 1942). The incidence of 6th nerve palsy is probably more frequent than the reports indicate, and many a case of slight paresis is likely to have been overlooked when a patient complains of blurred vision which clears in a few days. Blatt (1929) reviewed 97 cases of cranial nerve palsy, 6 of which occurred after lumbar puncture alone. There were 6 cases in which the 3rd nerve and 4 cases in which the 4th nerve was involved, the remainder being of the 6th nerve. The highest incidence is 1 palsy in 100 spinals (Terrien, 1923). Fairclough (1945) reports 1 in 202 cases, and Maxson (1938) records 10 in a series of 2,500. It is interesting to note that Woltmann (1936) reported two cases following ether anaesthesia.

The recorded facts about 6th nerve palsy largely point towards a low C.S.F. pressure being the cause of the condition. In the majority of cases diplopia is preceded by severe headache and often dizziness and photophobia. The time of onset of the palsy varies from anything between 3 to 21 days (uncomplicated spinal headaches may be delayed for as long as 7–10 days)—a factor which would account for many missed cases, as a lot of patients would have been discharged from hospital by three weeks after the original lumbar puncture. Dripps and Vandam (1951) claim to have correlated the incidence of the condition with the size of lumbar puncture needle used. In a total series of 6,147 patients they used a 16-gauge spinal needle in 637, and found an incidence of headache of 22 per cent and diplopia in 5 patients. In the remaining patients a fine needle was used and no further cases of 6th nerve palsy occurred. Low pressure is assumed to result in descent of the medulla and pons and to cause stretching of the nerve —since it is anchored between its position in the cavernous sinus and origin from the pons—as it passes over the apex of the petrous temporal bone.

In the past alternative theories have been put forward. Fairclough (1945) suggested that the 6th nerve fails early in cerebral lesions, due to the instability of binocular vision—one of the latest acquisitions of primates. The introduction of a toxic drug into the C.N.S. may thus upset this recently acquired function. He points out that many patients suffer from latent ocular muscle imbalance—the commonest being lateral convergent squint—and this is compensated for by extra tonic nerve impulses being sent to the external rectus muscle to preserve parallelism of the eyes and to prevent diplopia. Only slight trauma would be required to block these extratonic impulses and convert a latent squint into a manifestly convergent one. This, however, could be accounted for by the low pressure theory rather than some vague toxic effect on the nerve. Toxic causes have been invoked as the principal cause, however, based on the known susceptibility of some nerves to particular toxins, e.g. the radial nerve to lead. If such a theory were correct, the condition might be expected to be bilateral, but this is rarely so. Moreover, since 6th nerve palsy follows lumbar puncture alone, toxic causes can be ruled out (Blatt, 1929; Dattner and Thomas, 1941). Harris (1951) has developed a theory to account for all nerve lesions after spinal analgesia, but reference to this will be made later (p. 1238).

The treatment of the lesion is to cover the affected eye to eliminate diplopia and prevent nausea. Spontaneous recovery can be expected in 50 per cent of cases in about a month, but muscle exercises and fusion training may help. Any surgical correction should be postponed for two years as spontaneous recovery has been known to be delayed for as long as this.

Permanent Neurological Sequels to Spinal Analgesia

That permanent neurological damage may occur as a direct consequence of spinal analgesia has been shown beyond doubt, but whether this is due, as is the opinion of neurologists such as Walshe and Critchley, to the analgesic agent or to some error in technique is still debated. Before passing to a more detailed discussion of this important subject the lesions themselves must be classified.

The cauda equina syndrome.—Transient lesions of the cauda equina characterised by retention of urine, incontinence of faeces, loss of sensation in the perineal region and loss of sexual function are not uncommon. Some cases do not recover and the residual lesions persist for years, often until the death of the patient from other causes. For this reason the precise pathology has not been described in a great many cases. Three fatal cases reported by Ferguson and Watkins (1938) showed at autopsy local congestion of the pia arachnoid of the lumbar and sacral cord and vacuolation of the nerve fibres of the cauda equina.

Courville (1955) describes a case operated on in error for spinal tumour, which ultimately came to autopsy, in which the arachnoid at operation was very congested and adherent to the roots of the cauda equina. At autopsy only a mild arachnoiditis was found, but the nerve roots showed advanced degenerative changes. Another case described by Courville was operated on 27 days after a spinal analgesia which had resulted in a cauda equina syndrome, and the arachnoid found to be thickened and congested and the nerve roots bound together with adhesions. At a subsequent operation in the upper dorsal region 4 years later a similar state of affairs was found. Courville concludes from a review of the literature and his own personal experience, that the cauda equina syndrome constitutes the most common permanent neurological sequel to spinal analgesia.

Chronic adhesive arachnoiditis.—The basic pathological lesion is a congestion and thickening of the arachnoid mater with adhesions to the pia and dura. Loculated cysts containing C.S.F. may form and secondarily compress the cord. Nerve roots and blood vessels are strangulated in the adhesive process and secondary ischaemic changes of the spinal cord follow. It seems as if the toxic effect is primarily on the meninges, while cord changes follow from pressure and ischaemia. Sir Victor Horsley in 1909 reported 21 cases diagnosed at laminectomy for supposed spinal cord tumour, but in patients who had not had spinal analgesia. There were dense adhesions obliterating the subarachnoid space and in many cases the cord was shrunken and compressed from cystic accumulations of C.S.F. Elkington (1936) reviewed 41 cases, and in 18 was unable to demonstrate any possible cause.

Spinal cord changes.—These are essentially secondary to the pathological changes in the meninges from chronic adhesive arachnoiditis. Cord changes vary from diffuse shrinkage of the cord with loss of distinction between grey and white matter proceeding in some cases to actual softening of the cord, to simple peripheral demyelination. On microscopy extensive replacement gliosis can be seen. Various names have been attached to these spinal cord changes, such as "transverse myelitis", "meningo-myelitis" and "ascending myelitis". Compression by thickened membranes, arachnoid cysts, and degenerative changes in the blood vessels of the cord all contribute to the spinal cord damage which varies in detail from case to case.

Courville (1955) describes two cases of *acute* spinal cord damage where death followed shortly after the spinal analgesia. In one case there was acute softening of the grey matter of the cord, and in another peripheral necrosis: presumably due to direct action of the spinal analgesic on the cord. These cases must, however, be rare: the great majority of spinal cord lesions are secondary to adhesive arachnoiditis.

Theories of causation.—There is now a large number of published cases where adhesive arachnoiditis following spinal analgesia has been verified at spinal exploration or autopsy (Hewer, 1933; Kennedy *et al.*, 1945; Thorsen, 1947*b*; Woods and Franklin, 1951) and Courville (1955), reviewing the subject, dogmatically states: "It seems quite obvious that the lesions in cases of post-spinal chronic adhesive arachnoiditis are to be considered as a result of the irritative effect of the anaesthetic. It is very likely that a number of the 'idiopathic' cases of chronic adhesive arachnoiditis are actually post-anaesthetic in aetiology."

There is evidence from animal experiments that spinal analgesic drugs can produce pathological changes in the meninges and spinal cord. Davis and his associates (1931) demonstrated inflammatory changes in the arachnoid of dogs following intrathecal cinchocaine and procaine. Lundy and his co-workers (1933) showed that increasing concentrations of procaine in the subarachnoid space produced irreversible damage to the spinal cord of dogs when the concentration reached 20 per cent. Macdonald and Watkins (1937) working with cats, confirmed Lundy's work and also showed that 10 per cent amylocaine ("Stovaine") could produce similar cord changes. Clinically, "light cinchocaine" has been incriminated as causing chronic adhesive arachnoiditis; Hewer reported a case in 1933 and Thorsen (1947*b*) reported 6 in 744 patients given this drug for spinal analgesia. Out of five cases reported by Terp (1950), four had been given a light cinchocaine spinal, while Payne and Bergentz (1956) reported a case of chronic adhesive arachnoiditis following the same drug and confirmed at laminectomy.

Continuous spinal analgesia has been associated with a high incidence of neurological sequelae. Willauer *et al.* (1950) reported two cases in a series of 574 continuous spinal analgesias, and Kennedy and his colleagues (1950) have reviewed the history of five cases.

Harris (1951) has produced an ingenious theory to account for the haphazard incidence of nerve root and cauda equina lesions. It is known that when spinal analgesic solutions come into contact with the C.S.F., analgesic base is liberated in the same way as when local analgesics are injected into other body tissues. *In vitro* experiments with C.S.F. and spinal analgesic solutions show that cloudiness occurs on mixing and thin crystals of free analgesic base settle out of the solution. The size of the crystals varies with the concentration of the local analgesic solution. Crystals liberated from a 1 in 200 solution of cinchocaine are four times as large as those from a 1 in 1,500 solution. These crystals are insoluble in water and very soluble in lipoid. Harris likens the introduction of a spinal analgesic drug into the subarachnoid space to a shower of crystals of analgesic base precipitated out of solution and impinging in a haphazard way on individual nerve roots. He uses this theory to explain 6th nerve palsy, since, apart from the 4th, this nerve has the longest intracranial course and is therefore more likely to be affected by any crystals which might be swept into the cerebral subarachnoid space by currents of C.S.F. The delay in onset of the palsy (3–21 days) could be explained by the time taken for such crystals to reach the cerebral subarachnoid space. Attractive though this theory is, if it were true one would expect fewer neurological sequelae from dilute solutions of spinal analgesic drugs such as 1 in 1,500 cinchocaine, than from heavy solutions, but this is not the case.

The possibility exists that some cases of chronic adhesive arachnoiditis may be due to some unidentified virus infection; indeed Horsley described a case of paraplegia following an attack of herpes. This fact and the fact that adhesive arachnoiditis can occur in the absence of a drug introduced into the subarachnoid space, has given anaesthetists a convenient and attractive theory to account for paraplegia following spinal analgesia. Brock and his associates (1936) described 3 cases of paraplegia and attributed them to the effects of a virus infection plus spinal analgesia. Terp (1950), in spite of using the same technique for years, had 5 cases within a period of 6 months which he explained on the basis of a virus infection.

Another theory suggests that contaminants may be introduced into the subarachnoid space at the time of the lumbar injection. In the now famous Roe and Woolley case (*Times*, 1953), the court accepted the view that paraplegia resulted from phenol that had reached the local analgesic solution through minute cracks in the ampoules during their sterilisation by immersion in a solution of this disinfectant.

Other workers have attempted to explain post-spinal analgesic paralysis on the basis that the injection has exacerbated a pre-existing neurological disease. Lundy and his colleagues (1933) wrote: "Judging from our experiments, it seems probable that when paralysis follows the use of an ordinary dose of spinal anaesthetic agent, the spinal cord was previously diseased". It must be noted, however, that he found cord damage after administering 20 per cent procaine, a concentration unlikely to be used in clinical practice. But clinical cases of this nature do undoubtedly occur, and Dripps and Vandam (1951) report a case in which lumbar puncture and removal of C.S.F. caused vascular engorgement and oedema of a pre-existing spinal cord tumour with resulting paralysis. The tumour was removed subsequently with significant recovery. Such cases must be very rare and could not possibly explain all the cases of paralysis that have occurred.

To summarise, therefore, the theories of the causation of permanent paralysis following spinal analgesia can be divided into four main groups.

1. The effect of the local analgesic agent on the meninges and spinal cord.

Eminent neurologists, such as Walshe and Critchley, strongly support this view, and Walshe has summed up the position by saying that the only common factor to permanent neurological damage is the introduction of a spinal analgesic drug into the subarachnoid space.

The review by Courville (1955) of the pathological changes in the meninges and spinal cord after spinal analgesia lends strong support to this opinion.

2. A sub-clinical virus infection. In the absence of an identified virus this view cannot be taken too seriously.
3. Introduction of contaminants at the time of spinal analgesia. The role of such causes is well brought out by the Roe and Woolley case (*Times*, 1953), the details of which the reader is advised to read carefully, and then to form his own opinion.
4. Exacerbation of pre-existing neurological disease. This could account for a few cases, but as a significant factor in most cases is of doubtful value.

Comment.—The neurological sequelae of spinal analgesia are still a controversial subject. Large series of spinals without major complications are often quoted in an attempt to prove that the technique is free from such dangers—one such series of 10,000 cases has been analysed by Dripps and Vandam (1954). These figures, while impressive, and indicative of what can be achieved, must not distract anaesthetists from the essential fact that major neurological sequelae do in fact occur after spinal analgesia.

Incidence of Complications of Epidural Analgesia

Dawkins (1969), in a survey of the world literature, has summarised the complications and their incidence that may follow epidural analgesia as follows:

Lumbar and thoracic epidural analgesia

	Number of recorded analgesias	*Number of times complication occurred*
Dural puncture	43,152	1,090 (2·5 per cent)
Accidental spinal	48,287	102 (0·2 per cent)
Blood vessel puncture	6,578	189 (2·8 per cent)
Toxic reaction	66,366	144 (0·2 per cent)
Massive epidural	16,644	28 (0·1 per cent)
Severe hypotension	42,900	797 (1·8 per cent)
Backache	9,107	185 (2·0 per cent)
Transient paralysis	32,718	48 (0·1 per cent)
Permanent paralysis	32,718	7 (0·02 per cent)

Sacral epidural analgesia

	Number of recorded analgesias	*Number of times complication occurred*
Dural puncture	13,639	171 (1·2 per cent)
Accidental spinal	6,334	9 (0·1 per cent)
Blood vessel puncture	639	4 (0·6 per cent)
Failure to find sacral hiatus	2,803	87 (3·1 per cent)
Toxic reaction	3,332	6 (0·2 per cent)
Sepsis	3,767	8 (0·2 per cent)
Breakage of needle	850	12 (1·4 per cent)
Breakage of catheter	5,379	6 (0·1 per cent)
Severe hypotension	3,189	201 (6·3 per cent)
Transient paralysis	22,968	5 (0·02 per cent)
Permanent paralysis	22,968	1 (0·005 per cent)

Permanent Neurological Sequels to Epidural Analgesia

Such complications following epidural analgesia are certainly rare; indeed until recently it was thought that they did not occur. As with subarachnoid analgesia, large series of cases have been published without serious neurological sequels. Cyriax (1961), who has used epidural injections for the past 23 years in over 20,000 cases, states he has had no permanent complications. In two patients an aseptic meningitis was produced but both recovered within a week and the complications were attributed to contamination of the syringes used for injection by acriflavine that had found its way into the steriliser (see p. 1209). Paraplegia has, however, been recorded following an epidural (Davies *et al.*, 1958), the signs being those normally associated with thrombosis or spasm of the anterior spinal artery and often referred to as the anterior spinal artery syndrome. This may be caused by the hypotension that follows any degree of epidural analgesia. Other factors that could account for neurological sequels following epidural analgesia are inadvertent puncture of the dura and subsequent subarachnoid injection of some of the local analgesic solution, diffusion of local analgesic solution through the dura and even into the central nervous system itself, pressure on the spinal cord by a large haematoma in the epidural space and spasm of the anterior spinal artery from the effects of adrenaline, when this vasoconstrictor is added to the local analgesic solution.

Spinal and Epidural Analgesia against General Anaesthesia

The conflicting views on the subject of permanent paralysis have been presented and in the last analysis only the individual anaesthetist with the anaesthetic problem before him can decide whether he will use a spinal or not. If he adopts the view of neurologists such as Kennedy, Critchley and Walshe, then only very rarely will he give a spinal. If he takes the view of Macintosh that a patient has no more tendency to develop paralysis after spinal analgesia than he has to die after thiopentone, then he may use a spinal frequently. The notoriety given to these complications is undoubtedly one of the principal reasons for the decline in popularity of spinal analgesia in Great Britain. But equally important are the muscle relaxants, hypotensive and newer anaesthetic agents, and the general availability of trained anaesthetists who are able to satisfy the needs of most patients and surgeons by general methods and with few troubles. The swing away from spinal analgesia has, however, produced a situation in which anaesthetists undergoing their training are unable to learn the basic technique—yet there are undoubtedly individual patients who are better anaesthetised by spinal (or epidural) analgesia than by general methods. Here it must be emphasised that the only advantage of spinal over epidural analgesia is the greater ease with which it can be accomplished. Thus, provided trained personnel are available, no absolute indications for spinal analgesia remain.

Three cases are quoted to illustrate the types of strong indication that at times occur for epidural analgesia.

Case I.—Male aged 60 with extensive bronchiectasis—2 cupfuls of sputum per day. Admitted as an emergency with bleeding papilloma of bladder which required blood transfusion. The papilloma had been diathermied on a previous occasion under spinal analgesia, but the patient had developed a severe headache post-operatively because of the coughing associated with the bronchiectasis. Papilloma diathermied under epidural analgesia—no post-analgesia complications.

Case II.—Male geriatric patient aged 80 with large fungating carcinoma of tongue. Fell out of bed and fractured femur. General anaesthesia out of the question because of the carcinoma of tongue. Femur plated under epidural block.

Case III.—Male aged 60 at limit of respiratory reserve from chronic bronchitis and emphysema with heart failure. A bleeding rectal polyp was preventing compensatory polycythaemia. Polyp removed under epidural analgesia with patient semi-sitting up.

Comparison of Spinal and Epidural Analgesia

Technique

There is no doubt that spinal analgesia is technically far easier to produce than epidural analgesia. Indeed the difficulties of identifying the epidural space have limited many anaesthetists in their desire to produce this form of analgesia. The technique is, however, far more easily learnt than most anaesthetists suspect, and those who have the interest and patience to do so can render considerable service to their patients.

Onset of Action

In general, local analgesic drugs exert their effect more quickly when used in the subarachnoid space than in the epidural space—and this is an advantage for long operating lists since it minimises delay between cases. The newer local analgesic drugs—lignocaine and 2-chloroprocaine—in some measure overcome this difficulty. With lignocaine, only 10 minutes is required for the development of a satisfactory epidural block.

Extent of Spinal and Epidural Blocks

With an epidural injection the ultimate height of the block is not as predictable as with most spinal analgesic techniques, and the full extent of the block may not develop for as long as 30 minutes. Factors governing this have already been discussed (see p. 1197).

Analgesic Complications

Complications of injection.—Accidental intravascular injections and systemic reactions from absorption are more likely with epidural than spinal analgesia, and massive subarachnoid injection can occur with epidural injections. With normal doses of local analgesic, systemic toxic reactions are almost unknown following subarachnoid injections.

Blood pressure.—There is little or no difference in the fall of blood pressure for comparable heights of block with spinal and epidural analgesia.

Post-analgesic complications.—The greatest advantage of an epidural over a spinal block is the virtual elimination of post-analgesic complications. Post-spinal headaches, the bugbear of spinals, are eliminated though there is probably a greater incidence of backache after epidural injections. Although it is stated to be less frequent after epidural blocks, the relative incidence of post-operative urinary retention with the two techniques is difficult to determine, since this complication is never very common with either.

The question of permanent neurological sequelae must await the publication of the results of further large series of epidural blocks. Epidural analgesia has not yet enjoyed the wide popularity of spinal analgesia, and it will therefore take some time to obtain information that can be truly compared with that for spinal analgesia. Certainly, however, this technique should eliminate infective meningitis.

REFERENCES

AHEARN, R. E. (1948). Management of severe post-lumbar puncture headache. *N. Y. St. J. Med.*, **48,** 1495.

BLATT, N. (1929). Neuropathie und neuropathische Konstitution als prädisponierende Faktoren für Augenmuskellähmungen nach Lumbaranästhesie. *Wien. med. Wschr.*, **79,** 1391.

BONICA, J. J., BACKUP, P. H., ANDERSON, C. E., HADFIELD, D., CREPPS, W. F., and MONK, B. F. (1957). Peridural block: analysis of 3,637 cases and a review. *Anesthesiology*, **18,** 723.

BONNIOT, A. (1934). Note sur la pression épidurale négative. *Bull. Soc. nat. Chir.*, **60,** 124.

BRIDENBAUGH, L. D., MOORE, D. C., BAGDI, P., and BRIDENBAUGH, P. O. (1968). The position of plastic tubing in continuous-block techniques. An X-ray study of 552 patients. *Anesthesiology*, **29,** 1047.

BROCK, S., BELL, A., and DAVIDSON, C. (1936). Nervous complications following spinal anesthesia; clinical study of seven cases, with tissue study in one instance. *J. Amer. med. Ass.*, **106,** 441.

BROMAGE, P. R. (1954). *Spinal Epidural Analgesia.* Edinburgh: E. & S. Livingstone.

BROMAGE, P. R. (1962). Spread of analgesic solutions in the epidural space and their site of action: a statistical study. *Brit. J. Anaesth.*, **34,** 161.

BROMAGE P. R. (1967). Extradural analgesia for pain relief. *Brit. J. Anaesth.* **39,** 721.

BROMAGE, P. R., BURFOOT, M. F., CROWELL, D. E., and PETTIGREW, R. T. (1964). Quality of epidural blockade. I. Influence of physical factors. *Brit. J. Anaesth.*, **36,** 342.

BROOKS, W. (1957). An epidural indicator. *Anaesthesia*, **12,** 227.

BRUNNER, C., and ILKÉ, A. (1949). Beitragzen peridural anästhesia. *Schweiz. med. Wschr.*, **79,** 799.

BRYCE-SMITH, R. (1950). Pressure in the extra-dural space. *Anaesthesia*, **5,** 213.

BRYCE-SMITH, R., and WILLIAMS, E. O. (1955). The treatment of eclampsia (imminent or actual) by continuous conduction analgesia. *Lancet*, **1,** 1241.

BURN, J. M. B. (1963). A method of continuous epidural analgesia. *Anaesthesia*, **18,** 78.

CATHELIN, F. (1901). Une nouvelle voie d'injection rachidienne. Méthode des injections épidurales par le procédé du canal sacré. Applications à l'homme. *C.R. Soc. Biol.* (*Paris*), **53,** 452.

COLE, P. V. (1964). Continuous epidural lignocaine—a safe method. *Anaesthesia*, **19,** 562.

COOMES, E. N. (1961). A comparison between epidural anaesthesia and bed rest in sciatica. *Brit. med. J.*, **1,** 20.

COURVILLE, C. B. (1955). Untoward effects of spinal anesthesia on the spinal cord and its investments. *Curr. Res. Anesth.*, **34,** 313.

CURBELLO, M. M. (1949). Continuous peridural segmental anesthesia by means of a urethral catheter. *Curr. Res. Anesth.*, **28,** 12.

CYRIAX, J. H. (1957). *Textbook of Orthopaedic Medicine*, 3rd edit. London: Cassell & Co.

CYRIAX, J. H. (1961). Lumbar disc lesions. *Acta orthop. belg.*, **27,** 442.

DATTNER, B., and THOMAS, E. W. (1941). Bilateral abducens palsy following lumbar puncture. *N.Y. St. J. Med.*, **41,** 1660.

DAVIDSON, I. M. (1947). *Pseudomonas pyocyanae* meningitis following spinal analgesia. *Lancet*, **2,** 653.

DAVIES, A., SOLOMON, B., and LEVENE, A. (1958). Paraplegia following epidural anaesthesia. *Brit. med. J.*, **2,** 654.

DAVIS, L., HAVEN, H., GIVENS, J. H., and EMMETT, J. (1931). Effects of spinal anesthetics on spinal cord and its membranes; experimental study. *J. Amer. med. Ass.*, **97,** 1781.

DAWKINS, C. J. M. (1954). The present position of spinal and extradural analgesia. *Proc. roy. Soc. Med.*, **47,** 311.

DAWKINS, C. J. M. (1956*a*). Extradural analgesia in obstetrics and gynaecology. *Postgrad. med. J.*, **32,** 544.

DAWKINS, C. J. M. (1956*b*). Relief of post-operative pain by continuous epidural drip. *Proc. 4th Congr. Scand. Soc. Anaesthetists, Helsinki*, p. 77.

DAWKINS, C. J. M. (1957). Location of epidural space. *Anaesthesia*, **12**, 225.

DAWKINS, C. J. M. (1963). The identification of the epidural space. A critical analysis of the various methods employed. *Anaesthesia*, **18**, 66.

DAWKINS, C. J. M. (1969). An analysis of the complications of extradural and caudal block. *Anaesthesia*, **24**, 554.

DE SARAM, M. (1956). Accidental total spinal analgesia. A report of 3 cases. *Anaesthesia*, **11**, 77.

DEUTSCH, E. V. (1952). The treatment of postspinal headache with intravenous ethanol: a preliminary report. *Anesthesiology*, **13**, 496.

DICKSON, W. E. C. (1944). The cerebro-spinal fluid in meningitis. *Postgrad. med. J.*, **20**, 69.

DOGLIOTTI, A. M. (1931). Eine neue Methode der regionares Anästhesia: "Die peridurale segmentäre Anästhesia". *Zbl. Chir.*, **58**, 3141.

DOGLIOTTI, A. M. (1932). Un nuovo metodo di anestesia tronculare: la rachianestesia peridurale segmentaria. *Arch. ital. Chir.*, **38**, 797.

DOGLIOTTI, A. M. (1933). A new method of block anesthesia; segmental peridural spinal anesthesia. *Amer. J. Surg.*, **20**, 107.

DOGLIOTTI, A. M., and CIOCATTO, E. (1953). Our method of selective antalgic block for the therapy of intractable pains. (Presented at the Annual Meeting of the Amer. Soc. of Anesthesiologists in Seattle, Washington. Oct. 7th, 1953.)

DRIPPS, R. D., and VANDAM, L. D. (1951). Hazards of lumbar puncture. *J. Amer. med. Ass.*, **147**, 1118.

DRIPPS, R. D., and VANDAM, L. D. (1954). Long-term follow-up of patients who received 10,098 spinal anesthetics; failure to discover major neurological sequelae. *J. Amer. med. Ass.*, **156**, 1486.

EATON, L. M. (1939). Observations on negative pressure in the epidural space. *Proc. Mayo Clin.*, **14**, 566.

ELKINGTON, J. ST. C. (1936). Meningitis serosa circumscripta spinalis (spinal arachnoiditis). *Brain*, **59**, 181.

ERDEMIS, H. A., SOPER, L. E., and SWEET, R. B. (1965). Studies of factors affecting peridural anesthesia. *Curr. Res. Anesth.*, **44**, 400.

EVANS, F. T., Ed. (1954). *Modern Practice in Anaesthesia*, 2nd edit. London: Butterworth & Co.

EVANS, W. (1936). Intrasacral epidural injection in the treatment of sciatica. *Lancet*, **2**, 1225.

EVERETT, A. D. (1941). Lumbar puncture injuries. *Proc. roy. Soc. Med.*, **35**, 208.

FAIRCLOUGH, W. A. (1945). Sixth-nerve paralysis after spinal analgesia. *Brit. med. J.*, **2**, 801.

FERGUSON, F. R., and WATKINS, K. H. (1938). Paralysis of the bladder and associated neurological sequelae of spinal anaesthesia (cauda equina syndrome). *Brit. J. Surg.*, **25**, 735.

FOLDES, F. F., COLAVINCENZO, J. W., and BIRCH, J. H. (1956). Epidural Anesthesia: a reappraisal. *Curr. Res. Anesth.*, **35**, 33 and 89.

FRANKSSON, C., and GORDH, T. (1946). Headache after spinal anesthesia and a technique for lessening its frequency. *Acta chir. scand.*, **94**, 443.

GALLEY, A. H. (1949). Continuous caudal analgesia in obstetrics. *Anaesthesia*, **4**, 154.

GALLEY, A. H. (1952). Caudal analgesia—clinical applications in vasospastic diseases of the legs and in diabetic neuropathy. *Proc. roy. Soc. Med.*, **45**, 34.

GLESNE, O. G. (1950). Lumbar puncture headaches. *Anesthesiology*, **11**, 702.

GORDH, T. (1949). Xylocain—a new local analgesic. *Anaesthesia*, **4**, 4.

GORDON JONES, R. G. (1953). A complication of epidural technique. *Anaesthesia*, **8,** 242.

GREEN, R., and DAWKINS, M. (1966). Postoperative analgesia. The use of continuous drip epidural block. *Anaesthesia*, **21,** 372.

GREENE, N. M. (1958). *Physiology of Spinal Anesthesia.* Baltimore: Williams and Wilkins Co.

GUTIERREZ, A. (1933). Valor de la aspiracion liquida in el espacio peridural en la anestesia peridural. *Rev. Cir.* (*B. Aires*), **12,** 225.

GUTIERREZ, A. (1939). *Anestesia Extradural.* Buenos Aires.

HARALDSON, S. (1951). Headache after spinal anesthesia: experiments with a new spinal needle. *Anesthesiology*, **12,** 321.

HARGER, J. R., CHRISTOFFERSON, E. A., and STOKES, A. J. (1941). Peridural anesthesia: a consideration of 1,000 cases. *Amer. J. Surg.*, **42,** 25.

HARMEL, M. H., HAFKENSCHIEL, J. H., AUSTIN, G. M., CRUMPTON, C. W., and KETY, S. S. (1949). The effect of bilateral stellate ganglion block on the cerebral circulation in normotensive and hypertensive patients. *J. clin. Invest.*, **28,** 415.

HARRIS, T. A. B. (1951). *The Mode of Action of Anaesthetics.* Edinburgh: E. & S. Livingstone.

HAYMAN, I. R., and WOOD, P. M. (1942). Abducens nerve (VI) paralysis following spinal anesthesia. *Ann. Surg.*, **115,** 864.

HELDT, T. J., and MOLONEY, J. C. (1928). Negative pressure in the epidural space: preliminary studies. *Amer. J. med. Sci.*, **175,** 371.

HESS, E. (1934). Epidural anesthesia in urology. *J. Urol.* (*Baltimore*), **31,** 621.

HEWER, C. L. (1933). Discussion of nervous sequelae of spinal anaesthetics. *Proc. roy. Soc. Med.*, **26,** 507.

HORSLEY, V. (1909). Chronic spinal meningitis: its differential diagnosis and surgical treatment. *Brit. med. J.*, **1,** 513.

HOWE, Y. L., and CHEN, C. E. (1951). Headache following spinal anesthesia. *Chin. med. J.*, **69,** 251.

JANZEN, E. (1926). Der negative Vorschlog bei lumbal Punktion. *Dtsch. Z. Nervenheilk.*, **94,** 280.

JARMAN, R. (1937). Combination of intravenous with spinal anaesthesia, using pentothal and percaine. *Brit. J. Anaesth.*, **15,** 20.

KELMAN, H. (1944). Epidural injection therapy for sciatic pain. *Amer. J. Surg.*, **64,** 183.

KENNEDY, F., SOMBERG, H. M., and GOLDBERG, B. M. (1945). Arachnoiditis and paralysis following spinal anesthesia. *J. Amer. med. Ass.*, **129,** 664.

KREUGER, J. E. (1953). Etiology and treatment of postspinal headaches. *Curr. Res. Anesth.*, **32,** 190.

KUNKLE, E. C., RAY, B. S., and WOLFF, H. G. (1943). Experimental studies on headache. Analysis of the headache associated with changes in intracranial pressure. *Arch. Neurol. Psychiat.* (*Chicago*), **49,** 323.

LEE, J. A. (1962). A new catheter for continuous extradural analgesia. *Anaesthesia*, **18,** 66.

LLOYD, J. W., CRAMPTON SMITH, A., and O'CONNOR, B. T. (1965). Classification of chest injuries as an aid to treatment. *Brit. med. J.*, **1,** 1518.

LUNDY, J. S., ESSEX, H. E., and KERNOHAN, J. W. (1933). Experiments with anesthetics. Lesions produced in the spinal cord of dogs by dose of procaine sufficient to cause permanent and fatal paralysis. *J. Amer. med. Ass.*, **101,** 1546.

MCCORD, J. M., EPPERSON, J. W., and JACOBY, J. J. (1951). Headache following spinal anesthesia in obstetrics. *Curr. Res. Anesth.*, **30,** 354.

MACDONALD, A. D., and WATKINS, K. H. (1937). Experimental investigation into the cause of paralysis following spinal anaesthesia. *Brit. J. Surg.*, **25,** 879.

MACINTOSH, R. R. (1950). Extradural space indicator. *Anaesthesia*, **5,** 98.

MACINTOSH, R. R. (1953). Extradural space indicator. *Brit. med. J.*, **1,** 398.

MACINTOSH, R. R. (1957). *Lumbar Puncture and Spinal Analgesia*, 2nd edit. Edinburgh: E. & S. Livingstone.

MACINTOSH, R. R., and MUSHIN, W. W. (1947). Observations on the epidural space. *Anaesthesia*, **2,** 100.

MARSHALL, J. (1950). Lumbar puncture headache. *J. Neurol., Neurosurg., Psychiat.*, **13,** 71.

MAXSON, L. H. (1938). *Spinal Anesthesia.* Philadelphia: J. B. Lippincott Co.

MELZACK, R., and WALL, P. D. (1965). Pain mechanisms: a new theory. *Science*, **150,** 971.

MORRIS, D. D. B., and CANDY, J. (1957). Anaesthesia for prostatectomy. *Brit. J. Anaesth.*, **29,** 376.

MORRIS, G. C., Jr., MOYER, J. H., SNYDER, H. B., and HOYNES, B. W., Jr. (1953). Vascular dynamics in controlled hypotension: study of cerebral and renal hemodynamics and blood volume changes. *Ann. Surg.*, **138,** 706.

MUSHIN, W. W. (1943). Gravity control in spinal anaesthesia. *Postgrad. med. J.*, **19,** 175.

NASH, T. G., and OPENSHAW, D. J. (1968). Unusual complication of epidural anaesthesia (C.). *Brit. med. J.*, **2,** 700.

ODOM, C. B. (1936). Epidural anesthesia. *Amer. J. Surg.*, **34,** 547.

PAYNE, J. B., and BERGENTZ, S. E. (1956). Paraplegia following spinal anaesthesia. *Lancet*, **1,** 666.

PICKERING, G. W. (1948). Lumbar puncture headache. *Brain*, **71,** 274.

POGES, F. (1921). Anaesthesia metamerica. *Rev. Sanid. milit. argent.*, **11,** 351.

REDLICH, F. C., MOORE, B. D., and KIMBELL, I., Jr. (1946). Lumbar puncture reactions; relative importance of physiological and psychological factors. *Psychosom. Med.*, **8,** 386.

RICE, G. G., and DOBBS, C. H. (1950). The use of peridural and subarachnoid injections of saline solutions in the treatment of severe post-spinal headache. *Anesthesiology*, **11,** 17.

SCHEINBERG, P. (1950). Cerebral blood flow in vascular disease of brain, with observations on effects of stellate ganglion block. *Amer. J. Med.*, **8,** 139.

SHANBROM, E., and LEVY, L. (1957). The role of systemic blood pressure in cerebral circulation in carotid and basilar artery thromboses: clinical observations and therapeutic implications of vasopressor agents. *Amer. J. Med.*, **23,** 197.

SICORD, A. (1901). Les injections médicamenteuses extradural par voie sacrococcygienne. *C.R. Soc. Biol. (Paris)*, **53,** 396.

SIMPSON, B. R., PARKHOUSE, J., MARSHALL, R., and LAMBRECHTS, W. (1961). Extradural analgesia and the prevention of postoperative respiratory complications. *Brit. J. Anaesth.*, **33,** 628.

STRINGER, R. M. (1954). Epidural anesthesia with xylocaine. *Curr. Res. Anesth.*, **33,** 195.

TERP, A. (1950). Paraplegia following lumbar anesthesia; chronic hypertrophic arachnoiditis; 5 cases. *Nord. Med.*, **43,** 1026.

TERRIEN, F. (1923). Les accidents oculaires tardifs de la rachi-anesthesia. *Bull. méd. (Paris)*, **37,** 147.

THORSEN, G. (1947*a*). Neurological complications after spinal anaesthesia and results from 2,493 follow-up cases. *Acta chir. scand.*, **95.** Supp. *121*, 1.

THORSEN, G. (1947*b*). Injuries due to the anaesthetic agent, through an effect on the nervous substance. Injuries via an assumed perineal effect of the anaesthetic agent. *Acta chir. scand.*, **95**, Supp. *121*, 146.

TIMES (1953). Law Report. November 13th.

TUOHY, E. B. (1945). Continuous spinal anesthesia: a new method utilising a urethral catheter. *Surg. Clin. N. Amer.*, **25**, 834.

WEINTRAUB, F., ANTINE, W., and RAPHAEL, A. J. (1947). Postpartum headache after low spinal anesthesia in vaginal delivery and its treatment. *Amer. J. Obstet. Gynec.*, **54**, 682.

WIBERG, G. (1949). Back pain in relation to the nerve supply of the intervertebral disc. *Acta orthop. scand.*, **19**, 211.

WILSON, W. E. (1934). Intrathecal nerve root block; some contributions and new technique. *Brit. J. Anaesth.*, **11**, 43.

WOLFF, H. G. (1948). *Headache and Other Head Pain.* New York: Oxford Univ. Press.

WOLTMANN, H. W. (1936). Postoperative neurologic complications. *Wis. med. J.*, **35**, 427.

WOODS, W. W., and FRANKLIN, R. G. (1951). Progressive adhesive arachnoiditis following spinal anesthesia. *Calif. Med.*, **75**, 196.

WYKE, B. D. (1960). *Principles of General Neurophysiology, relating to Anaesthesia and Surgery*, pp. 98–9. London: Butterworth & Co.

ZELENKA, L. (1956). A new indicator for spinal epidural analgesia. *Anesthesiology*, **17**, 210.

ZWEIFEL, E. (1920). Die Todesfälle bei Sakrolanästhesie. *Zbl. Gynäk.*, **44**, 140.

Chapter 44

LOCAL ANALGESIC TECHNIQUES

by

D. D. B. Morris

This chapter is not meant to be comprehensive. The object has been to present some of the ways in which local analgesia can be usefully and simply produced. Local analgesia is not commonly practised in the United Kingdom but there are occasions, typically for unprepared out-patients and certain very poor risk patients, when it may be preferable to general anaesthesia. It is also useful for diagnostic and therapeutic reasons.

Spinal and epidural analgesia are described in Chapters 42 and 43. Some local analgesic techniques not described here are discussed in other parts of the book.

Stellate Ganglion Block

The cervical sympathetic normally consists of three ganglia, called the superior, middle, and inferior, according to their position in the neck, which are connected and through which the sympathetic supply to the upper limb, the neck, and the head is transmitted. A branch also runs to the cardiac plexus of nerves. The superior cervical ganglion is formed by the fusion of four sympathetic ganglia corresponding to the first four cervical nerves. The middle cervical ganglion represents ganglia of the fifth and sixth cervical nerves and the inferior cervical ganglion the seventh and eighth. The inferior cervical ganglion is frequently joined with that from the first thoracic nerve and is then known as the stellate ganglion. Sometimes the second thoracic ganglion is also included and occasionally either the fifth or sixth cervical ganglion, or both, are also incorporated, in which case the middle cervical ganglion is correspondingly smaller or absent.

The stellate ganglion is situated on the anterior surface of the neck of the first rib behind the origin of the vertebral artery just superior to the dome of the pleura.

Technique

The anterior approach to the ganglion is satisfactory in practice. The patient lies supine with the head fully extended at the atlanto-occipital joint. The two important landmarks for palpation are the carotid artery and the trachea. A needle is inserted just above the sterno-clavicular joint in the median plane of the neck and passed between the trachea and the carotid artery—which should be rolled laterally during the procedure—down to the lateral aspect of the body of the seventh vertebra (Pitkin, 1953). If the needle is now withdrawn slightly, its point will lie in the tissue plane anterior to the fascia which covers the prevertebral muscle and in which the sympathetic fibres run (Macintosh and Ostlere, 1955). After aspiration, 10 ml. of 1 per cent lignocaine should be injected.

The signs of a successful block have been recapitulated by Macintosh and Mushin (1954). They are enophthalmos, ptosis, myosis (the original triad of Horner's syndrome), unilateral blockage of the nose due to congestion of the nasal mucosa, flushing of the skin, and absence of sweating, all of which occur on the side of the block.

Indications

Stellate ganglion block may be of diagnostic and prognostic value in the treatment of Raynaud's disease of the upper limb. It is also useful in assessing a phantom limb, and as an emergency measure in the treatment of accidental intra-arterial injection of thiopentone. It is worth a trial in the treatment of severe angina at rest, and if successful may be repeated with a neurolytic agent such as phenol. Successful block does not produce dilatation of cerebral vessels, and its value for patients with cerebral thrombosis or embolism has not been proven.

Brachial Plexus Block

The brachial plexus arises from cervical roots 5, 6, 7 and 8 and the greater part of thoracic 1. It may also receive some supply from cervical 4. Brachial plexus block is useful for fractures, dislocations, and skin and muscle injuries of the forearm and hand, and—provided it is complete—will suffice for the reduction of a dislocated shoulder. It also provides analgesia of the skin over the outer side of the upper arm, but not of the superior part of the inner side which is supplied by thoracic 2. Should analgesia of the latter be required, the block must be combined with an intradermal and subcutaneous infiltration of local analgesic solution in the form of a ring around the top of the upper arm.

Supraclavicular Technique

The simplest technique for injection of the plexus is to approach it by the supraclavicular route as described by Macintosh and Mushin (1954). Lignocaine 1 per cent should be used and adrenaline may be added (on the basis of 0·5 ml. of adrenaline 1:1,000 to each 100 ml. of local analgesic solution) if analgesia lasting more than 45 to 60 minutes is required. The patient lies in the dorsal position with a pillow under his shoulders and his head turned away from the side to be injected. The affected arm must be by his side and the shoulder lowered so that the subclavian artery can be easily palpated above the clavicle. A skin weal is raised about a third of an inch above the midpoint of the clavicle just lateral to the area where the subclavian artery can be felt, and avoiding the external jugular vein. A 5 cm. (2 inch) 22-gauge needle is then introduced through the skin weal in a backward, inward and downward direction toward the upper surface of the first rib over which the plexus runs (Fig. 1). While inserting the needle with one hand, it is helpful to push the subclavian artery medially with the first two fingers of the other, thus avoiding the risk of arterial puncture. Paraesthesia in the hand or forearm will most likely be felt by the patient as the point of the needle enters the plexus; at this stage 30 ml. of local

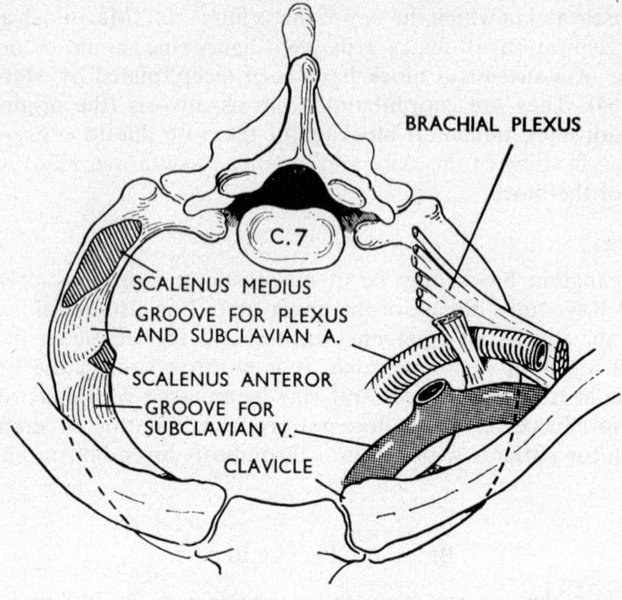

44/FIG. 1.—The first rib.

analgesic should be injected. If no paraesthesia is elicited, then the point of the needle must be advanced until it touches the upper surface of the first rib and local analgesic solution injected as it is withdrawn towards the skin. Repeated injections made in this manner, and with the needle point gradually moved along the upper surface of the first rib towards the subclavian artery, will block the plexus.

Puncture of the subclavian artery is not harmful provided local analgesic solution is not injected, but pressure should be temporarily applied to the vessel after removal of the needle to prevent the formation of a haematoma. The pleural cavity may also be entered if the direction of insertion of the needle is wrong.

Ball (1962) has recently described a modified supraclavicular approach to minimise the risk of accidental puncture of the pleura. In this technique the needle is inserted and advanced *vertically downwards* and *inwards*. This is a two-dimensional approach compared with the three-dimensional backward, inward and downward one previously described. Should the rib be missed the needle's position is anterior to the rib and outside the thoracic cage. If contact with the rib is not achieved at the first placing of the needle, it is withdrawn and re-introduced slightly more posteriorly but still vertically downwards.

Axillary Technique

The axillary approach to the brachial plexus is rapidly gaining in popularity. Using it, the success rate is equal to that by the supraclavicular route, and the complications of pneumothorax and phrenic paralysis are completely avoided. It is therefore particularly valuable when a bilateral block of the plexus is needed. It does not, however, produce analgesia of the shoulder. If this is required, the supraclavicular route must be used.

The arm is abducted at a right angle from the body and the axillary artery palpated. The highest part in the axilla at which pulsation can be felt is the site for injection of local analgesic solution through a short, fine needle of 24 S.W. gauge. Such a needle lessens the risk of damage to the division of the plexus in the axillary sheath, and makes a haematoma unlikely should the axillary artery or vein be accidentally punctured. A finger is placed over the axillary artery, and after raising a skin weal the needle is advanced to one side of the artery until a definite and sudden "give" is experienced as the needle passes through the fascial wall of the axillary sheath. After aspiration, 15–20 ml. of 1 per cent lignocaine are injected. The needle is then withdrawn as far as the subcutaneous tissues and then reinserted on the other side of the axillary artery where a further 15–20 ml. of 1 per cent lignocaine are injected. The axillary sheath is effectively filled by 40 ml. of solution and failure or partial block can follow the use of too small a volume of solution.

Intravenous Regional Analgesia

Holmes (1963) has described a useful method of producing analgesia of either an arm or leg by a modification of Bier's (1908) original intravenous analgesia technique.

Technique

A Gordh needle is placed in a suitable vein toward the extremity of the limb. The limb is then elevated and an Esmarch bandage applied from the fingers or toes inwards to reach a sphygmomanometer cuff on the upper arm or leg. This is now blown up to a level above the patient's systolic blood pressure, the Esmarch bandage is removed, and a solution of 0·5 per cent lignocaine is injected intravenously through the Gordh needle. About 40 ml. of solution are required for an adult arm and up to 100 ml. for an adult leg. The onset of analgesia is rapid and accompanied by paraesthesia and a feeling of warmth in the limb. Muscular paralysis occurs. The technique can usually be carried out successfully without an Esmarch bandage provided the limb is elevated long enough to allow some drainage of blood. The sphygmomanometer must be kept above the level of the systolic blood pressure until the operation is completed. Holmes suggests that if this is uncomfortable for the patient, a second cuff should be used below it on the analgesic part of the limb, and the original cuff removed. The use of a double-ballooned sphygmomanometer cuff has been advocated as a refinement of this technique (Hoyle, 1964).

The manner in which local analgesia and muscle paralysis are produced by this technique is unknown, but sensation and muscle power return within a matter of minutes after release of the sphygmomanometer cuff.

The safety of this technique with lignocaine is doubted by Kennedy *et al.* (1965) who describe a high incidence of severe neurological and cardiovascular side-effects following the release of the tourniquet. One patient developed cardiac arrest, but then responded successfully to external cardiac massage. Sorbie and Chacha (1965) encountered no serious toxic reactions in a series of

128 patients who were anaesthetised in a busy casualty department by house surgeons. The difference in these two series probably lies in Kennedy and his co-workers' detailed investigation of each patient by electrocardiography.

Digital Nerve Block

The digital nerves to a finger or toe can be blocked by infiltration of local analgesic solutions on either side of the base of the proximal phalanx. Lignocaine, 0·5 per cent, should be used, but without the addition of adrenaline in case marked vasoconstriction of the digital vessels should lead to gangrene.

Splanchnic Nerve Block

The posterior approach of Kappis (1919) is described here, the object being to deposit local analgesic solution in the vicinity of the coeliac ganglia and plexus of nerves as they lie in the retroperitoneal tissues anterior to the body of the first lumbar vertebra.

Technique

The needle can be inserted on either side of the body since bilateral block is unnecessary, the solution spreading from one side to the other. With the patient lying on his side, a skin weal is raised below the twelfth rib, four fingers breadth from the midline at the level of the spine of the first lumbar vertebra. A 12 cm. needle is directed through the weal, at an angle of approximately 45° to the median plane of the body, until the lateral border of the body of the first lumbar vertebra is reached. The needle is then withdrawn slightly and redirected more laterally to slip past the body of the vertebra. The needle point should now be near the crus of the diaphragm, and must be advanced a further short distance to pierce the crus and enter the retroperitoneal space. The use of a marker on the needle is of considerable help in estimating the distances. After careful aspiration, a single injection of 40–50 ml. of 0·5 per cent lignocaine is injected. The close proximity of the inferior vena cava on the right side not infrequently results in a bloody tap. The needle must then be reinserted and a careful aspiration test performed again. A successful block is always followed by some fall in systemic blood pressure due to dilatation of the splanchnic vessels.

Splanchnic block is required when upper abdominal surgery is performed under local analgesia alone. It is nowadays principally of value to relieve the severe pain of acute pancreatitis and of carcinoma of the pancreas. For the latter, block with phenol or alcohol is necessary.

Blocks for Abdominal Operations

Paravertebral and intercostal blocks for abdominal surgery are now rarely used. This is directly due to improvements in general anaesthesia, and, where a strong indication for local analgesia exists, to the many advantages of epidural block. To prepare a patient for an upper abdominal operation under intercostal combined with splanchnic block requires fifteen separate injections which in a psychologically unsuitable subject is difficult and not devoid of the risks of accidental pneumothorax and toxic reaction. However, as recently as 1962, Moore and Bridenbaugh listed seven reasons why this technique, or intercostal block with light general anaesthesia, might be considered the anaesthetic of choice for upper abdominal surgery.

For purposes of discussion, these seven reasons are quoted below:

1. Relaxation is equivalent to spinal or epidural analgesia or general anaesthesia plus relaxants.
2. Hypotension does not result unless the coeliac plexus is blocked, and even so, the hypotension is easily corrected.
3. The extent of analgesia is more predictable than that due to spinal or epidural block.
4. The duration of analgesia using amethocaine with adrenaline is longer than single-dose epidural or spinal block. Analgesia for 5–7 hours can be achieved.
5. The technique is ideal for a patient in a poor physical state, as it produces the minimum of physiological disturbance.
6. There are no neurological sequelae.
7. There are unlikely to be medico-legal objections on the part of the patient.

If each of these reasons is taken in turn and compared with modern general anaesthetic techniques using muscle relaxants, it is difficult to find any distinct or great advantage in their favour. When light general anaesthesia is used in addition to the intercostal nerve blocks, the morbidity of the local technique compared to that of the muscle relaxant is likely to be greater. Moore backed his opinions with a successful series of 4,333 patients and a low incidence of pneumothorax of only 0·092 per cent. This implies that the blocks were done by experts, but similar considerations would apply to the morbidity of relaxants given by experts.

Intercostal and other nerve blocks may in special circumstances still have a useful part to play. In some parts of the world few specialist anaesthetists are available and reliance must be placed on regional analgesic techniques performed by the surgeon himself. Farman and his colleagues (1962) describe a technique suitable for a single-handed surgeon. After inducing anaesthesia and intubating the patient, the general anaesthetic management of the patient is handed over to a relatively unskilled person by the surgeon, who then performs the intercostal nerve blocks.

Very occasionally a patient for whom general anaesthesia is technically impossible presents with an abdominal emergency. The author recalls such a one with acute intestinal obstruction and ankylosing spondylitis affecting the cervical spine which made intubation impossible. Here a regional block was the ideal solution to a very difficult problem.

A local nerve block technique may be useful in a very aged or poor risk patient with a strangulated hernia to avoid hazards of regurgitation and vomiting under general anaesthesia.

Technique of Intercostal Block

Upper abdominal operations require bilateral intercostal block of the 6th–12th segments and lower abdominal operations the 7th to the 12th segments.

Angle intercostal block, four fingers breadth from the midline of the back, is the author's choice. At this point the rib is free from the cover of the erector spine muscles and is easily palpable. The patient is placed in the lateral position with the shoulder blade of the side to be blocked drawn as far as possible away from the midline. For patients in very poor condition for whom the minimum of movement is desirable, intercostal block can be performed with the patient supine. The arms are drawn up to expose the axillae and the injections performed just posterior to the mid axillary line to include the lateral cutaneous branches of the intercostal nerve. The lower border of the rib is palpated and a skin weal raised. A 5-cm. needle is passed down to the lower border of the rib, and a rubber marker on the needle is then adjusted so that it indicates the exact depth the shaft has penetrated. The needle is then withdrawn and redirected to pass just below the rib to the depth of the marker. After aspiration, 5 ml. of 1 per cent lignocaine with adrenaline solution are injected, and a further 5 ml. while the needle is withdrawn. The nerve is blocked as it lies between the intercostalis internus and intimus muscles (Fig. 2) and the injection flows with a characteristic freedom when the needle is in the correct plane. It is essential to use markers for this block, as it is impossible to gauge the depth with an unmarked needle and it is all too easy to advance the needle too far and pierce the pleura. These blocks are often performed in poor risk patients and the whole value may be lost by the production of a bilateral pneumothorax.

Lignocaine 1 per cent with adrenaline produces satisfactory analgesia for up to two hours. For operations of longer duration amethocaine should be used.

Local Block for Herniorraphy

This can be very useful for a strangulated hernia in an aged or otherwise poor risk patient.

A single epidural injection will do just as well in many cases, but in some circumstances it may be particularly desirable to avoid a fall in blood pressure or the risk of dural puncture in, for example, a severe bronchitic where repeated coughing may lead to severe post-spinal headache.

An iliac crest block of the twelfth thoracic, the ilio-inguinal and ilio-hypogastric nerves (Fig. 3), as they lie between the transverse abdominis and internal oblique muscles, is performed as follows. A skin weal is raised two fingers breadth from the iliac crest along a line joining the anterior superior spine to the xiphisternum. A needle is then passed through this to strike the inner surface of the ilium just below the crest. Ten ml. of 1 per cent lignocaine solution are deposited as the needle is slowly withdrawn. The injection is then repeated with the needle reinserted at a slightly steeper angle. The contents of the inguinal canal are catered for by a separate injection into the neck of the peritoneal sac one finger's breadth above the mid-inguinal point. The needle is inserted perpendicularly until it pierces the aponeurosis of the external oblique, and the needle then advanced a further 2–3 cm. through the extra-peritoneal fat in this region. Ten ml. of solution are deposited at this depth and a further 10 ml. as the needle is withdrawn over 2 cm. (Macintosh and Bryce-Smith, 1953). This ensures block of the neck of the peritoneal sac and the genital branch of the genito-femoral nerve. The block is then completed by a subcutaneous infiltration of the line of the surgical incision.

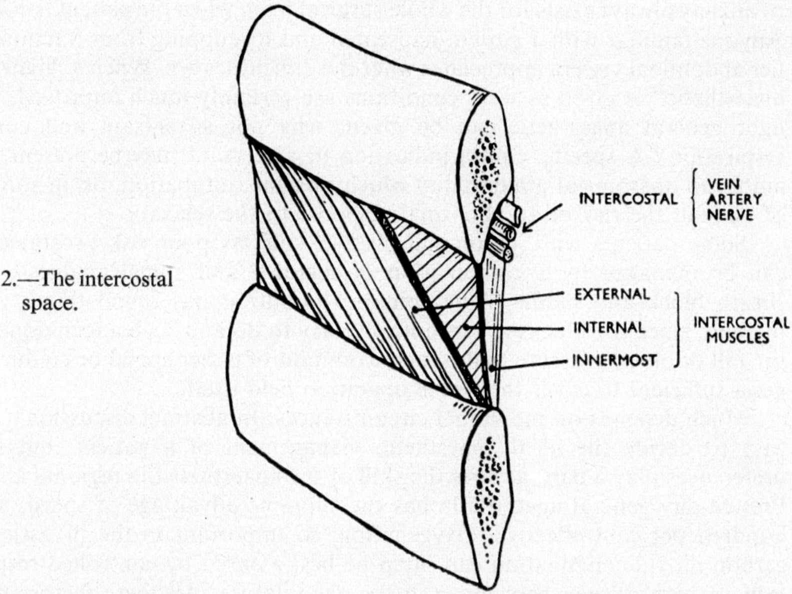

44/FIG. 2.—The intercostal space.

Discussion

At the time of writing, it is extremely difficult to define precisely the place of regional analgesia for abdominal surgery. Some points have already been touched on in the general description of the blocks. Undoubtedly, in the whole field of regional analgesia, its use for abdominal surgery has suffered the greatest decline. Several factors contribute to this. The techniques are exacting for anaesthetist and patient, and are time-consuming. A considerable element

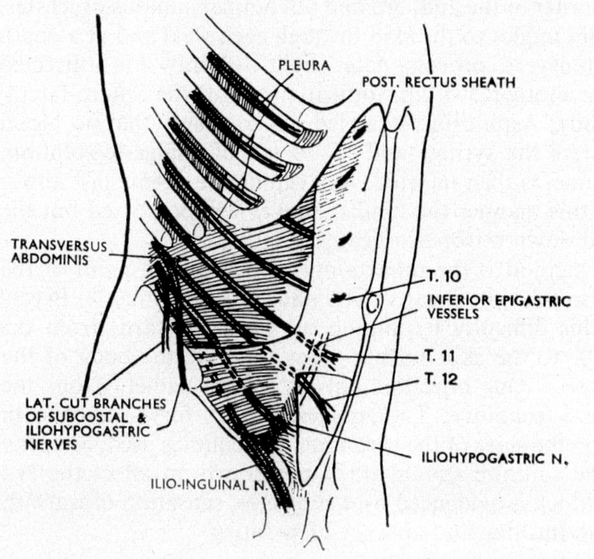

44/FIG. 3.—The lower intercostal, subcostal and first lumbar nerves.

of anxiety always exists for the whole surgical team when the patient is conscious. Anyone familiar with a patient nauseated and hiccupping from traction on upper abdominal viscera appreciates what the difficulties are. When a "light general anaesthetic" is given as well, conditions are certainly much improved, but if a light general anaesthetic can be given, why not a relaxant and controlled respiration? A specific contra-indication to a relaxant may be present, for example an anatomical abnormality which prevents intubation, or, in some types of patient, the risk of an abnormal response to the relaxant.

Some patients with abdominal disease, such as poor risk prostatectomies, can be managed by a combination of regional and spinal analgesia—rectus sheath block and saddle block spinal. The author has found this a valuable method, since the blocks are technically easy to do and such a technique avoids the fall of blood pressure that is a concomitant of either spinal or epidural analgesia sufficient to cover the whole operation field itself.

Much depends on individual circumstances. In abstract discussion it is often easy to decide the ideal anaesthetic management of a patient, but surgical preferences play a part, as does the skill of the anaesthetist in regional analgesia. Present-day general anaesthesia has the supreme advantage of speed, and is a hundred per cent effective. Oxygenation, so important in the ill patient, and carbon dioxide elimination can often be best assured by controlled respiration using a high oxygen percentage in the gas mixture. All these factors must be assessed by the individual anaesthetist in the circumstances in which he finds himself.

Lumbar Sympathetic Block

The lumbar sympathetic ganglia can be blocked where they lie against the vertebral bodies. The conventional approach was described by Mandl in 1926. The patient lies on his side and skin weals are raised 3 fingers' breadth or 5 cm. lateral to the upper border of the 2nd, 3rd and 4th lumbar spinous processes. A needle is inserted at right angles to the skin through each weal and at a depth of 4–5 cm. it strikes the transverse process. After slight withdrawal it is directed inwards and upwards for another 3–4 cm. until it slides off the antero-lateral aspect of the vertebral body. Aspiration is carried out to ensure that no blood or cerebrospinal fluid enters the syringe and 15–20 ml. of analgesic solution, such as 1 per cent lignocaine, is then injected. By keeping the needle just above the transverse process in this manner the lumbar nerves will be missed but the solution will track up and down retroperitoneally.

The objection to this method is the uncertainty of placing the point of the needle at the right depth to miss the great vessels and the psoas muscle. Bryce-Smith (1951) overcame this difficulty by aiming the needle inwards from the start at an angle of 60–70° to the skin surface so as to strike the body of the vertebra on its lateral aspect. One injection only is made, namely from the middle weal in the original technique. The analgesic tracks forwards beneath the tendinous arch bridging the sides of the vertebrae. If alcohol is used, Mandl's approach is better lest the solution should track posteriorly to affect the 3rd lumbar nerve. Successful block is evidenced by a subjective sensation of warmth in the lower extremity with flushing and absence of sweating.

Chemical lumbar sympathectomy with alcohol or phenol is sometimes of value in patients with chronic vascular disorders of the lower limb who are unfit for operation on general grounds. Temporary blocks with a local analgesic solution are not helpful in assessing the place for surgical sympathectomy, since the maximum benefits of operation are often not apparent for a long time—months in some patients. Temporary lumbar sympathetic block is useful when deciding whether sympathectomy will benefit phantom limb pain.

REFERENCES

BALL, H. C. J. (1962). Brachial plexus block. A modified supraclavicular approach. *Anaesthesia*, **17,** 269.

BIER, A. (1908). Ueber einen neuen Weg Localanasthesie an der Gliedmasse zu erzeugen. *Verh. dtsch. Ges. Chir.*, **37,** 204 (Part II).

BRYCE-SMITH, R. (1951). Injection of the lumbar sympathetic chain. *Anaesthesia*, **6,** 150.

FARMAN, J. V., GOOL, R. Y., and SCOTT, D. B. (1962). Intercostal block in abdominal surgery. A method for the singlehanded surgeon. *Lancet*, **1,** 879.

HOLMES, C. McK. (1963). Intravenous regional analgesia. A useful method of producing analgesia of the limbs. *Lancet*, **1,** 245.

HOYLE, J. R. (1964). Tourniquet for intravenous regional analgesia. *Anaesthesia*, **19,** 294.

KAPPIS, M. (1919). Sensibilität und lokale Anästhesie im chirurgischen Gebiet der Bauchohle mit besonderer Berücksichtigung der Splanchnicus-Anästhesie. *Bruns' Beitr. klin. Chir.*, **115,** 161.

KENNEDY, B. R., DUTHIE, A. M., PARBROOK, G. D., and CARR, T. L. (1965). Intravenous regional analgesia: an appraisal. *Brit. med. J.*, **1,** 954.

MACINTOSH, R. R., and BRYCE-SMITH, R. (1953). *Local Analgesia; Abdominal Surgery*. Edinburgh: E. & S. Livingstone.

MACINTOSH, R. R., and MUSHIN, W. W. (1954). *Local Analgesia: Brachial Plexus*, 3rd edit. Edinburgh: E. and S. Livingstone.

MACINTOSH, R. R., and OSTLERE, M. (1955). *Local Analgesia: Head and Neck*. Edinburgh: E. and S. Livingstone.

MANDL, F. (1926). *Die Paravertebrale Injektion, Anatomie und Tecknik, Begründung, und Anwendung*. Wien: J. Springer.

MOORE, D. C., and BRIDENBAUGH, L. D. (1962). Intercostal nerve block in 4,333 patients: indications, technique and complications. *Curr. Res. Anesth.*, **41,** 1.

PITKIN, G. P. (1953). *Conduction Anesthesia*, 2nd edit. Philadelphia: J. B. Lippincott Co.

SORBIE, C., and CHACHA, P. (1965). Regional anaesthesia by the intravenous route. *Brit. med. J.*, **1,** 957.

Chapter 45

NEUROLOGICAL AND OPHTHALMIC COMPLICATIONS OF ANAESTHESIA

HYPOXIA AND THE CENTRAL NERVOUS SYSTEM

WHATEVER the cause of hypoxia, the end results in the central nervous system appear to be the same, differing only in extent, which is in direct relation to the degree and duration of the period of sub-oxygenation. An acute anoxic episode caused by a period of cardiac arrest is dramatic enough to draw attention to any sequelae should the patient survive. Equally important are the equivalent degrees of acute hypoxia that can occur without cardiac arrest in some anaesthetic mishaps and certain disease states. Less obvious but just as potentially detrimental to the patient are the effects of prolonged but subacute hypoxia. Ancillary factors are the state of the brain prior to sub-oxygenation and repeated bouts of hypoxia. The normal brain will tolerate a moderate degree of oxygen lack for quite long periods without apparently being harmed, but the presence of disease, or even the ordinary changes associated with ageing, markedly increase its vulnerability. On the other hand, young babies have more resistance than adults. Repetitive bouts of moderate hypoxia may be cumulative (Lucas, 1946; Lucas and Strangeways, 1952), while once hypoxia of any degree has produced changes in the brain, a vicious circle effect leads to further sub-oxygenation. Ischaemic hypoxia is more dangerous than that associated with a normal flow of blood.

Clinical Picture

The clinical results are immensely variable, depending, as would be expected, on the severity and duration of the episode. Bedford (1955) describes the occurrence of adverse cerebral effects in old people following operations under general anaesthesia. These may vary from extreme dementia, through personality changes, to lesser degrees of incapacity which are only noticeable to the patient and his relatives, and range from inability to concentrate to simple impairment of memory. Here the sub-oxygenation, whatever its primary cause, is likely to have been slight though protracted. Acute and total anoxia may be followed by coma and death, although a period of decerebrate rigidity often intervenes. Cope (1960) emphasises that following an anoxic or hypoxic episode a patient may recover consciousness completely, only to lapse into coma soon afterwards. But far short of this, a whole series of clinical pictures, sometimes singly and sometimes together, may be portrayed. Convulsions, various paralyses—spastic and flaccid—Parkinsonism, total or partial blindness, dysphonia and multiple defects of intellectual function have been recorded (Allison, 1956). Finally, any period of hypoxia—although not marked enough to cause objective neurological sequelae—may yet bequeath to the patient a severe headache with associated sickness for several hours.

Physio-pathology

The higher centres are more vulnerable than the lower. Nerve cells have a much higher metabolism than nerve fibres so that reflex excitability is abolished if the centres are deprived of oxygen for even short periods.

Lesions due to general brain anoxia are commonly widely distributed but may vary according to the cause—hypotension, hypoxaemia, circulatory arrest, etc. Measurements of regional cerebral blood flow in patients with focal occlusive (anoxic) lesions have demonstrated a vasomotor paralysis of the blood vessels supplying the anoxic area giving rise to a "luxury perfusion syndrome" in which the rate of flow is increased above the post-anoxically lowered metabolic demands (Ingvar, 1968). This hyperaemia may lead to oedema. The same sequence may occur in generalised cerebral anoxia but there is some doubt as to whether major cerebral oedema can occur unless there is accompanying hypocapnia. Post-anoxic hyperaemia occurs within minutes and its duration is probably dependent on the duration and severity of the tissue hypoxia. Should generalised cerebral anoxia occur, this may set up a vicious circle which leads to raised intracranial pressure which ultimately diminishes the perfusion pressure gradient giving rise to generalised ischaemia and in severe cases to global brain ischaemia and necrosis.

Preventive Treatment

Although it may be considered elementary to write of prevention in relation to a complication of anaesthesia such as anoxia, which is generally regarded as obvious in its clinical manifestation, the work of Bedford (1955 and 1957) has drawn attention to the innumerable occasions during and following anaesthesia when a mild but insidious degree of sub-oxygenation of the patient may take place. Such occasions occur with moderate hypotension from the effects of anaesthetic drugs or in the immediate post-operative period almost as a reaction to surgery and anaesthesia—occasionally because the patient has been sat up too soon (Bourne, 1957). Premedicant and post-operative sedative and analgesic drugs—badly selected and prescribed in unnecessarily high dosage—can cause marked depression in the elderly whilst toxaemia, fever, fluid and electrolyte imbalance may further aggravate the situation. The use of low oxygen concentrations, often practised in dental anaesthesia, is to be condemned and there is ample evidence to show that oxygen concentrations during all anaesthetics should be above that of air. Consideration and avoidance of adverse factors and repeated appraisal of each patient with respect to the adequacy of oxygenation is the duty of the anaesthetist. Great care must be taken in the selection of patients for whom a deliberate reduction in blood pressure is intended. Incipient hypoxia may not be easy to diagnose. Lucas (1946), however, has restated the objective signs which individually are of limited significance, but taken together become very important. They are an increased respiratory rate with possibly dyspnoea, tachycardia, restlessness and sometimes delirium, and excessive sweating with pallor.

Active Treatment

Active treatment may save a patient who remains unconscious after an acute hypoxic episode. A complete neurological examination should be made at the earliest convenient time.

Ventilation.—Whether a patient should be allowed to breathe spontaneously or should have intermittent positive-pressure respiration instituted must depend on the degree of unconsciousness and on the adequacy of spontaneous ventilation assessed clinically and by acid-base measurements. An enriched oxygen mixture is essential. The presence of hypercarbia increases the risk of cerebral oedema, and intubation followed by moderate controlled passive hyperventilation will reduce intracranial pressure caused by hypercarbia. It remains to be proved that this technique is of value in the presence of a normal Pa_{CO_2} (Rosomoff, 1963). Secretions are more easily removed in an intubated patient. Tracheostomy may be necessary at a later stage.

Hypothermia.—Advantages claimed for its use include a decrease in cerebral blood flow, a corresponding reduction in cerebral metabolism, induced hypotension, decrease in brain volume and a fall in intracranial pressure. Rosomoff (1968) advocates lowering the temperature to 30–32° C for up to three weeks. Shivering is controlled by using an infusion of pethidine 100 mg., promethazine 100 mg. and phenobarbitone 100 mg. in 5 per cent dextrose in 0·2 per cent saline. Whilst induced hypothermia undoubtedly modifies the immediate reaction of the brain to injury, it has not yet been clearly shown that the ultimate degree of injury can be modified by lowering the body temperature (Strong and Keats, 1967). It is quite possible that the major benefit is derived from the prevention of hyperpyrexia rather than from the institution of hypothermia. Whatever method of cooling is used, it is essential that shivering be prevented.

Dehydrating agents.—These should be administered as soon as possible on the basis that if cerebral oedema or brain swelling occur, a reduction in brain volume, even if only temporary, is likely to be of benefit. There is less rebound with mannitol than urea but its administration intravenously should be restricted to 1 g./kg. body weight in not less than 20–30 minutes. More rapid administration may cause a dangerous increase in blood volume and result in pulmonary oedema (Coleman and Buckell, 1964). Although both mannitol and urea are contra-indicated in the presence of severe renal disease, it is perhaps wise in the presence of such a complication to err on the side of treatment by giving a small intravenous dose of mannitol such as 12·5 g., to assess the effect on the patient, rather than to do nothing and risk the onset of a vicious circle of anoxia. For long term administration, glycerol may be given by a gastric tube in a 50 per cent solution 1–2 g./kg. body weight and may be repeated 6–8 hourly even up to a week; its use is contra-indicated where there is a suspicion of a peptic ulcer.

Steroids.—Steroid therapy has been used increasingly in recent years both for the prevention and treatment of cerebral oedema. Its action is a paradox since it appears to induce a loss of sodium and water in cerebral oedema in contrast to its usual action of sodium and water retention. Dexamethasone is the agent of choice: it causes no significant changes in the sodium and water content of normal brain but appears to prevent its accumulation in experimental oedema (Taylor *et al.*, 1965). An initial dose of 10 mg. intramuscularly may be given with subsequent doses of 4 mg. 6 hourly for 2–3 days.

Fluid balance.—This is best maintained by the use of intravenous Ringer lactate solution or 5 per cent dextrose in 0·2 per cent saline. The use of 5 per cent dextrose in water, although isotonic, is potentially dangerous if it is given faster than water is lost (normally 1000–1200 ml./sq. metre/24 hours). This is because it is initially distributed throughout the total body water which includes the brain and cerebrospinal fluid. Subsequently the fall in blood glucose is more rapid than that in the brain and this leads to a movement of water from a relatively hypotonic plasma into a hypertonic brain and cerebrospinal fluid, thereby increasing cerebrospinal fluid pressure and possibly the cerebral oedema. These changes are exaggerated in the presence of water retention (Fishman, 1953).

Posture.—Keeping the head raised will lessen the cerebral venous pressure but hypotension may ensue.

Sedation.—There is evidence that barbiturates exert a protective action against the effects of hypoxia (Secher and Wilhjelm, 1968). Thiopentone infusion may well be beneficial (Holmdahl, 1969) but its use is still in an experimental stage.

General.—Other measures such as the passing of a nasogastric tube to avoid gastric distension or for feeding should follow those for the management of unconscious patients.

Prognosis

Although the immediate prognosis for life after a severe and protracted bout of cerebral hypoxia is undoubtedly poor, that for morbidity in patients who survive is very difficult to assess. It has long been known the the duration of cerebral anoxia or hypoxia is the most important factor determining the outcome but in clinical situations this is often unknown and the causes may be complex. Even when the period of cardiac arrest is known, it may have been preceded by an unknown period of circulatory insufficiency. Prognosis in the early post-anoxic period can be very difficult and in an unconscious patient anything other than a gross alteration in the level of the central nervous system function may not be detectable.

Pampiglione and Harden (1968) consider that the electro-encephalograph may be helpful at a very early stage in assessing the chances of survival, possible severity, occurrence of complicating factors and impending seizures, as well as "death of the brain". These workers made a prognostic evaluation of early E.E.G. findings following resusciation after cardiovascular arrest. They found that the best timing for E.E.G. studies for early prognosis was between 2–12 hours after resuscitation and that these should be repeated at 2–3 hourly intervals. They emphasized that before any prognostic evaluation was attempted, the E.E.G. should be recognised as only one physical sign to be interpreted in the context of the patient's history and other physical signs.They warned against misleading information where inadequate E.E.G. studies were performed and suggested that at least four different areas of each hemisphere should be simultaneously studied with appropriate leads.

Peripheral Nerve Palsies

Peripheral nerve palsies occuring during general anaesthesia are usually due to the effects, singly or combined, of pressure upon, or stretching, a nerve at some vulnerable point along its course. Occasionally such complications may result from the injection of an irritant substance into or near the nerve, or more simply from the trauma of a needle point. Evidence has accumulated to show that special conditions, such as induced hypothermia or hypotension, may themselves cause a neuropathy—while they will certainly aggravate any of the more common causes.

Stephens and Appleby (1956) and Swan and his co-workers (1955) describe the onset of nerve palsies following the use of hypothermia for cardiac operations. They were able to measure temperatures of 4° C in the gastrocnemius muscle of a patient who had a rectal temperature of 28° C. Exposure to cold in an ice water bath for periods of longer than thirty minutes led to peripheral nerve palsies in a number of patients.

In the assessment of any post-operative nerve palsy, a knowledge of the pre-operative neurological condition is of considerable importance. Not only is a diseased nerve more susceptible to trauma but the debilitating effects of both surgery and anaesthesia, even without any localised factor in the nerve itself, may accentuate pre-existing neurological disease. Diabetes mellitus, peri-arteritis nodosa and alcoholism are known pre-disposing causes.

Compression and Stretching

Brachial plexus palsy.—A combination of factors is most commonly the cause of trouble. Clausen (1942) described a case of brachial plexus palsy due to the effects of pressure alone, when a patient was maintained in the Trendelenburg position with inadequately padded shoulder supports. Presumably the supports were also badly positioned, because direct pressure upon the roots of the plexus is impossible if they are placed opposite the acromion processes.

The principal factors are weight bearing through the shoulder girdle in the Trendelenburg position, stretching of the plexus by moving the arm away from the side of the body, and abnormal relaxation of the muscles in this area. Weight bearing through the shoulder girdle leads to compression of the plexus between the first rib and the clavicle. When the arm is abducted from the side it is usually extended with some external rotation so that the plexus is put on the stretch. This may easily be accentuated to more than 90° by the unintentional and unnoticed movements of the surgeon, his assistants, or bystanders during the course of the operation. A further aggravating factor consists of placing the abducted arm at a lower horizontal level than the rest of the body (Jackson and Keats, 1965). This may occur if the arm drops away from the side of the body. Moreover the ill effects of this manoeuvre, which pushes the head of the humerus up into the already tightened plexus, are increased by raising the body still higher with a gall-bladder rest. The importance of the position of the arm, and hence of stretching as the principal cause of brachial plexus palsy, is illustrated by Kiloh's (1950) description of four cases, all of which occurred during gall-bladder operations. Kiloh also stresses the fact that individual variations of anatomy and idiosyncrasy, such as cervical ribs, the size of the cervico-axillary canal, the shape of the first rib and the slope of the shoulder may all play a part sometimes in rendering the brachial plexus more vulnerable. Brachial plexus palsy as a result of faulty posturing during surgery was described long before relaxant drugs were introduced into anaesthetic practice, but there is little doubt that the extreme degrees of muscle relaxation they induce renders this complication much more likely in certain circumstances than with general anaesthesia alone.

Compression

Facial nerve palsy.—The buccal branch of the facial nerve normally arises from the main stem in the substance of the parotid gland and emerges at the anterior edge of this gland to supply the lateral part of the orbicularis oris muscle. Occasionally this branch may arise more proximally and run superficial to the gland, in which case it is susceptible to pressure. Paresis of it may then be caused by compression when the jaw of an unconscious patient is held forward, or due to a firmly fitted head harness (Morris, 1959).

Radial nerve palsy.—The nerve is vulnerable as it winds round the mid-part of the inner surface of the humerus. In the lateral position—particularly with the arm placed away from the side of the body—it can easily be subjected to pressure.

Ulnar nerve palsy.—The ulnar nerve is unprotected as it passes superficially and inferior to the medial epicondyle of the humerus. Typically it may be compressed between the bone and the edge of the operating table should the arm not be placed close to the side of the body in the horizontal position. The surgeon, or his assistant, is likely to add further pressure during the operation as he stands up against the table.

Common peroneal nerve palsy.—This nerve, in a similar manner to the ulnar, may easily be compressed against the head of the fibula when the patient lies in the lateral position or from compression against the stirrups in the lithotomy position.

Saphenous nerve.—This nerve may be compressed against the stirrups on the medial side of the knee when the patient is in the lithotomy position (Schmidt and Lincoln, 1966).

Injection

Median nerve palsy.—The median nerve lies in close deep relationship to the basilic and median cubital veins at the medial side of the antecubital fossa. An extravenous injection of thiopentone in this area can easily reach the nerve. Pask and Robson (1954) have drawn attention to the difficulty of appreciating the injection of very small quantities of fluid from a 10 ml. syringe, and have shown that 0·2 ml. of 1 per cent lignocaine can affect the median nerve significantly. Should the patient move after the needle of a syringe containing thiopentone has been successfully placed in the basilic vein, the point might easily advance sufficiently for some of the irritant fluid to reach the nerve.

Lateral and median cutaneous nerves of the forearm.—Either of these nerves may inadvertently come into contact with thiopentone solution should an attempted intravenous injection lead to some extravasation outside the vein, or the nerve itself be pricked.

Radial nerve palsy.—The radial vein, and its tributaries lying about one to one and a half half inches above the wrist on the radial side of the forearm, are popular not only for intravenous injection but also for intravenous infusion. Injudicious attempts at either of these procedures may lead to trauma of the radial nerve as it lies deep to but not far from the veins.

Sciatic nerve palsy.—Intramuscular injection into the buttock is always fraught with the potential hazard of traumatising the sciatic nerve, especially in infants. The upper and outer quadrant of the buttock should be used, but a preferable and safe site for injection is the antero-lateral aspect of the mid-thigh.

Prevention

General awareness of these dangers on the part of anaesthetists, surgeons, nurses, and all who care for unconscious patients is the best safeguard against their occurrence. Special precautions must be taken in particular instances where the risk of a certain posture must be accepted in the general interest of the patient. Thus it may be essential to use shoulder supports to maintain a patient in the Trendelenburg position, with the legs in the lithotomy position at the same time, during the operation of synchronous combined abdomino-perineal resection of the rectum. In such an instance well-padded supports placed at the acromion processes are essential, and the arms should be placed by the side of the body. In all other inclined planes the body is more safely prevented from sliding by the use of a non-slip matress (Fig. 1; Hewer, 1953).

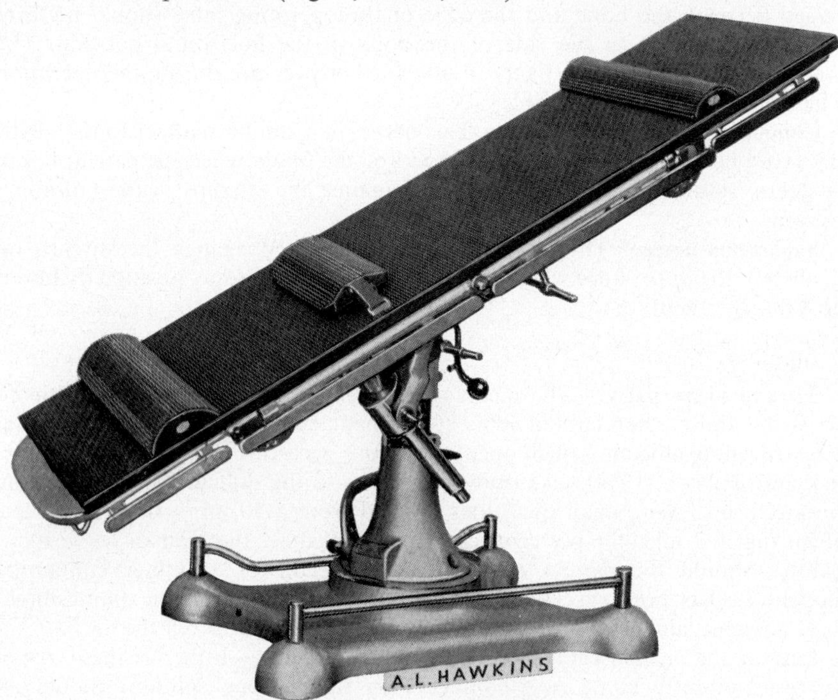

45/Fig. 1.—Non-slip mattress.

If an arm is to be abducted from the body for the purpose of intravenous injections or infusions during an operation—and this is frequently essential—it should be maintained at a higher horizontal plane from the body, and the use of a right angle lock will help to ensure it is never abducted beyond this. In the "hands up" position, elevation of the upper arm 6 inches off the table prevents injury (Jackson and Keats, 1965).

Treatment

This should consist of splinting to prevent deformities, and active exercises. Analgesics may be needed for a day or two after the onset of paresis.

Prognosis

The greater the pressure and the longer it is applied, the more severe is the injury. Provided there is no pre-existing neurological disease the prognosis for peripheral nerve palsies of the types described is good. They may be slow to recover completely but the majority will clear within six months. The only notable exceptions are those due to hypothermia, which may take considerably longer. As a rule power returns quickest in large muscles and more slowly in those concerned with fine movements. Thus patients who rely upon their fingers for everyday work and pleasure are more handicapped than manual workers.

The **neurological sequelae of spinal analgesia** are discussed in Chapter 43.

Convulsions During Anaesthesia

Convulsions may occur during local or general anaesthesia. Those due to local analgesic drugs are discussed in Chapter 41. Convulsions during the administration of general anaesthesia have often been associated with ether but are by no means limited to the use of this agent; indeed, accumulated experience suggests that they may be the result of a combination of factors. These may be divided into three groups:

1. *Physical predisposition.*—Children undoubtedly have a greater propensity to convulse than adults, and this is presumably due to the lability of their central nervous systems. A fit may be induced in a true epileptic by various stimuli—such as hypoxia or hypercarbia—but the evidence for believing that all patients who convulse during general anaesthesia have an epileptic tendency is inconclusive.

2. *Disease.*—Sepsis with its associated high temperature and increased basal metabolism leads to some tissue hypoxia of the histotoxic type and frequently to dehydration. An excessively high body temperature may be produced by an overheated operating theatre or the injudicious use of surgical drapes on the patient.

3. *Anaesthesia.*—The contribution of anaesthesia lies primarily in its ability to accentuate the other factors. Hence excessive premedication with atropine raises the patient's temperature by increasing both metabolism and dehydration, while deep inhalational anaesthesia adds to the tissue hypoxia. Moreover, unless respiration is at least assisted at this stage, some carbon dioxide retention occurs. Convulsions in children following premedication with "Pamergan SP100", a proprietary name for a combination of promethazine 50 mg., pethidine 100 mg. and hyoscine 0·4 mg., have been recorded (Waterhouse, 1967) and an idiosyncratic reaction to the promethazine element has been postulated. Convulsions have also followed premedication in children with papaveretum and hyoscine (Holmes 1968), and the opiate held responsible.

"Malignant hyperthermia", well documented in recent years, may be a cause of convulsions (Britt and Gordon, 1969). Its features and treatment are described elsewhere (Chapter 33).

Prevention should consist of a reasoned appraisal of the risk in likely subjects and the avoidance of all controllable and predisposing factors. The immediate treatment should be to ensure oxygenation; this is best achieved by paralysing the patient with a muscle relaxant and performing intermittent positive-pressure respiration with 100 per cent oxygen. Particular care must be taken to ensure that the carbon dioxide tension of the blood is kept within normal limits, and steps should be taken to lower the patient's body temperature. Prolonged treatment—on the lines suggested on p. 1259—may be needed should a period of acute anoxia occur before the convulsion can be controlled.

Ophthalmic Complications

Most ophthalmic complications follow direct trauma or the irritant effect of anaesthesic vapours, soda-lime dust, or sterilising solutions. Conjunctivitis, corneal abrasion and ulcers may also be caused in this fashion, and it is particularly important to ensure that the eyelids are covering the eye at all times. In certain postures, such as the prone position in neurosurgery, and when the eyes are especially vulnerable, as in exophthalmos, it is a wise precaution temporarily to strap the eyelids together with adhesive plaster. Indeed, in the latter case it is occasionally necessary to perform a tarsorrhaphy.

Less common complications affecting the eye as a result of anaesthesia and surgery are thrombosis of the central artery of the retina, acute glaucoma and pain in the region of the supra-orbital nerve. Thrombosis of the retinal artery, which causes blindness, is only likely to occur in those patients with pre-existing disease. Shock states, and excessive induced hypotension, could be a contributory cause. Post-operative blindness may also be part of a general syndrome caused by acute or sub-acute anoxia (see p. 1258). Givner and Jaffe (1950) suggest that compression of the eye by an anaesthetic mask may cause indirect pressure on the central artery of the retina. If the patient suffers from arterial disease then ischaemic changes in the retina may be produced. Difficulties of accommodation are not uncommon immediately after anaesthesia and can usually be related to the varying effects of the drugs used—including pre- and post-operative medicants and the relaxants—upon the ciliary and ocular muscles. Any agents which produce dilatation of the pupil and impede the circulation of the aqueous humour will accentuate a tendency towards glaucoma. Acute glaucoma, precipitated in a myopic patient, is a well-recognised post-operative complication, but its direct connection with either operation or anaesthetic is not always apparent. It has been suggested that the pressure of a face mask on the eye, and its subsequent release, is an important factor, but cases occur in which a mask has not been used. Certainly atropine and scopolamine should be used with caution for known cases of glaucoma, but the occasional acute case that occurs is more likely to be related to the general metabolic disturbance than to any single and specific factor.

Supra-orbital pain—a very rare complication—is almost certainly related to undue pressure in the area of the nerve.

The ocular complications of spinal analgesia are discussed in Chapter 43.

REFERENCES

Allison, R. S. (1956). Clinical consequence of cerebral anoxia. *Proc. roy. Soc. Med.*, **49,** 609.

Bedford, P. D. (1955). Adverse cerebral effects of anaesthesia on old people. *Lancet*, **2,** 259.

Bedford, P. D. (1957). Cerebral damage from shock due to disease in aged people with special reference to cardiac infarction, pneumonia and severe diarrhoea. *Lancet*, **2,** 505.

Bourne, J. G. (1957). Fainting and cerebral damage. A danger in patients kept upright during dental gas anaesthesia and after surgical operations. *Lancet*, **2,** 499.

Britt, B. A., and Gordon, R. A. (1969). Three cases of malignant hyperthermia with special consideration of management. *Canad. Anaesth. Soc. J.*, **16,** 99.

Clausen, E. G. (1942). Post-operative ("anaesthetic") paralysis of brachial plexus; review of literature and report of nine cases. *Surgery*, **12,** 933.

Coleman, D. J., and Buckell, M. (1964). The effect of urea and mannitol infusions on circulatory volume. *Anaesthesia*, **19,** 507.

Cope, D. H. P. (1960). Dehydration therapy in cerebral hypoxia. *Proc. roy. Soc. Med.*, **52,** 678.

Fishman, R. A. (1953). Effects of isotonic intravenous solutions on normal and increased intracranial pressure. *Arch. Neurol.* (*Chic.*), **70,** 350.

Givner, I., and Jaffe, N. (1950). Occlusion of the central retinal artery following anaesthesia. *Arch. Ophthal.*, **43,** 197.

Hewer, C. L. (1953). Maintenance of the Trendelenburg position by skin friction. *Lancet*, **1,** 522.

Holmdahl, M. H. (1969). Personal communication.

Holmes, R. P. (1968). Convulsions following pre-operative medication. *Brit. J. Anaesth.*, **40,** 633.

Ingvar, D. H. (1968). The pathophysiology of cerebral anoxia. *Acta anaesth. scand.*, Suppl. **29,** 47.

Jackson, L., and Keats, A. S. (1965). Mechanism of brachial plexus palsy following anaesthesia. *Anesthesiology*, **26,** 190.

Kiloh, L. G. (1950). Brachial plexus lesions after cholecystectomy. *Lancet*, **1,** 103.

Lucas, B. G. B. (1946). Anoxia and the central nervous system. An experimental and clinical study. *Thorax*, **1,** 128.

Lucas, B. G. B., and Strangeways, D. H. (1952). The effects of intermittent anoxia on the brain. *J. Path. Bact.*, **64,** 265.

Morris, P. M. (1959). Personal communication.

Pampiglione, G., and Harden, A. (1968). Resuscitation after cardiovascular arrest. Prognostic evaluation of early electroencephalographic findings. *Lancet*, **1,** 1261.

Pask, E. A., and Robson, J. G. (1954). Injury to the median nerve. *Anaesthesia*, **9,** 94.

Rosomoff, H. L. (1963). Distribution of intracranial contents with controlled hyperventilation: implications for neuro-anaesthesia. *Anesthesiology*, **24,** 640.

Rosomoff, H. L. (1968). Cerebral oedema and brain swelling. *Acta anaesth. scand.*, Suppl., **29,** 75.

Schmidt, C. R., and Lincoln, J. R. (1966). Peripheral nerve injuries with anaesthesia: a review and report of three cases. *Anesth. Analg. Curr. Res.*, **45,** 748.

Secher, O., and Wilhjelm, B. (1968). The protective action of anaesthetics against hypoxia. *Canad. Anaesth. Soc. J.*, **15,** 423.

Stephens, J., and Appleby, S. (1965). Polyneuropathy following induced hypothermia. *Trans. Amer. neurol. Ass.*, p. 102 (80th Meeting, 1955).

Strong, M. J., and Keats, A. S. (1967). Induced hypothermia following cerebral anoxia. *Anesthesiology*, **28,** 920.

SWAN, H., VIRTUE, R., BLOUNT, S. G., JNR., and KIRCHER, L. T., JNR. (1955). Hypothermia in surgery: analysis of 100 clinical cases. *Ann. Surg.*, **142,** 382.

TAYLOR, J. M., LEVY, W. A., HERZOG, I., and SCHEINBERG, L. C. (1965). Prevention of experimental cerebral oedema by corticosteroids. *Neurology* (*Minneap.*), **15,** 667.

WATERHOUSE, R. G. (1967). Epileptiform convulsions in children following premedication with Pamergan SP100. *Brit. J. Anaesth.*, **39,** 268.

Section Four

THE METABOLIC, DIGESTIVE AND EXCRETORY SYSTEMS

Chapter 46

HIBERNATION AND HYPOTHERMIA

IDEALLY, many operations upon the heart and brain require that the flow through these organs is arrested for a short time whilst the surgeon visualises and repairs the defective part. Apart from the use of the tourniquet and posture, hypotensive anaesthesia was the first deliberate attempt to reduce the blood flow through the operative field, but in many cases this alone is not sufficient. If the surgeon has to look inside the chambers of the heart or has to remove a complex vascular tumour of the brain, the circulation must sometimes be stopped completely. Although the myocardium itself is not very susceptible to hypoxia provided it has no work to do, the brain cells are extremely sensitive and cannot go without an adequate blood supply for more than about three minutes without showing some signs of damage. Progress in this field demands either that an artificial system be used to replace the work of the heart and lungs (i.e. an extracorporeal circulation) or that cold be used to depress the metabolism of the vital cells. If the metabolism is curtailed then less blood supply is required and consequently the cells can endure far longer periods of hypoxia. This is the basic conception of hypothermia, i.e. a reduction in general body temperature.

Hypothermia opens up a whole new field of physiological study. Much can still be learned from the animal kingdom, where certain species possess the remarkable ability to lower their body temperature upon the approach of the cold season. This process is called "hibernation".

HIBERNATION

The dormant state into which certain animals enter at the approach of winter has been termed "hibernation". This function is possessed only by certain rodents, such as the hamster, the hedgehog, the squirrel, and the groundhog. In earlier days the ability of an animal to survive a body temperature of 19° C or below was taken as evidence for the ability to hibernate (Horvath's test), but recent experimental evidence has shown that this criterion is no longer valid.

The marmot (a species of Canadian groundhog) is believed to be the largest animal capable of undergoing hibernation; since this animal rarely exceeds 3 kilogrammes in weight, the state of hibernation would appear to be limited to small animals. At one time it was seriously believed that the Canadian brown bear (weighing many hundreds of pounds) was capable of reducing its body temperature at will, and an expedition set out to study this matter. Since this animal is particularly ferocious it was not possible to measure the oral or rectal temperature! During winter it normally sleeps in caves or sheltered places, but these investigators were fortunate enough to find one that could be seen lying under a tree. After noting that snow rapidly melted when it fell upon the bear's nose, and also that it could be roused to violent activity in a matter of seconds, it was generally agreed that the brown bear should not be classed as a hibernating animal.

Physiological Changes in Hibernation

During the warm summer months all hibernating animals are *homothermic*. That is to say, like man they can maintain a uniform body temperature despite fluctuations in the temperature of their environment. During this period the sexual cycle is in full swing and the animal arrives at the beginning of winter in a fat and sleek condition. As the temperature of its surroundings grows colder, so the animal prepares to hibernate. The actual process takes only a few hours. The animal merely lies down as if to sleep, but by some unknown mechanism it is able to abandon the homothermic state and become a *poikilotherm*—in other words, like the reptiles and other cold-blooded animals, it adapts itself to the temperature of its environment. It is wrong to believe that the temperature of the hibernating animal falls so low that it equals that of the air around it, for in some cases this would necessitate a body temperature below 0° C. There appears to be some basic mechanism at work, even during hibernation, which prevents the animal's temperature falling below 3–4° C. The necessity for this base-line is probably connected with the fact that nerve conduction ceases at temperatures below this level and the animal would lose all ability to rewarm itself if danger threatened. Laboratory experiments, however, have shown that these animals may be cooled to temperatures well below 0° C without harm, provided adequate artificial means of rewarming are available.

As the body temperature of the animal falls, so the blood pressure, pulse rate, respiratory rate, and all other functions of metabolism gradually subside until the basic state is reached. At this level the pulse rate may be only two or three beats per minute, yet one of the outstanding features is the normality of the electro-cardiographic recording. Except for the enormously prolonged interval between individual beats the actual PQRS complex looks remarkably normal and there is no evidence of the disturbance of myocardial function which is such a common feature in other non-hibernating animals under hypothermia. Systole occupies only about one half of the time taken by diastole, so that the heart is allowed ample time for relaxation and filling. Respiration may fall to less than one per minute, yet the animal does not seem to be cyanosed. Trusler and his colleagues (1953), in a study of the blood chemistry in the hibernating animal, made four important observations:

1. *The oxygen and carbon dioxide content of whole blood was increased.*—The dissociation curve for oxygen of the hibernating animal, measured *in vitro* in the laboratory, was found to be shifted to the left. The effect of this would be to make it more difficult for the blood to give up its oxygen when it reaches the tissues. However, this detrimental action is compensated for by a reduction in demand for oxygen by the tissues, by an increase in the total amount of oxygen physically dissolved in the plasma, and also by an increase in the carbon dioxide content of the blood. This last effect may have a potent influence in offsetting the shift of the oxygen dissociation curve.

2. *The haematocrit values are increased.*—The most likely cause of this change is haemoconcentration due to an increased uptake of fluid by the tissues. Svihla and Bowman (1952) found a reduction in the circulating blood volume in hibernating squirrels. Thus, the increased concentration of red cells together

with a rise in the oxygen and carbon dioxide content of the blood, may be a finely-adjusted mechanism designed to prevent tissue hypoxia and at the same time allow a great reduction in the work of the heart and lungs at these low temperatures.

3. *The serum magnesium and potassium levels rise.*—The exact significance of these findings is unknown and, as in hypothermia, is not generally accepted by all workers in this field.

4. *The blood sugar level falls.*—This occurs despite the increased concentration of the blood and is caused by the animal slowly consuming the carbohydrate and fat storage deposits in the body.

The Hibernating Gland

A close anatomical study of all the known hibernating animals reveals the presence of pads of brown fat in certain parts of the body. It can be found on the internal aspect of the thoracic and lumbar vertebrae lying directly underneath the pleura and peritoneum upon the muscle tissue in these areas. It can also be found directly behind the sternum in the position occupied by the thymus in man, or between the scapulae. This tissue is richly supplied with nerves and blood vessels. Histologically it is similar to the adrenal cortex. Bigelow, in Toronto, has made many attempts to establish the exact significance of this tissue in the role of hibernation. It maintains its size during hibernation and diminishes rapidly as the animal arouses, thus suggesting some function other than simple food storage. It appears to be directly related to the ability to hibernate, since those animals with the largest amount of this tissue hibernate most readily. Despite these findings, attempts to isolate an extract which will induce a state of hibernation in the same species of animal from which the extract was taken have failed.

Theories of Hibernation

There are two main conceptions of how the hibernation process is brought about. The first is based upon endocrine activity, believing that there is a decrease or increase of substances that are ordinarily present in the body. This theory does not easily explain why the animal should spontaneously rewarm at the approach of spring. The second concept postulates that the central nervous system acts as the controlling mechanism and that the whole process is analogous to turning down the thermostat in a centrally-heated house.

HYPOTHERMIA

Historical Note

Over the centuries only brief references have been made to the use of cold as a therapeutic agent in medicine, and most of these were confined to cooling local areas of the body. One of the most significant contributions first appeared in 1862, when Walther described the effect of cooling rabbits down to 20° C. It was not until nearly eighty years later, however, that Lawrence Smith and Temple Fay (1940) reported upon the use of general hypothermia in the treatment of malignant disease. The rationale of this therapy was based upon their histological finding that cold led to signs of retrogression and degeneration of neoplastic tissue—similar to that seen after radiotherapy. On the other hand, normal tissue was believed to be relatively insensitive to the effects of cold. Each patient was anaesthetised with intermittent doses of barbiturate and cooled by surrounding the nude body with ice. The body temperature was lowered to between 35°–29° C for 4–5 days and then rewarmed. After a rest period of two days a further treatment was given. The importance of this contribution did not lie in its effectiveness as a cancer cure but rather that it revealed the essential secret of hypothermia—namely, that sedation or anaesthesia (including muscle relaxants) must be used to control shivering.

In 1950, in Canada, Bigelow, Callaghan and Hopps drew attention to the advantages of the use of hypothermia in cardiac surgery, and since that time it has spread to nearly every large medical centre in the world. A further impetus to this was given by the report from New York of a negro girl who was admitted to hospital with a rectal temperature of 18° C (Laufman, 1951). This is the lowest body temperature so far reported in a supposedly unanaesthetised subject. Reassessing the available evidence, it appears that this girl had been drinking heavily and then lay unconscious upon the waterfront for many hours. Upon admission to hospital the respiratory rate was found to be three to five per minute and the pulse rate varied between twelve and twenty beats per minute. On rewarming she became conscious around 30° C but later had to have all four extremities amputated for frostbite. From 1952 onwards reports of the experimental and clinical use of hypothermia began to increase in number.

Physiology of Hypothermia

Although much work still remains to be done, many of the essential changes taking place in hypothermia have already been revealed. Clearly no detailed description of the fall in pulse rate, respiration rate, blood pressure and metabolism in relation to the drop in temperature of the body is required, since these all become reduced in an approximately linear fashion. On the whole all bodily functions slow down or are reduced *pari passu* with the degree of hypothermia. This statement, however, presupposes that the act of shivering has been suppressed.

Heat production in the body comes largely from two sources—the metabolism of the ordinary cells using glucose to supply nourishment, and the muscle fibres which produce large quantities of heat when they are in full contraction. Basal metabolism suggests that the muscle cells are quiescent but there is still a certain amount of heat coming from vital processes throughout the body. If shivering starts then there is an immediate and dramatic rise in the heat production.

Shivering.—The thermo-regulating mechanism in the conscious subject is a fairly complex one, which is essentially in two parts. A peripheral mechanism controlling the calibre of the blood vessels makes adjustments for minor variations in skin temperature. If, at any one moment, the temperature of the air in contact with skin alters, these vessels will dilate or constrict in an attempt to maintain an even body temperature. One of the most potent drugs in frustrating this mechanism is alcohol—hence the time-honoured warning against going out into the cold after a convivial evening. A more recent clinical method of producing vasodilatation is to use chlorpromazine. Major changes in the external temperature call for a more powerful protective mechanism. Thus, when the temperature of the blood reaching the brain falls about 0·5° C the *thermal nucleus* in the hypothalamus is stimulated. In lower animals this nucleus consists of two separate and distinct centres, one stimulated by a rise in body temperature (heat centre) and the other by a fall (cold centre). The exact site of the thermal centre in man is still unknown, but it is believed to lie in the grey matter of the posterior portion of the hypothalamus. However, afferent pathways pass from the hypothalamus to another important centre in the region of the thalamus—namely the shivering centre. The thermal nucleus is concerned with co-ordinating the peripheral response to changes in skin and blood temperature and is thus the principal thermo-regulating mechanism in the body. In this manner the body can suddenly increase heat production by as much as 400 per cent in a few seconds. In other words, the basal metabolic rate shoots up, and at the same time the pulse rate and blood pressure are increased. Although shivering is not a direct form of autonomic activity, it is closely linked with this part of the nervous system.

The shivering reflex can be inhibited in one of two ways. First, by depression of the thermal nucleus of the hypothalamus with anaesthetic drugs—any agent capable of producing a moderate depth of anaesthesia is suitable. Secondly, the muscle movements of shivering can be prevented by giving a small dose of a muscle relaxant. The shivering reflex, therefore, holds the key to the successful application of hypothermia. If this muscle activity can be prevented, then under the influence of anaesthesia a homothermic man can be converted to a poikilotherm.

Metabolic rate.—The fall in metabolism runs *pari passu* with the fall in body temperature if shivering is prevented. Animal studies have suggested that when the body temperature reaches levels as low as 15° to 10° C metabolism has reached negligible proportions (Lynn *et al.*, 1954). This has not been borne out in clinical practice because Benazon (1960), using deep hypothermia (15–10° C) in man, found evidence of a steadily falling venous oxygen saturation during a period of circulatory arrest. This emphasises that even at these very low temperatures some cellular metabolism is still persisting and that for any given temperature there is clearly a limit for the period of circulatory arrest. These times have never been officially prescribed but the figures given below are an approximate guide (based on oesophageal temperatures) for the human body (Table 1).

46/Table 1

Body temperature	°C	*Safe period of circulatory arrest*
Normal	37	3 minutes
Mild hypothermia	30	10 minutes

Carbohydrate metabolism.—Hypothermia is believed to interfere with the intracellular enzymatic reaction concerned with glucose metabolism (Wynn, 1956). A rise in the blood sugar occurs partly due to decreased insulin liberation and partly to reduced liver metabolism. This situation can be further aggravated by infusion of a glucose solution. The increased concentration of glucose in the extracellular fluid leads to water being withdrawn from the interior of the cell by osmosis; in turn, the increase in the size of the extracellular fluid compartment leads to a dilution of the serum sodium level, which can lead to an increase in myocardial irritability. Thus dextrose infusions are used sparingly and in dilute concentrations in the hypothermic patient.

Oxygen dissociation.—As blood cools, whether it be *in vitro* or *in vivo*, the dissociation curve for oxygen shifts to the left (Fig. 1). This means that for any given tension of oxygen the haemoglobin can carry less oxygen than it does at

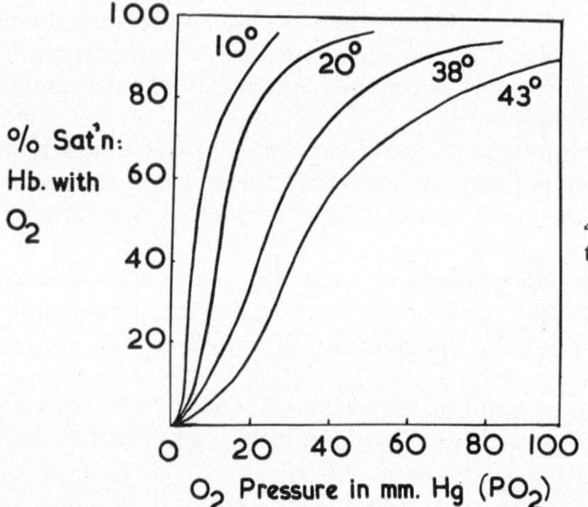

46/Fig. 1.—The effect of temperature on the oxygen dissociation curve.

normal temperatures. The result of this is to slow down the liberation of oxygen at the tissues. However, as can be seen in the hibernating animal, certain other compensatory actions take place—namely, an increase in the amount of carbon dioxide carried in the blood, haemoconcentration, and an increase in the amount of oxygen physically dissolved in the plasma.

On the whole, the shift of the curve to the left, which normally would prejudice the release of oxygen from haemoglobin, is counteracted by the increased amount of carbon dioxide dissolved in the plasma. This tends to move the curve back towards the right again so that the tissues do not suffer from hypoxia. Despite all these theoretical considerations, it is now well established that hypothermia *per se* does not lead to an oxygen debt or deficit in the tissues if the perfusion of that organ is adequate.

Changes in respiratory function.—Severinghaus and Stupfel (1956) have demonstrated in animals that several changes take place in respiratory function during hypothermia. At 25° C the anatomical dead space is increased by 70–90 per cent. Since a similar increase can be obtained in warm animals by blocking vagal activity with atropine, it is suggested that deep hypothermia removes the inherent bronchoconstriction from vagal stimulation. The physiological dead space is also increased by this bronchodilatation, but the alveolar dead space remains unchanged. The arterial and alveolar carbon dioxide tension ratio is unaltered.

Body water.—During the initial stages of hypothermia, particularly when associated with the muscular activity of shivering, there is a shift of water out of the vascular system and a concomitant increase in interstitial and intracellular water. As hypothermia progresses, and after all shivering has ceased, these water shifts are reversed (Horvath and Spurr, 1956). The available evidence indicates that at low body temperatures the reduction in blood volume is the result of loss of plasma from the circulation, either by stagnation in the peripheral vessels or by loss of whole plasma into the extravascular space.

Acid-base balance.—Few other aspects of hypothermia have evoked such interest as the changes in the acid-base balance produced by cold. There is no doubt that as the temperature falls, so the perfusion of the tissues steadily diminishes until finally cardiac action ceases completely. In some cases, therefore, the reduction in blood flow is even greater than the fall in cellular metabolism so that a metabolic acidosis develops. During a period of complete circulatory arrest this whole situation is even further aggravated. Furthermore, hypothermia increases the perfusion difficulties of the tissues by raising the viscosity of the blood, and the poor peripheral perfusion may lead to intravascular agglutination ("sludging") in the capillaries (Keen and Gerbode, 1963). All these factors tend to increase the tissue ischaemia.

The problem of the metabolic acidosis of deep hypothermia has been approached in two different ways. First, there is no doubt that the augmentation of the circulation by an artificial pump will improve the peripheral circulation. The advocates of this approach have stressed the close relationship between the amount of the blood flow and the size of the metabolic acidosis—the greater the flow, the less the acidosis (Rehder *et al.*, 1962; Daw *et al.*, 1964; Michenfelder *et al.*, 1964). On the other hand, Burton (1964) has stressed the importance of the carbon dioxide level of the blood. He points out that if a patient is hyperventilated during the process of hypothermia then the P_{CO_2} will fall to a much lower level than can be achieved at normal temperatures. The combination of a low body temperature and a low P_{CO_2} will push the oxygen dissociation curve far to the left and may impair the availability of oxygen for the tissues (Callaghan *et al.*, 1961). If, however, hyperventilation with carbon dioxide absorption is not practised, but the P_{CO_2} is maintained at around 40 mm. Hg at all temperatures, then Burton claims that this method "enables the body spontaneously to correct any metabolic imbalance caused either by the addition of acid to the circulation or by the procedure of cooling." He found that the adoption of this technique has been accompanied by an improvement in the clinical condition of the patient and the avoidance of brain damage which had been seen in those cases in which the P_{CO_2} was allowed to fall.

The available evidence does not support the hypothesis that hypothermia *per se* interferes in any way with the essential oxidative enzyme processes, so that variations in the peripheral blood flow and the carbon dioxide tension of the blood appear to be the principal factors causing the metabolic acidosis of hypothermia.

Electrolyte changes.—There has been much controversy about the conflicting data concerning serum-electrolyte levels in animals during hypothermia.

46/Table 2

Summary of Possible Causes of Increased Irritability of Myocardium under Hypothermia

1. Developmental. Increasing incidence in adult life.
2. Hypoxia of myocardium.
3. Electrolyte changes (particularly calcium).
4. Alterations in the pH of blood.
5. Increased sensitivity to endogenous catecholamines (adrenaline and noradrenaline)

significantly increase the depth of hypothermia that can be reached with safety, it tends to lead to cardiac asystole rather than ventricular fibrillation.

Electrocardiographic changes.—It is of paramount importance that the heart action of any patient undergoing hypothermia should be continually monitored by the electrocardioscope. In the majority it is extremely rare to observe any abnormality in rhythm until a temperature of 28° C or below is reached. From this point onwards the incidence of arrhythmia gradually increases until at 25° C and lower it is common to observe some abnormality. The commonest is the ventricular extrasystole, but in the early stages some signs of atrioventricular block may be seen. As the temperature falls there is a gradual lengthening of the QRS interval, followed by depression of the S–T segment and inversion of the "T" wave. These changes signify a gradual "breaking up" of the contraction until at very low temperatures the PQRST complex as such is hardly recognisable. Once the zone of myocardial irritability has been reached, ventricular fibrillation or standstill may occur at any moment. Very often ventricular fibrillation starts with no premonitory sign, but sometimes it follows a burst of ventricular extrasystoles. (For normal E.C.G. patterns see p. 565 *et seq.*)

Osborn (1953) has drawn attention to a secondary wave that can sometimes be seen immediately following the "S" wave. It is believed to be a "current of injury" and is often observed in deep hypothermia. Similarly, a high take-off for the RS complex is also recognised, and when this occurs at normal temperatures it signifies coronary insufficiency or damage to the myocardium.

The cerebral circulation.—The cerebral blood flow and oxygen consumption decrease during hypothermia at approximately the same rate. The reduction in cerebral flow averages 6·7 per cent per degree of Centigrade fall, whereas the mean blood pressure falls at a slightly slower rate, i.e. 4·8 per cent per degree of Centigrade fall. Thus the cerebral vascular resistance increases as the temperature falls (Rosomoff, 1956).

In man, "cold narcosis"—a state where the body metabolism is so depressed that anaesthetic drugs are no longer required—is believed to occur around 28° C. However, Cooper and Kenyon (1957) have pointed out that many of their patients were acutely aware of their surroundings and discomforts during rewarming when their body temperature was only 29° C. It appears, therefore, that though the anaesthetic requirements of a patient at this temperature are minimal, some cerebration is still possible. A figure of 26–25° C for cold narcosis (without drugs) in man would seem more realistic.

The hepatic circulation.—Hypothermia reduces splanchnic blood flow and liver metabolism in direct proportion to the fall in body temperature. Thus, the detoxication of drugs such as narcotics or hypnotics can be seriously disturbed.

For example, Gray and his associates (1956) have pointed out that the half-life of free morphine in the plasma is increased from 3–4 minutes at 37° C to 94 minutes at 24° C. Similarly, prothrombin formation is also reduced so that the coagulation time of the blood is prolonged. Furthermore, Brewin and his colleagues (1955) have emphasised the deleterious effects caused by a period of circulatory arrest combined with a high venous pressure; the intense congestion tends to produce serious hepatic cellular damage.

The renal circulation.—As the body temperature falls so there is a progressive reduction in both renal blood flow and glomerular filtration rate. Andjus (1956) working with rats, found that hypothermia had a direct inhibitory effect upon the reabsorption of the renal tubules. In the range 23–18° C sodium reabsorption was completely inhibited, while glomerular filtration and urinary flow were still present. Gil-Rodriguez and O'Gorman (1970) studied the effects of profound hypothermia on renal function in 41 adult patients undergoing cardiac surgery. They observed that the glomerular filtration rate increased, and attributed this to increased blood flow secondary to profound vasodilatation at temperatures below 20° C. Urine flow, as might be expected under these circumstances, was also high and this was partially due to a reduction of sodium re-absorption by the proximal tubules. Potassium was excreted in exchange for sodium by the distal tubules. The period of cardiac arrest included in this technique lead to signs of renal damage during rewarming. In fact, normal renal function had not recovered even 36 hours after operation. This finding lead the authors to recommend including some extracorporeal circulation in this technique during the period of cardiac arrest.

Blood coagulation.—As hypothermia progresses, the clotting time of blood becomes prolonged. When the temperature reaches 25° C the coagulation time may be increased to twelve or fifteen minutes (Ross, 1954*a*). The cause of this prolongation of the coagulation time is clearly related to a fall in the platelet count, since during hypothermia at 20° C in dogs the level of platelets may fall to 10,000 or lower. On rewarming they rapidly reappear (Villalobos *et al.*, 1956). Apart from a reduction in platelets, there is also a reduction in the prothrombin time, a fall in the white count, and an increase in the bleeding time. Experimental evidence suggests that the spleen, liver and bone marrow are responsible for sequestrating the blood platelets during hypothermia.

On theoretical grounds, therefore, one might expect that increased bleeding would be one of the principal dangers of hypothermia. However, the whole slowing down of the circulation (i.e. reduced blood pressure, heart rate, or cardiac output) is such that there is usually less bleeding than at normal temperatures. One of the principal advantages of the prolonged coagulation time is that when an extracorporeal circulation is used during the cooling process it is no longer so necessary to use heparin to prevent the blood from clotting.

Stress and Hypothermia

The exposure to cold of a conscious subject produces a series of reactions which are commonly referred to as the stress syndrome. The changes that take place throughout the body are briefly reviewed below, viz.:

1. Increased secretion of ACTH.
2. Release of adrenaline from the adrenal medulla.

3. Increased excretion of adrenal cortical steroids.
4. Depletion of adrenal cortical lipoids.
5. Neutrophilic leucocytosis, eosinopenia and lymphopenia.

(Sarajas *et al.*, 1958.)

The exact significance of these changes is incompletely understood but various attempts have been made to study the effect of hypothermia on the stress response. Since cold itself is known to be a typical stressor it is clearly important to differentiate the effects of the anaesthetic drugs from those due to deep hypothermia before forming an opinion. In the anaesthetised state the changes of the stress response depend largely on the method of cooling used (surface or blood), the depth of the anaesthesia, and the presence or absence of shivering. In a well-conducted case there is a reduced output of antidiuretic hormone and the secretions of the adrenal glands—both cortical and medullary—fall in relation to body temperature.

No one knows whether or not hypothermia actually protects the body against stress. Certainly cold, surgical trauma, shivering and even anaesthesia can induce the stress response, while such drugs as halothane and chlorpromazine, which are commonly used during hypothermia, tend to mask the common changes of stress.

The output of 17-hydroxycorticoids in the adrenal venous blood of hypothermic dogs decreases as the temperature falls (Ganong *et al.*, 1955; Egdahl *et al.*, 1955). Similarly, the urinary excretion of total steroids and 17-ketosteroids remained virtually unaltered in both dogs and human beings subjected to hypothermia (Gray, 1955). This evidence suggests that hypothermia does not elicit a stress response. On the other hand Sarajas and his associates (1958) found that the induction of hypothermia may evoke fundamentally different adrenal cortical reaction patterns, depending upon the type of anaesthesia used. Barbiturates alone appeared to inhibit the stress response to progressive cooling. When the barbiturates were used in conjunction with ether or a nitrous oxide/oxygen/muscle-relaxant sequence, the hypothermia consistently induced the stress response.

It has been suggested that chlorpromazine in conjunction with hypothermia exhibits an anti-shock mechanism by inhibiting the adrenocortical response to stress (Courvoisier *et al.*, 1953). In fact some of the earliest reports of the use of this drug claimed that the mortality of severely injured personnel could be reduced if this technique was employed. Certainly many of the signs of "shock" and "stress" cannot be recognised in the presence of chlorpromazine because it is an extremely potent dilator of peripheral vessels.

In view of the widely contradictory reports upon this matter the relationship between hypothermia and the stress response remains unsolved. Furthermore, if it could be proved that hypothermia inhibited stress, it still remains to be seen whether this protection is beneficial or not.

Deep Hypothermia and Super-cooling

Drew and his colleagues (Drew *et al.*, 1959; Drew and Anderson, 1959) have obtained temperatures of 15° C for intracardiac operations with full recovery of patients following periods of circulatory arrest for as long as 45 minutes.Their technique makes use of blood-stream cooling and, during the process, establishes satisfactory pulmonary and systemic circulations by means of two pumps which take over the functions of the ventricles. The cooling process can then be continued below temperatures at which the heart would normally have ceased to function efficiently.

Using a technique of anaesthesia combining oxygen lack with carbon dioxide accumulation, Andjus and his associates (1956) have succeeded in cooling rats to 0° C and lower. The technique includes the sealing of the animals in glass jars together with cooling of the container. When the body temperature has fallen to about 15° C the animals are removed and partially immersed in an ice-cold water bath. Respiration ceases around 12° C, and the heart-beat stops around 7° C. On reaching zero Centigrade some of the animals continue to cool if the temperature of the water bath is below 0° C. These animals enter a state of super-cooling and the lowest recorded temperature with subsequent survival is – 5° C. This temperature has been maintained for as long as 70 minutes; during this time the animal remains limp. More commonly, the body temperature will not fall below 0° C, and the animal becomes stiff and solid. If an ear or a tail is accidentally knocked it just breaks off. Under the microscope actual ice crystals can be seen forming in the tissue spaces and the red cells can be seen rupturing on rewarming.

The results of this work are extremely impressive, but the grossly unphysiological mode of anaesthesia makes it difficult to see how it could be adopted for use in man.

Methods of Lowering the Body Temperature in Man

The secret of the induction of hypothermia lies in the abolition of the shivering reflex. In the conscious subject exposed to cold there is first a widespread vasoconstriction in the skin and then, if this is insufficient to maintain the normal body temperature, a tremendous increase in heat production takes place by using violent unco-ordinated muscle tremors—i.e. the act of shivering. Death, if it occurs, is probably due to circulatory failure long before there has been a significant fall in the body temperature. If shivering is prevented, however, the temperature of the body falls until it reaches that of its environment. Consequently, most anaesthetised patients will show some slight degree of cooling, but as operating theatres are usually warm and the patients well covered during operation, this is seldom more than 1 or 2° C. However, if adequate precautions are not taken during long operations, and particularly for paediatric patients, the body temperature may fall to a dangerously low level. Patients who are subjected to a long thoracotomy or laparotomy will lose heat more rapidly than those undergoing a simple operative procedure upon a limb. Nevertheless, it must be remembered that anaesthesia *per se* does not necessarily produce the conditions for hypothermia. The depth of anaesthesia must be sufficient to prevent shivering. This reflex arc involving brain, spinal cord, and muscle fibres can be inhibited either by a moderate depth of anaesthesia or by light anaesthesia coupled with a muscle relaxant.

Hypothermia has now become so much a routine part of anaesthetic technique that the methods available have resolved themselves into two main groups. First, *surface* cooling, which is used primarily to attain mild hypothermia (30° C) for cardiac, vascular and cranial surgery in which only a short period of circulatory arrest is required. Secondly, *blood* cooling which is principally used in association with the extracorporeal circulation to attain deep hypothermia (15–10° C) for more prolonged periods of cardiac standstill.

Surface cooling.—There are three principal methods of surface cooling:

1. *Immersion* (Fig. 2).—The direct contact of cold water with the skin is the simplest, most rapid and efficient method of cooling the body. Following induction of anaesthesia the patient is stripped and then placed in a bath of cold water (4–10° C). The speed of cooling will depend principally on the temperature gradient between the patient's body temperature and that of the surrounding bath. It will also be strongly influenced by the amount of insulation the patient possesses in the way of subcutaneous fat.

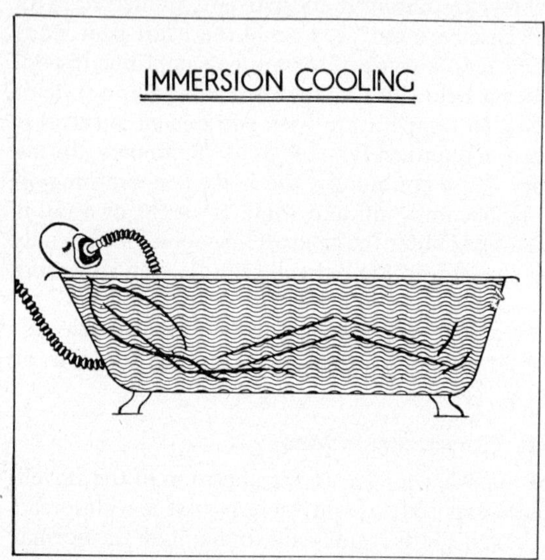

46/Fig. 2.—Method of immersion cooling.

The principal disadvantage of this method is the difficulty of transporting the unconscious patient into and out of a bath of water. Many ingenious devices, including a collapsible canvas bath, have been described in an attempt to overcome these difficulties. During removal of the patient from the bath it is particularly important not to raise suddenly the lower limbs, as this may lead to the immediate arrival of some very cold blood in the thorax, thus increasing the risk of ventricular fibrillation. Using this technique, the average adult body can be cooled within one hour from 37 to 30° C. As a general rule muscular males cool more quickly than fat females.

2. *Evaporation* (Fig. 3).—Although less efficient than immersion cooling, this technique is easier to perform. The patient can be positioned for surgery before commencing the hypothermia and therefore does not require any movement once the desired level of cooling has been reached. First, the skin is thoroughly wetted, then evaporation is achieved by creating a wind-tunnel around the patient with the aid of electric fans. As evaporation and heat loss proceed, so more water must be applied to the skin. In order to speed cooling,

ice-bags are placed at strategic points where the main vessels lie close to the skin surface, e.g. neck, axilla and groin. Using this technique, the average adult body can be cooled from 37 to 30° C in 1½–2 hours.

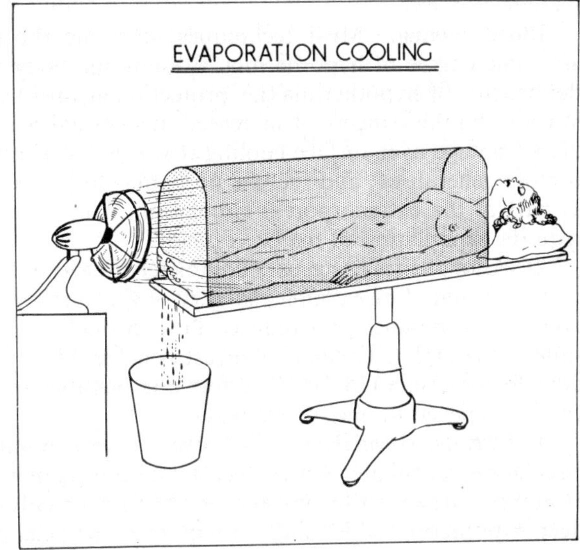

46/FIG. 3.—Method of evaporation cooling.

3. *Cooling blanket.*—Specially constructed blankets are available which consist of a long length of malleable tubing incorporated in a blanket. Very cold water or solutions are pumped through the tubing. This system is the most convenient yet the least efficient of all the methods of surface cooling. Not only must the solution in the blanket first cool the outer covering, but where this covering is not in direct contact with the skin the intermediate gap of air will tend to act as an insulator, preventing the fall in body temperature. Since the fluid perfusing the blanket is usually at a temperature less than 0° C, it is most important that no part of the skin should remain in direct contact with one part of the blanket for a prolonged time, lest an ice-burn be formed. Using this technique, the average adult body can be cooled from 37 to 30° C in 2–2½ hours.

One of the principal dangers of surface cooling is the "after-drop" or "overshoot" that occurs when the cooling process is withdrawn. When the ice-bags or the blanket are removed it is understandable that the neighbouring skin and tissues are extremely cold. In fact, they are much colder than the temperature of the circulating blood. Thus as the blood reaches these parts it continues to cool long after the active processes have been withdrawn. In using surface cooling, therefore, allowance for this "after-drop" must always be made. The extent or size of this overshoot depends upon the speed of cooling. If the body temperature has dropped rapidly, i.e. from 37–32° C in one hour—then one might well anticipate a drop of at least another 2° C, if not 3° C, during the next half hour if no direct steps to rewarm are taken. On the other hand, if the cooling has been slow—i.e. 37–32° C in two hours—then there will be only a small after-drop.

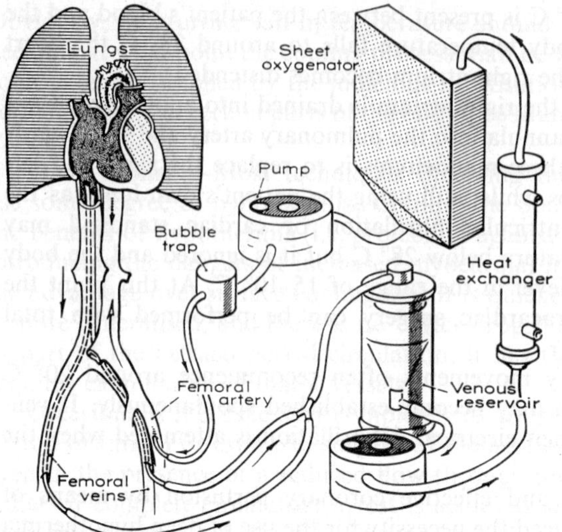

46/FIG. 5.—Method of closed-chest deep hypothermia for neurosurgery.

directly to the brain. In this manner they have achieved a temperature in the brain of 20° C whilst the general body temperature was still 30° C. Daw and his associates (1964) report on the use of a similar technique in one patient in whom a cerebral temperature of 15° C was attained. This method has possibilities for development in the future since the higher body temperature reduces the risk of cardiac arrhythmia yet the maximum degree of cerebral cooling is also obtained.

Anaesthesia for the Hypothermic Patient

Premedication for a patient about to undergo hypothermia should be light and respiratory depressant drugs should be restricted as far as possible because they tend to arrest respiration at a much higher temperature than usual. Chlorpromazine is a particularly useful premedicant drug because not only does it produce widespread peripheral vasodilatation which aids cooling, but it also sedates the patient without depressing respiration.

The choice of anaesthetic drugs is based upon the knowledge that the metabolism and renal excretion of the hypothermic patient is severely depressed, and at temperatures of about 26° C and below a state of "cold anaesthesia" exists where the patient no longer requires anaesthetic drugs. It is important, therefore, not to use large doses of the barbiturates, which are only slowly eliminated in such circumstances, whereas the volatile agents, such as ether, can satisfactorily be used. Cyclopropane has the disadvantage that it increases the myocardial irritability at normal temperatures, so is best avoided in the hypothermic patient.

Ether produces both peripheral vasodilatation and a stabilising effect on myocardial activity but cannot be used in the presence of diathermy for fear of causing an explosion. Halothane, on the other hand, is non-inflammable and leads to intense peripheral vasodilatation so that it has gained great popularity as the anaesthetic agent of choice for surface cooling. However, it can only be used in low concentrations because its hypotensive action tends to reduce the systemic pressure to an abnormally low level and this increases the risk of ventricular fibrillation. The final choice of anaesthetic depends upon the operation. For a thoracotomy or laparotomy a technique using thiopentone, halothane, nitrous oxide, oxygen sequence in combination with a muscle relaxant is employed. The induction dose of thiopentone should rarely exceed 200–400 mg. in such cases. Halothane in a concentration of 0·5 per cent augments nitrous oxide and oxygen. *d*-Tubocurarine has been found the most satisfactory relaxant drug for prolonged paresis, as its effects appear to be readily reversible with an anticholinesterase drug even at a temperature as low as 30° C. The effect of the cold, together with the reduced peripheral blood flow, tends to prolong the action of the muscle relaxants (see Chapter 30, p. 833). Nevertheless, the use of a muscle relaxant during the induction of hypothermia is particularly beneficial because it can abolish shivering if given in an adequate dose, but good ventilation must then be maintained by intermittent positive pressure. Small intermittent doses of chlorpromazine (5–10 mg.) are sometimes given in the early stages to promote vasodilatation and speed the cooling process.

When the continuous use of muscle relaxants is not essential for the operation, a moderate depth of inhalational anaesthesia (Stage III, Plane II) from ether or halothane, is satisfactory. Indeed the rate of cooling is probably quicker with these agents than with a technique primarily dependent upon the muscle relaxants. There is, therefore, much to be said for their use in the first place during the induction of hypothermia for all operations, followed by the judicious substitution of a muscle relaxant (if needed for the operation) when a satisfactory temperature has been reached, and just prior to the start of the surgical procedure.

Management of the Hypothermic Patient

This is similar to that of any other patient undergoing cardiac, cranial or general surgery, but there are certain points which require special attention.

Body temperature measurements.—These are best made with a standardised thermometer graduated to one-tenth of a degree Centigrade covering the range 0–45° C or with a suitable thermocouple. A thermometer is often chosen in preference to a thermocouple largely on the grounds of reliability and accuracy. It is particularly important during hypothermia that a true reading of the patient's body temperature is always readily available so that it is not allowed to fall too low. Thus, any thermocouple reading must be regularly checked with a standardised mercury thermometer.

The oesophageal temperature is the most frequently used since this site is close to the heart and great vessels. If a glass thermometer is used, in order to guard against breakage, the shaft of the thermometer is closely surrounded by a metal tube which extends from just above the mercury-filled bulb to a point just outside the mouth. This leaves the range 25–45° C exposed and easily visible. In cranial surgery the nasopharyngeal temperature is probably more reliable as a guide than the oesophageal because it is closer to the brain temperature. The rectal temperature is less useful because it lags by at least 1–2° behind the oesophageal temperature both during the cooling and the rewarming process. Further, if there is any interference with the blood supply of the lower part of the body—

as may occur during operations for an abdominal aneurysm—the rectal temperature figures will be misleading.

Level of hypothermia.—It is now generally accepted that 30° C is the optimum level for surface cooling. Lower temperatures can be used but these should always be combined with an extracorporeal circulation. Young children tolerate lower temperatures better than adults, and in these patients the optimal level is usually taken as 28° C. There is no fixed time that the cerebral cells can withstand circulatory arrest at 30° C, but it is generally agreed that at normal temperatures about three minutes total occlusion is sufficient to produce signs of damage, whereas under hypothermia (30° C) a time interval of at least three times that duration has elapsed without signs of injury. However, in these circumstances it would be unwise to exceed an interval of eight minutes.

Maintenance of hypothermia.—Once a satisfactory temperature level has been reached the patient can usually be stabilised at a given temperature without difficulty. Care must be taken not to influence the body temperature adversely by using very hot theatre lamps, cold packs or ice-cold infusions. The room temperature in the theatre is usually only a little below that of the patient's body, so that there is small chance with the poor skin circulation of the body losing much heat. The usual practice is to lay the patient on an electric blanket covered by macintosh sheeting. In surface cooling if the temperature shows signs of falling too fast or too low, the heating-blanket is turned on for a short time. In this technique it is important to be thinking and planning well ahead, since the application of warmth under such conditions is rarely followed by a rise in body temperature for at least half an hour. On the other hand, it may slow down the cooling process more quickly. If the temperature is found to be rising, further cooling must be carried out. Towards the close of the operation steps should be taken to commence rewarming.

Movement of the hypothermic patient.—Changing the patient's position can be particularly dangerous, because the sudden raising of the lower limbs may return a large quantity of very cold blood into the main circulation. Since the heart muscle is very sensitive to sudden changes in temperature this sudden transfusion may be sufficient to provoke ventricular fibrillation. If the patient is placed upon the operating table in the correct position for surgery before cooling is commenced this risk is obviated. The most likely cause of trouble in this connection is when immersion cooling is used for infants, because when the child is lifted out of the bath extra cold blood may enter the main circulation.

Speed of cooling.—The optimum rate of cooling has never been determined. A rapid method of dropping the body temperature is only dangerous if it permits the heart suddenly to receive much colder blood. Some blood cooling methods with the extracorporeal circulation maintain a drop of body temperature of 1° C per minute without apparent harm. Slow cooling, on the other hand, offers no particular advantage. It is important that whatever method of cooling is used, the fall in temperature should be spread as evenly as possible throughout the body. If the circulation is sluggish then widespread temperature differentials are achieved when surface cooling is used. In fact, it is possible to create a situation where the temperature in the big toe is 4° C whereas that of the brain is still 37° C. Thus an optimum time for a fall of body temperature from 37° C to 30° C would appear to be 1–1½ hours.

Precautions.—Safety control largely depends upon the use of continual electrocardiographic monitoring. The first sign of a persistent cardiac arrhythmia in a patient who previously had normal rhythm is an indication for rewarming to a higher temperature. In such a case it is not necessary to abandon hypothermia altogether, but rather to select a higher temperature as the base-line.

Infusions.—During hypothermia the whole metabolism is depressed and therefore the burning of exogenous glucose is slowed up. If 5 per cent dextrose is infused in large quantities over a period of a few hours, the blood sugar may rise to an astronomical figure. Wynn (1954) has shown that when hyperglycaemia develops under such conditions the plasma sodium and plasma total protein levels fall. The reason for this fall, together with that of the other electrolytes, is the haemodilution caused by the osmotic action of the glucose withdrawing water into the circulation from the cells and tissue spaces. Similarly the low renal function of hypothermia means that salt solutions will not be readily excreted. It is advisable, therefore, to use only half-strength solutions in hypothermia and to limit these to the body's requirements. A generous fluid intake of water is beneficial because it causes a water diuresis during the rewarming period and rapidly re-establishes a good urinary flow. Any haemorrhage is best treated by blood transfusion, and with a careful check on blood loss (using a swab-weighing technique) it should be possible to keep the blood volume at a normal level, after allowing for the slight tendency to haemoconcentration under hypothermia. High plasma citrate levels may occur during the infusion of citrated blood during hypothermia, since the metabolic destruction of this compound is reduced (Ludbrook and Wynn, 1958).

Temperature of infused solutions.—Particular attention must be paid to the temperature of infused solutions, since it is easy to lower a patient's body temperature too much by the rapid transfusion of blood taken straight from the refrigerator. In certain cardiac and aortic operations large quantities of blood may be urgently needed; during the operation a sufficient quantity of the correct blood should therefore be present in the operating theatre and this blood must be kept at a temperature close to that of the hypothermic patient. In practice, it is wise to keep the blood temperature a few degrees higher than the patient's in case of an accident when rapid rewarming might be required.

Heat exchanger.—These instruments have now become so efficient that it is important to consider the temperature differential if one of them is used in conjunction with the extracorporeal circulation for deep hypothermia. A difference of 12° C between the temperature of the water in the exchanger and that of the incoming blood is recommended. A much greater differential can lead to bubble formation when blood emerges from the apparatus so that there is a risk of gas emboli. Furthermore, very cold blood suddenly reaching the heart increases the risk of ventricular fibrillation.

Blood coagulation.—Despite the fact that hypothermia increases the clotting time, it has still been found necessary to heparinise the patient if cannulation of vessels is attempted. Daw and his colleagues (1964) have recommended repeating one-half the original dose about an hour after the start of the perfusion. This suggestion is based on some evidence that part of the original heparin is destroyed in the apparatus resulting in the formation of microclots of fibrin which are deposited both in the apparatus and in the body.

Metabolic acidosis.—This is sometimes encountered in patients with a prolonged perfusion time or in which only a low flow has been used. Alterations in the acid-base balance obviously occur following a period of circulatory arrest, but severe disturbances arising in the post-operative period are considered to be due mainly to a poor perfusion rate during the cooling process. Frequent monitoring of the pH and the buffer base concentration should be undertaken in all patients undergoing deep hypothermia; if necessary the change in the acid-base balance should be remedied by the infusion of sodium bicarbonate in suitable quantities.

Carbon dioxide.—Although it is common practice to use a carbon dioxide absorption technique in association with artificial hyperventilation for anaesthesia at normal temperatures, evidence is accumulating that this practice may be harmful when the body temperature is reduced (Zinn and Warnock, 1960; Burton, 1964; Broom and Sellick, 1965). The combination of cold and a low carbon dioxide tension of the blood can seriously reduce the availability of oxygen to the tissues and by reducing systemic blood pressure it can increase the risk of ventricular fibrillation. Furthermore, a low carbon dioxide tension reduces the cerebral blood flow.

Although these factors are not of great significance in mild hypothermia, it would appear to be more satisfactory to try to maintain a normal carbon dioxide level (P_{CO_2} of 40 mm. Hg) at all levels of body temperature. In order to achieve this in the presence of deep hypothermia it is necessary to add carbon dioxide to the gases exposed to the blood ; the exact amount is best determined by careful monitoring of the pH and P_{CO_2} levels of the perfusing blood.

Rewarming

Since the anaesthetised patient is poikilothermic, any rise in the temperature of his environment will be reflected in his body temperature. The simplest method, therefore, of rewarming the hypothermic patient is first to apply warmth to the skin and then when the patient has reached a reasonably safe temperature (i.e. 32–33° C) to withdraw the anaesthetic and allow him to regain consciousness and become homothermic once again. As the anaesthetic wears off, so muscle movements and internal heat production are resumed. In many instances shivering does not occur in the rewarming phase, presumably because the effects of external warmth upon the skin inhibit the stimulus of the cold blood bathing the shivering centre. In some cases, however, shivering does occur, and it is most important—particularly after cardiac operations—that it should be inhibited as soon as possible by sedation, otherwise it will throw an extra burden upon the myocardium and may lead to circulatory failure.

Skin rewarming.—The principal danger of any form of surface rewarming is that the skin blood flow in the hypothermic patient is extremely low, and for this reason a hot water bottle which would be considered merely to be warm by a normothermic patient, might be likened to red hot coal by a hypothermic one. Great care should be taken to avoid localised areas of heating as these may ultimately lead to burns. The most satisfactory technique is to surround the patient with warm blankets and then, over these to place a warm electric blanket, and finally to cover the whole with further blankets to prevent the heat escaping into the atmosphere. In the early stages a deliberate attempt is made to reverse the hypothermic process, but once the body temperature has reached 33–34° C it is safe to turn off all active forms of heating and merely permit the patient to rewarm himself slowly during the next few hours. In practice, once the anaesthetic has been withdrawn and consciousness has been regained the patient rapidly reaches a normal body temperature. Occasionally, owing to the instability of the temperature-regulating mechanism, a hyperpyrexia may develop and this may necessitate tepid sponging of the patient.

Blood rewarming.—This method can be employed if a cannulation technique has been used, but great care must be taken to keep the blood circulating in order to avoid coagulation. The cannulae are usually withdrawn once the body temperature has reached 33° C.

Complications of Hypothermia

Far and away the most important complication of hypothermia is the sudden and spontaneous onset of ventricular *fibrillation* or *cardiac standstill.* In cardiac surgery such an occurrence is generally not serious, since normal rhythm can usually be easily restored. In cranial surgery or in other patients without an open thoracotomy it may, however, prove fatal. Provided the body temperature is not allowed to fall below 30° C this complication can usually be avoided unless the heart is actually handled.

During an intracardiac procedure arrhythmias are usually ignored until the lesion has been repaired. In any event, if fibrillation ensues the myocardial temperature must be raised before attempting to restore a normal rhythm. This is best done by repeatedly filling the pericardial cavity with warm saline at a temperature not greater than 38° C. Cardiac standstill must be treated by continuous massage until normal rhythm is resumed, or at worst fibrillation intervenes. The occurrence of ventricular fibrillation demands the use of an electrical defibrillator, but only when the fibrillation is vigorous and the tone of the cardiac muscle is good (see Chapter 28).

Ice-burns are a common feature if solutions colder than 0° C are allowed to remain in contact with the skin for any length of time. Similarly, *heat-burns* may occur from over-enthusiastic rewarming. In this respect hot water bottles are particularly likely to lead to trouble, and care should be taken to see that they are not filled with water at more than 40° C.

Haemorrhage due to the prolongation of the coagulation time has also been suggested as a complication of hypothermia, and therefore great care must be taken to arrest all bleeding points before closing the wound.

Following deep hypothermia (30° C or lower) and prolonged hypotension, certain psychological changes have been noted. These consist mainly of a slight euphoria with confusion. As yet it has not been possible to determine the exact role—if any—played by the fall in body temperature.

Indications for the Use of Hypothermia

Any operation which requires the interruption of the circulation to any of the vital organs—the brain in particular—should be considered for hypothermia. Thus, some intracardiac, cranial and vascular procedures require the lowering of body temperature to prevent hypoxic changes in the vital tissues. Of the intracardiac group, closure of an atrial septal defect under direct vision commonly calls for this treatment. Similarly, open operations for the correction of pulmonary or aortic valve lesions often require this form of anaesthetic technique although the current tendency is to use cardio-pulmonary by-pass for these procedures. The kidneys can rarely stand more than twenty minutes without blood and therefore hypothermia adds a useful protection to these organs. Similarly, the hepatic cells are extremely susceptible to hypoxia. It is unnecessary however, to use hypothermia if the aorta is to be clamped below the level of the superior mesenteric and renal arteries, since the tissues below this level can withstand up to two hours or more of reduced blood flow without showing signs of injury afterwards.

In cranial surgery the commonest operations requiring the use of hypothermia are those in which excessive bleeding is anticipated, as, for example, in certain vascular tumours or aneurysms (see also Chapter 39). Some neurosurgeons favour the use of hypothermia for almost all large intracranial procedures, on the basis that when combined with hypotension the brain is smaller and there is less oozing. Certainly, hypothermia can readily be combined with ordinary hypotensive techniques, and theoretically it is better to lower the metabolism of the cells (hypothermia) than to run the risk of merely reducing their blood supply (induced hypotension).

Aneurysms of the carotid artery or of the thoracic and abdominal aorta often require the use of hypothermia. In man the occlusion of even one carotid artery for a short period of time is sometimes followed by signs of cerebral damage. It may be advisable, therefore, to incorporate hypothermia in the anaesthetic technique if such a procedure is contemplated during the operation.

Mild hypothermia has been used extensively in the treatment of traumatic cerebral injuries. However, such cases are difficult to control and the possible beneficial action of body cooling is difficult to determine. Rosomoff and his colleagues (1960) working with animals subjected to an experimental brain injury found that hypothermia improved the survival rate if it was started within three hours of the injury. No advantage was claimed if it was delayed for 7 to 8 hours. On the basis of this evidence, many clinicians feel there is sufficient justification for the immediate institution of hypothermia following the onset of cardiac arrest associated with anaesthesia (see also Chapter 45). Hendrick (1959) used hypothermia to treat children suffering from decerebrate rigidity due to a severe head injury. The advantage claimed for the lowering of the body temperature is that not only does it lower cerebrospinal fluid pressure and metabolism, but that it also partially protects the brain against the deleterious effects of the trauma.

REFERENCES

ADOLPH, E. F. (1951*a*). Some differences in response to low temperatures between warm-blooded and cold-blooded vertebrates. *Amer. J. Physiol.*, **166,** 92.

ADOLPH, E. F. (1951*b*). Responses to hypothermia in several species of infant mammals. *Amer. J. Physiol.*, **166,** 75.

ANDJUS, R. K. (1956). Effect of hypothermia on the kidney. *Proc. nat. Acad. Sci.* (*Wash.*), **451,** 214.

ANDJUS, R. K., LOVELOCK, J. E., and SMITH, A. U. (1956). Resuscitation and recovery of hypothermic, supercooled and frozen mammals. *Proc. nat. Acad. Sci.* (*Wash.*), **451,** 125.

BENAZON, D. (1960). The experimental and clinical use of profound hypothermia. *Anaesthesia*, **15,** 134.

BIGELOW, W. G., CALLAGHAN, J. C., and HOPPS, J. A. (1950). General hypothermia for experimental intracardiac surgery. *Ann. Surg.*, **132,** 531.

BREWIN, E. G., GOULD, R. P., NASHAT, F. S., and NEIL, E. (1955). An investigation of problems of acid-base equilibrium in hypothermia. *Guy's Hosp. Rep.*, **104,** 177.

BROOM, B., and SELLICK, B. A. (1965). Controlled hypercapnia in open heart surgery under hypothermia. *Lancet*, **2,** 452.

BURTON, G. W. (1964). Metabolic acidosis during profound hypothermia. *Anaesthesia*, **19,** 365.

CALLAGHAN, P. B., LISTER, J., PATON, B. C., and SWAN, H. (1961). Effects of varying carbon dioxide tensions on the oxyhaemoglobin dissociation curves under hypothermic conditions. *Ann. Surg.*, **154,** 903.

CHURCHILL-DAVIDSON, H. C. (1957). Personal communication.

COOPER, K. E., and KENYON, J. R. (1957). A comparison of the temperature measured in the rectum, oesophagus, and on the surface of the aorta during hypothermia in man. *Brit. J. Surg.*, **44,** 616.

COURVOISIER, S., FOURNEL, J., DUCROT, R., KOLSKY, M., and KOETSCHET, P. (1953). Propriétés pharmacodynamiques du chlorohydrate de chloro-3(diméthylamino-3-propyl)-10 phénothiazine (4,560 R.P.); étude experimentale d'un nouveau corps utilisé dans l'anaesthésie potentialisée et dans l'hibernation artificielle. *Arch. int. Pharmacodyn.*, **92,** 305.

COVINO, B. G., MARGOLIS, N., and D'AMATO, H. E. (1959). Effects of various drugs on spontaneous and surgically induced ventricular fibrillation in hypothermia. *Amer. Heart J.*, **58,** 750.

CURRIE, T. T., CASS, N. M., and HICKS, J. D. (1962). The scope of surface cooling. An experimental study using quinidine as a prophylactic against ventricular fibrillation. *Anaesthesia*, **17,** 46.

DAW, E. F., MOFFITT, E. A., MICHENFELDER, J. D., and TERRY, H. R. (1964). Profound hypothermia. *Canad. Anaesth. Soc. J.*, **11,** 382.

DELORME, E. J. (1951). Arterial perfusion of the liver in shock. An experimental study. *Lancet*, **1,** 259.

DREW, C. E. and ANDERSON, I. M. (1959). Profound hypothermia in cardiac surgery. Report of three cases. *Lancet*, **1,** 748.

DREW, C. E., KEEN, G., and BENAZON, D. B. (1959). Profound hypothermia. *Lancet*, **1,** 745.

EGDAHL, R. H., NELSON, D. H., and HUME, D. M. (1955). The effect of hypothermia on 17-hydroxycorticosteroid secretion in adrenal venous blood in the dog. *Science*, **121,** 506.

ELLIOTT, H. W., and CRISMON, J. M. (1947). Increased sensitivity of hypothermic rats to injected potassium and the influence of calcium, digitalis, and glucose on survival. *Amer. J. Physiol.*, **151,** 366.

GANONG, W. F., BERNHARD, W. F., and MCMURREY, J. D. (1955). The effect of hypothermia on the output of 17-hydroxycorticoids from the adrenal vein in the dog. *Surgery*, **38,** 506.

GIL-RODRIGUEZ, J. L., and O'GORMAN, P. (1970). Renal function during profound hypothermia. *Brit. J. Anaesth.*, **42,** 557.

GOLLAN, F., PHILLIPS, R., GRACE, J. T., and JONES, R. M. (1955). Open left heart surgery in dogs during hypothermic asystole with and without extracorporeal circulation. *J. thorac. Surg.*, **30,** 626.

GRAY, I., RVECKERT, R. R., and RINK, R. R. (1956). Effect of hypothermia on metabolism and drug detoxification in the isolated perfused rabbit liver. *Proc. nat. Acad. Sci.* (*Wash.*), **451,** 226.

GRAY, T. C. (1955). Discussion on induced hypothermia. *Proc. roy. Soc. Med.*, **48,** 1083.

HEGNAUER, A. H., and D'AMATO, H. E. (1954). Oxygen consumption and cardiac output in the hypothermic dog. *Amer. J. Physiol.*, **178,** 138.

HEGNAUER, A. H., SHRIBER, W. J., and HATERIUS, H. O. (1950). Cardiovascular response of dog to immersion hypothermia. *Amer. J. Physiol.*, **161,** 455.

HENDRICK, E. B. (1959). The use of hypothermia in severe head injuries in childhood. *A.M.A. Arch. Surg.*, **79,** 362.

HORVATH, S. M., and SPURR, G. B. (1956). Effects of hypothermia on general metabolism. *Proc. nat. Acad. Sci.* (*Wash.*), **451,** 8.

JENSEN, J. M., PARKINS, W. M., and VARS, H. M. (1956). Possibilities and limitations of differential brain cooling in dogs. *Proc. nat. Acad. Sci.* (*Wash.*), **451,** 271.

JOHNSON, P., LESAGE, A., FLOYD, W. L., YOUNG, W. G., and SEALY, W. C. (1960). Prevention of ventricular fibrillation during profound hypothermia by quinidine. *Ann. Surg.*, **151,** 490.

KEEN, G., and GERBODE, F. (1963). Observations on the microcirculation during profound hypothermia. *J. thorac. cardiovasc. Surg.*, **45,** 252.

KHALIL, H. H., and MACKEITH, R. C. (1954). A simple method of raising and lowering body temperature. *Brit. med. J.*, **2,** 734.

LANGE, K., WEINER, D., and GOLD, M. M. A. (1949). Studies on the mechanism of cardiac injury in experimental hypothermia. *Ann. intern. Med.*, **31,** 989.

LAUFMAN, H. (1951). Profound accidental hypothermia. *J. Amer. med. Ass.*, **147,** 1201.

LUDBROOK, J., and WYNN, V. (1958). Citrate intoxication. A clinical and experimental study. *Brit. med. J.*, **2,** 523.

LYNN, R. B., MELROSE, D. G., CHURCHILL-DAVIDSON, H. C., and MCMILLAN, I. K. R. (1954). Hypothermia: further observations on surface cooling. *Ann. roy. Coll. Surg. Engl.*, **14,** 267.

MCMILLAN, I. K. R., CASE, R. B., STAINSBY, W. N., and WELCH, G. H. (1957). The hypothermic heart. *Thorax*, **12,** 208.

MCMILLAN, I. K. R., MELROSE, D. G., CHURCHILL-DAVIDSON, H. C., and LYNN, R. B. (1955). Hypothermia: some observations on blood gas and electrolyte changes during surface cooling. *Ann. roy. Coll. Surg. Engl.*, **16,** 186.

MICHENFELDER, J. D., MACCARTY, C. S., and THEYE, R. A. (1964). Physiologic studies following closed-chest technique of profound hypothermia in neurosurgery. *Anesthesiology*, **25,** 131.

MICHENFELDER, J. D., TERRY, H. R., DAW, E. F., MACCARTY, C. S., and UIHLEIN, A. (1963). Profound hypothermia in neurosurgery: open-chest versus closed-chest techniques. *Anesthesiology*, **24,** 117.

OSBORN, J. J. (1953). Experimental hypothermia: respiratory and pH changes in relation to cardiac function. *Amer. J. Physiol.*, **175,** 389.

PENROD, K. E. (1951). Cardiac oxygenation during severe hypothermia in dog. *Amer. J. Physiol.*, **164,** 79.

REHDER, K., KIRKLIN, J. W., MACCARTY, C. S., and THEYE, R. A. (1962). Physiologic studies following profound hypothermia and circulatory arrest for treatment of intracranial aneurysm. *Ann. Surg.*, **156,** 882.

ROSOMOFF, H. L. (1956). Hypothermia and the central nervous system. *Proc. nat. Acad. Sci.* (*Wash.*), **451**, 253.

ROSENHAIN, F. R., and PENROD, K. E. (1951). Blood gas studies in the hypothermic dog. *Amer. J. Physiol.*, **166,** 55.

ROSOMOFF, H. L., SHULMAN, K., RAYNOR, R., and GRAINGER, W. (1960). Experimental brain injuries and delayed hypothermia. *Surg. Gynec. Obstet.*, **110**, 27.

ROSS, D. N. (1954*a*). Physiological observations during hypothermia. *Guy's Hosp. Rep.*, **103,** 116.

ROSS, D. N. (1954*b*). Venous cooling. A new method of cooling the blood-stream. *Lancet*, **1,** 1108.

SARAJAS, H. S. S., MYHOLM, P., and SOUMALAINEN, P. (1958). Stress in hypothermia. *Nature* (*Lond.*), **181** (4609), 612.

SEVERINGHAUS, J. W., and STUPFEL, M. (1956). Respiratory physiologic studies during hypothermia. *Proc. nat. Acad. Sci.* (*Wash.*), **451,** 52.

SMITH, L. W., and FAY, T. (1940). Observations on human beings with cancer, maintained at reduced temperatures of 75–90° Fahrenheit. *Amer. J. clin. Path.*, **10,** 1.

SVIHLA, A., and BOWMAN, H. C. (1952). Oxygen carrying capacity of the blood of dormant ground squirrels. *Amer. J. Physiol.*, **171,** 479.

SWAN, H., ZEAVIN, I., BLOUNT, S. G., Jr., and VIRTUE, R. W. (1953*a*). Surgery by direct vision in the open heart during hypothermia. *J. Amer. med. Ass.*, **153,** 1081.

SWAN, H., ZEAVIN, I., HOLMES, J. H., and MONTGOMERY, V. (1953*b*). Cessation of circulation in general hypothermia. I. Physiologic changes and their control. *Ann. Surg.*, **138,** 360.

TRUSLER, G. A., MCBIRNIE, J. E., PEARSON, F. G., GORNALL, A. G., and BIGELOW, W.G. (1953). A study of hibernation in relation to the technique of hypothermia for intracardiac surgery. *Surg. Forum*, **4,** 72.

VILLALOBOS, T. J., ADELSON, E., and RILEY, P. (1956). The effect of hypothermia on platelets and white cells in dogs. *Proc. nat. Acad. Sci.* (*Wash.*), **451,** 186.

WALTHER, A. (1862). Beiträge zur Lehre von der thierischen Wärme. *Virchows Arch. path. Anat.*, **25,** 414.

WOODHALL, B., SEALY, W. C., HALL, K. D., and FLOYD, W. L. (1960). Craniotomy under conditions of quinidine-protected cardioplegia and profound hypothermia. *Ann. Surg.*, **152,** 37.

WYNN, V. (1954). Electrolyte disturbances associated with failure to metabolise glucose during hypothermia. *Lancet*, **2,** 575.

WYNN, V. (1956). The metabolism of fructose during hypothermia in man. *Clin. Sci.*, **15,** 297.

ZINN, W. J., and WARNOCK, E. H. (1960). Safe hypothermia. *J. Amer. med. Ass.*, **174,** 284.

Chapter 47

ANAESTHESIA AND THE GASTRO-INTESTINAL TRACT

Some Aspects of the Anatomy and Physiology of the Oesophagus and Stomach

Valves and Sphincters

The oesophagus extends from the crico-pharnygeal sphincter at the level of the sixth cervical vertebra to the gastro-oesophageal junction which is called the cardia. The whole organ receives its nerve supply from the vagi and the sympathetic, but the function of the latter is unknown. The muscle layer at the top of the oesophagus, at the crico-pharyngeal sphincter, is composed of striated muscle, and is partly under voluntary and partly reflex control. The muscles of the lower two thirds of the oesophagus, including the gastro-oesophageal junction, consist of smooth muscle and are reflexly controlled. Dornhorst and his co-workers (1954) demonstrated that when liquid barium is drunk, the normal cardia offers practically no resistance to its forward passage, but prevents retrograde flow. They considered it to have a valve mechanism and they were also able to disprove the old notion that the contracting diaphragm plays a principal part in forming a sphincter at this area. Fyke and his associates (1956) illustrated, from pressure measurements, a sphincter at the bottom of the oesophagus where it joins the stomach and, in this area, a localised point. Fyke named this the pressure barrier since it seals off the sphincter area below it from changes in oesophageal pressure associated with normal conditions of respiration. The apparent contradiction in these findings appears to have been reconciled by Creamer and Pierce (1957), who, using cineradiography and pressure measurements simultaneously have demonstrated both a valve and a sphincter action at the gastro-oesophageal junction. They differentiate swallowing and drinking into two separate physiological processes, since with the former barium is momentarily held up at the gastro-oesophageal junction, while with the latter it passes straight through. Creamer and his colleagues (1959) have shown that in normal people the level of the pressure barrier coincides with the level of the oesophageal hiatus of the diaphragm and that below it there is a segment of oesophagus of about 2 cm. in length lying within the abdominal cavity and subject to intra-abdominal pressure. This abdominal part of the oesophagus is kept as a narrow tube by virtue of the sphincter area that surrounds it. Creamer suggests that a flaccid tube (the oesophagus) running from a chamber of low pressure (the thorax) to one of high pressure (the abdomen) would behave in the area of high pressure like a "flap" valve and collapse, only opening to allow forward flow when the pressure gradient has been overcome (Fig. 1).

The pressure within the resting stomach is a measure of the general intra-abdominal pressure, but significant intragastric pressure changes may result from the muscular activity of the stomach itself (Marchand, 1957). As Creamer suggests, a general rise in intra-abdominal pressure should act against reflux from the stomach to the oesophagus by closing the "flap" valve mechanism, while a rise in intragastric pressure *above* intra-abdominal would overcome the valve action—unless the sphincter area of the oesophagus is caused to constrict by the same forces as affect the stomach. Thus, although a rise in intra-abdominal pressure will lead to a rise in the intra-gastric pressure, it should not, in a normal person, lead to reflux.

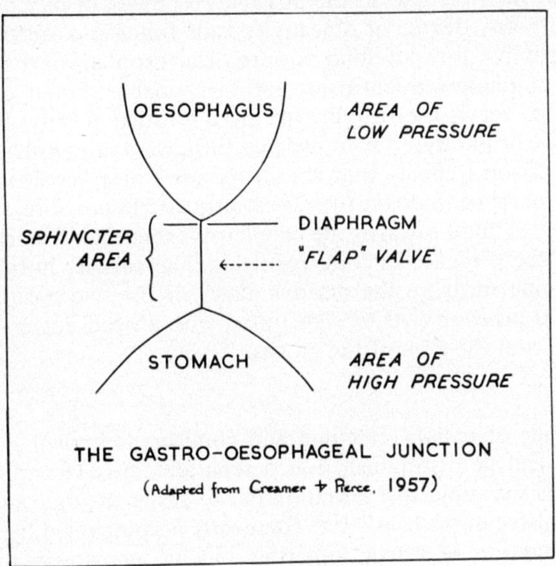

47/FIG. 1

Abnormalities.—Marked malfunction at the gastro-oesophageal junction may be associated with an anatomical distortion such as that caused by hiatus hernia, a distended stomach (Robson and Welt, 1959), the presence of an oesophageal tube, or with a physiological abnormality produced during the induction of anaesthesia. Airway obstruction during induction will reduce the intrathoracic pressure considerably during each attempted inspiration, and may make the valve mechanism incompetent (O'Mullane, 1954; Sinclair, 1959), and attempted inflation of the lungs by positive pressure following paralysis, before intubation of the trachea, can precipitate reflux from the stomach or oesophagus through the relaxed cricopharyngeal sphincter. Coughing and straining may precipitate reflux, if the mechanism to prevent it be weak or abnormal (Marchand, 1957).

Dinnick (1961) has drawn attention to the part that inspiratory obstruction during the induction of anaesthesia may play in causing regurgitation from the stomach of a patient with a previously unsuspected hiatus hernia, a condition which is common in pregnant women. It is tempting to speculate on the part that progesterone may play at the gastro-oesophageal junction during pregnancy. A high level of this hormone is present in the body during late pregnancy, and the relaxing effect that this produces on smooth muscle might conceivably affect the efficiency of the sphincter mechanism, and hence the functioning of the "flap" valve even when the diaphragmatic hiatus is normal.

Posture.—Although changes in position from supine to foot-down or to head-down produce alterations in intragastric pressure, they do not in a normal, unanaesthetised person, affect the proper functioning of the gastro-oesophageal junction. The effects of the position of a patient during the induction of anaesthesia and paralysis must be considered in relation to the action of the drugs administered at the time and to the possible responses of *that* patient. All that can be said with any degree of objectivity is as follows: a steep foot-down tilt prevents the passive flow of fluid towards the oropharynx once paralysis is complete, but it renders tracheal aspiration probable should gastric or oesophageal contents reach the oropharynx by any other means, either before or during the onset of paralysis. A foot-down tilt lowers intragastric pressure, and enhances any adverse effects that the drugs used may have on the patient's circulation. A steep head-down tilt raises intragastric pressure and encourages the passive flow of fluid towards the oropharnyx, but makes tracheal aspiration improbable in the presence of total paralysis. The supine, horizontal position combines in some measure the disadvantages of the two positions described, while the lateral position (left or right) used with a head-down tilt assists fluid to drain away from the area of the glottis.

Sickness

The syndrome of nausea, retching and vomiting is known as sickness, and each part of it can be distinguished as a separate entity (Knapp and Beecher, 1956). Nausea is the subjective sensation of the desire to vomit but without any attempt at expulsive movements. It is frequently accompanied by such objective signs as the secretion of saliva, sweating and an increase in pulse rate, and variations in the rate, depth and regularity of respiration. Retching and vomiting, both active expulsive mechanisms, are differentiated by the results of the process, the latter always producing some gastric contents, the former nothing. The mechanism consists of a series of movements designed to squeeze the relaxed stomach between the descending diaphragm and contracting abdominal muscles. The gastro-oesophageal junction and the crico-pharyngeal sphincter are open and the oropharynx is enlarged, the palate raised and the larynx held forward with the glottis closed. The act of vomiting is controlled by the vomiting centre situated near the respiratory centre in the medulla.

Discussion.—A knowledge of these mechanisms is important to the anaesthetist, particularly when dealing with patients who are likely to have fluid or food in either the oesophagus or stomach when anaesthesia is essential. The crico-pharyngeal sphincter is affected both by anaesthetic drugs and muscle relaxants, becoming progressively incompetent as anaesthesia deepens or muscle paresis increases. A fully relaxed sphincter aids the surgeon during oesophagoscopy. Any degree of relaxation, should the position favour it or the intrathoracic pressure be high, may allow fluid retained in the oesophagus to flow or be forced into the pharynx. Pulmonary inflation with high pressures or coughing may cause oesophageal reflux of this type under anaesthesia. The gastro-oesophageal junction is not affected by anaesthetics, muscle relaxants, local infiltration with analgesic solutions, or autonomic blocking agents (O'Mullane,

1954). The use of suxamethonium is associated with a rise in intra-gastric pressure in some patients (Andersen, 1962; Roe, 1962). Since there is no evidence to suggest that suxamethonium has a direct effect on the smooth muscle of the stomach, this rise in intra-gastric pressure is presumably secondary to a rise in intra-abdominal pressure caused by the fasciculations of skeletal muscles during depolarisation. Quite remarkable pressures can be applied directly to the stomach when it is full of air or fluid without evidence of reflux into the oesophagus in normal patients. During anaesthesia, provided the active processes of retching or vomiting are entirely suppressed and the gastro-oesophageal valve is not made incompetent, stomach contents will not enter the oesophagus in normal patients, even when postural changes, which would normally aid their movement, are taking place. Should a patient, however, be able to bring into action any part of the active mechanism of vomiting, then aspiration of stomach or oesophageal contents into the respiratory tract is always a potential danger due to the depressant effect of the anaesthetic or relaxant drugs upon laryngeal activity.

The syndrome of sickness may be initiated centrally by the effects of drugs or of hypoxia, or by stimulation of afferents throughout the body. Typically, these impulses arise from the stomach or other parts of the gastro-intestinal tract, and, during light anaesthesia, they may be started by surgical manipulation or by the anaesthetist inserting an airway or trying to introduce an irritant vapour too quickly. Afferent impulses can arise from almost any part of the body, and an important source is in the vestibular apparatus of the labyrinth.

Gastric Emptying Time

The time that the stomach takes to empty after a meal is very variable, even in a normal person. It is influenced principally by the following factors (Best and Taylor, 1955): the consistency of the gastric contents, their quantity and osmotic pressure, and the motility of the stomach itself.

The more fluid the meal, the quicker it leaves the stomach, so that a slow emptying time is usually associated with food such as meat which contains proteins and can only slowly be rendered fluid or semi-fluid. Large quantities need a long time, and if the meal follows soon after a previous one, a full duodenum may delay stomach emptying.

Hypertonic solutions are delayed in the stomach until they are rendered more nearly isotonic. A marked prolongation of emptying time has been demonstrated by Hunt and his colleagues (1951) who added sucrose in varying concentrations up to 25 per cent to a standard test meal.

The motility of the stomach is affected by numerous factors, such as disease, fear, many drugs and foods containing fats. King (1957) demonstrated the influence of some of these factors by comparing a group of fasting but healthy young adults with a series of patients (diabetic and non-diabetic), none of whom had any clinical or radiological evidence of delay in stomach emptying. A volume of 200 ml. of fluid containing 50 g. of glucose and a little phenol red was given to the young adults. Gastric aspiration was then performed at intervals of 15 minutes up to 2 hours. On average the meal was diluted to about twice the volume, but after two hours an average of 46 ml. of fluid containing 0·3 g. of glucose remained. Similar solutions, but containing no phenol red, were given to twenty patients two hours before operation and gastric aspiration performed just before anaesthesia was due to be induced. These patients were prepared in the normal manner and premedicated. In ten of them volumes ranging from 100 to 265 ml. (average 146 ml.) and containing 2–10·2 g. of glucose were removed from the stomach, thus demonstrating the influence of such factors as anxiety and premedication upon gastric function.

An easily digested meal will have left the stomach of a normal person in from one and a half to three hours, whereas a more solid one may take as long as four hours. Water, on the other hand, will pass into the duodenum almost as quickly as it is drunk.

It is probable that the stomach is never truly "empty", since normal secretions are continuously produced, although only in very small quantities—up to approximately 50 ml. in one hour—unless stimulated by food, by the presence of a gastric tube, or by emotion. Gastric secretions contain, amongst other things, about 0·5 per cent free hydrochloric acid.

Discussion.—The interplay of fear, disease and drugs on gastric emptying must at all times be present in the mind of an anaesthetist. Normality in this respect is so variable that the potential risk of even a small quantity of gastric secretion entering the respiratory tract must always be borne in mind when a patient's normal protective reflexes are depressed or abolished.

Although the risk of pulmonary aspiration is widely appreciated to be a potential complication of anaesthesia, it is less widely known as a hazard of feeding or vomiting in severely ill patients. Yet Gardner (1958), who has investigated the problem in both the living and the dead, considers that aspiration of food or vomit is often the *coup de grâce* in an ill patient who might otherwise recover. When such a complication arises it is usually labelled an agonal phenomenon, and very often the subsequent discovery of vomit in the lungs at a post-mortem is ignored. There is, in fact, no doubt that the gastric contents can reach the lungs after death, so that the trachea must be blocked at death if autopsy evidence of ante-mortem aspiration is to be considered conclusive. Gardner not only demonstrated such facts, but also studied a series of adult patients of both sexes who were either debilitated for a variety of reasons or who had undergone a recent major operation. He was able to show that about 9 to 10 per cent of the patients studied aspirated food while feeding and about 1 to 2 per cent aspirated vomit. Some of the patients died as a result of aspiration, but most did not, although a few developed a pulmonary complication. Gardner found it difficult to diagnose aspiration clinically—his investigation was carried out radiographically and with the aid of barium sulphate, which was placed in the patient's stomach or added to the food or fluid—but he thought that the aspiration of fluid was facilitated by the use of standard hospital feeding cups. These have a spout, which enables fluid to be poured into the trachea, and a hood that prevents the patient from seeing the level of the contents. An ordinary cup or glass is safer, and—for patients in the recumbent posture—the addition of a straw is helpful.

Preparation for Anaesthesia

Patients for elective operations should be prepared for anaesthesia—local or general—by pre-operative starvation for five hours. The last meal taken prior to this period should be light, preferably containing very little protein, and small in quantity. When the patient is to be anaesthetised as an out-patient, these instructions must be carefully explained, and it may be advisable to emphasise them by enlarging upon the unpleasantness, and perhaps even upon the danger, of sickness if they are not observed. Children need special care since they are unlikely to co-operate. When they are out-patients it is safest to give the parent or responsible person written instructions so that no doubt can exist, and to stress that starvation includes both food and fluid. Out-patient operations are best performed in the early morning.

Unless the patient is known to have been prepared in the manner described, it must be assumed that the stomach is not empty and all non-urgent operations must be postponed until it is. An exception may be made for relatively minor operations which can be easily performed with local analgesia. If an operation is delayed, the physical condition and mental state of the patient must be taken into account when estimating how long to wait for normal emptying to be completed.

A surprisingly large number of factors can be responsible for the presence of material in the oesophagus or stomach of a patient presented for anaesthesia. The anaesthetist must be aware of these possibilities, which are listed in Table 1 (Morton and Wylie, 1951).

The Hazards of Vomiting or Regurgitation

The active process of vomiting has already been described. Regurgitation can be considered as a passive process (Morton and Wylie, 1951), so that when the patient is horizontal or in the head-down position fluid will come out of the oesophagus and the stomach—if the gastro-oesophageal junction has been rendered incompetent by the presence of a tube—as a gravitational effect. Vomiting or regurgitation are dangerous when the patient is unconscious or the protective glottic reflexes are depressed. Edwards and his colleagues (1956), in an investigation of anaesthetic deaths, record 110 deaths as due to this hazard. These represent about 18·6 per cent of a total of 589 patients in whom anaesthesia was thought to be responsible for death.

Mechanism of Death

This may be due to respiratory obstruction caused by an overwhelming quantity of vomit. In an ill patient, unless pre-induction oxygenation has been carried out, sudden vomiting—even though no material enters the respiratory tract—may cause a sufficient duration of anoxia to kill the patient. Commonly, quantities of fluid vomit are aspirated into the trachea and major bronchi. Relatively small quantities of vomit may induce laryngeal spasm in lightly anaesthetised patients, and this may cause sufficient hypoxia to harm the patient. This situation is often accentuated on the one hand by attempted removal of the vomit with sucker, largyngoscope or perhaps bronchoscope, and on the other, by the addition of intravenous anaesthesia or a muscle relaxant in an endeavour to enable this treatment to be carried out more easily. Death may be delayed and follow the late results of aspiration into the lungs. Broncho-pneumonia, collapse of lung tissue and abscess formation are well-known; the condition of acute

47/Table 1

Conditions in which the Stomach may not be Empty

Material in the oesophagus	Oesophageal obstruction or pouch. Pyothorax with oesophageal fistula.
Material introduced into the stomach from above	Food and drink given, i.e. lack of pre-operative "preparation". Fluids given for medical reasons, e.g. to diabetics, or stomach washouts not completely removed. Swallowed blood. Bleeding from nose, mouth or pharynx, due to accident or operation.
Material introduced into the stomach from below	Intestinal obstruction. Ileus.
Material from the stomach itself	Normal or hypersecretion. Bleeding from ulcer, neoplasm, or site of operation.
Prolonged emptying time of the stomach	A. Pyloric obstruction (including congenital pyloric obstruction). B. Dilatation of the stomach. C. Reflex I. Emotional states. Pain. Parturition. Shock. Accidents—e.g. cuts, fractures, burns. II. Peritoneal irritation, e.g. perforated ulcer, twisted ovarian tumour. D. Abdominal distension, e.g. large tumours, pregnancy at term. Gross ascites. E. Severe illness. Toxaemia. Near-moribund patients. F. Drugs. Morphia, papaveretum, pethidine, scopolamine, atropine. Most anaesthetic agents.

Several causes are often present together, e.g. a patient brought to the theatre for resuture of a "burst abdomen" may be in poor general condition and may have taken food or fluids just before the incident. There will be shock, emotional disturbance, and peritoneal irritation, and morphine may have been given.

exudative pulmonary oedema described by Mendelson (1946) may also occur (see Chapter 14).

Vomiting or regurgitation may occur during the induction of anaesthesia, while the operation is in progress, or during the immediate recovery period while the patient emerges from anaesthesia.

Preparation for Emergency Operations

It is possible to differentiate surgical emergencies into those which are true and will brook no delay in their treatment, or at the very most a short period for essential preparation, and those which are relative in their acuteness and can safely be delayed while the essential points of normal preparation are carried out. The final decision upon the time for operation can only be taken by the surgeon, but part of the responsibility for adequate preparation must fall upon the anaesthetist. The importance of this division of emergency cases lies in the increased safety that goes with adequate preparation before anaesthesia and operation—and furthermore in the greater comfort for the patient. In the true emergency, when there is any doubt about the oesophagus or stomach being empty, steps must be taken to drain them.

In most patients—92 out of the 110 patients investigated by Edwards and his colleagues (1956)—the material is likely to be liquid, so that a small bore stomach tube is helpful. A 6-gauge (4 mm.) tube or a Ryle's tube (4 mm.) which has not become flabby from repeated boiling, will cause little discomfort to the patient and enable a lot of information to be gleaned about the stomach contents. Moreover, the surgeon may well require such a tube for the post-operative period. It should be passed before the premedication is given. Gentle suction is used and, if necessary, small quantities (10–20 ml.) of water are injected and aspirated with the patient supine. Then, after the washings have become progressively clearer and smaller in quantity, the process is repeated with the patient lying upon his right side to move any fluid from the cardia area. Finally, the tube is pulled up a little and the whole performance repeated. In this manner fluid can be removed from the stomach. A larger tube—gauge 12, or 7 mm.—is more unpleasant for the patient, but if well lubricated it can usually be passed through the nose and enables aspiration to be performed more quickly. It is doubtful whether a very large bore tube—24-gauge, or 13 mm.—has any advantage over the 12-gauge, unless a washout is necessary, and this can often be predicted from the material aspirated through the smaller one. A very small tube cannot be expected to drain fluid away as quickly as will be necessary in some cases of intestinal obstruction or during the surgeon's intra-abdominal manipulations. In cases of haematemesis or perforated peptic ulcer only very small quantities of water, if any, should be injected down the tube, and then only to keep the end clear.

Patients with early acute appendicitis and women in labour are often treated as exceptions to the general rule for gastric lavage—the former because nausea, vomiting and then a period of anorexia are typical of the disease, so that the patient is usually presented for anaesthesia with an empty stomach. If the inflammation has progressed to peritonitis, however, there may be some ileus, when full precautions must be taken. Obstetrical patients are considered in greater detail in Chapter 53.

Even after apparently successful preparation, an anaesthetic technique must be chosen so as to lessen any risk of aspiration into the respiratory tract should any material remain in the oesophagus or stomach.

Whenever it is proposed to induce anaesthesia with the risk of vomiting or regurgitation present, the essential apparatus must be checked beforehand. This must include an efficient suction apparatus. The patient should be induced on the operating table or a trolley which can be rapidly tilted either head-down or head-up.

General Anaesthesia

Safety during general anaesthesia for these cases can only be assured by a cuffed endotracheal tube. Nitrous oxide-oxygen-ether, with carbon dioxide if required, is the safest anaesthetic sequence for an inexperienced anaesthetist, though, needless to say, it is always preferable for patients who are likely to vomit or regurgitate during anaesthesia to be dealt with by anaesthetists who are well versed in the subject. Cyclopropane and oxygen has the advantage of ensuring a higher oxygen concentration than the nitrous oxide sequence during any period of vomiting, should one occur, but it is less easily administered by the inexperienced to a degree sufficient for intubation. Neither of these anaesthetic sequences for induction is markedly depressant for an ill patient, and once intubation is completed other drugs can be substituted. Halothane and oxygen usually ensure a smooth induction without any tendency to vomiting, but there may be some circulatory depression. Anaesthesia should be induced with the patient tilted head-down and in the lateral position, and must be deepened slowly to a stage when intubation can be carried out. The merit of this type of technique is that laryngeal reflexes are active during the time when active vomiting is possible, and laryngeal spasm, if it occurs, will not be as protracted as after thiopentone.

An alternative technique is to induce anaesthesia rapidly, follow it immediately by total paralysis from suxamethonium, and then intubate the trachea. Suxamethonium is indicated because it works quickly and must be given in a dose which produces total paralysis. Partial paresis of the patient at this stage is extremely dangerous. There are three main variations of this technique depending upon the posture of the patient during induction; namely the head-down and lateral position, the foot-down position, and the horizontal position with cricoid pressure. With the patient in the left lateral position and tilted head-down (Bourne, 1958), tracheal aspiration—should vomiting or regurgitation occur—is unlikely, but laryngoscopy is sometimes difficult, so that rapid intubation may be hard to achieve. Laryngoscopy is easier to carry out in the right lateral position. These positions tend to encourage fluid to flow to the oropharynx in some circumstances. In the presence of total paralysis active vomiting cannot occur, and passive regurgitation can be prevented by placing the patient in a foot-down tilt (Morton and Wylie, 1951). Snow and Nunn (1959) recommend a 40° foot-down tilt from the horizontal so that the larynx is raised 19 cm. above the cardio-oesophageal junction, assuming a distance between these two points in an adult of 25 cm. and a 10° inclination of this line to the vertical axis of the body. Their calculation of the degree of tilt is based on O'Mullane's (1954) finding that, even with distention of the abdomen, intragastric pressure did not rise above 18 cm. of water. If fluid or food does reach the oropharynx during induction in the foot-down position it is very likely to enter the trachea. Sellick (1961) suggests that during the induction of anaesthesia with the patient supine and horizontal, and the head and neck fully extended, backward pressure should be exerted on the cricoid cartilage by an assistant to occlude the oesophagus against the cervical vertebrae. Sellick warns that this technique may be dangerous in the presence of vomiting, since the oesophagus might be damaged under high pressure.

For all these variations intravenous thiopentone can be used for induction, but it must be preceded by the patient inhaling 100 per cent oxygen for two to three minutes, since inflation of the lungs must not be carried out before passing the endotracheal tube in case a reflux from the oesophagus or stomach is caused.

An alternative to thiopentone is 50 per cent cyclopropane with oxygen as described by Bourne (1954). Cyclopropane in such concentration works swiftly, is less depressant than thiopentone, particularly in the foot-down position, and the amount of oxygen in the induction mixture enables intubation to be carried out without previous inflation of the lungs provided the anaesthetist is speedy. Bourne (1962) advocates halothane and oxygen for the induction of anaesthesia, but with the patient in the left lateral position and tilted head-down.

Discussion.—No technique of anaesthesia is fool-proof but the use of a muscle relaxant following a rapid induction of anaesthesia is particularly hazardous, in the presence of a full stomach, if the rationale of this method is not fully understood by the anaesthetist. Snow and Nunn (1959) and Hodges and his colleagues (1960) report large series of patients for whom a rapid induction with thiopentone and suxamethonium has been successfully combined with a foot-down tilt and without complications from vomiting or regurgitation. The lack of complications may be due to the fact that an oesophageal tube was passed on any patient thought to be particularly likely to have a distended stomach. It seems certain, however, that despite a steep foot-down tilt, fluid may reach the oropharynx during induction and may enter the trachea. Active vomiting may take place before paralysis is complete (Sellick, 1961). In a reported series of 428 obstetric patients for whom a rapid induction of anaesthesia in the foot-down position was followed by paralysis with suxamethonium, three patients (0·7 per cent) were found to have fluid in the oropharynx at the time of laryngoscopy, and in one of these some fluid entered the trachea (Wylie, 1961). Whether this complication is initiated by an attempted vomit, partial respiratory obstruction, an abnormality at the gastro-oesophageal junction, the effects of the drugs administered, or to some other factor or factors, cannot yet be proved. It is, however, a risk which must be set against the advantages of the technique, and must be compared with the difficulties encountered when a passive flow of fluid follows the onset of paralysis in a patient placed either supine or in the lateral position with a head-down tilt. After paralysis is complete any undue delay in intubating the patient and ventilating the lungs may be disastrous. Laryngoscopy and endotracheal intubation cannot always be carried out easily, even when the patient is fully relaxed. Rarely, intubation may be impossible. Difficulties of this kind are commonly associated with malformation of the jaws or teeth and should therefore be visible to the discerning anaesthetist before the form of anaesthetic induction is chosen.

There is little doubt that the pre-operative administration to the patient of oral alkalis, to prevent the sequelae that can follow the pulmonary aspiration of acid gastric contents, and the use of cricoid pressure are the most valuable preventive measures.

Treatment of Vomiting or Regurgitation Occurring during Anaesthesia

If stomach or oesophageal contents enter the pharynx when the trachea is unprotected, urgent treatment is necessary. The patient must be quickly tilted into the head-down position, if not already in it, the obstructing material aspirated to clear the airway, and oxygen given. Priority for oxygen or suction will depend upon the particular state of affairs—obviously it will be a waste of time giving oxygen if the airway is completely blocked. Nevertheless, when the patient is breathing, and there is some sort of airway, it may be wiser to oxygenate first, with intermittent or continuous suction beneath the mask when possible, rather than risk death from anoxia. An oral airway will be a help if the jaw is relaxed. Attempts to intubate the patient before oxygenation, can be helpful only when the obstruction cannot be relieved by other methods or when the trouble arises in a paralysed patient. Attempted intubation in the presence of laryngeal spasm aggravates the situation; deliberate paralysis at this stage runs the risk of death before intubation and oxygenation can be completed.

Tracheal toilet down a bronchoscope may be necessary but should only be considered after the emergency treatment has been carried out, and the patient restored to a state in which the procedure can be justified. As an immediate measure it is very dangerous; an endotracheal tube is quite adequate for suction. As soon as the patient improves, bronchoscopy should be considered if it seems likely that material has been aspirated. Obvious food or fluid should be removed by suction and, if the fluid portion is considerable, 20 to 30 ml. of a weak solution of bicarbonate or saline should be squirted into the bronchi and, if possible, sucked back again, repeating the procedure two or three times in an endeavour to neutralise or dilute any hydrochloric acid that may remain. (Further treatment is discussed in Chapter 14.)

When possible the proposed operation should be postponed if the patient has suffered a long period of hypoxia or has aspirated material into the lungs.

Local Analgesia

Many emergency operations can be performed under local analgesia, and those on the extremities often lend themselves well to nerve block procedures. Operations upon, or within, the abdomen can be performed under more extensive blocks, such as epidural analgesia, and the risk of the dangers associated with a full stomach can usually be circumvented, but other dangers and considerations must then be assessed. Other factors besides the risk of aspiration alone—a bad chest, for example—may suggest a local technique, but provided precautions are taken general anaesthesia matches up to local analgesia in safety and is most often preferred by the patient and the surgeon.

Intubation of the trachea with a cuffed endotracheal tube may be undertaken with local analgesia and, once effected, general anaesthesia can be induced with safety. But this, like other local analgesic technique in the presence of a full stomach, does not guarantee that vomiting or regurgitation will not occur, so that the risk of tracheal aspiration persists until intubation is accomplished.

Children

The general principles of preparation and anaesthesia for children in whom the risk of vomiting or regurgitation is present, should be exactly the same as for adults. Neither the size of the child nor the apparent urgency of the condition is an excuse for avoiding unpleasant and difficult procedures, but in the very young local analgesia is rarely practicable. In children, however, many emergencies are relative rather than true. A short delay may enable the anaesthetist to avoid many difficulties by allowing the child to digest the last meal. For safety, neonates and babies up to three or four weeks of age are best intubated without either anaesthesia or relaxant.

Treatment

Carefully selected and administered anaesthesia, including both pre- and post-operative medication, will limit both the incidence and severity of sickness. Specific anti-emetics can be used routinely to prevent sickness or more selectively to treat the severer cases, but since none of the powerful anti-emetics is without side-effects, their routine use can only be justified if these other actions are thought to be reasonable and acceptable in the circumstances.

Drugs of the phenothiazine and associated groups are the most effective anti-emetics. A specific effect on the vomiting centre in the medulla is claimed for them, while their general sedative action also plays a part. Prevention of sickness is most usefully attempted by combining the chosen drug with the premedication, and then administering further doses at 3 to 4-hourly intervals in the post-operative period. Alternatively, they can be used as the main component of premedication instead of an opiate or one of its analogues, and only combined with atropine or scopolamine. Yet another way is to give a dose intramuscularly just before the patient leaves the operating theatre, and then to repeat the dose at intervals during the next 24 hours. All these methods will tend to prolong the period of unconsciousness or semi-consciousness which follows general anaesthesia, while the selective effect on the respiratory tract reflexes and autonomic ganglia may increase the hazards of the immediate post-operative period. It is therefore probably safer, and not much less effective, to use them when indicated in the post-operative period and only after the initial recovery of consciousness—though even then the induced hypotension is not without its dangers. Occasional patients who are known to have a severe sickness after anaesthesia might be accounted the exceptions and treated more thoroughly.

The effectiveness of these anti-emetics can be gauged from the published results of large investigations. Burtles and Peckett (1957) were able to reduce their incidence of post-operative sickness by approximately 50 per cent, using either chlorpromazine or promethazine in the premedication, while Knapp and Beecher (1956) converted an overall incidence of 82 per cent to 59 per cent, using a single intramuscular injection of chlorpromazine at the end of the operation.

Many drugs are useful anti-emetics, but the choice of a particular preparation depends upon a knowledge of its relative effectiveness in different circumstances and of its side-effects (Riding, 1963). These drugs are described in Chapter 36, but those most favoured are promethazine in a dose range of from 25–50 mg. and perphenazine in 5 mg. doses. Other similar compounds have their advocates for the prevention and treatment of post-operative sickness. Dimenhydrinate ("Dramamine") and promethazine-8-chlorotheophyllinate ("Avomine") are best used for cases of motion sickness typified in the post-operative period after operations on or near the labyrinth. The dose is from 25 to 50 mg. They are not of great use for other types of sickness. N-benzhydryl-N-methyl piperazine dihydrochloride ("Marzine") is said to have fewer side-effects than other antihistamines, but to have an equally effective control of sickness, and should be used in single doses of up to 50 mg. intramuscularly.

The relative mildness of much post-operative sickness suggests that some of the old-fashioned remedies may still have their place in treatment. Moreover, even the special drugs fail to control sickness in some patients, so that less specific and homely, but none the less practical, procedures may be helpful. Sips of cold water to which a little bicarbonate or a minim or two of iodide has been added are often beneficial, while pineapple is remarkably refreshing and settling to the stomach when sucked.

A small bore tube (Ryle's or similar type of 4 mm. diameter) for gastric suction is often a useful ancillary in the treatment of severe cases, and can also be helpful if used prophylactically in cases known to be liable to this complication. Occasionally, especially in episodes following operations upon children, intravenous replacement of fluid, food and electrolytes may be an essential part of treatment.

No case of persistent or severe post-operative vomiting should be treated by routine therapy until a surgical cause has been excluded.

REFERENCES

ANDERSEN, N. (1962). Changes in intragastric pressure following the administration of suxamethonium: preliminary report. *Brit. J. Anaesth.*, **34,** 363.

BEST, C. H., and TAYLOR, N. B. (1955). *The Physiological Basis of Medical Practice,* 6th edit. Baltimore: Williams & Wilkins.

BOURNE, J. G. (1954). General anaesthesia for out-patients, with special reference to dental extraction. *Proc. roy. Soc. Med.*, **47,** 416.

BOURNE, J. G. (1958). Maternal anaesthetic deaths. *Brit. med. J.*, **1,** 1064.

BOURNE, J. G. (1962). Anaesthesia and the vomiting hazard. A safe method for obstetric and other emergencies. *Anaesthesia*, **17,** 379.

BURTLES, R., and PECKETT, B. W. (1957). Postoperative vomiting. Some factors affecting its incidence. *Brit. J. Anaesth.*, **29,** 114.

CREAMER, B., HARRISON, G. K., and PIERCE, J. W. (1959). Further observations on the gastro-oesophageal junction. *Thorax*, **14,** 132.

CREAMER, B., and PIERCE, J. W. (1957). Observations on the gastro-oesophageal junction during swallowing and drinking. *Lancet*, **2,** 1309.

DAVISON, G. (1946). Incidence of congenital pyloric stenosis. *Arch. Dis. Childh.*, **21,** 113.

DENT, S. J., RAMACHANDRA, V., and STEPHEN, C. R. (1955). Post-operative vomiting: incidence, analysis and therapeutic measures in 3,000 patients. *Anesthesiology*, **16,** 564.

DINNICK, O. P. (1961). Hiatus hernia: an anaesthetic hazard. *Lancet*, **1,** 470.

DORNHORST, A. C., HARRISON, K., and PIERCE, J. W. (1954). Observations on the normal oesophagus and cardia. *Lancet*, **1,** 695.

EDWARDS, G., MORTON, H. J. V., PASK, E. A., and WYLIE, W. D. (1956). Deaths associated with anaesthesia. A report on 1,000 cases. *Anaesthesia*, **11,** 194.

FYKE, F. E., Jr., CODE, C. F., and SCHLEGEL, J. F. (1956). The gastroesophageal sphincter in healthy human beings. *Gastroenterologia* (*Basel*), **86,** 135.

GARDNER, A. M. N. (1958). Aspiration of food and vomit. *Quart. J. Med.*, **27,** 227.

HODGES, R. J. H., TUNSTALL, M. E., and BENNETT, J. R. (1960). Vomiting and head-up position. *Brit. J. Anaesth.*, **32,** 619.

HUNT, J. N., MACDONALD, I., and SPURRELL, W. R. (1951). The gastric response to pectin meals of high osmotic pressure. *J. Physiol.* (*Lond.*), **115,** 185.

KING, R. C. (1957). The control of diabetes mellitus in surgical patients. *Anaesthesia*, **12,** 30.

KNAPP, M. R., and BEECHER, H. K. (1956). Postanesthetic nausea, vomiting and retching. Evaluation of the antiemetic drugs dimenhydrinate (Dramamine), chlorpromazine, and pentobarbital sodium. *J. Amer. med. Ass.*, **160,** 376.

MARCHAND, P. (1957). A study of the forces productive of gastro-oesophageal regurgitation and herniation through the diaphragmatic hiatus. *Thorax*, **12,** 189.

MENDELSON, C. L. (1946). Aspiration of stomach contents into lungs during obstetric anesthesia. *Amer. J. Obstet. Gynec.*, **52,** 191.

MORTON, H. J. V. (1957). Intestinal obstruction and anaesthesia. *Brit. med. J.*, **2,** 224.

MORTON, H. J. V., and WYLIE, W. D. (1951). Anaesthetic deaths due to regurgitation or vomiting. *Anaesthesia*, **6,** 190.

O'MULLANE, E. J. (1954). Vomiting and regurgitation during anaesthesia. *Lancet*, **1,** 1209.

REES, G. J. (1958). Neonatal anaesthesia. *Brit. med. Bull.*, **14,** 38.

RIDING, J. E. (1963). The prevention of postoperative vomiting. *Brit. J. Anaesth.*, **35,** 180.

ROBSON, J. G., and WELT, P. (1959). Regurgitation in anaesthesia; report on some exploratory work with animals. *Canad. Anaesth. Soc. J.*, **6,** 4.

ROE, R. B. (1962). The effect of suxamethonium on intragastric pressure. *Anaesthesia*, **17,** 179.

SELLICK, B. A. (1961). Cricoid pressure to control regurgitation of stomach contents during induction of anaesthesia. *Lancet*, **2,** 404.

SINCLAIR, R. N. (1959). The oesophageal cardia and regurgitation. *Brit. J. Anaesth.*, **31,** 15.

SNOW, R. G., and NUNN, J. F. (1959). Induction of anaesthesia in the foot-down position for patients with a full stomach. *Brit. J. Anaesth.*, **31,** 493.

WATERS, R. M. (1936). Present status of cyclopropane. *Brit. med. J.*, **2,** 1013.

WATERSTON, D. J., BONHAM CARTER, R. E., and ABERDEEN, E. (1962). Oesophageal atresia: tracheo-oesphageal fistula. *Lancet*, **1,** 819.

WYLIE, W. D. (1961). "Anaesthesia for operative obstetrics." *Proc. 3rd World Congr. of Federation of Obstetricians and Gynaecologists, Vienna* (printed privately).

Chapter 48

ANAESTHESIA AND THE LIVER

Anatomy

The liver, the largest organ in the body, is situated below the right costal margin just under the diaphragm. It usually weighs between 1 and 4 kg. and is imperfectly divided into two lobes—a large right and a small left one. On the inferior and posterior surface between the right and left lobes are two smaller lobes—the caudate and the quadrate. The falciform ligament consists of two layers of peritoneum which are closely united until they reach the upper surface of the liver, where they part company to cover the peritoneal surface of the right and left lobe. This ligament joins the liver to the diaphragm and the anterior abdominal wall. In its free edge stretching from the umbilicus to the lower border of the liver is the ligamentum teres containing small para-umbilical veins. At its upper end the two layers of the falciform ligament separate widely to expose a small triangular area—the bare area of the liver. The right fold of the ligament joins the upper layer of the coronary ligament and the left fold sweeps away to become continuous with the anterior layer of the left triangular ligament.

The porta hepatis is found on the inferior surface of the liver lying between the quadrate lobe in front and a process of the caudate lobe behind. This structure is important because it consists of a deep fissure containing most of the essential structures of the liver. Viewed from below these structures, from right to left, are the common hepatic duct, which gives off a branch—the cystic duct—leading to the neck of the gall-bladder, the bile duct, the portal vein and finally the hepatic artery with a plexus of hepatic nerves.

The minute structure of the liver comprises a whole mass of neatly arranged lobules. Each lobule consists of numerous cells arranged in columns which radiate from around a central vein. Irregular blood vessels or sinusoids can be found between the columns of cells. The blood supply to these lobules comes from the hepatic artery and the portal vein. Both these vessels, soon after entering the porta hepatitis, divide into right and left branches. Each branch then undergoes dichotomy many thousands of times to supply all the lobules. The hepatic artery brings fresh oxygenated blood for the liver cells almost directly from the aorta, whereas the portal vein carries all ingested material in the venous blood from the gastro-intestinal tract and spleen. These two vascular supplies are carried throughout the liver on the periphery of the lobules. Small branches are given off from both vessels which encircle the lobule as the interlobular plexus and from these plexuses small capillary-like vessels (sometimes described as sinusoids) run between the column of cells of the lobule and finally drain into the vein in the centre of the lobule—the central vein. All the central veins join up to form the hepatic veins which finally drain into the inferior vena cava.

The nerve supply of the liver consists mainly of non-medullated sympathetic fibres which ramify around the vessels and bile ducts and finally terminate in the liver cells. It arises from the coeliac plexus.

Physiology

The blood flow to the liver is about 1,500 ml. per minute. Of this total, about 80 per cent (1,200 ml.) reaches the liver through the portal vein and the remaining 20 per cent (300 ml.) passes along the hepatic artery. However, the blood in the hepatic artery is about 95 per cent saturated with oxygen whereas that in the portal vein is around 85 per cent.

It has been estimated that the liver normally requires about 60 ml. of oxygen per minute, of which about 17 ml. are supplied by the hepatic artery and the remainder by the portal vein. The total amount of oxygen available to the liver cells can be reduced by a number of conditions:

1. Anaesthesia. Due to (*a*) reduced hepatic blood flow;
   (*b*) reduced arterial oxygen saturation through pulmonary shunting.
2. Lowered cardiac output, as in shock, haemorrhage or hypotension.
3. Inhalation of a low inspired concentration of oxygen.
4. Hypermetabolic states, e.g. pyrexia.
5. Hepatotoxic substances.
6. Obstruction of the portal vein or hepatic artery.

It is clear, therefore, that as the cells surrounding the central lobular vein are the last to receive nourishment, then they are the first to suffer from any deprivation. With toxic substances such as chloroform one might expect the cells surrounding the hepatic artery to receive the worst damage, but it is liver toxins which cause the hepatic cells to swell, and it is their swelling which further interferes with the blood supply of the central cells and causes them to suffer the worst damage.

Functions of the Liver

General metabolism.—Carbohydrate is converted into glycogen by the liver and stored there until required. The process of forming the glycogen is a complex one involving the reaction between glucose and adenosine triphosphate in the presence of the enzyme hexokinase to form glucose-phosphate, and then glycogen.

$$\text{Glucose} \xrightarrow[\text{Adenosine triphosphate}]{\text{Hexokinase}} \text{Glucose-6-phosphate} \rightarrow \text{Glucose-1-phosphate} \rightarrow \text{Glycogen}$$

Fats pass from the depots throughout the body to the liver and are broken down, almost as fast as they arrive, into glycerol and fatty acids under the influence of the enzyme liver lipase.

The end-products of protein digestion are amino-acids which play such an important part in cellular structure. The "amino-acid pool" is composed not only of the fresh supplies from the gut, but also from the continual breakdown and rebuilding of the tissues. The amino-acids number about twenty and each protein molecule is a composite group of most of them. Amongst the more important of these amino-acids are glycine, cystine, methionine, tyrosine and leucine. About one half of the body protein synthesis and resynthesis takes place in the liver and it is here that the surplus amino-acids undergo oxidative deamination. In this process the amine group (NH_2) is released as ammonia (NH_3): the latter substance is either excreted as urea or is used again for building other amino-acids. The remainder of the molecule (the non-nitrogenous part) is broken down to produce energy for the general metabolism.

The amino-acid methionine is of special interest because it is concerned in the synthesis of choline; it generously donates three methyl groups to ethanolamine to form choline, and this may then become acetylated in the presence of the enzyme choline acetylase to form the essential substance of neuromuscular transmission—acetyl choline. Another of methionine's important functions is to supply a methyl group to noradrenaline to synthesise adrenaline.

Storage.—Fats, protein and glycogen and likewise certain vitamins—such as vitamin B which plays such an important part in pernicious anaemia—are all stored in the liver.

Production and destruction.—Amongst its tasks the liver synthesises plasma proteins, prothrombin, fibrinogen and heparin. In early life it plays an important part in red blood cell formation and later becomes one of the principal places where the breakdown products of old red blood corpuscles are dealt with.

Formation of the bile secretion.—This is carried out in the liver.

Detoxication of drugs.—The liver is able to remove many foreign substances by oxidation. For example pethidine is removed in this manner and, therefore, liver function is important in any assessment of drug activity.

Liver Function Tests

Galactose Tolerance

The basis of this test is that when galactose is taken by mouth it is rapidly absorbed from the intestine, taken to the liver, and there converted to glycogen from whence it finally reaches the tissues as glucose. If the liver is severely damaged it is unable to form glycogen from galactose, thus forcing this polysaccharide to be excreted unchanged in the urine.

The test, therefore, is based on an analysis of the amount of galactose found in the urine. Normally a small amount is present. Following the ingestion of 40 g. of galactose the urine concentration in milligrams is measured four times at half-hourly intervals—i.e. after ½, 1, 1½ and 2 hours. The concentrations in each of these four specimens are then added together to produce the galactose index. The normal range of galactose index is 0–160. Abnormal figures are 160 or more and suggest liver damage. Such high readings of the galactose index are most commonly seen in cases of jaundice, or hyperthyroidism which is often associated with hepatic damage due to the excessive demands of metabolism.

Prothrombin Test

Vitamin K is responsible for the synthesis of prothrombin by the liver; in the presence of liver damage, therefore, the plasma prothrombin concentration falls, the coagulation time of the blood is prolonged, and sometimes haemorrhage may occur.

The prothrombin time is normally measured in seconds and is taken as the clotting time of oxalated plasma after the addition of calcium and thromboplastin (Quick's method). Normally the prothrombin time is about 12 to 30 seconds.

Hippuric Acid Test

When sodium benzoate is taken by mouth it is rapidly absorbed and then taken to the liver and kidneys where it is conjugated with glycine to form hippuric acid. This test, therefore, will show a low hippuric acid excretion in both liver and kidney disease and so must be associated with other tests before any conclusion can be made. The test is carried out by giving 6 g. of sodium benzoate. A normal patient should excrete 3 to 3·5 g. of hippuric acid in the urine in 4 hours. An excretion of 2·7 g. or less is abnormal.

Bromsulphthalein Test

This dye, consisting of phenol and tetrabromphthalein disodium sulphonate, is taken up by the liver cells and excreted unchanged in the bile. The test is based upon a study of the concentration remaining in the blood after the intravenous injection of this dye and is expressed as a percentage of the control value. The patient is given 2 mg./kg. body weight of bromsulphthalein intravenously, and if normal, should have 0 to 5 per cent of it left in the blood after forty-five minutes.

Flocculation Tests

These are widely used for determining liver damage, and are particularly useful for distinguishing between toxic and obstructive jaundice. A positive result is only shown when the liver cells have actually undergone destruction, as in hepatitis, and no change occurs when the bile ducts are choked by the obstruction. The underlying mechanism is still obscure but is due—it is thought—to alteration in the distribution of plasma proteins. The γ-globulins are believed to be increased in the presence of liver cell damage and these may be responsible for the specific changes found in these tests. Amongst the most useful of these tests is the *thymol turbidity*.

Thymol turbidity. Normal = 0–2 units.
Abnormal = 3 units and above.

Pseudo (Plasma) Cholinesterase Test

Pseudocholinesterases are responsible for the breakdown of acetylcholine and also suxamethonium. These esterases are believed to be formed mainly in the liver, and in the presence of damage to this organ low values may be expected. Nevertheless, a low pseudocholinesterase level may be present in otherwise healthy subjects and this is one of the first points that comes to mind if a prolonged apnoea follows suxamethonium. It must be assumed, therefore, that there are other causes of a low pseudocholinesterase reading besides liver damage; and it is known that merely altering the protein intake in the diet is rapidly reflected in the level of the esterase in the blood.

Pseudocholinesterase (*Michael's Method*).—40 to 100 units per 100 ml. (For details of the paper test see Chapter 32.)

Enzyme Tests

The multiplicity of tests for liver function is evidence of the individual inadequacy of each in the diagnosis of hepatic dysfunction, but recently a number of enzyme tests have been introduced which are now regarded as extremely sensitive and useful in the study of liver disease. Enzymes are present in most of the cells of the major organs throughout the body and the serum of the blood contains a steady level of each, since there is a constant small breakdown of cells. However, if an organ such as the heart or liver suddenly undergoes an ischaemic episode, then cellular breakdown will increase precipitously and this will be reflected in a dramatic elevation of the serum level of the corresponding enzymes. For this reason these enzyme tests play an important role in distinguishing jaundice due to hepatic cellular damage and that following early obstruction of the common bile duct.

The enzymes in question are either transaminases or dehydrogenases.

(*a*) **The transaminases.**—Transamination is a chemical reaction in which the α-amino group of an amino-acid is exchanged for the α-keto group, resulting in the synthesis of a new amino-acid (Sherlock, 1968). There are two principal transaminase enzymes:

1. Serum glutamic oxaloacetic transaminase (SGOT) which is present in large quantities in the liver, heart, kidney and skeletal muscle. High serum values for this enzyme are found in both hepato-cellular necrosis and myocardial infarction.

Normal values for SGOT:

Spectrophotometric method (Sherlock, 1968) 5–17 units per 100 ml.
Colorimetric method (Reitman and Frankel, 1957) 8–40 units per 100 ml.

2. Serum glutamic pyruvic transaminase (SGPT) is also present in many organs but there is relatively less in the liver cells as compared with the heart and skeletal muscle.

Normal values for SGPT:

Spectrophotometric method (Sherlock, 1968) 4–13 units per 100 ml.
Colorimetric method (Reitman and Frankel, 1957) 5–30 units per 100 ml.

In severe liver disease such as infective hepatitis, the level of these enzymes in the serum may rise to 800 units or more (per 100 ml.) whilst in the presence of simple obstructive jaundice the level is usually in the region of 50–100 units.

(*b*) **The dehydrogenases.**—These enzymes catalyse an oxidation-reduction reaction in the presence of a co-enzyme which serves as a hydrogen donor or acceptor (Sherlock, 1968). The principal enzyme of this group is lactic dehydrogenase (LDH), which is found in many parts of the body, especially liver, heart muscle, skeletal muscle and erythrocytes.

Normal values for LDH are up to 500 units per 100 ml.

This figure is considerably raised in infective or toxic hepatitis but is usually within normal limits in early obstructive jaundice.

Jaundice and Its Differential Diagnosis

The cause of the yellow tinge in the skin, which is so characteristic of jaundice, is an increase in the concentration of bilirubin in the blood. This may occur for a variety of reasons:

(*a*) **Haemolytic jaundice** is due to an excessive destruction of red blood cells with the consequent accumulation of large quantities of haemobilirubin. This haemobilirubin is formed so fast that the liver cells are simply unable to remove it quickly enough, so that the concentration in the blood rises. This type of jaundice most commonly occurs after the transfusion of incompatible blood, the injection of haemolytic drugs or sera, and as a congenital condition (acholuric jaundice).

(*b*) **Toxic jaundice** follows damage to the liver cells. The cells surrounding the central part of the lobule are the most susceptible to damage because they are supplied with the lowest saturation of oxygen and are thus the first to suffer. Damage to these central cells often introduces an element of "obstruction" into this type of jaundice.

(*c*) **Obstructive jaundice** signifies some form of blockage in the biliary system preventing the outflow of bile. A rare type of this condition occurs in the newborn where the congenital abnormality is some failure in the cannulation of the bile duct system. More commonly it is seen in adults as an acquired condition following obstruction of the common bile duct by a stone or by carcinoma of the head of the pancreas.

Bilirubin being the essential cause of jaundice, a description of its formation and fate is important in any attempt to differentiate between the various types of jaundice described above.

Normally the red blood cells are broken down by the reticulo-endothelial system to form protein-bound bilirubin and other products. This protein-bound bilirubin cannot be excreted unchanged by the liver and is the form in which it is commonly found circulating in the blood. A rise in red cell destruction, therefore, will lead to a corresponding rise in the protein-bound bilirubin or haemobilirubin, as it is sometimes called. This latter substance is altered by either the liver or the reticulo-endothelial cells, so that by the time it has passed through the liver lobule the protein is now either loosely attached or completely separated from the bilirubin. This type of bilirubin, which is found in the bile ducts, is sometimes referred to as cholebilirubin. It then passes down the bile duct to the intestines where it is acted upon by bacteria and forms urobilinogen. Some of this is then reabsorbed and passes into the bloodstream, but about half passes on down to join the faeces and in contact with air it becomes oxidised to form urobilin. Of that part of urobilinogen that is reabsorbed some returns to the liver to complete the cycle, whilst the rest passes to the kidney and is excreted in the urine. Ultimately it is likewise oxidised in the presence of air to form urobilin.

In haemolytic jaundice the total quantity of protein-bound bilirubin (haemobilirubin) and of bilirubin loosely attached to protein (cholebilirubin) are both greatly increased. The liver cells just cannot manage to deal with the huge quantities that are reaching them and a rise in concentration is inevitable. In obstructive jaundice the total quantity of bilirubin in the blood increases rapidly, but since there is no increase in the destruction of red cells in this case the protein-bound bilirubin concentration remains unchanged. Similarly it proceeds to bilirubin loosely attached to protein at a normal rate but cannot reach the gut through the obstructed bile channels.

The *Van den Bergh* reaction depends upon differentiating between the relative concentrations of haemobilirubin and cholebilirubin. There are two kinds of reaction:

1. *Direct reaction.*—When the serum is treated directly with the reagents a characteristic violet colour develops either rapidly or within ten minutes. If no colour has developed within this time the test is considered negative. Cholebilirubin gives a positive direct reaction which signifies that the bile has passed through the liver cells and that the jaundice is obstructive.

2. *Indirect reaction.*—The serum and reagents are mixed in the presence of alcohol which precipitates the serum protein. A positive result is given by haemobilirubin and is therefore indicative of a haemolytic jaundice. This test can be used quantitatively as well as qualitatively to measure the respective concentrations of haemobilirubin and cholebilirubin.

The *serum alkaline phosphatase* reaction is also useful in helping to diagnose the cause of jaundice, since a low figure in King Armstrong units (0–15 units) suggests either a normal response or the presence of inflammation of the liver cells. A high figure (35 or more units), on the other hand, signifies an obstruction to the flow of bile.

The *Icteric index* is used as a measure of the depth of jaundice present. It is made by comparing the degree of yellowness produced by bilirubin and biliverdin in the serum with a standard potassium dichromate solution.

Normal = 0 to 10 units.
Abnormal = 15 units and above (first signs of jaundice).

Liver Blood Flow

The splanchnic vascular system supplies all the blood passing to the intestines from which it finally drains into the portal system and is carried to the liver. The liver blood flow, however, receives another contribution in the hepatic artery so that variations in the splanchnic flow and in that of the hepatic artery are reflected in the final amount of blood which passes through the liver.

Measurement of Liver Blood Flow

This is a complex procedure based on the extraction of bromsulphthalein by the liver cells (Bradley *et al.*, 1945). This technique has been adapted for use in anaesthetised patients by Shackman and his associates (1953). The conscious patient is first screened and a radio-opaque catheter is passed under vision by an arm vein via the superior vena cava into the inferior vena cava and from there into a branch of the right hepatic vein. This provides samples of portal blood *after* it has passed through the liver. Bromsulphthalein is injected intravenously, first as an initial priming dose and then as a continuous infusion of a 3 per cent solution in saline at an average rate of about 1·4 ml./minute. Once stabilisation has been reached the concentration in a peripheral artery is taken to equal that in the blood reaching the liver cells. A comparison between this concentration and that in the hepatic vein will reveal a relative drop due to the extraction by the liver cells. Since the arterio-venous difference can also be determined for similar samples, the actual amount of blood flowing through the liver can be calculated. More recently, Caesar and his colleagues (1961) have described a technique using indocyanine green in order to measure the splanchnic blood flow.

Flow in the Conscious State

Measurements made on conscious subjects suggest that the average liver blood flow is about 1·25 to 1·5 litres per minute. As the normal cardiac output for a patient at rest is about 5 litres/minute this means that about 25 per cent of this output passes to the liver. Under certain conditions, however, the liver has to sacrifice some of this flow in order to protect the homeostatic mechanism, maintain the systolic pressure, and ensure a blood supply to the most "vital" centres. Haemorrhage, congestive heart failure and severe exercise are amongst these causes.

Flow in the Anaesthetised Patient

The induction of a light plane of anaesthesia is sufficient to produce a drop of about 25 per cent in the amount of blood flowing through the liver. As the average flow in the conscious patient is about 1·25 litres it follows that the onset of anaesthesia reduces this flow to around 880 ml./minute (Shackman *et al.*, 1953). Deeper planes of anaesthesia produce an even greater fall. Price and his colleagues (1965) used indocyanine green to measure the splanchnic blood flow during anaesthesia in a group of volunteers who were not undergoing surgery. When cyclopropane was the anaesthetic used, the liver blood flow was significantly reduced by splanchnic vasoconstriction. If, at this point, a small dose of hexamethonium (i.e. one insufficient to lower the blood pressure yet capable of some ganglion blockade) was also given, then both the hepatic and the splanchnic flow could be returned to normal. On the basis of these findings the authors concluded that the reduced liver blood flow of cyclopropane anaesthesia is probably secondary to increased sympathetic activity in the splanchnic vascular bed.

In contrast, halothane anaesthesia produced a fall in liver blood flow without any change in the splanchnic vascular tone. In this case the reduced hepatic flow is probably secondary to a fall in blood pressure.

This reduction in hepatic blood flow must be considered in the light of the tremendous increase in flow that takes place in the skin and muscle vessels at the same time. Since there is no compensatory increase in the cardiac output in most forms of general anaesthesia, it follows that the liver—ably helped by the kidney—is the source for this extra amount of blood passing to the periphery. In fact, active vasoconstriction takes place. There is no evidence to suggest that this reorganisation of the blood flow is in any way beneficial to the patient, and certainly it is extremely troublesome for the surgeon.

Flow during Hypotension due to Autonomic Blockade

This leads to a fall in the liver blood flow and thus increases the risk of any damage to the liver cells. The mechanism of this fall in blood pressure is peripheral vasodilatation which includes the splanchnic bed. The reduced hepatic blood flow is secondary to the fall in systemic pressure and cardiac output. This follows whether the paralysis of the autonomic system is brought about by spinal or epidural analgesia, or by the use of ganglion-blocking drugs.

Flow during Hypotension associated with Vasoconstriction

This follows oligaemia from severe blood loss. The splanchnic bed attempts to compensate for this alteration in the haemodynamics by vasoconstriction which, in turn, results in a drop in the portal flow. When the systemic pressure falls the flow through the hepatic artery also drops. Thus the combination of vasoconstriction in the splanchnic bed with hypotension—as occurs after severe haemorrhage—may lead to a severe depletion of liver blood flows.

Flow during Hypothermia

Hypothermia causes both a fall in blood pressure and a reduction in liver blood flow, but it has the great advantage that in this case the metabolism (oxygen requirements) of the hepatic cells are reduced *pari passu* with the fall in temperature and blood pressure. There is little evidence to suggest that the liver cells suffer any damage from hypothermia alone, but if a period of cardiac arrest is also included then severe congestion of the liver cells may result from temporary occlusion of the inferior vena cava.

Flow and Vasoconstrictor Drugs

The administration of such drugs may reduce the liver blood flow. The local action of adrenaline upon the liver is one of vasoconstriction, but the systemic effect of raising the blood pressure by increasing the cardiac output predominates and the result is that the hepatic flow rises. Noradrenaline, on the other hand, is such a powerful vasoconstrictor that the liver flow usually shows a slight fall despite the rise in systemic pressure. Cases of damage to the liver cells following the infusion of noradrenaline have been reported. Other vasopressors, like methylamphetamine, which stimulate cardiac output increase the hepatic flow.

Anaesthesia and the Hepatic Cells

Liver cells can be affected in a number of ways. Hypoxia or the accumulation of carbon dioxide both cause damage. Sims and his co-workers (1951) undertook a clinical study in which patients were intentionally exposed to an atmosphere containing 15 per cent oxygen or less but with a normal alveolar carbon dioxide level. Other patients were deliberately exposed to an atmosphere containing 10 per cent carbon dioxide but with a very high oxygen content. By this manner it was hoped to study the effects of hypoxia and hypercarbia separately. In all, eighty patients were investigated mainly under ether and chloroform anaesthesia. They concluded that liver damage (as evidenced by function tests) occurs in a high proportion of all patients anaesthetised with these agents, even when the concentration of the inspired gases is normal. The presence of either hypoxia or hypercarbia, however, considerably increased the incidence of damage to the liver cells. A sharp fall in blood pressure was also found to be a potent cause.

Most anaesthetic drugs can be classed as protoplasmic poisons of lesser or greater degree, so that it is not surprising that they figure prominently in any study of liver function. As has already been mentioned, the liver cells surrounding the central lobular vein are working with a low oxygen saturation; it is hardly surprising, therefore, that they are the first to suffer damage if the saturation falls even lower. This, if coupled with the action of any anaesthetic drug used, may be sufficient to produce signs of liver damage. In essence the two causes—hypoxia and drugs—are inseparable and complementary.

Sherlock (1964) has pointed out that therapeutic agents may affect the liver cells in one of three ways:

1. *Direct toxic effect.*—Carbon tetrachloride is an example of this group. The incidence is strictly dose-dependant and such lesions can easily be reproduced in animals. Death is due to kidney failure with anuria rather than to hepatic failure.

2. *Hepatitis-like effects.*—Iproniazid and its derivatives are an example of this group. The incidence is unrelated to the dose though it is more common after multiple exposures suggesting a sensitivity reaction. Furthermore, the liver lesion cannot be reproduced in animals. Pathologically, there is a centrizonal hepatic necrosis with minimal fatty changes and a severe inflammatory (mononuclear) reaction predominating in the portal zones. However, this picture is indistinguishable from acute viral hepatitis. Death is due to liver failure and kidney involvement is slight.

3. *Cholestatic* (*obstructive*) *effect.*—Chlorpromazine is believed to be an example of this group.

Recently, great interest has centred on the suggestion that halothane might very rarely produce a hepatitis-like effect. This matter has already been discussed in full elsewhere (see p. 332), but it is interesting to consider this theory against the background of the action of anaesthetic drugs as a whole on liver function. For example, Rollason (1964) in a study using serum transaminase activity (SGPT) could find no evidence that either chloroform or halothane produced damage to liver cells. Green and Mungavin (1964) reached the same conclusion, as also did Griffiths and Ozgug (1964). Bløndal and Fagerlund (1963) using trichloroethylene, were also unable to demonstrate any obvious liver cell damage even when the highly sensitive serum enzyme estimations were used. Nevertheless, most of these authors have emphasised the importance of the surgical procedure itself. Many patients who have intra-abdominal or retroperitoneal operations show some evidence of liver cell damage regardless of the anaesthetic agent used.

Sargant (1963), in a discussion of mono-amine oxidase inhibitors and liver damage, has pointed out that although some authorities have readily accepted such an association, some patients on recovery from jaundice have actually received further doses of these drugs without ill effect. On this basis he argues that many of the cases of liver damage are due to the coincidental occurrence of viral hepatitis.

The muscle relaxants and liver damage.—The exact relationship between *d*-tubocurarine and the metabolism of the liver is still obscure. Dundee and Gray (1953) drew attention to the observation that patients with liver dysfunction required more *d*-tubocurarine to produce complete muscular paralysis than was normally required in similar healthy subjects. It has been suggested that *d*-tubocurarine is partly broken down in the liver, but the percentage of the total dose given that is removed in this way is probably small. Nevertheless, if the liver were damaged one might anticipate that these patients would require less *d*-tubocurarine rather than more. Dundee and Gray have suggested that the reason for this relationship may be associated with the pseudocholinesterase level. It is first assumed that if this is low, the cholinesterase at the motor end-plates is likewise affected; in this event it is reasonable to suppose that the concentration of acetylcholine ions is higher than normal because it is not being destroyed so rapidly. Thus, more *d*-tubocurarine than usual will be required to bring about paralysis (see also Chapter 31, p. 876).

The relationship between suxamethonium and pseudocholinesterase is now firmly established. Since the pseudocholinesterase level is a test of liver function it follows that it will be low in cases of hepatic failure. In this event the action of suxamethonium may be prolonged.

Acute Liver Failure in Relation to Anaesthesia and Surgery

In clinical anaesthesia there are two important occasions on which the signs and symptoms of liver damage may be recognised. First is after the use of chloroform, particularly if its administration is combined with the inhalation of a low percentage of oxygen and severe depletion of the liver glycogen. Such an occurrence is uncommon today. Secondly, the signs of liver failure may be seen in patients who have undergone a period of severe hypotension during anaesthesia. Most occur during major abdominal surgery in the absence of deliberate abolition of vasoconstriction by special drugs. The hypotension follows excessive haemorrhage which is not adequately replaced by transfusion and usually a systolic pressure of less than 40 mm. Hg is recorded for a short time. Post-operatively the patient is drowsy and lethargic, but the first definite signs of trouble are a persistent oliguria leading possibly to complete anuria within 24–48 hours of the operation. These renal signs occur so soon after operation and are so intense that they mask the concomitant signs arising from the damage to the liver (see below). This syndrome is called *hepato-renal failure* and it is nearly always fatal.

The symptoms and signs of hepatic failure are rather vague and indefinite at first but gradually become more obvious. At the start the patient complains of lassitude, malaise, anorexia and headache. Vomiting and pyrexia are often prominent. At about the third day vomiting is persistent and at the end of a week jaundice may be present. This heralds the final stages when the mental state becomes confused, with periods of delirium, and finally drifts into coma and death. Some patients may show a type of Parkinsonian rigidity.

Laboratory data are listed below (Table 1).

Treatment

The general principles of treatment—as advocated by Sherlock (1968)—are to eschew or treat any factor that might accentuate failure or precipitate coma, and to give the patient a suitable diet. Narcotic and sedative drugs are best avoided unless the patient is uncontrollable, when a small dose of a long-acting

48/TABLE 1

SOME LABORATORY DATA TO BE FOUND IN A CASE OF ACUTE LIVER FAILURE

	Normal	*Liver failure*
Serum bilirubin . .	Less than 1·7 mg. per cent.	20 mg. per cent or more.
Icteric index . .	3–6 units.	100 units or more.
Plasma fibrinogen .	200–500 mg. per cent.	100 mg. per cent or less.
Prothrombin time .	12–30 seconds.	10 per cent or more of normal.
Blood urea . .	15–40 mg. per cent.	10 mg. per cent or less.
SGOT . . .	5–17 units* 8–40 units†	500–800 or more.
SGPT . . .	4–13 units* 5–30 units†	500–800 or more.
LDH . . .	Up to 500 units.	1,000 or more.

* Spectrophotometric method.
† Colorimetric method.

barbiturate may be tried. Anaemia must be treated—if need be by blood transfusion. Provided the patient is not in pre-coma or coma, a small quantity of protein (100 g.) can be included in the daily diet, which should approximate to about 2,500 calories and to which vitamins must be added. Amino-acids accumulate in liver failure and their administration is more likely to be dangerous than useful. In the presence of pre-coma or coma, protein must not be given and it is usually best to administer carbohydrates as intravenous glucose to preserve an adequate caloric intake. Fluid and electrolyte balances must also be maintained.

HEPATIC DISEASE AND ANAESTHESIA

The reserves of the liver are so great that unless the patient is rapidly approaching hepatic failure, there are few agents that cannot be used in small dosage. Two factors, must, however, always be kept in mind. First the extent to which any particular agent depends upon liver function for its breakdown and removal from the body, and secondly the effect of the agent, and indeed of the anaesthetic and surgical procedure as a whole, on liver function. In practice, for minor surgical procedures in patients with severe disease a choice between cyclopropane, nitrous oxide or local analgesia can be made. Bearing in mind the part the liver plays in the detoxication of all local analgesics, only small quantities are safe. When a local technique is used, however, care should be taken to avoid covering it with opiates and their analogues or the phenothiazine derivatives, since these are unlikely to be tolerated in anything but minimal doses. Not only do nitrous oxide and cyclopropane have an insignificant effect upon liver function, but they do not rely upon it for their elimination. Provided they are suitable to produce the surgical conditions needed, and hypoxia or marked circulatory changes, such as hypotension, are avoided, they are the general anaesthetics of choice. For extensive operations such as a portacaval anastomosis then an induction of anaesthesia with cyclopropane and oxygen is satisfactory. If a non-explosive technique is required this can be followed by a nitrous oxide/oxygen and gallamine sequence. Gallamine triethiodide is chosen as the muscle relaxant because it is believed to be excreted unchanged by the kidney.

REFERENCES

BLØNDAL, B., and FAGERLUND B. (1963). Trichloroethylene anaesthesia and hepatic function. *Acta anaesth. scand.*, 7, 147.

BRADLEY, S. E., INGLEFINGER, F. J., BRADLEY, G. P., and CURRY, J. J. (1945). The estimation of hepatic blood flow in man. *J. clin. Invest.*, **24,** 890.

CAESAR, J., SHALDON, S., CHIANDUSSI, L., GUEVARA, L., and SHERLOCK, S. (1961). The use of indocyanine green in the measurement of hepatic blood flow and as a test of hepatic function. *Clin. Sci.*, **21,** 43.

DUNDEE, J. W., and GRAY, T. C. (1953). Resistance to *d*-tubocurarine chloride in the presence of liver damage. *Lancet*, **2,** 16.

GREEN, K. G., and MUNGAVIN, J. M. (1964). Halothane and the liver. Retrospective studies. *Proc. roy. Soc. Med.*, **57,** 311.

GRIFFITHS. H. W. C., and OZGUG, L. (1964). Effects of chloroform and halothane anaesthesia on liver function in man. *Lancet*, **1,** 246.

PRICE, H. L., DEUTSCH, S., COOPERMAN, L., CLEMENT, A. J., and EPSTEIN, R. M. (1965). Splanchnic circulation during cyclopropane anaesthesia in normal man. *Anesthesiology*, **26,** 312.

REITMAN, S., and FRANKEL, S. (1957). A colorimetric method for the determination of serum glutamic oxalacetic and glutamic pyruvic transaminases. *Amer. J. clin. Path.*, **28,** 56.

ROLLASON, W. N. (1964). Chloroform, halothane and hepatotoxicity. *Proc. roy. Soc. Med.*, **57,** 307.

SARGANT, W. (1963). Antidepressant drugs and liver damage. *Brit. med. J.*, **2,** 806.

SHACKMAN, R., GRABER, I. G., and MELROSE, D. G. (1953). Liver blood flow and general anaesthesia. *Clin. Sci.*, **12,** 307.

SHERLOCK, S. (1964). The hepatotoxic effects of anaesthetic drugs. *Proc. roy. Soc. Med.*, **57,** 305.

SIMS, J. L., MORRIS, L. E., ORTH, O. S , and WATERS. R. M. (1951). The influence of O_2 and CO_2 levels during anesthesia upon post-surgical hepatic damage. *J. Lab. clin. Med.*, **38,** 388.

FURTHER READING

SHERLOCK, S. (1968). *Diseases of the Liver and Biliary System*, 4th edit. Oxford: Blackwell Scientific Publications.

Chapter 49

ANAESTHESIA AND THE KIDNEY

Anatomy

The two kidneys are situated retroperitoneally in the abdomen, lying on either side of the vertebral column with the upper poles at the level of the twelfth thoracic vertebra. The lower poles reach to the level of the third lumbar vertebra but the right kidney is always slightly lower than the left. The approximate weight of the kidney is 150 g. in the male and 135 g. in the female.

The anterior surface of each kidney bears important relationships to many intra-abdominal structures, the upper pole is closely attached to the suprarenal gland, and the renal vessels and ureter join the hilum upon the medial border. The kidney itself is ensheathed in a fibrous capsule which may easily be removed, exposing a layer of smooth muscle fibres beneath. A cross section of the kidney substance reveals the outer cortical and the inner medullary substance.

Vascular System

The renal artery divides into four or five branches as it enters the hilum and each one of these gives off a small vessel which runs to the suprarenal gland. The main branches then proceed to divide into lobar arteries which run to the renal papillae, and each of these forms two or three interlobar arteries which pass towards the cortex of the kidney. On reaching the point of junction between medulla and cortex at the base of the pyramids each interlobar artery divides into two, and in a T-shaped fashion each branch runs at right angles to the parent stem between cortex and medulla. These vessels do not anastomose with their opposite number in the neighbouring lobe, but they give off important branches which pass into the cortex to supply the glomeruli (glomerular arteries). The venous drainage is similarly arranged.

Urinary System

The glomerulus consists of a mass of capillary vessels surrounded by the blind end of an expanded renal tubule called the glomerular capsule. This apparatus is concerned with filtering substances other than protein from the blood stream. The glomerular tubule leads to the first convoluted tubule, down the spiral part to the descending loop of Henle and then up again through the ascending loop to the irregular or zig-zag tubule. From there it leads to the second convoluted part whence it finally drains into the collecting tubule. The function of this tubular system is selective reabsorption so that the material that finally reaches the ureters is urine.

Nerve Supply

This is derived from the renal plexus which is composed of branches from the coeliac and aortic plexuses, the lower part of the coeliac ganglion, and from the lesser and lowest splanchnic nerves. All the nerve fibres which run to the kidney arise from the 10th to 12th thoracic segments.

Physiology

Under normal resting conditions about 20–25 per cent of the total cardiac output passes through the renal circulation each minute. In other words, the two kidneys between them receive a blood flow of 1,100–1,200 ml./minute. Approximately half of this total consists of plasma and the rest is made up of cells. Despite the fact that various "shunts" have been described it is generally believed that all this blood passes sooner or later to the glomerular capsule. Here the hydrostatic pressure of the systemic circulation, opposed only by the osmotic pull of the protein content of the blood, drives the fluid across the glomerular membrane to reach the renal tubules. Thus, of the original total of about 1,000 ml. of blood that enters the kidneys every minute, about 1/10th or 100 ml. passes down the tubules. At this point the selective reabsorption mechanism plays a major role and almost all the fluid content passes back into the circulation again. Of each 100 ml. of fluid entering the tubules, 99 ml. is reabsorbed. Put in another way, this means that 1 ml. of urine is formed from every 1,000 ml. of blood that goes to the kidneys.

Glomerular Filtration

The glomerular membrane is permeable to both fluid and electrolytes, but not to protein or cells. The driving force across this membrane is the systemic pressure and opposing it is the osmotic tension of the protein content of the blood. The fraction that passes across the glomerular membrane is normally about one-sixth of the renal plasma flow or one-tenth of the renal blood flow.

Thus:

If the renal blood flow is 1,200/minute,
and the renal plasma flow is 750/minute,
the total reaching the tubules is one-sixth of 750/minute, i.e. 120 ml./minute.

If the mean blood pressure is 80 mm. Hg and the osmotic pressure of the protein element is 25 mm. Hg, the effective filtration force will be 80–25 = 55 mm. Hg. There are a number of factors which influence this force and the most important is clearly fluctuations in the systemic blood pressure. For example, if the blood pressure fell to 25 mm. Hg there would be no filtration pressure at all. Clinically, it is known that in cases of severe hypotension during or immediately after surgery renal excretion ceases altogether, and this may be associated with signs of renal damage in the post-operative period. Other factors affecting the filtration pressure are alterations in the osmotic pressure of the plasma proteins or back-pressure reaching the glomeruli from obstruction to the tubules lower down.

In renal disease there is a close relationship between the severity of the damage and the number of functioning glomeruli, so that any further damage by anaesthetic agents or the like becomes of prime importance. The glomerular membrane itself is particularly susceptible to damage by hypoxia, ischaemia and drugs. Normally molecules with a weight of 70,000 and over cannot pass through the membrane, but those of 68,000 and below traverse it with ease. For example, albumin, with a molecular weight of 70,000, cannot permeate through the normal glomerular membrane, whereas gelatin, with a molecular weight of 35,000, passes without difficulty. Ischaemia of the glomerulus destroys this semi-permeability, hence the value of albumin in the urine as a guide to renal damage.

Tests of glomerular filtration.—In normal circumstances the glomeruli filter the plasma contents without showing any favours. Substances with large molecules pass across more slowly than those with small ones. The glomerular filtration rate is described as the amount of fluid passing from the capillaries in the glomerular tuft into the lumen of the glomerulus every minute.

I. *Creatinine test.*—As creatinine is a normal constituent of the blood which is filtered rapidly by the glomeruli yet is not reabsorbed in the tubules, it has become a popular means of assessing glomerular function. Unfortunately a very small quantity is secreted by the tubules, but this can be taken into account in the final assessment. Fortunately the blood level of creatinine remains remarkably constant, so that a long period of study can be contemplated yet it is only necessary to measure the blood level once during this period. The concentration of creatinine is determined spectroscopically, based on the intensity of the orange colour produced in the sample by picric acid.

Details of test.—The patient first empties his bladder thoroughly and this specimen is discarded. A 24-hour save of all the urine passed is then commenced. During this time a sample of venous blood is taken. If the concentration of creatinine in the blood and in the urine is known, together with the total volume of urine passed during the period, then the total quantity of glomerular filtrate can be calculated.

Although this test is not quite as accurate as that with inulin (see below), its simplicity makes it much more convenient in routine clinical practice.

The normal value in an adult patient of the creatinine clearance (i.e. glomerular filtration rate) is approximately 120 ml./minute.

There is a wide variation of about ± 15 ml./minute, and as the age of the patient increases so the glomerular filtration rate declines steadily until by the time the age of 90 or over is reached, the flow has fallen by approximately 50 per cent to 60 ml./minute.

II. *Urea clearance test.*—Like creatinine, urea is a normal constituent of the blood and therefore it is easy to do a clearance simply by determining its blood and urine concentrations and measuring the total volume of urine passed. Since some of the urea that enters the tubules is reabsorbed into the circulation an allowance must be made for this and if the glomerular filtration rate is 120 ml./minute, then the urea clearance is 40 per cent of 120, or 75ml./minute. Furthermore, the urea clearance is very dependant on the rate of urine flow and when the flow drops below 2 ml./minute the inaccuracies are considerable. Then a figure can only be calculated with the use of a complex formula and is sometimes referred to as the *standard urea clearance*, but in clinical practice it is rarely used. Under normal conditions of the test, the fluid intake of the patient is so adjusted that the total quantity of urine passed exceeds 2 ml./minute. The result may then be termed a *maximal* urea clearance.

As the concentration of urea in the blood is subject to wide fluctuations it is essential that the total duration of the test is limited.

Details of test.—Prior to the test all food is withheld for a number of hours. Half an hour before it is due to begin the patient is asked to drink two glasses of water. At zero hour the bladder is emptied and the specimen discarded. At the end of the first and second hours the bladder contents are collected, measured, and their urea content determined. Also, at the end of the first hour the blood urea level is measured.

The calculation is made from the following formula:

$$\frac{\text{Concentration of urea in urine} \times \text{volume of urine}}{\text{Concentration of urea in blood}} = \text{urea clearance in ml./minute.}$$

Normal value: 75 ml./minute (when urine flow exceeds 2 ml./minute). Clinically this value is often expressed as 100 per cent of normal:

A fall to 50 per cent of normal denotes renal damage.
A fall to 20 per cent of normal denotes severe renal damage.
A fall to 5 per cent of normal denotes that uraemic symptoms are present.

III. *Blood urea and creatinine levels.*—As both urea and creatinine clearance values are useful methods of assessing glomerular filtration rates, so the level of these substances in the blood gives some indication of renal function.

The normal blood values for:

Urea are	15·0–40·0 mg. per cent.
Creatinine are	0·7– 2·0 mg. per cent.

A rise in blood urea is a relatively late sign of renal damage, for by the time this stage has been reached the urea clearance values may have fallen to 20 per cent of normal. Unfortunately, as both urea and creatinine are produced in the body their concentrations in the blood can be altered by other factors, such as dehydration, haemorrhage and low or high protein diets. Nevertheless a blood urea concentration of 60 mg. per cent, or a creatinine level over 2 mg. per cent usually denotes severe depression of the glomerular filtration rate (de Wardener, 1968).

IV. *Inulin clearance.*—The most accurate method of assessing glomerular filtration rate is by the use of inulin, as this substance is filtered unchanged by the glomeruli but is not reabsorbed by the tubules. Despite this, such measurements are usually reserved for estimations requiring great accuracy, as the continuous infusion of inulin and the repeated blood sampling make this method unsuitable for routine clinical testing.

V. *Proteinuria.*—The presence of significant quantities of protein in the urine denotes the presence of glomerular or tubular damage. Normally about 10–20 mg. per cent of protein passes across the glomerular membrane, but almost the entire quantity is reabsorbed by the tubules.

The method of detection of protein in the urine depends either on simple precipitation by boiling or by flocculation with 25 per cent salicyl sulphonic acid.

Salicyl Sulphonic Acid Test

Trace of precipitate—approximately equivalent to a concentration of 0·2 g. protein/litre.

Heavy precipitate—approximately equivalent to a concentration of 5·0 g. protein/litre.

The significance of a positive result to this test is influenced by the dilution of the urine. Thus a positive response in a very concentrated urine is of less importance than the same result in a dilute one. Macroscopic blood or pus will be responsible for some precipitate and care should be taken to avoid this error.

The exact type of proteins excreted is sometimes of significance in diagnosis of the underlying renal disease. Thus electrophoretic separation can distinguish between albumin and globulin. In acute nephritis both protein types are excreted in the same proportions as in the plasma, whereas in myelomatosis the globulin fraction may appear without albuminuria (de Wardener, 1968).

VI. *Blood cells and casts.*—Small amounts of blood cells (red and white) and hyaline casts may be found in the urine of normal subjects. Nevertheless, if a 4-hour save of urine is taken and the phosphates in it precipitated by glacial acetic acid, then when the resultant fluid has been centrifuged, the number of cells recognised microscopically in a counting chamber can be determined:

Normal urine contains 50,000 cells with a range of 0–200,000 red cells per hour.

Abnormal urine contains over 200,000 red cells per hour (de Wardener, 1958).

The only casts that are of any clinical importance are the blood and granular types. Both these denote renal damage.

Tubular Reabsorption

The contents of the glomerular filtrate are identical with that of the plasma lying across the glomerular membrane inside the tuft of capillaries. But although this liquid starts out on its journey through the tubular system resembling plasma, by the time it reaches the end it bears no relation to it at all. On its way down, enormous quantities of water and certain electrolytes are reabsorbed. This process is selective, so that the kidney tubules play an important part in controlling the electrolyte balance of the body. For example, for every 100 litres of water that enters the tubules less than 1 litre (0·9 litres, to be precise) reaches the urine. Any glucose which passes through the glomerular membrane is completely reabsorbed so that none enters the urine; nearly all the sodium, chloride and calcium ions are reabsorbed, and likewise 8 per cent of the potassium ions, 25 per cent of the phosphate, and 60 per cent of the urea (Wright, 1965). There are believed to be specific mechanisms controlling the reabsorption of salts and water. In the latter case the water content of the body is controlled through the antidiuretic hormone of the posterior pituitary, and it is well known that nearly all anaesthetic drugs stimulate the release of this substance. Adrenal corticoid excretion controls sodium and chloride levels and again this would appear to be slightly stimulated by anaesthetic drugs.

Tubular Excretion

This suggests that certain substances are actively excreted across the tubular membrane, and this concept replaces the rather controversial tubular secretion theory. In man none of the normal plasma constituents is so excreted, with the doubtful exception of creatinine. Injected dyestuffs such as diodrast may be treated in this manner.

Tests of tubular function.—As the role of the tubules is largely one of selective reabsorption, most of the tests are based on the concentration of solids in the urine. Similarly, as the primary function of the tubules is to withdraw most of the water from its lumen, the ability to pass a concentrated or dilute urine under different conditions can be used as a gauge of tubular activity.

I. *Urine concentration test.*—The specific gravity of the urine can be measured with a hydrometer. Normally, the range lies between 1,010–1,020 but much will depend on the fluid intake. In diabetes, when large quantities of glucose are reaching the urine, the specific gravity is high, whereas tubular damage leads to a very dilute urine.

The ability of the kidney to concentrate urine may be studied in two ways: (*a*) complete abstinence from fluids for a 24-hour period has been used. This method is extremely unpleasant for the patient. A normal kidney should produce one specimen during this period with a specific gravity of 1,020 or more. (*b*) An intramuscular injection of pitressin tannate (5 mg.) in oil is found to be a much more satisfactory alternative because it does not interfere with the patient's normal fluid intake. The action of the pitressin is to inhibit diuresis, so again a 24-hour urine save is instituted. The patient is allowed to eat and drink in a normal manner. One sample during this period should have a specific gravity of 1,020 or more if normal tubular function is present.

II. *Urine dilution test.*—For this test the patient consumes a known quantity of water (1 litre) and the ability of the kidney to excrete most of this intake is then studied. First the bladder is emptied and the contents discarded in the usual manner. Samples are then taken hourly for the next four hours. Normally at least 750 ml. out of the 1 litre drunk by the patient should be recovered in the urine and the specific gravity will be less than 1,004 in at least one specimen. Smoking and extreme emotion, however, may limit the diuresis.

Other methods that are used to study tubular function are more complex and involve the measurement of sodium, potassium, calcium, phosphate, and ammonium excretion (de Wardener, 1968).

Measurement of Renal Blood Flow (R.B.F.)

The renal blood flow is the total quantity of blood passing to the kidneys each minute. In order to measure this amount of blood it is necessary to find a substance which is completely removed from the plasma during a single passage through the glomerular tuft yet is neither reabsorbed nor excreted by the tubules. Then the plasma flow can be measured, and from this the blood flow to the kidney can be calculated. Diodrast and para-amino-hippuric acid (P.A.H.) nearly fulfil these criteria, but P.A.H. is technically easier to use. In fact only 90 per cent of it passes across the membrane and the remaining 10 per cent recirculates. Nevertheless allowances can be made for this fraction in the final calculation. The exact proportion of P.A.H. that is removed by a normal kidney has been confirmed in patients by simultaneous sampling of the concentration in the renal artery and vein during a steady infusion. Theoretically, if this substance was completely removed the concentration in the renal vein would be nil. In practice it was found that a small percentage (10 per cent) eluded filtration. The route that this proportion takes is not clear but it may pass through diseased or non-functioning areas and so avoid the glomeruli altogether. In the final calculation the *effective* renal plasma flow (as measured) is converted to the *true* renal plasma flow by multiplying the figures obtained by 1·1.

Measurement of renal plasma flow is made by first giving the patient a priming dose of P.A.H. followed by an infusion of it given at a rate which just compensates for its loss in the urine. In these circumstances the concentration of P.A.H. on the venous side is practically the same as that on the arterial side, so that venous samples may be used in the estimation.

Thus:

P.A.H. clearance × 1·1 = Renal plasma flow in ml./minute.

The plasma flow can be converted to blood flow if the value for the haematocrit is known:

R.B.F. = 1,100 – 1,200 ml./minute.

Renal Blood Flow in the Conscious Patient

In normal circumstances the flow through the renal vessels does not vary widely. This constancy is maintained largely by alteration in the calibre of the renal arterioles. The kidney has its own "regulating" mechanism which ensures that it receives as adequate a supply of blood as possible despite variations in the systemic pressure. There are many factors which can reduce the renal blood flow in a conscious patient and prominent amongst them are haemorrhage, fainting, asphyxia and the effects of spinal analgesia or ganglion blockade.

The mechanism by which these various conditions reduce the renal blood flow is not the same in each case.

(*a*) *In hypovolaemia*, as is evidenced by haemorrhage, the mechanism is complex. In man there is a profound fall in renal blood flow and glomerular filtration. This fall is out of all proportion to the drop in blood pressure and is caused by severe renal vasoconstriction. One of the principal features of this condition is that even if the patient is thoroughly transfused and the blood volume and pressure returned to normal levels, the vasoconstriction does not wear off for several hours (Lauson *et al.*, 1944).

The cause of this vasoconstriction has been thoroughly investigated and is now believed to be one of two factors—one nervous, the other humoral. Following severe haemorrhage with renal ischaemia, transfusion will slowly reverse the vasoconstriction if it is given within the first four hours. During this period the vasoconstriction is believed to be nervous in origin.

After four hours of renal ischaemia produced by hypotension the vasoconstriction may take many days to pass off even after suitable transfusion therapy; alternatively it may be irreversible. This persistent vasoconstriction is thought to be humoral in origin. Various substances have been suggested, and the most likely are renin (Wright, 1965) or vaso-excitory material (V.E.M.) (Shorr *et al.*, 1948).

(*b*) *In the faint reaction*, there is essentially a slowing of the heart rate with marked peripheral vasodilatation. The cardiac output falls and the renal blood flow is reduced.

(*c*) *When a high concentration of carbon dioxide or a low oxygen tension* occurs in the blood reaching the kidneys the renal vessels tend to constrict. The precise mechanism of this action is unknown.

(*d*) *In denervation*, as in autonomic block due to spinal analgesia or to the use of ganglion-blocking drugs, the renal vessels are dilated and the renal flow closely follows any changes in the systemic blood pressure. If the pressure remains unchanged the renal flow will do likewise: if it falls, so will the flow through the kidney. This merely emphasises the part played by the autonomic system in controlling the renal blood flow.

Renal Blood Flow in the Anaesthetised Patient

Effect of Anaesthesia

The induction of anaesthesia with ether, cyclopropane or thiopentone is followed by an almost immediate fall in the renal blood flow. The degree of depression of the flow will depend upon the depth of anaesthesia. Thus, under very light anaesthesia the flow will be about 800 ml./minute (*cf* conscious = 1,200 ml./minute), but under deep anaesthesia it falls to 200 ml./minute or even less. So fine and rapid is this change in flow in relation to alterations in the depth of anaesthesia with both ether and cyclopropane, that the renal blood flow could easily be used as an accurate sign of anaesthetic depth. During a long operation with a constant level of anaesthesia the flow remains unaltered, and as soon as the anaesthetic is withdrawn the blood flow starts to return to normal.

The mechanism of this reduction in flow has been studied in animals (Miles and de Wardener, 1952) using ether and cyclopropane. Dogs were anaesthetised by a continuous intravenous infusion of pentobarbitone sodium, which produces little change in the renal circulation. The kidney was then perfused with a constant volume pump. The inhalation of ether and cyclopropane resulted in a pronounced and sustained rise in the perfusion pressure. Since this effect no longer occurred after denervation of the kidney it was concluded that the fall in blood flow was due to neurogenic vasoconstriction. Halothane, like most other general anaesthetic agents, brings about a fall in renal blood flow in premedicated patients (Mazze *et al.*, 1963). However, at comparable depths of anaesthesia the reduction with cyclopropane and ether is greater than that with halothane. This could be explained on the basis that halothane produces less catecholamine excretion (leading to renal vasoconstriction) than either ether or cyclopropane.

Chloroform, halothane and trichloroethylene are all believed to produce renal vasoconstriction—the degree depending upon the concentration used.

Effect of Surgery

Habif and his co-workers (1951) have shown that most operative procedures do not produce any change in the renal circulation. de Wardener (1955) has confirmed these findings, but referred to one case where severe traction upon the large bowel had produced temporary vasoconstriction. Since there is considerable difficulty in obtaining adequate data on patients undergoing major surgery, it would at present seem advisable to conclude that major surgical stimulation—

particularly under very light anaesthesia—may lead to depression of renal blood flow.

Effect of Ganglion-blocking Drugs

Since the introduction of the hypotensive technique many authors have strongly condemned this method of reducing bleeding during surgery, on the grounds that it leads to increased damage to the kidney. It is difficult to gather from a simple comparative study of patients under anaesthesia with and without hypotension whether any renal damage occurs. Hampton and Little (1953) stated that the incidence of renal complications following the use of hypotensive drugs during anaesthesia was no greater than in a comparable control series. Evans and Enderby (1952) in a similar study based upon fluid excretion, proteinuria and the appearance of casts and red cells in the urine found, in a small series of 50 patients, that although the incidence of damage was slightly greater in the hypotensive group it was statistically insignificant. Miles and his colleagues (1952) produced valuable evidence by measuring the renal blood flow and glomerular filtration rate of patients undergoing hypotension without surgery. They used pentamethonium bromide and found in a series of 10 patients that although the systemic pressure fell by an average of 34 per cent, the average fall in the renal blood flow was only 5 per cent. In one of their cases the mean blood pressure fell below 40 mm. Hg yet the renal blood flow—though depressed—was still greater than they had found under deep anaesthesia in the absence of ganglion-blocking drugs.

From these observations it is concluded that renal vasodilatation must occur in the presence of hypotensive anaesthesia due to ganglion-blocking drugs. The experimental evidence available suggests that as the systemic pressure falls, so the renal vessels dilate to keep an almost steady flow of blood. On this basis it can be said that the normal kidney does not suffer damage from relatively short periods of hypotensive anaesthesia. It must be emphasised, however, that no data are available for very long periods of hypotension or the pathological kidney.

Moyer and McConn (1956), in a group of anaesthetised patients receiving pentamethonium, hexamethonium, and trimetaphan, were unable to confirm these results obtained by Miles and his colleagues. In their patients the fall in blood pressure was followed by a reduction in the renal blood flow and the glomerular filtration rate in both normal and hypertensive patients. Associated with the fall in glomerular filtration rate was a marked reduction in the excretion of water and sodium. This was so great that they emphasised the dangers of overloading such a patient with fluids. Wakim (1955), using a flow meter inserted into the renal vein of dogs, also found a fall in their renal blood flow during hypotension with hexamethonium.

This evidence completely contradicts that of Miles and his colleagues (1952), but on close scrutiny of the figures the actual reduction in blood flow is not very great. Most significant of all, little or no mention is made by Moyer and McConn of steps taken to prevent any fluctuation in depth of anaesthesia or to prevent a rise in the carbon dioxide tension of the blood. Since the smallest change in anaesthetic depth or carbon dioxide tension is sufficient to produce marked changes in the renal blood flow, variations in either of these measurements may account for the fundamental differences in these results.

Effect of Haemorrhage

On purely theoretical grounds it might be reasoned that the renal vessels would constrict in the presence of increasing blood loss. de Wardener and his associates (1953) have shown that this is not the case. In the anaesthetised subject the renal vessels dilate as the systemic pressure falls, so that they maintain an even flow of blood to the renal tissue despite the obvious paucity of flow in other parts of the body.

In their study these investigators measured the cardiac output, right auricular pressure, forearm blood flow, systemic pressure, heart rate, glomerular filtration and renal blood flow in a series of patients under light anaesthesia. The anaesthetic agents used were ether and cyclopropane. Haemorrhage was produced by venesection in amounts varying from 800–1,500 ml. at a rate of 70–200 ml./minute. In the whole group the average fall in the estimated blood volume was 23 per cent. The only frequent change that they observed was a small reduction in renal flow during the actual venesection, but this rapidly returned to the previous level after the bleeding was completed. In twelve out of their fourteen patients venesection produced no *significant* change in the renal blood flow. In the two remaining patients the blood pressure fell to such a low level (below 40 mm. Hg) that the flow of urine ceased. When it started again the data available suggested, however, that the renal blood flow had continued during the period of anuria and that this flow had been reduced far less than would have been expected. The severe hypotension and bradycardia that occurred in these two patients was corrected immediately by rapid transfusion.

There are two important facts that emerge from this work on haemorrhage in the anaesthetised patient. First, the normal kidney does not apparently suffer acute ischaemia from severe hypotension under anaesthesia, and any reduction in flow that may occur can quickly be restored by transfusion therapy. Secondly, it is possible for the normal anaesthetised patient to lose up to 25–30 per cent of his total circulating blood volume without showing any significant changes in blood pressure or heart rate. This finding is of particular importance in any discussion upon the aetiology of post-operative renal failure.

In man, complete renal ischaemia lasting longer than 30 minutes is usually followed by tubular damage and such an event is most likely to occur during the removal of an aortic aneurysm. This damage can be largely prevented by hypothermia; periods of up to two hours of total occlusion with only minor signs of renal damage at a body temperature of 28° C have been reported (Churchill-Davidson, 1955).

Auto-regulating mechanism.—In the conscious subject even a relatively small haemorrhage is followed by a vaso-vagal attack where the blood pressure falls largely due to widespread dilatation of the muscle vessels. At the same time the renal vessels dilate (de Wardener and McSwiney, 1951). Under anaesthesia, even after a relatively massive haemorrhage, the renal vessels still dilate, but now the muscle vessels are found to be constricted. It was originally thought that the renal dilatation that occurred on fainting might be part of a widespread neurogenic vasodilating mechanism. The finding that under anaesthesia the muscle vessels constrict whilst the renal vessels dilate supports, however, the concept that the kidney has its own auto-regulating mechanism which tends to maintain an even level of renal blood flow despite alterations in the cardiac output and systemic pressure. The presence of such an intrinsic mechanism has been confirmed in animals (de Wardener and Miles, 1952). Phillips and his associates (1945), working with dogs, also commented upon the relative stability of the renal circulation after haemorrhage, and they stated "the kidneys appear now to be favoured at the expense of the other peripheral circulation". Severe renal vasoconstriction occurred, however, after 4 to 6 hours of oligaemia.

Therefore, on the basis of all this evidence, it seems improbable that a transient reduction in blood volume, as may occur during surgery, can be responsible for the ischaemic renal damage that occasionally follows operations. Nevertheless, it is important to stress that all these measurements were made upon people with good kidney function and these deductions certainly do not hold when severe renal disease is already present.

Effect of Vasopressor Drugs

When hypotension develops during anaesthesia a vasopressor drug is often used to restore the systemic pressure to a normal level. Two assumptions are usually made when considering the injection of these drugs. First, that the low blood pressure is necessarily associated with a reduced flow to the vital organs, and secondly, that raising the blood pressure by pressor drugs will automatically improve the flow. When considering the kidney both these assumptions may be unwarranted.

In the conscious patient, raising the blood pressure either with adrenaline (Smith, 1943) or noradrenaline (Barnett *et al.*, 1950) is associated with a pronounced renal vasoconstriction and fall in renal blood flow.

In the anaesthetised patient, the action of adrenaline, noradrenaline and methylamphetamine upon the renal blood flow have been studied (Churchill-Davidson *et al.*, 1951). These pressor drugs were given to both a group of patients with a normal blood pressure and a group with induced hypotension produced by pentamethonium bromide. The effect of the drugs upon the renal vessels was essentially the same, whether a low blood pressure was present or not. Adrenaline and noradrenaline both produced a rise in blood pressure accompanied by a consistent fall in the renal blood flow. On the other hand, methylamphetamine led to a rise in blood pressure and an overall increase in renal blood flow. No information is available about the action of these drugs upon the renal circulation in cases of hypotension due to haemorrhage. Moyer and McConn (1956) studied the effects of vasopressor drugs on a group of hypertensive patients. Their results showed an increase in renal flow when the blood pressure was raised by noradrenaline after an injection of pentamethonium.

To summarise, the available evidence on the action of vasopressor drugs on the renal circulation is contradictory. Nevertheless, the change produced by these drugs, whether it be an increase or a decrease in blood flow, is not severe. The use of these drugs, therefore, should not be withheld (when they are necessary) on the grounds of possible damage to the renal tissue. In the presence of oliguria or anuria methylamphetamine would appear to be a more favourable pressor drug than noradrenaline.

Renal Failure in Relation to Anaesthesia and Surgery

Following major surgery it is commonplace to find traces of albumin, red cells and casts in the urine during the first three post-operative days. In fact, Evans and Enderby (1952) found that 78 per cent of a small series of normal patients developed proteinuria on the day after operation and in 34 per cent this persisted for more than three days. Cases of severe renal damage are fortunately rare, but when they occur they are often attended by a fatal result. The term "hepato-renal" failure has now been virtually abandoned, since it does no more than draw attention to the fact that what damages one organ also affects the other. The clinical picture of post-operative renal damage may be classed as either mild or severe.

In the mild condition the patient passes a plentiful supply of water in the first few days after operation. If it were accurately measured a polyuria would be noticed. Around the 7th–10th day the patient becomes mentally difficult or drowsy, and it is this change in the patient's mental attitude that often draws attention to the underlying condition. A blood urea taken at this stage reveals a level of 250 mg. or more. In all probability these patients had underlying renal damage before operation and a careful history usually reveals that they had polyuria at the same time. This can most easily be ascertained by a history of rising in the night to pass water with the absence of any prostatic enlargement on examination.

The severe type is the commoner condition and usually oliguria or anuria are noticed on the first post-operative day. Anuria is exceptional. The blood urea shows a steadily rising value and the rate of this rise is often taken as an indication of the severity of the condition. Vomiting and diarrhoea are early signs, together with restlessness, a wandering mind, and severe headache. Insomnia may be a marked feature and in the later stages muscle twitches and cramps may occur. By the third day the signs of hepatic failure with jaundice are usually present as well, and in such a case the prognosis is grave.

Causative Factor

Many factors have been blamed in the past, but at the present time the general opinion favours a prolonged period of hypotension leading to renal ischaemia as the principal cause. Anaesthesia, surgery, and even haemorrhage hardly affect the normal kidney, but then it is rare for the patient with normal kidney function to suffer failure post-operatively. During major surgery, particularly on the heart, a period of severe hypotension may occur. The resulting hypoxia of the renal cells is believed to lead to damage which is only revealed during the post-operative period. In the immediate post-operative period, when consciousness has been regained, a low blood volume state—as occurs after blood loss—is the most likely cause of intense renal vasoconstriction. Experimental data have shown that it is possible for a patient under light anaesthesia to lose 25 per cent of his blood volume without obvious circulation signs. When consciousness has been regained, however, a hypovolaemia of this extent may be sufficient to cause intense renal vasoconstriction while producing only a slight fall in blood pressure.

Under normal circumstances the renal blood flow in the conscious patient remains remarkably constant despite considerable fluctuations in the perfusion pressure. This intimate control is believed to be exerted through neural and hormonal influences as part of the homeostatic mechanism controlling the extracellular fluid volume. In severe haemorrhage there is an immediate increase in intrarenal vascular resistance, presumably due to vasoconstriction (Parsons *et al.*, 1963). In turn, this leads to a decrease in renal blood flow, a fall in the amount of sodium and water excreted and possibly a reduction in glomerular filtration rate. These changes, which are at first reversible but eventually lead to tubular damage, are more severe in those patients with pre-existing renal disease.

The induction of general anaesthesia causes a fall in the renal blood flow which is roughly proportional to the depth of unconsciousness. The exact mechanism of renal ischaemia in the surgical patient is still unknown but it is probably similar to that in the conscious state. The most widely held view is that it is related to a period of hypotension either during or immediately after the operation, and on this basis, during the period of ischaemia, the renal tubular cells are damaged. On the re-establishment of a normal blood flow these cells either recover completely or their permeability is damaged so that they swell with oedema and partially or totally occlude the lumen of the tubule. This theory is the basis for the use of mannitol in the prophylactic treatment of suspected cases of renal damage. As mannitol is excreted virtually unchanged it is presumed that a hypertonic solution not only tends to keep the lumen of the tubules patent but may also withdraw some of the water from the tubule cells, thus diminishing the effects of the oedema.

Evidence to support the hypotensive theory of post-operative renal failure is mostly clinical. Certainly oliguria and anuria are very rare complications in patients undergoing routine minor surgery with general anaesthesia. Yet in major surgery—particularly in association with the extracorporeal circulation with a poor total perfusion—the signs of renal damage are frequently observed.

Diagnosis

The first indication of renal damage in the post-operative period is oliguria. This is a term used to denote a total urinary output in twenty-four hours of less than 720 ml. (i.e. 0·5 ml./minute). Nevertheless, oliguria in the post-operative period is not always due to renal failure for it is commonly brought about by dehydration. If a patient's fluid intake by mouth is curtailed or abandoned for many hours before operation, yet the "insensible" loss of sweating, humidification and alimentary secretions continues, it is not surprising that dehydration rapidly occurs. The "insensible" loss is usually estimated at about 1 litre per 24 hours. To this must be added any haemorrhage at the time of operation together with the extrusion of fluid into the lumen of bowel during surgical manipulations. If adequate precautions are not taken to maintain the circulating fluid volume by infusion then dehydration will result. This will lead to haemoconcentration with a raised haematocrit and haemoglobin level.

The distinction, therefore, between a low urinary output due to dehydration and one due to renal failure can be made in two ways. First, the specific gravity of any urine voided is measured. If the circulating blood volume is low (as in dehydration) yet renal function is normal, then the kidney will pass out very concentrated urine. The specific gravity in the presence of dehydration will be above 1,018 and probably in the region of 1,020–1,030. On the other hand, if renal function is failing then the kidney loses its power to concentrate urine by the reabsorption of water in the tubules so that the specific gravity cannot rise above about 1,010.

Thus:	*Specific gravity*
In presence of dehydration	Over 1,018
In presence of renal failure	1,010 or less.

The second method of distinguishing between oliguria due to dehydration and that of renal failure is to measure the amount of urea present in the urine. In acute renal failure a value of less than 1,100 mg. of urea in 100 ml. of urine is a good indication of damage to tubular excretion (Molloy, 1962). This measurement is more helpful than that of the blood urea which often rises only as a late manifestation of renal damage, because essentially it depends on the amount of protein breakdown that is taking place.

Treatment

A patient with severe, acute post-operative renal failure rarely survives for more than ten days unless effective treatment is employed quickly. Even then the prognosis is poor. In the less severe type of case which responds fairly rapidly to therapy the oliguria gives way to polyuria. The onset of polyuria has often been regarded as due to some change in the excretory mechanism, but the more recent conception holds that it is due to the excess fluid that the patient has ingested during the period of oliguria.

The basic principle, therefore, of any treatment of this condition is twofold. First, since the cells of the collecting tubules are damaged, the fluid intake of the patient must be kept as nearly as possible equal to the fluid output. This latter figure must take into account any insensible loss from sweating, vomiting and diarrhoea, besides any small amount of urine that is passed. Secondly, the diet must be so arranged that protein metabolism is kept as low as possible, because the waste products of nitrogen metabolism soon mount to toxic levels. In normal subjects it is known that a high carbohydrate intake depresses protein metabolism and it is assumed that the same process takes place under the conditions of acute renal failure.

Bull and his associates (1949) were amongst the first to point out the advantages of conservative treatment in this condition. Their regime—designed to depress metabolism—consisted of restricting the fluid intake combined with a high carbohydrate intake.

However, this form of therapy has now been virtually abandoned for two reasons. First, the total fluid intake was excessive in that it made no allowance for the water produced as a result of tissue metabolism or from the metabolism of any ingested carbohydrates. It is estimated that as much as 450 ml. per day are added to the total body fluids simply due to tissue metabolism, and a further 150 ml. are obtained from the metabolism of carbohydrate. This means that the body itself can produce as much as 600 ml. of water per day. If this quantity is ignored and the patient is given a total fluid intake equivalent to the whole of his "insensible" loss, then he will rapidly become waterlogged.

The present-day management of patients with early post-operative renal failure is based on a strict surveillance of body weight and the biochemical changes in both blood and urine.

Preliminary measures.—1. The *weight* of the patient is accurately determined, as this will give an indication of gain or loss of fluids in the future treatment.

2. *Biochemical data* are also obtained as a baseline for the effectiveness of the therapy. The measurements made are:

(*a*) Blood. Values for urea, calcium, potassium, sodium, chloride and bicarbonate are obtained. The haematocrit is also measured.

(*b*) Urine. Values for urea, sodium and potassium are estimated.

3. *An indwelling catheter* is inserted into the bladder so that a close watch can be kept on the exact amount of urine that is excreted.

4. *Restriction of fluids.*—The vital importance of the water obtained from metabolism within the body has already been mentioned. This sum amounts to approximately 600 ml. daily. The total fluid required for a perfect balance of fluid therapy is composed of the sum of fluid lost by "sensible" and "insensible" loss. The "sensible" loss is the fluid which leaves the body either as urine or vomit. The "insensible" is the amount of fluid used up in sweating, humidification of the air in the lungs, and secretions into the bowel lumen which are lost in the faeces, and is usually taken as 1 litre per day. Thus a patient's fluid requirements will be 400 ml. of sugar solution which together with the 600 ml. produced within the body will provide for the 1,000 ml. lost from "insensible" sources. To this total intake must also be added exactly the amount lost through urinary excretion and vomit.

The basis for restricted fluid therapy in acute renal failure can be expressed as:

$$
\begin{array}{l}\text{Insensible}\\ \text{loss 1,000 ml.} + \\ \text{sensible loss}\end{array} = \begin{array}{l} 400\text{ ml. of sugar solution}\\ \left.\begin{array}{l}+\ 450\text{ ml. from tissue metabolism}\\ +\ 150\text{ ml. from carbohydrate metabolism}\end{array}\right\} = \begin{array}{l}\text{600 ml. from}\\ \text{body}\\ \text{metabolism}\end{array}\\ +\ \text{sensible loss}\end{array}
$$

In this way fluid intake and output can be finely balanced. However, a small steady weight loss of 200–500 g. daily will occur when a balance has been achieved, presumably due to a loss of body proteins.

Further measures.—1. *Carbohydrate* in the form of laevulose is most commonly used because not only is the sugar more easily metabolised than the others but it is also believed to be the least nauseating when given by mouth in high concentration. Normally 100 g. of laevulose are added to 400 ml. of water, and this can be taken orally. If vomiting occurs as a complication, then a sterile solution of fructose can be infused into a large vein. As high concentrations of sugar solutions produce a severe reaction with thrombosis in small veins, it is advisable to insert a polythene catheter into the lumen of the vena cava (inferior or superior) before starting the infusion. Nevertheless the oral route is preferable because of the risk of infected emboli from the use of intravenous catheters.

2. *Anabolic steroids* (i.e. testosterone) are given to reduce the breakdown of protein within the body.

3. *Antibiotics* and *Anticoagulants* must only be used with caution as many tend to accumulate in the circulation if renal function is poor. For example,

streptomycin is contra-indicated in such circumstances as even small doses may lead to VIIIth cranial nerve damage. Similarly, the sulphonamides should not be used as they tend to form crystals in the renal tubules, thus increasing the renal damage. Crystalline and the various oral penicillins have been found to be satisfactory.

Most of the long-acting anticoagulants (e.g. dicoumarin) tend to accumulate in the presence of renal failure but heparin can be used with safety because it is detoxicated in the liver.

4. *Ion-exchange resins* can be used to control the serum potassium level which tends to rise steadily in the presence of acute renal failure. These resins are in powder form and can be given either orally or rectally. They act by accepting potassium and releasing sodium in exchange. Using "Resonium" 15 g. four times a day, it is often possible to keep the serum potassium level between 3·5 and 4·0 mEq/litre. Alternatively in an emergency the administration of glucose (40 g.) and insulin (20 units) tends to lower the serum potassium level by holding the electrolyte within the cell.

Once this regime has been fully established it is then only necessary to observe closely the effects of this therapy. The future progress will reveal the extent and severity of the renal damage. If it is clear that restriction of fluids alone is not preventing a gradual deterioration in the patient's state then the question of dialysis must be considered.

Indications for dialysis are:

(*a*) Worsening of the clinical state of the patient—particularly the appearance of pre-uraemic features together with mental retardation.

(*b*) Blood urea nitrogen (BUN) over 150–170 mg. per cent or a blood urea over 300 mg. per cent.

(*c*) A rise in the serum potassium level over 7·0 mEq/litre.

(*d*) A fall in the plasma bicarbonate to 12 mEq/litre or below.

Dialysis.—There are two principal methods of trying to remove the waste products of metabolism from the circulation in the presence of poor renal function.

(*a*) *Peritoneal dialysis* necessitates the introduction of a large volume of fluid of known composition into the peritoneal cavity. Those electrolytes and nitrogenous substances which are in excess in the circulation can then diffuse out into the fluid and so finally be removed. This technique requires an intraperitoneal catheter with numerous fine holes in the terminal 4 cm. The tubing is inserted under local analgesia about one-third of the way along a line drawn from the umbilicus to the pubic symphysis; 2·5 litres of either an isotonic (if the patient is not overloaded already with water) or hypertonic (if waterlogged) solution are run in and left *in situ* for about 40 minutes, after which it is all drained out again. Antibiotics and heparin are added to the solution to prevent infection and the formation of fibrin clots. The whole technique is simple and effective in mild or moderate cases. It can be repeated frequently without much trouble. The only disadvantage is that it removes the plasma proteins and also exposes the patient to the risk of infection.

(*b*) *Haemodialysis* is based on the principle of passing the blood through semi-permeable cellophane tubing in its passage from an artery to a vein. The tubing is surrounded by a solution of known concentration so that during the passage of the blood the electrolytes and other waste products can diffuse out. Such an apparatus is often described as an "artificial kidney". The development of these machines has now progressed to a stage where it is perfectly feasible to keep a patient alive indefinitely without renal function provided his blood is dialysed at least twice weekly.

Histological Findings in a Fatal Case of Post-operative Renal Failure

The glomerular membrane is less sensitive to hypoxia and ischaemia than is the tubular system, so that it is not surprising that the latter structures suffer most in cases of acute post-operative renal failure. The distal convoluted tubules show dilatation with flattening of the epithelium, and pigmented casts may be found in the lumen of these tubules and also in that of the loop of Henle and the collecting tubule (Brun and Munck, 1957). Necrosis of the tubules is not a common finding in this condition, but the cells of the tubules show cellular infiltration and oedema. The anuria or oliguria is clearly not due to any damage to the glomerular apparatus but rather to alteration in the function of the tubules. Biopsy specimens have failed to confirm that swelling of the tubules occurs and blocks the flow of urine. The most acceptable explanation is that the tubules lose their semi-permeability and almost all the water passing down the lumen is reabsorbed.

Renal Disease and Anaesthesia

Like the liver, the kidneys have such large reserves that contra-indications are related more to the possible end-results of anaesthetic practice, such as hypotension or hypoxia, than to particular agents. The non-inhalational (and some inhalational) agents depend upon the kidneys for their removal from the body either as unchanged or as inactive end-products. A very extensive degree of renal failure must be present before they are likely to accumulate. Occasional cases of prolonged paralysis following the use of a non-depolarising relaxant in the presence of a marked reduction in renal function have been recorded. None of the non-inhalational agents *per se* affects the kidneys. The inhalational agents, with the exception of chloroform, cause so little damage by direct action that this can usually be ignored when moderate doses are administered.

TISSUE TRANSPLANTATION

For many years it has been established that in man tissues can easily be transferred from one region of the body to another, yet great difficulty is experienced if an attempt is made to transfer this same tissue to another person. This failure to accept the tissues of other human beings is due to the immune response. A significant advance in our knowledge of the mechanism of this response has been made by the contributions of Medawar (1958) and Burnet (1959) both of whom were jointly awarded the Nobel Prize for Medicine in 1962. These authors demonstrated that the immune reaction is a protective mechanism possessed by every animal and is most easily illustrated as the inflammatory response to an invading organism or the allergic reaction to a foreign protein. Without this protection, man would have succumbed to the microbe many centuries ago.

The treatment of chronic renal failure by means of renal transplantation has now become a well established practice. The use of regular haemodialysis enables patients to be maintained in a relatively normal physiological state in a dialysis unit or at home until the opportunity arises of receiving a transplanted kidney from a related or unrelated donor who on tissue typing is shown to be closely matched to the recipient.

The Immune Response

This is generated mainly by lymphoid tissue. It is most easily studied by observing the reaction to a homologous skin graft, though the same principle applies to transplanted organs such as the kidney. At first the new graft thrives, so that during the initial five days or so it becomes vascularised and pink with a really healthy appearance. On about the 5th to 7th day, the homograft takes on a discoloured appearance, and soon the evidence of necrosis begins to appear, until by the 12th day it is obviously dead. Pathological examination of the grafted region will reveal a lymphocytic reaction with also, but to a lesser degree, a proliferation of plasma cells. If a second attempt is now made to repeat the grafting process then the time taken for the rejection phenomenon to reveal itself is even faster.

It is clear, therefore, that the immune response is a fundamental law permitting the body to recognise self from non-self and involves two factors, cellular and humoral. The cellular factor is believed to be more important than the humoral one. The whole process is intimately linked with the lymphoid tissue throughout the body, and this system is known to be closely concerned with the production of antibodies. Burnet (1962) has suggested that the probable role of the thymus gland is to organise the immune response and this takes place around the time of birth. Once achieved, the thymus no longer has a function to fulfil so that it atrophies and shrinks. In mice, if the thymus gland is removed soon after birth this immune response does not develop. Thus it is established that if a successful homologous tissue transplantation is to be achieved in man, it is vital that first the immune response is suppressed.

Suppression of the Immune Response

The methods have been reviewed in detail by Richards (1963). Although numerous, the principal difficulty is to achieve a delicate balance between a lethal dose on the one hand and yet an adequate one on the other.

Genetic compatibility.—A number of successful kidney transplant operations have been reported between identical twins. Because of the genetic compatibility between these two beings, the immune response is not present. However, some of these patients have developed glomerulo-nephritis (the initial disease of the host) in the grafted kidney, but this complication is less likely to occur if the diseased kidney is removed first. The genetic relationship between children and parents and between siblings enhances the chance of successful transplantation in these groups.

Current methods of treatment.—1. *Cortisone and A.C.T.H.* Both agents are known to suppress or postpone the onset of the immune response in animals. However, alone they are insufficient to permit homologous transplantation but cortisone forms an essential part of current therapy.

2. "*Imuran*" (*azathioprine*). Many drugs, such as nitrogen mustard and 6-mercaptopurine, are known to have properties capable of mimicking irradiation. They bring about a marked suppression of bone marrow activity along with lymphopenia, and whilst under the influence of these drugs the immune response can be obtunded. The balancing of the exact dose, however, is very delicate: too little leads to rejection of the graft, yet too much leads to complete suppression of bone marrow activity. There is no doubt that more specific drugs will be found and at the moment the most satisfactory is "Imuran", most of which is excreted in an active form as thio-uric acid.

Other methods.—1. *Total body irradiation.* The immune response can be suppressed by adequate radiation therapy, but this is so close to the lethal dose that the management of the patient becomes extremely difficult. Bone marrow function is so depressed that the patient is at the mercy of any infection, necessitating extreme care in nursing. Attempts to combine renal transplantation with bone marrow transplants after a massive dose of irradiation therapy have not been wholly successful. Selective radiation of lymphoid tissue using yttrium 90 has proved more satisfactory.

2. *Thymectomy.* Since the thymus is intimately concerned with the organisation of the immune response, its removal may increase the chance of survival of a transplanted organ.

3. *Anti-lymphocytic serum.* It is thought that the development of anti-lymphocytic serum which suppresses the cellular response to transplantation will improve the clinical results.

The Rejection Phenomenon

The success or failure of a graft to "take" is determined by histocompatibility factors which are inherited. For this reason it follows that the nearer the donor tissue is to that of the recipient in such factors as red blood cell groups, leucocyte groups, and genetically determined plasma protein fractions, the more likely is the grafting to be successful. Ideally, therefore, the most suitable donor tissue is that taken from an identical twin. Next comes a close family relationship such as the mother for her son. Finally, a donor with as many genetically determined factors as possible in common with the patient should be selected.

The rejection response is a very complicated process and the signs can first be observed at any time from a few days to even months after the grafting. Sometimes the process can be halted and even reversed by local irradiation or increasing the dose of drugs if the diagnosis is established sufficiently early.

Diagnosis of the rejection response (Calne, 1964) of a renal homograft is made on the following basis:

(*a*) Impairment of renal function as shown by a fall in urine volume and its chemical constituents, especially the sodium concentration. This is the most important guideline to the development of the rejection response.

(*b*) Pyrexia, tachycardia, leucocytosis and a rise in blood pressure.

The following factors are of less significance:

(*c*) Appearance of cells in the urine.

(*d*) The grafted area (e.g. kidney) becomes very tender.
(*e*) Changes in enzymes in the urine, such as the lactic dehydrogenase, may prove significant but at present they are not very informative.

Management of the Patient

Chronic renal infection and uraemia are likely to be present, so that in most instances the patient is seriously ill. Uraemia can be satisfactorily treated by dialysis and most patients presenting for transplantation will have been attending a dialysis unit twice weekly or more frequently in the acute stage. Dialysis will ensure normal fluid balance as well as correcting electrolyte disturbances and eliminating urea. Haemodialysis, is performed through an arteriovenous shunt placed on the forearm or lower leg. The Scribner teflon shunt has been widely used for this purpose but recently the Cimino-Brescia shunt has become increasingly popular. This involves the establishment of a direct arteriovenous fistula between the radial artery and an adjacent vein by open operation. The marked dilatation of the veins in the forearm that results from this shunt enables frequent and easy access to be established with the circulation using needles of sufficient calibre to carry the blood flow required for haemodialysis. Once a satisfactory shunt has been established, dialysis can be performed whenever required but the whole process is time-consuming and costly as it takes about twelve hours to produce a satisfactory result.

Almost all patients presenting for transplantation are severely anaemic, as the anaemia associated with uraemia is very resistant to treatment. The infusion of large volumes of blood carries a risk of precipitating pulmonary oedema and moreover could stimulate the production of antibodies in patients who are awaiting a transplanted kidney. Blood is only added sparingly during dialysis as the stimulus to the patient's own erythrocyte production would be thereby reduced and moreover each transfusion carries the risk of introducing serum hepatitis, an infection liable to spread rapidly in dialysis units.

Most patients will have a haemoglobin level in the region of 7 g. per cent when they present for operation, a figure which would be regarded as totally unacceptable for other operative procedures. Nevertheless patients undergoing renal transplantation seem to survive surgery and anaesthesia remarkably well despite this severe degree of anaemia.

Because of the frequency of infections during chronic renal failure many patients having renal transplants will be receiving antibiotic therapy. The potentiation of the action of non-depolarising muscle relaxants following the intra-peritoneal administration of polymyxin, streptomycin and neomycin is well known. This phenomenon may also become manifest in patients with a low urinary output who are receiving these antibiotics by injection because their requirements for these drugs is considerably reduced (Samuel and Powell, 1970).

Anaesthesia for Kidney Transplantation Operations

The anaesthetist's services are required on two principal occasions. First, at the removal of the damaged kidney, because evidence is accumulating that the most satisfactory results of grafting are obtained in those patients in whom the influence of the affected kidney is removed before transplantation. Often a separate abdominal operation with removal of one or both of the patient's own kidneys is performed prior to transplantation. During the intervening period the onset of uraemia is prevented by frequent dialysis and this, together with removal of the diseased kidneys, may result in a considerable improvement in the patient's physical condition.

Once the recipient of a donor kidney has been selected by tissue typing, the time interval during which the donor kidney is without a blood supply should be reduced to a minimum.

The particular type of anaethesia selected, i.e. general, local or regional, will depend on the anaesthetist's preference. In many cases, general anaesthesia will be preferred. Clearly, drugs which are believed to be eliminated unchanged entirely through the renal tract should be avoided in favour of those which are either metabolised or excreted unchanged through some other channel, such as the respiratory system. Gallamine triethiodide would appear to be contra-indicated in these cases. Churchill-Davidson *et al.* (1967) describe a case in which following the administration of gallamine triethiodine for exploration of a kidney transplant, apnoea persisted for three days until the drug was removed by dialysis. Prior to induction of anaesthesia, intravenous atropine should be administered, and also oral mist. magnesium trisilicate. Great care should be taken to maintain the integrity of the shunt upon which vital dialysis may depend during the post-operative period. The other arm should be utilised for intravenous infusions and the application of the sphygmomanometer cuff. Adequate preoxygenation should be carried out because of the severe anaemia and be followed by a barbiturate induction with intubation under suxamethonium, taking full precautions, including the use of crycothyroid pressure, to minimise the risk of regurgitation and aspiration of gastric contents.

Intermittent suxamethonium has been advocated for these operations, but in the presence of hyperkalaemia it may predispose to cardiac irregularities, bradycardia and cardiac arrest. Samuel and Powell (1970), on the basis of experience gained in 100 transplantation cases, prefer to use intermittent *d*-tubocurarine in combination with nitrous oxide and oxygen and positive pressure ventilation. These authors quote the work of Cohen *et al.* (1967) who, using tritiated *d*-tubocurarine in dogs, were able to demonstrate that in the absence of renal function up to 40 per cent of a dose of the drug was excreted in the bile by the liver in a few hours. The absence of prolonged action of *d*-tubocurarine or of any difficulty in reversing its effect is attributable to this alternative route of excretion. The caution with which *d*-tubocurarine has hitherto been used in this field because of its supposed dependence on renal excretion for its elimination appears to be unnecessary.

Halothane has been advocated for renal transplantation (Strunin, 1966) but the use of a concentration sufficient to achieve adequate muscular relaxation may be associated with an undesirable degree of hypotension. As a supplement to nitrous oxide in a concentration of up to 0·5 per cent halothane is useful in combating any tendency to hypertension. An epidural technique combined with light general anaesthesia can also be used for renal transplantation.

Serum Hepatitis

The outbreak of serum hepatitis in dialysis and transplant units has become a recognised hazard in recent years. It affects both patients and staff working in these units although the clinical manifestation of the disease may be considerably modified in patients if they are immuno-suppressed by uraemia. The severity of this form of hepatitis varies but serious outbreaks have been reported and every effort must be directed to its prevention. Each patient on dialysis must have his own personal dialysis machine and as it appears that it can be spread by droplet infection and faecal routes as well as by blood, strict barrier precautions with the use of masks, gowns and gloves are advisable in treating and nursing these patients. The use of blood transfusions should be kept to a minimum to avoid the introduction of the virus which is endemic in the normal population. Blood should not be given unless it has been screened for the Australian S.H. related virus.

REFERENCES

Barnett, A. J., Blacket, R. B., Depoorter, A. E., Sanderson, P. H., and Wilson, G. M. (1950). The action of noradrenaline in man and its relation to phaeochromocytoma and hypertension. *Clin. Sci.*, **9,** 151.

Brun, C., and Munck, O. (1957). Lesions of the kidney in acute renal failure following shock. *Lancet*, **1,** 603.

Bull, G. M., Joekes, A. M., and Lowe, K. G. (1949). Conservative treatment of anuric uraemia. *Lancet*, **2,** 229.

Burnet, F. M. (1959). *The Clonal Selection Theory of Acquired Immunity.* (Abraham Flexner Lectures). Nashville: Vanderbilt University Press.

Burnet, F. M. (1962). Role of the thymus and related organs in immunity. *Brit. med. J.*, **2,** 807.

Calne, R. Y. (1964). Renal transplantation in man. *Brit. J. Surg.*, **51,** 282.

Churchill-Davidson, H. C. (1955). Hypothermia. *Brit. J. Anaesth.*, **27,** 313.

Churchill-Davidson, H. C., Way, W. L., and De Jong, R. H. (1967). The muscle relaxants and renal excretion. *Anesthesiology*, **28,** 540.

Churchill-Davidson, H. C., Wylie, W. D., Miles, B. E., and de Wardener, H. E. (1951). The effects of adrenaline, noradrenaline and methedrine on the renal circulation during anaesthesia. *Lancet*, **2,** 803.

Cohen, E. N., Winslow Brewer, H., and Smith, D. (1967). The metabolism and elimination of *d*-tubocurarine H^3. *Anesthesiology*, **28,** 309.

de Wardener, H. E. (1955). Renal circulation during anaesthesia and surgery. *Anaesthesia*, **10,** 18.

de Wardener, H. E. (1968). *The Kidney. An outline of normal and abnormal structure and function*, 3rd edit. London: J. & A. Churchill.

de Wardener, H. E., and McSwiney, R. R. (1951). Renal haemodynamics in vasovagal fainting due to haemorrhage. *Clin. Sci.*, **10,** 209.

de Wardener, H. E., and Miles, B. E. (1952). The effect of haemorrhage on the circulatory autoregulation of the dog's kidney perfused *in situ. Clin. Sci.*, **11,** 267.

de Wardener, H. E., Miles, B. E., Lee, G. de J., Churchill-Davidson, H. C., Wylie, W. D., and Sharpey-Schafer, E. P. (1953). Circulatory effects of haemorrhage during prolonged light anaesthesia in man. *Clin. Sci.*, **12,** 175.

Evans, B., and Enderby, G. E. H. (1952). Controlled hypotension and its effect on renal function. *Lancet*, **1,** 1045.

Habif, D. V., Papper, E. M., Fitzpatrick, H. F., Lowrance, P., Smythe, C. McC., and Bradley, S. E. (1951). The renal and hepatic blood flow, glomerular filtration rate and urinary output of electrolytes during cyclopropane, ether and thiopental anesthesia, operation and the immediate postoperative period. *Surgery*, **30,** 241.

Hampton, L. J., and Little, D. M. (1953). Complications associated with the use of "controlled hypotension" in anesthesia. *Arch. Surg. (Chicago)*, **67,** 549.

Lauson, H. D., Bradley, S. E., and Cournand, A. (1944). Renal circulation in shock. *J. clin. Invest.*, **23,** 381.

Mazze, R. I., Schwartz, R. D., Slocum, H. C., and Kevin, G. B. (1963). Renal function during anesthesia and surgery. 1. The effects of halothane anesthesia. *Anesthesiology*, **4,** 279.

Medawar, P. B. (1958). *The Immunology of Transplantation*, p. 144. (Harvey Lectures No. 52). New York: Academic Press Inc.

Miles, B. E., and de Wardener, H. E. (1952). Renal vasoconstriction produced by ether and cyclopropane anaesthesia. *J. Physiol. (Lond.)*, **118,** 141.

Miles, B. E., de Wardener, H. E., Churchill-Davidson, H. C., and Wylie, W. D. (1952). The effect on the renal circulation of pentamethonium bromide during anaesthesia. *Clin. Sci.*, **11,** 73.

Molloy, P. J. (1962). The early diagnosis of impaired post-operative renal function. *Lancet*, **2,** 696.

Moyer, J. H., and McConn, R. (1956). Renal hemodynamics in hypertensive patients following administration of pendiomide. *Anesthesiology*, **17,** 9.

Parsons, F. M., Blagg, C. R., and Williams, R. E. (1963). Chemistry, therapy and hemodialysis of acute renal failure. *Biochem. Clin.*, No. **2,** p. 457.

Phillips, R. A., Dole, V. P., Hamilton, P. B., Emerson, K., Jr., Archibald, R. M., and van Slyke, D. D. (1945). Shock and renal function. *Amer. J. Physiol.*, **145,** 314.

Richards, V. (1963). Basic concepts in homologous tissue transplantation. *Amer. J. Surg.*, **105,** 151.

Samuel, J. R., and Powell, D. (1970). Renal transplantation: anaesthetic experience of 100 cases. *Anaesthesia*, **25,** 165.

Shorr, E., Zweifach, B. W., and Furchgott, R. F. (1948). Hepato-renal factors in circulatory homeostasis; influence of humoral factors of hepato-renal origin on vascular reactions to hemorrhage. *Ann. N.Y. Acad. Sci.*, **49,** 571.

Smith, H. W. (1943). *Lectures on the Kidney*. (Porter Lectures, Series IX, and the William Henry Walch Lectures.) Lawrence, Kan.: Univ. of Kansas Press.

Strunin, L. (1966). Some aspects of anaesthesia for renal homotransplantation. *Brit. J. Anaesth.*, **38,** 812.

Wakim, K. G. (1955). Certain cardiovasculorenal effects of hexamethonium. *Amer. Heart. J.*, **50,** 435.

Wright, S. (1965). *Applied Physiology*, 10th edit. London: Oxford Univ. Press.

FURTHER READING

de Wardener, H. E. (1968). *The Kidney. An outline of normal and abnormal structure and function*, 3rd edit. London: J. & A. Churchill.

Shaldon, S., and Cook, G. C. (1964). *Acute Renal Failure*. Oxford : Blackwell Scientific Publications.

Section Five

THE ENDOCRINE SYSTEM

Chapter 50

ANAESTHESIA AND THE ENDOCRINE GLANDS

THE STRESS RESPONSE

THE concept that the body possesses a defence mechanism with which to combat aggression is not new. Claude Bernard placed emphasis upon the maintenance of a *status quo* or the *milieu intérieur* of the bodily functions; Cannon talked of "homeostasis", and Hartman advanced the theory that the corticoids were responsible for a general tissue hormone which controlled the breakdown and building up of cells. The concept of the stress response also owes much to the work of Hans Selye, which will be discussed in more detail later.

Almost any kind of initial stimulus—infection, trauma (surgical or accidental), burns or even anaesthesia alone—can be considered as an aggression upon the body tissues, and thus constitutes a form of stress. The body's response to this wide range of stimuli is remarkably constant and, although the functional changes set in motion are complex, they may be summarised as occurring in the following sequence:

1. Immediate circulatory adjustment.
2. The metabolic response
   (*a*) The catabolic phase
   (*b*) The anabolic phase.

The immediate circulatory changes are considered more fully elsewhere. Briefly, they may be seen as a generalised increase of adrenergic activity, resulting in tachycardia and vasoconstriction most marked in the splanchnic and cutaneous vascular beds. The apparent aim of these changes is to maintain adequate perfusion of vital centres.

The ensuing catabolic phase of the metabolic response is characterised by breakdown of the body proteins and negative nitrogen balance. Potassium is also lost, presumably being released from the cells as protein is metabolised. Oliguria with sodium retention—disputably obligatory—occurs and the blood picture shows a polymorphonuclear leucocytosis with lymphopenia and eosinopenia. The duration of this phase is variable, depending chiefly on the severity of the initial injury, but is usually about 48 hours. In the subsequent anabolic phase, there is nitrogen retention and restoration of the body proteins.

Mechanism of the Stress Response

The initial vascular response appears to be neurogenic, mediated by the sympathetic system, whose post-ganglionic nerve endings release noradrenaline as a chemical transmitter. The adrenal medulla may be regarded as a modified sympathetic ganglion, and it is believed that it participates in this increased sympathetic activity by releasing catecholamines, both noradrenaline and adrenaline, into the circulation. The principal actions of adrenaline and noradrenaline are summarised in Table 1 and their biosynthesis and metabolism in the diagrams (Figs. 1 and 2).

The mechanisms underlying the catabolic and anabolic phases are not fully understood, but it is generally considered that, in the former at any rate, the release of hormones from the adrenal cortex plays an important part. It is appropriate, therefore, to consider the functions of these hormones at this point.

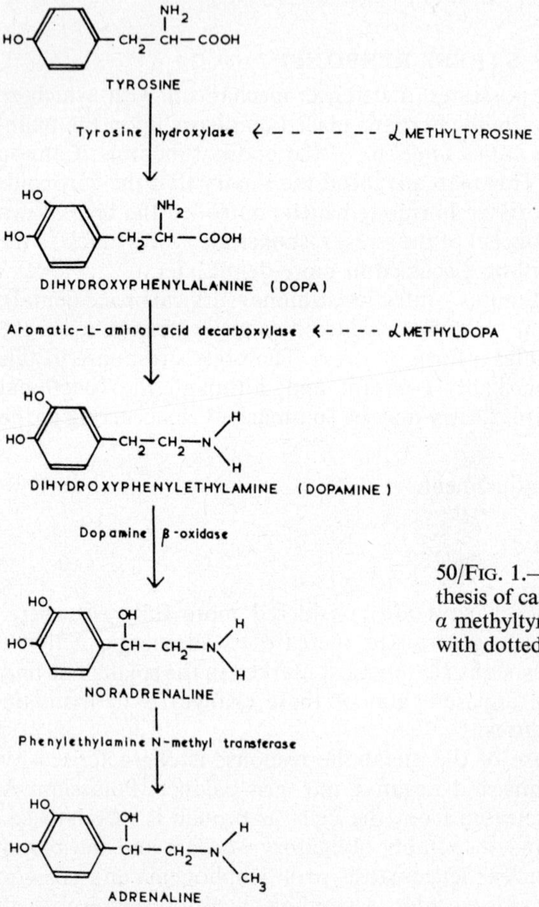

TYROSINE

Tyrosine hydroxylase ← – – – – – – α METHYLTYROSINE

DIHYDROXYPHENYLALANINE (DOPA)

Aromatic-L-amino-acid decarboxylase ← – – – α METHYLDOPA

DIHYDROXYPHENYLETHYLAMINE (DOPAMINE)

Dopamine β-oxidase

NORADRENALINE

Phenylethylamine N-methyl transferase

ADRENALINE

50/FIG. 1.—Diagram to illustrate the biosynthesis of catecholamines. The sites of action of α methyltyrosine and α methyldopa are shown with dotted arrows.

Functions of the Adrenal Corticoid Hormones

These hormones are usually divided into three groups:

1. **Mineralo-corticoids.**—The principal naturally-occurring hormone is aldosterone. It promotes the retention of sodium and excretion of potassium by the kidneys, its secretion being stimulated by a fall in extracellular fluid volume.

2. **Gluco-corticoids.**—Hydrocortisone is the principal gluco-corticoid produced by the adrenal cortex. It has an effect on carbohydrate metabolism opposed to that of insulin. In excess, it stimulates gluconeogenesis and produces a negative nitrogen balance associated with muscle-wasting, osteoporosis and atrophy of

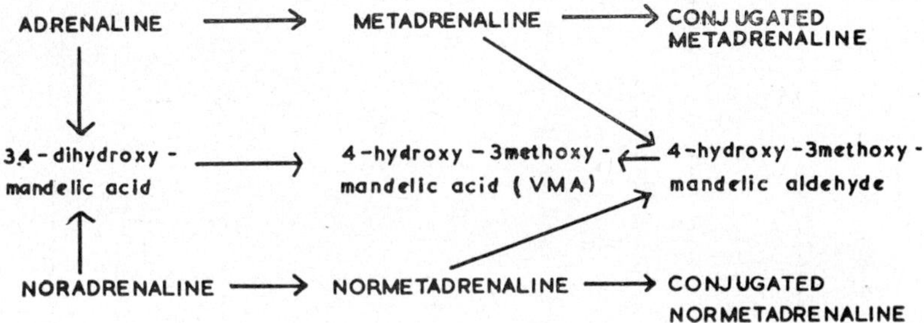

50/FIG. 2.—The metabolic pathways of adrenaline and noradrenaline.

the skin. It also has an anti-inflammatory effect, associated with lymphopenia and eosinopenia. Both hydrocortisone and other gluco-corticoids also possess weak mineralo-corticoid properties.

3. **Sex hormones.**—Adrenal androgens have weak virilising activity compared with testosterone, which is secreted by the testes. They are also believed to have anabolic effects. Progesterone and oestrogens are possibly secreted in small amounts by the adrenal cortex in women.

Relationship of the Adrenal Cortex to the Stress Response

It is clear from the above that the catabolic phase of the metabolic response to injury is closely simulated by excess of gluco-corticoid hormones. Further evidence that the secretion of the hormones is involved is shown by the finding that the adrenals enlarge after injury. Adrenalectomy and hypophysectomy in animals abolish the negative nitrogen balance.

Selye in 1950 presented a unifying concept of both neurogenic and hormonal factors in the response to stress, under the title of the general adaptation syndrome. He believes that the adrenaline released immediately after trauma activates the hypothalamus, which in turn causes the adrenohypophysis to release ACTH. This stimulates the production and release of gluco-corticoids from the adrenal cortex, thus bringing about the catabolic phase. Selye has also claimed that the ensuing anabolic phase is due to the subsequent predominance of mineralo-corticoid secretion, or possibly to the release of growth hormone (somatotrophin) from the pituitary. There is experimental evidence that the synthetic mineralo-corticoid desoxycortisone acetate (D.O.C.A.) augments the inflammatory response and produces hypertension and renal damage in toxic doses, but this is by no means conclusive support for Selye's views. His whole painting has many artistic qualities, and to some of the viewers it possesses rather more imagination than realism.

ANAESTHESIA AND STRESS

Traina and his associates (1953), in an investigation based upon eosinophil counts and designed to determine the exact extent of the response produced by anaesthesia alone, concluded, that although anaesthesia delayed the onset of this response, it did not prevent it. Virtue and Helmrich (1956), using plasma corticosteroid levels, found that thiopentone, cyclopropane and nitrous oxide

50/TABLE 1
PRINCIPAL ACTIONS OF ADRENALINE AND NORADRENALINE

	Adrenaline	*Noradrenaline*
Blood vessels	Total peripheral resistance decreased	Total peripheral resistance increased
A. Cerebal	Slight vasoconstriction	Slight vasoconstriction
B. Skin	Vasoconstriction	Vasoconstriction
C. Muscle	Vasodilation	Vasoconstriction
D. Splanchnic	Vasodilation	Vasoconstriction
E. Veins	Vasoconstriction	Vasoconstriction
Heart		
A. Rate	Increased	Decreased
B. Output	Raised	Raised by small doses; lowered by high doses
C. Rhythm	Arrhythmias likely	Unaffected
D. Coronary vessels	Vasodilation	Vasodilation
Blood pressure	Systolic raised slightly; diastolic unchanged	Systolic and diastolic raised
Smooth Muscle		
A. Bronchioles	Relaxed	
B. Stomach and intestine	Relaxed	As for adrenaline, but less active (A–C)
C. Fundus of bladder	Relaxed	
D. Parturient human uterus	Inhibited	Stimulated
Sphincters (intestine and bladder)	Contracted	Contracted
Central Nervous System		
A. Mental state	Anxiety with tremors	No obvious effect
B. Eyes	Pupils dilated; tears formed	As for adrenaline but less active
C. Anterior pituitary	ACTH production stimulated	No effect
Metabolism		
A. Oxygen consumption	Large increase	Small increase
B. Blood sugar	Raised	Unaffected

could not be classed as stressor agents, but that deep ether could, though only to a moderate extent. They emphasised that the surgical trauma over-shadowed any of the effects of anaesthesia, and that the plasma level of corticosteroid rose for several hours after operation. They were also able to establish a direct relationship between this level and the degree of surgical trauma. This relationship is a little misleading, however, because Virtue and Helmrich did not correlate it with blood loss. Blood loss may well bear a relationship to the degree of response, and it will be recalled that, in the stress syndrome, the signs of a decreased blood volume are always present. The work of Flear and Clarke (1955) does, in fact, suggest that with adequate transfusion the metabolic response to trauma does not occur. Carnes and his associates (1961) have shown that adrenocortical responses are depressed during halothane anaesthesia and for at least four hours afterwards. Carnes (1963) also states that local block analgesia prevents adrenocortical stimulation.

Anaesthesia itself can be regarded, at the most, as no more than a minor form of stress. The general tendency during it is for a reduction in hormone output, which a special technique such as hypothermia may enhance. Experimental evidence suggests that during hypothermia this may be related to depression of hypothalamic-pituitary activity (Khalil, 1954). However, MacPhee and his colleagues (1958), also in animal experiments, did not find any significant reduction in the production or excretion of corticosteroids during hypothermia in the range 26–30° C. Their results show that prolonged hypothermia and operation lead to an increase in corticosteroid excretion that is greater than after operation alone, and that the maintenance of hypothermia after an operation or an injury will depress the normal post-operative rise in excretion.

A normal patient can be expected to respond in a normal manner, but physical disease affecting the pituitary or adrenals, or the results of previous hormone therapy, can upset the balance. Specific treatment may then be required if the patient is to survive the anaesthetic, the operation and the post-operative period. (See also Stress and Hypothermia, p. 1281.)

Unexpected Reactions

Patients at the extremes of age—neonates and the very old especially—and those with chronic illness of long standing, may respond inadequately to the demands of a major operation. Adrenal insufficiency has been suggested as a possible cause of the subsequent general deterioration in their condition, which is progressive and relatively slow, but the evidence for this is not altogether convincing. The administration of corticosteroid to such patients, either routinely to cover the operation period or merely when the relapse is evident, is at the best empirical. Corticosteroids have also been recommended for the treatment of persistent hypotension in severely ill patients—due to such diseases as tetanus, poliomyelitis or coronary thrombosis.

Interest in pituitary-adrenocortical deficiency has also resurrected the old myth of status lymphaticus. Although he does not suggest that hormone deficiencies are associated with sudden death in all apparently fit children, Ucko (1954) has drawn attention to their association with thymic and lymphoid hyperplasia. Other workers have at various times remarked upon the relative hypoplasia of adrenal tissue in children dubbed as dying of status lymphaticus.

Again the evidence is inconclusive, but in this case there is little doubt that many more likely causes of death are often discovered when the episode is considered without bias and with all the clinical facts available.

Treatment with Hormones

As previously described, aldosterone and hydrocortisone are the principal natural steroids produced by the adrenal cortex, but for therapeutic purposes a number of substances are available, most of which have been produced synthetically and with chemical changes in their structure designed to increase their clinical value. The steroids that are commonly used therapeutically are classified in Table 2.

Corticotrophin (ACTH) may be given to stimulate adrenal cortical activity either when this has been suppressed by previous steroid administration or more

50/Table 2

Some Hormones in Common Use, and Their Dosage

Corticotrophin (ACTH)	Administered by subcutaneous or intramuscular injection, but as this hormone is very short acting when continuous therapy is indicated, the total dose must be divided and given at four-hourly intervals. Dose from 20 to 200 mg. a day.
Hydrocortisone Sodium Succinate	Prepared immediately before use for intramuscular or intravenous injection. Dose 50 to 100 mg. or larger as required.
Cortisone Acetate	Can be administered orally in tablet form or intramuscularly as a suspension. Dose 25 to 400 mg. a day.
Prednisone and Prednisolone	Derivatives respectively of cortisone and hydrocortisone, but five times more potent in respect of gluco-corticoid activity and with similar potency for mineralo-corticoid activity. Administered orally in a dose of from 10 to 100 mg. daily.
Dexamethasone and Betamethasone	Approximately thirty-five times more potent than cortisone but with virtually no mineralo-corticoid activity. Administered orally in a dose of from 0·5 to 10 mg. daily. For therapeutic purposes probably have no advantages over prednisone and prednisolone.
Deoxycortone Acetate (DOCA)	A synthetic steroid with approximately 1/100th potency of aldosterone and a similar action in controlling electrolyte and water balance. Administered intramuscularly in a dose range of from 2 to 10 mg.
Fludrocortisone Acetate	This is a fluorinated hydrocortisone with enhanced mineralo-corticoid activity, and is used in place of deoxycortone. Administered orally in a dose range of from 0·1–0·2 mg. daily.

simply as a means of treatment in some inflammatory and allergic disorders. It is, however, not commonly used for these purposes, but rather as a test of adrenal cortical activity (see p. 1365).

The principal indications for therapy with cortisone and similar corticosteroids are physiological replacement of the secretions of the adrenal cortex, suppression of some inflammatory and allergic disorders, and depression of adrenal cortical function. Prednisone and prednisolone are most commonly used for these purposes, but for emergency use hydrocortisone sodium succinate should be injected intravenously. When a specific control of water and electrolyte balance is required deoxycortone or fludrocortisone acetate are often preferred. The requisite dose depends on the therapeutic indication, the degree of urgency and the size of the patient. Although a relatively large initial dosage may be justified in certain circumstances, graded doses may be necessary to find the patient's essential requirements, and it is important to bear in mind that there are disadvantages in prescribing corticosteroids, particularly too much for too long a time.

The normal physiological output of the adrenal is put at about the equivalent of 20–25 mg. of cortisone a day, so that routine therapy in the absence of any adrenal function need rarely exceed this dose or its equivalent in terms of other steroids, and can be administered by mouth. Cortisone can, if necessary, be supplemented by 0·1 mg. of fludrocortisone a day. When replacement therapy is planned for either the removal of a pituitary or both adrenal glands it is usual to provide a larger initial dosage to cover the possible immediate and post-operative stress of the surgical and anaesthetic procedures. On such occasions it is best to start replacement with cortisone about twenty-four hours before the operation, maintain a high level for the day of operation and the day that follows it, and then gradually reduce the dose until a maintenance level is achieved. A variety of schemes are advocated but there is often little to choose between them and they usually represent individualistic opinions. The following is suggested as one possible method:

Day before operation:	Cortisone acetate 100 mg. i.m.
Day of operation:	Cortisone acetate 100 mg. i.m.
	Hydrocortisone sodium succinate 100 mg. either i.m. 2–3 hours before operation or i.v. during or immediately after operation.
Day after operation:	Cortisone acetate 100 mg. i.m.

On the second day after operation a start is made to reduce the dose of cortisone acetate, and if the patient can drink, it is given by mouth twice daily. A maintenance dose should be followed after about a week.

The important points to remember are that cortisone acetate given orally is rapidly absorbed into the blood stream but relatively quickly excreted, that cortisone acetate injected intramuscularly forms a depot and is slowly absorbed, giving a good blood level after about twenty hours and maintaining it for a day or more, and that hydrocortisone sodium succinate given intramuscularly provides an adequate level after one to three hours but only maintains it for two or three hours.

Effects of Corticosteroid Therapy

Apart from the useful results of treatment with corticosteroid, side-effects may occur, especially when large doses are used. Several are of particular importance and of interest to the anaesthetist. The patient frequently has a marked sense of well-being and is inclined to euphoria, which may mask the true physical state of affairs. There is evidence that corticosteroids produce a tendency to thrombosis and delayed wound healing, and that they diminish the normal response to infection. Thus they should not be given to patients suffering from tuberculosis. These effects are, however, very slight in clinical surgical practice, but when an operation is contemplated they must be weighed against the benefits of the steroid, though they do not contra-indicate their essential use. The effect of corticosteroids on the electrolytes is, as already described, weak, but they quite commonly produce glycosuria and they may lead to water and salt retention. This is especially likely to occur when they are used for replacement therapy during and after an operation on a patient already receiving treatment with the same or similar acting steroids. In such circumstances the dose must be adjusted accordingly, and if a large dose is considered necessary to cover the operative period, it must be reduced as soon as possible post-operatively. Long continued therapy causes some osteoporosis and weakening of the bones.

Cortisone and barbiturate poisoning.—Dhunér and Nordquist (1957) have drawn attention to the danger of administering cortisone to patients recovering from an overdose of a barbiturate, since this may result in the reinduction of unconsciousness. The danger also exists with promethazine poisoning. A similar phenomenon has been known to occur following the injection of hypertonic glucose into animals awakening from barbiturate narcosis (Lamson *et al.*, 1949). The explanation of this action of cortisone and glucose is not known. It may, however, have clinical importance not only when patients are treated for over-dosage of barbiturates or promethazine, but also in routine anaesthesia.

Hormone suppression of adrenal cortical activity.—The therapeutic use of adrenal cortical hormones in doses that are equivalent to or more than the patient's normal physiological requirements, will lead to suppression of this part of the gland's function. Ingle and Kendall (1937) showed that this effect is due to decreased secretion of the ACTH and similar hormones by the anterior pituitary—a form of pituitary inhibition—and that it eventually leads to adrenal cortical atrophy. This effect may outlast the original treatment for a considerable period of time—perhaps for as long as a year or more (Salassa *et al.*, 1953; Slaney and Brooke, 1957)—and does not necessarily only follow heavy or prolonged treatment with cortisone or similar compounds. A week of treatment may be long enough. The clinical significance of such a reduction in the function of the adrenal cortex is variable, but it is always potentially important. Such a patient's response to a period of stress—say, even to a minor anaesthetic and operation—may be inadequate, and acute adrenal insufficiency will then occur. This is characterised by sudden and severe hypotension, progressing to other signs of shock, coma and anuria, and may lead to death. It usually takes place in the immediate post-operative period, but there seems no reason why it should not occur during the operation and anaesthetic.

Nowadays, very many patients—particularly those suffering from one or other of the collagen diseases, such as rheumatoid arthritis—receive a course of corticosteroid therapy, and despite the fact that many of them are in all probability subjected to many differing forms of stress after treatment ceases, very few indeed go into acute adrenal failure. It is, however, important to remember the possibility when faced with sudden circulatory failure during or following an operation, particularly if the response to treatment with intravenous fluids and drugs is unexpectedly poor, or when the operative procedure seems unlikely to have been the major cause of the collapse.

Pre-operatively it is rational and wise to consider carefully any history of treatment with corticosteroid during the previous twelve months, the more so if the proposed operation is likely to be extensive. Certain facts may support the possibility of adrenal cortical inactivity in a patient. Fatigue, weakness and irritability are the typical symptoms which become more suspect with the history of corticosteroid treatment previously. Objectively a low urinary excretion of 17-ketosteroids is additional evidence. Some confirmation may also be sought in the results of a stimulant dose of ACTH; a continued low output of 17-ketosteroids is abnormal after this. The eosinophil response to ACTH is of doubtful value, but the count should not fall if the output of the adrenal cortex is poor. These tests are too cumbersome for routine use, nor are they necessary, since the risk of acute adrenal insufficiency in those patients who have had corticosteroid therapy and cannot be assessed or treated pre-operatively on clinical grounds, is very small. Moreover, the only really adequate test is the response of the patient to the anaesthetic and operation. If in doubt the patient should always be covered by a course of corticosteroid therapy for the period of operation and a day or two afterwards. Many authorities advocate this routinely for all patients who have had treatment with it within one year of the proposed operation, especially when this is of any magnitude. But an alternative approach is to bear in mind the risk, deliberately omit a routine cover and keep hydrocortisone available at the patient's bedside, so that it can be given intravenously if needed (Nelson, 1963) or to give an injection of hydrocortisone hemisuccinate (100 mg.) with the premedication and further doses only if required. Bearing in mind that very few patients who have been previously submitted to steroid therapy are, in practice, at risk, this method has at least the merit of objectivity and avoids any potential complications from the routine use of corticosteroids. When corticosteroid treatment is already being given to a patient—either for surgical reasons or because of some incidental disease—and an operation is contemplated, the dose should be increased to cover the period of stress in case the physiological response is inadequate. A safe rule is to double the patient's normal daily dose. A very dangerous collapse may follow discontinuing corticosteroid therapy during this critical period.

The treatment of acute adrenal insufficiency should be by intravenous hydrocortisone since the patient is usually collapsed, and often semi-conscious. For less urgent occasions, and provided the patient can tolerate it without sickness, a corticosteroid can be given by mouth, since it will be very rapidly absorbed from the stomach. Both glucose and sodium usually need replacement in this condition, and should be combined and given intravenously as a 5 per cent dextrose, 0·9 per cent saline drip.

The Adrenal Glands

Adrenal Cortex

Addison's disease.—This disease is usually caused by simple atrophy or by tuberculosis affecting both the cortex and medulla of the adrenals. The symptoms and signs, however, result from the absence of cortical secretions and principally consist of pigmentation, weakness, hypotension, and electrolyte changes due to the patient's inability to retain sodium. Many such patients are maintained by means of a high salt diet, cortisone (or a more potent equivalent) and, if necessary, fludrocortisone, but this may be inadequate for cases of more than average severity, or in the presence of exceptional stresses. A patient with Addison's disease who is to be submitted to anaesthesia and an operation should always be prepared with cortisone and fludrocortisone. Cortisone itself does little to maintain a normal electrolyte balance, so that it cannot be regarded as a substitute for fludrocortisone. There are no special points concerning anaesthesia, other than the intolerance of these patients to more than minimal doses of potent agents. Thiopentone is especially likely to precipitate an acute hypotensive episode, while its metabolism is slower than normal.

An Addisonian crisis may occur after operation. Typically, acute and marked hypotension is associated with nausea, vomiting, vague pains, hypoglycaemia, coma, and unless rapidly treated, death. Treatment of a crisis should consist of the intravenous injection of 50 to 100 mg. of hydrocortisone, the infusion of glucose saline and the intramuscular injection of 20 mg. of deoxycortone (DOCA). The hydrocortisone will have to be repeated possibly at three to four-hourly intervals for the first twenty-four hours, and the deoxycortone at daily intervals. The intravenous glucose saline must be continued until fluids are taken by mouth, unless there is evidence of a swing towards salt and water retention. In the early stages of the crisis, vasoconstrictors may be necessary to assist in maintaining a reasonable blood pressure level.

Adrenal Medulla

The adrenal medulla consists largely of chromaffin cells which are the equivalent of post-ganglion nerve fibres. Indeed, the medulla can be considered as a post-ganglionic nerve since it receives only preganglionic fibres from the sympathetic nervous system and it is activated by the release of acetylcholine at the synapse. The chromaffin cells can be divided into two types, those which store adrenaline and those which store noradrenaline. In humans the normal adrenal medulla contains about 80 per cent adrenaline and 20 per cent noradrenaline.

Phaeochromocytoma.—This is a tumour of chromaffin tissue which usually arises in the adrenal medulla, but may also be found in any part of the body where there is sympathetic nervous tissue. Thus, it may be found on the sympathetic chain in the abdomen or chest, and in the bladder wall. The tumours are most frequently benign in the sense that only about 10 per cent behave in a malignant manner by producing secondaries elsewhere in the body. They are, however, not necessarily single, since in about 10 per cent of cases more than one tumour is found. Most phaeochromocytomata are physiologically active, though this may be intermittent in occurrence, and nearly all secrete noradrenaline and adrenaline in varying proportions. Tumours arising outside the adrenal medulla are less likely to secrete adrenaline.

Clinical symptoms and signs.—The classical picture is of paroxysmal hypertension, but this may take the form of a maintained high blood pressure with intermittent episodes when it rises even higher. In an attack, and apart from having a very high blood pressure, the patient will complain of sweating, palpitations and headache. But the symptomatology may be unusual, and phaeochromocytomata have presented in bizarre ways with features suggesting primary renal disease, oligaemia with hypotension, toxaemia of pregnancy and even a cerebral tumour (Leather *et al.*, 1962). The presence of a phaeochromocytoma may only be suspected at operation for some incidental disease or during parturition when the blood pressure becomes markedly unstable (Ross, 1962). A phaeochromocytoma may present unexpectedly during aortography for the differential diagnosis of hypertension. It may also initially be mistaken for such other diseases as thyrotoxicosis and anxiety state, and it may cause glycosuria, but this is not of clinical significance (Robertson, 1965).

When undiscovered, the presence of a phaeochromocytoma eventually leads to a permanently sustained high blood pressure, which makes the disease difficult to differentiate from essential hypertension on clinical grounds. Structural changes in the heart and vessels occur sooner or later and death may follow from cardiac failure or cerebrovascular accident.

Diagnosis.—The history is frequently suggestive of the diagnosis, but the sight of a conscious patient during a bout of hypertension from the sudden liberation of catecholamines into the circulation may be diagnostic. The patient is anxious, pallid, sweating and complaining of headache and palpitations. Indeed, one clinical test for a tumour is to compress the area of the patient's loins in an attempt to induce such an attack. An alternative, but dangerous, method that is not commonly used nowadays is to inject intravenously a very small dose of histamine (0·025 to 0·05 mg.). A safer test is to try the effect of a blocking drug such as phentolamine during a period of hypertension. The intravenous injection of 5 mg. should produce a marked fall in blood pressure in a matter of two or three minutes, if the raised blood pressure is due to circulating catecholamines. Phentolamine has no effect on the level of blood pressure in patients with essential hypertension.

The best method of establishing a diagnosis is the assay of the patient's urine for excess excretion of either the catecholamines or the breakdown products. The plasma level of catecholamines can also be measured.

The following figures are quoted by Sheps *et al.* (1966).

A. Urine tests.

1. Catecholamines. Normal values are 119–338 μg./24 hours, but false positive results can occur in renal failure, jaundice or during therapy with methyldopa, phenothiazines, tetracyclines and vitamins. Normal people may under the conditions of considerable stress excrete more than the normal quantity, and a patient with a phaeochromocytoma may give a normal level unless the blood pressure is raised during the time of urine collection. Many authorities quote much lower figures than Sheps.

2. The stable metabolite of adrenaline and noradrenaline—3 methoxy, 4 hydroxy-mandelic acid (VMA). Normal values are 2·6–6·5 μg./24 hours.
3. Metanephrines. Normal values are 0·5–1·3 mg./24 hours.

B. Plasma catecholamines.
Normal values are 2·4–5·7 μg./litre.

Values for VMA and metanephrines are more reliable than those for catecholamines. The value for metanephrines changes more than those for VMA in patients with phaeochromocytoma, making this the screening test of choice.

The diagnosis can also be established by radiological techniques, but these are most useful for localisation of the tumour. The range of procedures is large and includes straight X-rays of the thorax and abdomen, and intravenous pyelography which, though simple, may yet be helpful. Presacral injection of carbon dioxide or oxygen (the former is safer, but is absorbed so quickly that the series of X-rays necessary may not be possible) will outline the kidneys and the adjacent adrenals, and the presence of a tumour may be demonstrated either on account of its size or, in the case of a small tumour, because of an alteration in the normal shape of the adrenal (Edwards, 1962). Retrograde catheterisation of the aorta with the injection of a dye to delineate the tumour, which is vascular, is also of value (Edwards, 1962). Catheterisation of the inferior vena cava with sampling for plasma catecholamines at different levels is a safe manipulation and helpful in the localisation of a tumour.

Preparation for operation.—Surgical removal is the only method of treatment but before it is attempted certain investigations must be carried out to determine the general physical state of the patient, particularly in relation to the heart and circulation, and the patient must be prepared for operation.

Apart from routine examination of the heart, electrocardiographs must be taken and blood volume studies may well be of considerable value. When the phaeochromocytoma is of long standing the patient may have a marked reduction in blood volume due to continuous vasoconstriction (Brunjes *et al.*, 1960), but this is the exception rather than the rule (Sjoerosma *et al.*, 1966; Walters, 1969). If the blood volume is low, removal of the tumour may be followed by acute hypotension due to vasodilatation in the presence of chronic hypovolaemia. Leather and his colleagues (1962) have drawn attention to the high haemoglobin values that may be found during and for a day or two after a hypertensive crisis. They explain them on a similar basis to the reduction in blood volume, since catecholamines reduce plasma volume and raise the venous haematocrit (Kalreider *et al.*, 1942; Finnerty *et al.*, 1958).

Preparation for operation should include special consideration of the administration of α and β blockers or of drugs that prevent catecholamine synthesis. In 1959, Ahlquist noted that in animal experiments nearly all sympathomimetic effects of the catecholamines could be prevented by the simultaneous use of α and β blockers, but the use of these agents in man is not yet fully elucidated. Of the α blockers phentolamine is most popular, and its pre-operative administration to control symptoms and blood pressure levels is recommended by many. Johns and Brunjes (1962) consider that if it is administered for a sufficiently long period of time pre-operatively the blood volume of the patient may be restored to normal and acute hypotension following removal of the phaeochromocytoma avoided. Although Sjoerosma and his colleagues (1966) consider the blood volume to be normal in most patients with a phaeochromocytoma they recommend adrenergic blockade to stabilise the blood pressure and to prevent arrhythmias. This can be done either by the use of an α and a β blocker for two to three days pre-operatively, or by the use of α-methylparatyrosine which blocks the hydroxylation of tyrosine to dopa. Clinical experience suggests that an α blocker is only rarely needed pre-operatively, though the case for a β blocker is more problematical. Now current practice is towards the use of complete adrenergic blockade pre-operatively with α-methylparatyrosine, supplemented by a β blocker when there is a specific indication, such as a tendency to cardiac arrhythmia.

Anaesthesia and operation.—There is no particular merit in using a phenothiazine drug in the premedication and there may be a disadvantage if it produces hypotension. Most of the anaesthetic drugs are likely to cause some change in systemic arterial pressure, but the essential prerequisite is a smooth induction and maintenance without straining, hypoxia or carbon dioxide retention. Our experience favours thiopentone, nitrous oxide and oxygen with the addition of muscle relaxants. Some of the latter can be faulted on account of their individual side-effects and the potential effects of these on the patient's heart and circulation, but we have not found any material disadvantages. Pancuronium for both intubation and maintenance would appear to be the relaxant of choice (James, 1970). Rollason (1964), Etsten and Shimosato (1965), Watson and Hansen (1967) and others have advocated halothane as the anaesthetic of choice since it can be administered in a dose sufficient to control any excessive hypertension. Although the addition of halothane in a low concentration to supplement too light a level of anaesthesia from nitrous oxide or as a substitute for nitrous oxide but combined with a muscle relaxant is unlikely materially to affect the blood pressure or to increase significantly the incidence of arrhythmias, we prefer to control the blood pressure more specifically—when this is necessary—with small intravenous doses of phentolamine (2·5 to 5 mg.). Cardiac arrhythmias present a special problem, but unless they arise in the ventricles and are continuous, suggesting the likelihood of the onset of ventricular fibrillation, they are probably best left untreated, since they usually subside. Indeed, the pre-operative use of propranolol make the occurrence of more than a minimal disturbance of this nature unlikely. Treatment, when necessary, should be with an intravenous injection of 2·5 mg. of propranolol but the drug must be used with great caution during anaesthesia.

Measurement of the arterial and central venous pressures should be performed throughout the operation and in the post-operative period until stability of the circulation is ensured. Similarly a continuous electrocardiograph should be monitored. Blood loss must be measured and replacement carried out. Hypotension is likely to occur soon after the tumour is removed, or in the immediate post-operative period, but it is not by any means invariable. Just occasionally persistent hypertension may suggest a second tumour in the patient. Almost always hypotension can be combated by the administration of a blood transfusion, and such treatment, usually in excess of the actual quantity of blood lost during the operation, is the best therapy for the low blood pressure. Noradrenaline is best avoided but may occasionally be required. It is as well to note that this agent may be ineffective if the patient's α receptors have been previously blocked, or that its effect may be greatly enhanced in the presence of α-methyl-paratyrosine. When a noradrenaline infusion is used, care must be taken to ensure that this does not cause or mask any persistent haemorrhage from the operation site, particularly in the post-operative period. The patient must be weaned as quickly as possible from the noradrenaline as the blood pressure stabilises itself. Patients who have had a phaeochromocytoma for a long time—particularly if structural changes have developed in their vessels—may well retain their hypertensive blood pressure level and never revert to normal.

Bilateral Adrenalectomy

Bilateral adrenalectomy is usually undertaken for the treatment of Cushing's syndrome or of patients with metastases from a breast carcinoma. For the former it can be expected to ensure remission of the disease whether the hyperadrenalism is due to a cortical tumour or to hyperplasia. Hypophysectomy is certainly the more logical treatment for hyperplasia and is becoming more popular. For the latter it is combined with bilateral oophorectomy, either at the same or another operation, in an attempt to remove all the hormone-producing tissue on which these tumours to some extent depend. A successful operation is usually associated with marked symptomatic improvement, particularly when pain has been a severe factor, and in many patients there is evidence of tumour regression.

The anaesthetic problem is created by the general state of the patient, who is usually seriously ill, often emaciated, and generally with multiple secondaries. A pleural effusion, not infrequently bilateral, often complicates the situation and may hamper respiration sufficiently to warrant aspiration before operation. Even small effusions create mechanical difficulties during anaesthesia when the patient is postured. When anaesthesia can be safely induced in spite of their presence, it is kinder, however, to aspirate as soon as the patient is anaesthetised rather than in the ward. The patient's tolerance for anaesthetic drugs is likely to be reduced, and, when large doses of opiates or other analgesics have been administered, great care is needed to avoid overdosage. Unless the patient is moved into the necessary position for operation with caution, bones may be broken at the site of secondary deposits.

A course of cortisone on the lines previously suggested must be given. Although hypotension may occur in this type of patient, both during and after operation, it appears to be more an indication of the weak general condition than of loss of adrenal medullary secretions. Provided blood loss is adequately replaced and the anaesthetic sequence and dosage are chosen to avoid circulatory depression, vasoconstrictors such as noradrenaline are unnecessary.

Bilateral adrenalectomy alone has also been advocated and performed for the treatment of malignant hypertension, but with a singular lack of success in improving the symptoms or course of the disease, and for this condition the operation carries a high mortality in spite of supportive therapy for the circulation.

The Pituitary Gland

Although the pituitary is frequently attacked by disease, by the surgeon and by the radiotherapeutist with yttrium, it is only when near-total loss of function occurs that acute complications, due to lack of corticotrophin stimulation of the adrenal cortex, are likely to be troublesome, and then seldom unless exogenous replacement of hormones has been omitted. Replacement is essential because once the pituitary has been totally removed, the adrenal cortices will atrophy away. Total removal may be performed for the treatment of Cushing's syndrome or of secondary carcinomata; since it is an elective operation, a course of cortisone should be administered as described on p. 1363.

Hormonal replacement must include not only corticosteroids but also thyroxine and pitressin. Thyroid hormone replacement is not necessary during or immediately after surgery, but usually at about the second or third week. Polyuria is controlled by pitressin tannate and is indicated by the quantity of urine passed following the operation, but it may be needed in the immediate post-operative period when it is best given by intramuscular injection. Hypophysectomised patients do not all develop marked polyuria, and many of those who do can ultimately be controlled by occasional rather than routine administration of pitressin. For long-term use pitressin can generally be satisfactorily administered as a nasal spray or as snuff. Removal of the pituitary causes little or no upset of carbohydrate metabolism in patients who are not diabetic, but in those who are there is a marked sensitivity to insulin. It is essential in the latter to reduce the insulin dosage, omitting it altogether on the day of operation despite the covering course of corticosteroids, and match subsequent doses against the patient's measured level of blood sugar.

Acute adrenal insufficiency following the removal of a pituitary tumour is very rare (Northfield, 1955), but has been described when a very thorough eradication has been attempted. Nevertheless persistent hypotension may be present in an occasional patient for several days after operation and, unless other factors suggest an alternative cause than lack of hormones, the low blood pressure should be an indication for cortisone. Another cause of hypotension following pituitary removal is disturbance of the hypothalamus during the operation. Congestion or thrombosis of small vessels in the neighbourhood of this organ may be the essential factors at fault, and if these are sufficiently marked the patient may never recover consciousness, but gradually succumb with a rising temperature. Less severely affected patients may be unduly sleepy and have a bradycardia associated with the hypotension for several days. The routine use of a cortisone cover for pituitary operations does not appear to be warranted, unless there is pre-operative evidence of an endocrine imbalance.

Chronic hypopituitarism may develop irrespective of surgery, and takes many forms, depending upon the extent of the destructive process and the age of the patient at the start of the illness. Different syndromes are often produced and these depend upon the number of hormones that are affected. Very frequently the whole lot are involved, as in panhypopituitarism or Simmond's disease. These patients are liable to sudden attacks of coma. The cause is endocrine failure, but the precipitating factors are often comparatively minor, thus emphasising the border-line level at which consciousness is maintained in such people. Analgesics and anaesthetics, even in small doses, can precipitate coma. The diagnosis of hypopituitarism need not be difficult if it is remembered that, at such a severe state of the disease, pubic and axillary hair will probably have long since disappeared, and the sexual organs atrophied. Immediate treatment should be with intravenous hydrocortisone, but any associated hypoglycaemia must be rectified. Occasionally coma in hypopituitarism is associated with marked hypothermia, in which case simple warming may restore consciousness.

The Thyroid Gland

Thyroidectomy for thyrotoxicosis no longer taxes the ingenuity of surgeon, physician and anaesthetist as it did just over twenty years ago before the introduction of thiourea and, subsequently, thiouracil and its derivatives. Nowadays, a very large proportion of patients suffering from this disease are cured by planned medical treatment with radio-active iodine or one of the antithyroid drugs, but some, on account of a relapse, intolerance to the specific drugs, secondary thyrotoxicosis in an adenoma, progressive exophthalmos, general enlargement of the gland with medical therapy, and perhaps obstructive symptoms, or more simply for personal reasons, need the surgeon's aid.

None should be operated upon until the thyrotoxicosis has been controlled to the fullest extent. This is usually done with one of the antithyroid drugs,* but when it is mild, simple iodine alone for a week or two immediately before operation may suffice. Iodine can be given as Lugol's solution which is an aqueous solution of 5 per cent w/v of iodine and 10 per cent w/v of potassium iodide; 10 minims are usually given q.d.s. Antithyroid compounds tend to enlarge the thyroid gland and make it more vascular—disadvantages for the surgeon—but a ten-day course of iodine before operation after the antithyroid drug may be useful to offset these by its involuting effect. If preparation of the patient by such means is carefully carried out, the risk of a thyroid crisis following the operation is extremely slight. Kadis and his colleagues (1966) claim that a thyroid crisis is most likely to be seen nowadays if a patient with previously undiagnosed and therefore uncontrolled thyrotoxicosis has to have an emergency operation for some unrelated condition. In such circumstances the thyrotoxicosis may be recognised pre-operatively and treatment should consist of sedation, adrenergic blockade and deep anaesthesia.

* Carbimazole (Neo-mercazole) is the drug of choice for the treatment of thyrotoxicosis. It is ten times more potent than methyl- and propylthiouracil and is used in an initial dose of from 30 to 45 mg. daily in divided doses, reducing to a maintenance dose of about 5 to 15 mg. daily.

Propylthiouracil and methylthiouracil are nowadays rarely, if ever, used. The initial dose required is about 100 mg. q.d.s., but this can be gradually reduced as the thyrotoxicosis is controlled. If long-continued medical therapy is indicated a small maintenance dose of from 50 to 100 mg. o.d. may suffice. Toxic symptoms are not common with these drugs, but the patient should be carefully observed for them, particularly during the first month of treatment.

The thiouracils and carbimazole prevent the synthesis of thyroxine, but potassium perchlorate stops the thyroid from taking up iodine. This drug is sometimes used to control thyrotoxicosis when toxic reactions are produced by the other drugs. It is not, however, free from side-effects and can cause aplastic anaemia when used for a long time continuously. The initial dose is 800 mg. daily in divided doses, reduced to a maintenance dose of about 200 to 400 mg. daily.

Radioactive iodine (I^{131}) has the advantage of being very simple to use since a single dose given by mouth is often effective, though further doses are sometimes needed at intervals of not less than three to four months. After absorption the iodine is concentrated in the thyroid gland; nevertheless, this form of therapy is usually reserved for elderly patients who are past the childbearing age.

Because these patients tend to be excitable, special consideration must be given to the pre-operative sedation, which may with benefit be started days, rather than hours, before the expected time. Usually a small dose of phenobarbitone (30 to 60 mg.) for a day or two is sufficient, but the choice of drug and its dose depends upon the patient, who may have been tried on several during medical treatment. Phenothiazine drugs have a special application and may be particularly useful for immediate premedication.

Anaesthesia

Although the operation can be very satisfactorily performed under local analgesia provided the surgeon is gentle, general anaesthesia is preferable for all concerned. The choice of anaesthetic depends very much on personal preference, but deep anaesthesia is unnecessary, and badly administered anaesthesia, particularly with sub-oxygenation, may be more hazardous than usual. Thiopentone, nitrous oxide-oxygen with supplementation either by inhalational agents such as trichloroethylene or halothane, or a judicious use of an intravenous analgesic, and with spontaneous respiration is satisfactory. But many anaesthetists prefer to control respiration throughout with a muscle relaxant and avoid the use of a potent inhalational agent. After induction an oral endotracheal tube should be passed with the aid of suxamethonium, not forgetting to oxygenate the patient and spray the trachea and glottis with 4 per cent lignocaine first. Intubation may increase the severity of the post-operative tracheitis but this is hardly a contra-indication. Infiltration in the area of the proposed incision with a solution of 1:200,000 adrenaline, or 1:400,000 noradrenaline, in saline markedly reduces the vascularity of the skin flaps, but must be carried out before the introduction of a volatile agent to the anaesthetic mixture. Induced hypotension is not recommended, since—merely to prevent bleeding—the advantages do not seem to outweigh the potential hazards for this type of operation; bleeding from the gland and its immediate surroundings depends very much on the adequacy of the surgical technique and, in competent hands, is surprisingly small. A little foot-down tilt will assist the venous drainage.

Three further points should be noted. It is not necessary to over-extend the patient's head upon a sandbag or hard pillow to give the surgeon good access; hyperextension puts the strap muscles on the stretch and produces occipital headache post-operatively. It may be helpful to the surgeon to watch the vocal cords during extubation and make certain that the recurrent laryngeal nerves are not damaged.* A patient at rest even with bilateral palsies may yet have an adequate airway, but returning consciousness with pain stimuli can lead to obstruction. Abductor palsy is even more dangerous (see also Chapter 1, p. 16 *et seq.*). A little care at this stage may save an acute emergency later. Finally, the patient's eyes must be carefully protected during the operation.

* Riddell (1970) believes that the vocal cords should be observed by the anaesthetist by direct laryngoscopy during thyroidectomy after resection of the first lobe, with the object of assessing the integrity of the recurrent laryngeal nerve on that side *before* resection of the second lobe. This necessitates a special technique of anaesthesia not only to allow direct laryngoscopy midway through the anaesthetic but to ensure that at that time there is no neuromuscular block to impair the value of stimulation of the recurrent laryngeal nerve.

Post-operative Care

This is normally routine, but the immediate progress of the patient must be observed in case a thyroid crisis or respiratory obstruction develop. The patient should be kept at a moderately cool temperature and be adequately sedated. A rapidly rising pulse rate, pyrexia, sweating, hypertension followed by hypotension with cardiac failure and excessive restlessness are the predominant signs of a crisis. Treatment is still largely empirical and supportive. Iodine intravenously, thiouracil, and digitalis for the heart are the most specific. Hypothermia would appear to have a special value here.

Respiratory obstruction is uncommon, but may be caused in several ways. Damage to the recurrent laryngeal nerves has already been mentioned, but laryngeal oedema, tracheal collapse and reactionary haemorrhage can lead to respiratory obstruction, each of which will require urgent treatment.

The Pancreas

The greater part of the pancreas consists of alveoli in which acinous cells secrete a digestive juice, but situated between the alveoli are occasional groups of epithelial cells known as the Islets of Langerhans, in which insulin is formed. The islets contain three distinguishable types of cell, A, B, and C. The B cells secrete insulin, the C cells are thought to be progenitors of the other two, and the A cells produce glucagon.

Insulin is intimately concerned with carbohydrate metabolism. Its more important function is the promotion of glucose utilisation by the tissues, probably by stimulating the transfer of the carbohydrate across the cell wall by activating enzymes concerned in its metabolism. Insulin increases the process of glycogen formation in the liver (glycogenesis), its storage in both the liver and other body tissues—principally the muscles—and the rate of formation of fatty acids from glucose in the liver. It inhibits the breakdown of glycogen to glucose (glycogenolysis) in the liver, and also the formation of both glycogen and glucose from the end products of protein metabolism (gluconeogenesis). Finally, the ultimate breakdown of glucose in the tissues, to provide energy for the body, is increased by insulin.

Many other factors are concerned in the metabolism of carbohydrates. Hormones from the anterior pituitary and the adrenal cortex tend to antagonise the effect of insulin on peripheral glucose utilisation and to increase the breakdown of glycogen to glucose and the formation of glucose from protein metabolism. They are, therefore, antagonistic to insulin. Thyroid and posterior pituitary hormone, and adrenaline from the adrenal medulla, have a similar effect—the mobilisation of sugar. Glucagon causes hyperglycaemia by promoting hepatic glycogenolysis, and catecholamines may block insulin secretion in response to rises in blood sugar. A rising blood sugar inhibits the liver's action in producing more glucose, while a falling blood sugar stimulates this. The blood sugar, in a normal person, represents the balance between these several factors. When insulin is absent, diabetes mellitus results; when it is present in excess, as may be the case in certain tumours of the pancreas, spontaneous hypoglycaemia occurs.

Diabetes Mellitus

The primary result of the absence of insulin is a rise in blood sugar caused by the liver failing to make and store glycogen, and increasing the production of glucose from protein metabolism. Sugar eventually appears in the urine. The secondary result is a rise in the level of ketones in the blood, caused by the liver's failure to break down glucose to fatty acids, with a consequent increase in fat metabolism to aid the body's energy requirements. The amount of ketones (aceto-acetic acid and β-hydroxy-butyric acid) produced by this process are more than the body needs. Ketones, like sugar, appear in the urine sooner or later. A subsidiary result of the body's failure to break down carbohydrate is that ingested carbohydrate food merely adds to the already raised blood sugar.

The clinical syndromes associated with insulin lack are variable, but the classical immediate results of a high blood sugar (hyperglycaemia) are thirst, and marked polyuria, due to the high osmotic pressure exerted by the sugar in the urine preventing tubular reabsorption. The effect of a rising ketone level in the blood (ketosis) is to produce acidosis. This leads to hyperventilation (in its extreme the classical Küssmaul respiration), loss of sodium due to the combination of these acids with body base and, as a result, more loss of fluid. Ultimately the patient becomes comatose, the blood pressure falls, and death follows. Peripheral neuritis and peripheral vascular disease are often associated with long-standing diabetes, and are probably the end results of associated metabolic deficiencies brought about by the absence of insulin.

The diagnosis of diabetes mellitus rests on the history, on examination of the urine and the blood sugar level.* The urine must be tested for sugar and for ketone bodies;† while a glucose tolerance curve will give evidence of the glucose metabolism (see Fig. 1). The normal renal threshold for glucose in blood is about 180 mg. per 100 ml. Patients with a low renal threshold may leak glucose into the urine, even though their carbohydrate metabolism is normal. An alimentary lag in the absorption of glucose from the blood into the liver accounts for an abnormally high rise in the blood sugar with glycosuria in some people after a glucose meal, but the level falls to normal as rapidly as it rises.

Diabetic patients broadly form two distinct types; those who are young, tend to be thin, are sensitive to insulin and easily made ketotic, and those who are elderly, perhaps well covered, insensitive to insulin and rarely ketotic. This is an important differentiation for purposes of treatment, since the first group need insulin and are easily controlled with it, enabling them to lead a normal life with few, if any, restrictions in diet. The second group are better controlled by

* *"Dextrostix" and the Blood Sugar*

An approximate blood sugar level can be gauged simply and quickly by the use of "Dextrostix". These consist of a buffered mixture of glucose oxidase, peroxidase and a chromogen system covered with a semi-permeable membrane on the end of plastic strip. A large drop of blood is spread over the reactive area on the strip, and washed off exactly one minute later by a jet of cold water. The presence of glucose is shown by the formation of a blue colour, and the quantity of glucose can be gauged by comparison with a colour chart.

† Urine Tests for Glucose and Acetone Bodies

Benedict's Test for Glucose. Eight drops of urine are added to about 5 ml. of Benedict's reagent in a test tube, the mixture is boiled and allowed to cool. A positive test is shown by

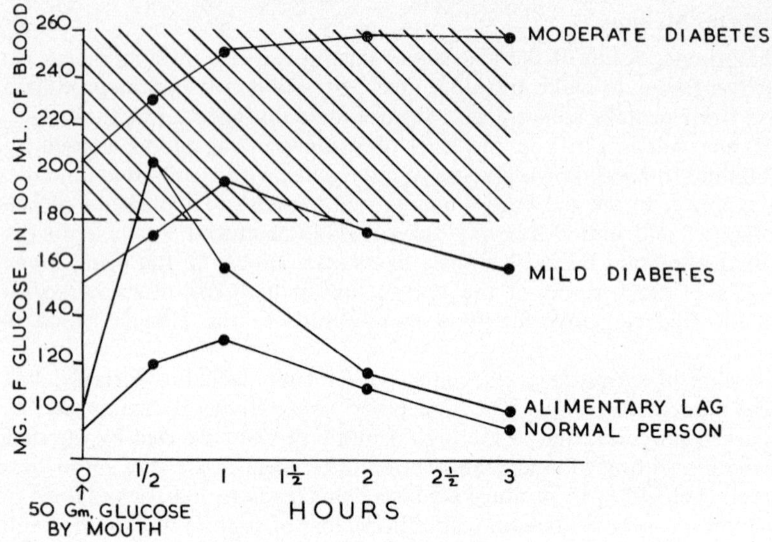

50/Fig. 3.—Glucose tolerance curves.

a colour change with a precipitate, from the original blue, through green, yellow and orange to a dark orange to red. The amount of sugar in the urine conditions the extent of the progression—a full change signifies over 1 per cent glucose in urine. Benedict's test is more sensitive than Fehlings, and reduced by few other substances than glucose.

Rothera's Test for Acetone and Aceto-acetic Acid. The ketone bodies aceto-acetic acid and hydroxybutyric acid are always present together. Aceto-acetic acid breaks up to form acetone in both the urine and in the blood of the lungs (this accounts for the smell of patients in diabetic coma). A test tube is half filled with urine, which must be saturated with ammonium sulphate crystals. Two or three drops of ammonia are then added, followed by a drop or two of freshly prepared sodium nitroprusside solution, when a positive result will be shown by the formation of a purple ring where this solution meets the urine. Alternatively, crystals of sodium nitroprusside can be shaken upon the urine mixture and the whole watched for a colour change.

Other tests. Several commercial tests are available for reducing substances, glucose and ketone bodies. All of these are conveniently set up and simple to carry out. The "Clinitest" for reducing substances is a tablet of copper sulphate and sodium hydroxide. Five drops of urine are placed in a dry test tube, ten drops of water are added and are followed by a tablet of the reagent. An alkaline solution of copper sulphate is produced, and this boils—provided the quantity of water is correct—due to the heat of the sodium hydroxide solution. After boiling has ceased, the test tube is shaken and the colour of its contents is compared with the colour chart supplied. When no reducing substances are present, the solution will be blue. Colours ranging from dark green, through yellow green and brown, to orange, and finally to dark green brown, correspond to increasing percentages of reducing substances in the urine. The presence of glucose itself can be ascertained by the use of either "Clinistix" or "Testape", both of which make use of the enzyme glucose oxidase. This will only oxidase glucose, and it produces hydrogen peroxide. "Clinistix" and "Testape" contain glucose oxidase and a reagent to detect any hydrogen peroxide that is produced. When "Clinistix" is dipped in urine containing glucose it turns blue, while "Testape" goes green in the presence of glucose. Reducing substances can be detected by "Acetest". This is a tablet of sodium nitroprusside with other reagents that control pH. A drop of urine is put on an "Acetest" tablet. If there are no ketone bodies present, the tablet will stay white, but if there are some then colour changes ranging from lavender to purple will take place. The presence of ketones can also be detected by a "Ketostix" which is a strip impregnated with sodium nitroprusside and glycine. It is dipped in urine and will develop a lavender colour at fifteen seconds when ketones are present. The depth of colour varies with the degree of ketosis.

some restriction of diet, since insulin is not always necessary and extremely large doses of it rarely have little effect upon them. Oral hypoglycaemic compounds* may have a part to play in the treatment of patients in the second group.

Excess of insulin in the sensitive patient may lead to symptoms of hypoglycaemia. These are sweating and tachycardia due to the release of adrenaline in an attempt to mobilise more glucose, and irritability of the central nervous system, due to lack of glucose. This takes the form of excitability, anxiousness, tremor, hunger, occasionally twitching, and rarely a fit. When treatment with intravenous glucose is not instituted quickly marked mental changes occur, followed by coma and death. Hypoglycaemic and hyperglycaemic coma are contrasted in Table 3 as the differential diagnosis is important to the anaesthetist, and may have to be dissociated from the effects of anaesthesia postoperatively.

Treatment.—It is not proposed to discuss the details of treatment, but only to stress the working principle that a young diabetic is best controlled with adequate doses of insulin—preferably a long-acting preparation such as protamine zinc insulin†—and allowed a free diet. Such treatment is amply justified by

50/TABLE 3

THE CLINICAL SIGNS OF HYPERGLYCAEMIA AND HYPOGLYCAEMIA

	Hyperglycaemia	*Hypoglycaemia*
General .	Cold, dehydrated, smell of acetone, sunken eye-balls, pupils not specific, may be vomiting. Reflexes all sluggish.	Sweating, pallor, large pupils generalised twitching and reflexes hyperactive (unless terminal).
Respiration .	Deep, sighing hyperventilation.	Unaffected.
Circulation .	Low blood pressure, tachycardia.	Blood pressure normal in early stages, but tachycardia marked.

A blood sugar always establishes the diagnosis. Sugar may be present in the urine in hypoglycaemic coma if there has been a sudden swing due to insulin. Ketone bodies signify hyperglycaemia, but it should not be forgotten that other causes than diabetes can account for it, i.e. ether or chloroform anaesthesia and prolonged vomiting.

* Oral hypoglycaemic compounds are of two types—sulphonyl ureas and diguanides. They are valuable in the treatment of mild diabetic patients who do not have ketosis. Most patients in this group develop diabetes late in life and tend to be fat, and many of them can be controlled by dietetic measures alone. It is only as a supplement to dietetic control that oral hypoglycaemic agents should be used.

The sulphonyl ureas are tolbutamide (Rastinon) and chlorpropamide (Diabinese), the former having a short action and necessitating twice daily dosage, while the latter is usually effective for twenty-four hours. Both are thought to produce hypoglycaemia by causing the release of insulin from the β cells of the pancreatic islets.

The diguanides are not often used, nor is their mode of action fully understood.

† There are many types of insulin available, the three commonly used being soluble insulin (S.I.), protamine zinc insulin (P.Z.I.) and insulin zinc suspension (I.Z.S.). S.I. has a short action

the large number of diabetic patients who lead normal lives without restriction of activity and without being any more upset by everyday illnesses than non-diabetic patients. Treating the diabetic patient as a normal patient is also the key to safe anaesthesia when it is needed. The fat, probably elderly patient is usually controlled by a restricted diet in terms of both calories and carbohydrate but if this does not succeed, and provided there is no ketosis, an oral hypoglycaemic agent should be tried. All diabetics must be maintained with ketone-free urine; a trace of sugar is satisfactory.

The blood sugar and anaesthesia.—Three sets of facts need consideration:

1. The Effects of the Anaesthetic Drugs and Technique.
2. The Effects of Operation.
3. The Effects of Pre- and Post-operative Complications.

1. *The effects of anaesthetic drugs and techniques.*—At one extreme are drugs such as chloroform and ether which produce hyperglycaemia in some degree, and at the other, thiopentone and nitrous oxide, with sufficient oxygen, which have no effect worth considering. Between them are halothane, trichloroethylene, cyclopropane and many other agents which tend to cause a slight, though varying, rise in blood sugar. A badly administered anaesthetic—particularly if associated with hypoxia—is very likely to produce hyperglycaemia.

The increased blood sugar is due to the liver breaking down more glycogen than under ordinary conditions, partly owing to the direct effects of certain anaesthetic agents—subsidiary points here are the concentration of the drug, its duration of action and, of course, the state of the liver—and partly owing to sympathetic stimulation and the release of pituitary-adrenocortical hormones. Factors which lead to the release of adrenaline are fear, a tiresome induction, hypoxia, and, indeed, the ability of an agent like ether to cause sympathetic stimulation.

The risk of hypoglycaemia is considerably increased by the administration of drugs which block the autonomic nervous system (Griffiths, 1953), since they potentiate markedly the action of insulin. Non-diabetics tend to get a fall in the blood sugar level after such drugs, but then remain stable. The diabetic patient is particularly susceptible and may have a severe hypoglycaemic reaction, the signs of which will be largely masked by the autonomic block. The reactions that occur during hypoglycaemia are in part due to the adrenaline that is released. Griffiths points out that the less complete the autonomic block is, the smaller will be the fall in blood sugar; he also draws attention to the presence of a persistent tachycardia as the only constant sign of hypoglycaemia in the presence of autonomic block. It could be argued that autonomic blocking drugs

of up to twelve hours, while P.Z.I. is effective for twenty-four hours or longer. The duration of action of I.Z.S. varies from about twelve to thirty-six hours depending upon the particular suspension used.

A mild or moderately severe case of diabetes can usually be controlled with a single dose of P.Z.I. given in the morning, or by a morning and evening dose of S.I. A severe case is unlikely to be completely controlled by P.Z.I. alone and may need S.I. as well in the morning to limit glycosuria during the day; both these insulins can, however, be combined in the same syringe and injected together. A suitable suspension of I.Z.S. may be as effective as a combined injection of P.Z.I. and S.I.

provide the logical preventive treatment to those anaesthetic agents and techniques which primarily raise the blood sugar through sympathetic stimulation. Their danger predominates, and the effect of a well chosen and carefully administered general anaesthetic upon blood sugar levels is negligible, just as it is in triggering the stress syndrome (see p. 1360).

2. *The effects of operation.*—These may be more profound than those of the anaesthetic, but are surprisingly slight. Griffiths (1953) showed a statistically significant, but clinically unimportant, maintained rise in blood sugar during upper abdominal sections, when sympathetic stimulation might be expected to be the cause. In superficial operations the blood sugar was not affected. On the other hand, removal of the cause of a hyperglycaemic response, such as the baby from a pregnant diabetic woman, may result in a hypoglycaemic tendency—particularly if the insulin dosage is not modified post-operatively (Foster and Francis, 1955).

3. *The effects of pre- and post-operative complications.*—The severity of the surgical condition, and any associated disease, are most important here. Acute infective processes in particular lead to an increased blood sugar as the energy requirements of the patient rise. Post-operatively similar considerations hold, but vomiting may be an additional complication. Protracted vomiting, pre- or post-operative, can, of course, lead to ketosis in otherwise normal people, but even moderate nausea and emesis may lead to hypoglycaemia in a diabetic patient by preventing an adequate carbohydrate intake.

The diabetic patient, operation and anaesthesia.—People with diabetes live normal lives. For them the risks associated with anaesthesia and operation are very little more than for a normal person, but certain essentials must be assumed for such a statement to be substantiated. The anaesthetic must be properly chosen and administered, adequate facilities for blood and urinary sugar estimations must be available, and the state of the diabetes at the time when the operation is proposed must be understood.

Diabetic patients needing an anaesthetic can be divided into two groups—those who are controlled and those who are not.

1. *The controlled diabetic patient.*—This is essentially the patient who lives a normal life and whose diabetes has not been upset by the surgical disease. When the operation is *elective*, there is no reason to expect that the normal balance will be upset, and no special preparation is necessary. The best time for the operation to be performed is at midday or thereabouts. Then, morning insulin, and a normal but early morning breakfast should be given, the patient prepared for anaesthesia and operation in the routine manner with five hours' starvation, and an anaesthetic sequence chosen which has least effect upon the blood sugar. There is no necessity to switch patients in this group from a long-acting to a short-acting insulin. Provided the operation is a minor one and both it and the duration of anaesthesia (these are not necessarily synonymous) brief, the immediate post-operative state of the patient will not preclude early fluid intake, so that hypoglycaemia is unlikely. In clinical practice such a regime has amply justified itself for several years. It is only necessary to add that even on those occasions when the operation has been performed early in the morning after a period of starvation lasting the night, and despite the administration of the usual dose of insulin, no harm has followed. A sudden change of surgical

plan, which either necessitates delaying the operation or enhancing its magnitude, post-operative vomiting, or any suspicion of hypoglycaemia—unexpected delay in the recovery of consciousness—should be covered by setting up an intravenous infusion of 5 per cent dextrose in water (a 500 ml. flask contains 25 g. of dextrose).

Although the same regime of preparation may be used when the operation is a major one, an intravenous infusion of 5 per cent dextrose in water should be set up automatically, and there is something to be said for transferring the patient to soluble (short-acting) insulin for quicker immediate control of the situation. Should this be advisable, it must be carried out a day or two before the operation to ensure adequate stabilisation. A controlled diabetic undergoing surgery and anaesthesia after the basis of treatment suggested is most likely to become hypoglycaemic, if indeed his blood sugar varies markedly at all.

When the operation is an *emergency*, an intravenous infusion of 5 per cent dextrose in water is always advisable, and during the post-operative period soluble insulin may need to be given in divided doses at four or six hour intervals to control the patient's response.

These are general rules, which must to some extent depend upon the individual patient and the severity of the diabetes. Oral glucose should, however, never be given an hour or so before a proposed operation. Not only is it dangerous as it may be vomited during anaesthesia and then aspirated into the lungs (see Chapter 47, p. 1303), but there is very little evidence that it helps the patient. The course of all these patients should be checked by frequent urine tests. Blood sugars are helpful but not always essential.

2. *The uncontrolled diabetic patient.—Elective* operations must never be performed on patients with uncontrolled diabetes. For *emergency* operations, a more empirical approach to the problem will probably be necessary. When both sugar and ketones are present in the urine, it may even be wiser to delay operation until the latter can be controlled—the risks of delay being balanced against those of ketosis. In either event, intramuscular soluble insulin and intravenous 5 per cent dextrose are needed, and the water and electrolyte balance of the patient must be carefully observed. The urine must be checked for sugar and ketones at regular intervals, and the blood sugar level frequently measured. The dose relationship between soluble insulin and dextrose will depend upon the degree of ketosis. When no ketones are present, 1 unit for every 2 g. of glucose is reasonable—about 25 units of insulin are given intramuscularly and the dextrose run in slowly. The presence of ketones will be an indication for an initial dose of insulin of about 50 units, followed by repeated doses as suggested by the urine or blood sugar tests.

Discussion.—Too great an emphasis is usually laid upon the danger of anaesthesia causing hyperglycaemia. The drugs and technique must always be chosen to avoid this. Thiopentone, nitrous oxide-oxygen, and muscle relaxants when necessary, is the best sequence, but a local analgesic technique may often be more expedient and, properly conducted, will have no effect upon the diabetes. Diabetic patients are put in danger when oral glucose is administered shortly before operation, or when the state and progress of their diabetes has not been considered pre-operatively by the anaesthetist.

Pancreatic Tumours

A rare tumour of the pancreas, arising from the Islets of Langerhans, may cause symptoms of hypoglycaemia due to the excessive secretion of insulin. These tumours may be benign or malignant, and the attacks they cause tend to be paroxysmal. They are frequently amenable to surgery. Hypoglycaemia may occur as a result of fasting during the pre-operative period (Fraser, 1963; Bourke, 1966) and if untreated can lead to circulatory collapse during the induction of anaesthesia and before the tumour is handled. The blood sugar level should therefore be gauged, at least approximately, just before induction of anaesthesia. An intravenous infusion of 5 per cent dextrose should be used throughout the operation, which may be associated with hypoglycaemia during the handling of the tumour. The only clinical evidence of this is likely to be an increasing tachycardia with perhaps sweating. Autonomic blocking agents should not be used because they potentiate the action of insulin. Removal of the tumour may be associated with some post-operative suppression of insulin formation by the remaining normal pancreatic tissue, so that a temporary hyperglycaemia occasionally results.

HYDROXYDIONE: A STEROID ANAESTHETIC

History

The anaesthetic properties of seventy-five steroids of varying structure were first demonstrated by Selye (1941 and 1942) in rats. He noted that some compounds had a high anaesthetic potency with minimal hormonal activity, and subsequently other workers showed experimentally that one, 21-hydroxypregnanedione succinate, or hydroxydione, has a wide margin of safety, a therapeutic index which is greater than that of thiopentone, and no hormonal activity (Laubach *et al.*, 1955; P'an *et al.*, 1955). Hydroxydione ("Viadril") was first used clinically during 1955 (Murphy *et al.*, 1955).

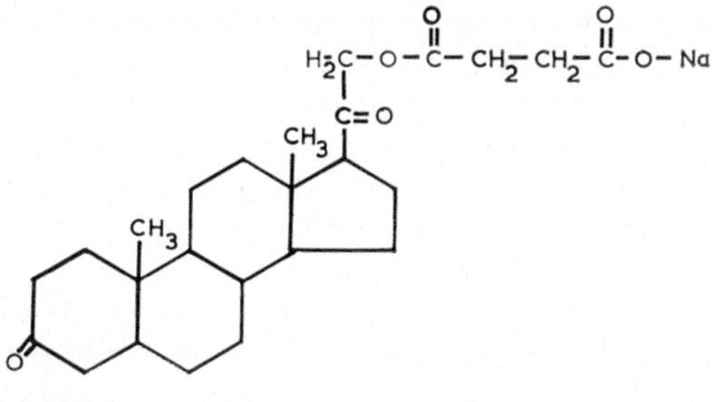

Physical Properties

Hydroxydione is a water soluble steriod, which is supplied as a white powder. Dissolved in water, saline or 5 per cent dextrose in water, the resulting solutions are all strongly alkaline, but the marked irritant effect that all hydroxydione solutions possess is due to the properties of the compound itself.

Pharmacological Actions

Loss of consciousness occurs very slowly, even when large doses are rapidly injected intravenously, and closely resembles the onset of natural sleep. The electro-encephalographic pattern is exactly the same as that produced by the thiobarbiturates such as thiopentone (Bellville *et al.*, 1956); a factor which favours the classification of hydroxydione as a hypnotic rather than a narcotic.

Respiration is slightly depressed in volume and the rate increased, but apnoea, such as typically occurs with the intravenous use of thiobarbiturates, is uncommon and of only brief duration. A specific suppressant effect upon respiratory tract reflexes is claimed. The blood pressure falls, probably due to a combination of central vasomotor depression, direct vasodilator effect upon the peripheral vessels, and some effect upon the ventricular muscle (Taylor and Shearer, 1956). Tachycardia results. The effect of hydroxydione upon the liver, kidney and uterus, and the exact mode of its breakdown and removal from the body, are incompletely known. The duration of action is variable, but 1 g. may be expected to exert some effect upon the patient for about two and a half hours (Harbord and Wild, 1956).

Clinical Use

The irritant properties of hydroxydione make considerable dilution essential if venous thrombosis is not to occur. Galley and Rooms (1956) recommend dissolving 0·5 g. of the powder in the usual 540 ml. bottle of saline; with the resulting solution, which has a concentration of less than 0·5 per cent, they have had no case of venous thrombosis. This dilution necessitates about 150 to 200 ml. of intravenous fluid to get a patient to sleep. Even then, the induction of anaesthesia may not be complete for 10 to 15 minutes after the injection. The long delay between the injection and unconsciousness does not reduce the incidence of respiratory depression or hypotension. Hunter (1957) has stressed the potential danger of such complications occurring several minutes after the induction dose of the anaesthetic has been given.

Hydroxydione is not satisfactory as the sole anaesthetic agent for any surgical operation. It can be conveniently compared with thiopentone, but—apart from the depressant, in place of the latter's stimulant, action upon respiratory tract reflexes—hydroxydione has little in its favour for routine clinical use. Relaxation is not sufficient for surgical access and other supplements must be added to it, even for procedures such as laryngoscopy. Galley and Rooms (1956) have commented upon the mental state of the patient in the early post-operative period, which they liken to that after cortisone—a sense of well-being and lack of fatigue. The incidence of sickness following hydroxydione is low.

Although hydroxydione does not itself appear to be a satisfactory substitute for existing agents, steroid anaesthetics do suggest interesting possibilities in anaesthesia. When further compounds can be produced without the side-effects and the disadvantage of a prolonged induction, the clinical anaesthetist may well find them useful tools.

REFERENCES

AHLQUIST, R. P. (1959). The receptors for epinephrine and norepinephrine. *Pharmacol. Rev.*, **11**, 441.

AXELROD, J. (1960). N-methyl-adrenaline, a new catechol amine in the adrenal gland. *Biochim. biophys. Acta* (*Amst.*), **45**, 614.

BELLVILLE, J. W., HOWLAND, W. S., and BOYAN, C. P. (1956). Comparison of the electroencephalographic pattern during steroid and barbiturate narcosis. *Brit. J. Anaesth.*, **28,** 50.

BOURKE, A. M. (1966). Anaesthesia for the surgical treatment of hyperinsulinism. *Anaesthesia*, **21,** 239.

BRUNJES, S., JOHNS, V. J., Jr., and CRANE, M. G. (1960). Pheochromocytoma: post-operative shock and blood volume. *New Engl. J. Med.*, **262,** 393.

CARNES, M. A. (1963). "Anesthetic considerations in adrenocortical disease." In: *Anesthesia for Patients with Endocrine Disease*. Ed. Jenkins, M.T. Philadelphia: F. A. Davis Co.

CARNES, M. A., MCPHAIL, J. L., FABIAN, L. W., and HURDY, F. D. (1961). Adrenergic and adrenocortical responses to fluothane and cyclopropane. *Amer. Surg.*, **27,** 223.

DHUNÉR, K. G., and NORDQUIST, P. (1957). Sleep reinduced by cortisone and glucose in patients intoxicated with barbiturates and related drugs. *Acta anaesth. scand.*, **1,** 55.

EDWARDS, D. (1962). Radiological investigation of phaeochromocytoma. *Proc. roy. Soc. Med.*, **55,** 428.

ETSTEN, B. E., and SHIMOSATO, S. (1965). Halothane anaesthesia and catecholamine levels in a patient with pheochromocytoma. *Anesthesiology*, **26,** 688.

FINNERTY, F. A., BUCHHOLZ, J. H., and GUILLAUDEU, R. L. (1958). The blood volumes and plasma protein during levarterenol-induced hypertension. *J. clin. Invest.*, **37,** 425.

FLEAR, C. T. G., and CLARKE, R. (1955.) The influence of blood loss and blood transfusion upon changes in the metabolism of water, electrolytes and nitrogen following civilian trauma. *Clin. Sci.*, **14,** 575.

FOSTER, P. A., and FRANCIS, B. G. (1955). An operation for the diabetic? *Brit. J. Anaesth.*, **27,** 291.

FRASER, R. A. (1963). Hyperinsulinism under anaesthesia. *Anaesthesia*, **18,** 3.

GALLEY, A. H., and ROOMS, M. (1956). An intravenous steroid anaesthetic. Experience with viadril. *Lancet*, **1,** 990.

GRIFFITHS, J. A. (1953). The effects of general anaesthesia and hexamethonium on the blood sugar in non-diabetic and diabetic surgical patients. *Quart. J. Med.*, **22,** 405.

HARBORD, R. P., and WILD, W. N. (1956). Observations on steroid anaesthesia. A preliminary report. *Proc. roy. Soc. Med.*, **49,** 487.

HUNTER, A. R. (1957). The complications of hydroxydione anaesthesia. *Anaesthesia*, **12,** 10.

INGLE, D. J., and KENDALL, E. C. (1937). Atrophy of adrenal cortex of rat produced by administration of large amounts of cortin. *Science*, **86,** 245.

JAMES, M. L. (1970). Endocrine disease and anaesthesia. *Anaesthesia*, **25,** 232.

JOHNS, V. J., Jr., and BRUNJES, S. (1962). Pheochromocytoma. *Amer. J. Cardiol.*, **9,** 120.

KADIS, L. B., BENNETT, E. J., DALAL, F. Y., and ZAUDER, H. L. (1966). Anaesthetic management of thyrotoxicosis. A report of two cases. *Curr. Res. Anesth.*, **45,** 415.

KALREIDER, N. L., MENEELY, G. R., and ALLEN, J. R. (1942). The effect of epinephrine on the volume of the blood. *J. clin. Invest.*, **21,** 339.

KHALIL, H. H. (1954). Effect of hypothermia on the hypothalamic-pituitary response to stress. *Brit. med. J.*, **2,** 733.

LAMSON, P. D., GREIG, M. E., and ROBBINS, B. H. (1949). Potentiating effect of glucose and its metabolic products on barbiturate anesthesia. *Science*, **110,** 690.

LAUBACH, G. D., P'AN, S. Y., and RUDEL, H. W. (1955). Steroid anesthetic agents. *Science*, **122,** 78.

LEATHER, H. M., SHAW, D. B., CATES, J. E., and MILNES WALKER, R. (1962). Six cases of phaeochromocytoma with unusual clinical manifestations. *Brit. med. J.*, **1,** 1373.

MacPhee, I. W., Gray, T. C., and Davies, S. (1958). Effect of hypothermia on the adrenocortical response to operation. *Lancet*, **2,** 1196.

Murphy, F. J., Guadagni, N. P., and DeBon, F. (1955). Use of steroid anesthesia in surgery. *J. Amer. med. Ass.*, **158,** 1412.

Nelson, D. H. (1963). Present status of the problem of iatrogenic adrenal cortical insufficiency. *Anesthesiology*, **24,** 457.

Northfield, D. W. C. (1955). Endocrine aspects of pituitary surgery. (Discussion on pituitary syndromes.) *Proc. roy. Soc. Med.*, **48,** 879.

P'an, S. Y., Gardocki, J. F., Hutcheon, D. E., Rudel, H., Kodet, M. J., and Laubach, G. D. (1955). General anesthetic and other pharmacological properties of a soluble steroid, 21-hydroxypregnanedione sodium succinate. *J. Pharmacol. exp. Ther.*, **115,** 432.

Riddell, V. (1970). Thyroidectomy: prevention of bilateral recurrent nerve palsy. *Brit. J. Surg.*, **57,** 1.

Robertson, A. I. G. (1965). Pre- and postoperative care in patients with phaeochromocytomas. *Postgrad. med. J.*, **41,** 481.

Rollason, W. N. (1964). Halothane and phaeochromocytoma. *Brit. J. Anaesth.*, **36,** 251.

Ross, E. J. (1962). Phaeochromocytoma: Medical aspects. *Proc. roy. Soc. Med.*, **55,** 427.

Salassa, R. M., Bennett, W. A., Keating, F. R., Jr., and Sprague, R. C. (1953). Postoperative adrenal cortical insufficiency; occurrence in patients previously treated with cortisone. *J. Amer. med. Ass.*, **152,** 1509.

Selye, H. (1941). Studies concerning the anesthetic action of steroid hormones. *J. Pharmacol. exp. Ther.*, **73,** 127.

Selye, H. (1942). Correlation between the chemical structure and the pharmacological actions of the steroids. *Endocrinology*, **30,** 437.

Selye, H. (1950). *The Physiology and Pathology of Exposure to Stress.* Montreal: Acta, Inc.

Sheps, S. G., Tyce, G. M., Flock, E. V., and Maher, F. (1966). Current experience in the diagnosis of phaeochromocytoma. *Circulation*, **34,** 473.

Sjoerosma, A., Engelmann, K., Waldmann, T. A., Coopermann, L. H., and Hammond, W. G. (1966). Phaeochromocytoma: current concepts of diagnosis and treatment. *Ann. intern. Med.*, **65,** 1302.

Slaney, G., and Brooke, B. N. (1957). Postoperative collapse due to adrenal insufficiency. *Lancet*, **1,** 1167.

Taylor, N., and Shearer, W. M. (1956). The anaesthetic properties of 21-hydroxypregnanedione sodium hemisuccinate (Hydroxydione): a pharmacological and clinical study of 130 cases. *Brit. J. Anaesth.*, **28,** 67.

Traina, V., Burstein, C. L., Ciliberti, B. J., and Rovenstine, E. A. (1953). Pituitary-adrenal response to surgical trauma and anesthesia. I. The eosinopenic response. *Anesthesiology*, **14,** 449.

Ucko, H. (1954). Status lymphaticus. *Brit. med. J.*, **2,** 398.

Virtue, R. W., and Helmrich, M. L. (1956). Adrenal response to stress before operation, during anaesthesia and during surgery. *Proc. roy. Soc. Med.*, **49,** 492.

Walters, G. (1969). Secretory characteristics of phaeochromocytomata and related tumours: their diagnostic and clinical significance. *Ann. roy. Coll. Surg. Engl.*, **45,** 150.

Watson, R. L., and Hansen, H. R. (1967). Phaeochromocytoma; cardiac stability during methoxyflurane anesthesia for surgical removal. *Curr. Res. Anesth.*, **46,** 324.

Section Six

THE REPRODUCTIVE SYSTEM

Chapter 51

PRACTICAL CONSIDERATIONS IN CHILDBIRTH

by

ANDREW DOUGHTY

INNERVATION OF THE GENITAL TRACT (Fig. 1)

THE female pelvic viscera are under both nervous and hormonal control. The nervous control is derived primarily from the hypothalamus through the reticular formation where the descending pathways interact with ascending influences from the pelvis. Thus the higher centres are concerned with the control of the balance between the effects of the two peripheral autonomic divisions, the sympathetic and the parasympathetic systems. They should not be considered as antagonistic to each other as in many instances they are synergistic and work harmoniously under the control of the descending pathway to achieve their physiological function.

The sympathetic centres for the female pelvic viscera lie in the lower thoracic and upper lumbar segments of the spinal cord. From here pre-ganglionic fibres pass through the ganglia of the sympathetic trunk to the *aortico-renal plexus* where they finally synapse. A part of the aortico-renal plexus extends along the ovarian artery as the *ovarian plexus*. The *superior hypogastric plexus* or *pre-sacral nerve* is the continuation of the aortico-renal plexus passing down over the bifurcation of the aorta where it divides in front of the sacrum into two trunks, the *right* and *left hypogastric nerves*. Each hypogastric nerve is joined by the *pelvic splanchnic nerves* (parasympathetic; nervi erigentes) of the corresponding side to form the right and left *pelvic* (inferior hypogastric; Frankenhauser's) *plexuses*. The pelvic plexuses thus contain a mixture of sympathetic and para-sympathetic elements. The *paracervical* or *utero-vaginal plexus* on each side is an extension of the pelvic plexus along the course of the uterine artery within the base of the broad ligament.

Nervous Control of Uterine Activity

Jeffcoate (1969) states "There is difficulty in deciding to what extent autonomic nerves demonstrated in the pelvic organs carry impulses to and from the blood vessels and to what extent they are motor or sensory to other tissues . . . It is not known whether the uterus receives both parasympathetic (cholinergic) and sympathetic (adrenergic) nerves or whether it has only a sympathetic component". In a summary of the present state of knowledge on these matters Wendell-Smith (1970) states "The pharmacological events which follow the arrival of an impulse at post ganglionic sympathetic nerve endings are complex and not completely understood. The uterus was one of the first organs for which it was demonstrated that sympathetic stimulation releases acetylcholine as well as adrenergic substances. There is increasing evidence that the release of acetylcholine is the first event in the sequence that makes the membrane of the sympathetic fibre perme-

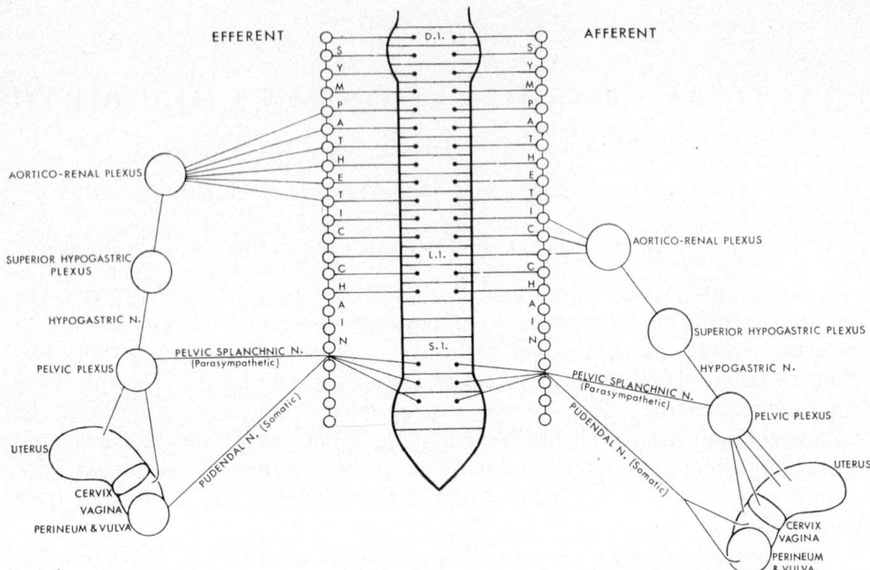

51/Fig. 1—Diagram of the principal innervation of the genital tract.

able to calcium ions. The calcium ions enter the fibre and release adrenergic transmitter substances from the bound form in which they are held. Furthermore the adrenergic transmitters are not pure substances but are mixtures of adrenaline, noradrenaline (the major component), probably dopamine and possibly other compounds. The proportions and amounts of these depend upon the intensity of nervous activity, and their synthesis, in the myometrium at least, is promoted by oestrogens".

From the welter of conflicting evidence concerning the motor innervation of the uterus, opinion seems to favour the view that the parasympathetic system contributes little to myometrial activity, and that the uterus is mainly affected by the stimulatory influences of the sympathetic system.

Hormonal Control of Uterine Activity

It is generally agreed that an intact nerve supply is not essential to the initiation and progress of labour. Quite apart from the number of paraplegic patients who have reached the second stage of labour without difficulty, there is the evidence of Vasicka and Kretchmer (1961) who showed that spinal block extending as high as the cervical region will not inhibit uterine activity unless there is a marked fall of blood pressure. When the blood pressure is restored there is a return to normal uterine activity.

Oxytocin, a hormone derived from the posterior pituitary, is the main factor in maintaining uterine activity during labour. It will not initiate contractions unless other hormonal systems have prepared the uterus for action.

Progesterone is the key factor in inhibiting uterine activity in pregnancy.

Although in the first few months it is produced by the corpus luteum, its site of production soon shifts from the ovary to the placenta. As the pregnancy nears term the influence of progesterone is superseded by other hormonal factors favouring the onset of labour.

In the non-pregnant uterus the effect of *noradrenaline* is preponderant over *adrenaline* and it is thought to be active in closing the isthmic canal during the late menstrual cycle to reduce the chance of abortion or low implantation of a fertilised ovum. During pregnancy the proportion of circulating adrenaline to noradrenaline increases fourfold.

The primary effect of adrenaline, whether liberated neurogenically or transmitted by the blood stream, is to inhibit uterine contraction. However if a beta-blocking agent, propranolol, is given with adrenaline, uterine activity is enhanced. This suggests that only the beta-activity is inhibitory while the less dominant alpha-activity is excitatory.

The myometrial inhibitory effect of specific beta-adrenergic stimulation has been put to clinical use in the treatment of premature labour with *orciprenaline*, but the effectiveness of this treatment is limited by the need to avoid undue maternal tachycardia (Baillie *et al.*, 1970).

Onset of Labour

These considerations suggest a possible explanation of the events leading to the onset of labour. During the first and second trimesters of pregnancy, uterine activity is normally inhibited by the stimulation of the beta-adrenergic receptors. As a result of other hormonal changes associated with the rise of oestrogen activity in late pregnancy, the myometrial inhibition by progesterone is reduced and the threshold of the beta-adrenergic receptors rises. The threshold of the alpha-adrenergic receptors falls, increasing the excitatory effect of adrenergic stimulation. The uterus is thus prepared for the production of the strong regular contractions in response to the release of oxytocin from the posterior pituitary or administered by the buccal or intravenous route.

Sensory Pathways

Sensory stimuli from the uterine body are transmitted through the pelvic, superior hypogastric and aortico-renal plexuses to the 11th and 12th dorsal and the first lumbar segments. It is also believed that a proportion of the afferent impulses emerge from the fundus in company with the tubo-ovarian vessels to the ovarian plexus thus bypassing the main sensory pathway through the pelvic and superior hypogastric plexuses.

Sensory stimuli from the *cervix* pass through the pelvic plexus along the pelvic splanchnic nerves to sacral segments 2, 3 and 4 and to the sacral portion of the sympathetic chain. The sensory supply of the *vagina* is derived partly from parasympathetic and partly from somatic nerves. Stimuli from the upper vagina run through the pelvic plexuses and the pelvic splanchnic nerves to sacral roots 2, 3 and 4. Those from the lower vagina pass via the pudendal nerve.

The *perineum* receives both a motor and a sensory innervation from sacral roots 2, 3 and 4 through the pudendal nerve. Other sensory pathways are derived from the terminal branches of the ilio-inguinal and genito-femoral nerves supplying the labia majora. The perineal branch of the posterior cutaneous nerve of the thigh communicates with the pudendal nerve in giving terminal branches to the perineal body.

Practical Implications (Fig. 2)

Sensation of the processes of labour are transmitted through dual pathways to the central nervous system. Uterine contraction is perceived via the sympathetic afferents entering at the lower dorsal and upper lumbar segments while the sensations of rectal pressure and vaginal, perineal and vulval distension are transmitted via sacral roots 2, 3 and 4. The significance of the afferent pathway from the cervix to sacral segments 2, 3 and 4 via the pelvic plexus and pelvic splanchnic nerves is less easy to determine but it is thought to be the route by which severe backache is felt in labours with inco-ordinate uterine action, cervical dystocia or a persistent occipito-posterior position of the infant's head. An explanation of the low backache of very early labour is that during a uterine contraction the fundus of the uterus comes forward causing pressure on the posterior segment of the pelvic brim. This sensation would therefore be transmitted by somatic nerves to sacral roots 2, 3 and 4 (Crawford 1965).

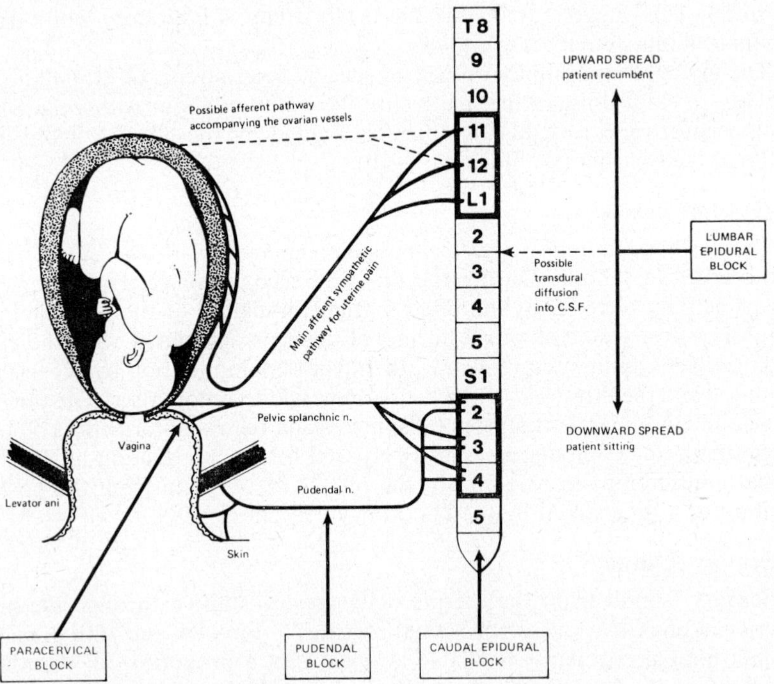

51/Fig. 2.—Schematic representation (simplified) of the effect of nerve blocks used in labour.

The degree of pain suffered in labour by individual women varies in intensity. For practical purposes it may be considered to be of *uterine* and *perineal* origin. Uterine pain is transmitted mainly by the lower dorsal and the upper lumbar roots and can be relieved by a blockade affecting these segments while perineal sensation, if it becomes painful, may be relieved by a block of sacral roots 2, 3 and 4. In the early part of labour, only uterine pain is felt but even when the head is pressing on the perineum and is distending the vulva the complaint may be only that associated with uterine pain. If the mother complains of perineal pain it will be relieved by a block affecting the sacral roots. Occasionally the severe backache associated with inco-ordinate action of the uterus or a posterior position of the occiput will only be relieved by a block affecting the sacral roots (Moir and Willcocks, 1967).

Caudal epidural block up to the 11th dorsal segment abolishes all sensation of labour by blocking both the sacral and the lower dorsal pain pathways—the sacral roots being blocked preferentially long before such block is needed by the mother. The muscles of the pelvic floor are paralysed predisposing to malrotation of the baby's head and in primigravidae the virtual inevitability of assisted delivery.

Pudendal block as is used for forceps delivery does not relieve the pain of labour but merely affords perineal analgesia and relaxation. Low subarachnoid (saddle) block would have a similar but more intense effect and in addition would relieve pain perceived via sacral roots 2, 3 and 4. It should not be forgotten that block of the pudendal nerve is insufficient by itself for episiotomy and forceps delivery. Perineal infiltration is needed to block the endings of the perineal branch of the posterior cutaneous nerve of the thigh. In addition infiltration of the labia majora may be required to block the labial branches of the ilio-inguinal and genito-femoral nerves.

Paracervical block blocks the nerve pathways by which uterine and cervical pain are felt but leaves perineal, vaginal and vulval sensation unimpaired. Its variable success may be due to the alternative afferent pathway from the fundus via the nerves accompanying the tubo-ovarian vessels.

Lumbar epidural block with large doses of local analgesic spreads up to the lower dorsal roots and down to the sacral roots thus obliterating all the sensations of labour. In smaller doses the effect can be made more selective (Doughty, 1969). If given with the mother in the horizontal position or with a slight head-down tilt the block can be limited to the lower dorsal and upper lumbar roots thus blocking uterine pain without affecting perineal sensation or the tone of the perineal muscles. If perineal analgesia is required later in labour a further injection may be directed to the sacral roots by placing the mother in a sitting position. Some degree of sacral block has been observed with a small-dose epidural block given at the 2nd–3rd lumbar interspace without any formal attempt being made to direct the solution caudally. This may be due to a direct transdural diffusion into the subarachnoid space affecting the cauda equina and is in accordance with the observations of Frumin *et al.* (1953) who found that procaine injected epidurally can be recovered in significant concentrations from the cerebrospinal fluid.

Implications of sympathetic blockade.—While it is necessary to block the sympathetic afferent impulses entering at the 11th and 12th dorsal and 1st lumbar segments to relieve the pain of uterine contraction, any extension of the block to a higher level will block the motor nerve supply to the uterus. Although the role of the motor nerves in the regulation of uterine activity in labour is very doubtful, any diminution of the strength and frequency of contractions following epidural block may be compensated by buccal or intravenous oxytocin.

Blockade of the sympathetic efferent impulses will cause arteriolar relaxation and fall of blood pressure which may be responsible for some diminution of uterine activity. This effect can be minimised by using doses just sufficient to produce relief of labour pain. The extent of the rise of the block in the dorsal region may be checked by testing the level of analgesia to pinprick on the anterior abdominal wall although it should be remembered that sympathetic block is likely to be effective for 2 to 3 segments above the level of sensory block.

A tendency to supine hypotension due to limitation of venous return to the heart caused by the backward pressure of the gravid uterus on the inferior vena cava will be magnified by even a small degree of sympathetic blockade (see p. 1431). A close watch should be kept for a sudden fall of blood pressure during caudal or lumbar epidural block which may be expected at any time up to 45 minutes from the initial injection or after any subsequent top-up.

Deliberate sympathetic blockade by epidural or subarachnoid injection has been used therapeutically in the management of pre-eclampsia, reflex anuria and femoral thrombo-phlebitis.

Pain in Labour

The uterus itself can be cut or compressed without discomfort but traction on the supporting ligaments is painful. During the latter part of pregnancy the uterus contracts rhythmically but without evoking any unpleasant sensation. Genuine labour begins when contraction of the muscles of the upper segment stretches the longitudinal fibres of the lower segment of the uterine body and cervix. Simultaneously the circular fibres of the cervix relax.

The pains are analogous to those produced by distension and stretching of other hollow viscera and are usually felt in the hypogastrium over the area supplied by the cutaneous branches of the 11th and 12th dorsal nerve roots. In other labours—particularly those in which the occiput is posterior—pain is felt in the back over the sacrum and occasionally on the posterior aspect of the thighs. Late in the first stage of labour the sensation of pressure on the rectum and levatores ani muscles may become painful as may the distension of the vagina, perineum and vulva in the second stage.

At the start of labour the contractions are ill-defined, infrequent and of short duration. As labour progresses they become more frequent, occur at fairly regular intervals, and persist for longer periods, until towards the end of the first stage they are likely to occur every three to four minutes and persist for about one and a half minutes. During the first stage there is normally little or no desire upon the part of the woman to bear down, but towards full dilatation of the cervix, a local pelvic reflex may come into play, making pain appear purposive although voluntary effort can be of no value and may result in oedema of the rim of the cervix. This is a most difficult pain for the mother to bear. With the onset of the second stage the contractions become more purposive and normally lead to active voluntary efforts to expel the infant. The purposiveness of the contractions now raises the threshold of the mother to their stimuli, so that by comparison with those of the late first stage they seem less severe. This may account for the observation (Doughty, 1969) that many mothers given an epidural block in the first stage of labour aimed at dorsal segments 11 and 12 for the relief of uterine pain will happily tolerate the purely somatic sensation of parturition even to tearing the perineum without complaint. The contractions are, in fact, not less intense but more so, especially as this stage progresses, and more frequent. They occur at approximately two minute intervals, and last for about a minute or less.

The intensity of pain bears no relationship to the strength of uterine contraction, nor to the consequent increased uterine pressure. Each uterine contraction slowly mounts to a maximum which is sustained for a few seconds and then rapidly falls away. Pain commences at a variable interval following the start of the contraction and the length of this interval depends on the individual mother's threshold to pain (Fig. 3).

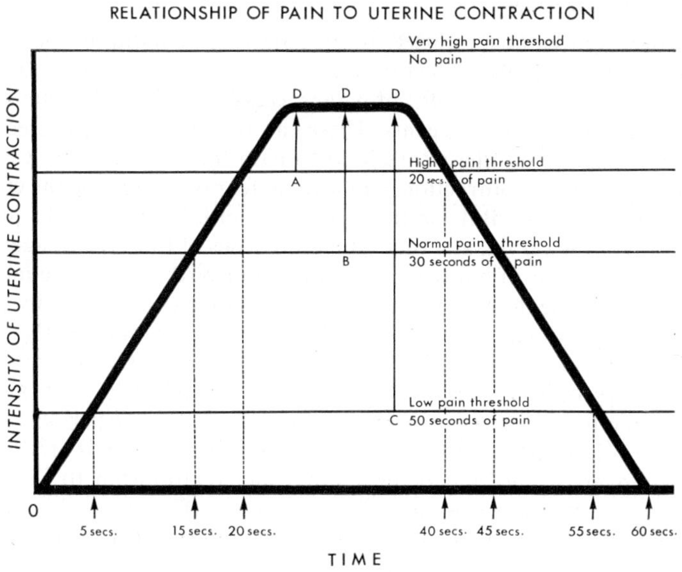

51/FIG. 3.—Relationship of pain to uterine contraction (see text).

In the diagram uterine contraction is represented by a curve ascending until maximum intensity is reached; it is held for a short time at maximum intensity and then diminishes until the contraction ceases at one minute from its commencement. At a variable degree of intensity of contraction the pain threshold is crossed. In the diagram the "normal" pain threshold is represented by a line which is crossed by the curve 15 seconds after the start of the contraction. The pain threshold is crossed again as the contraction diminishes in intensity 45 seconds from its start. Thus with the "normal" threshold to pain the mother would experience 15 seconds of painless contraction, 30 seconds of painful contraction followed by 15 seconds of painless contraction as its intensity dim-

Tunstall, 1968). Any apparatus designed for use in inhalational analgesia should be able to meet a demand of a peak inspiratory flow of 350 l./min. and tidal volumes up to 3 litres without imposing a resistance to inspiration.

The Foetus and Foetal Distress

With each uterine contraction the placental circulation is diminished, and the maternal placental blood pressure may fall to a very low level, even though the maternal blood pressure itself rises. Thus the transfer of oxygen to the foetal circulation falls with, and rises again after, each uterine contraction. Abnormal states of the placenta—such as partial or complete separation from the uterine wall or infarction with loss of surface area—diminish the oxygen-saturation level in the foetal circulation. The normal progress of the second stage of labour leads to a progressive diminution in the placental circulation, thus submitting the foetus to an increasing degree of hypoxia and acidosis. In ordinary circumstances this is compatible with the birth of a living child. Unduly prolonged labour or continuous uterine contractions may lead to such a degree of hypoxia in the infant as to produce permanent cerebral damage. This can be caused by the uncontrolled use of oxytocin particularly in the face of prematurity or other foetal abnormality.

The foetal heart rate.—The normal foetal heart rate varies from 120 to 160 beats per minute. Bradycardia is the response of the foetal heart and circulation to oxygen lack and may take the form of a sharp fall in rate to about 60 beats per minute or a less obvious but persistent slowing to about 110 beats per minute. To some degree the foetal heart may be expected to slow during uterine contractions but the failure to return rapidly to its normal rate between contractions may be a cause for concern. When hypoxia is particularly severe, irregularity may follow bradycardia.

Foetal tachycardia is sometimes noted as an early sign of distress but this has been thought unlikely to be due to hypoxia since, unlike bradycardia, it is not readily relieved by maternal oxygen inhalations. Nevertheless it should be taken as implying the need for a closer monitoring of the foetal heart rate as tachycardia has been shown to be associated with foetal acidosis and may be followed later by bradycardia (Coltart *et al.*, 1969).

The recent introduction of a foetal heart sound amplifier (Sonicaid) has facilitated the monitoring of the foetal heart in cases where it is inaudible through the usual simple stethoscope.

Amnioscopy.—The foetal heart rate is not the only means of monitoring foetal welfare. When the membranes are ruptured the appearance of meconium staining of the liquor amnii is taken as an early warning of asphyxia, although it is not regarded with the same significance when the breech is presenting. Before rupture of the membranes the liquor can be viewed with an amnioscope through the intact bag of forewaters. It should appear clear with visible flakes of white vernix floating in it. Foetal distress is probable if the liquor is discoloured by any appreciable quantity of meconium. The use of the amnioscope avoids the need to rupture the membranes prematurely merely for the purpose of inspecting the colour of the liquor but repeated aminoscopy may cause inadvertent rupture of the membranes and undesired induction of labour.

Foetal blood sampling.—In recent years the measurement of the pH of foetal blood has provided an additional means of assessing the condition of the foetus during labour. If the foetus is deprived of oxygen its glycogen metabolism proceeds anaerobically to the formation of lactic acid instead of through the normal aerobic metabolic pathway via pyruvic acid by the Krebs cycle to carbon dioxide and water. The accumulation of lactic acid in the foetal blood lowers its pH and results in metabolic acidosis. Thus a fall of the foetal blood pH can be an index of foetal asphyxia.

The mean range of variability of the foetal blood pH during labour is from 7·30 to 7·28. This should remain constant until shortly before delivery; then a fall in pH occurs due not only to the natural interruption of placental flow during the uterine contraction but also to an accumulation of lactic acid in the mother which is transferred to the foetus. In general a fall in foetal pH to below 7·25 would be considered abnormal and a fall in pH to 7·20 suggests that early delivery would be desirable.

Some caution is needed in the interpretation of these figures. An abnormally low pH value can be caused by errors in collecting the sample from the foetal scalp, its being taken from the caput succedaneum, contamination with liquor, inadequate mixing of the sample or a delay of more than a few minutes before making the measurement. Ideally, the pH measuring apparatus should be sited within the labour ward area, not only to avoid the delay in obtaining the result but also for the convenience of repeated tests, as clinical action on the basis of only one measurement may not be justified. Serial estimations at short intervals showing a steady fall in pH might suggest the need for some positive action to deliver the baby.

Before taking action on the basis of a low foetal pH it should be remembered that any degree of metabolic acidosis in the mother will be reflected in the foetus. For instance if the mother herself is acidotic as with dehydration and ketosis, a pH of below 7·25 in her infant may not be viewed as seriously as if her own acid-base status had been normal. In practice a maternal blood sample should be taken together with the foetal sample and any base deficit in the mother corrected with a bicarbonate infusion. Normally the maternal-foetal base deficit difference is 3 mEq/litre. A progressive increase of this difference in serial samples would indicate foetal asphyxia.

The benefits derived from foetal blood sampling are shown by the reduction in the number of Caesarean sections done for foetal distress at Queen Charlotte's Hospital from 86 cases in 1964/65 to 27 in 1966/67. It is now unusual to perform the operation solely because of the clinical signs of foetal distress if the pH remains within normal limits (Beard and Morris, 1969).

Placental Transfer of Drugs

The placental transfer of drugs is discussed in some detail in Chapter 3. This section is concerned with the clinical application of the present knowledge of the effects of drugs given to the mother on the foetus and neonate.

In their survey of the transfer of drugs from mother to foetus, Moya and Smith (1965) pointed out that the placental "barrier" is relative rather than absolute. It is now generally accepted that most drugs pass from the maternal to the foetal circulation but that the speed at which they do so is dependent on several factors. The most important is the concentration of drug presenting at the placental membrane at any particular time. Thus a dose given slowly to the mother is unlikely to reach as high a level in the foetus as the same amount given rapidly into the blood stream. The amount of drug available depends on the degree to which it is bound to the serum protein; only the unbound portion is free for transfer. The rate of transfer depends on the ease with which a drug is permitted to pass the placental membrane. Highly ionised substances pass very slowly because ions of opposite charge are attracted to the membrane while those of similar charge are repelled. The degree of ionisation of a substance depends to some extent on the environmental pH. Non-ionised substances, particularly those with a high lipid solubility, are readily passed. Volatile anaesthetic agents pass easily not only because of their affinity for lipoids but also in accordance with the gradient of partial pressures between the maternal and foetal blood.

The clinical significance of the placental transfer of drugs is whether or not they harm the foetus *in utero* during pregnancy, during labour or after birth. The teratogenic effects of thalidomide are too well-known to require further mention. The muscle relaxants, innocuous to the infant when used in a single dose at Caesarean section, may be reponsible for foetal deformities if used for prolonged therapeutic curarisation in pregnancy (Drachman and Coulombre, 1962). A case has been reported of a woman treated for status epilepticus with IPPV and prolonged curarisation who went into premature labour and was delivered of a paralysed infant whose serum was shown to have a curariform effect on a rat phrenic nerve diaphragm preparation (Older and Harris, 1968).

During labour the ready transfer of local analgesics can depress the foetal heart rate if given in high dosage or in the area of the uterine vessels as in paracervical block. Some of the cases of death *in utero* have been thought to be due not so much to placental transfer as to injection into the intervillous space. Narcotics given for the relief of pain in early labour cross the placenta but this has relatively little clinical significance as long as delivery is delayed until after the respiratory depressant effect on the foetus has passed.

The volatile general analgesics, being non-ionised and with a high lipid solubility, readily cross the placenta but the low concentrations given to the mother and the relatively short time for which they are usually administered ensures that the foetal blood level remains below that which would produce neonatal depression. A high alveolar concentration maintained for a long period would cause the infant to remain unduly sleepy after birth.

As a general rule it can be said that general anaesthetics and local analgesics readily pass the placental membrane, narcotics do so fairly readily and the muscle relaxants very slowly. What really matters is not whether a particular drug crosses to the foetus, but whether the transfer causes it harm *in utero* or affects its ability to survive independently of the mother after birth.

Neonatal Asphyxia and Neonatal Resuscitation

These subjects are discussed in Chapter 3, p. 116 *et seq.*

The Obstetric Anaesthetist and the Midwife

In the United Kingdom most women are delivered of their infants by midwives and it is customary for "medical aid" to be enlisted only when the management of the labour is beyond the midwife's competence. It follows that it is rare for an anaesthetist to assume personal responsibility for the relief of pain in a labour that is being conducted by a midwife. It is against the background of midwife-managed obstetrics that a variety of methods of pain relief have been developed, the over-riding consideration being that they should be safe for the single-handed midwife to administer in the mother's own home without interfering with her main task—that of delivering the baby.

The midwife's activities in England and Wales* are regulated by the Central Midwives' Board who prescribe her training, hold the examinations which she must pass before being allowed to practise and maintain the Roll of qualified midwives from which her name may be removed for serious breaches of professional conduct.

The anaesthetist has a part to play in the instruction of midwives concerning relief of pain and in the general supervision of the practice of analgesia in the labour wards of his hospital. The following extracts from the Handbook issued by the Central Midwives' Board suggest the range of responsibility of the anaesthetist in the training and practice of the midwife:

Section B

Rule 18*b* During either the first or second period of training a pupil-midwife shall receive theoretical and practical instruction in anaesthesia and analgesia in midwifery practice as follows:
(i) 3 lecture demonstrations by a specialist anaesthetist;
(ii) the administration of an analgesic to at least 15 patients in labour by means of an apparatus or method approved by the Board under the general supervision of a specialist anaesthetist and under the detailed supervision of a midwife who is experienced in the use of the apparatus or method or of a resident medical officer who is similarly experienced.

Rule 23*b* An institution shall not be approved in respect of instruction in analgesia unless:
(i) the institution is one training pupils or medical students or is providing post-certificate courses for midwives or holding postgraduate courses for medical practitioners, or is otherwise considered by the Board as suitable for approval;
(ii) the institution has attached to it a specialist anaesthetist;
(iii) the resident medical officer or the midwife who would undertake the detailed supervision of the practical work is experienced in the use of the apparatus or method on which the instruction at the institution will be based.

Rule 39 The Second Examination shall be oral, clinical and practical. A candidate may be required to answer questions on the following subjects:
(a) practical midwifery;
(b) analgesia in childbirth;
(c) etc. . . . . .

Section E

Treatment Outside a Midwife's Province

Rule 5 (a) A practising midwife must not, except in an emergency, undertake any treatment which is outside her normal province. The question whether in

*In Scotland and in Northern Ireland midwives are subjected to the regulations of separate authorities.

any particular case such treatment was justified will be judged on the facts and circumstances of the case.

(b) A practising midwife must not on her own responsibility use any drug, including any analgesic, unless in the course of her training, whether before or after enrolment, she has been thoroughly instructed in its use and is familiar with its dosage and methods of administration or application.

(c) A practising midwife must not, except on the instructions and in the presence of a registered medical practitioner, administer an inhalational analgesic otherwise than by means of an apparatus which is of a type approved by the Board for use by midwives, and, where the Board so directs in relation to particular types of apparatus, has been inspected and approved by or on behalf of the Board, within such a period before the date of administration as the Board shall from time to time determine, as fit for use by midwives.

(d) A practising midwife must not, except on the instructions and in the presence of a registered medical practitioner, administer an inhalational analgesic by means of an apparatus which is required by this rule to have been inspected and approved within a specified period before the date of use unless there is in the possession of the body or person by whom the apparatus is held a certificate signed on behalf of the Board, certifying that the apparatus was inspected and approved by or on behalf of the Board on a date falling within the appropriate period, as fit for use by midwives.

(e) A practising midwife must not, except on the instructions and in the presence of a registered medical practitioner administer an inhalational analgesic unless:

(i) she has, either before or after enrolment received at an institution approved by the Board for the purpose, special instruction in the essentials of obstetric analgesia and has satisfied the institution or the Board that she is thoroughly proficient in the use of the apparatus; and

(ii) the patient has at some time during the pregnancy been examined by a registered medical practitioner who has signed a certificate that he finds no contra-indication to the administration of the analgesic by a midwife and, if any illness which required medical attention subsequently developed during pregnancy, the midwife obtained confirmation from a medical practitioner that the certificate remained valid; and

(iii) one other person, being any person acceptable to the patient, who in the opinion of the midwife is suitable for the purpose, is present at the time of the administration in addition to the midwife.

(f) Unless special exemption is given by the Board to enable particular institutions to investigate new methods, a midwife must not administer any anaesthetic otherwise than on the instructions and in the presence of a registered medical practitioner.

Lecture Course to Midwives

The Central Midwives' Board offers the following suggestions as to the content of the prescribed lecture course:

First Lecture

Short history of the relief of pain in labour.

Definition of analgesia, amnesia and anaesthesia, and difference between sedation and analgesia.
Drugs commonly used in the first stage of labour, and methods of administration and dosage.
Effect of drugs on maternal and foetal condition, and on uterine contractions, and abnormal reactions which might occur.
Causes of failure to give relief.

Second Lecture

Inhalation analgesia or anaesthesia, with detailed description of approved apparatus and maintenance of such apparatus.
Principles of local infiltration, pudendal block and epidural block.
Choice of analgesic method and contra-indications.
Statutory rules and regulations relating to the use of drugs and analgesic methods of midwives.

Third Lecture

Preparation of patients for anaesthetics required for operative deliveries.
Care of the unconscious patient after deliver under anaesthesia.
Emergencies of anaesthesia, including the treatment of cardiac arrest.
Prevention and treatment of Mendelson's syndrome.
Resuscitation of mother and/or baby.

Comments

While many anaesthetists may be involved in giving pupil midwives their three statutory lecture demonstrations (Rule 18*b*, Section B) it may come as a surprise to find that they are expected to maintain a general supervision of the administration of analgesia in the labour wards of their hospitals. This provides a salutary opportunity to assess the effectiveness of their teaching and in this way they can help to maintain the standard of labour analgesia. They are able to introduce improved techniques for the administration of the permitted methods, and they are more likely than most to be familiar with new agents which become "approved" for use by the unsupervised midwife. Rule 5*b*, Section E, implies that the professionally qualified midwife relies on them for appropriate instruction in the use of such agents, and the recent introduction of methoxyflurane given with the "Cardiff" inhaler may be cited as a case in point.

In the ever-widening scope of subjects related to anaesthesia and analgesia in labour one may wonder with some justification whether the three prescribed lecture demonstrations are sufficient, not only to acquaint pupil midwives with all they should know but also to make sure that they really understand the basic principles of relieving pain in labour (Rule 5*b*, Section E).

The Central Midwives' Board obviously has in mind the likelihood of research into new methods of analgesia which might be given by the unsupervised midwife. Rule 5*f*, Section E, is a reminder that any such research involving the midwife's co-operation must have the Board's approval. This rule is also relevant against the background of the increasing popularity of epidural analgesia. A comprehensive service is only possible if the anaesthetist can be freed from the administration of the "top-up" doses and it is possible that the midwife could be trained to help in this field. This appears to be precluded by the rule that the midwife may only administer an anaesthetic in the presence of a registered medical practitioner. If the "top-up" dose were to be recognised as "any drug, including an analgesic" the practice might be permitted under Rule 5*b*, Section E, provided that a suitable code of safety could be drafted and that the midwife is "thoroughly instructed in its use and familiar with its dosage and methods of administration or application". Rule 5*f*, Section E could be interpreted as covering a midwife giving a simple anaesthetic under the supervision and on the responsibility of the doctor performing the delivery. As current practice has changed wisdom dictates that the Central Midwives' Board should be consulted before their rules are interpreted against the background of circumstances to which they were never intended to apply.

REFERENCES

BAILLIE, P., MEEHAN, F. P., and TYACK, A. J. (1970). Treatment of premature labour with orciprenaline. *Brit. med. J.*, **4,** 154.

BEARD, R. W., and MORRIS, E. D. (1969). *Modern Trends in Obstetrics*, p. 298. London: Butterworths.

CENTRAL MIDWIVES' BOARD (1962). Handbook incorporating the *Rules of the Central Midwives' Board*, 25th edit. London: Spottiswoode Ballantyne & Co.

COLTART, T. M., TRICKEY, N. R. A., and BEARD, R. W. (1969). Foetal blood sampling. Practical approach to management of foetal distress. *Brit. med. J.*, **1,** 342.

CRAWFORD, J. S. (1965). *Obstetric Anaesthesia*, 2nd edit., p. 23. Oxford: Blackwell Scientific Publications.

CRAWFORD, J. S., and TUNSTALL, M. E. (1968). Notes on respiratory performance in labour. *Brit. J. Anaesth.*, **40,** 216.

DOUGHTY, A. (1969). Selective epidural analgesia and the forceps rate. *Brit. J. Anaesth.*, **42,** 1058.

DRACHMAN, D. B., and COULOMBRE, A. J. (1962). Experimental clubfoot and arthrogryphosis multiplex congenita. *Lancet*, **2,** 523.

FRUMIN, M. J., SCHWARTZ, H., BURNS, J. J., BRODIE, B. B., and PAPPER, E. M. (1953). The appearance of procaine in the spinal fluid during peridural block in man. *J. Pharmacol. exp. Ther.*, **109,** 102.

JEFFCOATE, T. N. A. (1969). Pelvic pain. *Brit. med. J.*, **3,** 431.

MOIR, D. D., and WILLOCKS, J. (1967). Management of inco-ordinate uterine action under continuous epidural analgesia. *Brit. med. J.*, **3,** 396.

MOYA, F., and SMITH, B. E. (1965). Uptake, distribution and placental transport of drugs and anesthetics. *Anesthesiology*, **26,** 465.

OLDER, P. O., and HARRIS, J. M. (1968). Placental transfer of tubocurarine. *Brit. J. Anaesth.*, **40,** 459.

VASICKA, A., and KRETCHMER, H. E. (1961). Effect of conduction and inhalational anesthesia on uterine contractions. *Amer. J. Obstet. Gynec.*, **82,** 600.

WENDELL-SMITH, C. P. (1970). *Scientific Foundations of Obstetrics and Gynaecology*, p. 88. Ed. by E. E. Philipp, J. Barnes, and M. Newton. London: Heinemann Medical Books.

Chapter 52

THE RELIEF OF PAIN IN LABOUR

by

ANDREW DOUGHTY

ALTHOUGH drugs have an important part to play in the relief of pain in labour it must not be supposed that they are necessarily of greater importance than proper preparation and training for childbirth, or that they are invariably needed. Normal labour, can, for many women, be an easy, trouble-free and deeply satisfying experience provided a rational and understanding approach is made to the subject by the mother and her medical attendant.

The normal process of childbirth must be explained simply and the pain involved should be mentioned—but not stressed—and logically justified, so tha much of the dread that is so often associated with the word itself can be allayed. The mother must be told that pain can be controlled, and it is often worth while describing the methods by which this relief will be given. Since some women do not need analgesia, and others do not wish for it, it is important to mention that they are not obliged to have it unless they want it. Many women prefer to give birth to their child with their consciousness unclouded by drugs. The moment of birth is the climax of their months of pregnancy and they may regard as a disservice the imposition of heavy sedation or of a general anaesthetic merely for the crowning of the baby's head. Finally, relaxation during labour can be assisted by antenatal preparation with exercises designed to improve the voluntary control of the abdominal and pelvic muscles.

Successful preparation should create a bond of mutual confidence between the mother and her attendant so that in the subsequent confinement natural forces may have their way and ease the course of labour. Minimising the pain of labour depends to some extent upon the personality of the attending doctor or midwife. This may be half-way to hypnosis, and is certainly not outside the capacity of anyone prepared to spend the necessary time with the mother. Apart from drugs, she may be helped by such simple remedies as change of posture, changing a sodden sheet, rubbing of the lower part of the back and a few kind words of encouragement. The tendency to welcome husbands or other close relatives to stay with the mother during labour may help to avoid the loneliness which, to many women, is the most distressing memory of childbirth. The presence of any "outsider" may make the professional attendants more alert to the needs of the parturient for more adequate analgesia.

It is when the ordinary remedies fail that the obstetric anaesthetist may play a major role in saving the mother's morale.

HYPNOSIS IN CHILDBIRTH

The advantages claimed for hypnosis during childbirth—as compared with chemical agents—are, that the mother can be kept pain-free but awake and co-operative; if desirable, sleep can be induced; there are no complications attributable to the method; and post-hypnotic suggestion can help to prevent after-pains and the normal post-partum depression. The best results are undoubtedly achieved in selected patients, and, perhaps one should add, by selected hypnotists. Unfortunately the method is too unreliable to be considered as a satisfactory routine alternative to chemical analgesia.

Obstetrical patients sometimes make good subjects for hypnosis, being open to suggestion and needing only a light trance state to relieve their labour pains. There is moreover, a special value in the method since it enables the mother to remain awake and relaxed and consciously to participate in the birth of her child unaffected by depressant drugs.

To achieve a reasonable chance of success the mother must be trained by under-going hypnosis on a number of occasions during pregnancy. She is then prepared for the onset of labour when hypnosis can be induced immediately. This training is time-consuming, although after at least one personal interview a number of selected mothers may be hypnotised in antenatal clinics (Michael, 1952). During the course of the actual labour, personal attention is essential if the best results are to be obtained. It may be possible to teach a patient auto-hypnosis so that she can be independent of the hypnotist (Davidson, 1962).

GENERAL ANALGESIC DRUGS

The threshold for pain varies from patient to patient, so that each mother must be assessed individually. Some patients experience severe pain despite relatively weak uterine contractions—indeed it seems likely that, in some, the acuteness of the pain inhibits the normal relaxation of the cervix and the contractions of the uterus. For patients of this kind it is usually preferable to control the pain adequately and ensure sleep even if this involves a temporary depression of uterine action. A better alternative might be to use epidural analgesia and to enhance the uterine contractions with an oxytocin infusion.

Normal multiparous women are usually more rapidly delivered than the primiparous and generally need less analgesia particularly in the second stage owing to the added relaxation of the birth canal. This is not invariably so as many multiparae experience tumultuous, painful though rapid labours. The history of a previous childbirth may yield useful information as to what might be expected in the next.

The maturity of the child must be considered. Prematurity must be an indication for minimal doses of those drugs which cross the placenta. The small premature infant seldom causes difficulty at delivery, which generally enables adequate analgesia to be produced without undue quantities of any drug. In certain instances it may be better to dispense with general analgesia and to use some form of conduction block rather than to increase the risk of neonatal asphyxia—a risk much greater than in full-term infants irrespective of analgesic drugs.

First Period—Sedative and Analgesic Drugs

The practical implications of the control of pain in labour have been discussed in the previous chapter and—for the purpose of selecting a general analgesic drug—an artificial division of labour into two periods has been suggested. The pain of the first period, from the commencement of labour up to three-quarters dilatation of the cervix, is best controlled by non-inhalational agents, and that of the second period, from three-quarters dilatation to delivery, by inhalational agents (p. 1394).

At the commencement of labour, and often during the early part of the first period, the pain of the uterine contractions are rarely severe enough to warrant the use of a potent analgesic such as pethidine. Chloral is usually adequate to control the discomfort and induce sleep, when necessary. It may be given in a dose of 1–2 g. well diluted, by mouth. Chloral, besides being an efficient hypnotic, is also a weak analgesic and by long tradition has been used in the early part of labour. Unfortunately chloral is unpalatable and to many positively nauseating. A closely allied compound, dichlorphenazone (Welldorm), available in tablet form, is more acceptable and less liable to cause vomiting.

Other purely sedative drugs may be given by mouth at this time. Short-acting barbiturates such as pentobarbitone and quinalbarbitone are occasionally used in doses of 100–200 mg. while glutethimide—a non-barbiturate sedative—has also been recommended in a dose of 1 g. (Abbas, 1957).

The principal disadvantage of hypnotic drugs is their tendency to cause delirium in the mother if the pain becomes severe. Although this complication can be prevented by a small dose of an analgesic drug given with the sedative, it is better policy to use an adequate dose of pethidine or similar narcotic in the first place since this will both relieve the pain and sedate the patient.

Pethidine ("Demerol", "Meperidine")

Pethidine is the most generally used analgesic in the first period of labour. It is indicated when the discomfort of early labour merges into regular, frequent and painful contractions that are beginning to cause distress to the mother. The onset of genuine pain may be quite sudden and usually occurs at 3–4 cm. dilatation of the cervix. The initial dose of 100 mg. should be given by intramuscular injection; its effect will be apparent in 10–15 minutes and should last for two to three hours. When the pains are more severe or the woman unduly obese or anxious the initial dose should be raised to 150 mg.

The subjective effect of pethidine varies widely in different women. To some it gives a pleasurable euphoria coupled with relief of pain, to some a positive dysphoria with nausea and vomiting, while others will deny any analgesic effect at all.

The dose should be repeated as the effect of the first dose is beginning to wane rather than after waiting for the distress to become fully re-established. If the labour has reached the second period when inhalational analgesia would be more appropriate the administration of respiratory depressant drugs such as pethidine should be discontinued for fear of neonatal asphyxia.

The incidence of neonatal asphyxia severe enough to warrant active resuscitation is difficult to assess, and, in view of the almost universal acceptance of pethidine in labour for use by the unsupervised midwife, it must be assumed that the risk must be small enough to be outweighed by the benefits received. Nevertheless in comparing the condition of infants born of mothers receiving and not receiving pethidine during labour, the Medical Research Council's Committee on

Analgesia in Midwifery (1954) showed that while infant survival was unaffected, the use of pethidine was followed by an increased need for active resuscitation. Roberts *et al.* (1957) found some diminution of the respiratory minute volume of most babies for several hours after birth when the mothers have received pethidine. For this reason pethidine in combination with its pharmacological antagonist, levallorphan, has been recommended as a means of providing analgesia for the mother without fear of depressing the respiratory centre of her infant. Alternatively the combination of pethidine with phenothiazines or benzodiazepines as tranquillisers may reduce the amount of pethidine required to relieve the mother's discomfort without endangering the baby at birth.

Pethidine is believed to have an additional beneficial effect in labour quite apart from its analgesic action. Lindgren (1959) has shown that given when labour was well established, pethidine reduced uterine tone and the frequency of contractions but enhanced the amplitude of the contractions. In cases of lower uterine spasm the decreased frequency of contractions was associated with an increase in the rate of cervical dilatation. Jeffcoate (1961) has suggested that an infusion of pethidine 300 mg./litre often exerts an apparent anti-spasmodic effect and may resolve inco-ordinate uterine action. However, against the background of modern practice, epidural analgesia would probably be preferred in these circumstances.

Pethidine and its Antagonists

The allyl derivatives of morphine or levorphanol, nalorphine and levallorphan, can be used to offset the respiratory depressant effect of pethidine. A combination of pethidine 100 mg. with levallorphan 1·25 mg. in a 2 ml. ampoule is commercially available as "Pethilorfan". Bullough (1960) recommends this proportional admixture of the two drugs as providing maximal antagonistic effect to respiratory depression with minimal interference with the analgesic effect of pethidine. While nalorphine is considered to be an equally effective antagonist in a dose of 5 mg., levallorphan causes less drowsiness and is longer-acting. To achieve adequate analgesia, more frequent injections and larger pethidine doses are necessary when the narcotic-antagonist mixture is used than when plain pethidine is given. A working rule is that 100 mg. of pethidine in the narcotic-antagonist mixture has a similar analgesic effect to 60 mg. of plain pethidine, or 150 mg. of "Pethilorfan" has to be given to achieve the same analgesic effect as 100 mg. pethidine. Telford and Keats (1961) do not consider the value of a narcotic-antagonist mixture over plain pethidine proven. Nevertheless its place in the management of pain in labour is hallowed by widespread use over the past ten years.

These antagonists may be administered separately from pethidine either as an intravenous prophylactic to the mother ten minutes before delivery of the child or into the umbilical vein and massaged towards the infant immediately after birth. In the latter case the dose must be diluted and injected slowly. The type of infant for whom the antagonist is indicated is the one born when the mother has been given recent or repeated doses of narcotic. The child's muscle tone is good, it tends to open its eyes, it grimaces when stimulated but becomes progressively more cyanosed and makes only perfunctory efforts to breathe. If spontaneously breathing, the respirations are slow and deep and it should be distinguished from the gasping, pallid and flaccid infant associated with a traumatic delivery for whom immediate intubation and oxygenation is indicated.

Pethidine-Tranquilliser Combinations

The search for the ideal state of analgesia, somnolence and amnesia in labour has continued since the time when "twilight sleep" was in vogue. This involved the supplementation of the analgesic and soporific actions of an opiate with the cerebral sedative and amnesic effects of hyoscine. The disadvantages of hyoscine were firstly, the tendency to delirium in the mother when the analgesic effects of the opiate had worn off, and secondly, the discomfort of the dryness of the mouth due to its antisialogogue effect. More recently the combination of pethidine with the phenothiazines, chlorpromazine, promazine or promethazine have been used in the belief that they potentiate the analgesic action of pethidine without increasing its respiratory depressant effect. They also tend to produce, somnolence, mental detachment, anti-emesis and amnesia. Of the three phenothiazines mentioned, promazine ("Sparine") has become the most popular, possibly because it is said to be shorter-acting than chlorpromazine and because it has been found to have a mild analgesic effect in contrast to the anti-analgesic action found with promethazine by Dundee and Moore (1961). A further objection to promethazine is that it has been shown to have an inhibitory effect upon uterine contractions even in the presence of an oxytocin infusion.

In a double-blind trial using pethidine and promazine against pethidine and a placebo, Matthews (1963) showed that the potentiating effect of promazine, as measured by the reduced amount of pethidine given, was only evident in labours lasting more than 12 hrs. The retrospective maternal assessment of satisfaction showed no significant difference between the two groups. Even if a difference had been shown it could have been attributed to the amnesic effect of the promazine. Although no fall of blood pressure was recorded some tendency to tachycardia was observed.

A disadvantage of promazine and other phenothiazines is that, by virtue of their adrenolytic action, they tend to block the vascular response to loss of blood volume which may manifest itself in severe hypotension following quite a modest post-partum haemorrhage. Unexpectedly severe falls of blood pressure may occur with the subsequent induction of epidural analgesia or with halothane anaesthesia. A further disadvantage of promazine is that the mother may be so sleepy in the second stage of labour that she will be unable to summon up sufficient co-operation for the spontaneous delivery of her child. The disadvantages may be reduced by cautious dosage. While Matthews achieved his results by giving either 50 or 100 mg. promazine with 100 mg. pethidine, the more customary dose is only 25 mg. If the patient appears unduly sleepy when the next dose of pethidine is required, it should be given without promazine.

Fashions change in obstetric analgesia, and at the time of writing the use of the phenothiazines appears to be on the wane. In their place diazepam ("Valium") is becoming increasingly popular as a supplement to pethidine usually in a dose of 10–15 mg. It has sedative and amnesic properties but without the tendency to hypotension possessed by the phenothiazines. It is too early to assess its value or its disadvantages in this context, but it is worth noting that a myometrial relaxant effect has been reported by Cavenagh *et al.* (1966) and that Chalmers

(1967) used 30–60 mg./day in 51 cases of premature labour and found that labour was postponed for at least one week in 42 of the patients.

Other Analgesic Drugs

Despite the introduction of newer narcotic agents within the last decade such as alphaprodine, phenazocine, oxymorphone and recently, pentazocine, none has displaced pethidine as the analgesic for the routine relief of pain in the early part of labour. Mention should be made, however, of the place of morphine and diamorphine (heroin) in the management of prolonged labour with severe pain. Either morphine 15 mg. or diamorphine 10 mg. reliably relieve pain and induce sleep thus enabling an exhausted mother to rest and recover her morale. Despite clinical opinion to the contrary neither Caldeyro-Barcia *et al.* (1955) nor Eskes (1962) were able by intra-amniotic pressure tracings to demonstrate any depressant effect of morphine upon uterine contractility. By contrast, diamorphine was shown by the same technique to reduce the frequency and amplitude of the contractions (Tan and Wood, 1967). It should be remembered that when either of these drugs has been used the infant's respiratory centre could be affected if delivery occurred within five hours of their administration. In this event levallorphan given to the mother before delivery would guard against neonatal asphyxia.

It is doubtful whether morphine or diamorphine should ever be used in labour where facilities exist for epidural analgesia.

Second Period—Inhalational Agents

In 1934 Minnitt described his historic nitrous oxide/air apparatus which enabled the mother to administer analgesia to herself. It was approved in 1936 by the Central Midwives' Board, since when midwife-supervised self-administration has become the pattern of all the other "approved" methods of alleviation of the pain of the second period. From 8 cm. dilatation of the cervix in the primigravida and 6 cm. in the multigravida, narcotic analgesia should cease because of the risk of delivery of a depressed infant within the time of action of the drug. The gases and vapours in current use for the second period of labour should have a minimal effect on the neonate.

Nitrous Oxide and Air

This is given from a relatively simple type of intermittent flow apparatus of which the Minnitt, the Talley and the Jecta are examples and many thousands of these machines must now be in use all over the world. They are designed to deliver 50 per cent nitrous oxide in air with the result that the mother breathes a gas mixture containing 10·4 per cent oxygen. Since the introduction of oxygen-rich nitrous oxide mixtures and with the current concern for foetal welfare, the machines and the gas mixtures which they deliver must now be considered obsolete. The final seal has been set on the fate of nitrous oxide/air analgesia by the withdrawal of approval by the Central Midwives' Board in 1970.

It must be admitted that for over 30 years since its introduction nitrous oxide/air analgesia has been considered safe and satisfactory. It is surprising that there are so few published criticisms of the practice of allowing women in labour to respire an oxygen-deficient gas mixture particularly in view of the increasing preoccupation with the maintenance of adequate foetal oxygenation. Cole and Nainby-Luxmoore (1962) demonstrated a reduction of arterial oxygen saturation to 92 per cent while a mother was breathing 50 per cent nitrous oxide with air during the first stage of labour. Oxygen saturation fell to 88 per cent when the patient was breath-holding while bearing down in the second stage. These workers also showed that the reliability of the nitrous oxide machines in current use was suspect and that in the sample 35 machines tested, over half delivered mixtures containing nitrous oxide in excess of 50 per cent. The proportion of nitrous oxide delivered from individual machines varied according to the minute volume and could be changed easily by jolts, vibration and alteration of position.

Further work by Nainby-Luxmoore (1964) examined the performances of 14 machines of two different makes used at minute volumes from 3 to 40 litres. In Fig. 1 the line CMB represents the 10·4 per cent oxygen content of the mixture

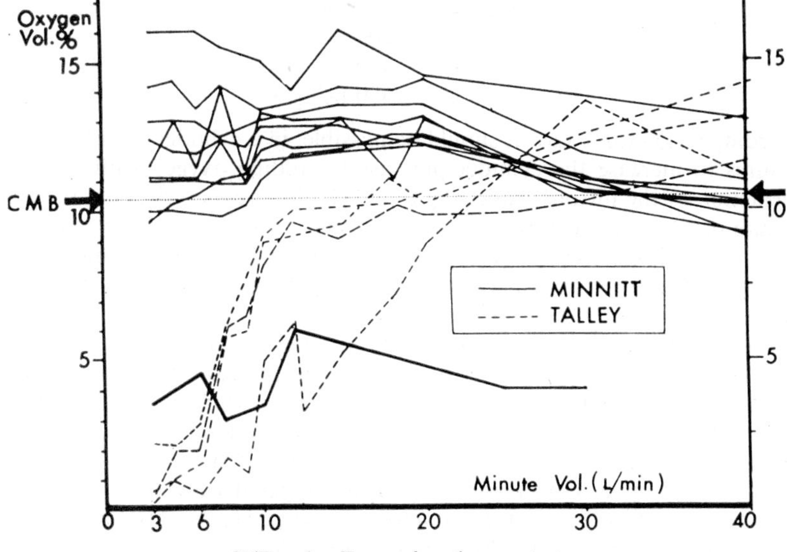

52/Fig. 1.—For explanation see text.

expected from the apparatus if it conformed exactly to the specification laid down by the Central Midwives' Board, namely, that the mixture should contain equal volumes of nitrous oxide and air at minute volumes between 3 and 9 litres. The performance of the machines was least reliable at low minute volumes while, with one exception, at minute volume in excess of 20 litres the oxygen percentage approximated to the prescribed level. Nitrous oxide air analgesia can therefore be considered an obsolescent method of relief of pain in labour not only because of the inescapable oxygen deficiency of the mixture but also because of the inherent defects in design of the available apparatus which result in the lack of reliability in composition of the mixture with changes in the minute volume of respiration.

observed with other gas mixtures including carbon dioxide and oxygen or nitrous oxide and nitrogen. It occurs most readily when the liquid phase is near its critical point, that is the temperature above which the gas can no longer be liquefied however great the pressure applied.

Pre-mixed nitrous oxide and oxygen is stable as long as the cylinder contents remain above the separation temperature of the mixture. Below this point some nitrous oxide liquefies and separates from the oxygen. Separation in a full cylinder originally at a pressure of 1980 psig occurs at −7° C with 50 per cent, at 1° C with 60 per cent and at 13° C with 70 per cent nitrous oxide. If the cylinder is used in the *vertical* position with the valve uppermost the early samples drawn off will be deficient in nitrous oxide and give inadequate analgesia while the samples taken when the cylinder is near exhaustion will be oxygen-deficient and cause hypoxia, undue sleepiness and loss of co-operation.

Excessive cooling of the cylinder is liable to occur in exceptionally cold weather while in transit from the factory to the consumer premises. Although records show that prolonged severe winter weather is unusual in the United Kingdom (Gale *et al.*, 1964) this takes no account of conditions which may occur in many other countries. The cylinders may also remain exposed to cold after delivery to the consumer who must accept the responsibility for taking them immediately into relatively warm storage.

Another cause of cooling is the fall of cylinder temperature while the gas mixture is running owing to the heat absorption which occurs when a compressed gas is released. However experiments have shown that even under conditions of high gas flow the temperature fall is never sufficient to change the composition of the emergent gas mixture (Crawford, *et al.* 1967). While cylinders containing nitrous oxide 50 per cent with oxygen would not contain separated gases until the temperature falls below −7° C, cylinders nominally of this composition have been found to contain mixtures with an oxygen content varying between 48 per cent and 56 per cent from cylinder to cylinder. Any increase in the proportion of nitrous oxide would raise the separation temperature of the mixture and therefore the frequency of occasions when the weather conditions would predispose towards separation. The manufacturers now take special precautions to ensure that the gas mixtures are reliable within a tolerance of ± 2 per cent.

Mere re-warming of the cylinder is insufficient to guarantee *immediate* adequate re-mixing of separated gases; the cylinders must be agitated by inverting them three times (Cole, 1964). This is reasonably practicable with the portable 500 litre cylinders, very difficult with the heavy hospital size 2000 litres cylinders and virtually impossible with the 5000 litre cylinders intended for pipeline use. However storage of cylinders in the *horizontal* position at a temperature above 5° C for 24 hours will re-constitute mixtures which have been separated by cooling down to −40° C. The more rapid distribution of the cylinder contents in the horizontal as compared with the vertical position is due to the larger area of interface between the liquid and the gaseous phase and the smaller distance between the surface of the liquid and the cylinder wall. This facilitates a more rapid evaporation and diffusion (Bracken *et al.*, 1968).

Because of the difficulty of handling the 5000 litre cylinder intended for pipeline use and because they are outside the direct control of the user the manufacturers have, as an added safety precaution, fitted them with dip-tubes extending from the valve to the further end of the cylinder cavity similar to that in a soda-water siphon. If storage and handling instructions have been ignored and some of the nitrous oxide is liquefied it will contain at least 20 per cent oxygen in solution and this sample would be drawn off first without serious danger to the patient. Without a dip-tube an oxygen-rich sample would be drawn off first with the risk of leaving a relatively hypoxic mixture when the cylinder is approaching exhaustion.

Apparatus.—The pre-mixed nitrous oxide and oxygen mixture is delivered by means of the "Entonox" apparatus (Fig. 3) which comprises a two-stage valve fitted to a cylinder head. A pressure gauge indicates the quantity of gas mixture

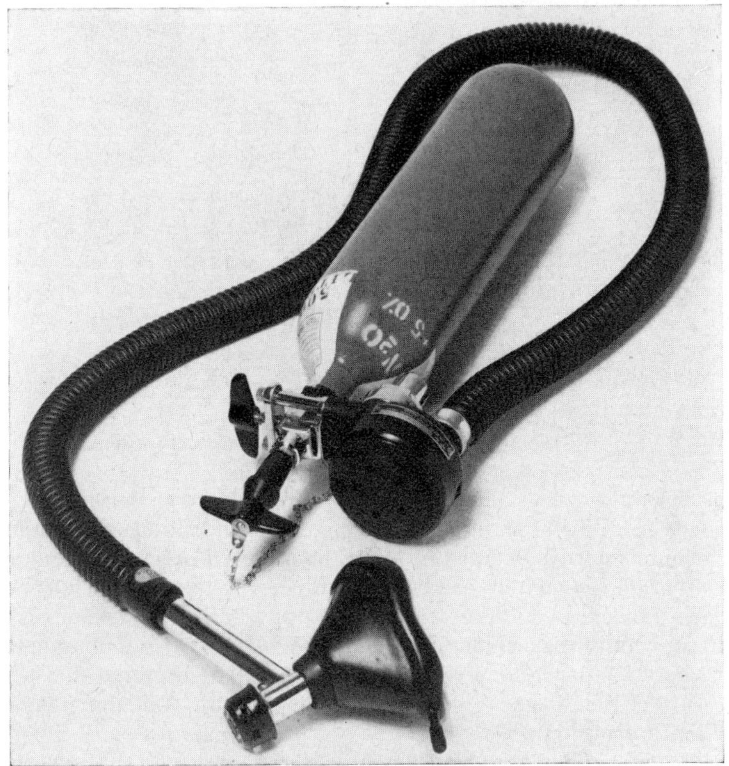

52/FIG. 3.—The "Entonox" apparatus.

in the cylinder and the gases pass on demand through a corrugated hose to a mask fitted with an expiratory valve.

The first stage consists of a simple reducing valve which decreases the full cylinder pressure of 138·6 kg/sq.cm. (1980 psig) to 13·9 kg/sq.cm. (200 psig) (Fig. 4). The slight negative pressure of inspiration opens the second stage tilting valve and the mixture is drawn into the corrugated hose. The slight positive pressure of exhalation pushes down the sensing diaphragm and the tilting valve connected with it closes the flow of gases from the reducing valve.

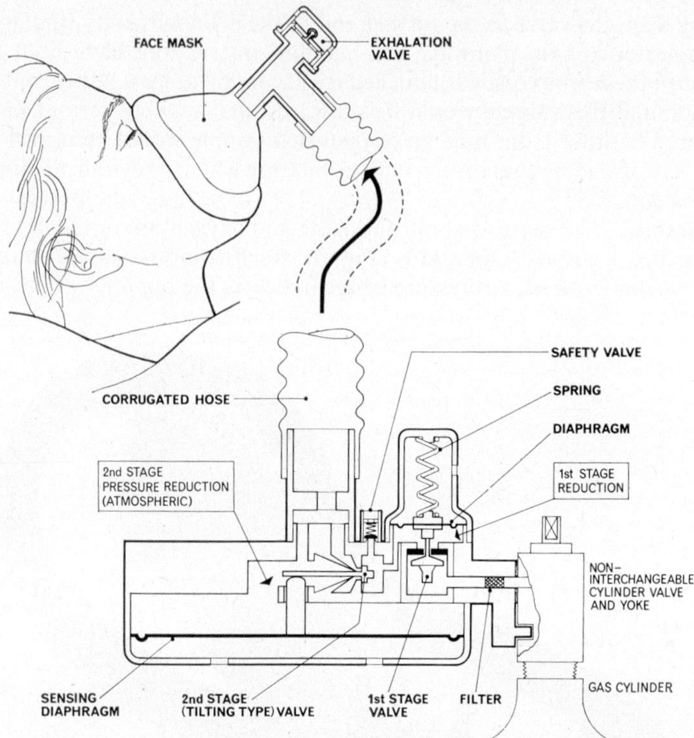

52/Fig. 4.—The "Entonox" nitrous oxide/oxygen analgesic apparatus.

The inspiratory resistance is extremely low; indeed if the corrugated hose is removed from the apparatus the gas mixture will continue to flow unless the outlet is momentarily occluded to make the tilting valve close. The design also ensures that no gas mixture can flow when the cylinder pressure falls below the first stage pressure of 13·9 kg/sq. cm. (200 psig). Although this means that the final 10 per cent of the cylinder contents is inevitably wasted it does represent an added safety factor. If some separation of gases has occurred due to cooling below —7° C the wasted gases would be a portion containing higher than 50 per cent nitrous oxide.

The Entonox machine, which was approved by the Central Midwives' Board in 1965, is very suitable for domiciliary practice, being compact and portable. It weighs 6·1 kg. (13½ lb.) with one full 500 litre cylinder. It is recommended that at least one spare cylinder should be carried for multiparous labours and two for primiparous (Crawford and Tunstall, 1968).

Not the least advantage of the pre-mixture of nitrous oxide and oxygen is that the mother, throughout the latter part of her labour, is breathing oxygen at a concentration near to that considered optimal for foetal welfare (Rorke *et al.*, 1968).

Nitrous oxide and oxygen from separate cylinders.—The advantages of a single concentration of nitrous oxide are less obvious in hospital practice where more bulky and less portable machines can be used to deliver nitrous oxide and oxygen either from separate cylinders or from a pipeline installation.

The "Lucy Baldwin" apparatus (Fig. 5) is a modification of the "Walton Five" dental gas machine (see Chapter 12) and is calibrated to deliver a range of mixtures from 80:20 nitrous oxide/oxygen to pure oxygen. The machine operates on demand only and has a stop at 70:30 nitrous oxide/oxygen so that mixtures stronger than this can only be obtained by using a special key. A safety device has been fitted so that when the supply of either nitrous oxide or oxygen fails the patient breathes room air only. Pressure gauges are provided for both oxygen and nitrous oxide and it should be remembered that while the pressure in an oxygen cylinder is proportional to its gas content, the pressure in a nitrous oxide cylinder remains constant until the liquid phase has evaporated. When the pressure begins to fall the cylinder is approaching exhaustion.

The advantage of this type of machine is that the inspired concentrations of nitrous oxide and oxygen can be changed not only to suit the needs of different patients whose responses to nitrous oxide may be variable but also to match the needs of an individual patient whose pain may vary with the changing intensity of the uterine contractions and to the waning influence of narcotic analgesics previously received.

In an attempt to determine the optimum proportion of the two gases, McAneny and Doughty (1963) gave either 50, 60, 70, 75 or 80 per cent nitrous oxide with oxygen to five groups each of 100 mothers. The numbers of those receiving satisfactory analgesia rose as the proportion of nitrous oxide increased from 50 to 70 per cent. Higher concentrations of nitrous oxide showed no improvement in analgesia but an increased tendency to cause unconsciousness. However, a trial conducted by the Medical Research Council (1970) showed little difference in analgesic effect between 50 per cent and 70 per cent in normal labours but that 70 per cent nitrous oxide appeared to be more effective in abnormal labours.

Variable mixture nitrous oxide/oxygen machines are not "approved" by the Central Midwives Board unless they are locked so that they cannot deliver concentrations in excess of 50 per cent nitrous oxide. The Board has given limited approval for midwives in hospital practice to use varying mixtures provided that the responsibility is accepted by a doctor.

Administration of nitrous oxide/oxygen analgesia.—In common with all inhalational agents the characteristics of nitrous oxide/oxygen analgesia depend on certain physical properties. Being gaseous at room temperature but relatively insoluble in blood, a high alveolar concentration and alveolar-blood equilibrium can be attained very rapidly. On discontinuing the inhalation the gas is rapidly eliminated. This means that nitrous oxide/oxygen can only provide intermittent analgesia unless it is respired continuously. Normally the mother breathes it in association with each uterine contraction and she should be instructed to start the inhalation as soon as the contraction is perceived and not to wait until the contraction becomes painful. It is important that she should understand that there is a time lag of about 15 seconds between the inhalation and the onset of analgesia. If the mother has a low threshold to pain the contraction becomes distressing too soon after its commencement and the mother would have no time to attain an analgesic blood level of nitrous oxide (51/Fig. 3). This type of patient

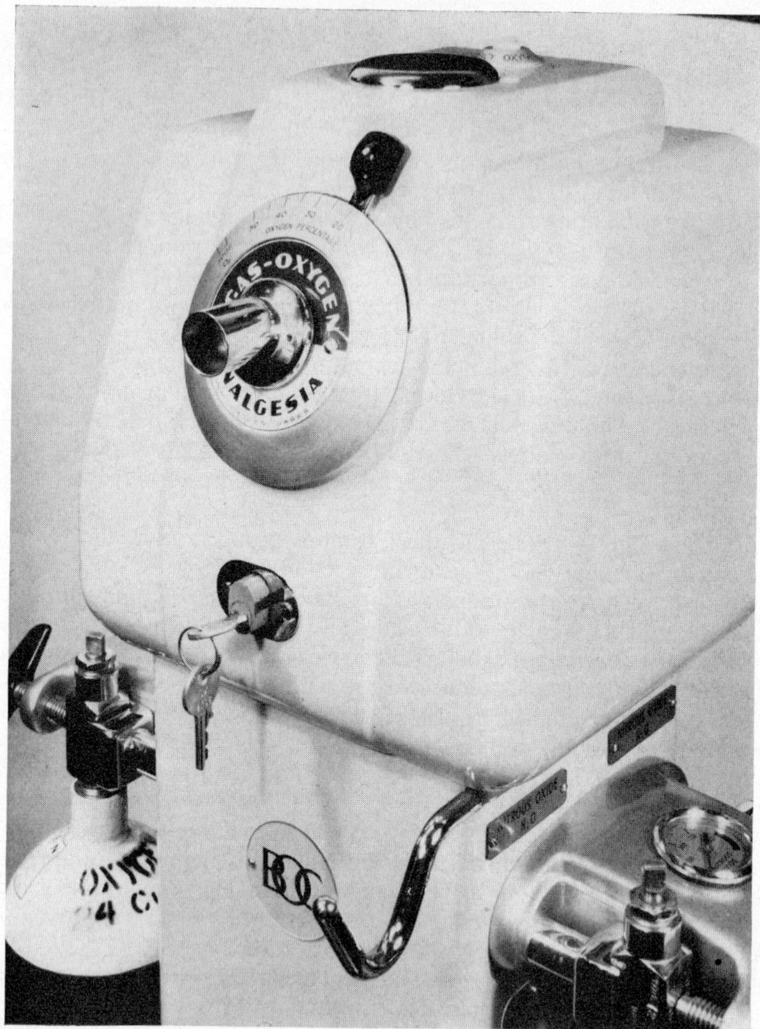

52/Fig. 5.—The head of the "Lucy Baldwin" apparatus.

is not satisfied by nitrous oxide and is probably better suited by trichloroethylene or methoxyflurane. On the other hand, nitrous oxide/oxygen analgesia may be started rather earlier in labour than trichloroethylene or methoxyflurane as there is no fear of a cumulative effect depressing the baby at birth.

Other points to be watched so as to get the best results from nitrous oxide analgesia are the importance of the immediate air-tight fit of the mask on the face followed by rapid deep respirations and the vigilant eye on the pressure gauge so that analgesia does not fail owing to cylinder exhaustion.

The disadvantages of nitrous oxide analgesia are that its efficacy depends on meticulous attention to the details of administration, its unsuitability for mothers with a low threshold to pain, the discomfort of the mouth and throat caused by the prolonged forced inhalation of dry gases and the exhaustion of the mother due to the muscular effort demanded by hyperventilation.

Trichloroethylene ("Trilene").

Trichloroethylene in a concentration of 0·5 per cent in air was approved by the Central Midwives' Board in 1955 for administration by the unsupervised midwife. Some ingenuity had to be employed in the design of the "approved" machines to ensure that the inspired vapour concentration does not exceed 0·5 per cent under all conditions of use despite changes in the ambient temperature, agitation of the apparatus and changes in the respiratory minute volume of the patient. The standards required of an approved inhaler drawn up by the Medical Research Council (1954) are as follows:

1. The concentration of trichloroethylene vapour delivered should be 0·5 per cent volume/volume in air with a permissible variation of $\pm$ 20 per cent. If possible, there should be available also a weaker setting, delivering 0·35 per cent of trichloroethylene, to allow for the increased susceptibility of some patients after prolonged inhalation.
2. The concentration of trichloroethylene vapour should remain within these limits with variations of room temperature from 12·5° C to 35° C (55° F to 95° F); a respiratory rate of 12–30 per minute; a tidal volume of 250–1,000 ml.; and a minute volume of 7–10 litres.
3. Where the respiratory minute volume falls to 7 litres or less, the concentration of vapour should also fall.
4. The resistance to air drawn through the apparatus should be not more than 1·25 cm. (0·5 inch) of water at a flow of 30 litres a minute.
5. The weight and bulk of the apparatus should be as small as possible. It should weigh not more than 6·1 kg. (15 lb.), should hold 60 ml. of liquid trichloroethylene, and should be sufficiently robust to stand up to reasonable wear and tear.
6. The apparatus must comply with these specifications in all working positions and after shaking and inversion. It must not be possible for liquid trichloroethylene to leak out.

In order to comply with the regulations of the Central Midwives' Board trichloroethylene inhalers must be checked annually by the British Standards Institution to ensure that they continue to function in accordance with specification. The date of testing is stamped on the machine and a certificate is issued to its owner.

The Automatic Emotril Inhaler (Fig. 6*a* and *b*).—This inhaler was designed by Epstein and Macintosh (1949). There are two separate entries for air, one directly into the vaporising chamber and the other through a by-pass to dilute the mixture of trichloroethylene and air emerging from the vaporising chamber. Changes in temperature are compensated by a bellows type thermostat which varies the size of the air exit. The surface from which the trichloroethylene evaporates consists of a wick which dips into the liquid agent below the chamber which is kept at a fairly constant temperature by means of a water jacket. The amount of trichloroethylene remaining in the inhaler may be estimated by the level in a gauge. The vapour passes to the patient through a non-return valve through an exit port. By opening a second bypass and allowing more air to be drawn into the machine, a weaker concentration of vapour—0·35 per cent in air—may be obtained if desired.

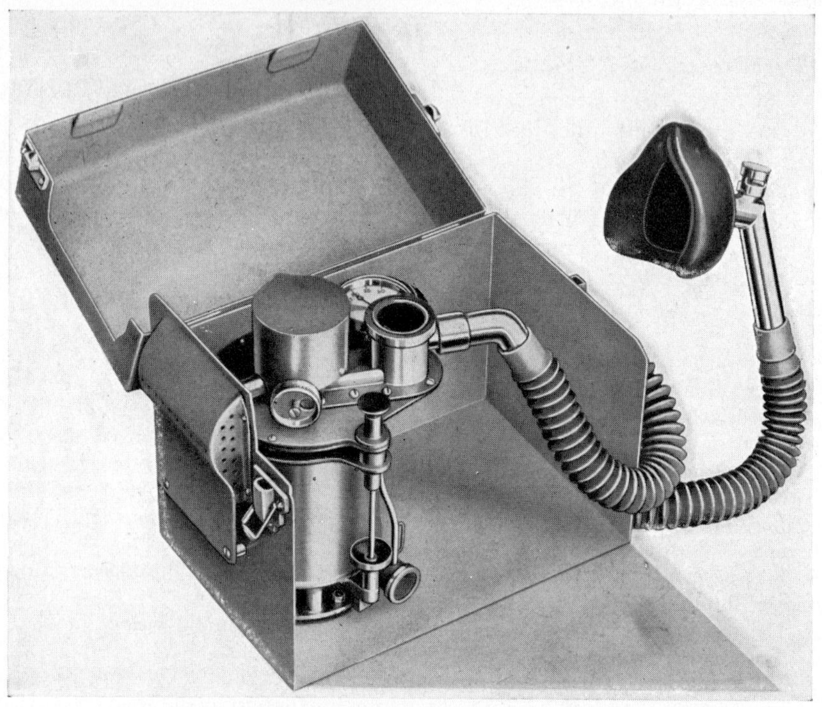

(*a*)

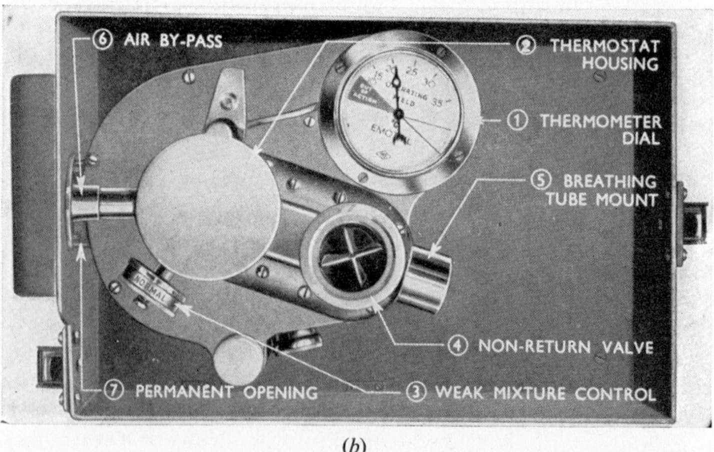

(*b*)

52/FIG. 6.—The automatic Emotril inhaler.

The Tecota Mark 6 Inhaler (Fig. 7).—Air is drawn through an opening where it divides into two streams. One stream passes through the vaporising chamber where it collects trichloroethylene vapour from the wicks and passes to an aperture, the size of which is controlled by a valve which is actuated by a bimetallic temperature-sensitive strip. The valve tends to open the aperture when the apparatus is cool and to close it when warm. Thus a greater or lesser proportion of vapour can leave the vaporising chamber according to the temperature. A constant bypass stream mixes with this and passes through a non-return valve to the patient. As with the Emotril inhaler the amount of trichloroethylene

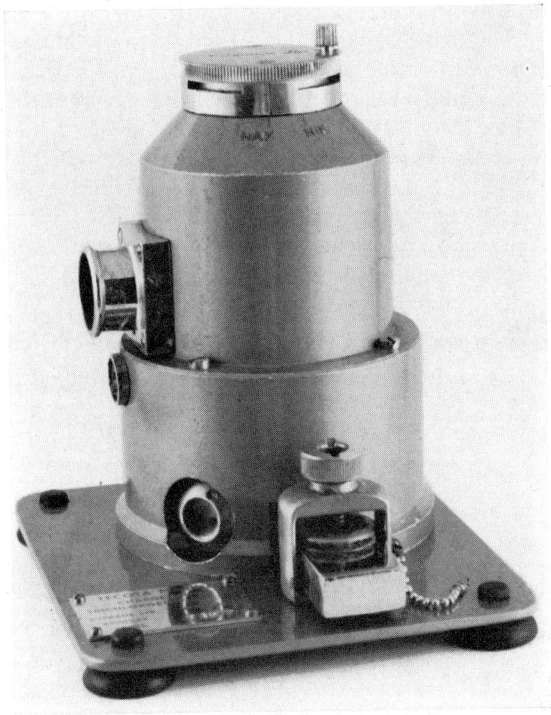

52/Fig. 7.—The Tecota Mark 6 Inhaler.

remaining in the inhaler can be estimated by the level in the gauge. A weaker mixture—0·35 per cent—may be obtained by increasing the flow of air through the bypass.

Administration of trichloroethylene analgesia.—Trichloroethylene has physical properties totally dissimilar to nitrous oxide. A liquid at room temperature, with a boiling point of 87° C, its vapour pressure is low but varies with changes in the ambient temperature. It is much more readily soluble in blood and has a high lipid solubility. Because of the low inspired concentration, uptake by the body is slow and because of its high blood solubility alveolar-blood equilibrium is unlikely to be reached in labour. This same property prevents a rapid recovery from its effects when inhalation ceases as the venous blood is not easily cleared of trichloroethylene during its passage through the lungs. With prolonged administration its accumulation in the body fats will further delay complete recovery.

When trichloroethylene is given in labour, the onset of analgesia is slow and inhalation in association with several uterine contractions is required before a satisfactory level of pain relief is achieved. However, the patient does not recover from the effects of the drug between inhalations so that trichloroethylene can be regarded as conferring continuous analgesia in contrast to the intermittent effect of nitrous oxide. It has therefore an advantage for mothers with a low threshold to pain for whom nitrous oxide is unsuitable.

Its cumulative effects are a disadvantage. The mother may become unduly sleepy with prolonged administration and while this effect may produce amnesia, the length of both first and second stages of labour tend to be prolonged. Because of the rapid placental transfer of trichloroethylene the infant is more likely to require resuscitation at birth, particularly after the use of pethidine earlier in the labour (Medical Research Council, 1954).

A further caution that should be mentioned is that mothers given trichloroethylene who subsequently require operative delivery must not be given an anaesthetic through a soda-lime absorber. Dichloracetylene may be formed by the reaction of trichloroethylene with soda lime and the re-inhalation from the absorber may result in cranial nerve palsies.

Nitrous Oxide Compared with Trichloroethylene

These two inhalational agents are compared in Table 1.

52/TABLE 1

COMPARISON OF NITROUS OXIDE AND TRICHLOROETHYLENE

	Nitrous Oxide and Oxygen	*Trichloroethylene and Air*
Analgesic Concentration	50 per cent with Oxygen	0·5 per cent with Air
Analgesic Effect	++ Intermittent	+++ Continuous
Onset of Analgesia	Rapid	Slow
Rate of Elimination	Rapid	Slow
Sedation	0	++
Amnesia	0	+
Prolongation of Labour	0	++
Foetal Asphyxia	0	+
Cost	Expensive	Cheap

Methoxyflurane ("Penthrane")

Methoxyflurane in a concentration of 0·35 per cent was approved by the Central Midwives' Board for use by the unsupervised midwife in 1970. It is given by means of the "Cardiff" Inhaler (Fig. 8) which is an adaptation of the Tecota Mark 6 trichloroethylene inhaler (Fig. 7). The only differences between the two

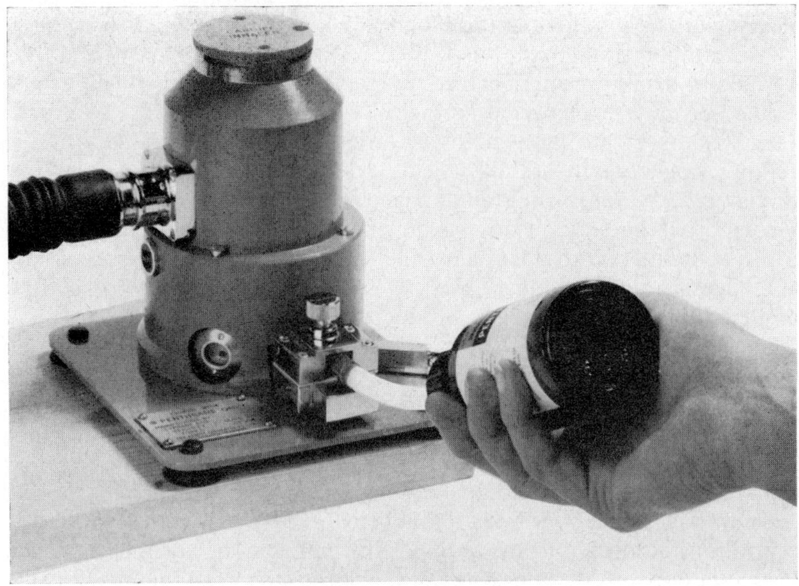

52/FIG. 8.—The "Cardiff" Inhaler.

machines are that the thermostat has been redesigned to suit methoxyflurane's vaporising characteristics, the control for the administration of a weaker strength has been removed and a charging device has been incorporated so that the inhaler can be filled only from the manufacturer's methoxyflurane bottle. As with the trichloroethylene machine, the "Cardiff" Inhaler must be subjected to an annual test by the British Standards Institution to ensure that it continues to function in compliance with the specifications which, apart from the difference in concentration of vapour delivered, are essentially similar to those which apply to trichloroethylene inhalers.

Like trichloroethylene, methoxyflurane is a liquid of low volatility (B.P. 104·8° C) and is administered in a low inspired concentration. It has a high blood and lipoid solubility and it might be expected to provide a similar type of analgesia with a relatively slow onset, slow recovery and a tendency to accumulation after prolonged administration.

Despite its approval by the Central Midwives' Board, opinions concerning its efficacy and its place in obstetrical analgesia remain confused. Boisvert and Hudon (1962) state that the intensity and rapidity of onset of analgesia is "remarkable" occurring within two minutes of the start of inhalation. On the other hand, Torda (1963) in tibial pressure studies, found a variable response with half his subjects showing an anti-analgesic effect after 4 minutes, which only disappeared after a further 8 minutes' inhalation. Dundee and Love (1963) in similiar experiments were unable to show any analgesic effect in sub-narcotic doses. In earlobe algesimetric studies Siker *et al.* (1967) found significant increases in pain threshold in 12 out of 14 volunteers inhaling variable concentrations of methoxyflurane up to 0·4 per cent. In two subjects however, there was little initial effect followed by minimal to marked falls in threshold at the point of onset of drowsiness. While the blood levels remained raised for some time after discontinuing administration 4 subjects during the recovery period showed a threshold to pain lower than before the start of the inhalations. These findings underline not only the expected biological variability of response to drugs but also the wisdom of having available a variety of analgesic agents rather than expecting a single one to suit all patients.

Bodley *et al.* (1966), using methoxyflurane 0·5 per cent as an analgesic in labour, reported that initially after six to ten breaths the mothers became relaxed and drowsy, indifferent to their pain and detached from the processes of labour. Later analgesia could be induced after two or three breaths. The possibility was raised that analgesia might not be produced in the absence of drowsiness.

Siker *et al.* (1968) reported that, as expected from the low degree of dissociation and high lipoid solubility, methoxyflurane crosses the placenta early and although there was significant foetal uptake there was a low incidence of foetal depression.

A detailed investigation of methoxyflurane in comparison with other inhalational analgesics is given in five publications from Cardiff:

(*a*) Major *et al.* (1966) compared methoxyflurane with trichloroethylene given continuously in labour by an anaesthetist who was able to vary the inspired concentrations according to the needs of the mother. They defined satisfactory analgesia not only by the suppression of the responses to painful uterine contractions, but also took account of the retention of consciousness and absence of restlessness between contractions. In the opinion of the anaesthetist, methoxyflurane appeared to maintain the more satisfactory state of objective analgesia for the period of the administration. The answers given by the mothers, when questioned directly, suggested that both drugs produced a comparably high standard of pain relief.

It was found that the mean inspired concentration of trichloroethylene necessary to give satisfactory analgesia fell from 0·4 per cent to 0·08 per cent over 85 minutes of administration while that of methoxyflurane fell only from 0·32 per cent to 0·16 per cent. The steeper slope of the trichloroethylene curve confirms the necessity for two fixed concentrations delivered by the inhalers, while the flatter slope obtained with methoxyflurane suggests that for intermittent administration only one fixed concentration is necessary.

(*b*) Major *et al.* (1967) reported that a single fixed concentration of 0·35 per cent methoxyflurane was superior to 0·25 per cent as a self-administered analgesic, not only in the opinion of the observing anaesthetist but also in the opinion of the midwives and the mothers concerned. A higher concentration of 0·45 per cent produced an unacceptable degree of drowsiness.

(*c*) Jones *et al.* (1969*a*) compared methoxyflurane with nitrous oxide/oxygen 50 per cent/50 per cent given continuously by an anaesthetist making adjustments to maintain the ideal analgesic state. Under these conditions the two agents were almost equally effective although nitrous oxide induced semi-consciousness too easily from which some patients awoke in confusion and distress complaining of unpleasant dreams. Nitrous oxide was also associated with a higher frequency of nausea and vomiting.

(*d*) Jones *et al.* (1969*b*) compared nitrous oxide/oxygen (50 per cent/50 per cent) with methoxyflurane 0·35 per cent in air self-administered by the mothers in midwife-conducted labours. From the observer's point of view methoxyflurane was the more satisfactory, mainly on account of its effect in suppressing the mothers' reaction to the uterine contractions. The previous administration of pethidine appeared to improve the efficacy of methoxyflurane, but not that of nitrous oxide/oxygen. When midwives and mothers were questioned no difference could be found between the two agents except for an association of nitrous oxide with nausea and vomiting.

(*e*) Rosen *et al.* (1969) reported on the results of a field trial on 1257 patients receiving methoxyflurane 0·35 per cent, trichloroethylene 0·5 per cent and nitrous oxide/oxygen (50 per cent/50 per cent) in eight maternity units. According to the mothers' opinions there was little difference between the three; the midwives' opinion was that both methoxyflurane and trichloroethylene gave better pain relief than nitrous oxide, but that mothers receiving nitrous oxide and trichloroethylene were more co-operative than those inhaling methoxyflurane. An association of nitrous oxide with nausea and vomiting was not confirmed.

The effect of pethidine in tending to produce neonatal asphyxia which has been so widely publicised in relation to trichloroethylene analgesia was apparent with all three agents; in fact the lowest Apgar scores were observed in those infants whose mothers had received nitrous oxide/oxygen.

General conclusions.—Apart from its smell, methoxyflurane is an acceptable and valuable analgesic which may be particularly useful in the later stages of labour or in rapidly progressing multiparous labours to relieve pain at a time when pethidine would not be given for fear of foetal depression. Nitrous oxide is a valuable analgesic which might be more effective if given in higher concentrations but the risk of unconsciousness in the mother is considered too great for general use by the unsupervised midwife. Trichloroethylene does not appear to have any advantage, apart from low cost, over the other two agents. It does not deserve the prejudice on the part of many midwives against it.

REGIONAL ANALGESIC TECHNIQUES

The methods of alleviation of pain so far considered in this chapter are essentially those practised against the background of midwife-supervised labours. These methods cannot ensure a painless childbirth nor can they make labour tolerable when the pain is exceptionally severe. It is on the occasions when the need for analgesia is beyond the midwife's ability to supply it that the obstetric anaesthetist can help by giving some form of regional analgesia. A previous edition of this book stated, "When complete pain relief is needed throughout labour, epidural analgesia is the safest and simplest method of procuring it. It is a weakness of anaesthetic practice in the United Kingdom that too few anaesthetists have either the time or the inclination to make use of this very valuable adjunct to normal and abnormal labour."

The need for the use of more effective methods was shown by a survey in Sheffield by Beazley *et al.* (1967) who made special efforts to ensure that the established sedative and analgesic drugs together with inhalational agents were given as soon as needed and with the closest possible attention to the details of their administration. Morphine, diamorphine and even paracervical block were freely used when the simpler methods failed. Despite this intensive effort only

23 per cent of women admitted having a pain-free labour and there remained 40 per cent whose childbirth was painful. The authors concluded that there might be a limit to the relief which can be obtained with techniques based mainly on central depression.

In view of the current interest in continuous lumbar epidural analgesia this technique will be described in some detail. Caudal epidural analgesia and paracervical block will be considered more briefly.

Lumbar Epidural Block

The anatomical basis of the practice of continuous lumbar epidural analgesia in labour has been discussed in Chapter 51 (51/Fig. 2), and numerous techniques for achieving it have been described. Duthie *et al.* (1969) aimed to block sensation from the 11th dorsal to the 4th sacral segments for the duration of labour. The dose given was 10–15 ml. 0·5 per cent bupivacaine with adrenaline or 15–20 ml. 0·25 per cent bupivacaine with adrenaline, the patient lying in the horizontal position. It was found that the weaker solution was as reliable as the stronger but with less liability to cause muscle paresis. Moir and Willocks (1968) performed epidural puncture in the sitting position to achieve greater spinal flexion and gave 6 to 10 ml. 2 per cent lignocaine as the initial dose. Bromage (1961) aimed to block the lower dorsal and upper lumbar segments with 7 ml. of local analgesic with the mother in the horizontal position and then to give a larger dose in the sitting position to block the sacral roots when the labour had reached the second stage. The object was to avoid relaxation of the muscles of the pelvic floor in order to facilitate the rotation and full flexion of the foetal head and avoid the undue frequency of assisted delivery. Doughty (1969*a*) observed that many mothers experienced no pain in the second stage of labour when the local analgesic had been aimed only at blocking the lower dorsal and upper lumbar segments. No formal attempt was made to block the sacral roots unless the mother specifically complained of vaginal or perineal pain. The intention was to provide relief of pain without depriving her of the sensations of labour and only when dictated by the mother's need was 10 ml. of local analgesic solution given in the sitting position. This techique was named "selective epidural block" and it was reported that as few as 19 per cent of mothers delivering spontaneously demanded a formal attempt to block the sacral roots owing to a fortuitous spread of the top-up doses producing some diminution of perineal sensation.

Advantages claimed for selective epidural analgesia include:

1. Preservation of the tone of the muscles of the pelvic floor and hence the normal mechanism of labour thus achieving a reasonably low incidence of assisted delivery.
2. Retention by the mother of the sensation of the baby's head in the vagina so that she preserved a sense of direction for her expulsive efforts.
3. The smaller doses of local anaesthetic given implied a reduced frequency of toxic side-effects, hypotension and paresis of the legs.
4. In the rare event of an inadvertent subarachnoid injection, recovery from a small dose would be more rapid than from a larger one.

Technique

The anaesthetist should first obtain the mother's consent to receive epidural analgesia and give her a brief explanation of what he proposes to do, the effect intended and the co-operation that he requires. The degree of dilatation of the cervix, the character of the labour pain, the mother's blood pressure and pulse and the foetal heart should already have been recorded by the labour ward staff.

The anaesthetist must take full aseptic precautions as for a surgical operation. The smooth running of all syringes must be checked and the patency of the Portex epidural cannula must be established, as must the ability of the cannula to pass through the Tuohy needle.

The mother lies horizontally on her left side with the knees drawn up towards the chest and the neck fully flexed. The back is swabbed with 1 per cent chlorhexidine in spirit. A weal is raised in the midline immediately caudal to the 2nd lumbar spine and some of the local analgesic injected up to 3 cm. deep to the skin weal. A puncture through the skin and supra-spinous ligament is made with a thick sharp needle to facilitate the passage of the blunter epidural needle. The Tuohy needle is passed through the skin and supra-spinous ligament and the 20 ml. syringe charged with about 15 ml. of 0·5 per cent bupivacaine is attached. The Tuohy needle is advanced in a slightly cephalad direction until the resistance of the ligamentum flavum is identified. The needle with attached syringe is very cautiously advanced through the ligamentum flavum, a slight pressure being maintained on the plunger of the syringe. As soon as the epidural space is entered the loss of resistance to injection will be appreciated. The syringe is detached from the Tuohy needle and a smoothly running 2 ml. syringe is attached and aspiration made for cerebrospinal fluid. The 2 ml. syringe is then filled with air and an attempt made to elicit a "pneumatic bounce' which would be apparent if the point of the needle were not in the epidural space. A dose of 5–7 ml. of 0·5 per cent bupivacaine without adrenaline is then slowly injected at the rate of 1 ml. per second. The smaller dose is given to mothers over 30, the larger to those under the age of 25. The syringe is then detached and the Portex marked epidural cannula (Fig. 9) is fed into the epidural space through the Tuohy needle until the 4-band (20 cm.) mark reaches the hub. The needle and cannula are then extracted together until the needle point emerges from the skin. The Tuohy needle is then slid up the cannula to its proximal end and the cannula is pulled out until the 2-band (10 cm.) mark is at skin level. The mother's back is sprayed with "Nobecutane", a dressing applied and the cannula strapped to the mother's back with waterproof adhesive tape. For the purposes of supplementary "top-up" doses the cannula can either be attached to a charged syringe enclosed in a plastic bag or led over the mother's shoulder and attached to a "Swinnex" millipore filter unit which enables top-ups to be done without cumbersome sterile precautions (Fig. 9).

The mother is then turned on to her back and positioned with a pillow under her left buttock to reduce the chance of a unilateral block (see notes below). The patient's blood pressure, pulse and the foetal heart rate are recorded at 15 minutes and 30 minutes following the induction of analgesia. Some tendency to a small fall of blood pressure of 10 to 20 mm. Hg is to be expected as severe pain tends to cause some hypertension above the level measured before the mother's distress becomes apparent. Any fall should be maximal after 30 minutes but as a precaution the patient should be turned to her side to counteract any degree of vena caval occlusion. Those in attendance on the mother should be warned that any tendency to supine hypotension should be treated immediately by

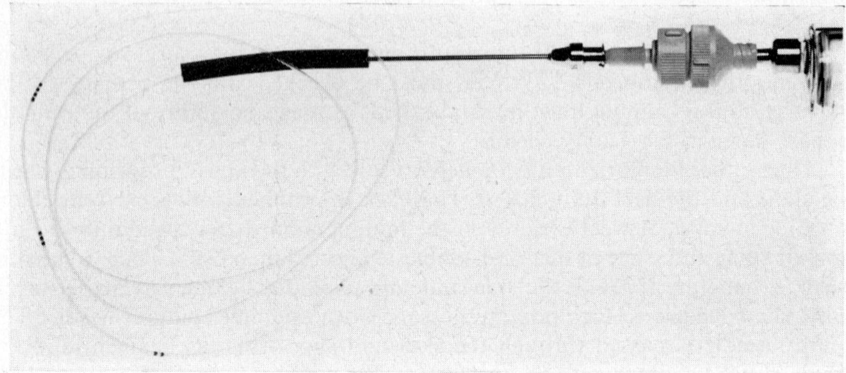

52/FIG. 9.—Plastic epidural cannula with "Swinnex" millipore filter.

turning her to the side with the onset of the premonitory symptoms of pallor, vertigo, nausea, faintness or ringing in the ears which may precede the actual measurable fall of blood pressure. On questioning, some mothers may volunteer that such symptoms have arisen in late pregnancy and they have found lying on the side more comfortable than on the back.

Topping-up

The duration of the effect of the initial dose of local analgesic is uncertain and hopes that the use of bupivacaine would guarantee at least 3 hours relief of pain have not been substantiated. Using the technique described the writer has noted a variability of length of action of 7 ml. of bupivacaine from 48 minutes to over 4 hours with a mean length of action of 135 minutes. Previous sedation particularly with phenothiazines seems to delay the return of complaints of pain.

If the complaint of returning pain is localised to the hypogastrium or over the sacrum, i.e. uterine pain, the top-up is given with the patient lying on her back. If the pain complained of is due to intolerable rectal pressure or is localised between the legs or to the perineum the top-up is given in the sitting position and the mother kept in this position for 5 minutes. Occasionally she may feel faint when sitting up and must not be kept in this position. In relatively few mothers delivering spontaneously has a block in the sitting position been indicated but a formal blockade of the sacral roots is needed for operative delivery.

The top-up must always be preceded by observations of blood pressure, pulse and foetal heart rate which must, as before, be repeated 15 and 30 minutes after the top-up.

Notes on technique.—1. Full sterile precautions are taken not only on general principles but also because there is always the remote possibility of dural puncture.

2. The importance of checking equipment cannot be overstressed. Sticky syringes detract from the delicacy of the loss of resistance test. Epidural cannulae have been known to be supplied kinked or without lumen. Tuohy needles may have been damaged by previous use and may not allow the cannula to pass. The bevel may be rough which could result in damage to the cannula.

3. The needle should not be advanced during a uterine contraction as the mother cannot be expected to co-operate at this time; the epidural veins are distended and dural pressure is raised; failure to observe this precaution may result in haemorrhage from the veins or in dural puncture.

4. The epidural injection must be made slowly and between contractions. An injection made rapidly or during a contraction may result in a widespread but patchy analgesia.

5. The epidural cannula should not be passed through the Tuohy needle during a uterine contraction owing to the risk of puncturing the temporarily tense dura or the congested epidural veins. It should always be filled with local analgesic solution before threading it through the needle as occasionally there is a reflex of blood from the epidural space which, if not diluted, would clot and block its lumen. If, during the course of labour a blood reflux is noted it should always be pushed back by a very small injection up the cannula.

6. The epidural cannula is fixed with the 2-band (10 cm.) mark at skin level so that the anaesthetist can be certain that analgesia will take effect from the level at which the cannula has been inserted. The depth of the epidural space from the skin varies from 3 cm. to 9 cm. and if the mean depth is about 6 cm. it can be expected that about 4 cm. will lie in the epidural space. Bromage (1954) has shown by radiography that a flexible catheter passed into the epidural space for any distance cannot be relied upon to travel according to the direction of the bevel of the Tuohy needle. He has demonstrated that it may pass out of the epidural space through an intervertebral foramen or be diverted by an obstruction and turn caudally.

7. The time between the injection of local analgesic and the turning of the patient on to her back must be kept as short as possible owing to the possibility of pooling of the drug on to the dependent side. This implies that the cannula must be passed and the dressing applied with the minimum of delay otherwise the pain relief may be only unilateral. To counteract this possibility Bromage (1961) suggests injecting 4 ml. only of local analgesic with the patient on her side and a further 3 ml. with the patient on her back. The writer's practice is to inject the full induction dose of 5–7 ml. with the patient on her side and then to turn the patient over on to her back as quickly as possible after the application of the dressing. After turning on to her back she is turned slightly to her right side with a pillow under the left buttock. Even so, unilateral pain relief was noted in 22 per cent of cases and paradoxically not always on the dependent side. To remedy this a further 3 ml. of local analgesic is given with the patient turned to the side on which pain persists. Where the epidural block is to be given electively the cannula can be put in place before labour becomes painful and the local analgesic injected through the cannula with the patient lying on her back (de Vere, 1969).

Difficulties

1. *Lack of co-operation by the mother.*—It has already been stated that epidural puncture should not be attempted during a uterine contraction. Occasionally the mother may be so distressed by pain and co-operation made impossible by sedatives and hypnotics that she could not be relied upon to lie still even between contractions.

In this case she should be given an effective dose of analgesic and the epidural puncture attempted when the drug becomes effective.

2. *Identification of bony landmarks.*—Occasionally the mother is so obese that the lumbar spines cannot be palpated with certainty. However, the 2nd and 3rd lumbar spines may be identified by seeking them by percutaneous exploratory puncture with fine hypodermic needles. It should be remembered that in such patients it may be necessary to advance the Tuohy needle into the patient as far as its hub before the epidural space is penetrated. The epidural cannula must be fixed at skin level at a point correspondingly further from its tip than with a normal woman.

3. *Difficulty in passing the cannula through the needle.*—The Tuohy needle is 9 cm. long. If the cannula will not pass to the 10 cm. mark the obstruction is at the tip of the needle and this should have been noted by the preliminary test of equipment before the epidural puncture. Needle and cannula should be withdrawn and the puncture attempted with another needle tested against the cannula. Once the 10 cm. mark has passed through the hub any obstruction to the passage of the cannula must be in the epidural space. Here the cannula may meet obstruction. Determined pressure on the cannula with a plain dissecting forceps rather than finger and thumb combined with rotation of the Tuohy needle usually succeeds but if obstruction is absolute the needle with cannula must be withdrawn and the puncture performed in a neighbouring space. On no account must the cannula be withdrawn through the needle as there is a risk of its end shearing off and remaining in the epidural space. Occasionally there is an absolute obstruction after the 3-band (15 cm.) mark has passed through the hub. In this case the needle can be withdrawn as the cannula is fed into it. After this manoeuvre sufficient cannula will be found to have been introduced into the epidural space.

4. *Prevention of top-ups by cannula obstruction.*—The possibility of damage to epidural vessels causing a reflux of blood up the cannula has already been mentioned. Pure blood remaining in the cannula will clot and if epidural analgesia is to be continued the puncture must be repeated and a new catheter inserted. Kinking of the cannula may also cause obstruction to the top-up. Inspection of cannulae that have become so blocked has shown that the kink is nearly always about 1 cm. below skin level, that is at the point where the cannula would pass through the supra-spinous ligament. When the patient's back is flexed as when the epidural puncture is done, the point where the cannula passes through the skin and the point where it passes through the supraspinous ligament are opposite each other. When the mother straightens her back the skin moves upwards in relation to the ligament, thus causing the cannula to bend sharply. The kink may be straightened out by asking the mother to flex her back, the skin of the back may be pushed caudally or the cannula may be withdrawn very

slightly. If none of these remedies succeed there is no alternative to repeating the epidural puncture.

5. *Failure of block.*—Occasionally, despite apparently impeccable technique, the single epidural injection given in the horizontal position fails to relieve the pain adequately. If the pain relief is unilateral the mother should be turned to the unaffected side and a further injection of 3 ml. of local analgesic solution given through the cannula.

If labour has been prolonged or the baby's head is in a posterior position or the cervix is near full dilatation a dose of 8–10 ml. should be given through the cannula in the sitting position to direct the solution towards the sacral roots. Following the injection the mother should remain upright for 5 minutes.

The pain relief may be patchy and small areas of the central hypogastrium continue to be painful. In this case the passage of a catheter to empty the bladder may bring relief. The possibility of a rupturing uterus may be considered and the pain of this and most other forms of pathological pain may not necessarily be masked by a small-dose epidural block.

If the block continues to be unsatisfactory it should be repeated through an adjacent lumbar interspace.

Indications for Epidural Analgesia

The primary effect of epidural analgesia is to relieve pain and thereby prevent exhaustion of the mother and preserve her morale. Indications for its use vary from hospital to hospital according to the availability, aptitude and enthusiasm of the anaesthetic service and the local predilections of the obstetricians and midwives. On the assumption that the service is readily available and the obstetricians would welcome the prospect of 30 per cent of mothers receiving epidurals in labour, the indications could be as follows:

Elective
- Trial of labour.
- Cardiac and respiratory disease.
- Premature or high risk foetus.
- Pre-eclamptic toxaemia.
- Fear of a repetition of a previous painful and harrowing experience.
- Expressed wish to have a painless labour.

Non-elective in labour
- Slow painful labour.
  - (*a*) Cervical dystocia.
  - (*b*) Uterine inertia when oxytocin stimulation causes insupportable pain.
  - (*c*) Inco-ordinate uterine action.
  - (*d*) Slow labour associated with persistent malposition of the foetal head.
  - (*e*) Cephalo-pelvic disproportion.
- Failure of conventional analgesia and impending loss of morale in an otherwise normal labour.
- Operative delivery when the stomach is known to be full.

Comment.—Most would agree that epidural analgesia given early can save the mother exhaustion in a trial of labour; she is then better able to withstand the stress of delivery by Caesarean section. With respiratory and cardiac disease

effaced and 3–4 cm. dilated, may be expected to proceed very rapidly particularly if stimulated with oxytocin. Here one would be prepared to induce epidural analgesia sooner rather than wait for 5–6 cm. dilatation of the cervix. A multipara with a previous history of rapid, tumultuous, painful labours should be given the epidural as soon as labour begins.

There is much to be said for the placing of the epidural cannula in position by the anaesthetist at his convenience before the mother requires pain relief. To guard against the chance that the cannula may have punctured the dura, he should stay to observe the effect of a test dose of 2 ml. of local analgesic solution given through the cannula. The main dose may then be safely injected when needed by any doctor trained in the management of patients receiving epidural analgesia.

When it is decided to give epidural analgesia to a patient because of obstetrical complications arising during labour it should be remembered that the mother may already have received a multiplicity of sedative drugs which may cause the effect of the initial dose of local analgesic to last considerably longer than if she had received little sedation. Following phenothiazines the tendency to hypotension may be more pronounced and if a mother has become demoralised with severe pain it may be difficult to obtain her co-operation in lying still for the injection. When distress is associated with cervical dystocia, inco-ordinate uterine action or a posterior position of the foetal head with severe backache, relief of pain may sometimes only be obtained by an injection given in the sitting position to block the sacral roots (Moir and Willocks, 1967).

The Care of Patients during Epidural Analgesia

It is particularly important that midwives and others in attendance should have been instructed in the special needs of mothers receiving epidural analgesia.

Change of position.—One of the advantages claimed for the small-dose or selective block is that the mother retains mobility on the labour-ward bed at least at first. In longer labours, when repeated doses have to be given, weakness and paresis of the legs may occur and, if not helped to change her position, the patient will lie passively and without complaint. She must be turned from one side to another at intervals. Scrupulous attention must be paid to smoothing out ridges in the bed linen which must be changed frequently when soiled. Duthie *et al.* (1968) have reported a pressure sore in a patient after 24 hours of epidural analgesia in spite of the retention of motor power in the legs.

Care of the bladder.—Care must be taken to ensure that the bladder does not become over-distended during labour as the desire for micturition is lost. The larger dose of local analgesic given for forceps delivery may cause prolonged loss of sensation in the immediate post-partum period and the bladder is liable to become over-filled owing to natural diuresis and the cessation of the anti-diuretic effect of synthetic oxytocin used in labour.

Diversion and nutrition.—Because the mother remains fully alert during labour some form of diversion is welcome including reading matter, portable radio and visits from close family relatives. Bland fluids should be given freely together with light food although the mother herself often refuses it. Occasionally she may be troubled by persistent nausea, which should be treated by intravenous perphenazine 2·5 mg. Larger doses are unnecessary and may cause undue sleepiness.

Top-up doses.—It is particularly important that top-up doses be given as soon as the contractions become painful: there is nothing to be gained by allowing the mother's morale to fail and she should be encouraged to draw attention at the first sign of returning discomfort.

Records.—Detailed records should be kept of all local analgesic doses given to the mother together with the effect on blood pressure, pulse rate and foetal heart rate before and after they are given. The effect of the doses and the height of the accompanying sensory blockade will help to determine the amount of the subsequent doses required. The occurrence of side-effects and the progress of labour should also be recorded. The use of a purpose-designed record card has the advantage not only of imposing a discipline on the labour ward staff to ensure the proper care of patients under epidural analgesia, but also of facilitating the handover should a change of clinical charge of the case be necessary.

The second stage.—It should be remembered that, with epidural analgesia, the mother may not notice a change of sensation when labour has progressed to the second stage. She may feel the uterus contracting and be able to push spontaneously in concert with it, but after prolonged epidural analgesia she may be unaware of the contractions and require constant reminders to bear down in compliance with her attendant's instructions. In multiparae particularly, the foetal head may be discovered on the perineum and while imperceptible spontaneous delivery is unlikely, those in attendance should be warned that an occasional visual and manual examination is needed to assess progress.

In short, mothers receiving epidural analgesia require little more than the application of the proper standards of care expected in any well-run labour ward. Epidural analgesia merely demands that there should be no relaxation of those standards.

Epidural Analgesia and the Forceps Rate

A possible discouragement to the more frequent use of epidural analgesia has been the belief that it inevitably leads to the need for operative delivery (Moir and Willocks, 1967). While this impression persists it is not surprising that hospital obstetricians see in it a source of increased pressure of work and midwives a cause of deprivation of the opportunity to practise their art and train their pupils.

In labours predominantly conducted by obstetricians, delivery by forceps may be elective and spontaneous parturition following epidural analgesia may be allowed to occur in only about 10 per cent of labours (Kandel *et al.*, 1966; de Vere, 1969). In other circumstances epidural analgesia may be used only in abnormal labours when assisted delivery would be anticipated irrespective of the type of pain relief employed.

The theoretical reasons why the use of epidurals should predispose to operative delivery are firstly, the abolition of the involuntary urge to bear down in the second stage of labour, secondly, the paralysis of the muscles of the pelvic floor which may cause malrotation and incomplete flexion of the foetal head and thirdly, the occasional diminution in the strength of uterine contractions possibly due to interruption of the motor innervation of the uterus above the 11th dorsal segment. However, the relief of maternal distress should eliminate one of the main indications for operative delivery.

Noble and de Vere (1970) reported that an increased use of epidural analgesia at the Westminster Hospital had not increased the rate of instrumental delivery. A satisfactory by-product of this policy was the virtual abolition of general anaesthesia for vaginal operative delivery.

Using a small-dose epidural technique mainly in obstetrician-managed labours, Doughty (1969*b*) reported a forceps rate of 24 per cent out of 425 cases —42 per cent in primigravidae and 11 per cent in multiparae. It was suggested that forceps delivery might be less frequently associated with epidural analgesia provided that:

1. The technique is employed in normal as well as in abnormal labours;
2. The strength of uterine contraction is augmented if necessary by an oxytocin infusion;
3. A selective technique is used involving minimal doses of local analgesic directed at the nerve pathways by which the mother is feeling pain at the time of injection;
4. The attending obstetrician is willing to allow the mother time and opportunity to deliver herself without unduly hasty intervention.

Practicability of Epidural Analgesia in Obstetrics

While the practice of epidural analgesia for the relief of pain in labour is growing there are undoubted difficulties in establishing a service in many major obstetric units. In some the obstetricians would like to see the service established but the anaesthetists are unable to supply it; in some the anaesthetists are able to offer the service but their obstetrician colleagues are unconvinced of its value, while in others local opinion is satisfied with the existing methods of pain relief and sees no reason for any change particularly if it implies an increase in the work of a busy department.

In establishing the service there must be the necessary skill available for the setting up of epidural analgesia. This is only obtained by constant practice and it is on the gynaecological operating list that the technique may be taught under general anaesthesia. Teaching on the conscious labouring mother should only take place when the anaesthetist has first acquired some competence in the operating theatre.

Fear of the complications tends to act as a deterrent. There are only three which assume practical importance. First is dural puncture, the frequency of which can only be reduced by meticulous technique and constant practice. Second is the unrecognised dural puncture followed by the injection of local analgesic into the subarachnoid space. This will cause a profound fall of blood pressure possibly leading to respiratory and cardiac arrest. No one should attempt epidural analgesia unless prepared to avoid this complication or to treat it efficiently and promptly. Third is the occasional fall of blood pressure due to the unmasking of the effects of vena caval compression. It is of the utmost importance that the midwives in attendance on the patient should be trained to recognise and treat, by turning the mother to her side, the early symptoms of supine hypotension which may follow the induction of epidural analgesia and the subsequent top-ups.

There has been a persistent suspicion that epidural analgesia may be responsible for neurological complications following parturition. The risks are minimal provided that the analgesia is managed with close attention to the precautions already described. It should not be forgotten that even normal labour without epidural analgesia may be followed by neurological damage (Chalmers 1949). Bladder disturbances, lumbo-sciatic pain and foot-drop are recognised as not uncommon sequelae of both normal and operative delivery. One should therefore keep an open mind as to whether epidural analgesia does or does not add to these risks.

It has hitherto been assumed that once epidural analgesia has been set up the anaesthetist is committed personally to stay with the patient until delivery. This is quite unnecessary as once he has satisfied himself that the block is effective and that there has been no undue fall of blood pressure he may leave the subsequent conduct of the analgesia in the hands of a resident doctor trained in the supervision of patients under epidural analgesia. In these circumstances it is wise to give the initial dose through the in-dwelling cannula to guard against the remote possibility that the cannula has punctured the dura (Moir and Hesson, 1965).

The key to the setting up of an epidural service is a united desire of midwives, obstetricians and anaesthetists to have it and to make it work. There must be the facilities for the training of all concerned in the technical skills involved and a standard routine must be evolved so that epidural analgesia becomes accepted as normal practice and is not associated with fuss, bother and a lot of extra work.

Caudal Epidural Analgesia

This technique for the relief of pain in labour was introduced by Hingson and Edwards in 1942. Local analgesic solution was injected through the sacral hiatus in quantities sufficient to rise within the epidural space to affect the sympathetic afferent pathways entering the central nervous system at the lower dorsal and upper lumbar segments (see 51/Fig. 2). In its passage up the epidural space the local analgesic also blocks the sacral roots producing perineal anaesthesia and relaxation of the muscles of the pelvic floor long before such a block might be indicated by the mother's need. The sacral block is reinforced with each successive top-up. A high rate of assisted delivery is considered a small price to pay for the benefit of total relief from pain (Stallworthy, 1969). In effect caudal analgesia is more specifically suited to operative delivery; relief of labour pain accrues as a secondary effect achieved by higher dosage.

Technique (Meehan, 1969; see also Chapter 43)

With the patient in the left lateral position and after full aseptic precautions the sacral hiatus is identified using the left thumb which then acts as a marker. The Hingson and Edwards malleable needle is inserted in front of the thumb at a right angle to the skin over the sacrum. A distinct "give" is felt as the needle pierces the sacro-coccygeal ligament. The hub of the needle is then depressed towards the natal cleft so that the needle lies at an angle of 40° to the skin and the needle is gently advanced into the sacral canal. The stylet is withdrawn and an aspiration test carried out to ensure that the needle has not pierced the dura or a dural vein. A length of polyvinyl catheter is introduced through the needle which is then withdrawn over the catheter. A test dose of local analgesic (1 per cent lignocaine with 1 in 200,000 adrenaline) is injected. If, after five minutes, the patient can still move her legs, inadvertent subarachnoid block can be excluded. The main therapeutic dose of 16 to 20 ml. of local analgesic is then injected through the catheter and relief of pain becomes fully established within 10 to 20 minutes.

Alternative techniques would include the use of a rigid wide-bore needle through which a marked plastic epidural cannula similar to that used for lumbar blocks could be passed. Bupivacaine rather than lignocaine might be injected to give more prolonged analgesia (Yates and Kuah, 1968).

Difficulties

Some trouble may be encountered in identifying and penetrating the sacral hiatus owing to obesity, possible oedema and anatomical abnormalities. With the mother lying on her side gravity causes the soft parts to fall thus giving a false impression of the midline of the body. Moore (1961) overcomes these problems by meticulous marking of the posterior superior spines and the sacral cornua on the skin and inserting the caudal needle with the patient in the knee-elbow position.

Other difficulties arise from misplacement of the needle. Its point may lie superficially to the sacrum and injection will be seen to produce swelling under the skin. Subperiosteal injection will cause severe pain as the periosteum is stripped from the bone. More serious but rare complications have been reported due to the passage of the needle past the body of the 5th sacral vertebra into the rectum or even into the foetus (Finister *et al.*, 1965). When the needle is correctly placed in the sacral epidural space, injection of air or fluid should encounter no resistance.

Comparison of the Techniques of Lumbar and Caudal Epidural Analgesia

The two techniques have much in common. The indications for and contra-indications to their employment are identical. Similar side-effects and complications occur, and the same precautions should be taken in caring for the patient with either form of epidural analgesia.

However, important differences arise mainly because of the contrasted sites of injection. The sacrum is well known for its anatomical abnormalities; it may be bifid, or the sacral hiatus may be too small or obliterated by ossification of the sacro-coccygeal ligament. In these cases an attempt at caudal analgesia is likely to fail. Although rare, anatomical abnormalities occur in the lumbar spine, but the anaesthetist has a choice of lumbar interspaces through which he may attempt a second puncture if the first is unsuccessful. Similarly dural puncture through the caudal canal is usually regarded as a reason for abandoning the technique, while this same complication in the lumbar region need not preclude lumbar epidural analgesia being given through an adjoining interspace.

An obese, oedematous patient who may defy the anaesthetist's attempt to identify the sacral hiatus may still have easily palpable lumbar spines and cause no difficulty with the induction of lumbar epidural analgesia.

A feature of the descriptions of the technique of caudal analgesia is the invariable recommendation to give a test dose as a precaution against the effects of inadvertent dural puncture. Although the dural sac within the sacral canal may occasionally extend below the level of the body of the 2nd sacral vertebra, it is usually considered safe to advance the needle up to 5 cm. without fear of dural puncture. In the lumbar region the epidural space may be from 3 to 9 cm. from the surface and the distance from the ligamentum flavum to the dura is only 0·3 cm. to 0·5 cm. One would expect a higher frequency of inadvertent dural puncture at the hands of the inexpert, yet practitioners of lumbar epidural analgesia rarely recommend a test dose believing that dural puncture is surely followed by an obvious flow of cerebrospinal fluid through the Tuohy needle.

The site of injection for epidural analgesia through the caudal canal also influences the size of the dose required to block the lower thoracic segments. Meehan's dosage (1969) of 16 to 20 ml. of local analgesic solution is conservative in comparison with that of other authors and even he mentions toxic reaction to local analgesics as one of the complications of the method. Lumbar epidural analgesia may be achieved with only 5 to 7 ml. and toxic reactions are unlikely to occur unless injection is made directly into an epidural vein. A dose adequate to reach the lower thoracic segments is essential for total relief of labour pain. Smaller doses given caudally will produce perineal anaesthesia without necessarily relieving the pain of uterine contractions. Selectivity of block is impossible with caudal analgesia and a high frequency of assisted delivery has to be accepted.

Lastly a caudal injection has to be made through a potentially unhygienic area, and whatever measures are taken to seal the site of entry of the cannula in the sacral hiatus the dressings are liable to become contaminated during the course of labour. Moore (1961) recognises this difficulty and maintains the hygiene of the area of injection by keeping the mother turned on to her side throughout labour. Lumbar epidural analgesia may be induced and maintained with a far higher standard of hygiene.

Whichever method is used will depend on the predilection and training of the practitioner. The curious fact remains that, as judged by recent publications at least in the United Kingdom, caudal epidural analgesia appears to be practised and written about by obstetricians despite its difficulties and disadvantages (Yates and Kuah 1968; Stallworthy 1969; Meehan 1969). Lumbar epidural analgesia appears to be the preserve of the anaesthetist who would use the caudal route only if the lumbar approach were impracticable.

Paracervical Block

This is a comparatively simple technique for the relief of the pain of uterine contractions in the first stage of labour. It may be given from 5 cm. dilatation of the cervix and can be repeated provided that a rim of cervix is identifiable lateral to the foetal head. Local analgesic solution is injected into the pelvic cellular tissue at the base of the broad ligament where it spreads in the utero-vaginal plexus to block both the sympathetic and parasympathetic afferent pathways to the central nervous system (51/Fig. 2). The fact that its success is variable may be due to the alternative afferent pathway from the fundus of the uterus via the tubo-ovarian vessels, well away from the site of injection.

Cooper and Chassar Moir (1963) used a specially constructed guard-tube 14 cm. in length, the tip of which is manipulated to the top of each lateral vaginal fornix. A needle is inserted through the tube and is of such a length that it protrudes beyond it for not more than 7 mm. It should, therefore, just penetrate the vaginal wall; any further extension beyond the base of the broad ligament carries the risk of injection into the uterine vessels, the placental site and even into the foetus itself. The dose originally recommended was 10 ml. 1 per cent lignocaine with adrenaline 1 in 200,000 on each side of the cervix; this has now been superseded by bupivacaine 0·5 per cent with adrenaline 1 in 200,000 which gives a longer period of action (Cooper *et al.*, 1968). Yates (1969) found that lignocaine/adrenaline gave pain relief for a mean time of only 88 minutes as compared with a mean time of 144 minutes afforded by bupivacaine/adrenaline. Even so, this relatively short period of action is a disadvantage and a technique has been described for inserting Teflon cannulae into the paracervical tissues so that supplementary doses can be given with the waning of effect of the previous dose (Baggish, 1964).

Some anxiety has been expressed concerning foetal bradycardia which has been noted shortly after the injection. Unexpected deaths *in utero* and the death of an infant—affected during labour—in the neonatal period have been reported (Stern *et al.*, 1969). Early speculation was that the adrenaline given with the local analgesic to reduce its toxicity and to prolong its action might be responsible for the effect on the foetus by reducing the blood supply to the placental site (Crawford, 1963). More recently it has been suggested that bradycardia is the direct effect of the local analgesic on the foetal myocardium. Cord blood studies have shown that the injected drug can rapidly reach the foetal circulation from the highly vascular paracervical tissues (Shnider *et al.*, 1968). They showed that normally the umbilical vein: maternal artery concentration ratio was about 1:2; in foetal-bradycardia cases the ratio tended to be reversed. This could be explained only by injection into or near the intervillous space and it was felt that foetal bradycardia was due more to technical errors than to the method itself. Gomez (1969) cites these errors as firstly, the alignment of the needle guide parallel with the vaginal wall on the side to be injected instead of at the correct inclination, and secondly the mistaken belief that the depth of injection is limited by the 7 mm. of needle projecting from the tip of the guard-tube. Light pressure on a yielding fornix may carry it beyond the safety limits. He emphasises that a small dose (4–5 ml. 1 per cent lignocaine) given by an accurate technique is quite sufficient to relieve pain and will help to avoid the dangers to the foetus. He also warns that foetal bracycardia ascribed to paracervical block may be due to associated obstetric causes.

In the interest of limiting the dose of local analgesic given to the mother, Gudgeon (1968) used 0·25 per cent bupivacaine with 1 in 400,000 adrenaline; pain relief was obtained for 135 to 245 minutes—average time 3 hours—and no case of foetal bradycardia was reported. The complication of parametrial haematoma was avoided by injecting into the posterior part of the base of the broad ligament, i.e. at 4 and 8 o'clock rather than the more usual 3 and 9 o'clock.

Although paracervical block may be used from 5 cm. dilatation of the cervix, it is most useful towards the end of the first stage of labour as a means of removing the desire to bear down before the cervix is fully dilated. It will only relieve the pain of uterine contraction and if the patient complains of perineal discomfort, a pudendal nerve block should be performed to block the somatic afferent pathway to the sacral segments.

Paracervical block could be given by the obstetrician to tide the patient over her distress while awaiting the arrival of the anaesthetist to give epidural analgesia; indeed it is surprising that it is not used more frequently for this purpose as the block is given within the genital tract, an anatomical area with which the obstetrician is familiar.

REFERENCES

ABBAS, T. M. (1957). Clinical trial of glutethimide in labour. *Brit. med. J.*, **1**, 563.

BAGGISH, M. S. (1964). Continuous paracervical block. *Amer. J. Obstet. Gynec.*, **88**, 968.

BARACH, A. L., and ROVENSTINE, E. Q. (1945). The hazards of anoxia during nitrous oxide anesthesia. *Anesthesiology*, **6**, 449.

BEAZLEY, J. M., LEAVER, E. P., MOREWOOD, J. H. M., and BIRCUMSHAW, J. (1967). Relief of pain in labour. *Lancet*, **1**, 1033.

BODLEY, P. O., MIRZA, V., SPEARS, J. R., and SPILSBURY, R. A. (1966). Obstetric analgesia with methoxyflurane. *Anaesthesia*, **21**, 457.

BOISVERT, M., and HUDON, F. (1962). Clinical evaluation of methoxyflurane in obste rical anaesthesia: a report on 500 cases. *Canad. Anaesth. Soc. J.*, **9**, 325.

BRACKEN, A., BROUGHTON, G. B., and HILL, D. W. (1968). Safety precautions to be observed with cooled pre-mixed gases. *Brit. med. J.*, **3**, 715.

BROMAGE, P. R. (1954). *Spinal Epidural Analgesia.* Edinburgh: E. & S. Livingstone.

BROMAGE, P. R. (1961). Continuous lumbar epidural analgesia for obstetrics. *Canad. med. Ass. J.*, **85**, 1136.

BULLOUGH, J. (1960). Obstetric analgesia based on pethidine-antagonist mixtures. *Proc. roy. Soc. Med.*, **53**, 509.

CALDEYRO-BARCIA, R., ALVARES, H., and POSEIRO, J. J. (1955). The action of morphine upon uterine contractility in late pregnancy. *Amer. J. Obstet. Gynec.*, **84**, 281.

CAVENAGH, D., ALBORES, E. A., and TODD, J. (1966). Comparative effects of two benzodiazepine compounds on isolated human myometrium. *Amer. J. Obstet. Gynec.*, **94**, 6.

CHALMERS, J. A. (1949). Traumatic neuritis of the puerperium. *J. Obstet. Gynaec. Brit. Cwlth.*, **56**, 749.

CHALMERS, J. A. (1967). Diazepam as a myometrial relaxant. In *Fifth World Congress of Gynaecology and Obstetrics.* Sydney: Butterworths.

COLE, P. V. (1964). Nitrous oxide and oxygen from a single cylinder. *Anaesthesia*, **19**, 3.

COLE, P. V., and NAINBY-LUXMOORE, R. C. (1962). The hazards of gas and air in obstetrics. *Anaesthesia*, **1**, 505.

COOPER, K., and CHASSAR MOIR, J. (1963). Paracervical block. A simple method of pain relief in labour. *Brit. med. J.*, **1**, 1372.

COOPER, K., GILROY, K. J., and HURRY, D. J. (1968). Paracervical nerve block in labour using bupivacaine (Marcain). *J. Obstet. Gynaec. Brit. Cwlth.*, **75**, 863.

CRAWFORD, J. S. (1963). Paracervical nerve block. *Brit. med. J.*, **2**, 119.

CRAWFORD, J. S., ELLIS, D. B., HILL, D. W., and PAYNE, J. P. (1967). Effects of cooling on the safety of premixed gases. *Brit. med. J.*, **2**, 138.

CRAWFORD, J. S., and TUNSTALL, M. E. (1968). Notes on respiratory performance in labour. *Brit. J. Anaesth.*, **40**, 612.

DAVIDSON, J. A. (1962). An assessment of the value of hypnosis in pregnancy and labour. *Brit. med. J.*, **2**, 951.

DE VERE, R. D. (1969). Painful labour: modern methods of management. *Proc. roy. Soc. Med.*, **62**, 186.

DOUGHTY, A. (1969*a*). Painful labour: modern methods of management. *Proc. roy. Soc. Med.*, **62**, 189.

DOUGHTY, A. (1969*b*). Selective epidural analgesia and the forceps rate. *Brit. J. Anaesth.*, **41**, 1058.

DUNDEE, J. W., and LOVE, W. J. (1963). Alterations in response to somatic pain with anaesthesia: XIV. Effects of subnarcotic concentrations of methoxyflurane. *Brit. J. Anaesth.*, **35**, 301.

DUNDEE, J. W., and MOORE, J. (1961). The myth of phenothiazine potentiation. *Anaesthesia*, **16**, 95.

DUTHIE, A. M., WYMAN, J. B., and LEWIS, G. A. (1968). Bupivacaine in labour. *Anaesthesia*, **23**, 20.

EPSTEIN, H. G., and MACINTOSH, R. R. (1949). Analgesia inhaler for trichlorethylene. *Brit. med. J.*, **2**, 1092.

ESKES, T. K. A. B. (1962). Effect of morphine upon uterine contractility in late pregnancy. *Amer. J. Obstet. Gynec.*, **84**, 281.

FINSTER, M., POPPERS, P. J., SINCLAIR, J. C., MORISHIMA, H. O., and DANIEL, S. S. (1965). Accidental intoxication of the fetus with local anesthetic drug during caudal anesthesia. *Amer. J. Obstet. Gynec.*, **92**, 922.

GALE, C. W., TUNSTALL, M. E., and WILTON-DAVIES, C. C. (1964). Pre-mixed gas and oxygen for midwives. *Brit. med., J.*, **1**, 732.

GOMEZ, D. F. (1969). Paracervical block in obstetrics. *Lancet*, **1**, 1163.

GUDGEON, D. H. (1968). Paracervical block with bupivacaine 0·25 per cent. *Brit. med. J.*, **2**, 403.

HINGSON, R. A., and EDWARDS, W. B. (1942). Continuous caudal analgesia during labour and delivery. *Curr. Res. Anesth.*, **21**, 301.

JEFFCOATE, T. N. A. (1961). Prolonged labour. *Lancet*, **2**, 61.

JONES, P. L., ROSEN, M., MUSHIN, W. W., and JONES, E. V. (1969*a*). Methoxyflurane and nitrous oxide as obstetric analgesics. I—A comparison by continuous administration. *Brit. med. J.*, **3**, 255.

JONES, P. L., ROSEN, M., MUSHIN, W. W., and JONES, E. V. (1969*b*). Methoxyflurane and nitrous oxide as obstetric analgesics. II—A comparison by self-administered intermittent inhalation. *Brit. med., J.*, **3**, 259.

KANDEL, P. F., SPOEREL, W. E., and KINCH, R. A. H. (1966). Continuous epidural analgesia for labour and delivery: review of 1,000 cases. *Canad. med. Ass. J.*, **95**, 947.

LINDGREN, L. (1959). Influence of anaesthetics and analgesics on different types of labour. *Acta anaesth. scand.*, Suppl. **2**, 449.

MAJOR, V., ROSEN, M., and MUSHIN, W. W. (1966). Methoxyflurane as an obstetric analgesic: A comparison with trichloroethylene. *Brit. med. J.*, **2**, 1554.

MAJOR, V., ROSEN, M., and MUSHIN, W. W. (1967). Concentration of methoxyflurane for obstetric analgesia by self-administered intermittent inhalation. *Brit. med. J.*, **4**, 767.

MATTHEWS, A. E. B. (1963). Double-blind trials of promazine in labour. *Brit. med. J.*, **2**, 423.

MCANENY, T. M., and DOUGHTY, A. G. (1963). Self-administered nitrous oxide/oxygen analgesia in obstetrics. *Anaesthesia*, **18**, 488.

McGarry, J. A. (1969). Management of patients previously delivered by Caesarean section. *J. Obstet. Gynaec. Brit. Cwlth.*, **26,** 137.

Medical Research Council (1954). *The Use of Trilene by Midwives.* London: H.M.S.O.

Medical Research Council (1970). Clinical trials of different concentrations of oxygen and nitrous oxide for obstetric analgesia. *Brit. med. J.*, **1,** 709.

Meehan, F. P. (1969). Painful labour: modern methods of management. *Proc. roy. Soc. Med.*, **62,** 185.

Michael, A. M. (1952). Hypnosis in childbirth. *Brit. med. J.*, **1,** 734.

Minnitt, R. J. (1934). Self administered nitrous oxide and air. *Proc. roy. Soc. Med.*, **27,** 1313.

Moir, D. D., and Hesson, W. R. (1965). Dural puncture by an epidural catheter. *Anaesthesia*, **20,** 373.

Moir, D. D., and Willocks, J. (1967). Management of inco-ordinate uterine action under continuous epidural analgesia. *Brit. med. J.*, **3,** 396.

Moir, D. D., and Willocks, J. (1968). Epidural analgesia in British obstetrics. *Brit. J. Anaesth.*, **40,** 129.

Moore, D. C. (1961). *Regional Block*, 3rd edit., p. 349. Springfield, Ill.: Chas. C. Thomas.

Nainby-Luxmoore, R. C. (1964). Further hazards of gas and air in obstetrics. *Anaesthesia*, **19,** 421.

Noble, A. D., and De Vere, R. D. (1970). Epidural analgesia in labour. *Brit. med. J.*, **2,** 296.

Roberts, H., Kane, K. M., Percival, N., Snow, P., and Please, N. W. (1957). Effects of some analgesic drugs used in childbirth with special reference to variations in respiratory minute volume of the newborn. *Lancet*, **1,** 128.

Rorke, M. J., Davey, D. A., and du Toit, J. H. (1968). Foetal oxygenation during Caesarean section. *Anaesthesia*, **23,** 585.

Rosen, M., Mushin, W. W., Jones, P. L., and Jones, E. V. (1969). Field trial of methoxyflurane, nitrous oxide and trichloroethylene as obstetric analgesics. *Brit. med. J.*, **3,** 263.

Shnider, S. M., Asling, J. H., Margolis, A. J., Way, E. L., and Wilkinson, G. R. (1968). High foetal blood levels of mepivacaine and foetal bradycardia. *New. Engl. J. Med.*, **279,** 947.

Siker, E. S., Wolfson, D., Ciccarelli, H. E., and Telan, R. A. (1967). Effect of Subanesthetic concentrations of halothane and methoxyflurane on pain threshold in conscious volunteers. *Anesthesiology*, **28,** 337.

Siker, E. S., Wolfson, D., Dubnansky, J., and Fitting, G. M. (1968). Placental transfer of methoxyflurane. *Brit. J. Anaesth.*, **40,** 588.

Stallworthy, J. (1969). Active labour. *Brit. med. J.*, **2,** 630.

Stern, L., Outerbridge, E. W., and Fawcett, J. S. (1969). Paracervical block in obstetrics. *Lancet*, **2,** 322.

Tan, B. H., and Wood, C. (1967). The effect of heroin upon uterine contractility. Unpublished data quoted by Wood, C. (1969) in: *Modern Trends in Obstetrics*, p. 93. London: Butterworths.

Telford, J., and Keats, A. S. (1961). Narcotic-narcotic antagonist mixtures. *Anesthesiology*, **22,** 465.

Torda, T. A. G. (1963). The analgesic effect of methoxyflurane. *Anaesthesia*, **18,** 287.

Tunstall, M. E. (1961). Obstetric analgesia. The use of a fixed nitrous oxide and oxygen mixture from one cylinder. *Lancet*, **2,** 964.

Yates, M. J. (1969). Painful labour: modern methods of management. *Proc. roy. Soc. Med.*, **62,** 183.

Yates, M. J., and Kuah, K. B. (1968). Bupivacaine caudal analgesia in labour. *J. Obst. Gynaec. Brit. Cwlth.*, **75,** 749.

Chapter 53

ANAESTHESIA FOR OPERATIVE OBSTETRICS AND GYNAECOLOGY

by

ANDREW DOUGHTY

INTRODUCTION

A woman in labour needing an anaesthetic constitutes one of the most difficult practical problems of anaesthesia. Not only are there two lives to be considered, but either or both of these may already be jeopardised by disease or abnormal labour while some of the precautions usually taken before anaesthesia will of necessity be impracticable. Furthermore, these hazards may be accentuated by the unsatisfactory environment in which the procedure takes place and the absence of proper equipment. Yet anaesthesia, as Beecher and Todd (1954) have so aptly written, is an adjunct to the care of the patient, hardly ever an end in itself. A maternal death, however infrequently it may occur, is a disaster, not only because of its tragic social consequences, but also because it is unexpected and frequently avoidable.

The most widely known feature of these deaths is their common association with aspiration pneumonitis following vomiting or regurgitation during anaesthesia. Ideally, with the requisite precautions and facilities, and the skill and experience of the anaesthetist, the frequency of this complication should be minimised. If unhappily it should occur the failure to realise that pulmonary aspiration is an indication for intensive therapy may cost lives that otherwise might have been saved (McCormick, 1966; Adams *et al.*, 1969).

The Ministry of Health's *Report on Confidential Enquiries into Maternal Deaths in England and Wales* shows (Table 1) that during the years 1952–54 at least 49 maternal deaths could be attributed to anaesthesia. Of these, 32 were due to inhalation of stomach contents, and the remainder to various causes, including the effects of individual drugs such as chloroform, which accounted for 6 deaths (Ministry of Health, 1957). In the years 1955–57 there were 31 deaths due to anaesthesia, 18 of which were associated with vomited or regurgitated stomach contents (Ministry of Health, 1960). During 1958–60, 30 women died due to complications of anaesthesia, in 17 of whom vomiting or regurgitation accounted for death (Ministry of Health, 1963). Three others died after receiving chloroform, and two after halothane. Some of the remainder died following the use of muscle relaxants, but the actual cause of death was not clearly specified.

In the Report for 1961–63 (Ministry of Health, 1966) 28 deaths were considered to be due to complications of anaesthesia of which 16 were associated with inhalation of stomach contents. The Report specifically states "failure to intubate the trachea seemed to be the commonest fault, though this procedure, alone, is not an absolute safeguard. Sellick's manoeuvre (cricoid pressure) might have prevented regurgitation which occurred before intubation could be per-

53/TABLE 1

DEATHS ASSOCIATED WITH COMPLICATIONS OF ANAESTHESIA COMPARED WITH ALL DEATHS IN THE ENQUIRY SERIES AND WITH TOTAL MATERNITIES

		Deaths				
	Total maternities	*Due to pregnancy or child-birth*	*Associated with pregnancy or childbirth*	*Deaths associated with complications of anaesthesia in the enquiry series*	*Rate per 1,000 maternal deaths in the enquiry series*	*Rate per million maternities*
1952–54	2,052,953	1,094	316	49	34·8	23·9
1955–57	2,113,471	861	339	31	25·8	14·7
1958–60	2,294,414	742	254	30	30·1	13·1
1961–63	2,520,420	692	244	28	29·9	11·1
1964–66	2,600,367	579	176	50	66·2	19·2

formed. Amongst 16 women whose death was either certainly or probably due to inhalation of stomach contents, in only 5 was it recorded that tracheal intubation was a planned procedure during the induction of anaesthesia". Concerning the acid aspiration (Mendelson's) syndrome the Report states: "This was often not treated energetically enough. In particular, the injection of hydrocortisone was often delayed until symptoms had appeared, by which time it appeared to be ineffective".

The Report for 1964–66 (Ministry of Health, 1969) shows a disturbing rise in the number of deaths associated with the complications of anaesthesia. 50 deaths were reported of which 26 were considered to be due to the inhalation of stomach contents. During this period anaesthesia accounted for 6·6 per cent of all reported maternal deaths as compared with 3 per cent during the previous 12 years. This trend seems particularly regrettable when viewed against the overall decreasing maternal mortality and the decreasing mortality of anaesthesia for all other purposes. By contrast with the period 1961–63 there was no reported failure to intubate the trachea as a planned procedure although the technical difficulties of intubation were considered to have contributed to some maternal deaths. The Report states that the practice of inflating the lungs after paralysing the vocal cords is likely to encourage the entry of regurgitated material into the lung; and it concludes: "Patients with obstetric emergencies are gravely at risk and require the knowledge and the skill of an experienced anaesthetist who must be readily available".

This is a matter concerning maternal anaesthetic deaths that is not always sufficiently appreciated. Most fatalities can be attributed to a failure on the part of the anaesthetist rather than to any intrinsic danger in the drugs used. Evidence from the official report shows that while some avoidable deaths happen with specialist anaesthetists, the majority occur when an inexperienced anaesthetist is giving the anaesthetic. As the Report for 1964–66 states "The consultant anaesthetist must assume responsibility for errors made by junior members of his team unless they disobey his instructions, and for seeing that obstetric emergencies are not left to unsupervised members of his team". Quite apart from the expected lack of knowledge, dexterity and expertise of the inexperienced anaesthetist, he may not possess the authority or the determination to resist the pressure of obstetrical urgency in order to ensure that the anaesthetic apparatus is in working order ready for use, that the patient is taken down from the lithotomy position and that a working suction apparatus and personal assistance is at hand at least for the period of induction of anaesthesia. A clearer and more sympathetic understanding of the anaesthetist's problems by all who work in the labour ward would be a contribution to the safety of obstetrical anaesthesia.

It is worth noting that while figures are available concerning maternal mortality due to anaesthesia, little is known about the incidence of maternal morbidity, nor indeed of neonatal mortality and morbidity following its use. Thus vomiting may lead to complications of pulmonary aspiration which, while not always fatal to the mother, will cause a state of hypoxia that is rapidly passed on to the foetus. As our knowledge of such hazards increases, so possibly will the justification for an entirely specialised approach to obstetric anaesthesia.

EMERGENCY OBSTETRICS

Anaesthesia for Forceps Delivery

Local analgesia avoids most of the dangers, and when both practicable and desirable from the obstetric point of view it should be the method of choice. Nevertheless, a patient vomiting in the supine position may aspirate stomach contents even though fully conscious (Moya, 1960), and a heavily sedated patient in the same position must be at a considerably greater risk. Local analgesia is particularly useful when an experienced anaesthetist is not at hand or when the unsuitable environment or the inadequacy of the equipment available prejudice the safety of general anaesthesia. However, local analgesia may be contra-indicated either because of the intended obstetrical manoeuvre—intra-uterine manipulation, for instance—or by the lack of co-operation of the mother, so that there will always be occasions when a general anaesthetic is required. The safest results are then only to be achieved by ensuring that all those called upon to anaesthetise obstetric patients are competent to do so. Even so, equipment must to some extent condition the choice of general anaesthetic technique, since some essentials, such as a suction apparatus—that should always be present in the comparatively ideal circumstances of the hospital labour ward—will most certainly not normally be available in domiciliary practice. There is a strong case for the mandatory admission to hospital of all obstetric patients requiring a general anaesthetic. Where this is not possible reasonable safety depends on arrangements being made to transport all the necessary equipment to the patient's home in specially designed portable containers (Argent and Evans, 1961).

Local Analgesia

Simple infiltration or pudendal nerve block is employed for many obstetric procedures. Infiltration is suitable for episiotomy and the subsequent perineal repair. Pudendal nerve block enables the majority of forceps deliveries to be successfully performed, but where rotation of the head or difficulty in extraction is anticipated general or epidural anaesthesia should be preferred. The techniques of local analgesia are usually carried out by the obstetrician and they should be acquired by all doctors likely to practise obstetrics.

Trans-perineal pudendal nerve block.—The pudendal nerve can be blocked behind the ischial spine before it enters its canal in the wall of the ischio-rectal fossa. A skin weal is raised over the right ischial tuberosity, and through this a 10 cm. (4 inch) needle is inserted. The fingers of the right hand are placed in the vagina and the needle guided through the ischio-rectal fossa until its point lies above and behind the ischial spine where 10 ml. of 1 per cent lignocaine are injected. Pudendal nerve block must be combined with infiltration of the labium majus and the base of the clitoris to anaesthetise the terminal branches of the perineal branch of the posterior cutaneous nerve of the thigh and the ilio-inguinal nerve. The injections must be repeated on the left side.

Trans-vaginal pudendal nerve block.—This technique is performed with a guarded needle similar to that used for paracervical block (see p. 1438) the tip

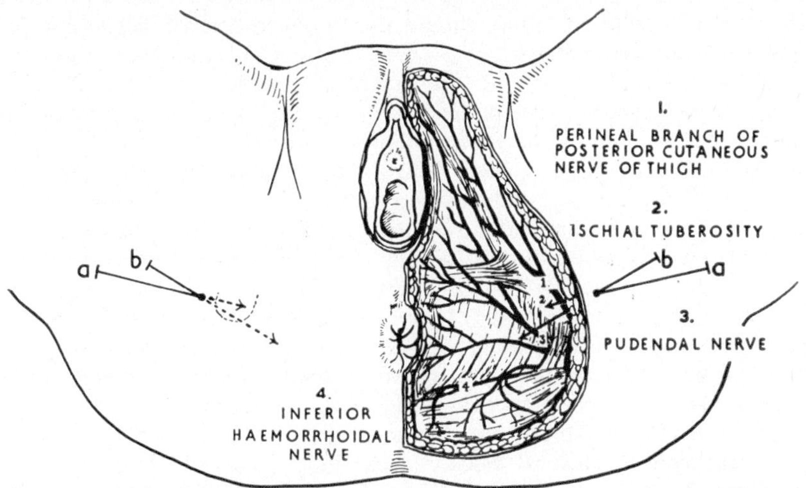

53/FIG. 1.—Diagram to illustrate nerve block of perineum and vulva.

of which is inserted just above and behind the ischial spine. The needle point is passed first through the vaginal mucous membrane and then through the sacrospinous ligament to the region of the pudendal nerve.

Infiltration analgesia.—As an alternative to nerve block, the branches of the pudendal nerve may be more simply infiltrated as they pass near the ischial tuberosity (Fig. 1). A skin weal should be raised over the tuberosity and the needle advanced on to its inferior aspect, where about 5 ml. of 1 per cent lignocaine solution should be injected to block the perineal branch of the posterior cutaneous nerve of the thigh. The needle is then passed medial to the tuberosity and, keeping close to the bone, into the ischio-rectal fossa for a distance of 2·5 cm. (1 inch), where a further 10 ml. of solution is placed so that it may diffuse around the inferior haemorrhoidal nerve and the termination of the pudendal nerve. The process is then repeated on the opposite side.

This form of local analgesic does not provide total block of all the sensation associated with forceps delivery and it does not relieve the pain of labour. Particular care must be taken to ensure that the pull of the forceps is synchronised with the mother's own voluntary efforts during the uterine contraction to avoid undue traction on the ligaments supporting the uterus. The whole procedure is best combined with inhalational analgesia, but as an alternative, a slow intravenous injection of 10 mg. diazepam ("Valium") with 30 mg. pentazocine ("Fortral") may be given until the mother becomes drowsy. However the full dose may be sufficient to induce brief unconsciousness in some mothers and even a moderate dose may lead to depression of the glottic reflex with consequent danger of pulmonary aspiration should vomiting occur.

Pethidine-phenothiazine mixtures given by slow intravenous injection have also been given to supplement local analgesia of the perineum. Holmes (1960) warns against this form of general analgesia in domiciliary practice for the single-handed obstetrician because of the occasional fall of blood pressure particularly in the hypertensive patient. The tendency of phenothiazines to block the vascular response to loss of blood volume should also be remembered if there is any degree of post-partum haemorrhage.

The fact that some form of supplementary general sedation and analgesia appears to be needed with pudendal block and local infiltration analgesia suggests that neither of these methods is adequate on their own to achieve comfortable conditions for forceps delivery. Scudamore and Yates (1966) found that only 36 per cent of pudendal nerve blocks achieved complete bilateral analgesia of the perineum and vulva and that of the two approaches, the trans-perineal route was far less successful than the transvaginal. They concluded that many so-called "pudendal" blocks must depend solely on local perineal and vulval infiltration for their effect. For operations involving more than a low forceps delivery they favour other forms of regional block or general anaesthesia. If this limitation of pudendal block were more widely appreciated, many mothers would be spared unnecessary pain when relatively complicated procedures are attempted under inadequate anaesthesia.

Subarachnoid or epidural block.—These blocks provide complete analgesia for forceps delivery without the need to sedate the mother. Both these techniques are relatively time-consuming and in practice the obstetric urgency rarely allows the anaesthetist the opportunity to carry out the injection with all the necessary aseptic precautions. Further delay is caused by the need to give the local analgesic time to act. The only advantage of subarachnoid over epidural block is the greater ease with which it can be performed by the inexperienced anaesthetist. Against this is the greater potential danger of a subarachnoid injection and the high incidence of headache that follows its use in obstetrics.

One of the attractive features of relieving labour pain by continuous epidural block is that the means of inducing analgesia for operative delivery is already present. The injection of a dose of local analgesic through the epidural cannula does not necessarily demand the presence of an anaesthetist. A wider use of the method simply for pain relief would diminish the frequency of the need for general anaesthesia.

General Anaesthesia

The problem might be summarised by saying that the anaesthetic technique, though comparatively simple in itself, is inevitably complicated by the need to guard against the aspiration of acid gastric contents into the lungs. The discussion of general anaesthesia for forceps delivery must centre around the numerous precautions which may be taken to reduce this risk.

Reduction of the quantity of stomach contents.—Normal pre-anaesthetic preparation by withholding food and drink for five hours is obviously impracticable for emergency obstetrical procedures, nor would it be good practice to attempt the enforcement of such a rule since the nutrition and hydration of the mother must be sustained. Moreover, most of the analgesic injections given to relieve pain exert a drying effect on the mucous membranes and the discomfort of a dry mouth is increased by the hyperventilation necessary to achieve successful inhalational analgesia. A sense of proportion must be maintained and only light and easily digested food given when labour is imminent and when labour has commenced small quantities of sweetened fluids only should be allowed. Even when no food has been taken for several hours the decreased gastric tone that occurs in labour may result in delay in the emptying of the stomach. Taylor and Pryse-Davies (1966) measured the quantity and pH of the gastric contents of 99 women who had been in active labour for at least 2 hours and who required general anaesthesia for obstetric surgery. In more than half of the patients the volume of gastric juice aspirated was in excess of 40 ml. The pH of the gastric contents even without artificial alkalinisation ranged from 1·25 to 8·20; neither the volume nor the pH of the gastric contents bore any relation to the length of labour. It follows that every woman needing an anaesthetic in labour must be assumed to have a full stomach of highly acid fluid contents.

To reduce the volume of gastric contents an attempt can be made to empty the stomach by the passage of a wide-bore oesophageal tube. Alternatively vomiting may be induced by the intravenous injection of 3 mg. of apomorphine (Holmes, 1957). This dose should be diluted in 10 ml. sterile water and injected slowly until just sufficient has been given to cause several effective vomits. It is rarely necessary to use the full dose and once vomiting starts atropine 1 mg. should be given intravenously. This not only antidotes the apomorphine but conveniently premedicates the patient for the subsequent general anaesthesia.

Both these methods of emptying the stomach have their advocates and one can respect the view of those who would use one or other on every patient needing general anaesthesia in labour as it is impossible to determine which patient has a full stomach and is liable to regurgitate or vomit during the induction. The protest that forcible emptying of the stomach by tube or by apomorphine-induced vomiting is distasteful and distressing to an already distressed mother may quite reasonably be countered by a reminder that these are precautions taken to protect the mother from avoidable death.

Although individual circumstances and experience may occasionally suggest otherwise, it is not our practice to empty the stomach of an obstetric patient before anaesthesia, but rather to regard her as an exception to the general rule regarding emergency operations and rely upon the technique of anaesthesia and the skill of the anaesthetist to avoid the hazards of pulmonary aspiration.

Alkalinisation of the gastric contents.—Taylor and Pryse-Davies (1966) repeated in rats the experiments originally carried out by Mendelson on rabbits (1946). They showed that lesions in the lungs comparable with those seen in Mendelson's syndrome could be produced by the instillation of hydrochloric acid or gastric juice into the trachea. The most severe damage was seen where the pH of the material instilled was below 1·75. Hydrochloric acid or gastric juice with a pH higher than this tended to produce only mild histological changes or in many cases no changes at all. Similar experiments were carried out on rats with hydrochloric acid and gastric juice neutralised with antacids. Magnesium trisilicate appeared to prevent severe pulmonary lesions while colloidal aluminium hydroxide did not give the same degree of protection. The reason for the difference was that the latter formed a gel which caused some bronchial obstruction.

In their investigations on emergency obstetric patients they found that in 42 per cent the pH of the gastric juice was less than 2·50 but that when given 14 ml. of magnesium trisilicate mixture (B.P.C.) the pH remained above this level for about 2 hours. Aluminium hydroxide was found to be less effective in maintaining the gastric juices at a pH above 2·50. It was therefore recommended that all patients requiring obstetric surgery under general anaesthesia should be given an oral antacid before operation to reduce the incidence of acid pulmonary aspiration. A dose of 14 ml. magnesium trisilicate mixture (B.P.C.) has been shown to be suitable for this purpose and should be given as soon as the decision is made to give the anaesthetic.

It should not be assumed that mere alkalinisation of the gastric contents renders their aspiration innocuous. The material may be solid and cause death by suffocation or to a lesser degree collapse of the lung, mediastinal shift and consolidation. Women delivered at the end of prolonged labour may have accumulated in the stomach large quantities of material with a high pH similar to that found in patients with bowel obstruction. Aspiration into the lungs may cause respiratory distress associated with severe endotoxin shock which may prove very difficult to treat successfully (Bosomworth and Hamelberg, 1962).

Anaesthetic technique and safety.—Faced with the problem of anaesthesia in a patient with a full stomach most anaesthetists instinctively turn to a technique which centres on the passage of a cuffed endotracheal tube to protect the lungs from the aspiration of gastric contents. It is therefore surprising that in the context of anaesthesia for emergency obstetrics the acceptance of an endotracheal technique is not universal especially in view of the criticisms made in the *Reports on Confidential Enquiries into Maternal Deaths*. However, Crawford (1965) states "We must soon seriously begin to question the applicability to newly developing countries of the methods of obstetric anaesthesia which we teach for 'home consumption' ". To some extent this counsel may apply more universally as long as experienced anaesthetists are not always available for emergency obstetrics. There may be circumstances where the occasional anaesthetist may be less dangerous using a simple technique rather than attempting to use methods which are safe only in the hands of the expert. The writer, while himself holding little brief for the avoidance of tracheal intubation, feels obliged to recognise that many responsible authors take an opposite view.

The safety of an intubation technique depends on three factors, the prevention of regurgitation or vomiting of gastric contents, the prevention of pulmonary aspiration and the intubation of the trachea as soon as possible following loss of consciousness. Unfortunately some of the precautions recommended are irreconcilable. While the theoretical and practical aspects of dealing with patients with a full stomach are dealt with in Chapter 47 their special application to women in labour is discussed in this chapter. Some repetition is therefore inevitable.

Prevention of regurgitation.—The force of gravity can be enlisted as an aid in the prevention of the passive regurgitation of gastric contents. Following O'Mullane's (1954) observation that even when the stomach is distended with fluid the intra-gastric pressure does not rise above 18 cm. of water, Snow and Nunn (1959) calculated that a 40° tilt from the horizontal would raise the larynx a vertical distance of 19 cm. above the cardio-oesophageal junction. This assumed that the distance between the two points in an adult is 25 cm. and that the oesophageal axis inclines 10° from the vertical axis of the body. This precaution presupposes that the patient is on a bed or operating table capable of being tilted to 40°. If regurgitation should occur the patient's safety depends on the table being tilted rapidly into the head-down position to enable the stomach contents to drain by gravity away from the larynx. Such tables have been designed by Wylie (1956), Steel (1961) and others. In the absence of such facilities there may be a tendency to pay only lip service to the need for a foot-down tilt and any tilt less than 40° would encourage regurgitated stomach contents to enter the trachea far more readily than if the patient were horizontal.

Another factor which may raise the intra-gastric pressure is the lithotomy position where the flexed thighs press against the gravid uterus (Spence *et al.*, 1967). The anaesthetist may find the patient in this position after the obstetrician has failed to extract the baby under a local anaesthetic. It often requires considerable persuasion to get the mother taken down from the lithotomy position before the anaesthetic is started. If regurgitation should occur in this position the delay involved in turning her to her side may prove fatal.

Clark and Riddoch (1962) observed that vagotomy increased the gastric opening pressure in 15 patients from 20 cm. to 55 cm. H_2O and a similar effect was found following intravenous atropine. This suggests that atropine given intravenously immediately before the induction of an obstetric anaesthetic may make a hitherto unappreciated contribution to its safety.

An important factor in the prevention of passive regurgitation of gastric contents into the pharynx is the use of backward pressure on the cricoid cartilage to compress the upper oesophagus against the cervical spine (Sellick, 1961). This implies the services of an assistant to apply the pressure while the anaesthetist is intubating the trachea. Unfortunately, in practice, there are occasions when this help is not readily forthcoming. The same assistant can contribute to the safety of the induction of anaesthesia not only by applying cricoid pressure with one hand but also by holding a working suction nozzle ready for use with the other.

Backward pressure on the cricoid cartilage has an incidental value in bringing the larynx into a better position for intubation, particularly in the patient with the more difficult oropharyngeal anatomy. However, if the manoeuvre is not correctly applied and the pressure is lateral rather than backward, intubation is made more difficult and the anaesthetist must guide the assistant's finger on the larynx into the position where it comes into view. Sellick has warned that should active vomiting occur during the manoeuvre the intra-oesophageal pressure may rise dangerously and tend to cause rupture of the oesophagus.

The muscle relaxant itself given to facilitate intubation is a factor which also facilitates passive regurgitation. In many women at the end of pregnancy it is thought that the cardiac sphincter becomes incompetent and when in the recumbent position the gastric contents are prevented from access to the pharynx solely by the tone of the cricopharyngeus muscle. Once this muscle relaxes there is no further obstruction to its flow into the pharynx. This fact underlines the importance of cricoid pressure, readily available suction and intubation without delay following the induction of anaesthesia when a relaxant technique is used.

It has been suggested that the muscular fasciculations caused by suxamethonium during the initial period of its action could temporarily raise the intra-gastric pressure. Whether this would be a significant factor with the abdominal muscles well stretched by the gravid uterus is a matter for surmise.

Prevention of vomiting.—Active vomiting of the stomach contents as distinct from their passive regurgitation is more frequently a hazard of the induction or recovery stage of inhalational anaesthesia without intubation. The anaesthetic agent, ether, trichloroethylene or cyclopropane, may be responsible as may the premature insertion of the oro-pharyngeal airway before the vomiting reflex has been suppressed. The anaesthetist's dilemma at this point is that the insertion of an oral airway may cause vomiting, coughing or laryngeal spasm during an inhalational induction, and yet the mother's nasal mucosa may be so congested as to block the airway through the nose. A shortened well-lubricated naso-pharyngeal tube of relatively small bore, say 5–6 mm., should be inserted as a temporary means of overcoming respiratory obstruction until the patient will tolerate an oral airway. A tube of larger bore inserted through the nose may cause considerable bleeding.

It must not be assumed that active vomiting on induction occurs solely with an inhalational non-relaxant technique. The hasty insertion of the laryngoscope into the pharynx before the relaxant has had time to become effective may also be responsible.

Prevention of aspiration of stomach contents into the lungs.—It has already been pointed out that although a head-up tilt to 40° may help to prevent regurgitation, this same posture will facilitate the access of gastric contents to the trachea if they should rise to the pharynx. By the same token the head-down position would tend to encourage the drainage of the regurgitated or vomited stomach contents from the pharynx away from the glottis and safety would be improved if the patient were also on her side. Adequate help for the anaesthetist and a working suction apparatus is of the greatest importance at this stage.

Deaths have occurred due to aspiration of stomach contents during recovery from the anaesthetic. To prevent this the passage of a wide bore stomach tube during anaesthesia is recommended. The patient should recover from the anaesthetic on her side on a tilting bed and under the personal supervision of the anaesthetist or an experienced nurse armed with a suction apparatus. Rapid return of consciousness and the shortening of the necessary period of close supervision of the patient is one of the advantages of a relaxant, intubation, nitrous oxide method as distinct from a purely inhalational technique with more potent agents.

Another cause of aspiration of stomach contents is the practice of oxygenating the patient by positive pressure following induction of anaesthesia and muscle paralysis. Any regurgitated stomach contents would then be pushed into the trachea through the relaxed vocal cords. When a relaxant technique is used the patient should be given pure oxygen to breathe for three minutes before induction of anaesthesia. Her apprehension at having a mask held over her face may be dispelled by telling her that she is breathing oxygen for the benefit of her baby.

Elimination of delay in intubation.—The main objection to an endotracheal technique is that the most dangerous period of the anaesthetic is that between the loss of consciousness and the attempt to intubate the trachea. Indeed some authors have been at pains to recommend an inhalational technique with a mask applied to the face and suggest that it is safe provided that the patient is anaesthetised in the lateral position with the head down, that the obstetrician can be persuaded to apply the forceps in this position, that the mask is not strapped on to the face and that the anaesthetic is continued until the operation is completed. It may be true that this could be the safest course where the anaesthetist is unskilled but in view of the criticisms implied in the *Report on Confidential Enquiries into Maternal Deaths* it might be legally difficult for a specialist anaesthetist to defend in court this choice of technique in an obstetric patient.

Where an intubation technique is used it is essential to take all possible steps to ensure that the interval between loss of consciousness and intubation is reduced to the minimum and that there is no avoidable delay in passing the endotracheal tube. At this point the anaesthetist may reflect whether gross anatomical abnormalities in the mother may cause a dangerous delay of intubation and unsuccessful attempts to pass the tube may result in greater hazard than a straightforward inhalational induction by mask alone. The short mandible, prominent teeth, high arched palate, the short, thick neck and the inability to extend the neck and open the mouth widely are warning signs of likely difficulty. Yet these are also the signs which warn the anaesthetist of difficulty with the airway if a tube were not passed. In short the patient with the well-recognised difficult anatomical features would give trouble with either method of anaesthesia, but once a tube is passed into the trachea most of the difficulties are solved. The temptation to opt for intubation is therefore overwhelming.

To minimise the hazardous induction-intubation time the patient should be given pure oxygen to breathe for three minutes before induction, a diaphragm needle fixed into a vein and atropine 0·6 mg. followed by 100 mg. methohexitone injected. Methohexitone is preferred to thiopentone because of its shorter recovery time. As soon as consciousness is lost suxamethonium 100 mg. is given. The relatively large dose is required to ensure total relaxation and hence near perfect conditions for an easy intubation. One must be certain that the potency of the suxamethonium has not diminished as a result of being kept unrefrigerated.

In an operating theatre the rapid turnover in the use of the drug ensures that the suxamethonium available is likely to be of near maximum potency. In an obstetric department, with its relatively infrequent use, suxamethonium kept in a multi-dose vial on the anaesthetic machine without the precaution of refrigeration is liable to serious deterioration in potency.

If the patient is to be intubated with the minimum of delay she should be placed in a position most advantageous and familiar to the anaesthetist. A steep head-up position to prevent regurgitation, a head-down or lateral position to reduce the chance of aspiration of stomach contents tend to make a rapid intubation more difficult. The relaxation of the cricopharyngeus muscle with the patient in the head-down position may result in a flood of gastric contents which will occupy the anaesthetist's whole attention before intubation is possible. If speed of intubation is considered important the patient should be in the horizontal position with the neck flexed and the head extended. Cricoid pressure should be applied and the laryngoscope inserted with the onset of muscular relaxation.

Selection of the correct size of tube is important for ensuring a rapid intubation. Owing probably to the retention of fluid in the tissues in late pregnancy, the size of the glottis appears to be reduced. While a 9 mm. cuffed tube would be expected to pass through the vocal cords in the non-pregnant woman, attempts to pass a tube of this size in the parturient woman may only lead to dangerous delay. Accordingly a 8 mm. tube should be selected initially and one of 7·5 mm. size should be ready for use if the larger size will not pass.

The failure of the laryngoscope light at the moment of intubation may be a further cause of delay. It follows that the instrument should be tested before use, and as a counsel of perfection a second tested laryngoscope should be immediately at hand. A further safety factor is the rapid inflation of the tube cuff as soon as possible after intubation and there is much to be said for the use of the self-sealing valve on the cuff. The tube can be passed with the inflating syringe attached to the pilot tube.

If any anatomical abnormality is likely to prevent the rapid passage of the tube, a malleable stylet may be useful and should be ready for use.

In an attempt to reduce the induction-intubation time it has been suggested that the intravenous barbiturate and the suxamethonium should be mixed and injected together rather than in succession. If the mixture is used freshly prepared there is no clinical evidence of loss of potency of the relaxant. However some patients may complain afterwards of the unpleasant sensation of the onset of paralysis before loss of consciousness.

Maintenance of anaesthesia.—Nitrous oxide and oxygen 50:50 with up to 0·5 per cent halothane normally suffices to maintain anaesthesia for a forceps delivery. If muscle relaxation with control of respiration is required intermittent injections of suxamethonium are given through the previously inserted diaphragm needle. Avoidance of a deeper level of anaesthesia ensures a rapid recovery of consciousness, thus diminishing the time that the mother is at risk.

Safety during recovery.—Anaesthesia must be continued until the operation has been completed and the patient has been taken down from the lithotomy position. The patient should recover under close supervision lying on her side on a tilting bed with a working suction apparatus at hand. A wise precaution against aspiration of stomach contents and difficulty with the airway is to leave the endotracheal tube in place until the recovery of consciousness. This should not be long delayed if anaesthesia has been maintained at a light level.

Recommended technique for general anaesthesia.—It cannot be too strongly emphasised that safety in operative obstetric anaesthesia lies in the wider use of local analgesic techniques so that the dangers of general anaesthesia can be avoided. In this connection Jamieson (1963) and Newland (1969) have reported a need for general anaesthesia in only 5 per cent and 8 per cent respectively of forceps deliveries. The diversity of sometimes irreconcilable opinions concerning general anaesthesia for forceps delivery is sufficient evidence that no single technique on its own can guarantee safety to the mother and baby. Nothing can substitute for the skill, judgment, experience and dexterity of the individual anaesthetist. Subject to these reservations the following standard technique is recommended. The patient lies horizontally on a bed capable of being tilted head-down. Following a dose of 14 ml. magnesium trisilicate mixture the patient is given pure oxygen to breathe for three minutes. An assistant is at hand to apply cricoid pressure and to hold a working sucker ready for use. A diaphragm needle is inserted into a convenient vein. Intravenous atropine 0·6 mg. is given followed by methohexitone 100 mg. and refrigerated suxamethonium 100 mg. The assistant applies cricoid pressure as consciousness is lost. The patient is intubated with an 8 mm. cuffed endotracheal tube and the cuff is inflated. Anaesthesia is maintained with nitrous oxide, oxygen and a trace of halothane. The patient is turned to her side at the end of the operation before anaesthesia is allowed to lighten. She recovers under close supervision and the cuffed tube is not removed until she regains consciousness.

Equipment.—The obstetric anaesthetist is expected to be both safe and speedy and much depends on his finding well-maintained equipment and the necessary drugs immediately to hand on his arrival in the labour ward together with an assistant prepared to help him during the critical first few minutes of the anaesthetic. A well-organised purpose-designed anaesthetic trolley cuts down unnecessary delay in finding and fitting together the necessary equipment. Indeed with such a system the patient can often be ready for the operation more quickly than if a simpler purely inhalational technique were used. In emergency obstetrics the anaesthetist is often under undue pressure to be speedy and this pressure is often accentuated by the fact that the obstetrician is necessarily present before the anaesthetist. Under no circumstances should the anaesthetist allow himself to be pressed into a hurried induction of anaesthesia without taking the time to check that all the equipment is ready and that safety precautions have been observed.

Treatment of Pulmonary Aspiration (Mendelson's) Syndrome

Diagnosis.—Acid pulmonary aspiration should be suspected following any obstetric general anaesthetic if the patient shows symptoms similar to those of an acute asthmatic attack with cyanosis, tachycardia, tachypnoea and hypotension with wheezes, rales and rhonchi heard over the affected areas of the lungs. Should the symptoms have arisen following vomiting or regurgitation of stomach contents during anaesthesia the diagnosis is seldom in doubt but severe symptoms requiring intensive therapy have been reported following an apparently uneventful anaesthetic (McCormick *et al.*, 1966). The onset of symptoms may be immediate or may be delayed until some hours later when a sense of false security may have been induced.

Management of aspiration of stomach contents.—If pulmonary aspiration is suspected the patient should be placed head down on her right side to provide postural drainage. Following intubation with a sterile cuffed tube and rapid suction of the trachea and bronchi, the lungs should be ventilated with pure oxygen. Hydrocortisone 300 mg. should be given intravenously followed by 100 mg. 6-hourly intramuscularly.

If symptoms and signs are minimal, no further treatment is required beyond careful surveillance against the later development of severe respiratory distress. If there is bronchospasm, semi-coma, persistent hypotension and peripheral cyanosis despite the inhalation of pure oxygen, the patient should be paralysed with pancuronium and mechanically ventilated with oxygen. Very high inflation pressures may be required owing to a greatly reduced lung compliance (Adams *et al.*, 1969). If pulmonary oedema develops, it must be treated by aspiration and diuretics. Cardiac failure may be improved by intravenous digoxin. The patient's acid-base state must be assessed and any base deficit corrected with intravenous sodium bicarbonate. As the use of hydrocortisone tends to prevent the normal response to secondary bacterial infection a broad spectrum antibiotic such as ampicillin should be given.

Bronchoscopy.—There may be a temptation to aspirate gastric contents from the lungs by bronchoscopy. In unskilled hands this procedure is extremely hazardous in a hypoxic patient and in any case the amount of material which can be aspirated is small as any liquid matter will already have been absorbed from the bronchial lumen. Bronchoscopic aspiration is only indicated where the bronchi are obstructed by solid matter, that is when the hazards of the procedure are outweighed by the danger of its omission.

Pulmonary lavage.—Lavage of the lungs with large volumes of bicarbonate or saline to neutralise or dilute the acid has been recommended as a valuable therapeutic measure. However Bannister *et al.* (1961) have shown that this may cause the further spread of acid to areas of the lung hitherto unaffected by increasing its volume, while Hamelberg and Bosomworth (1964) believe that the spread of the acid is so rapid that it would not be neutralised by the subsequent lavage with an alkaline solution.

In conclusion McCormick (1966) states "The emphasis should clearly be upon prevention of pulmonary aspiration. When aspiration occurs, a plan of management must be initiated to save the mother's life. If the initial asphyxia can be overcome, adequate therapy will ensure survival of most patients".

ANAESTHESIA FOR CAESAREAN SECTION

General anaesthesia for Caesarean section involves consideration of both maternal and foetal welfare. While preoccupation with the problems posed by the full stomach do not arise to the same extent in the elective operation, the precautions as detailed for a forceps delivery must be taken when the operation is performed as an emergency. A technique using an intravenous barbiturate, muscle relaxant and tracheal intubation followed by IPPV with nitrous oxide and oxygen is widely used. This method enjoys a well-merited popularity because it can provide light narcosis with minimal central depression and full oxygenation of the infant. Nevertheless over the past few years there have been reservations expressed concerning its uncritical acceptance.

The misgivings arise principally from the reports of return to consciousness of the paralysed patient under very light anaesthesia during the operation and the possible harm to the foetus of anaesthesia supplemented by deliberate hyperventilation of the mother.

Awareness during Anaesthesia

The occurrence of awareness under nitrous oxide-oxygen-relaxant anaesthesia for general surgery was reported by Hutchinson (1961). Enquiry was made of 656 patients and 8 appeared to have "dreams" connected with events in the operating theatre. Although no obstetric patients were included in the series all were women and all but one had received an opiate premedication. It was felt that the most likely causes were an inadequate nitrous oxide percentage in the inspired gas mixture and the failure to achieve the degree of hyperventilation necessary to produce the hypnotic effect of hypocapnia. Wilson and Turner (1969) reported factual recall by 3 out of 150 patients for elective and emergency Caesarean section. A larger number complained of disturbing dreams making a total of 26 who had an unpleasant recall of their experience. Hyperventilation did not reduce its incidence and oxygen "flushing" at the time of delivery surprisingly did not increase the frequency of unpleasant recall. The only significant factor was that it occurred more in the elective than in the emergency group. The elective patients had received no narcotic as premedication but a high proportion of the emergencies had received an opiate during labour before the operation. It was concluded that potent premedication was still appropriate in patients undergoing nitrous oxide-relaxant anaesthesia for Caesarean section. As respiratory depressant drugs are contra-indicated it was suggested that benzodiazepine drugs might be suitable although the same authors in a later publication showed that diazepam appeared to increase the frequency of unpleasant recall (Turner and Wilson, 1969).

An alternative approach in preventing unpleasant recall might be to use hyoscine as premedication and low concentrations of trichloroethylene during anaesthesia both of which have well-recognised amnesic properties (Lambrechts and Parkhouse, 1961). There seems little harm in supplementing nitrous oxide with *very low* concentrations of more potent volatile anaesthetics in order to make more sure of the mother's unconsciousness during the early part of the operation particularly if oxygen-rich gas mixtures are given for the benefit of the foetus.

Foetal Oxygenation during Caesarean Section

Oxygenation of the infant is the most important single factor bearing on its well-being following delivery by Caesarean section. While some degree of foetal hypoxia may on occasion be related to placental insufficiency, the anaesthetist is responsible for maintaining adequate oxygenation of the mother during the critical induction-delivery interval.

The effect of varying concentrations of oxygen in the inspired mixture given to 34 women undergoing Caesarean section has been examined by Rorke *et al.* (1968) (Table 2). The patients were divided into three groups according to

53/TABLE 2

Maternal Inspired O_2 Concentration	*Maternal Pa_{CO_2}*	*Umbilical Pv_{CO_2}*	*Umbilical Pa_{CO_2}*
33 per cent	25·8	38·8	46·3
67 per cent	29·0	42·6	48·8
100 per cent	31·7	48·7	59·1

The effect on carbon dioxide tensions in the maternal and foetal circulation of increasing the inspired oxygen percentages (after Rorke *et al.*, 1968).

whether they received 33 per cent, 67 per cent, or 100 per cent oxygen with a muscle relaxant and IPPV technique. These inspired concentrations of oxygen resulted in mean maternal P_{O_2} levels of 135, 255 and 439·5 mm. Hg respectively. Unconsciousness was assured by adding 2 per cent ether or 0·3 per cent methoxyflurane to the gas mixture. The mean induction-delivery time was over 45 minutes. Samples of blood for oxygen and carbon dioxide tensions together with acid-base values were taken from the maternal radial artery, from the foetal scalp immediately before delivery and from the umbilical artery and vein immediately after delivery. The findings can be summarised as follows:

1. The umbilical vein P_{O_2} increased as the maternal P_{O_2} rose to 300 mm. Hg. Further increase in maternal P_{O_2} resulted in a fall in the umbilical vein P_{O_2}. This supports the findings in animal experiments by Dawes and Mott (1964) that an increase in maternal oxygen tension may alter the blood flow in the placental vessels in order to protect the foetus against excessively high oxygen tensions.

2. Despite ventilation of the mother at 12 litres/minute the maternal P_{CO_2} only fell significantly from the pre-operative level in the group receiving 33 per cent oxygen in the inspired gases and then only by 4 mm. Hg. This correlates with the findings by Scott *et al.* (1969) that it is difficult to produce respiratory alkalosis by mechanical ventilation in obstetric patients.

3. Despite efforts to maintain comparable ventilatory control in all three groups, the maternal P_{CO_2} rose with the percentage of oxygen in the inspired mixture. The rise of P_{CO_2} in the umbilical vein and artery rose disproportionately more than the maternal arterial P_{CO_2}. This suggests that very high oxygen tensions in the mother interferes with the elimination of carbon dioxide by the placenta.

4. The Apgar scores of infants born of mothers given 67 per cent oxygen were significantly higher than of those given 33 per cent. There was no further improvement in the state of the infants born of mothers given 100 per cent oxygen, in fact a reverse tendency was noted.

5. The umbilical vein P_{O_2} and the Apgar score improved with a rise of the maternal P_{CO_2} to an optimal level of 32–34 mm. Hg, that is, approximately the pre-operative level. Above this level there was a decrease in the umbilical venous P_{O_2}.

The results of this work suggest that the ideal anaesthetic technique should attempt to achieve in the mother's arterial blood an oxygen tension of 300 mm.

Hg and carbon dioxide tension of 32–34 mm. Hg and that as long as the anaesthetic gas mixture is rich in oxygen there is no merit in oxygen "flushing" before delivery. The best results are obtained when the maternal P_{CO_2} is near the pre-operative level so that hyperventilation is contra-indicated. Unconsciousness in the mother is assured by the addition of low concentrations of volatile agents which appeared to have no adverse effect on the infant despite a background of relatively slow surgery.

Hyperventilation and Foetal Welfare

Some doubt has been cast on the safety to the foetus of hyperventilation of the mother during anaesthesia for Caesarean section. Holmes (1963) compared the CO_2 content of blood in the umbilical vein of 40 babies born by abdominal delivery in which the anaesthetic techniques were designed to produce:

Group 1. Respiratory acidosis without central depression, namely spontaneous respiration with sub-apnoeic doses of tubocurarine, nitrous oxide and oxygen.

Group 2. Respiratory acidosis with central depression, namely inadequate IPPV, with tubocurarine and cyclopropane.

Group 3. Respiratory alkalosis without central depression namely, hyperventilation, suxamethonium, nitrous oxide and oxygen with CO_2 absorption.

Group 4. Normal respiratory environment as a control. Local analgesia.

10 cases were allocated to each group.

As expected, it was found that the CO_2 content of the umbilical vein blood was higher in Groups 1 and 2 where the anaesthetic technique produced maternal respiratory acidosis than in the control Group 4. Where the anaesthetic technique produced respiratory alkalosis (Group 3) the umbilical vein blood CO_2 content was lower than the control. The time from delivery of the infant to establishment of spontaneous respiration was within 10 seconds in all cases in Group 1 but was considerably delayed in Group 3 in which only one infant out of 10 breathed spontaneously within one minute. Central depression accounted for some delay in Group 2 while in the control group the onset of respiration was immediate in 7 out of 10 cases. It was therefore concluded that respiratory alkalosis might be a factor in retarding the onset of regular respiration in the baby.

Motoyama *et al.* (1966) observed that the umbilical vein P_{O_2} was significantly lower when the maternal P_{CO_2} was low than when it was raised. This finding was confirmed by experiments on pregnant sheep by direct comparison of maternal arterial P_{CO_2} against samples taken from the foetal carotid artery. Moya *et al.* (1965) confirm that moderate hyperventilation with slight lowering of the maternal P_{CO_2} can reduce the degree of foetal acidosis but this did not improve the condition of the infant as judged by the Apgar score. Increasing degrees of hyperventilation interfered with the exchange of blood gases across the placenta, producing severe foetal metabolic acidosis and thus adversely affecting the state of the baby at birth. Moya *et al.* suggest that the critical level of maternal arterial P_{CO_2} is 17 mm. Hg; below this there is likely to be sufficient foetal acidosis to delay the onset of respiration.

Coleman (1967) questioned whether maternal hypocapnia was harmful to babies delivered by Caesarean section. Eighteen mothers in early labour were anaesthetised by a thiopentone, relaxant and hyperventilation technique. Immediately before delivery the mean maternal arterial pH was 7·618 and the mean arterial P_{CO_2} 15·7 mm. Hg. The mean pH of the umbilical vein blood at delivery was 7·31 and the mean P_{CO_2} 36·3 mm. Hg. In these cases therefore marked maternal respiratory alkalosis was not matched by a comparable foetal respiratory alkalosis. Three infants who were judged clinically to have respiratory depression at birth had blood values similar to those of their clinically normal fellows. It was concluded that there was no reason to forego the valuable technique of "hypocapnic enhancement" of nitrous oxide anaesthesia in obstetrics on the grounds of possible harm to the infant.

Scott *et al.* (1969), in seeking to reconcile these opposing views, found that while they could confirm that foetal acid-base status moved in the same direction as that of the mother, the high inflationary pressures required to produce hyperventilation during anaesthesia could cause a reduction in cardiac output by as much as 50 per cent. An additional factor in causing interference with placental circulation could be a coincidental tendency to inferior vena caval occlusion (supine hypotensive syndrome). They concluded that in spite of the possible dangers of a hypocapnic technique the method appeared in practice to be free from deleterious effects on the infants. This could be due to the fact that adverse effects, if any, were not operating for a sufficiently long time to produce irreversible foetal hypoxia. Light general anasthesia with controlled ventilation was a safe and useful method for Caesarean section, provided that excessive inflationary pressures were avoided, that the maternal P_{CO_2} did not fall below 20 mm. Hg, that delivery of the child was not unduly delayed by slow surgery and that allowance was made for other forms of coincidental circulatory embarrassment.

Moir (1970*a*) recognising the need to avoid depression of the foetus, excessive blood loss and awareness in the mother during operation compared the effects of anaesthesia with thiopentone, relaxant and nitrous oxide/oxygen unsupplemented and supplemented with 0·5 per cent or 0·8 per cent halothane. Extreme hyperventilation was avoided, the minute volumes imposed by the respirator being 7 to 8 litres/min.

The findings were that mothers given unsupplemented nitrous oxide/oxygen 70:30 were delivered of more depressed babies and lost more blood than those given nitrous oxide/oxygen 50:50 supplemented with halothane. In addition 2 out of 50 mothers given no supplement had definite unpleasant recall of events when they were supposed to be unconscious. The disadvantage of 0·8 per cent halothane as compared with 0·5 per cent was the higher frequency of maternal hypotension. In a parallel series of Caesarean sections epidural analgesia was given to 20 patients using 12 to 14 ml. of 2 per cent lignocaine with adrenaline. In these cases the blood loss was half that caused by operation under unsupplemented nitrous oxide/oxygen anaesthesia and the frequency of undue hypotension was not increased.

Recommended Technique

Following the precautions against the dangers of pulmonary aspiration of stomach contents detailed on p. 1447 *et seq.*, the patient should be pre-oxygenated for three minutes. Anaesthesia is induced with intravenous atropine, thiopentone

200–250 mg., followed by suxamethonium 100 mg. The mask is removed without positive pressure inflation of the lungs and the trachea intubated as soon as possible after the onset of relaxation. The patient is ventilated mechanically at an expired minute volume of 6–8 litres/min. with nitrous oxide/oxygen 50:50 supplemented with 0·5 per cent halothane. An infusion of compound sodium lactate solution is set up as a convenient channel for rapid transfusion and for the administration of drugs. A litre of cross-matched blood should have been prepared before the operation. Apnoea is maintained with intermittent or continuous suxamethonium or a dose of non-depolarising relaxant. As the baby's head is delivered 0·5 mg. ergometrine is given intravenously and once the cord is clamped 20 mg. papaveretum is given to obtain some post-operative analgesia. The anaesthetist may then resuscitate the infant if necessary. At this stage a blood loss of 300–500 ml. may be accepted as normal and should not require replacement owing to the autotransfusion by the contracting uterus. Undue alarm should not be taken at the quantity of bloody fluid in the sucker bottle as the major part of this is likely to be liquor amnii. On the other hand a massive blood loss must be restored by a massive transfusion with due regard to warming the transfused blood, central venous pressure monitoring, and replenishment of the loss of ionised calcium with calcium gluconate.

When epidural analgesia has been used for the relief of pain in labour, Caesarean section may be performed without any further action on the part of the anaesthetist as long as the level of loss of skin sensation extends above the umbilicus. The epidural cannula should remain in place and a further injection can be given at the end of the operation to ensure post-operative analgesia. Normally patients with an epidural block prefer to be unconscious during abdominal surgery and the simplest method of achieving this is by thiopentone, suxamethonium, endotracheal nitrous oxide/oxygen 50:50 and 0·5 per cent halothane with spontaneous respiration. However, epidural analgesia might be considered inadvisable if the patient has shown a marked tendency to supine hypotension during labour.

An elective Caesarean section may be carried out in the conscious patient following an epidural injection of 15 ml. 0·5 per cent bupivacaine in the horizontal position. A cannula should always be inserted for supplementary dosage in case the initial injection does not give complete analgesia.

ELECTIVE OBSTETRIC PROCEDURES

External Cephalic Version

Conversion of a breech presentation to a vertex is usually carried out between the 32nd and 36th week of pregnancy. This is nearly always achieved without an anaesthetic but success depends on the mother being able voluntarily to relax her abdominal muscles. After the 36th week of pregnancy the uterus becomes increasingly irritable until labour actually starts. Irrespective of the mother's ability to remain relaxed during the procedure the uterine contractions prevent the success of the procedure. Even with an anaesthetic, attempts at version may not succeed owing to intra-uterine causes such as extended legs of the foetus, an unduly short cord, a large fibroid, septate uterus or deficient quantity of liquor.

The anaesthetist must be prepared to provide complete relaxation of the abdominal musculature and, if uterine contractions impede the obstetrician's efforts, to relax the uterus with deep general anaesthesia. The patient should be premedicated with papaveretum-hyoscine and lie on a bed with a 15° downward tilt to help lift the breech out of the pelvis. Before induction of anaesthesia the obstetrician should check that the breech is still presenting and that a spontaneous version has not occurred. He may find that under the premedication version without anaesthesia may be possible. Anaesthesia is induced with methohexitone, suxamethonium and tracheal intubation. During the short period of skeletal muscle relaxation the obstetrician may succeed in turning the child or may decide that excessive uterine tone is frustrating his efforts. Uterine relaxation with halothane or ether is then provided although this may take 10–15 minutes to achieve if the uterus is particularly irritable.

Complications of external version include foetal distress or detachment of the placenta with ante-partum haemorrhage. The anaesthetist should remain in the vicinity for a short while in case an emergency Caesarean section is indicated.

Induction of Labour

When anaesthesia is required for this procedure no premedication is required and the membranes may be ruptured under methohexitone, nitrous oxide/oxygen and halothane. Normally simple amniotomy can be performed without an anaesthetic but its use is justified if the obstetrician wishes to stretch the cervix and "sweep" the membranes.

OPERATIVE OBSTETRICS AND HALOTHANE

In the early years of its use an anaesthetic, halothane gained a reputation as a potent myometrial relaxant and neonatal depressant when used for operative obstetrics. Experience showed that the uterine response to ergometrine was abolished and post-partum haemorrhage was increased. Infants born following halothane anaesthesia were more depressed than those delivered following a nitrous oxide/oxygen-relaxant sequence (Montgomery, 1961). Further work by Crawford (1965) led to the dictum: "There is absolutely no justification, other than the desire to produce uterine relaxation, for administering halothane to an obstetric patient."

Since then this opinion has been modified. Following their use of halothane-oxygen anaesthesia in elective Caesarean section, Johnstone and Breen (1966) showed that maternal narcotic requirements were well below the dose that would depress the contractility of the uterus or the foetal respiratory centre. This view is confirmed by Moir (1970*a*) who found that anaesthesia for Caesarean section based on nitrous oxide/oxygen 50:50 with halothane 0·5 per cent was associated with livelier infants and no more operative blood loss than after an unsupplemented nitrous oxide/oxygen sequence.

A more tolerant attitude towards halothane in obstetrics may be associated with a more rational approach towards its employment. Those who described its undesirable effects tended to give it with the vaporiser setting at 1·5 to 2 per cent in contrast to Moir's more cautious dosage of 0·5 per cent.

The place of halothane in operative obstetrics remains primarily as a myometrial relaxant. For external version high vapour concentrations are used because the anaesthetist is concerned neither with the dangers of post-partum haemorrhage nor of neonatal depression but solely with achieving the optimum conditions for the obstetrician. For the relaxation of a constriction ring, the release of an infant from a tonic uterus at Caesarean section, at breech delivery, or for the second of twins, a concentration of 1·5 to 2 per cent is given only until the desired effect is obtained. Halothane is then discontinued and washed out with unsupplemented nitrous oxide and oxygen so that uterine tone is restored as soon as possible.

Anaesthesia for the removal of a retained placenta implies producing just sufficient myometrial relaxation to facilitate the obstetrician's work. If the placenta is detached but trapped in the cervix less halothane will be required than if the obstetrician has to introduce his hand into the uterine cavity to detach it from the placental site. In these circumstances the anaesthetist must be guided by his colleague as to the degree of relaxation he requires. Excessive myometrial flaccidity may make it difficult for him to define the plane of cleavage between the placenta and the uterine wall. Following removal of the placenta, halothane is discontinued and washed out with unsupplemented nitrous oxide and oxygen. Ergometrine is given and any excessive loss of blood volume is replaced.

Halothane 0·5 per cent may safely be given for its purely narcotic effect as a supplement to nitrous oxide and oxygen for Caesarean section or for any of the various short but painful procedures in obstetrics such as perineal suture without fear of interfering with myometrial contractility.

SOME DANGERS DURING OBSTETRIC ANAESTHESIA

The Supine Hypotensive Syndrome

Postural hypotension with fainting and nausea may occur in pregnant women approaching term when they lie on their backs. Wright (1962) found that of 100 women lying supine in the ninth month of pregnancy 47 showed a fall of 10 per cent in their normal systolic blood pressure and 6 showed a 30 per cent fall with unpleasant symptoms. The hypotension is associated with a rise of venous pressure in the legs and is due to the compression of the inferior vena cava by the gravid uterus restricting the venous return to the heart. The hypotension is corrected and the symptoms relieved when the woman lies on her left side (Brigden *et al.*, 1950). Scott (1968) has shown by inferior vena cavograms that some degree of vena caval obstruction occurs in the majority of women in late pregnancy and yet comparatively few suffer severely from the effects. Normally there is a collateral circulation from the internal iliac through the paravertebral veins to the vena azygos and it is probable that those who are immediately intolerant of the supine position are those in whom the collateral circulation fails to maintain an adequate venous return.

The reduced venous return to the heart causes a fall in cardiac output of 20 per cent in those who are symptomatically unaffected by the supine position. This fall is not necessarily accompanied by an alteration in mean arterial pressure or in heart rate. It follows that compensation must be due to a considerable increase in peripheral resistance.

There are three situations in which inferior vena caval compression may be

haemorrhage which may exhaust the available blood transfusion resources.

A patient with presumed amniotic fluid embolism but without severe hypofibrinogenaemia survived with the following treatment by Willocks *et al.* (1966):

1. IPPV with 100 per cent oxygen to combat the severe hypoxia;
2. Tracheal aspiration to remove oedema fluid from the lungs;
3. Aminophylline to dilate the bronchi and reduce pulmonary vasospasm;
4. Low molecular weight dextran to increase pulmonary blood flow;
5. Sodium bicarbonate to correct metabolic acidosis;
6. Hydrocortisone to protect the patient in a severe stress situation;
7. Frusemide to reduce pulmonary oedema by diuresis;
8. Digoxin to strengthen the myocardium, reduce the pulse rate and for its diuretic effect.

It is clear that the successful management of this rare complication would be difficult in a maternity unit isolated from the laboratory and intensive care facilities normally found only in a large general hospital.

Pre-Eclampsia

Pre-eclampsia is characterised by hypertension, oedema and albuminuria which may be complicated by eclampsia which is defined as the occurrence of fits in a pre-eclamptic patient. It appears to be a kind of hypertensive encephalopathy, the immediate effect of which is to produce localised arteriolar spasm, leading to cerebral anaemia and cerebral hypoxia. Eclamptic fits may occur without warning and without severe symptoms of pre-eclampsia but they are most likely to be triggered by a sudden increase in the blood pressure due to muscular work or to any external stimulus.

Treatment

The essential treatment of pre-eclampsia is primarily a matter for the obstetrician. It consists of complete rest, restriction of fluid intake and is aimed at controlling the blood pressure and the prevention of eclampsia. Attempts may be made to reduce the blood pressure with various hypotensive agents but their value remains unproven particularly in terms of foetal salvage. Termination of the pregnancy by induction of labour or Caesarean section may be considered and the obstetrician has to choose between the risk of prematurity to the infant, and the risk of increasing placental insufficiency to the infant with the risk of eclampsia to the mother if the pregnancy is allowed to continue. It should be remembered that a fair proportion of cases of eclampsia occur in the puerperium.

As there is no general agreement as to the aetiology of the disease treatment is necessarily empirical. Sedation with large doses of morphia is common although this is criticised on the grounds that morphia stimulates the supraoptic nucleus and increases the output of anti-diuretic hormone and hence fluid retention. Amylobarbitone and phenobarbitone may be considered more suitable sedatives in preventing the onset of fits, as may mixtures of phenothiazines with pethidine. As an alternative bromethol ("Avertin") may be given by rectal infusion, this being the only field in which this drug now finds an application.

A promising method of treatment of pre-eclamptic toxaemia in labour has been described by Duffus *et al.* (1968) using the anti-convulsant chlormethiazole. It is given as an 0·8 per cent intravenous infusion and can be used to prevent eclampsia or for the treatment of the convulsion. The patient is maintained in a state of light sleep from which she can easily be aroused and the rate of infusion must be increased if the patient becomes restless or wakeful.

The anaesthetist is likely to be involved in the management of eclampsia or pre-eclampsia to assist in controlling the fits, sedation of the patient, the lowering of the blood pressure and in giving anaesthesia for delivery of the infant. In controlling the fit the minimum effective dose of thiopentone should be given possibly followed by suxamethonium as a muscle relaxant. As a matter of course facilities for intubation and artificial ventilation must be at hand.

Continuous epidural analgesia is an effective method of controlling the blood pressure. An injection of 8–10 ml. bupivacaine 0·5 per cent, preferably without adrenaline, should be given at the 2nd–3rd lumbar interspace and this should produce analgesia up to the 9th–10th dorsal dermatome. Further injections through the cannula may be given until the desired fall of blood pressure has been attained. Care should be taken to monitor the blood pressure closely as severe hypotension may occur necessitating the use of pressor drugs. These should be given well diluted and in minimal doses to avoid over-correction of the hypotension.

Despite initial success, attempts to control hypertension with epidural analgesia over long periods are often disappointing as the blood pressure may continue to rise even though the sensory block has reached a level well above the costal margin. It has therefore no place in treatment before labour has begun. Given during labour it will not only temporarily lower the blood pressure but will also relieve pain thus reducing afferent stimuli along with the darkened room and the hushed voices. The foetus, already at a disadvantage with prematurity and placental insufficiency, is given time to recover from the depressant drugs given to the mother and will stand a better chance of survival at birth.

ANAESTHESIA FOR GYNAECOLOGICAL OPERATIONS

Gynaecological operations performed through the lower abdomen present few problems different from those of general surgical procedures and the choice of anaesthetic should be made in accordance with the principles discussed in Chapter 47.

Operations for the repair of prolapse may occasionally demand a reduction of congestion in the surgical field particularly if the surgeon is exacting. While many surgeons are satisfied with a standard anaesthetic technique for pelvic floor repair, others will demand more complex techniques to reduce bleeding at the operation site especially in pre-menopausal patients in whom bleeding may be particularly troublesome. Induced hypotension with ganglionic blockade has been advocated; the head-down position helps to drain the blood from the site of operation and decreases the risk of an inadequate cerebral blood flow.

Epidural analgesia has been shown to provide the most effective and safe "bloodless field" in this area despite the maintenance of near normal blood pressure levels (Moir, 1968). With ganglionic blockade a comparably dry field can only be achieved by inducing hypotension. The aid of posture, an essential part of the technique, cannot be fully exploited unless the surgeon is prepared to perform the vaginal repair in the "jack-knife" position—an unusual and unlikely event.

Bond (1969) measured the blood loss on 45 patients undergoing major vaginal surgery some of whom had epidural analgesia with light sedation while others were given epidural analgesia with endotracheal halothane and oxygen. The fall of blood pressure was significantly less in those patients given an epidural with light sedation than in those who were given halothane anaesthesia in addition to the epidural. However the mean blood losses in the two groups were similar and there was no correlation between blood loss and the fall of blood pressure. The explanation is that an epidural affecting segments D10 to S3 causes sympathetic blockade only from D10 to L1, but because the pelvic viscera receive their vasomotor innervation from above the level of the epidural blockade, the baroreceptor response can produce a compensatory vaso-constriction at the site of operation and thus diminution of bleeding. If, in addition to the epidural, a general anaesthetic is given, the reflexly constricted vessels in the pelvic viscera become dilated. The blood pressure falls, no further reduction in bleeding is achieved and the impression of a blanched surgical field is lost.

The advantages of epidural analgesia in major gynaecological surgery are not confined to the reduction of blood loss. With an epidural cannula remaining in place effective post-operative analgesia may be maintained particularly in bronchitic patients in whom post-operative pain may hinder effective coughing.

The individual anaesthetist will decide for himself whether the benefits of epidural analgesia outweigh the disadvantage of using a time-consuming technique on a lengthy operating list. One might reflect that the time may be well spent if it results in an increase in the number of anaesthetists competent to perform epidural techniques in circumstances where they are more clearly indicated.

REFERENCES

Adams, A., Morgan, M., Jones, B. C., and McCormick, P. W. (1969). A case of massive aspiration of gastric contents during obstetric anaesthesia. *Brit. J. Anaesth.*, **41,** 176.

Argent, D. E., and Evans, M. D. (1961). Anaesthesia in domiciliary obstetrics. Experiences with a flying squad. *Lancet*, **1,** 994.

Bannister, W. K., Sattilaro, A. J., and Otis, R. D. (1961). Therapeutic aspects of aspiration pneumonitis in experimental animals. *Anesthesiology*, **22,** 440.

Beard, R. W., and Roberts, G. M. (1970). Supine hypotension syndrome. *Brit. med. J.*, **2,** 297.

Beecher, H. K., and Todd, D. P. (1954). A study of the deaths associated with anesthesia and surgery. *Ann. Surg.*, **140,** 2.

Bond, A. G. (1969). Conduction anaesthesia, blood pressure and haemorrhage. *Brit. J. Anaesth.*, **41,** 942.

Bosomworth, P. P., and Hamelberg, W. (1962). Etiologic therapeutic aspects of aspiration pneumonitis. Experimental study. *Surg. Forum.*, **13,** 158.

Brigden, W., Howarth, S., and Sharpey-Schafer, E. P. (1950). Postural changes in the peripheral blood-flow of normal subjects with observations on vasovagal fainting reactions as a result of tilting, the lordiotic posture, pregnancy and spinal anaesthesia. *Clin. Sci.*, **9,** 79.

CLARK, C. G., and RIDDOCH, M. E. (1962). Observations on the human cardia at operation. *Brit. J. Anaesth.*, **34,** 875.

COLEMAN, A. J. (1967). Absence of harmful effect of maternal hypocapnia in babies delivered at Caesarean section. *Lancet*, **1,** 813.

CRAWFORD, J. S. (1965). *Principles and Practice of Obstetric Anaesthesia*, 2nd edit. Oxford: Blackwell Scientific Publications.

DAWES, G. S., and MOTT, J. C. (1964). Changes in O_2 distribution and consumption in foetal lambs with variations in umbilical blood flow. *J. Physiol.* (*Lond.*), **170,** 524.

DUFFUS, G. M., TUNSTALL, M. E., and MCGILLIVRAY, J. (1968). Intravenous chlormethiazole in pre-eclamptic toxaemia in labour. *Lancet*, **1,** 335.

HAMELBERG, W., and BOSOMWORTH, P. P. (1964). Aspiration pneumonitis: experimental stu,dies and clinical observations. *Anesth. Analg. Curr. Res.*, **43,** 669.

HOLMES F. (1960). The supine hypotensive syndrome. Its importance to the anaesthetist. *Anaesthesia*, **15,** 298.

HOLMES, F. (1963). Neonatal respiration following abdominal delivery. *Brit. J. Anaesth.*, **35,** 433.

HOLMES, J. M. (1957). The prevention of inhaled vomit during obstetric anaesthesia. *Proc. roy. Soc. Med.*, **50,** 556.

HUTCHINSON, R. (1961). Awareness during surgery: a study of its incidence. *Brit. J. Anaesth.*, **33,** 463.

JAMIESON, R. (1963). Maternal deaths from aspiration asphyxia. *Brit. med. J.*, **2,** 1129.

JOHNSTONE, M., and BREEN, P. J. (1966). Halothane in obstetrics: elective Caesarean section. *Brit. J. Anaesth.*, **38,** 386.

LAMBRECHTS, W., and PARKHOUSE, J. (1961). Postoperative amnesia. *Brit. J. Anaesth.*, **33,** 397.

LOELIGER, E. A. (1966). *Coagulation Disorders in Obstetrics*, p. 89. Amsterdam: Excerpta Medica.

MCCORMICK, P. W. (1966). The severe pulmonary aspiration syndrome in obstetrics. *Proc. roy. Soc. Med.*, **59,** 66.

MCCORMICK, P. W., HAY, R. G., and GRIFFIN, R. W. (1966). Pulmonary aspiration of gastric contents in obstetric patients. *Lancet*, **1,** 1127.

MENDELSON, C. L. (1946). Aspiration of stomach contents into the lungs during obstetric anesthesia. *Amer. J. Obstet. Gynec.*, **52,** 191.

MINISTRY OF HEALTH (1957). *Report on Confidential Enquiries into Maternal Deaths in England and Wales, 1952–1954*. London: H.M.S.O.

MINISTRY OF HEALTH (1960). *Report on Confidential Enquiries into Maternal Deaths in England and Wales, 1955–1957*. London: H.M.S.O.

MINISTRY OF HEALTH (1963). *Report on Confidential Enquiries into Maternal Deaths in England and Wales, 1958–1960*. London: H.M.S.O.

MINISTRY OF HEALTH (1966). *Report on Confidential Enquiries into Maternal Deaths in England and Wales, 1961–1963*. London: H.M.S.O.

MINISTRY OF HEALTH (1969). *Report on Confidential Enquiries into Maternal Deaths in England and Wales, 1964–1966*. London: H.M.S.O.

MOIR, D. D. (1968). Blood loss during major vaginal surgery. *Brit. J. Anaesth.*, **40,** 233.

MOIR, D. D. (1970*a*). Anaesthesia for Caesarean section. *Brit. J. Anaesth.*, **42,** 136.

MOIR, D. D. (1970*b*). Ergometrine. *Brit. med. J.*, **1,** 563.

MONTGOMERY, J. B. (1961). The effect of halothane on the newborn infant delivered by Caesarean section. *Brit. J. Anaesth.*, **33,** 156.

MOTOYAMA, E. K., RIVARD, G., ACHESON, F., and COOK, C. D. (1966). Adverse effect of maternal hyperventilation on the foetus. *Lancet*, **1,** 286.

MOYA, F. (1960). Obstetric anesthesia: general principles. *Bull. Sloane Hosp. Wom. N.Y.*, **6,** 41.

MOYA, F., MORISHIMA, H. O., SHNIDER, S. M., and JAMES, L. S. (1965). Influence of maternal hyperventilation on the newborn infant. *Amer. J. Obstet. Gynec.*, **91,** 76.

NEWLAND, M. C. (1969). Massive aspiration of gastric contents during obstetric anaesthesia. *Brit. J. Anaesth.*, **41,** 715.

O'MULLANE, E. J. (1954). Vomiting and regurgitation during anaesthesia. *Lancet*, **1,** 1209.

RORKE, M. J., DAVEY, D. A., and DU TOIT, H. J. (1968). Foetal oxygenation during Caesarean section. *Anaesthesia*, **23,** 585.

SCOTT, D. B. (1968). Inferior vena caval occlusion in late pregnancy and its importance in anaesthesia. *Brit. J. Anaesth.*, **40,** 120.

SCOTT, D. B., LEES, M. M., DAVIE, I. T., SLAWSON, K. B., and KERR, M. G. (1969). Observations on cardiorespiratory function during Caesarean section. *Brit. J. Anaesth.*, **41,** 489.

SCOTT, J. S. (1969). Disordered blood coagulation in obstetrics. *Brit. J. Hosp. Med.*, **2,** 1847.

SCUDAMORE, J. H., and YATES, M. J. (1966). Pudendal block—a misnomer. *Lancet*, **1,** 23.

SELLICK, B. A. (1961). Cricoid pressure to control regurgitation of stomach contents during induction of anaesthesia: preliminary communication. *Lancet*, **2,** 404.

SHNIDER, S. M., and MOYA, F. (1961). Amniotic fluid embolism. *Anesthesiology*, **22,** 108.

SNOW, R. G., and NUNN, J. F. (1959). Induction of anaesthesia in the foot-down position for patients with a full stomach. *Brit. J. Anaesth.*, **31,** 493.

SPENCE, A. A., MOIR, D. D., and FINLAY, W. E. I. (1967). Observations on intragastric pressure. *Anaesthesia*, **22,** 249.

STEEL, G. C. (1961). A hydraulic-powered, foot-operated, tilting obstetric bed. *Brit. med. J.*, **1,** 963.

TAYLOR, G., and PRYSE-DAVIES, J. (1966). The prophylactic use of antacids in the prevention of the acid-pulmonary-aspiration syndrome (Mendelson's syndrome). *Lancet*, **1,** 288.

TURNER, D. J., and WILSON, J. (1969). Effect of diazepam on awareness during Caesarean section under general anaesthesia. *Brit. med. J.*, **2,** 736.

WILLOCKS, J., MONE, J. G., and THOMSON, W. J. (1966). Amniotic fluid embolism: case with biochemical findings. *Brit. med. J.*, **2,** 1181.

WILSON, J., and TURNER, D. J. (1969). Awareness during Caesarean section under general anaesthesia. *Brit. med. J.*, **1,** 280.

WRIGHT, L. (1962). Postural hypotension in late pregnancy. *Brit. med. J.*, **1,** 760.

WYLIE, W. D. (1956). Modified "Oxford" labour-ward bed. *Lancet*, **1,** 840.

Appendix I

AN INTRODUCTION TO STATISTICS*

by

I. Z. Roth

W. W. Holland

Introduction

Doctors frequently betray an innate prejudice against accepting results which are said to be "statistically significant". Traditionally medicine has been regarded as an art, and the value of a particular form of treatment has been "proved" only by the cure of the individual, when it is self-evident. With the recent advances in medical science, and in particular with the development of new drugs and methods of care, it has however become obvious that the assessment of results must have some numerical basis. The full significance of detailed experiments and investigations can only be appreciated by statistical analysis, and it is therefore becoming increasingly important for the doctor to have some knowledge of statistical terminology and techniques. Only then will he be in a position to make an independent assessment of results.

No very great knowledge of mathematical theory is needed to enable him to do this. The laboratory worker can frequently exclude variables in which he is not interested and confine his attention to one or more controlled factors at a time. The clinician has to use data which it is known may be influenced by many factors which cannot be controlled but which must be taken into account. The essence of the statistical method lies in the elucidation of the effects of the conditions under which the particular measurements were observed. Although the doctor does not need to have sufficient knowledge to perform the calculations himself, some familiarity with the implied assumptions and the logical steps involved in statistical analysis is essential.

To quote an analogous situation: no doctor is inhibited in prescribing an antibiotic, though he probably has no idea of the way in which it was produced. On the other hand, he would not consider using a drug which the dosage and toxicity were unknown.

This chapter is intended as a general introduction to the methods of statistical reasoning used in medical studies.

Descriptive and Medical Statistics

All statistical work is concerned with the examination of a number of subjects and the observation of one or more variables on each subject. Large aggregates

* Our thanks are due to Miss C. M. Watson for invaluable help in the preparation of this section.

of observations may very often present irregularities and patterns which are difficult to distinguish and explain. In order to draw any general conclusions from the data, the material collected must be presented in a form which will enable the investigator to determine the distribution of the values of different variables among subjects.

The word "statistics" is defined by the Oxford English Dictionary as "numerical facts systematically collected on a subject". This definition corresponds closely with the methods used in descriptive statistics, which involves the collection and tabulation of data. Demography and vital statistics are principally concerned with the descriptive method: an excellent example of this approach is provided by the Registrar-General's Annual Report on births, marriages and deaths. The collection and interpretation of such data do not present any great mathematical difficulties, though they do necessitate an intimate knowledge of the field of study.

If it is possible to observe all members of a population of interest, full information about the distribution of any observed variable will be provided by descriptive statistical analysis. In the great majority of medical studies this is not practicable, because only a small proportion of these relevant to the investigation can be examined. The intention is, however, to obtain results which would have general application to any individual in a given situation. In order to make this assumption the selection of subjects studied must be as wide as possible. A representative sample is therefore drawn from a much larger population and observation is concentrated on this group. The representative character of the sample is achieved by random sampling techniques. Random sampling implies that every individual in the population or with the disease has an equal chance of being included in the sample: that is, selection must be entirely unconnected with the qualities to be studied. For example, the choice of a sample for the study of the incidence of a particular disease must be unaffected by any factors, such as occupation or area of residence, which might be thought to contribute to the development of the disease.

Due to the effect of chance in sampling there is usually some difference between the sample and total populations in the distributions of the variables found; but the larger the sample, the closer are its characteristics to the characteristics of the "parent" or total population, and the smaller is the probability of deviation from the whole.

The parent population may be either real or hypothetical. The latter is more often found in medical research and experimentation, where the principal aim is to test a theory which may be applied to all individuals in a given situation and not to study a finite number of individuals at a particular point in time. The parent population is therefore taken to be all hypothetical individuals who would comply with the definition of those found in the sample or used in the experiment. This hypothetical parent population is assumed to be infinite in size. For example, a study of the duration of anaesthesia after the application of a given drug would provide the data necessary to generalise the mean duration in all men and women with the same characteristics. The characteristics considered in statistical analysis are essentially hypothetical rather than real, and form the basis for the construction of the so-called parent population.

Qualitative and Quantitative Variables

The aim of statistical analysis is as we have said the assessment of the distribution of one or more variables in the population of a study area. The character of the distribution depends on the type of variable, which is in turn determined by the values which the variable may acquire.

There are two basic types of variable, *qualitative* and *quantitative*. Sex, race and the presence or absence of a given symptom are all qualitative variables and share the same statistical characteristic: they cannot be expressed numerically. The reverse is true of quantitative variables. These may be expressed as a numerical quantity which is in correspondence with the real object measured. In some instances there is a direct correspondence between the object and the number used, as in the case of height measurement, where the number of length units conforms with the actual body length. At other times the correspondence shows no such direct relationship between object and measurement. The score for the depth of narcotic sleep is for example given according to an arbitrarily constructed scale of a few numbers, where 0 may represent no sleep and 5 deep sleep.

Quantitative variables may be further subdivided into *discrete* and *continuous* variables. The value of discrete variables can only be expressed in whole numbers (0, 1, 2, 3, etc.) or their multiples. These variables may be straightforward counts, for example the number of heart attacks, the number of teeth or the number of radiation impulses recorded on a counter. They may also be ordered variables, that is scores or ratings, and in this case a more exact measurement is given by making the basic step equal to a half (0, $\frac{1}{2}$, 1, $1\frac{1}{2}$, 2, etc.). For example the severity of symptoms shown by a subject may be recorded by a number of crosses (+++); if the results are dubious the symbol ± is used, and this is then interpreted as half the cross.

Continuous variables are those which may take any value from a given interval. Examples of such variables are weight, age, duration of narcotic sleep and skin conductivity. The values of these variables are said to have infinite range or interval, for although they must be positive, no fixed upper limit can be defined. There are however continuous variables which have a finite range. The concentration of a fluid substance can for example vary only between 0 and 100 per cent. When speaking of continuous variables it is important to remember that only the object phenomena are in fact continuous; the recorded measurements are expressed in numbers rounded to a given decimal place, thus becoming actually discrete. This is however explained by the inefficiency of the recording methods and not by the nature of the observed quantities.

Frequency Distribution

Quantitative Variables

Once a detailed description has been made of the values of observed variables in the sample group, one can calculate the number of times the value or values occur in each subject or relevant group of subjects (for example, one age group). In statistical terms, this is the calculation of the frequencies of observation. The frequencies are presented either in original numbers or in percentages of the total group of observed subjects. This numerical presentation of values is called frequency distribution.

A frequency distribution may be depicted visually in the form of a histogram in which the individual values or groups of values are given on the horizontal axis and the vertical axis shows a scale measuring the number of times these values occur in the sample (the observed frequency). The respective frequency of each value or group of values is represented by a column or bar, the area of which represents the observed frequency (see Fig. 1).

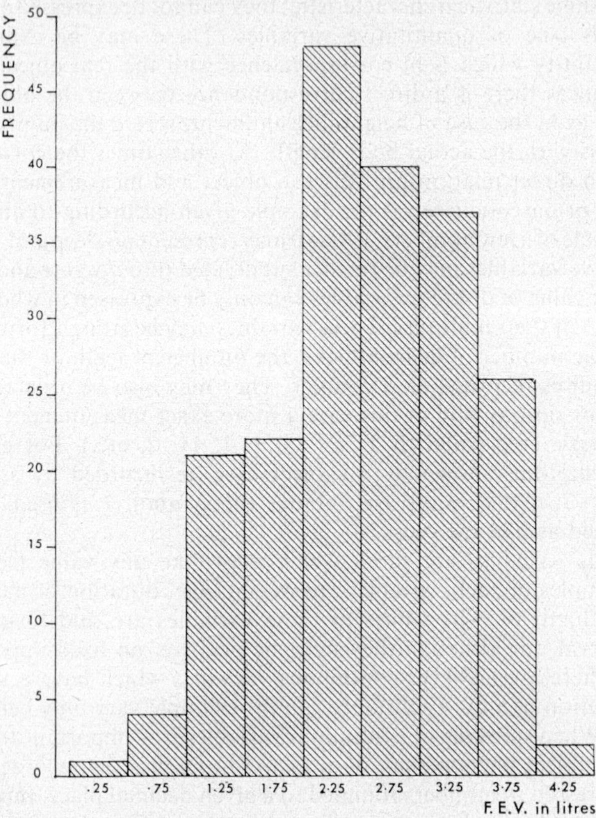

APPENDIX 1/FIG. 1.—Frequency distribution of 1 second forced expiratory volume for man (a sample). Unit is litre.

F.E.V. in litres	*No. of men with said F.E.V.*
0 –0·5	1
0·5–1·0	4
1·0–1·5	21
1·5–2·0	22
2·0–2·5	48
2·5–3·0	40
3·0–3·5	37
3·5–4·0	26
4·0–4·5	2
Total	201

The histogram has in many instances only one peak, and the distribution of values is then said to be "unimodal". The value of the variable associated with the peak is called the *mode*. The frequencies of a unimodal distribution usually decrease towards both ends of the histogram; these terminal parts are called "tails". If the peak occurs above the central point of the range of the variable and the frequencies decrease symmetrically on either side of the peak, the distribution is symmetric (Fig. 2). If the peak occurs at any other point the distribution is asymmetric and is called "skew".

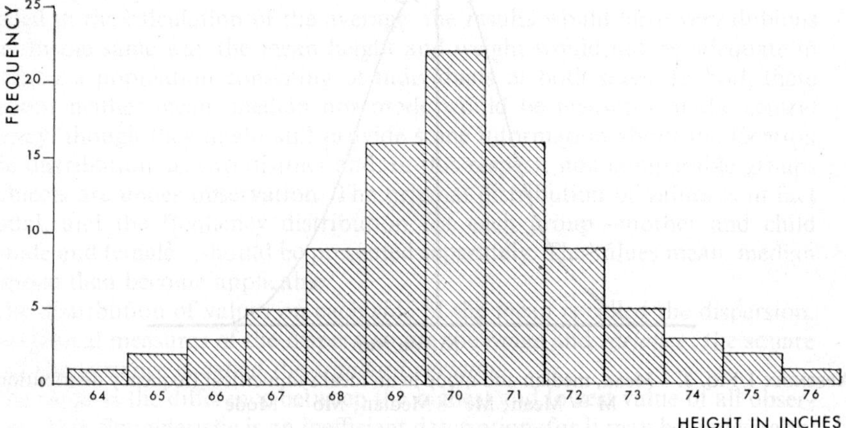

APPENDIX 1/FIG. 2.—Data for the symmetric distribution.

Height in inches	*Frequency*
64	1
65	2
66	3
67	5
68	9
69	16
70	22
71	16
72	9
73	5
74	3
75	2
76	1

For the purposes of calculation the main features of a histogram can be described statistically. The two features of main interest are its *width* and *location*. The width represents the scatter of individual observations; the location is sometimes called the central tendency and has three statistical measures, *mean*, *mode* and *median*. The mode has been defined in the previous paragraph. The mean is the average value of all individual observations and is computed according to the formula,

$$\bar{x} = \frac{\Sigma x_i}{n}$$

where n is the number of observations, x_i are the individual observations and $\bar{x}$ denotes their mean. From this formula it may be deduced that the sum of

Since variance is a function of squares of original data, its value is on the scale of the squares of the original units. For convenience the square root of variance is often used as the measure of dispersion. This is called standard deviation, in which the scale of the value complies with the scale of observed variables. The standard deviation is sometimes expressed as a percentage of the mean, which is called the coefficient of variation. This percentage is calculated according to the formula:

$$V = \frac{100s}{\bar{x}}$$

where V is the coefficient of variation, s is the standard deviation and $\bar{x}$ is the mean.

Qualitative Variables

Qualitative variables are recorded by their presence or absence. When dealing with the observed distribution of such variables the only characteristic used as the mean is the percentage. This expresses the relative frequency of each value of the observed variable in the group studied. To quote a very simple example: where 10 men in a group of 50 have blue eyes, this would be expressed by stating that 20 per cent of the observed population have blue eyes.

Probability Theory

A brief outline was given at the beginning of this chapter of the effect of chance in sampling and the probable difference between the distribution of variables in a sample and in the parent population. Probability theory enables any such difference to be calculated with reasonable certainty.

The essential element of probability theory is the random event. When this occurs the random variable associated with the event takes some value which has a specified probability. The probabilities for all the possible values of a random variable create the probability distribution. This concept of the probability distribution is used in random sampling and is directly comparable to that of the frequency distribution among observed subjects.

The principles involved in calculating the probabilities corresponding to the values of a random variable may be simply illustrated by a description of the situation found when tossing a coin or throwing a die. When tossing a coin the two possible values of the random variable are heads and tails, both having the same probability of 1/2. Random variables may also have different characters and different values. If the die has sides of different colours the random variable is qualitative and each colour has a probability of 1/6. If the sides are distinguished by different numbers of dots (1 to 6) the random variable is quantitative and discrete, taking the values of the integers between 1 and 6 inclusive. If the die has 3 dots on 3 faces, 2 on 2 faces and 1 on the last face, the probability of any face landing upermost is 1/6, but the probability of obtaining the value of each variable (1,2,3) is different. The probability of throwing a 3 is 1/2, of throwing a 2 is 1/3, and of throwing a 1 it is 1/6.

The situation found in random sampling differs only in the greater number of subjects and variables observed. The random event is the selection of a subject from the total population. The probability of drawing each individual is the same (if sampling is by replacement) and is equal in value to the fraction of the total population represented by one individual. Thus in a parent population of 100,000 the probability of each subject being chosen would be 1/100,000. The probability of drawing a particular value of any observed variable in a chosen subject is equal to the frequency of that value in the parent population. In other words, the frequency distribution in the parent population forms the sampling probability distribution. But, as we have said, real parent populations are rarely used in medical research and experimentation. Infinite hypothetical parent populations are generally used, and in these no real frequency distribution exists. However one assumes that the sampling probability distribution is present, and the probability theory provides some reasonable mathematical models for its calculation. These models vary with the character of the variable observed.

For continuous variables the symmetrical unimodal model is the Gaussian or so-called "normal" distribution. The mathematical form of the model is defined by only two parameters, the mean and the variance of the distribution. Almost all the classical "parametric" methods of statistical inference assume a "normal" distribution of the variable in the population, which produces the familiar bell-shaped curve when plotted.

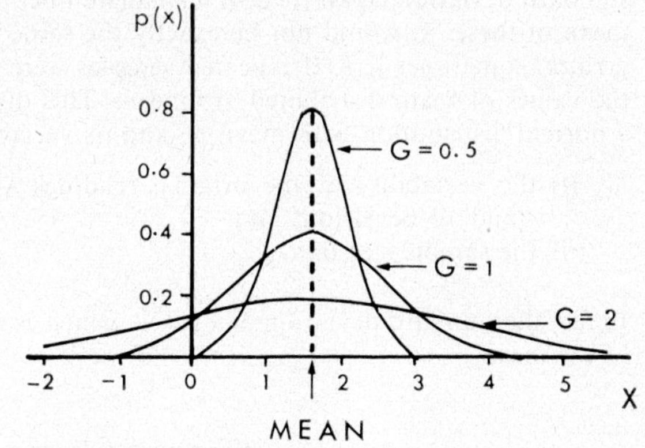

APPENDIX I/FIG. 5.—Normal distribution for several values of standard deviation (G). (Changing the mean merely shifts the curves to the right or left without changing their shapes.)
x is the random variable;
p(x) is the probability of x at given values

For discrete variables the model often used is the binomial or "Poisson" distribution.

For qualitative variables it is assumed that a fixed probability exists for each quality drawn from the parent population. This is expressed as a percentage equivalent to the frequency of this quality in the parent population.

Probability theory of sampling is used in experimental calculations. For example, any method of measuring the plasma cholesterol must involve a certain experimental error. If five readings were taken, they would differ slightly. What, then, is the correct value? It is assumed that if a large number of readings were taken (the readings may be regarded as a random sample of the normally distributed parent population of possible readings) their distribution would be normal, with a mean, *m*, equal to the true value of plasma cholesterol and a

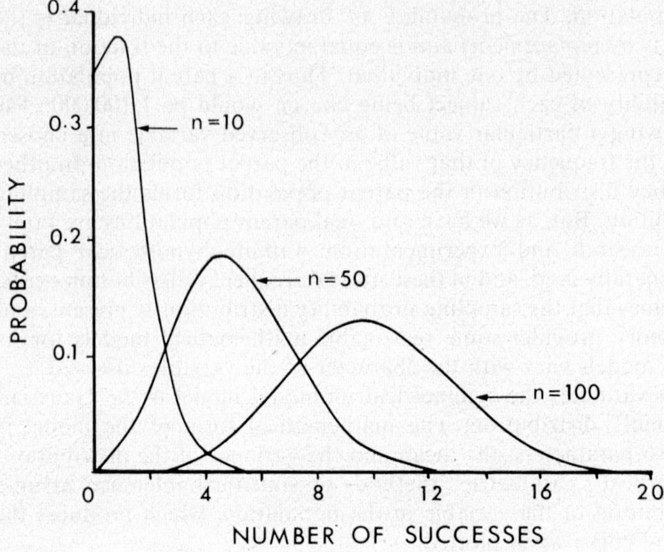

APPENDIX I/FIG. 6.—Binomial distribution for p = 0·9 and q = 0·1 for several values of n (number of observations).
p = probability of success or event occurring
q = probability of failure or event not occurring
n = number of observations or trials

standard deviation equal to Σ. If a small number of readings, n, were taken, the mean of these, $\bar{x}$, would not be exactly the same as *m*: sometimes it would be greater, sometimes less. If repeated samples were taken it would be found that the values of $\bar{x}$ are distributed around *m*. This distribution of means would be a normal distribution with mean *m*, and its variability will depend on:

(i) the variability of the original readings x_i, which is measured by the standard deviation; and
(ii) the sample size n.

In fact the standard deviation of $\bar{x}$ is $\frac{\Sigma}{\sqrt{n}}$ which is also called the standard error of the mean.

STATISTICAL INFERENCE

Statistical inference attempts to estimate the parameters of a parent population distribution and to assess the reliability of the estimates given by a sample. Alternatively, inference is used to test whether a sample distribution complies with an assumed hypothetical form of the distribution in the parent population. The first approach is called confidence interval estimation, the second, testing of hypotheses.

Interval Estimation

All statistical characteristics of the distribution in a parent population are generally estimated by the corresponding sample characteristics. When a given distribution function in a parent population is assumed, as in the case of a hypothetical parent population, the sample characteristics are used as estimates for the parameters of the distribution. In the case of the normal distribution, the parameters concerned are the mean and variance, estimated by the sample mean and variance. Mathematical statistics provides the method of constructing the *confidence intervals* for the estimated parameters. A confidence interval around the calculated value of the estimator (that is, a sample characteristic) is expected to cover the "true" value of the unknown parameter (or population characteristic) with a high probability, called the *confidence level.* The confidence levels generally used are 0·95 or 0·99, that is, 95 per cent or 99 per cent. When a 95 per cent confidence interval (for a confidence level of 0·95) for an arithmetic mean is constructed around the sample mean, then the result can be stated as follows: 95 per cent of the intervals obtained in this way will include the population mean. Thus when calculating the mean plasma cholesterol, it is also possible to provide a confidence interval for its "true" value.

When constructing a series of such intervals for different samples or experiments, on average the "true" population characteristics fall within the confidence intervals in 95 per cent of all cases; in 5 per cent of cases they fail to do so. In a given experiment it is unfortunately impossible to determine which of the two situations is found, and there is therefore always a probability of 5 per cent (that is, in 1 in 20 cases) that the population mean may be outside the calculated confidence interval. This possibility should always be borne in mind.

Testing of Hypotheses

In many cases the aim of analysis is not to estimate unknown values of population characteristics, but to test if some assumptions about the distribution of the variable in the population are in agreement with the results of the sample examined. Such an assumption may be concerned with one of the following characteristics:

(i) the type of distribution (a test of goodness of fit);
(ii) the differences between two or more distributions (a test of agreement);
(iii) the parameters (a test for differences between means, variances, etc.).

The statistical procedure starts with a definition of the *null hypothesis*, which expresses the tested assumption about the population distribution or distributions. In a test of difference between means and other characteristics of several groups, the null hypothesis generally takes the character of the negative or "undesired" situation. In such situations the null hypothesis states that there are no differences between the groups which are being compared. When testing the relation or even the effect of some concomitant variable on the mean of the distribution (for example, the effect of a dose of a particular drug on the basal metabolism) the null hypothesis states there is no such effect. However, in the case of the goodness of fit test, the null hypothesis takes a positive form, stating that the population distribution has a particular shape.

The statistical test then used is based on the assumption of the validity of the null hypothesis. All possible samples data are then classified into two groups:

(i) those in concordance (that is, with the null hypothesis having a relatively high probability of being true);
(ii) those in discordance (that is, with the null hypothesis having a low probability of being true).

The latter group is called *the critical* or *rejection region*. This group is chosen in such a way that the probability of a sample falling into the critical region is very low, in medical statistics usually 0·05 to 0·01. This is called the *significance level*. In practice a test criterion (for example the "t" test) is calculated, the distribution of which is known if the null hypothesis is valid, and the limits of its critical region are tabulated for a few convenient significance levels (usually 10 per cent, 5 per cent, 1 per cent and 0·1 per cent). These limits are called *critical values*. When the calculated test criterion falls beyond these limits (that is, into its critical region) the observed sample data have a very low probability of being observed if the null hypothesis were true. Therefore the null hypothesis is rejected at the given significance level. When, for example, comparing the sample means of two groups of normally distributed variables, the test criterion t is calculated according to the formula,

$$t = \frac{\bar{x}_1 - \bar{x}_2}{\sqrt{s^2(n_1 + n_2)}} \sqrt{n_1 n_2}$$

where $\bar{x}_1$ and $\bar{x}_2$ are the means to be compared, n_1 and n_2 the respective sample sizes, and

$$s^2 = \frac{\{\Sigma (x_1^2) - n_1(\bar{x}_1)^2 + \Sigma (x_2^2) - n_2(\bar{x}_2)^2\}}{n_1 + n_2 - 2}$$

If the absolute value of t exceeds the critical value for a given significance level and given number of "degrees of freedom" then the null hypothesis of the equal value of both population means is rejected and the difference between the two means is said to be statistically significant at the given significance level.* The conclusion follows that the two samples compared represent groups from parent populations with different population means.

For a test of difference between two percentages, the "chi-squared" test for a fourfold table is used.

APPENDIX I/TABLE 1

EXAMPLE OF FOURFOLD TABLE

Treatment	*Patients Improved*	*Patients Not Improved*	*Total*
A	12	12	24
B	8	16	24
Total	20	28	48

For a test of difference of variances the F-test is used. This F criterion is also used in the "analysis of variance" concerned with differences among more than two means. Most statistical textbooks give more detailed explanations of these tests.

In the discussion of interval estimation it was stated that there is always

* Values of t for different levels of significance and varying degrees of freedom are found in statistical books (for example, Dixon and Massey, 1957) and "Geigy" Tables.

a probability that the population mean will be outside the calculated confidence interval. In the same way, in the testing of an hypothesis there is a probability equal to the chosen significance level that the null hypothesis is true even if the test criterion falls into the critical region. Thus there is always a risk that the claimed deviation from the null hypothesis is not true. When using the 5 per cent significance level we would reject the null hypothesis on an average of 1 in 20 cases even if the null hypothesis were always true. The possibility of drawing such a false conclusion should always be kept in mind when considering the results of statistical analyses. It must also be emphasised that it would be wrong to accept without question the null hypothesis when it is not rejected. If for instance the difference between the means of two groups is not statistically significant, one cannot conclude that the two populations are necessarily the same, only that they might be. The power of a statistical test to recognise deviation from the null hypothesis depends on sample size and the amount by which the true distribution or distributions differ from that given by the null hypothesis. For the difference of two means the power of the t-test increases with the size of the sample, and with the true difference between the population means. If a study is planned and there is a desire to reject the null hypothesis for a particular difference in population means, the power of the test may be increased by increasing the sample size.

It is important to stress that one is never certain that the results of statistical analysis give a true picture of the whole situation. All one can deduce is that a certain distribution of values appears to exist, and can be assumed with a reasonable degree of probability.

Regression Analysis

The problems discussed so far have been concerned only with a consideration of separate variables. One of the principal concerns of statistical analysis is to determine whether values of observed variables are correlated with other variables observed concurrently. If for example the observed variable is basal metabolic rate, it is reasonable to expect that it is related to the age, weight and sex of the subject and possibly also to the other conditions. Even if individuals of the same age, weight and sex were found, their basal metabolic rates would not be equal, though the values of their metabolic rates would provide a statistical distribution with a certain mean value. The mean value is then regarded as a function of age, weight and sex, and perhaps of other variables. In this situation age and weight represent continuous variables and sex has the nature of a condition which may be represented with a dummy variable (for example a variable having the value 0 for men and 1 for women). The mean of the distribution is essentially regarded as a function of one or more so-called "independent" variables, and the variable whose distribution is observed is then called a "dependent" variable. Such a function is called the regression function.

In the applications of statistical analysis the regression function is often supposed to be a linear function of independent variables ($x_1, x_2, \ldots, x_n$) of the form

$$M = b_0 + b_1x_1 + b_2x_2 + \ldots + b_nx_n$$

where M represents the mean, n is the number of independent variables and $b_0, b_1, \ldots, b_n$ are the so-called regression coefficients.

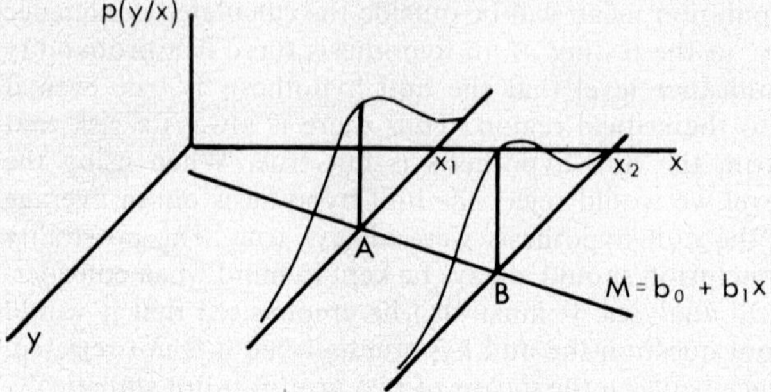

APPENDIX I/FIG. 7.—Representation of a simple linear model. For any given value of x, the random variable y is normally distributed with mean $b_0 + b_1x$
y = dependent variable
x = independent variable
p(y/x) = probability density function
A = mean of y at x_1
B = mean of y at x_2

In statistical analysis these regression coefficients are estimated and/or tested. The null hypothesis for absence of a regression on, say, the first independent variable is expressed as the assumption that b_1 is equal to zero.

CORRELATION ANALYSIS

In some cases more than one variable is observed on each subject. The correlation between the values of the two variables is then frequently of interest, and the extent to which the two variables are correlated is measured by means of the correlation coefficient. Its value is equal to 0 for uncorrelated variables, and less than +1 and greater than −1 in all other cases. It would be equal to +1 or −1 only if one of the variables were a linear function of the other. The correlation coefficient is positive if a higher value of one variable implies that a higher value of the other may be expected: it is negative if a lower value may be expected. The closer to 1 the correlation coefficient is, the more the two observed variables are linearly related (see Fig. 8).

It must however be stressed that the correlation coefficient can only be used if the values of both variables are observed on an otherwise homogeneous sample of subjects. If one of the variables is controlled (for example, dosage, in a trial of treatment by a particular drug, or, age of subjects, in a sample where the population is stratified according to age) the correlation coefficient loses its value as a measure of the correlation between two variables, since its value may be altered by rearrangement of the experiment or the sampling scheme.

CONTROLLED TRIALS

The statistical techniques used in the analysis of results of medical studies have been discussed at some length. Some of the difficulties involved in the organisation of one of the commonest methods of study, the controlled trial, should also be considered. The controlled trial is generally undertaken in order to compare the efficacy of some new form of treatment with that of the standard form. The problems encountered often relate to the difficulty of finding two groups of subjects which are directly comparable in all respects likely to affect the outcome of the trial. There are many factors which can invalidate the comparison if the situation is not properly controlled.

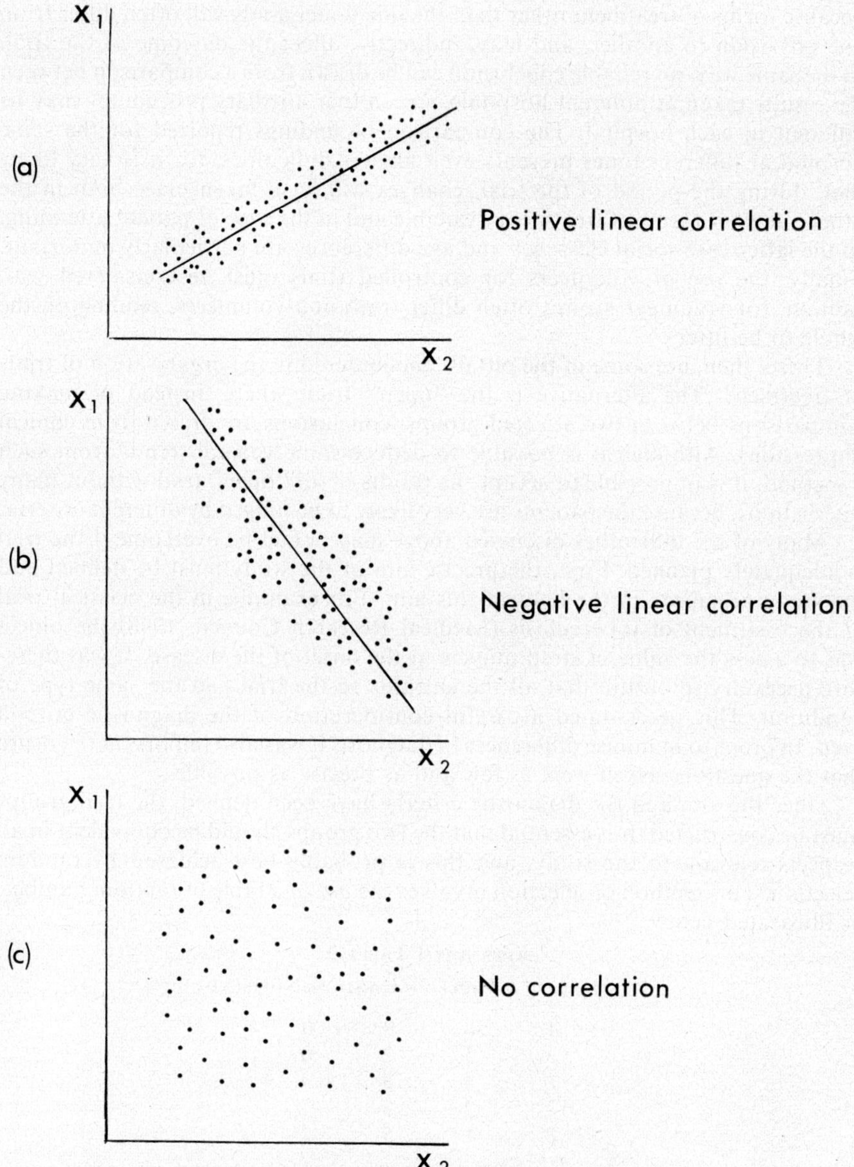

APPENDIX I/FIG. 8.—Scatter diagrams for positive and negative linear correlation and no correlation between two variables x_1 and x_2.

In the first place, a physician may well choose to limit a trial of a new method of treatment to those patients whom he considers will react successfully. The results of any comparison between those treated in the new and the traditional manners will therefore in all probability be biased towards the new method. A comparison between results reported by two different physicians is again invalid, because forms of treatment other than the one under study will often differ from one physician to another, and may, indirectly, affect the outcome of the trial. In the same way, no reliable conclusion can be drawn from a comparison between the results taken at different hospitals, since other ancillary procedures may be different in each hospital. The comparison of findings reported for the same hospital at different times presents even greater difficulties, for it is very likely that, during the period of the trial, changes will have taken place both in the other ancillary forms of treatment available and in the type of patient attending. In the latter case social class, sex and age differences are particularly important. Finally, the use of volunteers for controlled trials must be considered with caution, for volunteer groups often differ from non-volunteers, tending on the whole to be fitter.

These, then, are some of the pitfalls encountered in the organisation of trials of treatment. The alternative is the "open" trial, where, instead of making comparisons between two selected groups, conclusions are drawn from clinical impressions. Although it is possible to deduce some general trends from such a method, it is impossible to accept the results of an "open" trial without many reservations, because the patients are very likely to be judged by different criteria.

Many of the difficulties discussed above may in fact be overcome if the trial is adequately planned. First, the precise aim of the study must be defined and the study organised in the light of this aim. For example, in the classical trial of the treatment of tuberculosis (Medical Research Council, 1948) the object was to assess the value of streptomycin at the onset of the disease. It was therefore necessary to ensure that all the entrants to the trial had the same type of condition. This necessitated a careful consideration of the diagnostic criteria used. In order to minimise differences in diagnosis it was also important to ensure that the questions asked were as few and as precise as possible.

Once the aim and the diagnostic criteria have been defined, the trial groups must be constructed. It is essential that the two groups should be equivalent in all respects relevant to the study, and this is probably best achieved by random selection. This method of selection involves the use of a table of random number, as illustrated below.

Appendix I/Table 2

Example of a Table of Random Numbers

1	6	9	0
3	5	2	0
2	4	8	4
7	2	3	7
8	1	5	7

Further examples of such tables are found in all statistical text books. Suppose each of the numbers in Table 2 corresponds with one of 20 patients. Before the beginning of the trial it is decided that patients given an even random number will be treated by one method (A), while those given an odd number will be treated by an alternative method (B). A series of envelopes is prepared, numbered consecutively from 1 to 20, and a slip of paper showing the treatment to be administered is inserted into each envelope. Thus the first envelope (which corresponds to an odd number in the table) indicates that treatment B should be given; the second envelope indicates the same treatment; the third shows treatment A, the fourth B, and the fifth A. When the first patient appears, he is given the first envelope, and treatment B is administered. This procedure is repeated for each of the 20 patients. It will be seen from Table 2 that, although treatment is randomly allocated, at the conclusion of the trial half the patients will have received treatment A and half treatment B.

A further safeguard, which ensures complete objectivity of reporting, is the adoption of a double blind procedure, where neither the patient nor the doctor knows which form of treatment is being administered.

Before the trial begins it is essential to decide the method of assessment to be used: this should be carefully adhered to throughout the conduct of the trial.

The question of differential exclusion should also be considered. If for any reason any patients have been excluded after admission to the trial the careful balance secured by randomisation will be disturbed and the validity of the findings will be affected. There are several situations in which differential exclusion may occur. In a study of the effects of treatment by a particular drug, it may become apparent during the trial that certain patients cannot be retained on the drug owing to toxic side-effects. In a trial of the relative value of pneumonectomy and radiation in the treatment of cancer of the lung, there would undoubtedly be situations in which pneumonectomy would be impossible to perform. It would therefore appear sensible to exclude these subjects, though no such exclusion would be made in the group treated by radiation. But if patients from one group alone are excluded, it would be impossible to assert that the groups are comparable in everything but treatment. Unless the losses are few, and therefore unimportant, it may be necessary to retain all original patients in the comparison. The trial would then measure the intention to treat in a particular way rather than the effects of treatment. The question of the introduction of bias through exclusion for any reason, including that of disappearance, must be carefully considered throughout the trial. Any exclusion should be studied immediately in order to decide whether the subject should be retained in the enquiry for follow-up measurement.

In some situations the patient may be used as his own control. In many ways this is the ideal solution, because many possible factors which could affect the validity of the outcome of the trial are then excluded; but this is not possible where lengthy or drastic forms of treatment are involved.

In conclusion it is perhaps necessary to mention the ethical problems involved in the trial of new forms of treatment. This question has been discussed by the Medical Research Council (1963) and the World Medical Association (1962), and has been considered in some detail in the *British Medical Journal* (1955, 1962, 1963; Hill, 1963). The reader is referred to these publications for a full explanation of the problems involved.

REFERENCES

British Medical Journal (1955). Leading Article: Experiments on human beings. **1,** 526.

British Medical Journal (1962). Leading Article: Experimental medicine. **2,** 1108.

British Medical Journal (1963). Leading Article: Ethics of human experimentation. **2,** 1.

DIXON, W. J., and MASSEY, F. J. (1957). *Introduction to Statistical Analysis.* New York: McGraw Hill.

statistician Herman Hollerith developed the tabulating machine in its present form.

The first digital computer, ENIAC (the Electronic Numerical Integrator and Calculator), appeared in 1944. By comparison with present-day computers, ENIAC was a clumsy device, weighing some 30 tons and containing 18,000 vacuum tubes. It was capable of gross errors, caused by the generation of excessive heat after continued use. The decimal system of calculation was used. Despite the disadvantages of the machine it was nevertheless capable of rapid arithmetical calculation, and a whole new field of possible use was opened up when it was discovered to be capable of learning to read, write and memorise. The computer models of the next twelve years showed enormous improvements in both speed and accuracy. In 1952 the binary system replaced the decimal system for most scientific work, and four years later transistors were substituted for the numerous and unwieldy vacuum tubes. Thus a second generation of computers was developed, considerably reduced in size and capable of working ten times faster than ENIAC. These models were also easier to adapt and control and had greatly increased storage facilities. During the mid-1960s a third generation of computers emerged, further improved in speed, efficiency and adaptability. The modern computer can provide 10,000 operations per second for 100 users simultaneously; this concept of "time-sharing" has an important bearing on cost and availability as well as efficiency.

The skills and uses of the computer have shown an equally rapid development over the last twenty-five years. It was originally intended as a useful aid to mathematicians and scientists for performing repetitive and lengthy calculations, for example solving differential equations. It was however soon realised that the computer was capable of processing data with much greater speed and accuracy than the tabulator. Its potential value in business calculations was then accepted, and large organisations such as the Treasury, the Forces and the Post Office were soon investing enormous sums of money in computers to handle their accounts and payrolls.

The computer has proved capable of handling non-numeric symbols as quickly and easily as numbers. Beginning with the alphabet and other symbols used in business and scientific dealings, the computer has since been taught to imitate the grammatical structure of the language, and to write other languages. The linguistic ability of the computer has made it available to a substantial group of non-scientists, which has facilitated its widespread use in business and other fields.

In recent years the computer has crept into a wide variety of unlikely areas of study; it has been used to simulate engineering, production and other problems, to prove theorems, to test the practicability of military strategy, and even to play chess. It is now capable of reading handwriting and understanding spoken words, has been made a business partner, and has been used in the organisation of space projects. Its ability to operate without detailed instructions or supervision has led to its introduction into large organisations such as atomic plants, where the computer is now sometimes given sole responsibility for the supervision of routine chemical and other processes. Computer-written music has been produced, and the computer has been employed to investigate problems of literary criticism and linguistic analysis—for example, the authorship of different parts of the Bible.

Digital and Analogue Computers

There are two types of computer—digital and analogue—which differ in both construction and usage. The digital computer deals with discrete units which are represented by electronic impulses, rather like morse dots. Its basic function is to perform numerical or non-numerical symbol manipulations: in order to do this the computer must have facilities for data storage and retrieval, computation, the interpretation and performance of instructions, and logical decision-making. The mechanisms which enable the computer to perform these tasks are discussed in the following section. The decision-making ability of the computer is based on the comparison of two numbers, or symbols, alternate impulses being activated according to whether the data under examination is similar or dissimilar. Although the computer stores everything in the form of numbers, simple numerical codes can be used to represent letters or symbols held in the memory unit. This enables the computer to handle and store alphabetic data, to compare the data and to organise it for the construction of systematic files of information. The machine can therefore be used for compiling alphabetic lists of names, or tracing a particular individual or group of individuals with some common characteristic.

In the analogue computer, the problem to be solved is arranged as a model, in which the behaviour of the system under study is mimicked by a similar arrangement of electronic computing units. Because of the close correspondence between the model and its counterpart, measurements and ideas are easily translated from one to the other. The analogue is able to deal with variables that are continuously changing; these variables are represented by currents, voltages or some other physical quality. The earliest analogues were mechanical, but these have now been replaced by electronic assemblies. Analogue computers have been used in engineering for many years, and now play an important part in medical and biochemical research.

The analogue computer can be compared to a slide rule, while the digital computer resembles an abacus. Any calculation performed by the analogue can be done by the digital computer, which has much wider scope and flexibility. As the digital computer is now rapidly replacing the analogue, the latter will not be discussed further here.

Structure (Digital Computers)

Different makes of computer may vary in structure, but the main parts are the same in every machine. All computers include an *input device*, through which the instructions are read; these are then stored in the *memory unit* or *main store*. The required calculations are executed by the *arithmetic* or *processing unit*, and the results are released by the *output device*. In order to enable the computer to work independently of detailed external direction, the workings of these separate mechanisms are regulated and co-ordinated by a *control unit* or *supervisor*. Figure 1 shows the positioning of all these component parts.

The central memory unit, arithmetic unit, control unit and supervisor are all *central units*. These operate at a much higher speed than the *peripheral units*, which are the input and output devices and the magnetic tapes and discs used to supplement the central units.

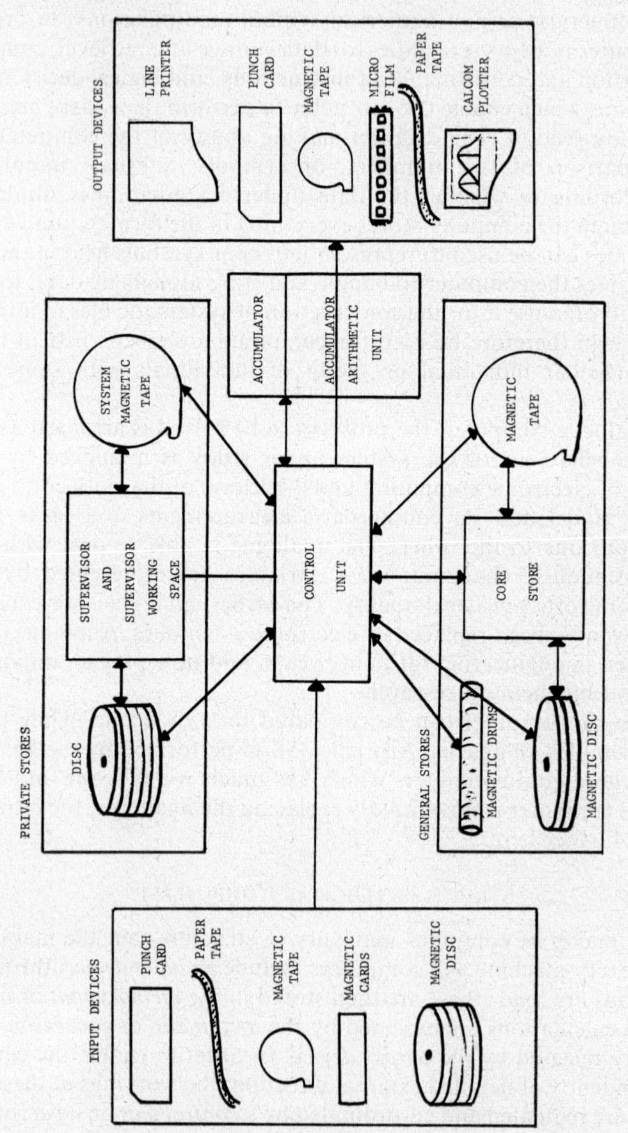

APPENDIX II/FIG. 1.—Design of the computer.

Figure 2 shows some of the peripheral units in a computer installation. In the forefront of the picture is a typewriter, used for feeding instructions and data into the computer. The machine on the extreme right is a disc unit (see also Fig. 5); against the far wall is a line-printer (an output device). On the left-hand wall there are magnetic tape drives and a 360 operator panel, used for direct control of the computer.

Input Devices

The input unit is required to read in data for processing, to transfer the data to its own store and to read in programs of instructions. The instructions indicate how the data is to be processed for a particular job, and may also tell the computer to perform checks on the validity and credibility of the data.

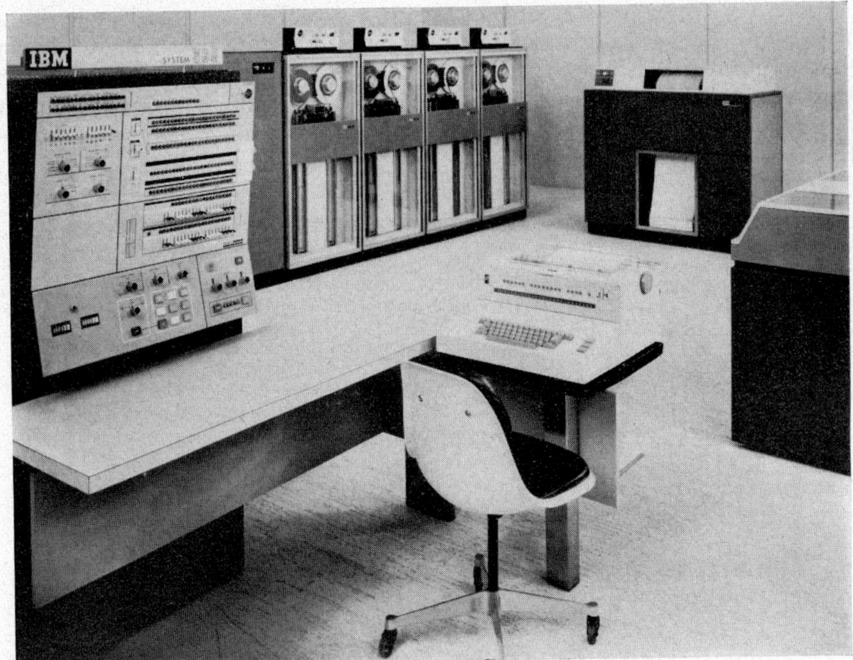

APPENDIX II/FIG. 2.—View of a computer installation.

All input must be in a medium comprehensible to the computer. At present written and spoken language cannot be used, though the recent technical advances which have been discussed earlier indicate the possibility of using computer input in these forms in the future. Input devices which can recognise some verbal command instructions have already been developed, but it will probably be some time before the computer will be able to cope with variations in intensity of sound or accent. The possibility of using handwritten input seems at present more practicable: devices have already been developed which enable the computer to read handwritten numerical information, but as yet the standard of this type of input is too poor for efficient usage.

The forms of input acceptable to the computer at its present stage of development are listed below:

(i) punch cards
(ii) punched paper tape
(iii) magnetic tape
(iv) magnetic discs
(v) magnetic cards
(vi) data written directly into the computer by typewriter
(vii) data directly interpreted by mark sense reader.

Of these, *punch cards* and *punched paper tape* are the most widely used. By comparison with the advanced techniques employed in the computer itself, the methods used for the preparation of these forms of input are slow and laborious. The data is recorded on the cards or tape by operating a keyboard similar to a typewriter's. Punched cards may be of varying size and design, though those in most frequent use measure $3\frac{1}{4}$ by $7\frac{3}{8}$ inches and are divided lengthwise into 80 columns, each column having 12 vertical positions. One character of the data is represented by a pattern of punched rectangular holes in one of the columns (Fig. 3).

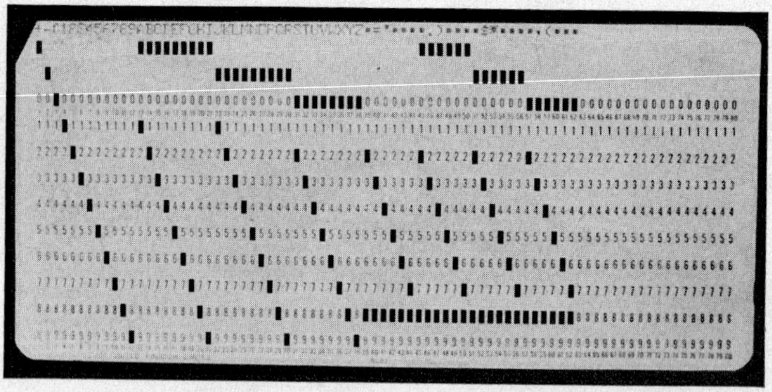

APPENDIX II/FIG. 3.—Example of an 80-column punch card.

Paper tape is generally between $\frac{3}{4}$ to 1 inch wide and is supplied in reels of about 1,000 feet. One character is represented on the tape by a pattern of circular holes in one row (Fig. 4).

Punched tape is particularly useful for large amounts of data, as it is not restricted to 80 characters per card. In comparison with cards it does however have two serious disadvantages. Firstly, rearrangement or correction of data is possible only by cutting and rejoining. With punch cards these are relatively simple operations, and there are machines available for sorting. Secondly, visual checking is impossible as data is represented only by hole patterns, whereas data may be printed along the top edge of the card while it is being punched. Paper tape is nevertheless the cheapest form of input, and is extremely compact and easy to store. The choice of input must however ultimately depend on the data and equipment available.

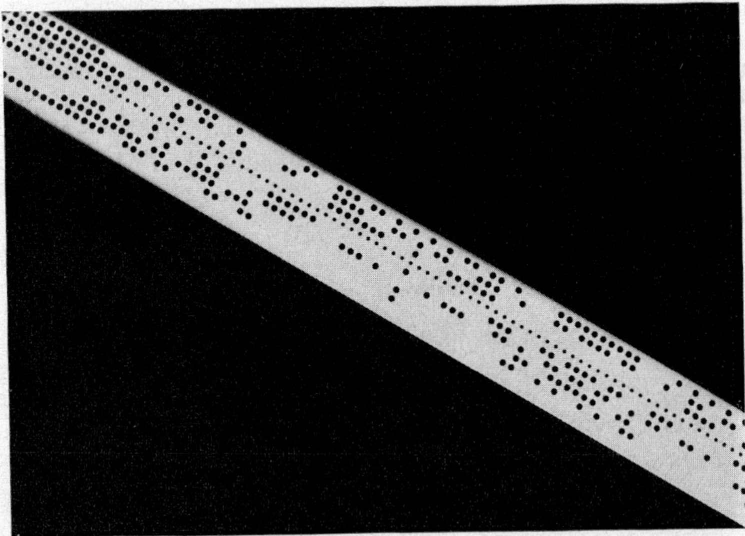

APPENDIX II/FIG. 4.—Example of paper tape.

The average speed of a punch operator is between 5 and 10 characters per second. This is too slow to feed a computer directly, and it is usual to pre-record the data in coded form. This is read later by the machine at a much higher speed. There is the additional problem of error in the transcription of data. It is at this initial stage that many of the mistakes in computer calculations are made, and it has been estimated that punch operators make between two or three errors per 1,000 characters punched. All input therefore has to be checked by a second operator who feeds the original tape or series of cards into a verifying machine. This reads the tape (or cards) and compares it character-by-character with the data. If the two agree, a second "verified" tape or card is produced; if there is any discrepancy the verifier automatically locks and the operator locates and corrects the error.

Punched paper tape is read by optical devices which illuminate the tape; small photo-sensitive cells then detect the holes by the light which shines through them. Punch cards may be read in a similar way, or by wire brushes which trace the position of the holes. Reading speeds of 2,000 cards per minute are possible, though the average is around 1,000. As defined by numbers of characters read, the reading speeds of both forms of input are similar, 500 to 1,000 characters per second.

Magnetic tape is a more recent form of input and is now becoming increasingly common. It consists of a thin ribbon of plastic material, $\frac{1}{2}$ to 1 inch in width, a few thousands of an inch thick and thinly coated on one side with plastic varnish containing oxides of iron. The method for recording data on magnetic tape is very similar to that used on punched paper tape: the oxide surface runs over a "read/write head" consisting of a group of small electromagnets. The speed of punched paper tape and magnetic tape are both about 100 inches per second, but the magnetic tape is able to transfer the data to and from the computer at a much higher rate (50 to 100 times faster) because it is possible to place the spots of magnetism on magnetic tape very much more closely than the holes in paper tape. Data can therefore be written onto or read from magnetic tape at speeds of between 50,000 and 150,000 characters per second.

Magnetic discs and *cards* operate on the same principle as magnetic tape, though in a different form. Figure 5 shows a disc unit used for input.

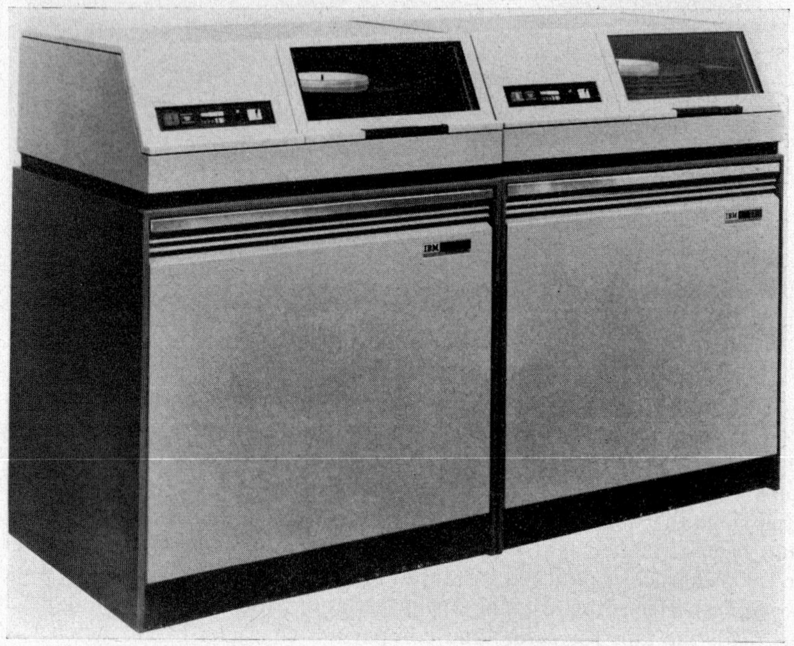

APPENDIX II/FIG. 5.—Disc unit (input).

If additional instructions or data are required during the process of calculation, these may be fed directly into the computer using a *typewriter*. The *mark sense reader*, or *optical character reader*, is a device for reading hand-written input. At present it is unreliable, but as it is a convenient method of input, it is likely to be widely used in future.

Memory Unit

This is the section of the computer used for the storage of instructions and input data required for calculations. It also retains intermediate results during the process of calculation.

The machines contained in the memory unit are shown in Fig. 1 immediately beneath the control unit. The main part of the memory unit uses small rings or cores of ceramic magnetic material, called ferrite, to store the information in binary code. A core can be magnetised in a clockwise or anticlockwise direction to represent the digit 0 or 1. The cores are threaded onto a rectangular matrix of wires which transfer information to and from the cores by means of electronic impulses. The coded instructions or data are generally written into a fixed number of consecutive cores, and a word is recognised irrespective of the size of the binary code. Thus the working capacity of the computer is limited, firstly by the word length and secondly by the number of words in the core store. The access time to and from the store is one of the factors determining the overall speed of the computer and can be as low as several tenths of a microsecond. Since the core store is the most expensive part of the computer, its size is limited by the money available. A *magnetic drum* is generally used to supplement the capacity of the core store. This consists of a cylinder coated with magnetic material which revolves at high speed. An electromagnetic read-write head, resting on this cylinder, transfers information to and from the cylinder. Drum capacity is much cheaper than core storage, but the access time may be a thousand times slower. The core store may also be supplemented by one or several *magnetic disc stores*: these take the form of stacks of discs and operate in the same way as drum storage, though at a slower speed (Fig. 6). *Magnetic tape* may also be used; this is both the cheapest and slowest form of additional storage. Input data is usually held on the tape or disc and instructions, programs and intermediate results in the core.

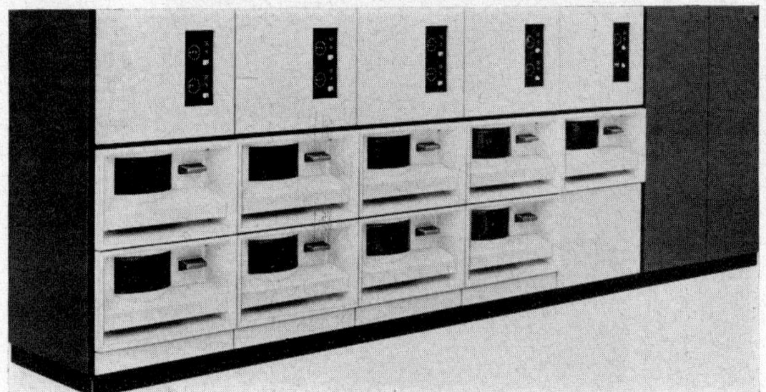

APPENDIX II/FIG. 6.—Disc unit (additional storage).

Arithmetic Unit

The cells in the central memory unit cannot perform arithmetical and logical operations on the data. These operations are carried out in cells, called *registers* or *accumulators*, in the arithmetic unit. Words, numbers or symbols required for a calculation are transferred from the central memory unit to the registers as they are needed, and when the operation is complete the result is transmitted to the memory unit.

Control Unit

This sophisticated mechanism co-ordinates the actions of the whole computer mechanism and is responsible for the interpretation and implication of the instructions given in the program. The control unit operates to a two-beat rhythm: in the first beat it obtains the next instruction from the store and places it in a special single-location store; in the second it decodes and examines the digits which make up the instruction and determines the appropriate electrical control for the required operation. When the operation has been completed, a signal is returned to the control unit, which then obtains the next instruction.

In addition to controlling the central processor, the control unit directs the transfer of data to and from peripheral units, such as card readers, magnetic tapes and printers. As these units work at a much slower speed than the central processor, this could involve considerable loss of time. In order to avoid this, several programs may be run concurrently, a process known as "time-sharing", which allows every unit in the machine to operate continuously at maximum speed. In practice fully efficient time sharing is very difficult to achieve.

The control unit enables communications between the operator and the computer via a display panel or teletyper and a keyboard (Fig. 7). The display panel indicates the point reached in the program and shows the location of errors; the keyboard is used to feed in additional information if necessary.

The control unit also governs the *compiler*, a complex machine language

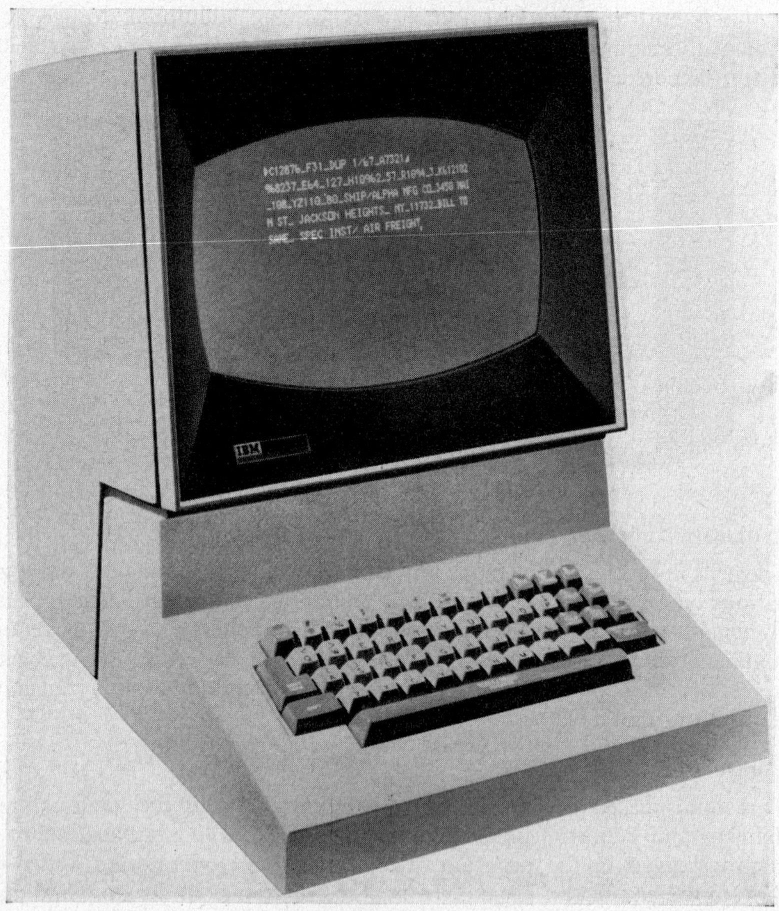

APPENDIX II/FIG. 7.—Visual display unit.

program contained within the memory unit. This breaks down a particular problem into the different processes required for its solution and translates the problem into language comprehensible to the computer. The introduction of the compiler is one of the most important recent advances in the development of the computer, and has enabled programs to be written in "English-like" words.

Output Devices

When the computer has completed a particular job, the results must be made available for use. This is most frequently done by automatic printers under the direct control of the supervisor. There are three different types of printer. The first is an *electric typewriter* which produces output at a slow speed, perhaps ten characters per second, and is primarily used for the control of the computer or for answering occasional enquiries. The second type of printer produces a line of output at a time (a *line-printer*); this is effected by a row of hammers which strike against revolving typewheels, inked ribbon or carbon paper being interposed between the two. The speed achieved ranges from between 300 and 1,800 per minute, 1,000 lines being typical. The third type of printer, called a *Xerograph printer*, displays characters to be printed on a cathode ray tube, rather like a television screen. An image of the output is focused into a revolving electrified drum where it produces an electric image which is then used to transfer pigment to paper. These machines can operate even faster than line-printers, achieving speeds of up to 3,000 lines per minute.

For scientific use, output may be presented in graphic rather than tabulated form. Output may also be written out on punch cards, punched paper tape, magnetic tape or magnetic cards, though these forms of output are less frequently found. Results not immediately required may be transferred to the external storage unit until required.

Programming

Repeated references have been made in the previous section to the importance of programs in the different stages of computer calculations. The computer performs many different operations at an extremely high speed, and the rapidity with which the results are produced may give the impression to the uninformed observer that the computer is working independently of external direction. The computer is however only capable of doing what it has been instructed to do. In the solution of any problem the computer must be given detailed instructions about the necessary procedure. These instructions must be presented to the computer in a formal manner which gives no scope for ambiguity. The formal list of instructions presented to the computer is called the *program*, and the translation of the problem into the language and format comprehensible to the computer is called *programming*.

The steps involved in programming a problem are numerous and complex, and the writing of a working program is usually time-consuming. When the problem is lengthy it is extremely difficult to formulate a procedure which is applicable in all eventualities.

The following situation illustrates the work involved in writing a simple program. A doctor with a list of blood pressure measurements for a group of 100 patients has to determine the number of subjects with diastolic values greater than 120 mm. Hg. If he were asked to explain the procedure he followed in this calculation, he would probably simply say that he read through the list and noted each diastolic value larger than 120 mm. Hg. A more detailed consideration of his actions reveals however that the procedure is longer than he imagines. It can in fact be divided into three separate stages:

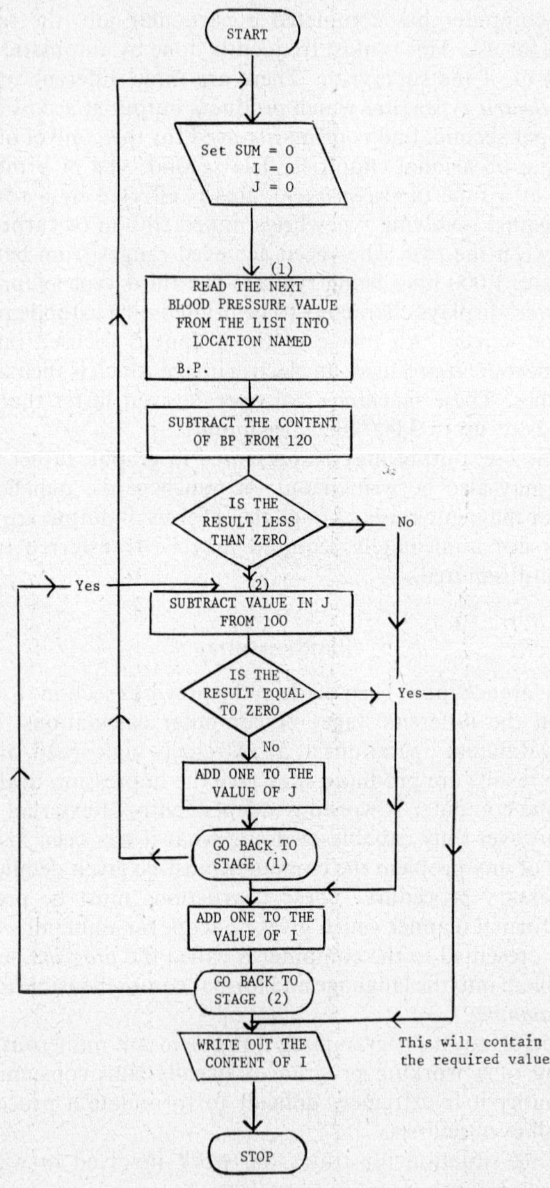

1. He reads a value from the list.
2. He asks himself if this is greater than 120, and
   (i) if the answer is "yes" he adds 1 to his sum (which is zero at the beginning of the calculation);
   (ii) if the answer is "no" he returns to his list and reads another value.
3. He repeats actions 1 and 2 until he reaches the end of the list.

If this calculation were being performed by computer the required procedure would be formally presented as shown in the diagram opposite

THE USES OF COMPUTERS IN MEDICINE

The foregoing description demonstrates that computers have two basic functions—performing mathematical operations and processing non-numeric information. It also emphasises that one of the computer's greatest assets is its ability to store large amounts of data, which may then be sorted and presented in a variety of different ways.

In addition computers may be programmed to absorb the output of many different machines, to detect patterns within these outputs and to perform the required operations on the data.

Computers have so far been developed principally for use in office work, but their value in different fields of medicine is now becoming increasingly clear.

Pathology

Pathology, and chemical pathology in particular, is one of the areas in which computers have been most successfully used. Pathological tests are readily automated using an auto-analyser (Fig. 8).

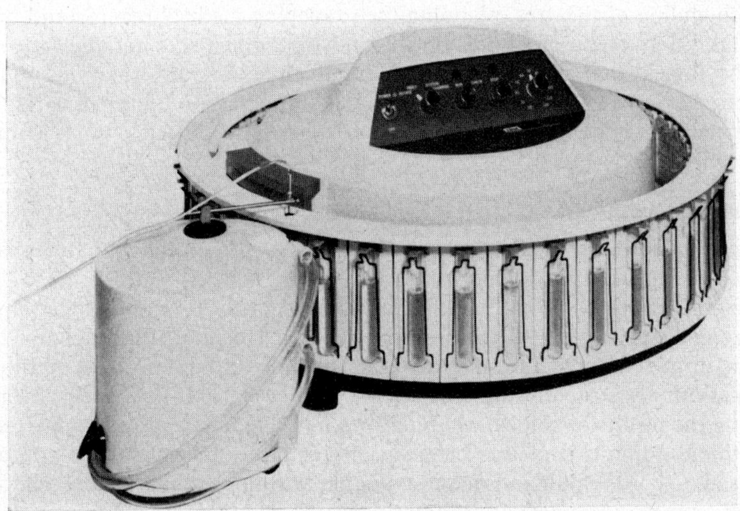

APPENDIX II/FIG. 8.—An auto-analyser.

The computer senses the output of the auto-analyser, performs the appropriate calculations on the output and presents a typed result. A description of such uses is given in a recent symposium (College of Pathologists, 1969).

The computer could be used in a similar way in haematology and bacteriology. In these studies systems could be developed for collecting data on punched paper tape and subsequently analysing these data by computer. Systems by which analytic equipment reads straight into a computer (an on-line system) are also possible. At present however both methods of recording and analysing data are still at the planning stage.

Radiotherapy

Computers are now being used for planning courses of radiotherapy (Parr and Newell, 1968; Emery, 1968; Clifton, 1970; Newell, 1970). The preparation of these plans is largely a matter of complex and lengthy arithmetic, for which the computer is ideally suited. The introduction of computers in this field should minimise delays in producing plans for treatment, and should also enable a wider range of treatment to be considered.

Physiological Signals

ECG, EEG and EMG recordings can also be readily adapted for computer analysis. The output from these machines consists of electric signals, which can be translated into signals intelligible to the computer. The computer is programmed to recognise and record particular patterns. Research into this use of computers has reached an advanced stage, and is described by Lawrie and Macfarlane (1968) and Adgey (1970).

Organisation of Patient Care

In the administration of a hospital a large volume of information must be sorted, stored and kept readily available for use. For example, patient registration, scheduling of theatres, planning diets, keeping medical records and ordering drugs, all involve a great deal of clerical work, which is essentially concerned with the logical and orderly presentation of alphabetic information. Various attempts have been made to process this information automatically, and several methods of handling the data have been developed (Bates, 1968; Kennedy *et al.*, 1968).

Clinical Records

Clinical records are used in four principal ways—for administrative, research, and medico-legal purposes, and for patient care.

A great deal of research into the handling of medical records by computer is at present in progress. At the Queen Elizabeth Hospital, Birmingham, basic data on in-patient registration, discharge diagnoses and results of pathology investigations are stored in the computer (Cross *et al.*, 1968). A wider coverage, including the results of clinical examinations and diagnostic X-rays and a record of treatment administered, has been suggested. If a sufficiently large computer were used, records could be made available within seconds at any one of a hundred or more terminals at different parts of the hospital. Thus communication between departments would be greatly improved.

There are however two basic problems involved in the automation of medical records. The first relates to the amount of information which should be stored. It is quite possible to store all the information recorded, but, if this is done, difficulties will arise in retrieving and presenting the data in a form suitable for analysis. Possible projects in this field are reviewed by Bennett and Holland (1968). The second problem is concerned with the difficulty of getting information into the system. Many members of the medical, nursing and clerical staff who are at present responsible for the preparation of medical records would be unable to use the typewriter-like keyboard which is necessary to feed the data into the computer. The obvious solution to this difficulty is for the computer to "interrogate" the user by asking a series of questions, displayed on a visual screen. A number of possible answers are similarly displayed, and the user has to point to the appropriate answer. A great deal of work however is still required before the question and answer sequences appropriate to every clinical situation are established.

General Practice and Local Health Work

Although few local authorities operate computers, the data recorded by health authorities is generally far simpler than that found in hospital clinical records, and would therefore be more easily adaptable for filing in a computer memory. Very little work has so far been attempted in this field, though a project undertaken by Galloway (1963) in West Sussex provides a notable exception. Here birth notifications are recorded on the local authority computer, and as the children reach the ages appropriate for the usual immunisations and vaccinations, they and their general practitioners are informed. Appointments and payment to general practitioners are also organised by computer. The introduction of this automated method has brought a considerable improvement in the immunisation rate for the area.

The use of a similar system has been proposed for the organisation of blood banks.

Record Linkage

The medical information required on an individual must be continuously stored, current records being linked with data already recorded for the same patient. Acheson (1967, 1968) has demonstrated the use of computers in record linkage, showing the advantages of an automated system.

Medical Research

A great deal of medical research necessitates the organisation of large amounts of data and lengthy arithmetical calculations, and the computer is invaluable in both tasks. In addition, the automation of medical records would make a much greater number of case histories available for study, since those relevant to a particular investigation could be easily extracted.

Patient Monitoring

Where computers are applied to patient monitoring, the machine may be used to collect, store and diplay the data. It can also be programmed to elucidate additional physiological information from the primary data, to sort through the data for values indicating significant changes in the patient's state and to provide a clinical interpretation of physiological observations. The value of the computer in this field is now becoming widely recognised.

REFERENCES

ACHESON, E. D. (1967). *Medical Record Linkage.* London: Oxford Univ. Press.

ACHESON, E. D. Ed. (1968). *Record Linkage in Medicine.* Proc. International Symposium. London: E. & S. Livingstone.

ADGEY, A. A. J. (1970). On-line patient monitoring. In: *Medical Computing—Progress and Problems.* Proc. Conference of British Computer Society. Ed. Abrams, M. E. London: Chatto and Windus.

BATES, J. A. V. (1968). Preparation of clinical data for computers. In: Computing in Medicine. *Brit. med. Bull.*, **24**(3), 199.

BENNETT, A. E., and HOLLAND, W. W. (1968). The medical record and the computer. Part I. In: *Computers in the Service of Medicine. Essays on current research and applications*, Vol. II. Eds. McLachlan, G., and Shegog, R. A. London: Oxford Univ. Press, for Nuffield Provincial Hospitals Trust.

CLIFTON, J. S. (1970). Developing a computer service for radiotherapy. In: *Medical Computing—Progress and Problems* (see above).

COLLEGE OF PATHOLOGISTS (1969). *Automation and Data Processing in Pathology.* Proc. Symposium of College of Pathologists. Ed. Whitehead, P. *J. clin. Path.*, **22,** Suppl. (Col. Path.), 3.

CROSS, K. W., DROAR, J., and Roberts, J. L. (1968). Electronic processing of hospital records. In: *Computers in the Service of Medicine*, Vol. I (see above).

EMERY, E. W. (1968). Computer applications in radiotherapy. In: Computing in Medicine. *Brit. med. Bull.*, **24**(3), 341.

GALLOWAY, T. McL. (1963). Management of vaccination and immunisation procedures by electronic computer. *Med. Offr.*, **109,** 232.

KENNEDY, F., COX, A. G., GLEN, A. I. M., ROY, A. D., and SUNDT, C. E. (1968). A computer-based system for handling clinical data. In: *Computers in the Service of Medicine*, Vol. I (see above).

LAWRIE, T. D. V., and MACFARLANE, P. W. (1968). Towards automated electrocardiogram interpretation. In: *Computers in the Service of Medicine*, Vol. I (see above).

NEWELL, J. A. (1970). Radiotherapy rotational treatment planning on a small computer. In: *Medical Computing—Progress and Problems* (see above).

PARR, R. F., and NEWELL, J. A. (1968). Radiotherapy treatment planning. In: *Computers in the Service of Medicine*, Vol. I (see above).

Appendix III

CARE AND STERILISATION OF APPARATUS AND INSTRUMENTS

Too little consideration is generally given to the cleanliness and sterility of apparatus used in anaesthesia, and particularly to those parts which indirectly or directly come into contact with the air passages. Absolute sterility is not always essential, since the upper air passages are in constant contact with the atmosphere but there is evidence that infections have been spread from patient to patient through the use of contaminated anaesthetic or respiratory apparatus. This has been shown to occur with the use of ventilators (see Chapter 16). For this reason those parts of the anaesthetic system through which rebreathing takes place, and apparatus such as an endotracheal tube, face-mask and laryngoscope which actually comes into direct contact with the patient, must be thoroughly washed after use and either sterilised or at least kept clean until required again. If the equipment has been used for a patient suffering from a known infection then washing *must* be followed by sterilisation.

Constant washing and sterilisation of apparatus, particularly of rubber or plastic components, leads to some wear, but a more potent cause of deterioration is to be found in the use of lubricants containing vaseline or greasy bases. The use of these, rather than repeated sterilisation, is the commonest cause of baggy rubber on cuffed tubes (Buckley, 1952). The lubricants should always be non-greasy and either alone or incorporated with an analgesic; a good example is the following:

PASTA LUBRICANS (ST. THOMAS'S HOSPITAL)

Tragacanth, powdered	12 gr. (0·78 g.)
Glycerin	28 ♏ (1·7 ml.)
Liquefied phenol	2·5 ♏ (0·15 ml.)
Distilled water (by weight) to . . .	1 oz. (28·4 ml.)

But even lubricants can harbour organisms, so that they are best dispensed in small tubes which can be discarded daily before they become infected.

STERILISATION OF ANAESTHETIC APPARATUS

Each piece of equipment should be thoroughly washed in soap and water, both internally and externally, then dried and finally sterilised. All anaesthetic apparatus which comes into contact, however remotely, with the exhaled gases of a patient with an infected respiratory tract, should be cleaned and sterilised. Everything, from the bag and corrugated tubing of a Magill semi-closed assembly, or from the narrow rubber tubing carrying the gases to an absorber, to the face-mask or endotracheal tube, should be treated. This means of necessity that when a technique involving carbon dioxide absorption is used on such patients the standard to and fro system should be chosen, since a circular system cannot be simply and quickly sterilised. When necessary, however, a circular absorber can be sterilised by gas (ethylene oxide) in the same manner as a ventilator (see Chapter 16).

Ideal sterilisation.—In ideal circumstances simple anaesthetic apparatus, such as face-masks, endotracheal tubes and pharyngeal airways, are sterilised in a central sterile supply department by autoclaving or (in respect of certain articles manufactured from heat labile materials) by gas sterilisation using ethylene oxide. The latter method is not suitable for all such equipment, but a recently developed technique using steam at sub-atmospheric pressure (80° C) with a small amount of formalin vapour creates sporicidal conditions without damaging the materials. All of these methods permit the presentation of the article in a "visible" pack. When it is available, the sub-atmospheric steam and formaldehyde technique should be used as the routine, since it can be used for most anaesthetic equipment. It is faster and cheaper than ethylene oxide and it is devoid of the toxic by-products that can be isolated from rubber and plastic materials after ethylene oxide sterilisation (Clinical Anaesthesia Conference, 1969).

Other methods.—In less sophisticated situations boiling for three minutes is satisfactory. This kills all bacteria, including those of tuberculosis, but is ineffective against the spores of certain organisms such as *Cl. tetani.* In all theatre work the assumption is made that spore-bearing organisms are unlikely to be present due to normal cleanliness in the care of apparatus and the surroundings.

Rubber, including the fine cuffs on endotracheal and endobronchial tubes, will tolerate this treatment, provided the steriliser boils gently and the duration of time does not exceed three minutes. Repeated sterilisation of cuffed tubes in a high-vacuum, high-pressure autoclave does not shorten the life of a tube provided that air is efficiently removed from the autoclave, thus preventing the risk of oxidisation. Face-masks must be deflated. Portex tubes are softened, but rapidly harden as they cool, while their shape—and indeed that of all endotracheal tubes—can be maintained by storing them in round tins.

Metal instruments such as bronchoscope and laryngoscope blades which are detachable from battery-carrying handles can also be sterilised by boiling, and the electrical bulbs will generally not be harmed. However, if the blade of either instrument cannot be detached, an alternative method is to stand it in a jar of 1:20 carbolic for 30 minutes after washing and then to rinse in water before use. Bronchoscopes are also commonly sterilised by storing in a formalin oven and rinsing in sterile water just prior to use, but there is no particular merit in this form of sterilisation over simple boiling—other than to avoid subjecting the small bulbs to heat.

The Macintosh spray (rubber type) for topical analgesia is one of the few anaesthetic instruments which will not tolerate boiling even for three minutes. This is because the internal tube in the nozzle is made of very fine rubber which expands slightly with boiling. The result is that instead of a fine spray, a jet of liquid is now delivered on use. A further factor which tends to accentuate the rapid deterioration of this rubber is the tendency for local analgesic solutions to form deposits in it after use, unless the whole instrument is carefully washed and blown through with cold water.

Sterilisation of Syringes

The most satisfactory syringes and needles for anaesthetic work are disposable and sterilised by either ethylene oxide or gamma radiation. In most countries their routine use can be justified on economic grounds, since their cost is less than that of a syringe service. When their routine use cannot be justified, the most satisfactory methods for sterilising syringes and needles are by autoclaving or dry heat. These are effective against all organisms and spores, and neither blunts the point of a needle, as does boiling. Boiling is an acceptable method of sterilisation in the absence of a better, provided the syringes are kept for anaesthetic purposes only and are boiled immediately before use. Sterilisation by immersion in a disinfectant is inadequate, and storage in one after sterilisation by another method is dangerous—disinfectants, besides being less than 100 per cent effective, are likely to become diluted with use, and have been known actually to harbour pathogenic organisms. Rinsing before use is also necessary to avoid passing some of the solution into the patient.

All types of syringe will stand boiling provided they are dismantled and placed in warm water and then slowly brought up to 100° C. The risk of breakage can be diminished by wrapping the glass portions in a piece of gauze. Record (glass-metal) types of syringe will also stand autoclaving, but for this method all-glass syringes are preferable, while for dry heat they are essential.

Whichever type of sterilisation is chosen, syringes and needles must be carefully cleaned both immediately after use and before sterilisation, so that all coagulated blood or foreign material is removed. Remnants such as these may form a nidus of protection for organisms even in the face of otherwise perfect sterilisation, and there is evidence that contamination of this sort is one of the sources of spread from one patient to another of virus hepatitis.

A sequence of events that is effective and makes use of dry heat sterilisation is as follows: After use the syringe is washed through with cold water, but, prior to sterilisation, washing is carried out by immersion in "Teepol" (a commercial detergent). The duration of time is unimportant provided the syringe is properly covered, and then cleaned internally and externally by a brush. "Teepol" effectively removes any grease, oil or protein. Needles are soaked in a similar manner and then blown through with a jet of water; they are also sharpened at this stage. After rinsing, the components are dried (a special oven is used for this purpose) and the barrel lubricated very slightly with silicone diluted in industrial alcohol. They are then reassembled and packed in individual containers. A glass tube makes an excellent container, since the state of cleanliness of its interior—and its contents—is easily apparent. It should be sealed with an aluminium cap ("Ideal Capsule") in which is incorporated a piece of string or strong thread. The best type of seal is simply applied and equally simply removed. Sterilisation is then carried out by dry heat after having achieved a temperature of 160° C. The total cycle time is likely to be $1\frac{3}{4}$ hours.

Sterilisation of Instruments for Local Analgesia

Special packs should be made up for each type of local analgesic procedure. Each pack should contain not only needles and all-glass syringes of the requisite size, but also some swabs and, for spinal and epidural analgesia, ampoules of local analgesic solution. The pack should be wrapped in a suitable porous wrapping material and autoclaved at a temperature of 134° C for 3½ minutes. The total time including pre- and post-vacuum phases will be about twenty minutes. Local analgesic solutions will stand autoclaving but not dry heat. However, if the process is repeated those solutions containing glucose—typically so-called "heavy" spinal mixtures—become ineffective due to precipitation of this substance. The sub-atmospheric steam technique described previously using formalin vapour has a place here since it avoids deterioration of analgesic solutions.

Tubing.—Rubber will stand boiling and autoclaving but not dry heat. Tubing made of portex or polythene can be sterilised by boiling, but its internal diameter and general shape is preserved best when shock cooling by immersion in cold water is practised. Tubing of very fine diameter made from portex or polythene becomes unsatisfactory after any kind of heat sterilisation; it also kinks very easily. Vinyl plastic tubing—even when of very fine bore—maintains its shape and size when autoclaved or boiled, but is likely to kink unless coiled up very loosely. It will not stand more than one sterilisation.

Most types of tubing for anaesthetic work can now be obtained commercially, and packed and sterilised by gamma radiation. Disposable sterile sets which include tubing, syringe and connection pieces, are also available for certain forms of local analgesic technique.

REFERENCES

Buckley, R. W. (1952). Danger from endotracheal tubes. *Brit. med. J.*, **2,** 939.

Clinical Anaesthesia Conference (1969). Hazards associated with ethylene oxide sterilisation. *N.Y.St. J. Med.*, **69,** 1319.

USEFUL FACTS

Blood

Normal Chemical and Physical Values

Alkali Reserve	53 to 77 ml. of CO_2 per 100 ml. of plasma (24 to 35 mEq/litre).
Amylase	Less than 200 units per 100 ml.
Amino acids	4 to 6 mg. per 100 ml.
Bicarbonate	21·2 mEq/litre
standard bicarbonate	24–34 mEq/litre.
Bilirubin (serum)	Less than 1·7 mg. per 100 ml.
Bromsulphthalein retention test	0 to 5 per cent at 45 minutes.
Calcium (serum)	9 to 11 mg. per 100 ml. (5 mEq/litre).
Cephalin—cholesterol flocculation test	0 to 1.
Chlorides (serum)	95 to 110 mEq/litre.
Cholesterol (serum)	150 to 300 mg. per 100 ml.
Circulation time:	
arm to tongue (saccharin, sodium dehydrocholate)	9 to 16 seconds.
arm to lung (ether)	4 to 8 seconds.
Congo red removal	0 to 35 per cent at 30 minutes.
Creatine phosphokinase (CPK) (serum)	0–35 International units/litre.
Creatinine (serum)	0·7 to 2·0 mg. per 100 ml.
Magnesium (serum)	3 mEq/litre.
Non-protein nitrogen (serum)	20 to 40 mg. per 100 ml.
pH (hydrogen ion concentration)	7·3 to 7·5.
Phosphatase:	
alkaline	3 to 13 King Armstrong units.
acid	0·5 to 5 King Armstrong units.
Phosphates (serum):	
adult	3 to 4·5 mg. per 100 ml.
child	4 to 6 mg. per 100 ml.
Potassium (serum)	3 to 5 mEq/litre.
Proteins:	
albumin	4·0 to 5·5 g. per 100 ml.
globulin	1·5 to 3·0 g. per 100 ml.
fibrinogen	0·2 to 0·5 g. per 100 ml.
Total	6·0 to 8·0 g. per 100 ml.
Pseudo (plasma) cholinesterase	40 to 100 units per 100 ml.
Sodium (serum)	135 to 150 mEq/litre.
Sugar:	
glucose (fasting)	70 to 110 mg. per 100 ml.
glucose (after meal)	Up to 180 mg. per 100 ml.
Thymol flocculation test	0 to 1.
Thymol turbidity test	0 to 4.
Transaminases	
SGOT (Spectrophotometric)	5–17 units per 100 ml.
SGOT (Colorimetric)	8–40 units per 100 ml.

SGPT (Spectrophotometric) . . . 4–13 units per 100 ml.
SGPT (Colorimetric) . . . . 5–30 units per 100 ml.
Urea . . . . 15 to 40 mg. per 100 ml.
Uric acid . . . . 2 to 5 mg. per 100 ml.
Volume (blood) . . . . . . 3·5 to 7 litres (6 to 12 pints).
(Adults—85 ml./kg. body weight.)
(Infants and children—90 ml./kg. body weight.)

Haematological Values

Haemoglobin is 100 per cent on the Haldane scale when 14·8 g./100 ml. of blood, and is 100 per cent on the Sahli scale when 14·0 g./100 ml. of blood.

	Red cells (millions/c.mm.)	*Haemoglobin (g./100 ml. of blood)*
At birth .	6·5 to 7·25	19·8
Men . .	5·0 to 6·4	14 to 17
Women .	4·2 to 5·6	12 to 15·5

Bleeding time (Duke's method) . . 2 to 5 minutes.
Coagulation time:
Wright (capillary) . . . . 10 to 15 minutes.
Lee and White (venous) . . . 5 to 7 minutes.

Colour index . . . . $= \dfrac{\text{Haemoglobin per cent.}}{\text{Red cell count (per cent of normal).}}$

Normal value is 1·0 (range 0·85 to 1·15).

Haematocrit (P.C.V. or packed cell volume) is the volume of red cells in 100 ml. of whole blood. Normal values:

Men: 40 to 54 ml. per 100 ml.
Women: 37 to 47 ml. per 100 ml.

Mean corpuscular diameter (M.C.D.) . 6·7 to 7·7μ.

Mean corpuscular haemoglobin (M.C.H.) $= \dfrac{\text{Haemoglobin in g./100 ml. of blood}}{\text{Red cell count in millions/c.mm.}} \times 10.$

Normal value is 27 to 32 micromicrograms.

Mean corpuscular haemoglobin concentration (M.C.H.C.) $= \dfrac{\text{Haemoglobin in g./100 ml. of blood}}{\text{Haematocrit value}} \times 100.$

Normal value is 32 to 38 g. per 100 ml. of blood.

Mean corpuscular volume (M.C.V.) $= \dfrac{\text{Corpuscular volume in 1,000 ml. of blood.}}{\text{Red cell count in millions/c.mm.}}$

Normal value is 78 to 94 c.μ.

Platelet count	250,000 to 500,000 per c.mm.
Prothrombin time. (The normal range varies with the technique used.)	
Quick (thromboplastin from brain)	12 to 30 seconds.
Reticulocytes	0 to 2 per cent of the red cells.
Sedimentation rate (Westergren):	
Men	1 hour—1 to 5 mm. 2 hours—7 to 15 mm.
Women and children	1 hour—4 to 7 mm. 2 hours—12 to 17 mm.
White cell count	5,000 to 9,000 per c.mm.
Neutrophils	65 to 70 per cent.
Lymphocytes	20 to 25 per cent.
Monocytes	5 to 6 per cent.
Eosinophils	0 to 4 per cent.
Basophils	0 to 1 per cent.

Body Water

	Body water as a percentage of body weight	
	Men	*Women*
Total water	60	55
Extracellular water	15	15
Intracellular water	45	40

Water intake (Adult):

As liquid	1,500 ml. per day.
As food	1,000 ml. (including 300 ml. water of oxidation) per day.
Total	2,500 ml. per day.

Water elimination (Adult):

Skin	500 ml. per day.
Lungs	400 ml. per day.
Faeces	100 ml. per day.
Urine	1,500 ml. per day.
Total	2,500 ml. per day.

Cerebrospinal Fluid

Cells	0 to 8 per c.mm.
Chlorides	700 to 750 mg. per 100 ml.

Colloidal Gold Curve . . . . . 000000.
Protein . . . . 10 to 45 mg. per 100 ml.
Sugar . . . . 40 to 70 mg. per 100 ml.

Faeces

Total fat (dried faeces) . . . 10 to 25 per cent.
Trypsin:
adults . . . . 0 to 40 units.
infants . . . . More than 40 units.

Gastric Juice

Fasting juice:
Volume . . . . 20 to 100 ml.
Free acid (as N/10 HCl) . . . 0 to 30 ml. per 100 ml.
Total acid (as N/10 HCl) . . . 10 to 50 ml. per 100 ml.

Metabolism

Basal metabolic rate . . . . + 14 per cent to — 14 per cent.

Respiration

Average values for adult male

Tidal volume . . . . . 500 ml.
Respiratory rate . . . . . 12/min.
Minute volume . . . . . 6 L./min.
Dead space . . . . . . 150 ml.
Alveolar ventilation . . . . 4,200 ml.
FEV in 1 sec. . . . . . 83 per cent of vital capacity.
Oxygen consumption . . . . 240 ml./min.
Carbon dioxide output . . . . 192 ml./min.

Neonatal values

Respiratory rate . . . . . 30–50/min.
Tidal volume . . . . . 15–19 ml.
Dead space . . . . . . 5–9 ml.
Minute volume . . . . . 650 ml./min.

Composition of dry inspired, alveolar and expired air in volumes per cent at N.T.P.

	Inspired (atmospheric) air	*Alveolar air*	*Expired air*
Oxygen	20·94	14·2	16·3
Carbon dioxide . . .	0·04	5·5	4·0
Nitrogen and inert gases .	79·02	80·3	79·7

Gas tensions in inspired and alveolar air, and in the blood, in mm. Hg.

	Inspired air (atmospheric)	*Alveolar air*	*Arterial blood*	*Venous blood*
Oxygen . .	158·2	103	100	40
Nitrogen . .	596·5	570	573	573
Carbon dioxide .	0·3	40	40	46
Water vapour .	5·0	47	47	47
Total .	760·0	760·0	760·0	706·0

Urine

Catecholamines
- Adrenaline in 24-hour save . . } 119–338 μg.
- Noradrenaline in 24-hour save . . } (see also p. 1367)
- 3 methoxy, 4 hydroxy-mandelic acid (VMA) in 24-hour save . . . 2·6–6·5 μg.

Calcium . . . . 0·1–0·3 g./24 hrs.

5-Hydroxytryptamine excreted as 5-Hydroxyindoleacetic acid in 24-hour save . . . . 2–9 mg.

Potassium . . . . 35–90 mEq/24 hrs.

Sodium . . . . 110–240 mEq/24 hrs.

Urea . . . . 10–35 g./24 hrs.

The Metric System and Conversion Factors

The reader is referred to a pamphlet titled *Metrication in Scientific Journals* produced by the Royal Society Conference of Editors and published by the Royal Society of 6, Carlton House Terrace, London, S.W.1. in 1968. In this pamphlet is a description of the Système International d'Unités or SI which is an extension and a refinement of the metric system.

The conversion factors that follow are a very limited number that may be of help in those areas of clinical practice where traditional but outdated systems of measurement are still in use.

Pressure

1 lb. per sq. inch = 0·070 kg. per sq. cm.
= 51·7 mm. of mercury
= 70·3 cm. of water
1 mm. of mercury = 1·36 cm. of water
1 cm. of water = 0·73 mm. of mercury
1 atmosphere = 760 mm. of mercury
= 14·7 lb. per sq. inch
= 29·9 inches of mercury
= 1·03 kg. per sq. cm.
= 33·9 ft. of water

Thermometer

Fahrenheit to centigrade. $°C = °F - 32 \times 5/9$
Centigrade to Fahrenheit. $°F = °C \times 9/5 + 32$

Volume

1 Imperial gallon = 1·201 U.S.A. gallons
1 U.S.A. gallon = 0·8327 Imperial gallons

Special Symbols*

— Dash above any symbol indicates a *mean* value.
. Dot above any symbol indicates *a time derivative*.

For Gases

Primary Symbols (Large Capital Letters)		Examples	
V	= gas volume	V_A	= volume of alveolar gas
$\dot{V}$	= gas volume/unit time	$\dot{V}_{O_2}$	= O_2 consumption/min.
P	= gas pressure	$P_{A_{O_2}}$	= alveolar O_2 pressure
$\bar{P}$	= mean gas pressure	$P_{\bar{c}O_2}$	= mean capillary O_2 pressure
F	= fractional concentration in dry gas phase	$F_{I_{O_2}}$	= fractional concentration of O_2 in inspired gas
f	= respiratory frequency (breaths/unit time)	D_{O_2}	= diffusing capacity for O_2 (ml. O_2/min./mm./Hg)
D	= diffusing capacity		
R	= respiratory exchange ratio	R	= $\dot{V}_{CO_2}/\dot{V}_{O_2}$

Secondary Symbols (small capital letters)		Examples	
I	= inspired gas	$F_{I_{CO_2}}$	= fractional concentration of CO_2 in inspired gas
E	= expired gas	V_E	= volume of expired gas
A	= alveolar gas	$\dot{V}_A$	= alveolar ventilation/min
T	= tidal gas	V_T	= tidal volume
D	= dead space gas	V_D	= volume of dead space gas
B	= barometric	P_B	= barometric pressure
STPD	= 0° C., 760 mm Hg, dry		
BTPS	= body temperature and pressure saturated with water vapour		
ATPS	= ambient temperature and pressure saturated with water vapour		

For Blood

Primary Symbols (Large Capital Letters)		Examples	
Q	= volume of blood	Q_c	= volume of blood in pulmonary capillaries
$\dot{Q}$	= volume flow of blood/unit time	$\dot{Q}_c$	= blood flow through pulmonary capillaries/min.

*This list of special symbols with examples is reproduced from *The Lung* by the kindness of Professor Julius H. Comroe and the Year Book Medical Publishers, Incorporated.

C	= concentration of gas in blood phase	Ca_{O_2}	= ml. O_2 in 100 ml. arterial blood
S	= % saturation of Hb with O_2 or CO	Sv_{CO_2}	= saturation of Hb with O_2 in mixed venous blood

Secondary Symbols (small letters)		Examples	
a	= arterial blood	Pa_{CO_2}	= partial pressure of CO_2 in arterial blood
v	= venous blood	Pv_{O_2}	= partial pressure of O_2 in mixed venous blood
c	= capillary blood	Pc_{CO}	= partial pressure of CO in pulmonary capillary blood

For Lung Volumes

VC	= Vital Capacity	= maximal volume that can be expired after maximal inspiration
IC	= Inspiratory Capacity	= maximal volume that can be inspired from resting expiratory level
IRV	= Inspiratory Reserve Volume	= maximal volume that can be inspired from end-tidal inspiration
ERV	= Expiratory Reserve Volume	= maximal volume that can be expired from resting expiratory level
FRC	= Functional Residual Capacity	= volume of gas in lungs at resting expiratory level
RV	= Residual Volume	= volume of gas in lungs at end of maximal expiration
TLC	= Total Lung Capacity	= volume of gas in lungs at end of maximal inspiration

Average Values for Lung Volumes

VC	4,800 ml.
IC	3,600 ml.
IRV	3,100 ml.
ERV	1,200 ml.
FRC	2,400 ml.
RV	1,200 ml.
TLC	6,000 ml.

INDEX

INDEX